65.00

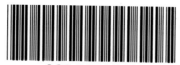

369 0289546

KU-627-848

Oxford Textbook of **Palliative Social Work**

Oxford Textbook of
Palliative Social Work

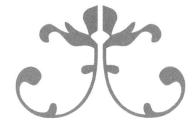

EDITED BY

Terry Altilio, MSW, LCSW, ACSW
Social Work Coordinator
Department of Pain Medicine & Palliative Care
Beth Israel Medical Center
New York, NY

Shirley Otis-Green, MSW, LCSW, ACSW, OSW-C
Senior Research Specialist
Division of Nursing Research and Education
City of Hope National Medical Center
Duarte, CA

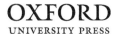

OXFORD
UNIVERSITY PRESS

OXFORD
UNIVERSITY PRESS

Oxford University Press, Inc., publishes works that further
Oxford University's objective of excellence
in research, scholarship, and education.

Oxford   New York
Auckland   Cape Town   Dar es Salaam   Hong Kong   Karachi
Kuala Lumpur   Madrid   Melbourne   Mexico City   Nairobi
New Delhi   Shanghai   Taipei   Toronto

With offices in
Argentina   Austria   Brazil   Chile   Czech Republic   France   Greece
Guatemala   Hungary   Italy   Japan   Poland   Portugal   Singapore
South Korea   Switzerland   Thailand   Turkey   Ukraine   Vietnam

Library of Congress Cataloging-in-Publication Data

Oxford textbook of palliative social work / edited by Terry Altilio and Shirley Otis-Green.
    p. ; cm.
  Includes bibliographical references and index.
  ISBN 978-0-19-973911-0 (alk. paper)
  1. Terminal care—Social aspects—Textbooks. 2. Palliative treatment—Social aspects—Textbooks.
  3. Social work with the terminally ill—Textbooks. I. Altilio, Terry. II. Otis-Green, Shirley.
  [DNLM: 1. Palliative Care--methods. 2. Social Work—methods. W 322]
  R726.8.T4647 2011
  362.17′5—dc22   2010026603

3 5 7 9 8 6 4 2
Printed in the United States of America
on acid-free paper

Dedication

To those whose voices are reflected in these pages;
Voices past & present
    heard & unheard
    halting & hesitant
    mellow & meek
    pleading & piercing
    raging & raucous
    soft & sorrowful
    tender & tremulous
    joyful & jubilant
    courageous & caring
May this work hone our listening and bring excellence to our response

CONTENTS

Section VI

Regional Voices from a Global Perspective

Section VII

Ethics

FOREWORD BY BETTY R. FERRELL

I began my career-long admiration of social workers with the start of my nursing career on an oncology unit. My initial years in oncology as a new graduate were in many ways best described as total chaos. Patients were very ill and the evolving field of oncology was struggling to develop use of chemotherapy, radiation therapy and to develop both inpatient and outpatient services.

Aggressive surgical techniques included drastic surgeries for patients such as radical mastectomies, incredibly invasive head and neck surgeries amid a care system that was ill prepared to manage the tremendous physical and psychological burdens on patients and families resulting from this emerging field of care.

In the midst of this chaotic and overwhelming world of oncology I was introduced to social work. These professionals were quite simply the calm in the storm. The oncology social workers were tranquil yet strong patient advocates; they were focused on the person and family surrounding the tumor and in many ways the social workers represented a solid anchor and in a clear sense of humanity in an environment otherwise void of such qualities.

From those early years, I learned a key lesson for survival as a nurse: Stay close to the social workers. I also learned that these social workers were equally attentive to nurses and other staff and that their influence extended to the broader systems of care. I observed that the common nursing or medical response amidst a crisis (a dying patient, an angry spouse, a dysfunctional family) was generally, "Has anyone called the social worker"?

In my own professional career journey to focus on palliative care, I have remained impressed by my social work colleagues. I don't fully understand the professional preparation or the culture of social work but I do know that their presence offers a consistent focus on patient and family needs, and is the embodiment of advocacy and a passion for whole person care. Social workers are often the conscience of an organization, the moral voice and the advocates for justice and compassion amidst an ever burdened system of care.

The field of palliative social work has emerged parallel to palliative nursing. It has been my privilege to witness the development of palliative social work, largely by observing the enormous commitment and passion of the two editors of this textbook, pioneers Shirley Otis-Green and Terry Altilio. My own passion and commitment has been inspired by observing their tireless efforts to advance palliative social work.

In 2001 my colleague Nessa Coyle and I published the first edition of the Textbook of Palliative Nursing. I realized then the importance of a book for a field. Far beyond a collection of chapters, a major Textbook represents the collective wisdom of a field; it sets the standard of what excellent care should look like and it holds all its members to a higher plane of practice.

Terry Altilio and Shirley Otis-Green have made a major professional contribution in the publication of this book. It is a work of art, quite fitting for the profession of social work, which is indeed a science and an art. The breadth and depth of content in this Textbook are monumental. They have defined the field and in doing so, there is no turning back.

Betty R. Ferrell, PhD, MA, FAAN, FPCN
Research Scientist
City of Hope Medical Center
Duarte, CA

FOREWORD BY KATHLEEN M. FOLEY

For all of those who have worked to build the interdisciplinary field of hospice and palliative care, the role of the social worker is recognized as central to our overarching goal of providing humane compassionate and competent care to patients and families with life-limiting illnesses.

This textbook marks an important stage in emphasizing the role of the social worker in palliative care. It sets the standard for the practice of palliative social work. Through its chapters, it defines a body of knowledge that outlines the field, describes its core curriculum and emphasizes its professional development.

The editors, Terry Altilio and Shirley Otis Green, are two professionals who bring to this task a breadth and depth of social work practice that is unparalleled. They have walked the walk and talked the talk. As practitioners and educators, they have helped to build the field and shape its domains. Their clinical experience, teaching and research efforts provide the critical background knowledge for framing the body of information that comprises the field of palliative social work.

They have both modeled the role of the social worker in interdisciplinary teams and in collaborative practices. They have team taught and led major educational efforts. Both have been in leadership positions in various organizations and have played important roles in supporting the development of standards in palliative social work and in advocating for formal certification programs. Both were supported as social work leaders in the Project on Death in America whose focus was to transform the culture of dying in the United States. Terry Altilio was our social worker on our Pain Service at Memorial Sloan-Kettering Cancer Center and our

team learned how to address and care for patients' and families' psychosocial needs from her.

The book begins with an historical perspective, which sets the stage for understanding how palliative care became a focus for social work practice and research. This section points out the challenges, struggles and current opportunities for social work's role in advocacy, treatment, care and support for patients with life-limiting illnesses.

Numerous chapters focus specific attention on the core competencies in training the social worker in palliative care; others describe the various settings and disease specific populations which invite social work expertise and which help to define their scope of practice. These chapters point out the wide range of opportunities for improving palliative care be it in the hospital, the hospice, the nursing home, the prison or the rural community. On the global perspective of palliative social work, a range of chapters by international faculty describe a rich array of culturally sensitive variations in social work practice in palliative care.

All of the chapters in the textbook are authored by experts in their topic area. Their writings reflect both a practical and theoretical knowledge of what are the important facts to know to provide palliative social work services.

This textbook has sufficient breath and depth that allows new social work students to learn the history and the basics of palliative social work and the expertise to refresh their knowledge and learn the field's potential, growth, development, international policy impact and future direction.

Professional and ethical issues are represented well and provide for the reader clear, balanced discussions of the challenges and complexities of caring for patients who are dying, coming to terms with a fatal illness, or trying to resolve complicated grief and bereavement issues.

Providing palliative care for all of those who need it is a daunting task. Such care requires an interdisciplinary team and the social worker is an essential team member. This textbook is a compendium of information that is authoritative, comprehensive and readable. It describes the elements of the field's core competencies and also the challenges of research, professional development and the integration of palliative care into health care policy. It joins two other *Oxford Textbooks*—in palliative medicine and nursing—expanding the body of knowledge and expertise in the field of palliative care and clearly describing the contributions and the role of the social worker and the domains of palliative social work.

Kathleen M. Foley, MD
Professor of Neurology, Neuroscience
& Clinical Pharmacology
Weill Medical College of Cornell University
Attending Neurologist
Memorial Sloan-Kettering-Cancer Center
Medical Director, International Palliative Care Initiative
Open Society Institute

FOREWORD BY RUSSELL K. PORTENOY

Whether driven by a sense of shared purpose to redress a distortion in medical care, or simply a sense of satisfaction that comes with helping others, health professionals of all types have begun to flock to the discipline of palliative care. In so doing, they are creating a great wave of good around the world. In many dozens of countries, professional caregivers have awakened to the importance of a competent and compassionate approach to patients with serious illness, and have targeted the delivery of high quality care to a set of primary goals, including the relief of suffering, lessening of illness burden, and retained quality of life, that have become the cornerstones of good palliative care for the ill and their families.

In the United States, the health professions are living through an exemplar experience. Following a period in the 1970s during which innovators developed early models of hospice or palliative care for the dying, US activists pushed the government to create a new national system of care delivery through the creation of the Medicare hospice benefit in 1983–1984. Although this benefit embodied many elements of a future construct—specialist palliative care—the early 1980s were a time of activism at the policy level which would much later be accompanied by operational frameworks that would define the specialty or position it in mainstream health care as a set of services to address the complex needs associated with advanced illness. Hospice quickly evolved into a very large and effective system for end-of-life care. The hospice industry serves more than one million patients and families each year, garners extraordinarily high rates of satisfaction by the families it touches, and saves the health system money. It has, however, remained largely outside of the mainstream health care system, usually accessed when death is less than a month away and disease-modifying therapies are stopped. The dedicated professionals who work in this US version of hospice have long understood that hospice needs integration into the larger system of health care, but the constructs that would provide a strategy for change were lacking for many years.

The term "palliative care" also entered the health-related lexicon in the 1970s, but there was no clear definition appropriate for the US system, the goals and objectives were not evident to most practitioners, and the distinctions between palliative care and the US version of hospice as a separate system for end-of-life care were indistinct. For most health professionals working in hospitals or in the community, the criterion that gave meaning to both these labels was the imminence of death and not the clinical need for management of illness burden in multiple domains. Take away the challenge of "dying well," and even the most compassionate physician, nurse or social worker was likely to doubt whether there really was a difference between palliative care and just good care of the sick.

The gradual, and quite extraordinary, change in this view is the context from which to understand the significance of this new tome devoted to specialist-level palliative care practiced by social workers. This book is more than a beautifully edited and much needed compendium of existing knowledge of theoretical and practical importance to social workers. It is yet another milestone along a path that is humanizing health care and establishing a set of specialist competencies without which a palliative care movement in the US and elsewhere would wither.

In the US, there have been many small but momentous steps along this path. Even as the Medicare benefit was the impetus for the development of a billion dollar industry to provide an interdisciplinary model of care for dying patients at home, expert committees were impaneled to define palliative care. Each of the US definitions, from the Institute of Medicine to the National Quality Forum, complemented those created by the World Health Organization and other international and national groups. All emphasized a set of core values and concerns targeting patients with any type of serious life-threatening illness and their families. It refers to patient-centered and family-focused care that addresses complex needs in any of the multiple domains that are affected by illness. It is care that is needed throughout the continuum of disease and in every venue of care. It overtly helps to define the goals of care and does so in the broadest terms, incorporating the objective of disease control to prolong life and limit the impact of pathology, but considering the appropriateness of this care when risks and burdens and true benefits are acknowledged. Medical decision making is grounded in culture and ethics, and refracted through the individual prism formed by the life experiences and the values, preferences and wishes of the patient and family.

Once the definition and the clinical objectives of palliative care were articulated, the important role of hospice became clearer and the need for better palliative care upstream from end-of-life became evident. Two simple observations provided subtext for this realization: Estimates of survival do not correlate well with clinical need, and in any case, prognostication is too inexact to rationalize access to care. Palliative care has become understood in the US as a model that supports the physical, psychosocial, and spiritual well being of the patient and family throughout the course of a disease that could require many years to progress. The focus on a clinical response to active dying is necessary, but not sufficient to address the burden of illness and its treatment. From diagnosis onward, the goals of care must be broadened to encompass expert symptom control, empathic and effective communication, management of psychological and psychosocial distress, help for spiritual and existential concerns, practical assistance and coordination of care, and other strategies to address the complicated and changeable scenario of illness. Palliative care accepts both the inevitability of death and the powerful desire to forestall it. When the disease is advanced and death is anticipated soon, palliative care acknowledges the potentially special nature of the care required by the patient or the family.

In the U.S. and a small number of other countries, this process of definition gradually overwhelmed an emerging controversy about the nature of palliative care—is it just good care, or is it something else? If palliative care is best understood as a therapeutic model targeting diverse populations with serious or life-threatening illnesses and pursued by diverse health professionals with common goals, it is undeniably part of the good care that should be offered by any professional, a best practice for physicians, nurses, social workers and others. This does not negate the alternative view, however. With validity endorsed by the success of the hospice industry, it is now axiomatic that some patients and families also need care delivered as a specialist practice by professionals with advanced training and specific resources.

The conceptualization of palliative care as a model that may be viewed through a lens that distinguishes generalist from specialist practice has had profound implications. It suggests to all types of health professionals that there is an affirmative obligation to understand the basics about this model of care and incorporate elements into practice whenever a patient with a serious or life-threatening illness requires treatment. All clinicians who provide services to patients with serious or life-threatening illness should have generalist-level skills in palliative care. They should understand and embrace the broad tenets of this discipline and perform core aspects, such as a multidimensional assessment. Each of these professionals can promote elements of good communication, such as advance care planning, or offer specific interventions that may address problems that undermine quality of life. Each should understand how to refer to other professionals or programs.

Generalist-level palliative care should be supported by systems of care, such as hospitals and nursing homes. These facilities can be encouraged to adopt specific programming, such as quality or performance improvement projects, patient or family education, or programs that reduce disparities related to language or culture. They should provide for accessible specialist services, like hospice.

Consensus about the parameters of generalist palliative care illuminates the nature of specialist care. More than 25 years ago, the federally-mandated hospice model required an interdisciplinary team for care delivered in the community, presaging an essential element of specialist practice. Specialists always try to work in teams, the core of which is the physician, the nurse, the social worker and the chaplain. Each member of the specialist team relies on the knowledge and skills of the others; ideally, each should have the advanced study, mentored training, and experience that are the foundations for specialist care. Together, the team offers continuous and comprehensive care with a level of sophistication and expertise that can handle complex problems and multiple sources of distress in any type of patient or family, in any venue of care. Although palliative care is inarguably not just end-of-life care, it is the setting of advanced disease and imminent death that often brings the type of complexity in goal setting and communication, and the management of symptoms and other sources of distress, that calls for the input of experts. In the US, institution-based palliative care teams rapidly evolved and now mirror in many hospitals and nursing homes the interdisciplinary approach to care for the dying pioneered by hospice.

The nature of specialist care places a very high value on professionalism. Indeed, it is the commitment to professionalism that may be one of the key drivers of the palliative care movement in the United States and other countries. "Professionalism" connotes an identity, supported by membership in a group defined by devotion to a core set of attitudes, deep knowledge, and a special set of skills. In health care, it implies a commitment to lifelong learning, quality work derived from standards of care, support for rational care based on evidence, and the promise of integrity and ethical practice.

Professionalism in the health professions also embraces the convention of certification. A certificate, earned by demonstration of knowledge and experience, is a tangible indicator that a discipline has defined itself, that committed practitioners exist, and that high standards will be applied as it evolves. In the US, the 2006 adoption by the American Board of Medical Specialties of a new medical subspecialty—Hospice and Palliative Medicine—gave new weight to the discipline for physicians. For these professionals, there was immediate mainstreaming, based on a long list of competencies that implicitly distinguished generalist from specialist care.

The acceptance of Hospice and Palliative Medicine as a medical subspecialty has been a very important milestone along the road to full integration of palliative care into the US system. It followed many positive events, which together gave support to an early vision of this change. Among these events were the earlier acceptance of palliative medicine's specialty status in United Kingdom and then several other countries, and the rapid growth of a medical literature devoted to the competencies required to specialize in this field. It was fitting that the first medical textbook devoted to palliative medicine, the Oxford Textbook of Palliative Medicine, originated from the UK. Published in 1993, this book assumed a role beyond a compendium of evolving knowledge. It awakened medical professionals to an emerging and rich literature in palliative care, and defined new medical reality of specialist practice by physicians.

Seventeen years following the publication of the first edition of the Oxford Textbook of Palliative Medicine, Altilio and Otis-Green have a similar accomplishment in producing the Oxford Textbook of Palliative Social Work. It is a signal to the broader professional community that palliative social work—specialist-level care provided to patients and families by social workers with specialist knowledge and competencies—is a reality. This book will add to the momentum for a formal specialty, support the professionalism of those already involved, and inspire younger colleagues to enter the field. Certainly important as a clinical resource, its good is likely to extend far beyond this, providing another essential step in the slow but inevitable shift in the priorities of a health care culture that remains in need of change.

Russell K. Portenoy, MD
Chairman, Department of Pain Medicine
and Palliative Care
Beth Israel Medical Center
New York, N.Y.

Professor of Neurology and Anesthesiology
Albert Einstein College of Medicine

PREFACE

Terry Altilio, MSW, LCSW, ACSW
Social Work Coordinator
Department of Pain Medicine & Palliative Care
Beth Israel Medical Center

Shirley Otis-Green, MSW, LCSW, ACSW, OSW-C
Senior Research Specialist
Division of Nursing Research and Education
City of Hope National Medical Center

"I've a feeling we're not in Kansas anymore" are the words spoken by Dorothy Gale, a curious, yearning, and adventurous young girl who, with her dog Toto, is magically transported during a tornado to a strange, unfamiliar place. These words from the novel *The Wonderful Wizard of Oz* (Baum, 1900) mark a transition from the sepia-toned landscape of a farm in Kansas to the technicolor, mystical Land of Oz, where Dorothy and Toto will encounter complex characters, some gentle, some harsh, some good, and some evil, and embark on an array of adventures infused with magic and beauty, fear and danger, mystery and humor.

In the movie *The Wizard of Oz* (1939), based on L. Frank Baum's classic novel, a range of human experiences are captured through words, songs, actions, conflicts, and allegories. For many, the story provides opportunities for philosophical and political analysis (Dirk, n. d.). We've chosen the phrase "we're not in Kansas anymore" to introduce this text because it marks a transition of sorts with implicit themes of self-realization and transformation, growth and collaboration, power and potential, loss and adaptation, magic and mystery. The adventures of Dorothy and Toto seize our attention because they involve unique characters, including witches, the Scarecrow, Tin Man, Lion, and the Wizard of Oz, who in curious ways synthesize necessary attributes of palliative care. The characters and their evolution serve as symbols for processes implicit in palliative social work, in the building of this text, and in the learning experience we have worked to create within these pages.

Themes and Characters

And what of the characters and themes that appear in the Land of Oz; how do they relate to the *Oxford Textbook of Palliative Social Work*? Almost immediately we are invited to consider a theme that is implicit in palliative care and has long been central to the focus of social work: the existential and emotional experience of feeling "unheard." Dorothy is rebuffed by the adults who surely care for her but are otherwise preoccupied. She chooses to run away both to save her dog Toto from potential harm and in reaction to having her fears and worries delegitimized and her needs minimized.

This theme of acknowledging the vulnerable and advocating for the needs of those who are unseen and unheard is pervasive throughout social work. Many persons who benefit from palliative services are vulnerable consequent to illness and the myriad of related bio-psychosocial-spiritual factors that impact their experience. This text reflects a focused voice for the profession and the populations that we serve—a voice asserted through the writings and lived experiences of over 130 authors.

This theme of impacting the lives of those with soft voices continues into the Land of Oz when Dorothy, through no conscious effort of her own, influences the social and existential experience of "little people" who have been enslaved by the powerful Wicked Witch of the West. Dorothy's house, lifted by the tornado, drops and ends both the life of this witch and her tyrannical powers. This precipitous death results in an unintended and unplanned consequence: The previously enslaved "little people" are freed and look to Dorothy as their heroine. This multidimensional and highly symbolic event is followed by the emergence of witches, both good and evil, who bring both guidance and threat to the world of Dorothy and Toto. It is in this complex setting of death, liberation, revenge, and serendipitous events that Dorothy begins to long for the comfort of her home and her caregivers, Auntie Em and Uncle Henry. She is guided by Glinda, a benevolent witch, and begins the trek down the yellow brick road in enchanted ruby red slippers to fulfill dreams and aspirations and seek the omniscient Wizard of Oz. Living in Emerald City, the Wizard purports to have mysterious powers that may transport Dorothy and Toto back to Kansas, to the familiarity and comforts of home.

The "yellow brick road" seems an appropriate metaphor for the evolving journey of social work into palliative care, while the magical "ruby slippers" are a symbol of endless potential to influence the care for patients and their families and the systems which are intended to serve them. The blend of the comforts implicit in Dorothy's longing for home and the mystery, uncertainty, and possibilities represented by Dorothy's beginning journey is for many a metaphorical representation of the illness experience that palliative care clinicians are privileged to join.

Here also is where the *Oxford Textbook of Palliative Social Work* has symbolic synergy with the lives and strivings of Dorothy and the companions who join her trek: the Scarecrow, the Tin Man, and the Lion. These allegorical figures represent essential aspects of clinical practice in palliative care. The Scarecrow desires knowledge, the ability to think; the Tin Man wants a heart to experience emotion; and the Lion searches for courage. They seek the Wizard of Oz, whose power and wisdom are thought to hold the answers to their

hopes, dreams, and self-realization. Of course, the trek is not without obstacles, danger, and challenges. Negotiations are necessary, hopes are enhanced and expanded, and the Wizard, while initially devious and insincere, eventually assists Dorothy and her colleagues to search for and discover their internal resources and abilities. Perceptions are reframed so that the pursuit for a brain stretches beyond an anatomical organ to the process of critical thinking, the need for a heart extends to the capacity to love and be loved, and pursuit for courage is woven with wisdom.

It is the intent of this text to integrate knowledge, thoughtfulness, heart, compassion, and courage as central components of palliative social work and to invite social workers to build on practice principles and values that are foundational and fundamental to this specialty. We invite readers on a journey to discover how the richness and depth of a sepia-toned world blends with the vibrance and excitement of technicolor. "We're not in Kansas anymore" is an invitation to honor and assimilate the range of concepts and values that are embedded in social work and palliative care and reflect that integrated experience in the manner in which we serve patients and families.

Blending: Sepia and Technicolor

We are privileged to present the *Oxford Textbook of Palliative Social Work* as a companion volume to the classic *Oxford Textbook of Palliative Medicine and the Oxford Textbook of Palliative Nursing*. This important addition to Oxford University's library of definitive palliative care textbooks reflects the unique synergy of palliative care and the social work profession, while honoring the interdisciplinary sharing that is fundamental to excellent care for patients and families. The need for this text grew concurrently with the global proliferation of palliative care and hospice programs, where social workers provide culturally respectful psychosocial-spiritual care for patients and families across a variety of settings and throughout the life span (Cadell, Johnston, Bosma & Wainright, 2010). It joins respected authors, educators, researchers, and practitioners to create a volume that integrates the best theory, research, and practice wisdom in a manner that both generalist and specialist clinicians and educators will find scholarly and practical.

Sepia tone for many evokes feelings of warmth and nostalgia, compelling a response that is significantly different than that elicited by the vibrant colors of a technicolor world. Many photographs printed with sepia tone evoke an older era. When our profession reflects on an "older era" we find traditions of service and advocacy on the individual, family, community, and policy level. Reflecting these historic roots, this text focuses on individuals, their families of origin, and families of creation, and it delineates the public policy and ethical issues that summon our participation and challenge us to intervene in such aspects of care as the undertreatment of pain, access to care, and the physical and psychosocial-spiritual impact of caregiving. We also see that early pioneers in social work articulated values and clinical perspectives that are essential to palliative care. As early as 1917, Mary Richmond emphasized a core value of providing the patient a "fair and patient hearing" and to establish, if possible, a sympathetic mutual understanding (1917, p. 114). Gordon Hamilton (1951) would later point to the importance of the person telling his or her own story and Helen Harris Perlman would reinforce the idea that the client's problem is best understood from his or her own perspective (1957). These principles are imminently transferable to palliative care because they encourage clinicians to search for and listen to the context in which illness occurs and to seek to understand the singular experience of each patient and family upon which to create a plan of care.

And what of the technicolor stimulus that set the stage for the publication of the *Oxford Textbook of Palliative Social Work*? These influences are many, emanating from within the profession of social work and from the evolution of palliative care as an interdisciplinary specialty. The initiative and advocacy for our text followed a period of intense and exciting growth of the specialty. In 2009, the National Consensus Project for Quality Palliative Care (NCP) issued the second edition of the *Clinical Practice Guidelines for Quality Palliative Care*, which included the following eight domains of care, each of which invites expert social work participation:

- Structure and processes of care
- Physical aspects of care
- Psychosocial and psychiatric aspects of care
- Social aspects of care
- Spiritual, religious, and existential aspects of care
- Cultural aspects of care
- Care of the imminently dying patient
- Ethical and legal aspects of care

Each domain is followed by specific clinical practice guidelines regarding professional behavior and service delivery (National Consensus Project for Quality Palliative Care, 2009, p. 14).

In 2006, the National Quality Forum (NQF), a private nonprofit organization that aims to improve the quality of health care for Americans, endorsed, adopted, and integrated the *Clinical Practice Guidelines for Quality Palliative Care* into their document *A National Framework for Palliative and Hospice Care Quality Measurement and Reporting*. The NQF reinforced that palliative care:

Refers to patient and family-centered care that optimizes quality of life by anticipating, preventing, and treating suffering. Palliative care throughout the continuum of illness involves addressing physical, intellectual, emotional, social, and spiritual needs and facilitating patient autonomy, access to information, and choice. Hospice care is a service delivery system that provides palliative care for patients who have a

limited life expectancy and require comprehensive biomedical, psychosocial, and spiritual support as they enter the terminal stage of an illness or condition. It also supports family members coping with the complex consequences of illness, disability, and aging as death nears. Hospice care further addresses the bereavement needs of the family following the death of the patient. Of particular importance, palliative care services are indicated across the entire trajectory of a patient's illness and its provision should not be restricted to the end-of-life phase. (NQF, p. VI)

The Framework document provides the foundation upon which to build a quality measurement and reporting system. As shown in Table I., it identifies the 12 structural and programmatic elements as essential to quality performance.

The Framework served as a guide for the development of 38 preferred practices, derived from the NCP eight domains of quality palliative and hospice care. These preferred practices are intended to serve as "building blocks for high quality programs across many practice settings and as the basis for developing performance measures" (NQF, p. VI). (For more information, please see Chapter 53).

The domains, guidelines, and preferred practices assist clinicians to serve persons who are living with life-threatening disease, responding to their needs and those of their families, over time and transitions, working to build continuity and coherence as patients and family move through the experience of illness. In addition to the essential synchrony of social work values with principles of palliative care, the profession has an existing opportunity to move palliative care beyond health care settings into the community. For example, social workers employed in senior centers may easily become advocates for pain and symptom management, assist participants who might wish to complete advance directives, and intervene when caregiver distress impacts older adults and their families. School social workers who work with families where illness exists or death occurs have the opportunity to intervene on an individual, family,

Table I. National Quality Forum: Elements of Quality Performance	
Interdisciplinary teams	Quality assessment/ performance improvement
Diverse models of delivery	Community outreach programs
Bereavement programs	Administrative policies
Educational programs	Information technology and data gathering
Patient and family education	Methods for resolving ethical dilemmas
Volunteer programs	Personnel self-care initiatives
Source: National Quality Forum, 2006, p. 8–11.	

institutional, or community level. Private practitioners will meet clients whose histories, current realities, or futures involve illness-, death-, or grief-related experiences, which often become the substance of therapeutic work. We hope that this text, while reflecting the learning and skill required of specialist providers, will also invite generalist clinicians to integrate an awareness of palliative social work. In this way, the profession actualizes a latent potential to enhance the care of patients and family members who may never require or request palliative care consultation.

The technicolor world of palliative care includes specific social work documents that are available to enrich and standardize practice excellence within the profession. For example, the National Association of Social Workers has established Standards for End-of-Life Care (NASW, 2009a) and in collaboration with the National Hospice and Palliative Care Organization (NHPCO, 2009) developed a social work credential in hospice and palliative care (NASW, 2009b) (for more information, please see Chapter 77). In Canada, palliative social workers established 11 practice competencies through a process of national consultation that included developing and validating the competencies and creating a plan for implementation (Bosma et al., 2009; Kelley et al., 2009). Available through the Canadian Hospice Palliative Care Association, these competencies are unique in that they evolved through a national consultation process which included interdisciplinary providers as well as recipients of services (for more information, see Chapter 55). Since the inception of the Project on Death in America Social Work Leadership Awards in 1999, there have been a plethora of projects, documents, and research validating professional values while enhancing the technicolor landscape within which the work of palliative care occurs (for more information, see Chapters 3, 76, and 77).

Oxford Textbook of Palliative Social Work:
A Sectional Overview

The *Oxford Textbook of Palliative Social Work* has many objectives. As an inaugural edition in a specialty that is essentially interdisciplinary, our challenge has been to reflect the unique social work contribution and potential while respecting the shared and collaborative nature of palliative care. Our primary goal was to create a text that honors the practice wisdom and compassion of social workers while simultaneously informing this work whenever possible with evidence. We have engaged authors with a passion for their work and specialties, some who are emerging leaders, as well as many who have contributed not only to the evolution of palliative social work but also to the growth and integrity of the profession as a whole. With this in mind, the first section of this text is devoted to the historical development of social work. Readers will find "Social Work and Palliative Care: The Early

History" a critical commentary focusing on palliative care pioneer Dame Cicely Saunders. This is followed by an informative chapter on the emergence of the field by inspirational leader Bernice Catherine Harper.

In conceptualizing the text we chose to integrate culture within the chapters to reflect the integrated nature of the cultural experience of patients, families, and clinicians. "Patient and family narrative" is the phrase we have selected to describe the clinical situations that exemplify the work of palliative social work and to emphasize the persons beyond the diagnosis and the dilemmas that they live and struggle with throughout the course of illness.

The setting-specific section of the text sends an implicit message to practicing clinicians who might discover the potential benefits that palliative care can provide to their setting and their population while at the same time stimulating a reciprocal contribution to the evolving palliative care knowledge base.

An overarching goal has been to provide clinicians, educators, researchers, and policy makers with a resource that delineates the range of screening, assessment, and intervention skills and perspectives that inform and enrich the practice of palliative social work.

Chapters focusing on population- and illness-specific practice reflect the generic and all-encompassing focus of palliative care principles irrespective of the diagnosis, age, or social circumstance of persons living with life-threatening illness. These chapters bring a variety of populations into focus, including children, elders, inmates, veterans, rural and urban dwellers, and many others. Authors worked to delineate the challenges of each disease and the needs of specific populations to assist readers in grasping the context in which palliative care may be helpful to patients, their families, the intimate network, and the larger social system in which they are cared for.

The collaborative practice section of the text reinforces the essential collective nature of palliative care, sometimes shared between social workers, across disciplines, settings, and systems, creating an ongoing challenge to ensure that care is not compromised and that patients and families are not abandoned as they move through the disease trajectory. These chapters are co-authored with colleagues across disciplines, and we invite you to use these chapters to foster thoughtfulness and discussion about interdisciplinary relationships and to consider how teams and individuals negotiate the communal aspects of the work while respecting the unique expertise of each professional. Social workers in health care settings have survived consequent to their ability to share, so the challenge for our profession may be essentially different from that of nurses, physicians, or spiritual care providers who have varied histories and relationships to health care settings and teamwork. To this end, the collaborative practice section reflects the experiences of clinicians who have worked together to provide narratives and models that may serve to enhance and amplify the relationships which often go unexplored day after day, month after month.

The global section offers readers a glimpse into the experience of patients and families living around the world and into the practice of the social workers who serve them. While the scope of palliative care involves interventions along the continuum of illness, we see in the global section that in many places in the world limited resources force a focus on the essential needs of the imminently dying and their families. The creativity, clinical work, and cultural nuance integrated into these chapters demonstrate a richness and resourcefulness that emanates not from funds and budgets, but from social workers passionately committed to giving voice to their patients and families.

The ethics chapters discuss ethical principles specific to social work and explore various topics that infuse health care debate and clinical decision making across settings, diseases, and populations. The aim of this section is to enhance critical thinking and shared decision making while acknowledging that the complexity and profound nature of the questions may provoke conflict and shared struggle, which are often essential elements of authentic interdisciplinary team practice.

The last section provides an overview of professional issues relevant to this emerging specialty with a closing chapter that reflects the accumulated wisdom gleaned from the lived experiences of patients, families, and practitioners.

We hope that readers will find the *Oxford Textbook of Palliative Social Work* a useful tool to navigate their own "yellow brick road." The text is a tribute to the values and principles that infuse the social work profession, to the patients, their families, partners, and friends whose lives and experiences are represented in the narratives and to the clinician wisdom presented within the chapters. Finally this is an invitation to our profession to integrate and build theory and research and enhance critical thinking both to inform and enrich current practice and advocacy and to contribute to the growth and capacity of palliative care to meet the common human needs of those who are impacted by life-threatening illness.

REFERENCES

Baum, L. F. (1900). *The wonderful wizard of Oz.* Chicago, IL: George M. Hill Company.

Bosma, H., Johnston, M., Cadell, S., Wainwright, W., Abernethy, N., Feron, A., . . . Nelson, F. (2009). Creating social work competencies for practice in hospice palliative care. *Palliative Medicine, 23,* 1–9. doi:10.1177/0269216309346596

Cadell, S., Johnston, M., Bosma, H., & Wainright, W. (2010). An overview of contemporary social work practice in palliative care. *Progress in Palliative Care, 18(4),* 205–211.

Dirk, T. (n. d.) The wizard of Oz (1939). Retrieved from http://www.filmsite.org/wiza4.html

Hamilton, G. (1951). *Theory and practice of social casework.* New York, NY: Columbia University Press.

Kelley, M. L., Kortes-Miller, K., Kerbashian, J., Cadell, S., Feron, A., Wainwright, W., . . . Thompson, M. (2009, May). *Palliative end-of-life care: A dialogue about social work practice competencies and educational strategies for implementation.* Panel presentation presented at the meeting of Canadian Association of Social Work Educators Annual Conference 2009, Ottawa, ON.

National Association of Social Workers. (2009a). *NASW standards for practice in palliative and end-of-life Care.* Retrieved from http://www.naswdc.org/practice/bereavement/standards/default.asp

National Association of Social Workers. (2009b). Certified Hospice and Palliative Social Worker (CHP-SW) and Advanced Certified Hospice and Palliative Social Worker (ACHP-SW). Retrieved from http://www.naswdc.org/credentials/credentials/chpsw.asp

National Consensus Project for Quality Palliative Care. (2009). *Clinical practice guidelines for quality palliative care* (2nd ed.). Retrieved from http://www.nationalconsensusproject.org/guideline.pdf

National Hospice and Palliative Care Organization. (2009). Join NHPCO. Retrieved from http://www.nhpco.org/i4a/pages/index.cfm?pageid=3307

National Quality Forum. (2006). *A national framework and preferred practices for palliative and hospice care quality: A consensus report.* Retrieved from http://www.qualityforum.org/Publications/2006/12/A_National_Framework_and_Preferred_Practices_for_Palliative_and_Hospice_Care_Quality.aspx

Perlman, H. H. (1957). *Social casework: A problem solving process.* Chicago, IL: University of Chicago Press.

Richmond, M. E. (1917). *Social diagnosis.* New York, NY: Free Press.

ACKNOWLEDGMENTS

This volume represents an emblematic collaboration that began in 2009 at the American Academy of Hospice and Palliative Care annual meeting. It was there that Betty Ferrell, PhD extended the invitation to meet with Tracy O'Hara, editor at Oxford University Press to propose a comprehensive palliative social work textbook. Since that fateful meeting, Betty's unwavering mentorship and inspiration have both nurtured and challenged us.

We are eternally grateful to Lisa Kilburn, BA, for her boundless energy, professionalism and commitment to improving these pages. We are indebted to our Oxford team for their support and to the dedication of all who have sustained this effort.

We are humbled by the expertise and passion expressed by the contributors to this text. The social work practice and perspectives reflected in these pages honor the patients, families and colleagues who have enriched our work and our lives. Our hope is that the lessons so arduously learned and so generously shared will enable future social workers to integrate palliative care principles within their practice, education and research.

We dedicate this work to our sons, Douglas and Manne, in the hope that future generations will have reliable access to equitable and integrated care delivered by competent and compassionate healthcare providers who embody a personal commitment to excellence.

CONTRIBUTORS

Terry Altilio, MSW, LCSW, ACSW
Social Work Coordinator
Department of Pain Medicine & Palliative Care
Beth Israel Medical Center
New York, NY

Becky A. Anderson, LMSW ACHP-SW
Palliative Care Fellowship
VA Hospice and Palliative Care Center
VA Palo Alto Healthcare System
Palo Alto, CA

Linda Anngela-Cole, MSW, PhD
Assistant Professor
School of Social Work
University of Nevada, Reno
Reno, NV

Amy Bauer, MSSA, LISWS
Cleveland Clinic Health Systems
Cleveland, OH

Diane Benefiel, MSW, LCSW
The University of Texas M.D. Anderson Cancer Center
Houston, TX

Laura Benson RN, MS, ANP, AOCN
Vice President, Medical Affairs
(OSI) Oncology
Melville, NY

Peter Beresford OBE, BA Hons Oxon, PhD, AcSS, FRSA,
    DipWP
Professor of Social Policy and Director of the Centre for
    Citizen Participation
Brunel University
Uxbridge, West London, United Kingdom

Mercedes Bern-Klug, PhD, MSW, MA
Assistant Professor, School of Social Work
Director, UI Aging Studies Program
John A. Hartford Geriatric Social Work
    Faculty Scholar
University of Iowa
Iowa City, Iowa

Susan Blacker, MSW, RSW
Director
Cancer Services Planning & Performance
St. Michael's Hospital
Toronto, Ontario, Canada

Joann N. Bodurtha, M.D., M.P.H.
Professor, Department of Human and
    Molecular Genetics
Virginia Commonwealth University
Richmond, VA

Tracy Borgmeyer, LCSW
St. John's Regional Medical Center
Joplin, MO

Harvey Bosma, MSW, PhD Candidate
University of British Columbia
Vancouver, BC, Canada

Karlynn BrintzenhofeSzoc, PhD, MSW, OSW-C
Catholic University of America
Washington, DC

Teri Browne, PhD, MSW
Health Social Work Services Research Assistant Professor
College of Social Work
University of South Carolina
Irmo, SC

David M. Browning, MSW, BCD
Senior Research Scientist
Education Development Center
Senior Scholar
Institute for Professionalism and Ethical Practice
Children's Hospital Boston
Boston, MA

Karen Bullock, PhD, LCSW
Associate Professor
John A. Hartford Scholar
North Carolina State University
Department of Social Work
Raleigh, NC

Susan Cadell, MSW, PhD
Associate Professor, Director Manulife
    Centre for Healthy Living
Wilfrid Laurier University
Ontario, Canada

John G. Cagle, MSW, PhD
Research Fellow
Cecil G. Sheps Center for Health Services Research
University of North Carolina at Chapel Hill
Chapel Hill, NC

Katharine M. Campbell, PhD, LCSW, OSW-c
Clinical Oncology Social Worker
Sylvester Comprehensive Cancer Center–Deerfield
UHealth: University of Miami Health System
Deerfield Beach, FL

Grace H. Christ, DSW, PhD
Professor, Columbia University School of Social Work
New York, NY

Nancy F. Cincotta, MSW, MPhil, LCSW, ACSW, BCD
Director of Psychosocial Services
Camp Sunshine at Sebago Lake
Casco, Maine
Adjunct Instructor
Department of Preventive Medicine
The Mount Sinai School of Medicine
New York, NY

Elizabeth J. Clark, PhD, ACSW, MPH
Executive Director
National Association of Social Workers
Washington, DC

Yvette Colón, PhD, ACSW, BCD
Director of Education and Support
American Pain Foundation
Baltimore, MD

Maura Conry, Pharm D, MSW, LCSW, LSCSW
Kansas City, KS

Suzy Croft, BA Hons, CQSW
Diploma in Applied Social Sciences
Senior Scholar
Senior Social Worker
St. Johns Hospice
London, United Kingdom

Ellen L. Csikai, MSW, MPH, PhD
Professor
Editor, Journal of Social Work in End-of-Life and
    Palliative Care
School of Social Work
The University of Alabama
Tuscaloosa, AL

Louisa Daratsos, LCSW, ACSW
Psychosocial Coordinator Oncology/Palliative Care
New York Harbor Healthcare System
Brooklyn Campus; Doctoral Candidate
Wurzweiler School of Social Work
Yeshiva University

Elena Davis-Stenhouse, LCSW
Palliative Care Specialist
Denver, CO

Csaba L. Degi, MSW, PhD
Babes-Bolyai University
Faculty of Sociology and Social Work
Cluj Napoca, Romania

Elena D'Urbano
Licenciada Trabajadora Social
Pallium Latinoamérica
Equipo de Cuidados Paliativos del Hospital del Gobierno de
    la Ciudad de Buenos Aires "Dr. Carlos B. Udaondo"
Buenos Aires, Argentina

Sheila R. Enders, MSW
Associate Clinical Professor
Department of Internal Medicine
University of California, Davis

Betty R. Ferrell, PhD, MA, FAAN, FHPN
Research Scientist
Division of Nursing Research and Education
Department of Population Sciences
City of Hope National Medical Center
Duarte, CA

Iris Cohen Fineberg, PhD, MSW
International Observatory on End of Life Care
School of Health and Medicine
Lancaster University
Lancaster, United Kingdom

Richard B. Francoeur PhD, MSW, MS
Associate Professor
School of Social Work
Adelphi University
Garden City, NY

Daniel S. Gardner, PhD, LCSW
Assistant Professor
New York University
Silver School of Social Work
New York, NY

Julie Garrard BSW, MSW with Merit
    (University of Sydney)
Senior Social Worker and Researcher
Calvary Health Care
Sydney, Australia

Les Gallo-Silver, LCSW-R
Associate Professor in Health Sciences/
    Program Director of Human Services
LaGuardia Community College
Long Island City, NY

Sarah Gehlert, MA, MSW, LCSW
E. Desmond Lee Professor of Racial and Ethnic Diversity
The Brown School
Washington University in St. Louis
St. Louis, MO

Susan Gerbino, PhD, LCSW
Clinical Associate Professor
Silver School of Social Work
New York University
Hartsdale, NY

Myra Glajchen, DSW
Director
Institute for Education and Research in Pain and
    Palliative Care
Department of Pain Medicine and Palliative Care
Beth Israel Medical Center
New York, NY

William Goeren, LCSW-R, ACSW, BCD
Director of Men's Cancers Program
Senior Clinical Supervisor
CancerCare National Office

Jaime Goldberg, MSW
Palliative Social Worker
VA Greater Los Angeles Healthcare System
Los Angeles, CA

Ellen Goldring, LPC, ATR-BC, CCLS
Hackensack University Medical Center
Hackensack, NJ

Julie Greathouse
Senior Social Worker
Pain Medicine and Palliative Care
Children's Hospital at Westmead
Sydney, Australia

Gary Gardia, MED, LCSW
President
Gary Gardia Inc.
Las Vegas, NV

Bernice Catherine Harper, MSW, MSc.PH, LLD, ACSW
Retired
Rockville, MD

Hollye Harrington Jacobs, RN, MS, MSW
Vice President of Programs
Dream Foundation
Santa Barbara, CA

Sue Hearn BSW (UNSW)
Grad Cert Palliative Care (Edith Cowan) & Loss & Grief
    (Univeritsy of Queensland)
Manager Social Work/Bereavement Coordinator
HammondCare Health & Hospitals Greenwich
Sydney Australia

Susan Hedlund, MSW, LCSW
Director of Social Services
Hospice of Washington County
Faculty-Portland State University
Graduate School of Social Work
Portland, OR

Christopher M. Herndon, PharmD, BCPS
Assistant Professor
Southern Illinois University School of Pharmacy
Edwardsville, IL

Philip C. Higgins, MSW, LICSW
Director of Palliative Care Outreach
Clinical Social Worker
Pain & Palliative Care Service
Dana Farber/Brigham & Women's Cancer Center
Boston, MA

Jimmie C. Holland, MD
Wayne E. Chapman Chair in Psychiatric Oncology
Attending Psychiatrist
Department of Psychiatry & Behavioral Sciences
Memorial Sloan-Kettering Cancer Center
New York, NY

Jennifer Jane Hunt, MA
Independent Palliative Care and
    Bereavement Consultant
Avondale, Harare, Zimbabwe

Barbara Ivanko
Chief Operating Officer
Hospice of Palm Beach County
West Palm Beach, FL

Diane R. Jackson, MSW, LCSW, BCPS, CPE
Major, US Air Force
Belleville Family Health Center
Belleville, IL

Aarti Jagannathan MA, M.PHIL
National Institute of Mental Health and Neurosciences
    (NIMHANS)
Koramangala, Bangalore, India

Meaghen Johnston, MSW, PhD Candidate
University of British Columbia
Calgary, Alberta, Canada

Barbara L. Jones, PhD, MSW
University of Texas at Austin School of Social Work
Austin, TX

Srilatha Juvva, PhD
Tata Institute of Social Sciences (TISS)
Deonar, Mumbai, India

Lana Sue Ka'opua, MSW, LSW(HI), DCSW
Associate Professor & Chair
Health Concentration Director
Ka Lei Mana'olana Breast Health Project
Honolulu, HI

Julia Kasl-Godley, PhD
Staff Psychologist
VA Hospice and Palliative Care Center
VA Palo Alto Health Care System (116B)
Palo Alto, CA

Sheila G. Kennedy, MSW, LCSW
Hospice Coordinator
VA Hospice & Palliative Care Center
Palo Alto, CA

Jeanne Kerwin, DMH, CT
Ethics & Palliative Care Coordinator
Overlook Hospital
Summit, NJ

Yukie Kurihara, LMSW, LMT
Division of Palliative Medicine
Shizuoka Cancer Center
Nagaizumi, Shizuoka, Japan

Cecilia Lai Wan Chan, BsocSc, MsocSc, PhD, RSW
Si Yuan Professor in Health and Social Work
Director, Center on Behavioral Health
University of Hong Kong
Hong Kong, China

Robin Rudy Lawson, LMSW
Tampa, FL

Carrie Lethborg, PhD, MSW, BSW
Oncology Department
St. Vincent's Hospital
Victoria Parade, Fitzroy, Victoria, Australia

John F. Linder, MSW, LCSW
Specialist, Department of Internal Medicine
Division of Hematology & Oncology
University of California, Davis

A. Marlene Lockey, MSSW, LCSW
The University of Texas M.D. Anderson Cancer Center
Houston, TX

Marie C. Lynn, MSW, LMSW
Borgess Visiting Nurse and Hospice
Kalamazoo, MI

Valerie Maasdorp, B Soc Sc (SW), CT (Adec)
Island Hospice & Bereavement Service
Belgravia, Harare, Zimbabwe

Louise E. Marasco, PhD
Palo Alto Veterans Affairs Healthcare System, Fellowship
Psychology 116B
Palo Alto, CA

Anne Martin, PhD, LCSW
Memorial Sloan Kettering Cancer Center
Department of Social Work
Clinical Supervisor/Program Manager
New York, NY

Lucia McBee, LCSW, MPH, CYI
Jewish Home Lifecare
New York, NY

Andrew J. McCormick, PhD, MSW
Harborview Medical Center
Seattle, WA

Kelly M. McHenry MSW
San Diego, CA

Patricia McKinnon, BA Dip Soc Wk Grad Cert Social Work
    (Dying, Death & Palliative Care) with Merit, DSW
    research student (University of Sydney)
Senior Palliative Care Social Worker
Sacred Heart Hospice
Sydney, Australia

Carolyn Messner, DSW, MSW, LCSW-R, BCD
Director of Education & Training
CancerCare
New York, NY

Margaret Meyer, MSW, MBA, LCSW
The University of Texas M.D. Anderson Cancer Center
Houston, TX

Jaclyn Miller, MSSW, LCSW, PhD
Associate Professor Emeritus
School of Social Work
Virginia Commonwealth University
Richmond, VA

Pamela J. Miller, MSW, PhD
Professor of Social Work
School of Social Work
Portland State University
Portland, OR

John Mondanaro, MA, LCAT, MT_BC, CCLS
Beth Israel Medical Center
New York, NY

Kennan Moore, MSW, LCSW
Palliative Care Specialist
Denver, CO

Teresa Moro, MSW, Phd(c)
University of Chicago
Glenview, IL

Colleen M. Mulkerin, MSW, LCSW
Director
Palliative Medicine Consult Service
Hartford Hospital
Hartford, CT

Susan Murty, PhD
School of Social Work
University of Iowa
Iowa City, IA

Rebecca Myers, MSW, ACSW
Director, External Relations
National Association of Social Workers
Washington, DC

J. J. Nadicksbernd, MSW
Institute for Palliative Medicine
San Diego Hospice
San Diego, CA

Stacey Needleman, MA, MSW, LCSW, ACSW
Senior, Licensed Clinical Social Worker
The Joseph M. Sanzari Children's Hospital
Hackensack University Medical Center
Hackensack, NJ

Holly Nelson-Becker, MSW, PhD, LCSW, ACSW, DCSW
Associate Professor
University of Kansas School of Social Welfare
Lawrence, KS

Becky Niemeyer, LCSW
Palliative Care Specialist
Denver, CO

Patricia O'Donnell, PhD, LICSW, MSW
Director, Center for Ethics
Inova Health System
Fairfax, VA

Stacy F. Orloff, EdD, LCSW, ACHP-SW
Suncoast Hospice
Clearwater, FL

Shirley Otis-Green, MSW, LCSW, ACSW, OSW-C
Senior Research Specialist
Division of Nursing Research and Education
City of Hope National Medical Center
Duarte, CA

Guadalupe R. Palos, RN, LMSW, DrPH
The University of Texas M. D. Anderson Cancer Center
Houston, TX

Debra Parker Oliver, PhD, MSW
Associate Professor, University of Missouri
Family and Community Medicine
Columbia, MO

Lissa Parsonnet, PhD, LCSW, OSW-C
Private Practice
Springfield, NJ

Malcolm Payne, BA, DipSS, PhD
Policy and Development Adviser
St Christopher's Hospice
London, United Kingdom
Visiting Professor, Opole University, Poland
Honorary Professor, Kingston University/St George's
    University of London

Judith R. Peres, LCSW-C
Supporting Successful Transitions
Private Clinical Social Work Practice
Expert Consultant in Long-Term Care and Palliative Care
Bethesda, MD

Shlomit Perry, PhD, MSW
Davidoff Center
Belinson Hospital
Petach-Tikva, Israel

Farya Phillips, MA, CCLS
Doctoral Student, School of Social Work
University of Texas at Austin
Austin, TX

Linda F. Piotrowski, MTS, BCC
Pastoral Care Coordinator
Palliative Care/Norris Cotton Cancer Center
Dartmouth-Hitchcock Medical Center
Lebanon, NH

Robin Pollens, MS, CCC-SLP
Western Michigan University
Department of Speech Pathology and Audiology
Kalamazoo, MI

Pamela Pui Yu Leung, BSW, PhD, RSW
Assistant Professor
Department of Social Work and Social Administration
Honorary Research Fellow; Center of Behavioral Health &
    Center on Aging
The University of Hong Kong
Hong Kong

Hanan Qasim
Senior Social Worker in the Oncology Day Care Unit
Social Work Coordinator, Breast Cancer Services
Shaare Zedek Medical Center
Jerusalem, Israel

John M. Quillin, PhD, MPH, CGC
Assistant Professor of Human and Molecular Genetics
Virginia Commonwealth University
Richmond, VA

Mary Raymer, LMSW, ACSW, DPNAP
Chief Clinician/President
Raymer Psychotherapy & Consultation Services, PC
Acme, MI

Dona J. Reese, PhD, MSW, LCSW
School of Social Work
Southern Illinois University Carbondale
Carbondale, IL

Margaret Reith, BA, CQSW, MPhil, AASW
Senior Social Worker
Palliative Care Team, Epsom and St Helier University
    Hospitals NHS Trust
Sutton, United Kingdom

Stacey S. Remke, MSW, LICSW
Children's Institute for Pain and Palliative Care Pain
Palliative Care Program Children's Hospitals and Clinics
Minneapolis, MN

Bernice Sandowski, MSW, MS
Doctoral Student
Adelphi University School of Social Work
Interim Administrator
Good Samaritan Nursing Home
Garden City, NY

Dame Cicely Saunders OM, DBE, FRCP, FRCN (1918–2005)
Director, St. Christopher's Hospice, UK

Michal Scharlin, MSW, MPH
Palliative Social Worker, Fellowship Trained
Veterans Integrated Palliative Program
VA Greater Los Angeles Healthcare System
Los Angeles, CA

Tracy A. Schroepfer, PhD
Assistant Professor
Hartford Geriatric Social Work Faculty Scholar
University of Wisconsin-Madison
Madison, WI

Sheryl Shermak, MSW, RSW
PhD Student
School of Nursing
University of Victoria
Victoria, BC, Canada

Nancy J. Sherman, MSW, MSM, LICSW
Center for Grief and Healing/Hospice of the North Shore
Danvers, MA

Kelsey Simons, PhD, MSW
Social Work Scientist
Baycrest
Kunin-Lunenfeld Applied Research Unit
Assistant Professor of Social Work
Factor-Inwentash Faculty of Social Work
University of Toronto
Toronto, Ontario, Canada

Kathryn M. Smolinski, MSW
Juris Doctor Candidate
Wayne State University School of Law
Detroit, MI

Judith Solomon, MSW, LCSW, MPH
Hackensack University Medical Center
Hackensack, NJ

Donna L. Soltura, MSW
Continuing Care Manager
Palliative Care Service
Dartmouth Hitchcock Medical Center
Lebanon, NH

Doretta Stark, MA, LICSW
Retired–University of Minnesota Medical Center Palliative
    Care Consultation Service and Clinical Manager,
    Oncology Social Work Department
Currently, Private Consultant
St. Paul, MN

Gary L. Stein, JD, MSW
Associate Professor
Wurzweiler School of Social Work
Yeshiva University
New York, NY

Kathryn Thornberry, LCSW
Doris A. Howell Service
John & Rebecca Moores Comprehensive Cancer Center
University of California, San Diego
San Diego, CA

Charles F. von Gunten, MD, PhD
Institute for Palliative Medicine at San Diego Hospice
San Diego, CA

Katherine Walsh, PhD, MSW, LICSW
Associate Professor
Westfield State University
Westfield, MA

Wendy Walters, LCSW, OSW-C
University of Alabama at Birmingham Hospital
Birmingham, AL

Cheng Wan Peh, MSocSci (Counseling) BA, RSW
Senior Medical Social Worker
Department of Medical Social Services
Assisi Hospice
Singapore

Karla T. Washington, MSW, PhD
Assistant Professor
University of Louisville
Kent School of Social Work
Louisville, KY

Dennis E. Watts
University of Alabama at Birmingham Hospital
Birmingham, AL

Tzer Wee Ng, MSW, RSW
Principal Medical Social Worker
Dept. of Care and Counseling
Tan Tock Seng Hospital
Singapore

Sherri Weisenfluh
Hospice of the Bluegrass
Lexington, KY

Yvonne Yim, MSW, LCSW(HI), DCSW
Private Consultant and Clinician
Director of Operation, HBI
Honolulu, HI

James R. Zabora, ScD, MSW
Dean, School of Social Service
National Catholic University
Washington, DC

Oxford Textbook of **Palliative Social Work**

I
Historical Context

"One must start somewhere. On the beginning of your journey in palliative care, I would strongly suggest to find yourself a supportive, knowledgeable and joyful mentor."

Sandy Chan LCSW, ACHP-SW
Stanford Hospital and Clinics
Palliative Care Inpatient Consult Service
Inpatient Medical Oncology

1   *Dame Cicely Saunders, OM, DBE, FRCP, FRCN*

Social Work and Palliative Care—The Early History*

Dame Cicely trained as a nurse, a medical social worker, and finally as a physician. Since 1948 she has been involved with the care of patients with terminal illness, has lectured widely on this subject, written many articles, and contributed to a great number of books. She founded St Christopher's Hospice in 1967 as the first research and teaching hospice linked with clinical care. This has been a pioneer in the field of palliative medicine, which has now been established worldwide.

Dame Cicely is recognized as the founder of the modern hospice movement and has received many honors and awards for her work. She holds over 25 honorary degrees, from both this country and overseas. Awards include the BMA Gold Medal for services to medicine, the Templeton Prize for Progress in Religion, the Onassis Prize for Services to Humanity, The Raoul Wallenberg Humanitarian Award, and the Franklin D. Roosevelt Four Freedoms for Worship Medal. She also holds the Freedoms of the London Boroughs of Bromley and Lewisham, the areas served by St Christopher's Hospice.

Dame Cicely was awarded the Order of Merit by Her Majesty The Queen, the highest personal honor the monarch can bestow.

The recent research of Professor David Clark (1998, 1999a, 1999b) make it clear that a hospice movement was underway in both the United Kingdom and the United States several years before 1967, the opening of St Christopher's Hospice in South East London[1]. Although that has frequently been given as the beginning of the modern hospice development, some of the earlier literature and much correspondence reveal how the basic concepts and principles came together long before its opening. From its beginnings during the 1960s, it brought together sound research and multidisciplinary education with care for people at the end of life, wherever they may be.

Much of the early correspondence was with social workers, psychiatrists, and sociologists in the United States, as well as with the early researchers in clinical studies of pain relief. The hospice emphasis on the whole family, its needs and role as part of the caring team in home care, stems from the first of these disciplines as well as my own training experience as a "Lady Almoner" or medical social worker, from 1946 through 1951. Home care and family and bereavement support were planned from the beginning, alongside the controlled drug studies and work on the general management of pain and other symptoms. Such an approach has had a strong influence on the ability of the movement to cross boundaries of culture and resources and to flourish in both industrialized and developing countries. This has rightly been recognized as a medical speciality, but because it ideally goes far beyond symptom control alone, it demands the whole multiprofessional team. Social workers, so early involved with the insoluble problems of lack of suitable support or facilities, produced a number of articles relating to this area of care which deserve wider recognition.

In July 1947 I joined the Lady Almoner's Department of St Thomas' Hospital in London. I was a member of the Northcote Trust Team founded in 1909 to support social work first begun in the hospital in 1905. In the days of cash-strapped voluntary hospitals, we had to collect vouchers and suggest possible contributions to patients. It was a huge relief when the National Health Service was introduced in 1948.

We also carried out a surprising amount of case work and family support. Our department kept a cancer register and followed up on patients who had been discharged with the help of an energetic home visitor. My own experience with the end-of-life problems of distressed patients and families and the many home visits this entailed had a lasting influence on the way the modern hospice developed with its regard for the family as both the unit of care and, frequently, the caring team. Social work input into the field owes much to several early pioneers whose writings merit renewed attention. The first of these was Ruth Abrams (Abrams, Jameson, Poehlman, & Snyder, 1945), senior social worker at Massachusetts General Hospital for many years, with whom I had a most stimulating visit in Boston in 1963 and who gave me two important articles at that time. In 1945 *The New England Journal of Medicine* published a study of 200 patients attending Boston clinics from the observations of their four senior social workers. They wrote:

Medical Social Workers who daily attempt to cope with the task of arranging for the terminal care of cancer patients have long been concerned with the fact that the combination of limited facilities for the care of chronic cases, hospital policies and human nature makes this an almost insurmountable problem. Because this situation

---

* This chapter originally appeared as Saunders, D.C. (2001). Social work and palliative care: the early history. *The British Journal of Social Work*. pp. 791-799. Reprinted by permission. Dame Cicely Saunders (1918-2005) founded the modern hospice movement.

[1] Adapted from a talk given at the Annual General Meeting of the Association of Hospice and Palliative Care Social Workers, 13th September 2000.

5

became increasingly difficult, four medical social workers representing as many tumour clinics in Boston, met to discuss the nature of the problem, to review the limitations of resources and to discover how they could obtain mutual help. (Abrams et al., 1945, p. 726)

They studied an unselected sample and found that:

Several elements are involved in providing adequate terminal care. These are the patient's medical and nursing needs, the family's acceptance of the medical situation and what it implies, the family's ability to care for the patient at home—both physically and emotionally—the patient's wishes referable to care at home or elsewhere and existing facilities that are available. (Abrams et al., 1945, p. 726)

Describing problems and often unsatisfactory outcomes because of paucity of provision, they concluded with this plea to doctors:

I have tried in this short paper to plead once more for the patient as an individual. For most of you such a plea is superfluous, but if a few of the younger graduates have been stirred into a renewed interest in this important subject, I shall not feel that your time or mine has been wasted. As Peabody stated, "The secret of the care of the patient is in caring for the patient."
(Abrams et al., 1945, p. 727)

Provision for these patients in the Holy Ghost (later Youville) Hospital, which I observed on that visit to the United States in 1963, was surely due to their persistent advocacy and the evidence they collected.

Ruth Abrams' later paper (1951) discussed the problem of working with patients "when one is not sure what the patient has been told" (p. 425). Referring to the potential for the resolution of some of the presenting problems as "rehabilitation" she writes:

If rehabilitation is to begin at the moment the patient comes to the hospital, we should realize the importance of making a plan as early as possible—a flexible plan that is subject to change and based on the sharing of pertinent information of those professional persons caring for the patient. In a hospital this includes the physicians, nurses and social workers. (Abrams, 1951, pp. 425–426)

After summing up the roles of physician and nurse, she adds:

The caseworker as another member of the professional group has by the very nature of his function and training the best opportunity to study and to contribute to the evaluation of the attitudes of the patient with cancer and to give him sustained and planned support where and when this is indicated. The worker's knowledge of the general reactions to cancer, and of the particular patient's attitudes, has long-range

possibilities for future help both to the patient and to his relatives. By learning how the individual reacts to his diagnosis and treatment, and how his illness affects those within the family group, the social worker has tangible leads for determining the strengths and for setting the goals for a suitable medical social plan. The social worker is the member of the medical team who can be called upon at any time for further planning, even in the terminal cases when the hospital no longer offers readmission or care. (Abrams, 1951, p. 426)

In her book *Not Alone with Cancer* (1974), Abrams gives much clear guidance for families and patients and ends with wise guidelines for caregivers:

1. Be available when needed. In particular, try to visit the patient regularly.
2. Accept the patient as he conducts himself: his silence and withdrawal, his resignation and dependence, his manner and place and time of dying.
3. Take the role the patient assigns you; do not expect too much from the patient or attempt to influence his emotional, social or spiritual outlook. Make it easy for him to accept or reject help.
4. Make sure that the needs of the patient and his family are available when called for, including advance preparation for the death. Be aware of where it may occur, whom to call, funeral arrangements.
5. Remember that everything said and done at this time should be appropriate to the real gravity of the situation. The atmosphere should be such that the patient and his family can grieve together and separately. It is appropriate also for caregivers, both professional and non-professional, to show sorrow. (Abrams, 1974, pp. 82–83)

The lack of control by patients of which she hints must surely reflect the less satisfactory symptom control of that era.

Before I met Ruth Abrams I had published a study of four dying patients (Saunders, 1957) and discussed some general problems of the management of dying more fully. In conclusion I wrote:

Patients always rely on their own hospital. It seems best that they should stay at home as long as possible and then go to a Home for the Dying if and when it becomes necessary. Continuity of treatment by the doctor in charge should somehow be combined with this. One has in mind some form of Home Care with a doctor visiting from the hospital and a Home in close contact with that hospital, all working in co-operation with the family doctor. (Saunders, 1957, p. 46)

This proved to foreshadow the later development of integrated hospice programs.

Only after this did I discover Alison Player's (1954) sensitive article "Casework in terminal illness." She wrote:

There are a few things I am sure of, some I have only questions about, and some I have not even begun to think of yet. We can learn an immeasurable amount from our association with our clients. We can learn that death and sorrow can be faced with courage and serenity which are an inspiration, that the companionship of two loving people facing them together can be enriching to both. We can learn that for some people they can bring disabling fear and bitterness. We can only try to see the ways of helping people to find in dying an ennobling experience rather than an ordeal beyond their strength to bear except by becoming less than their best selves.

We cannot over-estimate the value for the patient and relatives of the help with practical plans which the caseworker can give. The arrangements for financial benefits so that the patient may not want, facilities for medical treatment, pain relieving drugs, home nursing care, admission to a hospital if necessary, and all the other plans which may be helpful—these are essential. If the family can know in advance what sort of services are available, and can call on the social worker to arrange them as smoothly as may be, the security and comfort for them is immense.

The worker will often have to take a great deal of responsibility and initiative and assume direction because of the patient's weakness and suffering and the family's distress and bewilderment. This entails the social worker's sure and detailed knowledge of possibilities. (Player, 1954, pp. 477–478)

Player also emphasized the importance of giving patients themselves as much responsibility as possible. She refers to the lack of discussion in the ways of helping people face death and the need to help people find spiritual help and comfort which she believes of importance if they are to be sustained and comforted. She also emphasizes the value of support from the local community.

1959 was a year of several independent yet related initiatives. Feifel published his seminal book *The Meaning of Death* (Feifel, 1959). Renee Fox published *Experiment Perilus* (Fox, 1959), a participant observer's study of life in a ward where medicine carried out the first experimental work with steroids among patients with life-threatening illnesses. When I later discussed this with one of the nuns who nursed at St Joseph's Hospice in East London, we agreed that we found, among other similarities, that we too found somewhat black humor to be an essential element in our coping.

That same year, Margaret Torrie founded Cruse, the support service for widows, and the then editor of *The Nursing Times*, Peggy Nuttall, asked me to write a series of six articles on *Care of the Dying*, which, reprinted as a booklet a year later, sold many thousands of copies and was reviewed by the *Manchester Guardian* and *The Lancet* (Saunders, 1960). Two other social workers published articles in 1959. Aitken-Swan's "Nursing the late cancer patient at home" (1959) reports on interviews with the families of 200 patients to:

ascertain to what extent the relatives' account of their experience at this time could be a material factor in the spread of cancer fears. Did they think that terminal care was adequate? How many patients were admitted to hospital or Home? How many wanted to go but could not? Was home nursing considered difficult? Were they satisfied with the medical care received? Did they stress pain and suffering more than anything else? What impression were they left with, or rather, what sort of stories were they passing on to others?

Fears that a home visit paid a month or two after the patient's death would be felt to be an intrusion proved groundless. Many families were grateful for the hospital's continued interest and were glad of an opportunity to obtain information themselves. Their readiness to talk and to discuss events critically seemed to show they were speaking their minds. (Aitken-Swan, 1959, p. 64)

She went on to write:

Their impressions in these 200 interviews will be summed up by attempting to answer the seven questions asked at the beginning of this article.

Did the family think that "terminal care" was adequate? In all but approximately 15% of cases. How many patients were admitted to hospital or a cancer home? 14%

How many wanted to go but could not? 15% Was home nursing considered difficult? Many relatives described difficult home circumstances and one-third described them as intolerable.

Were they satisfied with the patient's medical care at home? Yes, in 77% of all cases—a magnificent tribute to general practitioners.

Did they stress the patient's pain and suffering more than anything else? Nearly half the relatives (48%) thought the patient had less pain than had been expected or considered that he had been adequately relieved. In 18% a qualified statement was made. In 20% of cases they described severe pain unrelieved by any measures taken.

Finally, what impressions were they left with? The predominant feeling was that all that could have been done had been done. The majority of the families gave the impression of stability and independence. They did not appear to expect much help and were prepared to carry on alone in spite of difficult circumstances. Where there was a good relationship with the family doctor, the difficulties were considerably lessened. His visit, which was spoken of with such appreciation by one third of the relatives, was valued for its moral support even more than for the purely medical aid given. In 16% of cases families clearly had not achieved this relationship with their doctor.

The many questions asked about the patient's illness, and sometimes the misconceptions expressed about treatment, indicated a need for a better system of communication between hospital doctor and relatives. This would be welcomed by the relatives. It might also help the cause of public education concerning cancer by reducing the amount of misinformation spread by them. (Aitken-Swan, 1959, p. 65)

Also Aitken-Swan and Easson (1959) (a radiotherapist) published an article concerning the reactions of people on being told their diagnosis. The conclusion reads:

A study is presented of the reactions of 231 selected patients who were told they had curable cancer. Two-thirds said they were glad to know the truth, 19% denied they had been told, while only 7% (all women) resented the consultant's frankness. The family doctors of 35 patients reported no untoward effects of this knowledge and none opposed the general policy of telling such patients their diagnosis.
It is concluded that since a sufficiently large majority of patients are able to accept the truth, and benefit from the knowledge, all patients with the more curable cancers, unless obviously unstable, should be told their diagnosis. This is considered an essential part of public education on cancer, aiming at earlier treatment and higher cure rates. (Aitken-Swan and Easson, 1959, p. 783)
They also quote from a television speaker, a Dr Khanolkar, who said, "I believe there is a very large fund of courage and resolution in human minds which we have not accounted for in the past."

In the same year Margaret Bailey (1959) carried out a survey of:

A group of 155 patients, roughly a third of whom had been treated by resection, were included in a survey of the social needs of patients with incurable lung cancer. Nearly half of the 155 patients who have died have been visited by the almoner at Home, generally during the last month of life. (Bailey, 1959, p. 390)

She concludes:

The timing and choice of terminal care arrangements could be precipitated by several factors; increasing medical problems, inadequate family care or the strain of long-term nursing. A patient's admission to a particular institution depended on the joint planning of the hospital, general practitioner and the family, the patient's and relatives' feelings about the special terminal homes, their faith in the original treating hospital and the uncertainty of obtaining vacancies. Adequate care at home was possible for nearly half of the patients. In these cases the family resources, the patient's and relatives relationship with the private doctor and the provision of certain material conditions,

together with the continued support and interest of the hospital, largely determined the practicability of nursing at home. (Bailey, 1959, p. 391)

The following year Margaret Birley (1960) wrote a prize-winning essay on "Terminal care." She said:

When we are about to discuss what is to be done about the final days of someone else, we are brought face to face with our own feelings about death. If it is something we fear, then I think, we are especially fearful of discussing it with others, particularly if we are aware that, while some patients are most fearful, others are quite unafraid. In this respect it may be the patient who leads us in the conscious examination of feelings. Patients who are not afraid to die have often given a great deal of thought to this matter. One who has known from what he has been suffering, especially a patient with a malignant condition, may have reached an adjustment to the idea of death which, in the fact of all that has gone before in the way of pain, may seem to a troubled worker sublime serenity. I do not mean that these patients want to die because they can bear no more, but that they have completely accepted incipient death and are prepared to make it the ultimate achievement of their life. (Birley, 1960, p. 87)

As she went on to observe:

Frequently, a patient who has for some time suspected a lack of progress has his suspicions confirmed by the sudden cessation of interest by the medical staff. The Consultant's round, particularly in large hospitals, is often a weekly event of major importance in the ward. Many patients of all sorts regard this as the time when their fate is determined, and the terminally ill patient's reaction to receiving only a cursory examination or even to being completely by-passed is likely to be one of depression coupled with a sense of failure. The mystery surrounding so many medical rites, and patients' primitive faith in the power of doctors, results in the ignored patient feeling that he has somehow displeased Omnipotence and incurred anger by not recovering. Being ignored is as much part of the punishment as the incessant discomforts of pain and weakness. (Birley, 1960, p. 89)

The often desperate needs of patients at home were revealed by the Marie Curie Memorial Foundation Survey (1952). "The physical and mental distress of the dying" in the wards of a London teaching hospital were documented in detail by Hinton (1963). What could be done by a social worker in influencing the management of fatal illness was recorded by Foster (1965). In a hematology service in a veterans' hospital in New York she encountered a group of men between 25 and 40 years old who were consistently denied true information concerning their illness. She writes:

The doctors developed and acted out a stereotyped view of [the patient's] behaviour. They suppressed questions, offered evasive answers, and provided direct reassurance to offset any patient doubts. For his own good, the patient was not encouraged to express feelings, reactions, or doubts. Thus, staff culture defined how the patient should respond to his illness. (Foster, 1965, p. 31)

And he goes on to write:

A result of this system was that the family and doctor bypassed the patient and excluded him from decision-making. Thus, the family became part of the ward culture, and found the role of relative clearly prescribed. They saw patients as helpless, dependent, and incapable of self-assertion. Therefore, they must take action on the patient's behalf. Financial matters, future planning, and concerns of children were not referred to the patient. Since these patients were generally married men who until recently fully supported their families, role reversal occurred suddenly—husband and father roles were cancelled out by the patient role. (Foster, 1965, p. 31)

However, she became involved in helping a man whose spouse also developed a fatal illness. She presented his need to plan for their infant child's future to the rest of the ward team. Two other similar cases were resolved with her input, and she wrote:

Three cases which occurred in a relatively short period of time were handled differently but this did not result in disaster. The patients appeared to be functioning well, talking more freely with their doctors, and obviously liked and trusted them and showed new self-reliance. These patients were successful in bringing about significant social change in the ward milieu. For the first time it became a matter of ward policy to consider the willingness and capacity of each patient to know his diagnosis. Furthermore, the majority of patients were considered capable of understanding the nature of their diseases. The ward culture was influenced strongly by this expressive, questioning, assertive and independent majority. The good patient was no longer one who silently submitted to his fate, but one who courageously faced his disease, and continued in his role as husband, father, and breadwinner. The improved communication system between doctor and patient fostered a mutual respect that had not existed previously. Patients were able to view the doctor more realistically and had less of a need to invest him with magical, omnipotent powers. (Foster, 1965, p. 34)

She concludes her discussion of these changes with a shrewd note:

It is recognized that modifications in ward culture inevitably raise new problems. Patients have varying capacities to recognise and integrate their poor prognoses, internalize their anxiety, and meet a complex of social roles. Although the new ward culture offers a broader range of coping patterns, it may not provide adequate protection for those patients in need of external supports to maintain essential defences of denial. Experience has shown that many patients can make successful adjustments to fatal illness based on a well-developed connection with reality. Some cannot. Better techniques are needed to provide a ward social system that can meet the needs of all. (Foster, 1965, p. 35)

Although most hospice units and home and hospital palliative care teams today have social workers involved with some of the issues presented here, their proper recognition is not always apparent in busy centers. Discharge plans are inadequate or even absent, and crises take the place of the continuity that should characterize end-of-life care. These voices from the past had much impact on the planning of St Christopher's Hospice, the first of the modern hospices and a catalyst for the original development of palliative care. The implications for the approach to diseases other than cancer are only now being appreciated and moving into action.

This chapter is a salute both to the many patients and families I met as a medical social worker and to the careful assessment and imaginative writing of those quoted, which proved an important catalyst to early teaching and planning and which largely escaped the attention of the public. They had a major impact on the concept of the "total pain" (Clark, 1999b), with its complex of physical, emotional, social, and spiritual elements—comprising a whole experience of profound suffering, often endured at the end of life. Their work thus provided considerable impetus to the now worldwide development of palliative care.

REFERENCES

Abrams, R. (1951). Social casework with cancer patients, *Social casework*, pp. 425–426, and 431.

Abrams, R. (1974). *Not alone with cancer*. Springfield, IL: Charles Thomas Publishing.

Abrams, R., Jameson, G., Poehlman, M., & Snyder, S. (1945). Terminal care in cancer, *The New England Journal of Medicine*, 232(25), 726–727.

Aitken-Swan, J. (1959). Nursing the late cancer patient at home. The family's impressions, *The Practitioner*, 183, 64–65.

Aitken-Swan, J., & Easson, E. C. (1959) Reactions of cancer patients on being told their diagnosis, *British Medical Journal*, I, 779–783.

Bailey, M. (1959). A survey of social needs of patients with incurable lung cancer, *The Almoner*, 11, 390–391.

Birley, M. (1960). Terminal care, *The Almoner*, 13, 86–97.

Clark, D. (1998). Originating a movement: Cicely Saunders and the development of St Christopher's Hospice, *1957–67*, *Mortality*, 3(1), 43–63.

Clark, D. (1999a). Cradled to the grave? Terminal care in the United Kingdom, *1948-67, Mortality, 4*(3), 225-247.

Clark, D. (1999b). Total pain, disciplinary power and the body in the work of Cicely Saunders, *1958-1967, Social Science and Medicine, 49,* 727-736.

Feifel, H. (1959). *The meaning of death,* New York, NY: McGraw-Hill Book Co. Inc.

Foster, Z. (1965). How social work can influence hospital management of fatal illness, *Journal of the National Association of Social Workers, 10*(4), 30-35.

Fox, R. C. (1959). *Experiment perilous.* Glencoe, IL: The Free Press.

Hinton, J. M. (1963). The physical and mental distress of the dying, *Quarterly Journal of Medicine, 32*(1), 1-21.

Marie Curie Memorial Foundation. (1952). *Report on a national survey concerning patients nursed at home.* London, England: Marie Curie Memorial Foundation.

Player, A. (1954). Casework in terminal illness, *The Almoner, 6,* 477-478.

Saunders, C. M. (1957). Dying of cancer, *St Thomas's Hospital Gazette,* pp. 37-47.

Saunders, C. M. (1960). Care of the dying. *Nursing Times Reprint.* London, England: Macmillan.

2 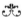 *Bernice Catherine Harper*

Palliative Social Work: An Historical Perspective

Ruth was dying in a hospital in Virginia, grieving for herself and not getting sufficient pain medication because she never asked for medication. The doctor said to me, "Your sister is not in any pain." I replied, "Yes, she is." The doctor questioned, "How do you know that? You just got here." I answered, "By her moans, groans, and 'oh me's." These words conveyed an urgent familial cultural dynamic, which meant "get and give me what I need."
—Bernice C. Harper (In Davidson & Doka, 2001, p. 148)

Key Concepts

This textbook on palliative social work is a companion volume to the Oxford Textbook of Palliative Medicine and the Oxford Textbook of Palliative Nursing. To that end, this chapter will accomplish the following:

- *Address the historical perspectives and foci relative to medical social work in health care and its evolving synergy with hospice care and palliative care*
- *Include a discussion of the legislative and political issues that affected both the social work profession and institutions in which social workers practice*
- *Give impetus to the importance of social work's contribution to the interdisciplinary aspects of helping patients and families confronting catastrophic diseases and life-threatening illnesses*
- *Contribute a personal and historic perspective that helps to build a foundation for the balance of the textbook*

Introduction

I deem it a professional honor to have been invited by my esteemed peers and colleagues to write this chapter. It gives me the opportunity to draw upon my many years of professional practice to help humanize the health care delivery system. It is my hope and belief that this complex system will become a seamless magic blanket, floating over blue skies and purple mountains—meeting needs of patients, families, communities, and health care providers from life's beginnings, life's endings, and in between life's processes.

A Beginning

The past, present, and future have important connections. It is necessary to explore the roots, foundations, fundamental policies, and procedures relating to social work in palliative care. It is important to briefly trace major developments in medical care programs that culminated in medical social work, hospice care, and palliative care. Roots are found in the public sector and the private arena, respectively. For example, the Marine Hospital Service (MHS), a precursor to the Public Health Service (PHS), was formed and operated by the federal government in 1798 to provide for the temporary relief and maintenance of sick and disabled seamen. This was the first prepaid medical program financed through compulsory employer tax and federally administered in the United States (Social Security Online "History," accessed 2009). The National Institutes of Health (NIH) and the Centers for Disease Control and Prevention (CDC) trace their origins to a one-room laboratory set up in 1887 on Staten Island to conduct research and help control the spread of disease (Office of History, National Institutes of Health, Retrieved 2009). These are two examples of early American medical care programs.

This has historical significance because in 2009–2010 U.S. President Barack Obama sought legislation to provide health care to all Americans. The genesis of this endeavor dates back to 1798. One can trace this historical significance and connect all the dots through the years and various presidential administrations. The current health care debate between the administration, Congress, a variety of health care agencies, and the American people gives impetus to the importance of health care for all Americans.

Medical social work was the term promulgated in the private sector between 1905 and 1912. Three private hospitals come to mind as early developers and employers of social work in their institutions: Massachusetts General in Boston, Massachusetts; Johns Hopkins in Baltimore, Maryland; and City of Hope National Medical Center in Duarte, California. It has been said that medical social work was founded at Johns Hopkins Hospital. It has also been said that medical social work had its beginning at the Massachusetts General Hospital, under the direction of Ida Cannon, a nurse, and Dr. Richard Cabot, a physician, who witnessed a relationship between the physical, social and environmental factors and had the foresight to bring social workers into the hospital setting. At the same time across the country, Minnie Kahn, one of the first social workers at the Los Angeles Sanatorium in Duarte, CA (currently known as the City of Hope National Medical Center), noted the significance of separation and illness in the life of a patient when she wrote the following: "For the past seven years an effort has been made to meet each individual at the train station, to welcome him, to try as far as possible to alleviate the feeling of being a 'stranger in a strange land'" (Kahn, 1934, p. 20).

Medical social work, later referred to as social work in health care, had a beginning like everything else in the world. Historically speaking, it is interesting to note that I have been involved, in some way, with these three institutions, all of which were involved in the building of the health care social work movement. After completing graduate school, I applied for a social work position at Johns Hopkins. Amy Green, director of social work, wrote me a letter which said, "Your credentials are excellent, but I have to tell you that we hire only one colored social worker at a time in our clinic and the position is currently filled." Segregation was the order of the day (1947). When I was at the Harvard School of Public Health, my major professor, Elizabeth Rice, took me to see Ida Cannon, who was in a nursing home. She was 80 years young. In her wonderful, animated conversation, she talked at length about social work. She envisioned that industry and labor would be areas for social work development (1959). I worked at the City of Hope National Medical Center as a home care coordinator (1959), assistant director (1959–1960), and subsequently as director of the Department of Social Work (1960–1976).

Major Institutional and Legislative Events

The following institutional and legislative events were public developments that helped set the stage for the growth of social work:

- 1912—The Children's Bureau was established to combat exploitation of children.
- 1920—After World War I, the Vocational Rehabilitation Act of 1920 provided education and help for disabled workers who had served on the home front.
- 1935—The Depression gave impetus to the first Social Security and Public Assistance Program under the Social Security Act.
- 1939—The Social Security Board was made part of the newly established Federal Security Agency (FSA), which integrated the Public Health Service, the Civilian Conservation Corps, the National Youth Administration, and the Office of Education into one administrative unit designed to administer existing federal programs relating to health, education, and welfare.
- 1949—A consolidated system of regional offices was set up that included additional programs, such as mental health, hospital programs, and dental health.
- 1953—President Dwight Eisenhower submitted to Congress his "Reorganization Plan No. 1," dissolving FSA and creating the Department of Health, Education and Welfare (DHEW). Congress approved the plan, which became effective April 11, 1953.
- 1960—Under the Kerr-Mills Amendment, medical care suppliers for the elderly surfaced, and the concept of the "medically needy" was promulgated and became the operative phrase that referred to persons who, though not financially eligible for public assistance, could not pay high medical expenses. All 50 states developed programs to pay suppliers of medical care for the elderly, and 47 states also paid for the care of the medically needy.

Medicare and Medicaid: The Early Years

"Medicare! Medicare! Medicare!" Public announcements hit all of the airwaves. President Lyndon Baines Johnson on July 30, 1965 in Independence, Missouri, and in the presence of his predecessor, Harry S. Truman, signed the Medicare Bill (H.R. 6675) at the Truman Library. Witnesses of the signing included Vice President Hubert H. Humphrey, Lady Bird Johnson, and Bess Truman (see Fig. 2.1).

Wilbur Cohen, secretary of the Department of Health, Education, and Welfare, and a *social worker* participated in drafting the Health Insurance Legislation. Much of the credit for startup went to Arthur Hess, director of the Bureau of Health Insurance of the Social Security Administration. Medicare went into effect on July 1, 1966, following nearly 25 years of often bitter debate between organized medicine and Medicare proponents. The program promised to pay hospital care, nursing home care, home nursing services, and outpatient diagnostic services for Americans 65 years of age and older. The original Medicare Bill also contained provisions for insurance to cover doctor bills and certain other medical expenses. The participants, in the beginning, agreed to pay $3 per month in premiums. Medicare was scheduled to serve approximately 19 million at the outset at a cost of $1 billion. In 2010, at the time of the writing of this chapter, there are approximately 43 million Medicare beneficiaries at a cost of $300 billion; 51 million Medicaid recipients at a cost of $200 billion from the federal government; and $180 billion matching funds from the states (Medicare/Medicaid, The first two decades 1965–1985. DHE, Healthcare Financing Administration. p. 3). This joint federal medical assistance program was designed to help the poor, indigent elderly and chronically ill disadvantaged. For millions of aging and disabled, a bed was made available in a licensed nursing facility. It may be said that Medicaid spawned today's nursing facility industry.

Countless children of the poor with disabling conditions have been diagnosed and treated through Medicaid immunization programs and an Early Periodic Screening, Diagnosis and Treatment Program (EPSDT) for children. Medicare and Medicaid split the notion of welfare from health care. The elderly were able to pay for health care through the Health Insurance program of Medicare. At the same time, the needy, whether elderly or not, could be aided by the Medical Assistance Program of Medicaid.

The Expansion of Medicare and Medicaid Programs

Shep Glazer appeared before the House Ways and Means Committee in the fall of 1971, with a large gadget the size of a commercial washing machine attached to his body by two tubes hooked up to one of his arms. It was a kidney dialysis machine and it kept him alive at a cost of $12,000 to $25,000 a year for treatment on artificial kidney machines. It was estimated that some 10,000 Americans needed this type of care. Mr. Glazer asked for Medicare benefits to pay for the treatment. The issue was financial: As more kidney disease patients would be kept alive, the cost of assistance would grow into billions of dollars. Congress and the President sided with Mr. Glazer. The End Stage Renal Dialysis (ESRD) bill was signed by President Nixon, expanding Medicare eligibility to individuals of all ages requiring renal dialysis.

August 6, 1971 was the historic date when the President of the United States of America expressed the administration's concern about the many nursing homes and related long-term care facilities that fell short in their capacity to provide quality care for their residents, the vast majority of whom

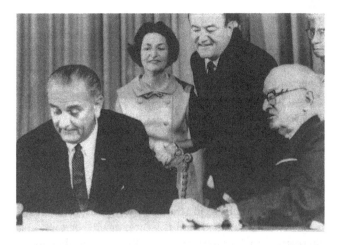

Figure 2.1. July 30, 1965: President Lyndon Baines Johnson signed the Medicare Bill (H.R. 6675) at the Truman Library in Independence, Missouri. Witnesses of the signing included: Harry S. Truman, Vice President Hubert H. Humphrey, Lady Bird Johnson and Bess Truman.

were older citizens. In his speech, entitled "Statement about Actions to Improve the Quality Care in Nursing Homes," President Nixon called for a "plan for action" to upgrade the quality of health care provided to these citizens. The President's message stated:

I have directed the Department of Health, Education and Welfare to institute a new program of short-term courses for physicians, nurses, dieticians, social workers and others who are regularly involved in furnishing services to nursing home patients. Appropriate professional organizations will be involved in developing plans and course materials for the program and the latest research findings in this complex field will also be utilized. In many cases, those who provide nursing home care—though they would generally be well prepared for their profession—have not been adequately trained to meet the special needs of the elderly. Our new program will help correct this deficiency. (Nixon, 1971)

Expressing concern about the need for positive action in the area of research and development, President Nixon said:

I am directing the Secretary of Health, Education and Welfare to undertake a comprehensive review of the use of long-term care facilities as well as the standards and practices of nursing homes and to recommend any further remedial measures that may be appropriate. Such a review is badly needed. Study tells us—compellingly—that many things are wrong with certain nursing home facilities, but there is not yet a clear enough understanding of all the steps that must be taken to correct this picture. (Nixon, 1971)

The Public Health Service accepted the challenge of the President's Nursing Home Initiatives and promised full implementation of the proposed plan of action. Specific aspects of the plan were assigned to appropriate programs in the Health Services and Mental Health Administration (HSMHA). During this period, Ruth Knee, a social worker, served as the Program Director of Long-Term Care. I was appointed director of the Division of Long-Term Care with a staff of 18 in the central office; there were 10 regional office long-term care education coordinators. A national Long-Term Care for the Elderly Research Review and Advisory Committee was appointed. Social workers were involved in these three program entities.

In August 1973, the Division was transferred to the National Center for Health Services Research. In the area of research and development, the Division expanded its thrust to learn more about systems of care, quality of care, and alternatives to long-term care. In the area of short-term training, the Division broadened its efforts in provider improvement, as demonstrated in the final analysis by the 787,000 individuals who participated in the short-term training courses (A Promise Kept/Annual Report).

On October 30, 1972, President Nixon signed a Social Security amendment, which expanded Medicare to previously ineligible aged, blind, and disabled people.

National Association of Social Workers, Inc.

Relative to provider training, the National Association of Social Workers (NASW) received a $200,000 contract in 1971. The project was entitled Project Provide: National Social Work Training Program to Meet Human and Social Needs of Long-Term Care Facility Patients. Its purpose was to train social work designees and consultants employed in long-term care facilities to provide appropriate social services to reduce the unmet social and human needs of residents and their families.

NASW conducted training programs in 39 different locations, covering 31 states in each of the 10 DHEW regions. Of the 2700 participants, 33% were social work designees; 44% were staff social workers; 9% were social work consultants; and 14% were primarily medical social workers and welfare workers who worked indirectly with many nursing home residents and their families. The evaluations showed that the training was highly beneficial and affected both social work practice and future directions in training of long-term care facilities' social service personnel. There was also a "spin-off" benefit in the increased cooperative efforts among NASW chapters and local, state, and regional agencies concerned with long-term care.

One recommendation was that a manual for social work consultants in long-term care facilities be developed. NASW received a $37,500 contract for this project, entitled A Guide for Social Work Consultation in Long-Term Care Facilities. The monograph covered the following areas:

- The role of the social work consultant
- Optimum utilization of social work consultations

- Experience and training needed by the consultant
- Teaching techniques with faculty staff
- Helping the long-term care facility utilize community resources effectively
- Measuring the effect of social work consultation with improved resident care
- The social work consultant's role in developing and participating in multidisciplinary approaches.

The 10th Anniversary of Medicare and Medicaid

By 1975 Medicare and Medicaid programs were well established in the American health care arena and had earned the right to stay. Medicare covered 21.8 million elders and 3 million disabled Americans. An estimated 95% of Medicare Part (A) hospitalization enrollees were also voluntarily enrolled in Medicare (B), which covered doctor bills. Wilbur J. Cohen, who became dean of the School of Education at the University of Michigan, referred to Medicare as a "breakthrough" and credited it with breaking "the back of its ideological opposition to the public role in health insurance" (Cohen, 1985).

The Health Care Financing Administration

President Carter's administration put new systems in place for the Medicare and Medicaid programs in 1977. I was in the audience when DHEW Secretary, Joseph A. Califano, Jr., presented and described the plan to "simplify" and "streamline" the Department (Califano, 1977). He placed Medicare and Medicaid under a new agency called the Health Care Financing Administration (HCFA). Previously, Medicare was operated by the Social Security Administration (SSA), under the Social and Rehabilitation Services.

HCFA was provided a $32 billion budget and policy responsibility for Medicare, while SSA continued to manage Medicare applications and payments in the field through its local SSA offices across the nation. Similarly, HCFA held policy responsibility for Medicaid, but local management and administration remained with the states.

Progress and changes in Medicare and Medicaid programs included the following:

- Medicaid reforms
- Medigaps and beneficiary costs
- Program cost increases
- Tightening of cost controls
- Prospective payment system
- Diagnosis-related groups (DRGs)
- Peer review organizations (PROs)
- Physician fee schedule
- Health maintenance organizations (HMOs)
- Home- and community-based Medicaid services.

In the autumn of 1981, the health and social care needs of a 3-year-old girl called attention to the need to evaluate Medicare and Medicaid programs. Her name was Katie Beckett, of Cedar Rapids, Iowa, and she was hospitalized with complications from viral encephalitis and inflammation of the brain. Katie's physician and her parents wanted her to be cared for at home. Home care would cost about $1000 per month. Medicaid was paying $6,000 per month for her hospital care. Mr. and Ms. Beckett's income disqualified them for Medicaid assistance outside of a hospital.

President Reagan brought Katie into the national spotlight on November 10, 1981, when he told news conference attendees how Katie, a Medicaid patient, had spent most of her life hospitalized more by government regulation than by medical need. Following the news conference, DHEW gave Katie a "waiver," which became regulation and allowed Katie to leave the hospital and receive less costly home care paid for by Medicaid (Reagan, 1981). It was a progressive endeavor in that the regulation increased the availability of home care under Medicare and Medicaid as well as created a workable alternative to institutionalization, hospitals, or nursing homes.

Hospice: An Historical Recapitulation

The word *hospice* was first used around the fourth century when Christian orders welcomed travelers, the sick, and those in many kinds of need. The term was first applied to the care of dying patients by Mrs. Jeanne Garnier, who founded the Dames de Calaire in Lyon, France, in 1842. The Irish Sisters of Charity adopted it when they opened Our Lady's Hospice in Dublin, Ireland, in 1879 and then again when they opened St Joseph's Hospice in Hackney, London, England, in 1905 (NHPCO, n. d.)

Hospice did not become more widely known until Dame Cicely Saunders founded St. Christopher's Hospice in 1967 (http://www.stchristophers.org.uk/). Dame Cicely had been a nurse, but she was working as a medical social worker when she came upon a patient by the name of David Tasma in 1948. David was suffering from inoperable cancer. Together they talked about her hopes for one day opening up a place that was more of a home environment to care for the terminally ill and that did a better job of focusing on pain management and preparing the patient for death. It is said that before David died he told her, "I will be a window in your home." With that said, after the opening of St Christopher's Hospice, her ideals have been adopted all over the world and she is known as the "founder of the modern hospice movement" (St Christopher's Hospice, n. d.).

In 1963 Dame Cicely Saunders visited the United States prior to the opening of the first modern hospice in 1967. She visited a number of facilities, including the City of Hope National Medical Center. At the City of Hope I served as her preceptor and we spent the day discussing the care and the needs of dying patients, those confronting life-threatening illnesses, and their families. I remembered that day whenever we met at subsequent meetings. As a nurse, social worker, and later, as a physician, Dr. Saunders had great expectations of health professionals who used their skills and expertise in caring for individuals who would not recover (St Christopher's Hospice, n. d.).

Two years after the opening of St. Christopher's Hospice in England, Dr. Elisabeth Kubler-Ross wrote a book she based on over 500 interviews with dying patients titled *On Death and Dying*. This now well-known book gave people a first-hand insight into the emotions and stages that people may face when they are terminally ill. In her book, Dr. Kubler-Ross pleaded for better home care as opposed to an institutional or hospital setting. She argued that patients should have a choice when it came to their health care and promoted their ability to participate as much as possible in the decisions that affected them (Hinds Hospice Web site, 2007).

Also inspired by Dame Saunders' ideals, students at Yale University in New Haven, Connecticut, invited her to speak. The year was 1974 and they were so inspired that they created and launched the U.S. hospice movement. In that same year a hospice nurse in Connecticut and an accompanying volunteer made their first home care visit to a hospice patient in their own home (Simms, 2007).

Moving forward in years to 1981, Nancy Hinds in Fresno, California, began caring for terminally ill patients in her own home. This inpatient hospice home allowed patients a place to die with dignity in a home setting when their family or caregivers were not able to care for them in their own homes (Hinds Hospice Web site, 2007).

In 1986, Congress made permanent the Medicare Hospice Benefit and various states were allowed to decide whether they wanted to include hospice in their Medicaid programs. As of 2008 in the United States there were 4,850 hospice programs serving approximately 1.45 million people (NHPCO, 2009). Hospices are currently located in all 50 U.S. states, as well as worldwide. (For more info on Hospice Care please see Chapter 8 or for more information on Home-Based Palliative Care please see Chapter 10)

Federal Intervention in Hospice Care

The rights of the terminally ill and dying patients and their families surfaced officially on May 29, 1978, when the Secretary of the DHEW asked Peter Libassi, Office of the General Counsel, to chair a task force to study hospice. Linda Miller was appointed the Secretary's representative on this group. I represented the HCFA and had prepared a briefing paper on Hospice for the Secretary. The task force method was utilized to include all individuals who could contribute to the knowledge base and the gathering of intelligence related to this new modality of care.

Hospice is an area in health care that lends itself to inclusion of all who want to help, share, and "love thy neighbor as thyself." For this reason, it was an unusual and exciting afternoon on June 14, 1978, when Peter Libassi chaired the first meeting of the Secretary's Task Force on Hospice Care. In addition to the special assignment, the important thing was that the Department's heart was pulsating with love, and had, for a brief moment, defied those who believe that institutions, bureaucracies, and government cannot express care and compassion for the people they serve. The end of the day came and went with no one rushing to go home or to "get" their carpool. There is a bond in hospice that links all men and women in our global world so closely and intimately that even differences of color, spiritual beliefs, culture, and daily activities are insignificant behind it. This bond captured those civil servants who already shared a variety of activities in progress within different programs in the government.

As a result of these meetings, in 1979, HCFA initiated a demonstration program that selected 26 hospices across the country to assess the cost effectiveness of hospice care and to help determine what a hospice is and what it should provide. The 26 sites were paid by Medicare for their services representing the first time hospice care had been reimbursed. The demonstration projects paved the way for legislation to be introduced to create a hospice benefit under Medicare.

Section 122 of the Tax Equity and Fiscal Responsibility Act (TEFRA) of 1982 (Pub. L. 97-248, enacted on September 3, 1982) contained what was considered the perfect piece of legislation: a provision that promised to cut federal spending, promote a humanitarian service, and provide comfort for thousands of terminally ill people. Sponsored by more than half of the Senate and two-thirds of the House, the provision for the first time permitted Medicare funding for hospice care, which supported the concept that those who were dying were best cared for in the loving atmosphere of their homes than they were in hospitals. Hospice advocates gathered on the Capitol steps in September 1982 to celebrate the passage of the legislation; the only social worker in the group was Judi Lund (see Fig. 2.2).

On August 18, 1983, the long-awaited proposed regulations that would provide a new benefit to pay hospice care costs for terminally ill Medicare beneficiaries were signed by Secretary Margaret Heckler. Carolyn Davis, Ph.D., was the Administrator of HCFA during the development of these regulations for the hospice Medicare benefit. In my capacity as medical care advisor, Office of Professional and Scientific Affairs, I reviewed and commented on the regulations before they were published in the Federal Register. This was an ideal opportunity to influence public policy. Hospice was promulgated as an approach to treatment that recognized that the impending death of an individual warranted a change in focus from curative care to palliative care. The goal was to help terminally ill individuals continue life with minimal disruption in normal activities. The regulation also specified that the hospice benefit would cover the following: nursing care, medical social services, physician's services, counseling,

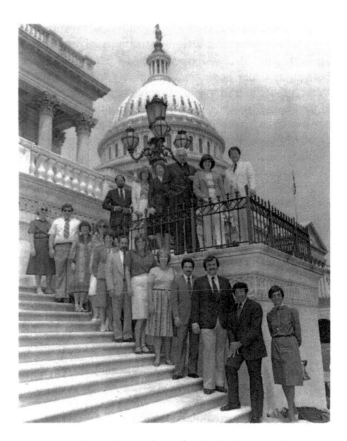

Figure 2.2. Photo taken in front of Capitol celebrating the Passage of the Medicare Hospice Benefit (September 29, 1982). Top row, from left to right: Jay Mahoney, Colorado; Kathleen Hart, New Mexico; Judi Lund, North Carolina; Don Armussen, Arkansas; Mary Dede, California; Don Gaetz, Florida Bottom row, from left to right: Dorothy Moga, Virginia; Dick Brett, California; Madalon Amenta, Pennsylvania; Judy Fox, Virginia; Ann Morgan Vickery, Washington, DC; Phil Decker, Pennsylvania; Linda Kilburn, Massachusetts; Barbara Ward, New Jersey; Michael Rosen, Florida; Hugh Westbrook, Florida; Congressman Leon Panetta, California; Mary Taverna, California

and other forms of care (US Department of Health and Human Services, 1983).

Palliative care is an approach that improves the quality of life of patients and their families facing the problems associated with life-threatening illness through the prevention and relief of suffering by means of early identification, assessment, and treatment of pain and other issues. (World Health Organization Web site. Retrieved 2009). Hospice care allows the patient to remain at home as long as possible by providing support to the patient and family and keeping the patient as comfortable as possible while maintaining his or her dignity. A hospice uses an interdisciplinary approach to deliver medical, social, physical, emotional, and spiritual services through the use of a broad spectrum of caregivers (NHPCO, 2009).

HCFA used the Medical Hospital Insurance (Medicare Part A) to help pay for hospice care if the following three conditions were met:

1. A physician certifies that the patient is terminally ill, which is interpreted as a life expectancy of less than 6 months if the disease runs its normal course.
2. A patient elects the hospice benefit or chooses to receive hospice care rather than the standard Medicare benefits for the terminally ill.
3. The care is provided by a Medicare-certified hospice program.

Relative to social work, in 1983, the hospice Conditions of Participation defined a social worker as "a person who has at least a bachelor's degree from a school accredited or approved by the Council on Social Work Education" (US DHHS, 1983). When the Conditions of Participation were updated in 2008, the definition of social worker was expanded and currently a social worker must meet one of the following qualifications:

- Have a master of social work (MSW) degree from a school of social work accredited by the Council on Social Work Education and 1 year of experience in a health care setting.
- Have a baccalaureate degree in social work (BSW) from a school of social work accredited by the Council on Social Work Education and 1 year experience in a health care setting.
- Have a baccalaureate degree in psychology, sociology, or other field related to social work and at least 1 year of social work experience in a health care setting. Services must be provided under supervision of a social worker with a MSW.

All Medical social services must be provided in a manner that is consistent with acceptable standards of practice.

A Change of Name and Medicare Part D

HCFA became the Centers for Medicare and Medicaid Services (CMS) under President George W. Bush in June 2001. Medicare Drug Prescription Benefit Part D was passed by the Congress in 2003, and CMS was given the responsibility for administration and implementation of this legislation, which became effective January 2006.

Social Work: The Public Sector and Private Arena

Social work has not, does not, and never will operate in a vacuum. The public sector made it possible for social workers to further their growth and development through the years. The U.S. Public Health Service has always included the provision of social work services in its numerous programs of health and social care for the citizens of this nation. Medicare was the major program that elevated and

highlighted the importance of medical social services under the supervision of the physician. Physician direction of medical social services was a statutory requirement when the Medicare hospice benefit was passed in 1982 and remains so today. The provision of social work in these health care programs was borne out of legislation mandated by Congress. Social services were woven into the federal regulatory processes and became part and parcel of the Medicare Conditions of Participation, guidelines and manuals, as well as surveying and certification in all health care programs. Social workers, including Ruth Taylor, Ruth Knee, Pearl Bierman, Eileen Lester, Mary Pope Byrd, Mary Gillis, Neota Lawson, and myself participated in these processes.

A wide variety of professional organizations, associations, and activities contributed to the growth and development of medical social work as it evolved to social work in health care, hospice care, and palliative care. For example, the Society of Social Work Directors initially under the aegis of the American Hospital Society in 1965 became an independent group called the Society of Social Work Leadership in Health Care. The goal of this organization was to improve and enhance social work in hospitals and other health care institutions. Beatrice Phillips was the first president of this organization and I became president in 1970.

In April 1973, Meg Jamison chaired a meeting of 75 medical social workers at a Veteran's Administration interdisciplinary meeting in Boston held in conjunction with the American Society of Artificial and Internal Organs. This group became the Association of Nephrology Social Workers (ANSW), which serves in an advisory capacity to the National Kidney Foundation. Dr. Norman Deane of the New York Nephrology Association contributed $250 toward getting the new organization started (Gammarino, Kammerer, & King, 1990). This was an important and sizeable contribution at the time from a physician who recognized the importance of social work in meeting the needs for patients with kidney disease.

The Medicare Renal Amendments took effect in the summer of 1973, thus removing the financial disincentives to providing chronic hemodialysis and thereby greatly improved patient access to treatment (Social Security Administration, 1972). ANSW had considerable input into the final federal regulations, which mandated that social workers in end-stage renal disease (ESRD) programs hold masters-level degrees (US DHHS, 1976).

The National Hospice Organization incorporated in April 1978 and became the National Hospice and Palliative Care Organization (NHPCO) in 1999. This organization developed the first standards for hospice programs, originally published in 1979, which detailed the important role of the social worker in hospice care. The organization played a signal role in the development and the defining of palliative social work through its many educational activities, research, policies, procedures, programmatic thrusts, committee assignments, task forces, and programs of its state organizations.

Oncology social workers contributed to defining the role and function of social work in caring for patients and families with life-threatening diseases. The Association of Oncology Social Workers (AOSW) is dedicated to the enhancement of psychosocial services for people with cancer and their families. Created in 1984 by social workers interested in oncology, AOSW has over 1000 members who embrace the organization's mission, "To advance excellence in the psychosocial care of persons with cancer, their families and caregivers, through networking, education, advocacy, research, and resource development" (AOSW, 2010). The members of AOSW practice in hospitals, outpatient clinics, home care, hospice agencies, and other settings.

In 1994, the Open Society Institute's Project on Death in America (PDIA) was launched under the leadership of Kathleen Foley, MD, with a mission to understand and transform the culture and experience of dying through initiatives in research, scholarship, the humanities, and the arts; to foster innovations in the provision of care, public education, professional education, and public policy. The PDIA Faculty Scholars Program was designed to provide participants with knowledge and skills necessary to take leadership roles at their institutions and nationally. The aim was to develop an intellectually vibrant, mutually supportive, and cross-fertilizing network of colleagues involved in multiple facets of work with the dying and survivors of loss. Interaction among the fellows would foster new interdisciplinary approaches to key issues related to death in America. The PDIA established a Social Work Leadership Development Awards Program led by Grace Christ DSW to promote innovative research and training projects that reflect collaboration between schools of social work and practice site (see Chapter 3 for more on this influential program).

End-of-life issues first surfaced with the American Hospital Association and came into full vogue with the Robert Wood Johnson Foundation sponsored, Study to Understand Prognoses, and Preferences for Outcomes and Risks Treatment (SUPPORT). The results of the study were reported on the front page of the *Washington Post*, November 22, 1995, under the headline, "US Hospitals' Way of Death Resist Change." The article states that the "Findings of the study of more than 9,000 acutely ill patients in five teaching hospitals present a pattern of depersonalized care near the end of life and poor communication among patients, families and doctors." The fact that the findings stunned and shocked researchers gave impetus to the notion that health care providers had not been talking with, listening to, or hearing patients. For me, the findings suggested a number of changes, including the following:

- Care at the end of life must be envisioned and accepted as the responsibility of health care institutions. Thus, hospice and palliative care must be built into the mission and goals of the institution.
- Life-threatening illnesses demand an interdisciplinary team, including the patient, family, and significant others.

- Medical and health education and all allied health programs must address end-of-life issues with experiential involvement.
- Patient management at the end of life must be based on the modality of hospice care and the treatment principles of palliative medicine. The caring component reflects a holistic approach that is maintained throughout the illness, up until the moment of death, and includes the family.
- End-of-life prognoses must be approached with meaning and understanding of cultural ramifications and practice implications.
- The attitudes toward patients who do not recover must be continually evaluated, and feelings of defeat, hopelessness, and despair replaced with positive and specific measures to eliminate pain, needless suffering, emotional isolation, and loss of dignity. All health care professionals must fully understand the importance of living well until death.

Social Work: Credentials and Standards

In 2001 the Society for Social Work Leadership published Care at End of Life; Best Practice Series (Taylor Brown, Blacker, Walsh-Burke, Christ, & Altilio, 2001). In 2005, Gwyther et al. published Competencies in Palliative and End-of-Life Care in the first edition of the *Journal of Social Work in End-of-Life & Palliative Care*, edited by Ellen Csikai. The NASW Standards for Palliative and End-of-Life Care (2004) is representative of practice. It is also a supportive and educational tool relative to palliative social work which served to inform the first Advanced Certified Hospice and Palliative Social Worker (ACHP-SW) credential. This credential is a product of collaboration between the National Hospice and Palliative Care Organization and the National Association of Social Workers.

Getting on the Same Page

Hospice care, palliative care, comfort care, end-of-life care, and *palliative medicine.* These terms are often used interchangeably in health care terminology, causing confusion for professionals and users of services. For future reference I have done some thinking:

- The term *hospice* is the modality.
- The diagnosis is the disease entity.
- The prognosis estimates the end of life.
- Treatment involves palliative care, comfort care, and/or palliative medicine.

It has been said that hospice cannot do all of the things that palliative care can do relative to the end of life.

- It is not the name. It is the care and the provision of services.
- It is not the name, but how will you die?
- It is not the name, but how did they handle the pain?
- It is not the name, but did they meet the needs of the patient and the family?

The World Health Organization (WHO) has described palliative care as an approach that improves the quality of life of patients and their families facing the problems associated with life-threatening illness, through the prevention and relief of suffering by means of early identification and impeccable assessment and treatment of pain and other problems, physical, psychosocial, and spiritual.

From the perspective of a social worker engaged for decades in the public and private response to the needs of patients and their families, palliative care may also be envisioned as follows:

P Represents the *patient* and the family.
A Is the *action* required to meet the needs of the patient, family, staff and community.
L Is the key to *love* and compassion needed for the patient and family confronting a life-threatening illness.
L *Leadership*, knowledge, and skills are necessary in the provision of care.
I Demonstrates the *interest* in caring for the patient and the family.
A Demands the total *acceptance* of the patient and family.
T Aggressive caring, appropriate *treatment,* and management of pain and suffering form the centerpiece for successful intervention.
I *Initiative* for and understanding of cultural factors that set the stage for the right assessment.
V Is for the *visionary mind* of the caregivers and providers of services.
E Supports the entering into an *effective contract* with the patient and family in the provision of a plan of care.
C Stands for the importance of *continuity of care.*
A Making the necessary *arrangements* for handling the grief.
R Utilization of appropriate *resources* for the patient and family.
E Understanding of the *empathy* required to provide the care for the patient and family.

Conclusion

This personal and historical perspective reflects the lived experience of a unique social work journey tracing medical social services from its early beginning in the public sector and the private arena to social work in health care to its present stance in hospice and palliative care:

1. Medical social services are part federal legislation.
2. Social work in health care is also a product of the private arena.
3. Social work in hospice care is an outgrowth of private initiative and federal legislation.
4. Palliative social work emerged from the body of knowledge that informs hospice care, pain management, and palliative medicine and focuses on meeting the needs of patients and families confronting life-threatening illness.

A physical disorder is the sum of many conditions and the end result of a long chain of processes. Seldom is there one single etiological factor; rather, there is always a constellation of them. There can be no question that the modern concept of medicine recognizes the importance of social and emotional factors in relation to disease; its etiology, treatment, and prevention require a wide variety of specialists. The social worker is one of these specialists who utilize special knowledge and skills in assisting and supporting patients and families confronting catastrophic diseases and life-threatening illnesses.

The public and private sectors have worked together to produce a health care delivery system with its strengths, weaknesses, connectedness, continuity, and interlocking and interfacing of skill, knowledge, and resources. From the standpoint of social work, a sound psychosocial diagnosis is of utmost importance as the basis for determining an individual's care plan. In fact, diagnosis and care are closely intertwined. There are many factors to be considered:

1. Patient's current needs
2. Relationship of current needs to past life experiences
3. Attitudes and behavior patterns
4. Interaction with other family members and the balance or lack of it in these relationships
5. Other interpersonal and mental status
6. Economic situation
7. Cultural and spiritual background.

These factors are significant in building care plans and enhancing the ongoing quality of life of the patient and family confronting life-threatening illnesses. Yet there is more. Social workers and other palliative care professionals, who would be successful in working with patients who do not recover, and their families, must come to grips with their feelings about their own immortality, life's end, and the in-between life processes. That is, professional anxieties related to working with catastrophic diseases are observable phenomena for which a coping mechanism can be developed. The health care professional who comes to accept his or her own feelings is enabled to provide sensitive caregiving and to give strength and support to patients and relatives. The patient can be helped to die with dignity and self-respect in a loving, caring, cultural context and atmosphere. Families and significant others can be helped to come through a traumatic experience with some semblance of mental health and the ability to cope with grief, mourning, and bereavement (Harper, 1977).

The stage has been set for appropriate, accessible, acceptable, coordinated, and quality care for all peoples of our global world. Social workers as experts are daily witnesses to the unmet needs of society in health and social care. Social workers and other health care professionals must develop the strategies to lead the way from hospital care, to managed care, home health care, to hospice care, palliative care and on to health promotion and preventive services for the next generation who will be utilizing the health care delivery system. Social workers will be needed more than ever to assist patients and families in a global world to live productive lives, to maximize the utilization of health, mental health, social care, financial, and spiritual resources during the various phases and stages of illness along life's continuum: the beginning phase of the illness, the middle phase of the disease, and the ending phase of life. Palliative social work requires social work to be performed at its most professional level.

LEARNING EXERCISES

1. Describe the emergence of palliative social work using the terms "public sector" and "private arena."
2. Health professionals do not enter practice academically, emotionally, and psychologically prepared to deal with death and dying. Think and then record your reaction to this statement.

REFERENCES

Association of Oncology Social Workers (AOSW). (2001). *AOSW Mission Statement.* Retrieved from http://www.aosw.org/html/mission.php

Califano, J. A. (1977). Office of Education reorganization. Memorandum: Secretary Califano to President Carter, April 8th. Department of Education, Box 195, Eizenstat, DPS, Jimmy Carter Presidential Library. Atlanta, GA.

Cohen, W. J. (1985). The twentieth anniversary of Medicare and Medicaid: The long, difficult road to enactment. The Report of the Committee on Economic Security of 1935; and other basic documents relating to the development of the Social Security Act with essays by Wilbur Cohen and Robert Ball. Washington, DC: National Conference on Social Welfare.

Davidson, J. D., & Doka, K. J. (2001). *Caregiving and loss: Family needs, professional responses.* Oregon, IL: Quality Books, Inc.

Gammarino, M., Kammerer, J., & King, K. (1990). *The National Kidney Foundation: The first forty years.* Councils of the National Kidney Foundation, 49th Anniversary Issue. Philadelphia, PA: WB Saunders Company.

Gwyther, L. P., Altilio, T., Blacker, S., Christ, G., Csikai, E. L., Hooyman, N., ... Howe J. (2005). Competencies in palliative and end-of-life care. *Journal of Social Work in End-of-Life and Palliative Care,* 1(1), 87–120.

Harper, B. C. (1977). *Death: The coping mechanism of the healthcare professional.* Greenville, SC: University Press, Inc.

Hinds Hospice. (2007). *History of Hospice.* Retrieved from http://www.hindshospice.org/hospice.htm

Kahn, M. (1934). *The work of social services.* 20th Anniversary of the Los Angeles Sanatorium and Expatients Home. City of Hope National Medical Center Archives. Duarte, CA.

Marine Hospital Health Care. (1978). *Financing Administration Newsletter,* 2(2).

National Hospice and Palliative Care Organization (NHPCO). (n. d.). *History of Hospice Care: A historical perspective.* Retrieved from http://www.nhpco.org/i4a/pages/index.cfm?pageid=3285

National Hospice and Pallitaive Care Organization. (NHPCO). (2009). *Facts and figures: Hospice care in America.* Retrieved from http://www.nhpco.org/files/public/Statistics_Research/NHPCO_facts_and_figures.pdf

Nixon, R. (1971). *Statement about actions to improve the quality care in nursing homes* (Public Papers of President Richard Nixon, No. 259 - 1971). Office of the Federal Register, National Archives and Records Service, General Services Administration. Public Papers of the Presidents of the United States. Washington, DC: United States Government Printing Office.

Reagan, R. (1981). *The President's news conference* (Public Papers of President Ronald Reagan, 1981). Office of the Federal Register, National Archives and Records Service, General Services Administration. Public Papers of the Presidents of the United States. Washington, D.C.: United States Government Printing Office.

Saint Christopher's Hospice. *History.* Retrieved from http://www.stchristophers.org.uk/

Simms, T. (2007). Hospice Care: The Modern Hospice Movement. *Topics in Advanced Practice Nursing ejournal,* Lighthouse Hospice, Cherry Hill, NJ. Retrieved from http://www.medscape.com/viewarticle/549702_2

Social Security Administration. (1972). *Public Law 92-603, Social Security Amendments of 1972* (86 Stat. 1329). Washington, DC: Government Printing Office.

Taylor Brown, S., Blacker, S., Walsh-Burke, K., Christ, G., & Altilio, T. (2001). *Care at the end of life; Best practices series.,* Philidelphia, PA: Society for Social Work Leadership in Health Care.

U.S. Department of Health and Human Services. (DHHS). (1976). *41 FR 22501, Medicare Program; Conditions for coverage for end stage renal disease facilities; Final rule* (Federal Register Doc). Washington, DC: Government Printing Office.

U.S. Department of Health and Human Services, Health Care Financing Administration. (1983). *42 CFR 418, Medicare program; Hospice care; Final rule* (Federal Register Doc. 83-1216). Washington, DC: Government Printing Office.

U.S. Department of Health and Human Services, Centers for Medicare and Medicaid Services. (2008). *42 CFR 418, Medicare and Medicaid programs: Hospice conditions of participation; Final rule* (Federal Register Doc. 08-1305). Washington, DC: Government Printing Office.

Washington Post, (1995) US Hospitals' Way of Death Resist Change, November 22.

3 *Susan Blacker and Grace H. Christ*

Defining Social Work's Role and Leadership Contributions in Palliative Care

If you would understand anything, observe its beginning and its development.

—Aristotle

Key Concepts
- *The historic legacy of the Project on Death in America (PDIA) Social Work Leadership Award program launched many projects that have enhanced the contribution of social work to palliative and end-of-life care.*
- *Included in this legacy is the development of the Social Work Hospice and Palliative Care Network (SWHPN).*

Introduction

The last decade has proven to be a time of tremendous growth and development in palliative care. This is generally attributed to advances in disease prevention, disease-modifying therapies, and medical technology in combination with the aging of the population that has resulted in a dramatic growth in the number of adults living with serious illness (Morrison, Maroney, Galin, Kralovec & Meier, 2005). Since the mid-1990s, concerns about the experience of patients with serious illness have heightened. A number of studies and reports noted that patients too often receive care that has not adequately addressed symptoms and suffering, has left personal and home care needs poorly met, and has neglected the burden on caregivers. Communication around goals of care, support for transitions in care, and support for psychosocial needs have been limited, causing low levels of patient and family satisfaction and underutilization of hospice care (Field & Cassell, 1997).

Palliative care, by definition, strives to improve quality of care for patients with advanced illness and for their families through an interdisciplinary approach. Clearly, many identified needs of patient and family require specific social work skills to provide better preparation and education, clarify goals of care, enhance communication, help with transition between care settings and connection to resources, and offer more timely alleviation of biopsychosocial-spiritual suffering (Altilio & Otis Green, 2007; Colon, 2007).

Growing Numbers of Social Workers in Palliative Care

Social workers comprise the largest group of mental health professionals providing psychosocial services in both hospice and palliative care (Connor, 2008). This is consistent with the historical presence of social work in other specialized care areas, like oncology. A 1995 national survey found that 75% of supportive counseling for all cancer patients at

National Cancer Institute (NCI) designated cancer centers was provided by social workers (Coluzzi, Grant, Doroshow, Rhiner, Ferrell, & Rivers, 1995). With the creation of many new palliative care programs in American hospitals, the number of social workers employed in this field has grown rapidly over the past decade. In 2005, there were over 1486 palliative care programs in hospitals; 75% of hospitals with over 300 beds had programs (Center to Advance Palliative Care, 2010). In the mid 1980s, there were only a handful in existence. In 2009, there were 520 inpatient hospice facilities and residences and approximately 4850 hospice programs in total in the United States (NHPCO, 2009). Both hospice and palliative care coordination models aim to improve quality of life for patients with advanced illness and their families through pain and symptom management, communication and support for medical decisions consistent with goals of care, and assurance of safe transitions between care settings (Morrison et al., 2008).

It is important to consider the impact that social workers can have for patients not yet referred for specialist palliative care services. The broad range of settings in which social workers provide care to those with serious or life-limiting illness includes the following: acute and subacute hospitals, skilled nursing and extended care facilities, hospice, home health care, hospital palliative care programs, community health and mental health clinics, and bereavement and funeral service settings. In summary, as stated in the National Agenda for Social Work Research in Palliative and End-of-Life Care, social workers have an important role to play in palliative and end-of-life care "given their work in varied and divergent practice settings across the lifespan, their role in addressing mental health needs, grief, and psychosocial aspects of well-being, and their commitment to promoting culturally competent, effective, and humane care, particularly for the most vulnerable and oppressed members of society" (Kramer, Christ, Bern-Klug, & Francouer, 2005, p. 418). When considering the impact of illness beyond the medical setting to include care of those touched directly or indirectly by illness and death, it can be inferred that almost all social workers provide services to individuals confronting loss, distress, and adaptation in their own lives.

While social workers have long functioned as core team members providing essential services to patients with advanced illnesses and their families (Colon, 2007), the establishment of a critical mass making focused contributions in education, research, administration/program development, policy, and leadership in palliative care is much more recent. Social work has become an active voice in the dialogue in this expanding field. It is imperative that social work continue to expand its knowledge base and incorporate this knowledge into all levels of professional education for medical social work, with the goal of continuing to influence the dialogue about how to ensure the highest quality of care for all patients and families living with life-limiting illness—at the bedside, in the classroom, and in the broader professional and public realms.

The Contributions of Social Work in Palliative Care

Social work plays a critical role in palliative care because of its unique perspective, knowledge, and skills, including (1) its expertise in navigation of medical and social systems; (2) its knowledge base in the support, education, and interventions with patients, families, and interdisciplinary teams; and (3) its commitment to social justice and alleviation of health disparities. The social work role encompasses a broad range of functions in addition to direct practice with patients and families. These include, for example, providing education for patients, families, communities, and other disciplines; advocacy for patients at all system levels; and increasing involvement in psychosocial research and institutional and broader policy issues.

The Need to Strive for Improvements in Care Delivery

A number of reports over the past decade have documented the state of care along the continuum of illness and at the end of life and recommended essential strategies to influence systemic improvements. Some have focused on unique populations such as cancer patients (*Improving Palliative Care for Cancer* by the National Cancer Policy Board, National Research Council, 2001) and children and families facing life-threatening illness (*When Children Die*, Institute of Medicine, 2003). Arguably one of the most pivotal was the Institute of Medicine report from 1997, titled "Approaching Death: Improving Care at the End of Life". This report had a significant impact on promoting professional research, education, training, as well as improving models for care delivery for the dying. It highlighted the following issues:

- Too many dying people suffer from pain and other distress that clinicians could prevent and relieve with existing knowledge and therapies.
- Significant organizational, economic, legal, and educational impediments to good care can be identified and, in varying degrees, remedied.
- Important gaps in scientific knowledge need serious attention from biomedical, social science, and health services researchers.
- Strengthening accountability for the quality of care at the end of life will require better data and tools for evaluating the outcomes important to patients and families.

Among other recommendations for improving care, the Institute of Medicine report advocated strongly for enhancement of palliative care education for health care

---

professionals at all levels of training. The Project on Death in America Social Work Leadership Awards program (discussed in the next section) was greatly informed by this report.

While not focused on palliative care specifically, the more recent Institute of Medicine report on psychosocial services to cancer patients, "Cancer Care for the Whole Patient: Meeting Psychosocial Health Needs" (2008) provides a critical discussion of the unmet psychosocial needs of this population. This report highlighted the large number of evidence-based practices and services that have been reported as helpful in meeting these needs, as well as the medical systems' failure to successfully integrate them. The committee noted the challenges and barriers to integrating evidenced-based services in the care of cancer patients within a system that often fails to recognize or value these needs and related services. The report found the following:

- Many of the recommendations that have been made over the years calling for more attention to the psychosocial concerns of cancer patients and their families have not been acted upon.
- Both cancer survivors and their caregivers report that their providers failed to understand their psychosocial needs and to recognize and adequately address depression and other symptoms of stress.
- Their providers also appeared to be unaware of available resources that could offer support or at least did not make any referrals.
- Providers generally did not consider psychosocial support to be an integral part of quality care for the oncologic patient.

This report illuminates the importance of advocating for and developing models that fully integrate social workers in the treatment setting to enable proactive identification of patient and family needs. For social workers focusing in the palliative care setting, it highlights the magnitude to which needs may have gone unrecognized or unmet earlier in the care continuum (Blacker, 2004).

Leading Social Work in the Quest for Better Care for the Dying: History of the Social Work Leadership Development Award

As a first step in considering specific opportunities to support social work, the Project on Death in America (a program of the Soros Foundation, Open Society Institute) supported a national survey in 1999 of the practice, research, education, and training needs of social work practitioners and educators who provided end-of-life and palliative care education and service. The findings of this survey were similar to those that examined the training of physicians and nurses; social workers were not receiving up-to-date education and training in palliative and end-of-life care either at the graduate or postgraduate level (Christ & Sormanti, 1999).

Beyond the educational context, it was also recognized that the social work contribution in end-of-life research and policy development was limited.

The Social Work Leadership Development Awards Program (SWLDA) was then established by PDIA. It provided a forum for social work experts to become visible and accessible leaders in both social work–specific and interdisciplinary arenas. Although many social workers were practicing in this specialty, and some had recognized practice and scholarly achievements, there was previously no forum for them to collectively exercise leadership and disseminate their knowledge and skill effectively within the profession or in interdisciplinary forums. A group of 42 social work leaders (see Table 3.1) were selected to promote development of social work in palliative and end-of-life care through innovative projects in practice, education, research, and in collaboration with other disciplines.

PDIA Social Work Leadership Development Award Recipients

Table 3.1 lists the awardees in each of the five cohorts funded during the Social Work Leadership Development Award program. Their projects resulted in new educational initiatives at both the preparatory and continuing education levels, research projects focused on enhancing understanding of the experience and needs of patients and their families, and innovative models for service delivery. Projects were developed in a range of settings, including schools of social work, health care organizations, and community agencies; they focused on specific populations, including cancer, HIV/AIDS, pediatrics, and the aged. Dissemination of the outcomes and findings from these projects resulted in a dramatic increase in the number of presentations and publications about social work in hospice and palliative care.

Social Work Leadership Development Awards: 2000–2003 Grantees and Projects by Cohort

The program aimed to identify leaders in practice and academia who would be supported to develop projects that would advance the field, create educational and practice models and resources, and provide more visible leadership for this growing specialty area. The challenge was to identify social work experts, draw together a network of leaders, integrate and expand the knowledge base, and begin the process of standard setting and developing an agenda for the future.

The accomplishments of this group over the 5 years of the program were significant and transformative. The short-term result was the creation of a broad range of initiatives, including training programs, publications, texts, research grants, innovative practice programs, and standards of practice. Postgraduate continuing education programs were

Table 3.1.
Award Recipients of the PDIA Social Work Leadership Development Award Program

Cohort I, 2000	Cohort II, 2000	Cohort III, 2001	Cohort IV, 2002	Cohort IV, 2003
Joan Berzoff *Developing a Certificate Program and Textbook in End-of-Life Care*	**Terry Altilio** *A Multidimensional Intervention for Social Workers in Palliative and End-of-Life Care*	**David A. Cherin** *The University of Washington's School of Social Work End-of-Life Care Knowledge Institute*	**Mercedes Bern-Klug** *Psychosocial Concerns at the End of Life for Nursing Home Residents: The Role of Social Work*	**David Browning** *Developing a Pediatric End-of-Life Care Curriculum for Social Workers*
Susan Blacker *Social Work and End-of-Life Care: An Educational Initiative*	**Elizabeth Mayfield Arnold** *Unmet Patient Needs at the End of Life: The Hospice Social Work Response*	**Ellen L. Csikai** **Mary Raymer** *The Social Work End-of-Life Care Educational Program (SWEEP)*	**Sheila R. Enders** *Creating a Handbook for Advance Care Planning and Decision Making at the End of Life in Populations with Low Literacy, Mild Learning Disabilities, or Mild Cognitive Deficits*	**Karen Bullock** *Resource Enrichment Center*
Iris Cohen *Multidisciplinary Care Tools: Teamwork and Family Conferences in Palliative Care*	**John F. Linder** *Fostering Interdisciplinary Cooperation in the Delivery of Enhanced End-of-Life Care Through a Collaborative Social Work/Clergy Graduate Curriculum*	**Judith Dobrof** *Caregivers and Professionals Partnership: Assessing a Structured Support Program*	**Richard B. Francoeur** *Palliative Care in an Inner-City Minority Population: The Impact of Chronic Disease, Material Deprivation, and Financial Burden*	**Elizabeth Chaitin** *Interdisciplinary Specialty Team Training in Palliative Care*
				Nancy Cincotta *A National Initiative to Unite Social Workers and Families in the Interest of Dying Children*
				Elizabeth J. Clark *Building Social Work Practice and Policy Competencies in End-of-Life Care*

Barbara Dane	Margo Okazawa-Rey Norma del Rio	Betty J. Kramer	Barbara L. Jones	Nancy Contro
University/Agency Collaboration to Advance Training in End-of-Life Care	Multicultural Social Work Practice with Clients at the End of Life	Strengthening Social Work Education to Improve End-of-Life Care	Psychosocial Protocol and Training Program for End-of-Life Care for Children with Cancer: A Social Work Curriculum	Latino Families in Pediatric Palliative Care
Jim Keresztury	**W. June Simmons**	**Shirley Otis-Green**	**Jane Lindberg,**	**Rita Ledesma**
Social Work End-of-Life Training — A Network Approach	End-of-Life Social Work Field Education Project	Proyecto de Transiciones: Enhancing End-of-Life and Bereavement Support Services for Latinos within a Cancer Center Setting	Social Worker Bereavement Training Program	Loss and Bereavement in an American Indian and Alaska Native Community
Mary Sormanti	**Susan Taylor-Brown**	**Amanda Sutton** **Yvette Colon**	**Susan Murty**	**Bonnie Letinich**
State-of-the-Art Psychosocial Care for the Dying and Those Who Love Them	Enhancing the Care of Families Living with HIV/AIDS: A Clinical, Educational, and Research Initiative in a Community-Based HIV Care Facility with a Family Camping Component	The End-of-Life Internet Forum	Developing Social Work Leadership in End-of-Life Services in Rural Communities	Pediatric Palliative Care Education for Social Workers
Gary L. Stein	**Katherine Walsh-Burke**		**Bruce A. Paradis**	**Aloen Townsend**
The Excellence in End-of-Life Care Fellowship for Social Workers	Internet-based Continuing Education Curriculum		End-of-Life Care: Birth through Old Age	Family Assessment Collaboration to Enhance End-of-Life Support
			Sherri Weisenfluh	**Terry A. Wolfer** **Vicki Runnion**
			The Kentucky Project, Enhancing End-of-Life Care: A Social Work Manual for Students and Practitioners	Casebook on Death and Dying for Social Work Education

created for local, state, and national audiences. The outreach of the collective training programs reached thousands of practicing social workers in the United States. (Details about these projects can be found at: http://swhpn.org/swlda/archive/)

Social Work Leadership Summits

In late 2001, The Social Work Leadership Development Awards Program of the Project on Death in America identified the establishment of a social work agenda in end-of-life and palliative care as an essential and strategic next step to propel the profession and the field forward. In March 2002, with support from Last Acts, the Project on Death in America, and the Duke Institute on Care at the End of Life, a 2-1/2 day summit was held in Durham, North Carolina. The intent was to formalize a collaborative and supportive effort within the social work profession. Participants from more than 35 organizations and institutions accepted the invitation and began with the question: *"What are anticipated challenges related to end-of-life and palliative care—within the policy, research, education, and practice domains of social work—that need to be addressed during the next decade?"* The more than 200 specific ideas generated reflected 10 key domains:

- Defining end-of-life care
- Role of social work in end-of-life care
- Attitudes and perceptions about death and dying
- Defining scope and standards of practice
- Policy change/improving care systems
- Social work foundation training
- Postgraduate training
- Funding and training for end-of-life care research
- Identifying a research agenda
- Leadership for social work

Using a guided decision-making process, the group developed goals and projects aimed toward actualizing the domains. The outcome of this meeting was the creation of "A Priority Map for Social Work in End of Life and Palliative Care." (Consensus-building exercises at both summits were facilitated by a team led by Benjamin Broome, PhD, of Hugh Downs School of Communication, Arizona State University.) The following priority areas were identified at the 2002 Summit.

- Develop a consensus statement for social work in end-of-life and palliative care
- Create a social work coalition of experts, institutions, and organizations
- Produce a concise document that integrates and synthesizes research and practice-based literature
- Develop competencies for social work in end-of-life and palliative care to guide and develop standards of practice

- Create an information clearing house to increase public and professional awareness
- Develop social work end-of-life and palliative care content for infusion into existing curricula
- Advocate for funding of research, training, and education in end-of-life and palliative care through federal and state authorizing legislation
- Develop research awards and grants
- Establish academic and clinical partnerships for collaborative research on social work interventions and best practices
- Identify, create, implement, and disseminate models for postgraduate continuing education about end-of-life and palliative care

Several short-term outcomes resulted. A number of the participating organizations included information about the summit in their communications to members, further extending the reach of this event and increasing awareness about this unique area of practice. A group of practitioners and educators also formed at the summit with the goal of producing a publication about competencies for social work practice in palliative and end-of-life care (Gwyther et al., 2005). This initiative also contributed to the development of the National Association of Social Workers (NASW) *Standards for Social Work in Palliative and End-of-Life Care*, published in 2004.

Social Work Summit, 2005

The second Social Work Summit on End-of-Life and Palliative Care was again sponsored by the Open Society Institute's Social Work Leadership Development Awards Program of the Project on Death in America. The summit was hosted at the NASW in Washington, DC. Participants came from the United States, Canada, the United Kingdom, and Singapore. Some 60 representatives of more than 35 social work and hospice palliative care–focused organizations collaborated on developing a focused action strategy on June 1–3, 2005. This included representatives from the Society for Social Work Research (SSWR), the Council on Social Work Education (CSWE), the NASW, the Association of Oncology Social Work (AOSW), the Society for Social Work Leadership in Health Care (SSWLHC), the Association of Pediatric Oncology Social Work (APOSW), the National Hospice Palliative Care Organization (NHPCO), and the Hartford Foundation.

This second meeting continued the dialogue initiated 3 years prior about the importance of social work's role in improving care for the seriously ill, dying, and bereaved, and it aimed to develop specific strategies to further build capacity within the profession. Specific goals of this meeting included the following:

- Continue momentum within the profession to make end-of-life and palliative care an important strategic area of focus

- Further develop a network of organizations and leaders, create a mechanism for collaborative efforts, and further the profession's evolution in the areas of policy/advocacy, practice, research, and education
- Identify key strategies, initiatives, and action plans that would build on the Priority Agenda for Social Work in Palliative and End of Life Care that was developed at the first summit (Christ & Blacker, 2005)

Participants focused on the areas of policy/advocacy, research, education, and practice and began the day with state-of-the-field presentations by teams of experts. The presenters were as follows:

- Betty Kramer, Richard Francoeur, and Mercedes Bern-Klug:
  - The state of social work research in end-of-life and palliative care
- Gary Stein, Pat Sherman, and Stuart Kaufer:
  - The state of social work policy in end-of-life and palliative care
- Katherine Walsh-Burke and Ellen Csikai:
  - The state of social work education and training in palliative, end-of-life, and grief care
- Terry Altilio, Gary Gardia, and Shirley Otis-Green:
  - The state of social work practice

Full papers related to these presentations were published in several journals (see the references included at the end of this chapter). Summaries of these reports can be found in *Charting the Course for the Future of Social Work in End-of-Life and Palliative Care: A Report of the 2nd Social Work Summit on End-of-Life and Palliative Care* (2007), edited by Susan Blacker, MSW, RSW, Grace H. Christ, DSW, and Sallie Lynch, MA, available at http://www.swhpn.org. Collectively the participants of the summit identified key priority initiatives related to each of these areas and then developed action plans that would move the field forward.

The Social Work Hospice and Palliative Care Network

Based on the outcomes of two Social Work Leadership Summits in Palliative and End-of-Life Care, the recommendation was made to develop a professional network to achieve the following:

- Build consensus within the profession about this field as a unique area of practice, research, and education
- Create intraprofessional and interprofessional partnerships
- Develop a social work–specific knowledge and skill base in this area of practice
- Disseminate information to the social work community (nationally and internationally)

- Collaborate with other organizations on program initiatives and resource sharing
- Further the development of capacity within social work in hospice and palliative care, and ultimately, advance the field

The Social Work Hospice and Palliative Care Network (SWHPN) was created in December 2007 and is an outgrowth of the Open Society Institute's Project on Death in America Social Work Leadership Development Program. This membership network is a tangible way to further the agenda developed at the leadership summits and to engage members of the profession. This has established a profession-specific entity focused on social work in hospice and palliative care. Formation of a membership-based organization parallels the similar organizational structures and their efforts to advance palliative care in nursing and medicine, including the Hospice and Palliative Care Nurses Association and the American Academy of Hospice and Palliative Medicine. This reflects that social work in hospice and palliative care has evolved as a field of practice with specialized knowledge and skill—and that having a professional association dedicated to the advancement and dissemination of this knowledge is essential. This profession-specific entity includes social work practitioners, educators, researchers, and policy advocates, with membership that is international. SWHPN also seeks to develop partnerships and connections to relevant social work and hospice palliative care leadership organizations through specific projects and preconference workshops. For example, the inclusion of social work leaders who also have awards as Faculty Scholars in the Hartford Social Work Geriatric Initiative has created a cadre of Researchers in SWHPN who are committed to further the social work research agenda in palliative care.

Member Benefits SWHPN has resulted in the creation of a dynamic "virtual community of practice" for social workers in practice, education, and research. Member services and initiatives now in place that have been designed to address the priority agenda include the following:

- Providing an online members-only networking space using a Web-based social networking platform for health care professionals that links SWHPN members and provides access to an online repository of resources, a discussion forum, and a "Hear from the Expert" interactive series
- Subscription to the electronic version of the *Journal of Social Work in End-of-Life and Palliative Care* (publisher: Taylor and Francis) as part of membership
- Electronic Newsletters and E-Blasts on current developments in the field and new resources of interest to clinicians and educators
- Alerts about upcoming professional conferences in palliative care and related topic areas, and encouragement of members to present at these forums

- Access to data collected on professional interests in the field
- Special access to state-of-the-field reports and teaching materials
- Special continuing education events (including preconference workshops at the *American Academy of Hospice and Palliative Medicine* annual assembly)
- A mentoring matching program for interested attendees at selected conferences
- Provisions to share selected conference presentation summaries for SWHPN members unable to attend.

The following are a sampling of events that mark the history of the evolution of the SWLDA Program and SWHPN.

Selected Key Milestones and Publications

1999 Need for education and training for social workers in end-of-life care documented (Christ & Sormanti, 1999)

1999 Project on Death in America Social Work Leadership Awards established and first cohort of awardees selected; first joint meeting with PDIA Scholars and social work leaders

2000 New PDIA supported certificate training programs at Smith College and New York University begin to accept first students. National conference held at Johns Hopkins Oncology Center; network established of social workers in palliative and end-of-life care with directory and online newsletter created

2001 Publications jointly created by PDIA social work leaders begin with a joint publication; Society for Social Work Leadership in Health Care Best Practices Paper (Brown, Blacker, Walsh-Burke, Christ, & Altilio, 2001)

2001–2004 PDIA Social Work Leaders' projects continue to launch, increasing the number and range of training programs, including fellowships, conferences, and research initiatives; PDIA funded listserv established at Beth Israel Medical Center, New York

2002 First Social Work Summit held at Duke University; outcomes of the meeting published in first issue of new journal: *Journal of Social Work in End-of-Life & Palliative Care*

2004 Presentation of summit priority agenda at 15th International Congress on Palliative Care in Montreal

2004 *Standards for Social Work Practice in End-of-Life and Palliative Care* produced by NASW (PDIA Social Work Leader: Betsy Clark); available at http://www.naswdc.org

2004 Publication of social work competencies in palliative care (Gwyther et al., 2005)

2004 PDIA SWLDA Award program comes to completion; planning for further development of ideas generated at the first Social Work Summit begins

2005 Second Social Work Leadership Summit on Palliative and End-of-Life Care held at NASW, Washington, DC; development of formalized network recommended as high priority. Presentations of "state of the social work field" in palliative and end-of-life care practice, education, research and policy were later published (Altilio, Gardia, Otis-Green, 2008; Csikai and Walsh, 2005; Kramer, Christ, Bern-Klug, & Francoeur, 2005; Stein & Sherman, 2005.)

2005 Publication documents social workers' continuing education and skill needs in end-of-life care (Csikai & Raymer, 2005)

2005 Special Social Work series launched in the *Journal of Palliative Care* (Guest Editors: Susan Blacker and Grace Christ)

2007 SWHPN was formed as a 501.c3 nonprofit entity, with Board of Directors and founding members; launch of the Web site and virtual community of practice. New PDIA Social Work Leadership Award recognizing outstanding leadership in social work within the field of hospice and palliative care created with financial support from PDIA

2007 Inaugural PDIA Social Work Leadership Award presented to Deborah Parker-Oliver at NHPCO Clinical Conference in New Orleans

2008 First SWHPN preconference institute for social workers held at American Academy of Hospice and Palliative Medicine (AAHPM)/ Hospice and Palliative Nurses Association (HPNA) in Tampa, FL. PDIA Social Work Leadership Award presented to Shirley Otis-Green at AAHPM/HPNA

2008 SWHPN Web site developed and discussion forum created, establishing a virtual community of practice for members; http://www.swhpn.org

2008 Certified Hospice and Palliative Social Worker (CHP-SW) and Advanced Certified Hospice and Palliative Social Worker (ACHP-SW) credentialing launched by NHPCO and NASW

2008 First regional SWHPN conference, *Social Work in Hospice and Palliative Care: The Emerging Landscape*, held in New York, NY, supported by Wurzweiler School of Social Work in collaboration with Columbia University School of Social Work

2008 The Journal of Social Work in End-of-life and Palliative Care adopted by SWHPN as a membership benefit

2009 Second SWHPN preconference institute for social workers held at AAHPM in Austin, where the PDIA Social Work Leadership Award was presented to Barbara Jones

2010 Third SWHPN preconference institute for social workers held at AAHPM in Boston, where the PDIA

Social Work Leadership Award was presented to Susan Blacker

Looking Forward

Much momentum has been created within the profession, through the initiatives described in this chapter, and beyond. Anticipating the future, the contributions of social work will be notable as the field of palliative care continues to evolve. They will include, but not be limited to, the following:

- Deepening expertise in understanding and responding to needs related to ethnic, cultural, and economic diversity
- Strengthening understanding and strategies for enhancing family and support networks
- Improving knowledge base about psychosocial-spiritual aspects of symptom management and suffering (Altilio, Otis-Green, Hedlund & Cohen Fineberg, 2006)
- Developing innovation in providing bereavement interventions
- Creating strategies for enhancing intra- and interprofessional team practice
- Advancing training in palliative care, for social work and other professionals (Walsh & Csikai, 2005)
- Enhancing understanding of unique interventions across the life cycle
- Identifying systems interventions that effectively address fragmentation, gaps, and inadequacies in health care and enhance quality of life along the continuum of illness and the dying process

Social work will continue to contribute expertise in analyzing, influencing, and implementing policy change at local, state, and federal levels to improve care of those living with life-limiting illness and those who are dying or bereaved. Social work research has the potential to address many previously overlooked areas of palliative and end-of-life care, such as issues concerning vulnerable populations, substance abuse, crises interventions and interventions at different life cycle stages and within varied community and organizational contexts (Christ & Blacker, 2005).

REFERENCES

Altilio, T., & Otis-Green, S. (2007). An Emerging Synergy: Pain and Social Work. Newsline: Quarterly Insights Edition, National Hospice and Palliative Care Organization, 18(6), 31.

Altilio, T., Gardia, G., & Otis-Green, S. (2008). Social work practice in palliative and end-of-life care: A report from the summit. *Journal of Social Work in End-of-Life and Palliative Care*, 4(4), 1–19.

Altilio, T., Otis-Green, S., Hedlund, S., & Cohen Fineberg, I. (2006). Pain management and palliative care. In S. Gehlert & T. A. Browne (Eds.), *Handbook of health social work* (pp. 645–673). New York, NY: John Wiley & Sons, Inc.

Blacker, S. (2004). Palliative care and social work. In J. Berzoff & P. Silverman (Eds.), *Living with dying: A handbook for health care practitioners* (pp. 409–423). New York, NY: Columbia University Press.

Brown, S. T., Blacker, S., Walsh-Burke, K., Christ, G., & Altilio, T. (2001). End of life care giving. *Society for Social Work Leadership in Health Care—Best practice series*. Philadelphia, PA: Society for Social Work Leadership in Health Care.

Center to Advance Palliative Care. (2010). Press release. "*Palliative Care Programs Continue Rapid Growth in U.S. Hospitals Becoming Standard Practice throughout the Country*" Accessed on Aug. 25/10 at: http://www.capc.org/news-and-events/releases/04-05-10

Christ, G., & Blacker, S. (2005). Setting an agenda for social work in end-of-life and palliative care: An overview of leadership and organizational initiatives. *Journal of Social Work in End-of-Life and Palliative Care*, 1(1), 9–22.

Christ, G., & Sormanti, M. (1999). Advancing social work practice in end-of-life care. *Social Work in Health Care*, 30(2):81–99.

Colon, Y. (2007). End-of-life care. In S. Gehlert & T. Browne (Eds.), *Handbook of health social work* (pp. 615–635). New York, NY: John Wiley & Sons, Inc.

Coluzzi, P. H., Grant, M., Doroshow, J. H., Rhiner, M., Ferrell, B., & Rivera, L. (1995). Survey of the provision of supportive care services at National Cancer Institute-designated cancer centers. *Journal of Clinical Oncology*, 13, 756–764.

Connor, S. R. (2007/2008). Development of hospice and palliative care in the United States. *Omega (Westport)*, 56(1), 89–99.

Csikai, E., & Raymer, M. (2005). Social workers' educational needs in end-of-life care. *Social Work in Health Care*, 41(1), 53–72.

Field, M. J., & Cassell, C. K. (Eds.). (1997). *Approaching death: Improving care at the end of life*. Washington, DC: National Academies Press.

Gwyther, L. P., Altilio, T., Blacker, S., Christ, G., Csikai, E., Hooyman, N.,…Howe, J. (2005). Social work competencies in palliative & end-of-life care. *Social Work in End of Life and Palliative Care*, 1(1), 23–32.

Institute of Medicine. (2003). When Children Die: Improving palliative and end-of-life care for children and their families. Eds. Field and Behrman. Washington, DC: National Academies Press.

Institute of Medicine. (2008). *Cancer care for the whole patient: Meeting psychosocial health needs*. Eds. Field and Cassell. Washington, DC: National Academies Press. Retrieved 2008, from: http://www.nap.edu/catalog/11993.html

Kramer, B. J., Bern-Klug, M., Christ, G., & Francoeur, R. B. (2005). A national agenda for social work research in palliative and end-of-life care. *Journal of Palliative Medicine*, 8(2), 418–431.

Morrison, S., Maroney, Galin, C., Kralovec, P., & Meier, D. E. (2005). The growth of palliative care programs in United States hospitals. *Journal of Palliative Medicine*, 8(6), 1127–1134.

National Cancer Policy Board (2001). Improving Palliative Care for Cancer. Eds. Foley and Gelband. Washington, DC: National Academy Press.

National Hospice and Palliative Care Organization (NHPCO).
(2009). *NHPCO facts and figures on hospice.* Retrieved from
www.nhpco.org/files/public/Statistics_research/NHPCO_facts_
and_figures.pdf

Stein, G., & Sherman, P. A. (2005). *Promoting effective social work
policy in end-of-life and palliative care.* Journal of Palliative
Medicine. (8)6, 1271–1281.

Walsh-Burke, K., & Csikai, E. L. (2005). The Project on Death in
America's social work leadership development awardee's
contributions to professional social work education in
end-of-life care. *Journal of Social Work in End-of-Life and
Palliative Care, 1*(2), 11–26.

World Health Organization. (2005). WHO definition of palliative
care. Retrieved from http://www.who.int/cancer/palliative/
definition/en/

4

Philip C. Higgins

Guess Who's Coming to Dinner? The Emerging Identity of Palliative Social Workers

Always be a first-rate version of yourself, instead of a second-rate version of somebody else.
—Judy Garland

Key Concepts

♦ *As palliative social work continues to develop as a specialty practice, it will be important to develop a clear sense of professional identity.*

♦ *Adaptation of Bronfenbrenner's ecological systems theory and Atkinson, Morten & Sue's minority identity development theory highlights challenges and opportunities in palliative social work identity development.*

Introduction

Palliative social workers are a people on the rise. The profession of social work has played a fundamental role in medicine since the mid-twentieth century and in the American hospice movement since its inception in the 1970s and 1980s (Foster, 1979). With the recent advent of hospital and other institution-based palliative care programs, however, clinical social workers have struggled to maintain a consistent foothold on specialist-level palliative care service delivery. This was recently illustrated in a study of palliative care teams at 96 U.S. cancer centers, only 55% of which were identified as having a team social worker (Hui et al., 2010, p. 1058). Palliative social workers possess the unique skill set needed to address the psychosocial aspects of coping with advanced illness, complex end-of-life decision making, and the myriad of other factors that arise throughout illness and bereavement. Possessing these skills and having the freedom, confidence, and position to employ them, however, are different matters. As social workers in palliative care, we face barriers—within our own discipline, within the palliative care teams of which we are a part, and within the larger institutions that employ us—that can make it difficult for us to do our jobs. Caught up in the daily task of balancing the clinical work that feeds our souls with the administrative and professional politics that threaten to drain them, we can easily forget another, more immediate barrier: ourselves. What is our own responsibility to the work we do, and to securing the freedom to do it? More to the point: as individual clinicians and as an emerging specialty group, *who are we*?

Many chapters in this book will address our most important obligation of all, that of providing thoughtful, expert palliative care to seriously ill patients and their families. This chapter will focus specifically on the development of palliative social work as a specialty. Even more specifically, this chapter will direct our focus on palliative social work in the acute care hospital setting. This is not to ignore the emergence of palliative and/or hospice social work in home- and other non-hospital-based settings; indeed, these settings present equally important and unique challenges and opportunities for palliative social work practice. While some of the issues addressed here are applicable across settings, attempting to explore the nuances of each practice setting would exceed the capacity of a single chapter and dilute the robust aspects inherent to hospital-based palliative social work.

A Question of Self-Concept

Toward the end of *Guess Who's Coming to Dinner?* Sidney Poitier tells his father, "I love you. But you think of yourself as a colored man. I think of myself… as a man." The implicit subtext of John's statement is the distinction between his father's choice to self-identify first and foremost according to the color of his skin, accepting an implicit message of inferiority based on the social rules and limitations of race in the 1960s, and John's own attempt at circumventing these limitations, refusing to play the subordinate. As we meet the daily systemic challenges of doing the work that we love to do, we as palliative social workers would also do well to think about how we self-identify. In the broader context of medical social work, palliative social workers may feel like "resident guests" in the hospital setting (Dane & Simon, 1991), or as though we are constantly "advocating for a seat at the table" within our field (Meier & Beresford, 2008). Far from arbitrary, such identifiers are strongly rooted in the reality of our lives. As clinicians within physician- and nurse-dominated institutions—institutions whose chief purpose is to address patients' physical health needs—the services that social workers provide may indeed seem to fall outside of the traditional function of the hospital. Historically, this has often resulted in a dynamic whereby social work seems poised at the bottom of the interdisciplinary food chain—a view that we ourselves may inadvertently sanction. Regardless of whether we truly occupy the lower rungs of the hospital hierarchy, our acceptance of this "truth" naturally leads us to question where we fit in and to seek a voice and a level of respect equal to that of our medical and nursing team members. Without lessening the importance of this endeavor, it is vital that we maintain a reciprocal respect for the unique responsibilities of our physician and nurse colleagues, who hold patients' lives in their hands in a way that we typically do not.

The facts are the facts. Often enough, we may feel like "guests" in our home institution, without a reserved seat at the table where discussions are held and decisions are made about our patients, their families, and the programs and policies that affect them. Less clear is how we respond to these facts. Do we play the victim, bemoaning the tribulations of life as the clinical underdogs in a hierarchical, medically focused world? Or do we splash cold water on our faces, fix our hair, and step back into the fray with a secure sense of *who we are* and *what we do*? Clearly, the choice is not as simple as this, for our lives as palliative social workers are a synthesis of many factors, both internal and external to our sense of identity. It also bears stating that there is no neat parallel between the struggles of our profession and those of black Americans or any other minority group fighting for their basic civil rights. There is no denying, however, that the professional world we inhabit is inherently political. We may not be Sidney Poitier knocking at the front door, but neither are we Spencer Tracy deciding who gets to cross the threshold.

It is a commonly held truth that social workers are not nearly as vigilant in advocating for our own needs as we are for those of the clients or patients we serve. Perhaps, then, it is time for palliative social workers to design a clinical intervention for *ourselves*. Perhaps it is time to adopt a strengths-based perspective about *us*, identify our *own* key resources, and strive for our *own* self-actualization. It is not too heavy handed to say that we as a group are at risk of being disenfranchised; indeed, many of us may already feel this way, whether on occasion or as a general rule. Without playing the victim, is there a way for us to acknowledge this inequity while also taking concrete steps toward dismantling it? Are we, as a group of specialist providers with unique skills, not entitled—even obligated—to claim primary responsibility and ownership over that for which we have been trained? At the same time, do we not have an equal obligation as responsible and conscientious clinicians to take a critical look at ourselves, our skill levels, the work we do, and the intersection of that work with our equally dedicated and skilled interdisciplinary colleagues? The time may be ripe for us to achieve class-consciousness and declare a palliative social work manifesto; such a manifesto must not be based solely on reclaiming our birthright, however, but also on our responsibilities to our social work and interdisciplinary colleagues, both within palliative care and without.

Our task, then, is two-fold. Palliative social workers—individually and collectively—must create opportunities for our integral contribution to patient and family care, a contribution that must itself be backed up by genuine clinical skill and expertise. We must do so, however, in a collaborative way that emphasizes respect for both our patients as well as our colleagues and avoids the adversarial tenor that serves none but our own insecurity.

An Emerging Identity

It takes courage to grow up and become who you really are.

—e.e. cummings

We can examine the emergence of palliative social work along two separate but related dimensions. The first is a cross-sectional dimension, representing the dynamics occurring between us and the systems that surround us—including our social work colleagues, our palliative care team members, and the hospital system at large—at any point in time. Simultaneously, we travel along a longitudinal dimension that plots the evolution of our individual and collective palliative social work identity over time. To gain the most accurate sense of who we are, what we do, and where we are headed, it is important to examine ourselves along both of these dimensions. Two conceptual frameworks that can assist in this endeavor are Bronfenbrenner's (1979) ecological systems theory and Atkinson, Morten, and Sue's (1998) minority identity development (MID) model. The first provides us with a systemic snapshot of palliative social work as it stands at the present time, amidst the dynamics occurring at four increasingly broad systems levels. While such a cross-sectional picture is informative, a longitudinal view is equally important as we study the stepwise identity development of palliative social workers. Owing to the innate politicization of our work, it is also important that the framework we adopt be sensitive to identity politics. MID theory provides us with such a lens, and it can be loosely adapted to illustrate how the emergence of palliative social work practice is impacted by the development of our professional identity.

An Ecological Systems Perspective

Bronfenbrenner's ecological systems theory identifies interactions occurring at four systemic levels. The microsystem consists of the smallest unit of activity or interpersonal relationships. Interactions between this microsystem and other microsystems occur at the mesosystem level. The microsystem interacts with and is indirectly influenced by surrounding organizational systems at the exosystem level, followed by interactions with the broader cultural, economic, or historical context at the macrosystem level. Adapting this systemic framework to our practice, we can study our internal dynamics and identity as a group, including the personal and collective parameters we establish as social workers in palliative care (microsystem); our interaction with other hospital social workers, as well as with our interdisciplinary palliative care team members (mesosystem); our role within the hospital system at large (exosystem); and the ways in which our work is influenced by current health care policy, cultural mores, and other overarching structures and policies (macrosystem).

Microsystem

Applying systems theory to our professional work, it may seem more intuitive to consider as our microsystem the palliative care team to which we belong, as this is likely to be the most basic "unit" of our day-to-day working lives. As this chapter focuses specifically on palliative social work, however, it is more helpful to conceptualize the palliative social worker him/herself as the basic unit of analysis. Taking some creative license with Bronfenbrenner's theory, it is even more helpful to consider as our microsystem palliative social

workers *as a specialty*, embodied in the palliative social worker *as an individual*. This is not to disregard our personal concepts of what it means to do palliative social work, or our own autonomous identities as clinicians. As the intent of this chapter is to explore our emerging identity as a collective, however, we must assume some level of coherent group identity in each of us as individual providers.

As a group, palliative social workers have formed an increasingly cohesive identity over the past decade. The early leaders in our field came from hospice, oncology, critical care and other more established fields of practice, and brought with them the unique skill sets exemplified by our social work peers who continue to practice in those areas. These clinicians have performed the necessary work of all pioneers, forging ahead through what must at times have felt like the wilderness, to create the relative bounty from which the rest of us continue to benefit. What they have wrought has resulted in a number of social work fellowships and certificate programs in palliative and end-of-life care, a transdisciplinary education program in palliative care, a peer-reviewed journal dedicated to our practice, an international online list-serv community, a hospice and palliative care specialist credential for social workers and, most recently, a national organization for social workers in hospice and palliative care that functions alongside sister organizations for physicians and nurses (see Chapters 76 & 77 for more information on all). These entities provide us with a means of reinforcing our cohesion as a group, as well as forums for internal dialogue and debate around present and future practice. A review of the professional literature reveals the significant work being done to clarify and strengthen the role of palliative social work (Altilio, Gardia, & Otis-Green, 2007; Altilio, Otis-Green, & Dahlin, 2008; Gwyther et al., 2005; Kramer, Christ, Bern-Klug, & Francoeur, 2005; National Association of Social Workers, 2004; Otis-Green et al., 2009; Raymer & Gardia, 2007). Despite the strong foundations that have been laid, however, it bears recognizing that we all very much remain pioneers. Ours is still a nascent field, ripe with opportunities for increased depth and breadth of evolution. Our emergence as a specialty field will only be enhanced as a growing number of new and seasoned clinicians choose to specialize in palliative social work and as we continue to produce data-driven evidence of our contributions to the broader field of palliative care.

Mesosystem

While maintaining the creative license we have taken with Bronfenbrenner's theory by adopting an individual-as-representative-of-the-whole view of the palliative social work microsystem, at the same time we recognize that individual palliative social workers also belong to other microsystems, including the larger group of hospital social workers and the palliative care team itself. Analyzing the interactions between the microsystems of palliative social work, hospital-wide social work and the palliative care team highlights the challenging dynamics of our work as well as opportunities for future growth.

As the number of palliative care teams increases, so, presumably, will the number of palliative social workers. The growth of our field presents unique challenges with respect to our inpatient social work colleagues who occupy the role of primary team- or unit-based social worker for many of the patients we see. While every relationship should entail mutual efforts at appreciation and compromise, it is ultimately our responsibility to communicate with the team or unit social worker regarding our involvement with a given patient or family. The relationships we develop will vary depending on the unique culture of each institution; even within our home institution, we are likely to have different relationships with different social work colleagues. In some hospitals palliative social work involvement is expected and welcomed, while in others it must be carefully negotiated from one patient to the next. Ultimately, we can assume that our collective goal is to establish some form of respectful, collaborative practice with our social work colleagues, whether working together on a particular case or determining that only one of us needs to be involved.

A greater challenge lies in social work as a profession achieving greater comfort with the notion of palliative and end-of-life care specialization. While inpatient specialties such as psychiatric, substance abuse, or HIV social work seem to have gained an appreciable level of acceptance, there remains an assumption in many hospitals that all social workers possess the necessary skills to provide expert intervention with seriously ill or dying patients and their loved ones. By supporting this assumption, we can easily rob our patients as well as ourselves of the opportunity to engage in the most appropriate and comprehensive level of psychosocial intervention.

At the same time, palliative social workers must allow for—indeed, *welcome*—the possibility that we are not always needed, or that this need exists along a sliding scale. Particularly in hospitals that do not have a dedicated palliative social worker, many team- or unit-based social workers have developed their own palliative care skills. This is especially true in specialized environments such as intensive care units or oncology floors. At the same time, because we may not be tethered to a particular unit or floor, it is important that palliative social workers highlight for our colleagues our ability to provide continuity if patients are expected to move from one team to another, for example, from the intensive care unit to a general medical floor. Even when primary team social workers do not possess strong palliative care expertise, we have an opportunity to enhance the overall delivery of patient care by educating and mentoring our social work colleagues around grief work, familiarity with palliative care concepts, multidimensional pain and symptom management, and facilitation of discussions around goals of care and complex medical and end-of-life decision making. We can achieve similar ends by assuming an active role in making our practices available to graduate-level social work interns,

many of whom receive little classroom education in the clinical and practical aspects of psychosocial care in life-threatening illness and at the end of life. A primary task, then, at the mesosystem level is to identify and advocate for opportunities to provide expert psychosocial palliative care intervention ourselves, while at the same time gauging how much of our involvement is needed and promoting the palliative care skills of our social work colleagues.

There are a number of ways in which we negotiate the dynamics that invariably arise at the intersection of palliative care social work and palliative care teamwork. In considering some of these, it is helpful to first acknowledge and temporarily set aside the fundamental unjustness of the medical system hierarchy. While the traditional hierarchical system may be fading on some level or in some locales, the fact remains that hospitals are first and foremost medical institutions and will be predominantly physician- and nurse-led. Concomitantly, there is bound to be some de facto, hierarchical trickle-down effect within the teams and services that populate the hospital, including palliative care teams. Even at their most egalitarian, then, palliative care teams nevertheless operate within a broader institutional culture, a culture whose values and priorities related to traditional hospital hierarchies may contrast with those of the team. If we are willing to operate within this framework—while at the same time challenging it when appropriate—palliative social workers have the opportunity to be vital team members.

The most significant challenge typically lies in helping our interdisciplinary team members to understand the specific training and skill set we possess that positions us as "resident expert" on the psychosocial aspects of palliative care. This is often complicated by the fact that many of our colleagues are drawn to palliative care based on the very opportunity to engage in more psychosocially oriented work, a complication that may be enhanced by the assumption that performing this work effectively is more dependent on personal motivation than training. Non-social work team members may perceive significant role overlap with their social work colleagues when it comes to the "psychosocial work to be done" and may also lack a clear understanding about the true scope of clinical social work practice (Lister, 1980). We may have the opportunity, then, to educate our interdisciplinary colleagues not only around the work that our roles do entail but also the work that our roles do not necessarily entail. For example, a physician colleague may mistakenly assume that we are experts at psychiatric illness or child welfare, and at the same time overlook the important role we should be playing in discussions around goals of care.

At the same time, as we inevitably encounter non–social work team members who demonstrate extraordinary skill in addressing our patients' psychosocial needs, we recognize that unique and valued relationships are sometimes formed regardless of skill set. This raises a peculiar concern, for it may very well limit our argument that we are the *most* skilled team member to address a particular psychosocial issue. Perhaps the best response in this situation is to celebrate having a colleague who can contribute to the overall psychosocial well-being of our patients, while at the same time highlighting the benefit of role division not only in terms of skill set but also efficiency. In other words, a physician colleague may well have the necessary skills to address a particular psychosocial need, but doing so may limit the time she or he has to address the medical needs of other patients requiring close physician input. Nevertheless, patients and families are drawn to different providers for countless and complex reasons, both related and unrelated to specific skills or expertise. When this occurs, the best choice is often to support the "chosen" team member, honoring the uniqueness of relationships while providing clinical insight when needed, suggesting joint visits if helpful, and working together to ensure that the team is adequately meeting patient and family needs.

Other team challenges and opportunities exist alongside role delineation. On a basic level, our mere presence on palliative care teams—preferably in a full-time capacity with devoted funding—provides us with a more secure place from which to engage our palliative care colleagues. Arming ourselves with a working vocabulary of the relevant medical and nursing concepts allows us to "speak the language," thereby gaining credibility, enhancing our own clinical work, and mitigating communication barriers with our colleagues. The opposite also holds true: By speaking up about the relevant psychosocial issues in a given case rather than assuming that our team members have also identified them, we not only help our colleagues to understand our own language but we also further position ourselves as resident experts. We cannot expect our colleagues to view our work as important if we do not feel that our work is important enough to share. Related to this role as educator, as well as to the question of who-does-what, palliative social workers can further model for our teammates by overtly balancing our own ego needs with the needs of our patients and families. Returning to our earlier example, by acknowledging that a palliative care colleague or a unit-based social worker is best suited to handle a psychosocial concern that would typically fall under our domain, we demonstrate a level of patient-centered care that the rest of the team might emulate. Based on the personal nature of our work as well as time efficiency, palliative social workers may gravitate toward solitary work rather than visiting patients and families as a team. While this is often appropriate, it may also result in missed opportunities to teach our colleagues as well as to learn from their own bedside interactions; finding a balance between team and solo work, then, is another way of negotiating social worker–team dynamics. Finally, we would do well to remember the exhortation, "Act like you belong!"—for indeed, we *do* belong at the table, and presenting ourselves as confident and skilled team members will only reinforce this for our palliative care colleagues.

Exosystem

As illustrated by the impact of the hospital hierarchy on our work, our microsystem is further influenced by the hospital culture at large. In thinking about the exosystem-level dynamics

that occur between palliative social workers and the larger hospital institution, we can consider the institution not only as an entity in and of itself but also as a conglomerate of all the individuals and groups that comprise it. As social workers gain a more predictable presence on palliative care teams, we have the opportunity to take on more prominent roles within the institution as educators, taskforce members, and specialist clinicians. Owing to our training in effective interpersonal communication and, perhaps, the "nonthreatening" position we may hold in contrast to our physician colleagues, a growing number of palliative social workers find themselves engaged in palliative care outreach, case finding, or "public relations" within various hospital units as we attempt to expand our programs and enrich care; this type of work not only broadens our visibility with the institution but also solidifies our "indispensability" to our teams.

While hospitals are bound to specific legislative as well as institutional policies and regulations regarding the role of the medical social worker, palliative social workers nevertheless have the opportunity to shape our work within those confines, or even to challenge those confines. The fact that our interventions remain bundled within the hospital's general provision of social work precludes us from billing independently for our services, but it does not prevent us from demonstrating the indirect financial impact of our work. By documenting our work clearly and efficiently, we can call the hospital's attention to the unique aspects of our clinical interventions and the significant influence we have on patient and family satisfaction as well as length of stay. We can also advocate to hospital leadership for data-driven research initiatives to further identify our impact on staff education and morale as well as patient and family care. While the issue of billing for our services may feel like an insurmountable obstacle, perhaps we can also call upon hospital and social work leadership to create a credentialing infrastructure and standardized curriculum that will help us to challenge these regulations as our nurse practitioner colleagues have successfully done.

Our medical and nursing colleagues in palliative care have made great strides in research and publishing; how often do we think about our own professional development in this vein, as well as our responsibility to contribute our own insights and experiences to the professional literature? While hospital culture is not conducive to providing social workers with the same protected administrative time that physicians typically receive, palliative social workers might advocate for this as a means of achieving better equity between disciplines and enhancing both our own professional development as well as the hospital's public profile. As with our interdisciplinary teams, one way for palliative social workers to be taken more seriously by our home institutions is to treat ourselves more seriously. Regardless of whether our home institutions provide protected time does not preclude our professional responsibility to grow and enhance our skills; this is inherent in the role of a professional and reinforced in the Social Work Code of Ethics:

Social workers should strive to become and remain proficient in professional practice and the performance of professional functions. Social workers should critically examine and keep current with emerging knowledge relevant to social work. Social workers should routinely review the professional literature and participate in continuing education relevant to social work practice and social work ethics. (NASW, 2008)

Macrosystem

Perhaps most daunting to consider are the interactions that occur at the broadest, macrosystem level between palliative social workers and the cultural, historical, and political forces around us. Few of us have escaped the cocktail party dialogue that begins with someone asking, "So, what do you do?" and ends with us explaining why our jobs are not completely depressing, or listening to an annotated history of our inquisitor's deceased relatives. In other words, we have a lot of work to do in educating the public about our profession. While we continue to address the issue one dreaded cocktail party conversation at a time, we can also engage in more wide-scale initiatives such as the National Hospice and Palliative Care Organization (NHPCO) document "What Social Workers Do: A Guide to Social Work in Hospice and Palliative Care" (Raymer & Gardia, 2007) or the National Association of Social Workers (NASW) "Helps Starts Here" image campaign (http://www.helpstartshere.org/).

Public perception of our work also stems from the historical role played by social workers in the United States in terms of public welfare. If people "know" anything about social work, it usually has something to do with removing children from their parents or administering to the poor. As the field of palliative care gains more prominence and greater familiarity within the lay lexicon, the public will have more direct experience with and appreciation of palliative social work. This, in turn, can only further enhance our work and the ability of the structures around us to support that work at the exo- and mesosystem levels. At the same time, increasing public familiarity with palliative social work may give rise to unexpected challenges for the profession. In a British study of patient and family perceptions of palliative social work, Beresford, Croft, and Adshead (2008) discovered that the very qualities most valued by service users—the ability to establish more equal partnerships characterized by trust, reciprocity, flexibility, accessibility, nonjudgment, respect, and general "ordinariness" or "humanity"—may also contribute to the profession's difficulty in establishing "external recognition" and respect by non–social work colleagues. This discrepancy should give us pause as a specialty, as we seek to reconcile the needs of our patients and their families with our own need for professional regard. In addition to navigating these questions around public perception, palliative social workers can also remain engaged at the macro level by advocating for legislative changes to current inpatient billing policies, as well as legislation related to graduate school loan

forgiveness that will make it more financially viable to continue our work.

A Minority Identity Development Perspective

Be what you are. This is the first step toward becoming better than you are.

—*Julius Charles Hare*

Social workers are a minority in palliative care. The origination of palliative care within the medical system, the innate immediacy of medical and nursing needs among patients with advanced illness, the historical hierarchy of disciplines within medical institutions, and a number of other factors all contribute to this fact. The position we occupy makes it plausible to apply a corresponding framework that highlights the process of minority identity development within a dominant culture. While we are by no means an *oppressed people* in traditional terms and should avoid overidentifying as such, the fact remains that we are a relative but distinct minority group within palliative care, subject to similar internal and external dynamics that other minority groups face as we negotiate the inherent politics of our work.

Atkinson et al.'s (1998) MID model "defines five stages of development that oppressed people may experience as they struggle to understand themselves in terms of their own minority culture and the oppressive relationship between the two cultures (p. 34)." The authors are quick to highlight that their model represents a fluid, permeable, continuous process rather than a literal stepwise transition from one stage to the next. As we will see, this flexible conceptualization makes the model more pertinent to the work we do and our own identity development over time, and it also allows us to focus on those stages most pertinent to our own experience and practice setting. While the model focuses on minority individuals, it also addresses the individual's relationship to the larger minority group, thereby allowing us to think about not only our individual identities as palliative social workers but also our collective identity.

The five stages of the MID model include *conformity*, in which a minority individual overidentifies with and desires to assimilate into the dominant culture to the extent that the minority culture of origin is depreciated or denied; *dissonance*, in which there is a gradual breakdown of denial and increased conflict between appreciation and rejection of both the minority and dominant culture; *resistance* and *immersion*, characterized by a complete endorsement of minority-held views and self- and group-pride along with rejection, dislike, and mistrust of the dominant culture; *introspection*, marked by growing autonomy and self-identity, discomfort with absolute endorsement or rejection of minority and dominant cultures, conflict between personal autonomy and group allegiance, and ability to identify both positive and negative aspects of the dominant culture and its individual members; and, finally, *synergy*, in which there is further refinement of objective examination of both minority and dominant cultural views, increased self-confidence and self-worth, strong group pride, and openness to the constructive elements of the dominant culture.

In adapting the MID model to palliative social work identity development, it is important to recall that the model is meant as a tool for thoughtful exploration rather than a hard-and-fast framework. Some stages may seem more relevant to a particular clinician's experience, or even to palliative social work in general, depending on our unique hospital environments, team constellations, and years of practice. Similarly, the model is most helpful when considered as a series of fluid, bidirectional transitions from one stage to the next. Indeed, it may be most helpful to think of these stages both in the long term, as we evolve as individuals and as a group over time, as well as the short term, wherein we may experience several of these stages over the course of one week. Finally, while the following sections highlight interactions between social worker and physician as a means of best illustrating the MID model's focus on the dominant–minority dynamic, the concepts may be applied in a similar fashion to relationships between palliative social workers and any other clinician or administrator where the task is to evolve an egalitarian environment.

Conformity Stage

The first stage outlined by Atkinson and his colleagues may seem the most remote to social workers who have identified palliative care as their specialty practice, but the dynamics present at this stage will nevertheless resonate with many of us. As it pertains to hospital social work in general, the conformity stage is one marked by complete buy-in to what has become the traditional "medical model" of social work practice. While masters-level social workers have always been trained to provide expert clinical intervention with patients and families, the social work identity in many hospital settings has developed into one based on case management and discharge planning. With increasing attention paid to limiting patient lengths of stay as a means of preserving a hospital's fiscal stability, social workers often assume primary responsibility for efficient and timely patient disposition. At the same time, many hospitals have cut social work lines to the bare minimum, resulting in unrealistically high caseloads. These dynamics place clear limits on social workers' abilities to perform the intensive psychosocial assessment and intervention for which we are trained and which ought to inform the clinical aspect of discharge planning. While the myriad of contributing factors are too complex for this chapter, one could argue that we as social workers have *allowed* ourselves to be relegated to this narrow and incomplete, albeit important, role. Physicians and others who train and work in settings that promote this view of social work, and who may not have experience with any other practice model,

will incorporate it into their own practice. Unless social workers advocate for a change in identity, rather than acquiescing to what the dominant medical culture assumes that identity to be, the model is perpetuated. This is not to disregard the importance of hospital discharge planning or the tremendous skill and passion with which many social workers perform this work; still, this restricted identity ignores many aspects of the graduate-level training that social workers bring with them, and it wastes countless opportunities for expert clinical intervention in the inpatient setting.

Dissonance Stage

Assuming they have the luxury of time and energy to do so, hospital social workers may take a step back from their work and begin to question the fate to which they have been resigned, or to which they have heretofore resigned themselves. As social workers transition into the dissonance stage, they may recall their graduate training and mourn their inability to fully utilize it. Feeling less like an autonomous, skilled clinician and more like another cog in the giant hospital wheel, they may start to reject the dominant culture's view of social work and develop or regain a sense of professional pride. If this pride grows strong enough, they may find success in advocating for policy change within their hospital, identifying ways of fostering greater respect for and utilization of clinical social work skills and training. Perhaps it is this type of catalyst that prompts some social workers to seek specialization in areas such as palliative care, oncology, or other disease-based practices where there may be greater opportunity to utilize their full range of clinical skills. Even those of us who are already on a palliative care team may find ourselves having a "dissonant" day or week, questioning our team's understanding of the social work role and feeling underutilized. Those of us who practice in relative isolation from other palliative social workers may join a supervision group or an online list-serv and, hearing about the experiences of our peers, realize that much of our practice has been based on what we are expected to do rather than what our own clinical and professional instincts tell us. The Dissonance stage can feel particularly uncomfortable as we begin to question our assumptions as well as those of the medical colleagues or program directors with whom we may have developed smooth-functioning relationships, dipping our toes into what can feel like dangerous waters as we experiment with and formulate a better sense of personal and group identity.

Resistance and Immersion Stage

As we get used to dipping our toes, those dangerous waters can start to feel quite nice, tempting us to plunge in headfirst. The resistance and immersion stage, however, may be the most dangerous of all, particularly because it can feel so good. To be fair, there are positive aspects that we might assign to this stage of identity development. As palliative social workers have developed a stronger sense of cultural identity, we have built a community that fosters group cohesion. We have our own scholarly journal, our own online resources, and our own professional association, in addition to the growing number of programs and fellowships mentioned earlier. All of these resources are critical to our growth and success as a specialty. Separation from the dominant ideology and development of our own identity, however, may lead to feelings of resentment or anger toward our medical colleagues, whether temporary or more longstanding. As we become aware of our relative lack of power in the medical hierarchy, or the ways in which our non–social work colleagues have entered our clinical territory, we may grow frustrated, angry, and territorial. Finding solace in the sympathetic ears of our palliative social work brethren—"Can you *believe* she did that!"—feels validating and comforting, but it can easily take on a life of its own. It may feel easier to huddle together with the people that understand us than to consider both sides of the equation. Resistance and immersion may be marked by complete disregard for the work that our physician and other colleagues do and for the unique skills and experiences that they bring. Our fear that they will undermine us or try to do our jobs may blind us to the ways in which we may be undermining or underappreciating them. This stage can be particularly present in teams that have not had a dedicated social worker before or who hire a social worker with a more defined prior sense of his or her palliative care practice. Feeling stifled, underutilized, or underappreciated by the team—feelings rightfully validated by the larger palliative social work community—may drive that social worker further away from his or her palliative care colleagues and into the depths of anger, isolation, and despair.

Introspection Stage

As palliative social workers continue to gain confidence in our team roles, as well as in our clinical skills specific to palliative care, we may begin to loosen the tight grip we have been holding on our self-centric identities. With security comes flexibility and as our egos feel less threatened they become less of a barrier. When we enter into the stage of introspection, we continue to gain strength from our palliative social work peers, but we also grow more autonomous as individual practitioners with unique styles and practice settings. Introspection is often sparked by experience. Despite all of our well-honed, well-intentioned efforts at separating ourselves from what may feel like the oppressor, we will inevitably be caught off guard by the realization that our interdisciplinary colleagues are in fact a talented group of people. Whether it is the team as a whole or one team member in particular, something will typically occur that proves to us that this clinician is our ally. Perhaps this colleague overtly expresses understanding or appreciation of our work, or perhaps a shared case leads to an "Aha!" moment in which both providers gain a deeper appreciation for the other. As long as our defenses are raised, it is virtually impossible to appreciate what our colleagues bring to the care of our patients because so much of our energy is focused on protecting our turf. As these defenses fall, we develop a gradual recognition of what is possible when we collaborate and combine our efforts; a similar process can occur in our collaboration with primary team social workers. At the same time that we start to appreciate our team members, we also look at the larger entity of palliative social work and become more discerning in terms of what does and does not resonate with our own practice, agreeing or disagreeing with the practice standards set forth by our group of origin. The introspection stage is, appropriately, marked by a great deal of introspection and reflection: What kind of palliative social worker do I want to be? What skills do I need to develop? What courage do I need to find? This exercise requires a fair amount of confidence as well as self-insight, a willingness to challenge our assumptions and beliefs at the same time as we begin to take risks as individual providers and assert ourselves more strongly on our teams.

Synergistic Stage

Regardless of whether we have been conscious of it, hopefully most of us have at least experienced a glimpse of the synergistic stage of identity development. Predictably this is the hardest stage to achieve and can feel equally difficult to maintain on a daily basis. The most realistic goal might not be to live in a perpetual state of synergetic identity, but to recognize how much better it feels and how much more effective we are as palliative care providers when we allow our identities to evolve in this direction. At the synergistic stage we develop an even greater sense of confidence and security, both in our own practice and position within the palliative care team, as well as those of our physician and other colleagues. Trust is a key concept at this stage. As we gain a sense of trust in our own clinical skills and insights, we learn to stand confidently behind our work. Concomitantly, it is a sign of true evolution when—continuing the work begun at the introspection stage—we also trust our team members enough to confidently acknowledge our own failures or weaknesses without fear of shame or reprisal. To be sure, this is a two-way process and requires that our teammates be equally self-evaluative, as well as supportive of the identity we have fostered. Still, as clinicians trained in interpersonal dynamics as well as the value of behavior modeling, the responsibility for taking the first step may be ours. When we do so, we are likely to find not only that we are able to perform our jobs more effectively but also that we have as much to learn from our non–social work colleagues as they do from us, particularly in the areas of research, publishing, education, and other academic pursuits. This is well exemplified in Payne's (2006) discussion of the "mutual engagement in a shared enterprise" that ideally occurs between palliative social workers and our interdisciplinary colleagues. As we allow for the gradual, "bottom-up" emergence of professional identities rather than a "top-down" adherence to "standard professional packages," "... the professional identity, social work, is still defined globally or generally, while what they are and do is defined locally or specifically by the joint history of learning" (p. 148).

Conclusion

There came a time when the risk to remain tight in the bud was more painful than the risk it took to blossom.
—*Anaïs Nin*

The emergence of palliative social work is not a simple process. Rather, it is one to be negotiated gradually and carefully between a number of vested parties, not the least of which is the palliative social work clinician him/herself. As we have seen, our evolution as a profession is one that takes place both crosswise as well as longitudinally, requiring that we remain vigilant of our personal and collective progress on both fronts. Studying our development from both perspectives, several guiding principles emerge. First, as we seek to define our specialty and garner the opportunity to employ it, palliative social workers must maintain a balance between confidence—courage, even—and diplomacy. As experts in the finer nuances of interpersonal dynamics, we can appreciate the value of collaboration over antagonism, while at the same time understanding the importance of standing one's ground. Of equal importance is our need to bolster our confidence with clinical expertise, so that there is true substance behind our contributions that warrants our colleagues' respect as we take our seat at the table. To do otherwise would not only quickly erode the confidence of our colleagues but would abuse their trust as well. Finally, as we have witnessed with so many of our clients, sometimes the most effective way to foster a desired behavior is to model that behavior ourselves. Social workers have the luxury of training that helps us to appreciate the very process of *process*. Recognizing that behavior change is a process, we know that modeling respect for and trust in our non–social work colleagues will likely result in reciprocal respect and trust. In asking the question, "Who are we?" then, the answers—or some of them, anyways—seem to lie within, as the old adage goes. By drawing upon our professional training and turning our clinical interventions upon ourselves, we can move closer to answering this question not only for our colleagues but, more important, for ourselves.

LEARNING EXERCISE

This chapter references the film *Guess Who's Coming to Dinner?* in exploring the emergence of palliative social work within the context of interdisciplinary teams and hospital hierarchies. After you finish reading the chapter, use this film as a vehicle for further thought and discussion. In what ways might you apply ecological systems and minority identity development theories to the film's storyline? What parallels or differences exist between the experiences of the film's characters and those of palliative social workers? What lessons might you apply from the film's ending to the future of palliative social work? Consider other films, novels, or plays that offer additional insights into the emergence of palliative social work.

REFERENCES

Altilio, T., Gardia, G., & Otis-Green, S. (2007). Social work practice in palliative and end-of-life care: a report from the summit. *Journal of Social Work in End-of-Life and Palliative Care, 3*(4), 68–86.

Altilio, T., Otis-Green, S., & Dahlin, C. (2008). Applying the national quality forum preferred practices for palliative and hospice care: A social work perspective. *Journal of Social Work in End-of-Life & Palliative Care, 4*(1), 3–16.

Atkinson, D.R., Morten, G., & Sue, D.W. (1998). *Counseling American minorities: A cross-cultural perspective* (5th ed.). New York, NY: McGraw-Hill.

Beresford, P., Croft, S., & Adshead, L. (2008). "We don't see her as a social worker": A service user case study of the importance of the social worker's relationship and humanity. *British Journal of Social Work, 38*, 1388–1407.

Bronfenbrenner, U. (1979). *The ecology of human development: Experiments by nature and design.* Cambridge, MA: Harvard University Press.

Dane, B. O., & Simon, B. L. (1991). Resident guests: Social workers in host settings. *Social Work, 36*, 208–213.

Foster, Z. (1979). Standards for hospice care: Assumptions and principles. *Health and Social Work, 4*(1), 117–128.

Gwyther, L. P., Altilio, T., Blacker, S., Christ, G., Csikai, E. L., Hooyman, N., ... Howe, J. (2005). Social work competencies in palliative and end-of-life care. *Journal of Social Work in End-of-Life and Palliative Care, 1*(1), 87–120.

Hui, D., Elsayem, A., De La Cruz, M., Berger, A., Zhukovsky, D., Palla, S., Evans, A., ... Bruera, E. (2010). Availability and integration of palliative care at US cancer centers. *Journal of the American Medical Association, 303*(11), 1054–1061.

Kramer, B. J., Christ, G. H., Bern-Klug, M., & Francoeur, R. B. (2005). A national agenda for social work research in palliative and end-of-life care. *Journal of Palliative Medicine, 8*(2), 418–431.

Lister, L. (1980). Role expectations of social workers and other health professionals. *Health and Social Work, 5*(2), 41–49.

Meier, D. E., & Beresford, L. (2008). Notes from the field: Social workers advocate for a seat at palliative care table. *Journal of Palliative Medicine, 11*(1), 10–14.

National Association of Social Workers (NASW). (2004). *Standards for palliative and end-of-life care.* Retrieved from http://www.socialworkers.org/practice/bereavement/standards/standards0504New.pdf

National Association of Social Workers (NASW). (2008). *Code of ethics of the National Association of Social Workers.* Retrieved from http://www.socialworkers.org/pubs/code/code.asp

Otis-Green, S., Ferrell, B., Spolum, M., Uman, G., Mullan, P., Baird, R. P., & Grant, M. (2009). An overview of the ACE Project–Advocating for Clinical Excellence: Transdisciplinary palliative care education. *Journal of Cancer Education, 24*(2), 120–126.

Payne, M. (2006). Identity politics in multiprofessional teams: Palliative care social work. *Journal of Social Work, 6*(2), 137–150.

Raymer, M., & Gardia, G. (2007) *What social workers do: A guide to social work in hospice and palliative care.* Alexandria, VA: National Hospice and Palliative Care Organization.

II
Social Work Practice: Setting Specific

I Am Not Dying Now

I am not dying now
I am living my life
the best that I can
Doing the things
that I always did
until the day I can do
them no more
Please don't take that
from me by tiptoeing
around and acting
like I am already gone.
Don't think I don't
care about what's
happening with you
what's happening out there
just because of
what's happening to me
There is more to my life
than thinking about dying
There are other things I want
to talk about today
Some day that may change
and I will ask you to sit with me
and be with me in my dying
but not today
I am not dying now
I am living my life
the best that I know how

Deb Kosmer MSW, CSW, CT
Bereavement Coordinator
Affinity Visiting Nurses Hospice

5 *Colleen M. Mulkerin*

Palliative Care Consultation

You are the only one who talked to me about dying. You helped my husband finally understand. Now when you see me when I'm in the hospital—I know you know, and you know I know.

—*an anonymous patient*

Key Concepts

- *Palliative care consultation is increasingly available to patients and their families in the hospital setting.*
- *Consultation etiquette guides the processes of referral and consultation.*
- *The roles and opportunities for social work range from direct clinical care to leadership responsibilities on the team.*

Introduction

Social workers are uniquely, in fact ideally, qualified to provide palliative care in the setting of hospital consult teams. The mission and vision of palliative care are aligned with the core values of the social work profession. This chapter explores how social work addresses patient and family needs in hospital-based palliative consult teams and in palliative care units. There are many opportunities within this specialty for social workers to provide clinical care, education, and leadership and to impact the systems to optimize integrated palliative care throughout health care settings.

Definition and Scope

Palliative care has grown in hospitals as inpatient consult teams, specialty units, and outpatient programs. "The number of U.S. hospitals offering palliative care services is growing rapidly. The American Hospital Association Survey of Hospitals 2007 reports that, of the 4,103 hospitals appropriate for palliative care, over 30% have a palliative care program" (Making the case..., 2010). Palliative care has been able to grow and develop as the definition has changed. *Palliative* historically had been used interchangeably with *hospice* and in some settings continues to be equated with end-of-life care. Now the mission of palliative specialists is to partner with clinicians to deliver integrated palliative care throughout the hospital to patients, their families, and valued friends to enhance the quality of living for those with serious, complex, or terminal illness. The palliative consult team brings expertise in symptom management, setting goals of care, communication, and support to patients, family, and caregivers who are asked to make difficult decisions in difficult circumstances. The World Health Organization (WHO) has defined palliative care as:

> *an approach that improves the quality of life of patients and their families facing the problems associated with life-threatening illness, through the prevention and*

relief of suffering by means of early identification and impeccable assessment and treatment of pain and other problems, physical, psychosocial and spiritual. Palliative care:

- *Provides relief from pain and other distressing symptoms*
- *Affirms life and regards dying as a normal process*
- *Intends neither to hasten nor postpone death*
- *Integrates the psychological and spiritual aspects of patient care*
- *Offers a support system to help patients live as actively as possible until death*
- *Offers a support system to help the family cope during the patient's illness and in their own bereavement*
- *Uses a team approach to address the needs of patients and their families, including bereavement counseling, if indicated*
- *Will enhance quality of life and may also positively influence the course of illness*
- *Is applicable early in the course of illness, in conjunction with other therapies that are intended to prolong life, such as dialysis, chemotherapy or radiation therapy, and includes those investigations needed to better understand and manage distressing clinical complications (World Health Organization, 2009)*

Palliative Care Consult Teams

Palliative care is a response to one challenging aspect of our health care delivery model that is marked by the many specialists often involved in the care of the patient. To make the situation of multiple specialists even more challenging, in some settings, the physicians cover hospitalized patients a week at a time with the result that patients and family may meet a new team of physicians each week. Consultants may be called in to contribute their expertise from specialties such as critical care, pulmonary, cardiology, and nephrology. Many families find that working with multiple physicians adds to their stress, because they struggle to understand who is in charge. They do not often experience the continuity that contributes to a rapport that may be helpful for decision making in complex health care issues. Palliative clinicians who work with patients and families over time are charged with helping the patient feel known and cared for in the health care system by carrying the patient's unique history, experiences, culture, preferences, and values across time, across units in the hospital, and across admissions.

A palliative consult service has the potential to be a flexible and inclusive model for providing care. It allows the care to be patient centered and family focused and *meets the patient where he or she is* literally and figuratively. The changing

perception of *palliative care* from end of life to care along the continuum provides access for the patients and families that are most in need. Patients with complex and/or life-limiting illness can be engaged without anyone—physician, patient, or family—being asked to discuss a potential dying process, changing a code status to do not resuscitate (DNR), or giving up access to life-prolonging therapy.

As a consult service, we need to be invited to be a part of the care of the patient. "The rules of consultation are known as consultation etiquette: A set of unwritten but important standards that define how the consultant is expected to behave in response to requests from attending physicians" (Meier & Beresford, 2007, p. 7). By following the rules of consultation etiquette, we find that we establish trust with our physician colleagues who consult us to share the care of their patients. A consult may be to answer a very specific question or to address a specific care need, and by respecting those boundaries you become established and trusted by your community. The reasons for consultation are many and can include developing well articulated, realistic goals of care; assisting in the process of advance directives; providing psychosocial care; enhancing communication through patient-family meetings; managing difficult symptoms; educating about the natural history of a disease; addressing spiritual needs; contributing to the process of decision making and planning for the next level of care. Often this work is best done in collaboration with the referring clinicians both to minimize a sense of abandonment for patients and families and because important medical and prognostic information is essential to the outcome.

Goals of Care

At times, in the current health care environment, physicians, patients, and their families can become caught up in the details of decision making before understanding the potential outcomes or the overarching goal. The dichotomous thinking about "winning" and "losing" a battle against disease or injury often dominates the hospital culture. This conceptual framework is reinforced in the high-tech environment of hospitals. (For further information, please see Chapter 75).

A ... feature of critical care culture is the supremacy of the "technologic imperative." This imperative serves as a default principle, which specifies that if a technology is available, it must be used. Thus the question, "Can we?" always takes precedence over "Should we?" to the point that evaluation of the rationale for intervention is often ignored. This norm continues to exist despite the recognition that an intervention is justified only if there is reason to believe that the intervention is likely to accomplish a defined goal and the burdens of the intervention are outweighed by the benefits, as evaluated by the patient or the patient's proxy. (Daly, 2001, p. 258)

Negotiating the "win-lose" environment and the technologic imperative requires consistent questioning as to which treatments and interventions produce effects but do not necessarily benefit the patient. By working with patients and their families to identify the parts of their life that define them, the elements that give their life meaning and joy, and what *states may be worse than death*, the consult team can help them negotiate these options, and formulate and reformulate the overall goals of care that guide decision making about medical interventions.

In the hospital environment, too often the discussion of goals, values, and meaning in life comes at the end of the hospital course. As palliative specialists join with primary teams the hope is to demonstrate how these conversations can come earlier. Within this collaboration, there may be ongoing attention to diagnosis and prognostication and discussion of advance care planning in a setting of inquiry and respect for the patients' values, culture, and preferences and evolving medical realities. It is vital to negotiate and renegotiate the goals of care with the patient–family system, and it is important that the primary teams engage in regular discussions as the clinical course develops. The *all*-or-*nothing* approach is too often the language used to discuss goals of care. Families may start with the *all*: "He wants everything done" and providers may feel that there is *nothing*: "There is nothing more we can do." With regular discussions and clinical social work interventions, we can bridge the gap of that type of dichotomous communication. At the same time that we seek to understand—"What do you think he meant when he said 'do everything?'"—we use supportive counseling and anticipatory guidance to help colleagues and families to move from "Nothing more to do" to the care that will be provided when disease-modifying treatment or technologic support is no longer beneficial or appropriate. Social workers are positioned to help patients and families clarify what gives life meaning and purpose, which combines with medical information to inform goals of care. This process is exemplified by the narratives in Box 5.1.

Box 5.1
Patient/Family Narratives: Goals of Care

Restorative/cure: *A 54-year-old white male was admitted to the hospital having been found unconscious at home for an unknown period of time. The head computed tomography (CT) scan showed a grade IV subarachnoid hemorrhage and aneurysm. He is now in the intensive care unit, intubated and sedated. He has been married for 15 years and works as a physical education teacher in the middle school. He has two children ages 9 and 11. He has no significant past medical history, and a week prior to admission ran in the local marathon. His spouse, as his legal surrogate, and his physicians have restorative goals of care.*

Return to baseline: *A 76-year-old female was admitted after a fall at an assisted living facility, and she sustained a subdural hematoma. She has a past medical history of a cerebral vascular accident, atrial fibrillation, and is on coumadin. She needed minimal assistance with her activities of daily living prior to admission. She is following simple commands and has begun to work with the rehabilitation team. Her daughter and the neurologists have established goals of care to support the patient in returning to her prehospital baseline.*

Improve survival: *A 66-year-old male presented to the hospital with difficulty breathing. He was found to have pneumonia and his breathing worsened to respiratory failure; he was intubated and sedated. He has been living with advanced lung cancer and has completed a course of chemotherapy and radiation therapy. He has been married for 39 years, and his daughter's wedding is next month. The patient and family understand his limited prognosis consequent to his cancer diagnosis but would like aggressive treatment of his pneumonia and to continue life-prolonging therapy because his goal is to walk his daughter down the aisle at her wedding.*

Improve function: *A 70-year-old African American male was admitted with a left middle cerebral artery infarct. His past medical history includes hypertension and a recent diagnosis of colon cancer. He lives with his daughter and son-in-law. His daughter promised that she'd never "put him in a nursing home," but the physicians are hopeful that with active rehabilitation he can make gains in his performance status. The therapist feels admission to a subacute rehabilitation facility would significantly improve his functional status, which would create the opportunity for active treatment of his colon cancer as well as his return home.*

Relieve symptoms: *A 54-year-old male was diagnosed 1 month ago with a glioblastoma, a rapidly progressing malignant brain tumor. He has a significant symptom burden, which includes headaches and psychomotor agitation. His family would like him to receive active treatment, but his symptoms and current performance status precludes his receiving additional disease-modifying treatments. The consulting neuro-oncologist would like help with symptom management and psychosocial care for the patient, wife, and children as they integrate the diagnosis and its impact on their lives.*

Allow natural death (Meyer, n.d.): *A 93-year-old Jamaican male was living independently at home when his knee gave out and he sustained a fall. He was transferred from an outlying hospital and diagnosed with a subdural hematoma. He had a rocky course in and out of the intensive care unit with sepsis, respiratory failure, and new mental status changes. During his hospitalization his neurological status declined and he was found to have a new stroke. His daughter said: "I know he wouldn't want this" and presented the team with his written advance directive. His goals of care were changed to aggressive symptom management and to allow a natural death. He was moved from the intensive care unit to the palliative care unit.*

Goals of care are established by discussing what is possible and ensuring that our patients and families have access to the medical information and can understand the relative benefits and burdens of interventions. Medical providers present their best information to assist patients and families to understand the scope and nature of the potential benefit. Burden is often a subjective valuation defined by the patient.

The principle of proportionality has been endorsed by ethicists. Their view is now quite widely accepted under the name of "the principle of proportionality." It expresses the view that the correct test of the ethical obligation to recommend or to provide an intervention is the estimate of its promised benefits over its attendant burdens … . It gives patients and surrogates the right to determine what they will accept as benefits and burdens. (van Bogaert, & Ogunbanio, 2005, p. 67)

The palliative consult service assists in maximizing opportunities to hear values and preferences expressed by the patient or by their surrogate if the patient is unable to participate. Goals of care are optimally negotiated and renegotiated between the caregivers, the patient, and often the patient's family, throughout the course of the illness as the lived experience continues.

Social Work Opportunities

Social workers encounter a lack of preparedness to deal with complex end-of-life care issues in their practice (Christ & Sormanti,1999; Csikai & Raymer, 2005). For the social work profession this impacts the ability to intervene on the micro and macro level.

Dealing with issues of death and dying may create a strong sense of helplessness among practitioners if they are not educationally prepared. In today's death-defying society, few may be aware or have confronted their own feelings and values regarding their own mortality. This may make it more difficult to assist individuals and their families to cope with the dying process. (Csikai & Raymer, 2005, p. 68)

Recent healthcare efforts aimed at supporting individuals facing advanced illness are marked by debate over assisted suicide, untimely referrals to hospice care, inconsistent adherence to advance directives, and substantive amounts of unrelieved pain in end-of- life…Social workers require a clear understanding of the current political and social climate if they are to navigate the ethical dilemmas as they are presented in end-of-life care. (Roff, 2001, p. 51)

Frequently, social workers are called on to intervene in complex illness and end-of-life issues, in many instances, with the same lack of preparedness and training as the rest of the team.

NASW has set forth a policy to help guide social workers dealing with end-of-life care decisions and the preservation of client self-determination in these

situations … However, the present study (N = 63) revealed that a majority (57%) of social workers were not aware of the existence of, or were only somewhat familiar with the policy. (Csikai & Bass, 2000, p. 1)

Social workers are motivated, as are their interdisciplinary colleagues, to understand how to minimize suffering along the continuum of illness and at the end of life. As a part of the health care team, the social worker often assesses suffering from multiple dimensions: for the patient, the family, and the health care providers. The patient's suffering can emanate from many sources and may be due to poor pain and symptom management, spiritual distress, conflict, and ambivalence related to complex decision making. The family may be suffering due to poor communication about diagnosis, prognosis, and the treatment plan. The family may not have any past experience with a sick or injured member and enters the unfamiliar health care environment in a time of crises. When patients have not discussed their end-of-life wishes, the family may feel unprepared or not empowered to act on behalf of the patient as a surrogate decision maker. As the social worker develops a biopsychosocial-spiritual understanding of suffering, it becomes possible to intervene effectively and engage the patient, family, and health care team to respond to and diminish reversible causes of suffering. The practitioner's suffering may be due to personalizing the enormous societal expectation that new health care technologies can fix everything. The tremendous push to "save" lives can create a feeling of failure and sadness among the health care providers when death occurs.

Social work opportunities come from our core competencies in comprehensive assessment, treatment planning, and interventions. "Multidimensional assessment enables the social worker to plan biopsychosocial-spiritual interventions with the patient/client/family/caregiver and support network in collaboration with care providers and/or interdisciplinary team" (Gwyther et al., 2005, p. 98).

Social Work in the Context of the Team

The National Association of Social Workers (NASW) Standards for Palliative and End of Life Care state that

Social workers should be part of an interdisciplinary effort for the comprehensive delivery of palliative and end of life services. Social workers shall strive to collaborate with team members and advocate for clients' needs with objectivity and respect to reinforce relationships with providers who have cared for the patient along the continuum of illness. (NASW 2005, p. 5)

In addition, there are leadership opportunities for social work both on a micro level and on the macro level. Leadership can be demonstrated in the context of the team, with a particular patient, and in the ways we impact institutional policy and program planning.

Within the palliative consult service there exists an enormous opportunity to develop and effectively utilize the role of social work on a myriad of levels from the most practical to crises intervention and psychotherapeutic assessment and interventions that help to guide a meaningful plan of care (Gwyther et al., 2005, p. 101). These may include the following:

1. Incorporating biopsychosocial-spiritual history into the plan of care
2. Exploring the cultural beliefs and values that require clinician adaptation and accommodation
3. Facilitating interdisciplinary family meetings
4. Clarifying advance directives and identifying an appropriate surrogate decision maker
5. Assessing literacy and language needs and providing appropriate education to inform discussions of treatment options, including code/resuscitation status
6. Assisting the team to monitor patient-family satisfaction with our care.

Indirect services can include promotion of healthy collaboration among the health care teams, identifying barriers to the plan of care, and diffusing stress among the health care providers. As social workers on a consultation team, the range of services and interventions we utilize impact direct care as well as the system in which patients and their families receive care. (Please see Chapter 6 for further information)

When death is the anticipated outcome:

Social workers have a key role as "context interpreters" in helping people at the end of their lives and their families: understand the natural course of the illness, the process of dying, the advantages and drawbacks of medical interventions, to comprehend the medical and social contexts within which they face end-of-life decisions. (Bern-Klug, Gessert, & Forbes, 2001, p. 38)

This context-driven perspective extends beyond end of life to context across the continuum of illness as the landscape against which patients and families integrate and adapt over time.

Palliative Consultation in the Intensive Care Unit

The idea of palliative care in the intensive care unit (ICU) has been seen as a contradiction in terms. The technology and the culture of the environment in critical care have promoted a model of aggressive life-saving treatment goals.

The original orientation of critical care units is perhaps most in evidence in the assumption that survival at all cost is the goal. This is sometimes evident in critical care staff's questioning of the appropriateness of having a patient admitted to the unit after a do-not-resuscitate (DNR) decision has been made. Again, when attempts to resuscitate in the event of a sudden arrest were all

that the ICU had to offer many patients, it was reasonable to equate DNR decisions in the ICU with inappropriate use of scarce critical care resources. Today, however, we know that treatment limitation decisions are much more complex than dichotomous all-or-nothing decisions. Rather, treatment limitation is best understood as existing on a continuum of aggressiveness with the level or extent of limitation stemming from individual patient goals. (Daly, 2001, p. 258)

As patients live for extended periods with serious illnesses and options for palliative treatments have expanded, ICUs will provide care to patients who have been offered interventions that were not available in the past. There are many examples of patients living with a chronic or terminal disease having an admission for a palliative surgery to relieve a symptom not well managed by other interventions. Palliative care clinicians may join with intensive care to assist patients and families when the outcome is uncertain and goals of care are in flux. Social workers are essential to this process because they intervene to mitigate the impact on family systems and create an environment of inclusion and collaboration as medical information is understood in the context of values, beliefs, hopes, and as decisions evolve. (For more information, see Chapter 6)

For example, if the goal is to facilitate a peaceful and inevitable death, withdrawal of all life-prolonging interventions may be indicated. If on the other hand, the goal is to maximize the chance of returning the patient to home once more without adding to the current burdens of treatment, withholding additional interventions might be indicated whereas withdrawing treatment and monitoring may not. (Daly, 2001, p. 267)

There is a range of experience among consumers of health care services, and the palliative social worker may be in a unique position to assist the health care teams to understand the importance of these experiences as they relate to the critical medical situation in the family. The patient-family's expectations may be shaped by television dramas that resolve medical emergencies in 30 minutes; it may be informed by a history of distrust of the health care system (Bullock, McGraw, Blank, & Bradley, 2005) or by cultural and generational factors that affect relationships with physicians (see narrative in Box 5.2). "Social workers should understand systems of oppression and how these systems affect client access to, and utilization of, palliative and end-of-life care. Many cultures maintain their own values and traditions in the areas of palliative and end-of-life care" (NASW, 2004, p. 25).

Palliative Interventions in High-Risk Surgery

Palliative care consults, in collaboration with the surgical team, may ensure a meaningful exchange related to the hopes and goals of patients in the face of a high-risk surgery. A focused conversation has the potential to support the goals of care while validating the uncertainty that infuses medical care of seriously ill patients. Psychosocial assessment and intervention can begin during preoperative consults and promote conversations with patients and families about "what ifs" and provide an environment to hope for the best and plan for the worst. Preparing patients and families may protect families from facing that awful not-knowing moment when the surgeon asks such questions as: "Did you ever talk about what he wanted in the case of kidney failure?" "Would he want artificial nutrition?" Our health care systems, including medical options and possibilities, create opportunities for patients and families, but as of yet they have not created systems to prepare them fully for the expected and unexpected outcomes. Palliative care consult teams can offer the surgical teams and patients and families the opportunity before important surgeries to consider advance directives that are culturally sensitive and support patient- and/or family-centered decision making.

Box 5.2
Patient/Family Narrative: Nonoperable Ischemic Colon

A 60-year-old Puerto Rican female was admitted to the intensive care unit (ICU) from the operating room when she was found to have a nonoperable ischemic colon. The family was told by the surgeon that there was no hope for survival. Goals of care changed to allow a natural death (AND) and aggressive symptom management. The ICU team prepared to withdraw the patient from all life support and to provide pain management and other comfort measures. The surgeon informed the family that she would not survive the day. When asked about the patient's spiritual needs, the family identified her as Roman Catholic and requested that she receive the Sacrament of the Sick. The out-of-town adult children were gathering and the priest was called to provide spiritual care to this patient and her family. Based on the surgeon's prognosis, the family anticipated a quick death when the life supports were discontinued. Several hours passed and the vigil at the bedside continued. The family was welcomed to be at the bedside, for as long or as brief a time as they needed; entering and exiting at will. The hours turned to days and the patient's family struggled to understand how she could survive despite her terminal diagnosis and the physician's predictions.

The family was with her around the clock for the long week it took for her body to react to the overwhelming source of infection from her ischemic colon. After the first 24 hours had passed the family was offered the option of transfer to the hospital's palliative care unit. The family felt comfortable in the ICU environment and was reluctant to explore other options. There were multiple reasons for their hesitation to move the patient to another unit. They expressed feeling well cared for by the ICU team, whom they had come to know during this very intense period of time. The historical context provided additional insight into their hesitation. The patient had a long illness without proper diagnosis. Previously the patient had been referred for psychiatric assessment because her

physicians could not find a medical source for her pain. She had a long stay at a small community hospital before she was transferred to a tertiary care environment and diagnosed correctly and eventually had the corrective surgery she required. She then had postoperative complications due to vascular disease, which caused poor profusion to her colon. The family distrusted physicians and felt it was easier to understand her current status if she was hooked up to monitors so they could see her vital signs. If she were moved to the palliative care unit they knew that they would not have access to monitors. On day four, the patient's daughters requested a tour of the palliative care unit.

The palliative consult team was integral to these processes and decisions joining the family as they considered transitions and sought to understand the fact that their patient had not died as predicted. Upon their arrival they were able to visualize their mother in that unit and to consider how a different environment could meet their own comfort needs and perhaps the current goal and needs of their patient. In an effort to create a therapeutic transition and respond to the fears and past experience of the family, the ICU nurse utilized a transport monitor to move the patient. The palliative care unit agreed to frequent vital signs to help the family mark her dying trajectory. The family was invited to request vital signs if they needed that information to add to their understanding of the dying process.

Teaching via interdisciplinary sessions and written material was provided to help further the families understanding of the dying process. The profound need to maintain and maximize trust of the health care team was recognized and integrated into the interventions, which allowed them to safely transition to a more comfortable environment. The change that occurred after the transition to the palliative care unit was visible in the family's relaxing body language, facial expressions, and tone. Although the plan of care did not change, the family was able to focus more on the patient and less on their anger about the delay in her diagnosis from the other institution. The patient died 9 days after admission to the ICU from the operating room. It was 20 minutes after her last sibling arrived from Puerto Rico.

Patient-Centered and Family-Focused Care

The National Consensus Project Clinical Practice Guidelines for Quality Palliative Care and the World Health Organization identify the needs of the patient and family as central to palliative care. Utilizing a systems approach, family care needs to be built into the care of the patient. "In order to begin to work effectively with the family system, the clinician must identify what constitutes the family's constellation. In the patient's definition, this may include both the family of origin and family of choice" (Blacker & Rainess Jordan, 2004, p. 551). In the setting of technological advances, family members, regardless of geographic distance can be invited and integrated into care through the use of Internet communication, video conferencing, and speaker phones.

Family members need information and access to the patient. The task is to provide accurate clinical information as it becomes available. Information needs are evaluated and assessed within the biopsychosocial model. Each individual patient and family system has its own unique history, culture, and values. How, when, and who we communicate with should be respectful of the patient's culture and needs. The families need to be engaged in a process that provides a supportive and safe environment as they integrate the diagnosis and prognosis, and participate in a planning process. Recent research with patients and families in focus groups:

> ... *identified four aspects of ICU palliative care that were most important to them: communication by clinicians about the patient's condition, treatment, and prognosis; patient-focused medical decision-making; clinical care of the patient to maintain comfort, dignity, personhood, and privacy; and care of the family.*
> (Nelson et al., 2010, p. 809)

These identified aspects of care are easily transferable from the ICUs to other venues in the hospital. Patients, their families, and their support systems are also helped by an orientation to the hospital environment and the health care team. This orientation to the hospital routine and environment may reduce some of the external stressors impacting the patient/families' experience. Amenities like parking, telephones, the family lounge, restrooms, the chapel, lodging, and the cafeteria can address a range of family needs and assist in the orientation to the unfamiliar.

Deepening the relationship between family members and clinicians is vital to develop therapeutic rapport and the trust that may enhance the relationship with palliative clinicians. This can be facilitated through assigning consistent caregivers and following through with telephone contacts as needed. Scheduling regular and proactive family meetings, with and without the primary provider, as determined by the patient's condition and the family's needs, ensures families that there will be regularly scheduled times to make inquiries and to express their thoughts and feelings about the patient's care and plan of care. Recent research supports that patients/families "placed high value on the ICU family meeting, which they believed improved communication and should be held proactively and frequently" (Nelson et al., 2010, p. 812). This active approach has the potential to diminish the confusion often created when numbers of specialists, such as cardiologists or nephrologists, talk to patients and families regarding their isolated interventions and outcomes which do not necessarily generalize from a specific organ to the overall condition of the patient.

Another focus is to identify the learning needs of the patient's family system. By providing individualized information, surrogates and family will learn about the relevant tests, procedures, and equipment involved in the care of their family member in a language and style that enhances the possibility for integration. Social workers can sometimes function as a link between family members and other health care providers. Helping the family join and adapt to the patient's

experience and the hospital setting and clarifying their preferences or style of visiting can individualize the needs of patient and family. Communicating those preferences and needs to the health care team can be invaluable to both meeting their needs and minimizing misunderstandings.

During transitions, patients may be approaching transfer or discharge to a different level of care, which may mean that progress has been made or may be an indication that no more progress is expected. Sometimes values and preferences dictate that another level or site of care is warranted. These are very different medical and emotional realities. If the health care teams, especially the palliative care clinicians who may follow patients through most transitions, are able to effectively acknowledge the meanings of these transitions, the family may maintain trust in the providers as they integrate the changing circumstances and prepare to move their patient to the next level of care. In a continuing effort to create seamless transitions, the palliative care team collaborates with the next group of caregivers and when possible organizes a tour of the new patient-care area both to meet the new providers and to enhance the family's understanding of what the next level of care may offer.

Social Work Skills and Team Process

Crisis intervention is a vital skill for palliative social workers. As with all interventions, effective active-listening is the foundation for the critical thinking that drives clinical decisions. Social work training in family systems and group dynamics is a unique and essential contribution to the work of palliative care teams. Palliative social workers assess family structure, strengths, and stresses and work to reflect the family's concerns and feelings in an affirming, empathetic, respectful, warm, and sensitive manner (Gwyther et al., 2005, p. 96). It is also a priority for social workers to be able to model appropriate behavior and empower family members to address their needs within the parameters of cultural and generational differences. At times social workers are able to support the family by asking clarifying questions of the physicians in family meetings and asking interprofessional colleagues to elucidate a complex medical concept. These interactions may model for families how to meet their communication needs within the hospital setting. Social workers, who are engaged in the uncertainty that pervades the work of palliative care, need to be flexible as they explore and clarify changing needs and normalize stress reactions. Flexibility allows the patient and family time and space to express their unique responses without rigid rules and institutional biases.

Another responsibility of the social worker is to assist in establishing and encouraging professional boundaries. Team members are responsible for monitoring appropriate self-disclosure and avoiding family splitting. It is possible to "side" with the family member that agrees with your assessment and to write off and label another family view as unreasonable. It is important to support differing family views and allow the process to unfold with support and communication.

Social workers' ability to effectively collaborate within the team and within their institution impacts care of patients and families and the relationships of the consult service within the hospital. It is vital for the social worker to help the team resolve differing clinical assessments to avoid splitting and fractured, confused care for patients and families. The process of discussing differing assessments and points of view within the team can greatly benefit the patient's plan of care and outcome and enrich the team process. It is assumed that each member will contribute to establishing an agreed-upon plan of care and carry out their role, an assumption that emanates from trust and mutual responsibility of team members. Where disagreements persist, a collaborative team will seek out and consult peers for problem solving and support. Social work training in group dynamics and systems theory is vital in observing and intervening with team dynamics and inviting team members to problem solve when conflicts arise (NASW, 2004, p. 17). The impact of team process on the patient-family system is profound. (For more information please see Chapter 38)

Conclusion

The do-everything-at-all-costs mentality of health care does not serve patients and families; the costs are too high financially and emotionally on patients, families, and our health care teams. Patients, families, and interprofessional caregivers are often left feeling that an outcome that includes an acceptance of end of life signifies giving up or failure of the patient, family, and/or professional provider. Social workers assist patients and their families to express their expectations of the hospital and medical care and discuss reasoned approaches for providing care. Palliative care along the continuum of life-threatening illness can join with patients and families and primary teams as goals evolve and treatments are explored. The continuity implicit in this collaboration can serve to mitigate the "either/or" perspective and positions palliative care as a contribution that enriches the care of patients and their families as they adapt to an evolving medical reality. Palliative social work can intervene on multiple levels, including the provision of psychosocial care and support, pain and symptom management, and honest communication. In collaboration with interdisciplinary colleagues, it is possible to impact many of the challenges embedded in our current model of health care delivery. There is a unique match between social work values, ethics, and core principles and the domains of palliative care that enhances our potential to lead, collaborate, and practice with our interdisciplinary colleagues the art and science of palliative care.

LEARNING EXERCISES

You are consulted to intervene with a patient and family who are considering high-risk cardiac surgery. The patient has a busy schedule with preoperative workup and multiple consultants in and out of the room.

- How do you plan your consultation? Who should be in the room?
- What facts do you need to understand prior to meeting the patient?
- What collaboration with interdisciplinary colleagues needs to occur?
- Describe therapeutic interventions you use to meet the needs of the patient-family system.
- Identify any outcomes that may be a part of this consultation.
- Identify the potential impact of a preoperative assessment on a patient-family experience.
- Identify the potential impact of a preoperative assessment on an ICU team's experience.
- Identify the potential impact of a preoperative assessment on a surgeon's experience.

ADDITIONAL SUGGESTED READINGS

Berzoff, J., & Silverman, P. (Eds.) (2004). *Living with dying: A handbook for end-of-life care practitioners.* New York: Columbia University Press.

Cairns, M., Thompson, M., Wainwright, W., & Victoria Hospice Society. (2003). *Transitions in dying and bereavement: A psychosocial guide for hospice and palliative care.* Baltimore, MD: Health Professions Press.

ADDITIONAL RESOURCES AND WEB SITES

ADEC: Association for Death Education and Counseling: http://www.adec.org/
An interdisciplinary organization in the field of dying, death and bereavement. ADEC offers educational opportunities through its annual conference, courses and workshops, certification program, and newsletter, *The Forum.*
Aging with Dignity: http://www.agingwithdignity.org/
A national nonprofit organization with a mission to affirm and safeguard the human dignity of individuals as they age and to promote better care for those near the end of life.
American Academy of Hospice and Palliative Medicine: http://www.aahpm.org/
The professional organization for physicians specializing in hospice and palliative medicine.
American Pain Society: http://www.ampainsoc.org/
A multidisciplinary community that brings together a diverse group of scientists, clinicians, and other professionals to

increase the knowledge of pain and transform public policy and clinical practice to reduce pain-related suffering.

CAPC: Center to Advance Palliative Care: http://www.capc.org/

Provides health care professionals with the tools, training, and technical assistance necessary to start and sustain successful palliative care programs in hospitals and other health care settings

EPERC: End of Life/Palliative Education Center: http://www.eperc.mcw.edu/

Continues to be a resource to End of Life/Palliative health care professionals through support from the Medical College of Wisconsin.

Growth House.Org: http://www.growthhouse.org/

Provides education about life-threatening illness and end-of-life care.

The Kenneth B. Schwartz Center: http://www.theschwartzcenter.org/

Strives to strengthen the patient–caregiver relationship.

The National Association of Social Workers (NASW): http://www.socialworkers.org/

The largest membership organization of professional social workers in the world, with 150,000 members. NASW works to enhance members' professional growth and development, create professional standards, and to advance social policies.

SWHPN: Social Work Hospice and Palliative Care Network: http://www.swhpn.org/

An emerging network of social work organizations and leaders who seek to further the field of end-of-life and hospice/palliative care.

REFERENCES

Bern-Klug, M., Gessert, C., & Forbes, S. (2001). The need to revise assumptions about the end of life: Implications for social work practice. *Health and Social Work, 26*, 38–48.

Blacker, S. & Rainess Jordan, A. (2004). Working with families facing life-threatening illness in the medical setting. In J. Berzoff & P. R. Silverman (Eds.), *Living with dying* (pp. 548–570). New York, NY: Columbia University Press.

Bullock, K., McGraw, S. A., Blank, K., & Bradley, E. H. (2005). What matters to older African Americans facing end-of-life decisions? A focus group study. *Journal of Social Work in End-of-Life and Palliative Care, 1*(3), 3–19.

Christ, G., & Sormanti, M. (1999). Advancing social work practice in end of life care. *Social Work in Health Care, 30*(2), 81–99.

Csikai, E., & Bass, K. (2000). Health care social workers' views of ethical issues practice and policy in end-of-life-care. *Social Work in Health Care, 32*(2), 1–22.

Csikai, E. L., & Raymer, M. (2005). Social workers' educational needs in end-of-life-care. *Social Work in Health Care, 41*(1), 53–72.

Daly, B. J. (2001). Organizational change and improving the quality of palliative care in the ICU. In J. R. Curtis & G. D. Rubenfeld (Eds.), *Managing death in the ICU: The transition from cure to comfort* (pp. 257–272). New York, NY: Oxford University Press.

Gwyther, L., Altilio, T., Blacker, S., Christ, G., Csikai, E. L., Hooyman, N., … Howe, J. (2005). Social work competencies in palliative and end-of-life care. *Journal of Social Work in End-Of- Life and Palliative Care, 1*(1), 87–120.

Making the case for hospital-based palliative care. (2010). *Center to Advance Palliative Care.* Retrieved from http://www.capc.org/building-a-hospital-based-palliative-care-program/case

Meier, D. E., & Beresford, L. (2007). Consultation etiquette challenges palliative care to be on its best behavior. *Journal of Palliative Medicine, 10*(1), 7–11. doi:10.1089/jpm.2006.9997

Meyer, C. (n. d.). Allow natural death—An alternative to DNR? Retrieved from the Hospice Patients Alliance website: http://www.hospicepatients.org/and.html

National Association of Social Workers. (2004). NASW standards for palliative and end of life care. [Brochure] Washington, DC: NASW Press.

Nelson, J. E., Puntillo, K. A., Pronovost, P. J., Walker, A. S., McAdam, J. L., Ilaoa, D., & Penrod, J. (2010). In their own words: Patients and families define high-quality palliative care in the intensive care unit. *Critical Care Medicine, 38*(3), 808–818.

Roff, S. (2001). Analyzing end-of-life care legislation: A social work perspective. *Social Work in Health Care, 33*(1), 51–68.

van Bogaert, G. A., & Ogunbanio, G. A. (2005). The principle of proportionality: Foregoing/ withdrawing life support. *South African Family Practice, 47*(8), 66–67.

World Health Organization (WHO). (2009). *WHO definition of palliative care.* Retrieved from http://www.who.int/cancer/palliative/definition/en/

6 *Andrew J. McCormick*

Palliative Social Work in the Intensive Care Unit

I know he would not want heroic treatment and would not want to be a vegetable. But he would want to fight. … I don't want him to suffer forever.
                    —Wife of 77-year-old man with burns on 44% of his body

Key Concepts

◆ *Palliative care in the intensive care unit (ICU) is part of both the rescue culture of critical care and the hospice culture of palliative medicine.*

◆ *Palliative care begins with admission to the ICU and continues as a patient's medical condition improves sufficiently to leave the ICU, stabilizes and no longer responds to ICU intervention, or declines toward death.*

◆ *The social worker's ecological approach is a unique contribution to palliative care.*

◆ *Social worker activities humanize the decision-making process for family members.*

Introduction

Like so many other family members in the ICU, the woman quoted in the epigraph is on the horns of a dilemma facing the difficult choice between continuing aggressive medical treatment intended to cure or at least stabilize her husband, and stopping some or all of the treatments with the goal of minimizing his suffering and with the likely possibility that death will occur. It is a contradictory situation that is now being recognized by medical professionals as a growing phenomenon in intensive care and one that because of our aging population may be acted out with increasing frequency. We are in an age when, "The challenge to clinicians and educators in this area is to span two cultures: the rescue culture of critical care and the hospice culture of palliative medicine" (Curtis & Rubenfeld, 2001, p. 4).

The Intensive Care Unit as a Setting for Palliative Care

The modern ICU is a foreign culture for patients and their family members. In emergency situations at the beginning of an ICU stay, physicians often make decisions quickly without consultation with either the patient or the family. Their focus is completely on life-saving interventions. In an emergency, consent is assumed. It is thought that every patient who arrives for emergency care wants to live and the staff does everything they can to make that possible. ICU medical techniques and interventions have accelerated in their complexity and power. Physicians called intensivists now manage the care of patients in the ICU because the care has become so specialized.

Critical care, as ICU care is also called, provides full life support, which now incorporates a number of highly specialized artificial means of preserving a patient's life, such as mechanical respiration with a ventilator, artificially delivered nutrition and hydration through a feeding tube, intravenous fluids, nutrition and medication, renal dialysis, cardiac and respiratory monitoring, and placement of a tracheostomy. Various combinations of these life-sustaining treatments are used with many ICU patients and create decision dilemmas for families and clinicians.

In the past 10 years there has been increasing specialization within intensive care units. In large teaching hospitals, the ICU is no longer housed on one unit. These large medical centers can have as many as six or seven ICUs each with a separate specialty. There are neurological ICUs with a focus on brain and spine injuries and disorders such as tumors, and hemorrhagic and occlusive strokes. Surgical ICUs specialize in injuries and illnesses of internal organs such as the liver, spleen, stomach, and pancreas. Medical ICUs treat pulmonary ailments such as chronic obstructive pulmonary disease (COPD) and lung neoplasms. Cardiac ICUs treat heart attacks and heart disease. Trauma ICUs treat multiple organ injuries combined with multiple fractures. Burn ICUs treat burns from flames, chemicals, and electricity. Pediatric ICUs treat all of these injuries and other illnesses of children 14 and under.

Death is quite common in the ICU, and it often results after a decision is made to limit specific treatments provided to a patient. Approximately 9%–10% of patients admitted to the ICU will die there or shortly after they leave the unit. A major national survey was conducted in 131 ICUs at 110 hospitals in 38 states over a 6-month study period in 1994 and 1995 (Luce & Prendergast, 2001). A total of 74,502 patients were admitted to these ICUs during the study period. Of these, 6303 (9%) of the patients died in the ICU. Of those who died, 794 (14%) had life support withheld and 2139 (36%) had life support withdrawn. Of the 5910 patients who died in the ICU and were not brain dead, 4366 (74%) received less than full support. It is clear that hospital staff and family members are making difficult decisions to determine the benefits and appropriateness of interventions for patients in the ICU who may be close to death.

Despite the frequency of death in the ICU, most patients, including many followed by a palliative care team, discharge from the ICU. In one medical ICU among 191 patients followed by palliative care, 111 (58%) died either in the ICU or elsewhere in the hospital, but 34 (18%) went home, 39 (20%) transferred to a skilled nursing facility, and 3 (2%) went to a hospital rehabilitation unit (Table 6.1) (Norton et al., 2007). The authors report they did not follow all of these patients through their hospital course but agreed the results support a need to examine the effect of identifying patients earlier in their hospital stay and continuing full follow-up until death or discharge for all patients. Palliative care social workers in the ICU need to be prepared to assist patients and family members for a variety of patient outcomes.

Because the threat of death in the ICU is so high and the environment often one of crisis, family members are typically quite anxious and worried about their loved one. Many express their fears and may also become quite sad, angry, or withdrawn. The parents of children in the ICU ride an especially emotional roller coaster. They want to be listened to and be considered experts regarding their child, yet they

Table 6.1.
Discharge disposition of patients followed by PC team (n = 191)

Discharge Disposition	N (%)
Death in hospital	111 (58)
Home	34 (18)
Skilled nursing facility	39 (20)
Rehabilitation/other hospital	3 (2)
Missing	4 (2)

Source: Adapted from Norton, S. A., Hogan, L. A., Holloway, R. G., Temkin-Greener, H., Buckley, M. J., & Quill, T. E. (2007). Proactive palliative care in the medical intensive care unit: Effects on length of stay for selected high-risk patients. Critical Care Medicine, 35(6), 1532. Copyright 2007 by Lippincott, Williams and Wilkins.

have to relinquish the care of their child to medical experts. In situations where ICU patients are parents or grandparents, families often need encouragement to move beyond the medical crisis and consider engaging children and adolescents to help them understand and possibly participate in the family process that ensues during an admission to the ICU. Families require accurate, clear, and timely information presented in a language that invites a beginning integration not only of the issues at hand but also of the potential outcomes. Other stressors such as financial matters, past conflicts between family members, problems at work, difficulty with transportation, and finding lodging close to the hospital complicate the life of families of patients in the ICU. Social workers address all of these problems on a regular basis.

Patient Populations in the Intensive Care Unit

Patient populations in the ICU vary. About 60% of all patients admitted to the ICU are age 65 or older (Nelson & Nierman, 2001). This percentage is expected to increase over the next several decades as will the proportion of those 85 and over whom authors call the "oldest old." Older adults in the ICU will have new options for treatment based on new technologies, and these will not only increase our ability to extend life but may also further complicate decision making.

The number of infants and children in ICUs is small by comparison to the number of older adults. Nevertheless, the admission of a child to an ICU is an important and often difficult experience for the family. About 200 per 100,000 children in the United States will be admitted to an ICU. Most of the admissions are due to premature birth, congenital malformation, acquired neurological problems due to head or spine injuries, and cancer and other diseases. About 5% of pediatric ICU patients will die in the hospital (Field & Behrman, 2003).

Many other patients move to the ICU for a short stay following a planned surgery. Most of these patients do well and are soon transferred to a regular hospital room. On some occasions a complication from a surgery may put a patient's life in danger and he or she will remain in the ICU receiving critical care. Young adults with traumatic injuries or exacerbations of chronic diseases make up most of the rest of the ICU population.

Many patients in the ICU are not able to communicate with staff, the social worker, or their family members. This may occur because they are unconscious, sedated with medication, intubated (an endotracheal tube is inserted into their mouth), or so severely injured that they cannot stay awake. Consequently, an important focus for ICU social workers becomes intervention with various combinations of the patient's intimate network of spouse or partner, family members, and close friends.

Palliative Care in the Intensive Care Unit

Palliative care in the ICU includes treatment for both the patient and the family and is usually provided concurrently with life-sustaining treatment and continues through treatment transitions. Treatment may shift from a focus on rescuing the patient and saving his or her life to stabilizing the patient, albeit sometimes at a very compromised or critical level. For some the emphasis will be on maximizing the patient's comfort and possibly planning for his or her death. Other patients may move to a step down unit or a regular hospital room and eventually discharge from the hospital.

Patients in the ICU can benefit from palliative interventions focused on symptom management almost immediately upon admission because they are exposed to pain resulting from their illness or injuries, and pressure on their body's tissues from a variety of procedures, including placement of the endotracheal tube, and long periods of time in bed. Patients need treatment to control pain and other symptoms of anxiety, nausea and vomiting, dyspnea (a feeling of suffocation), and agitation. Many patients report after discharge from the ICU that they had been anxious while in the ICU and particularly disturbed by the placement of the endotracheal tube or a face mask. Combinations of medications to treat pain and anxiety seem to work the best (Foley, 2001). Patients being treated with paralyzing agents to prevent unwanted movement do better when also treated with analgesic (pain-relieving) and anxiolytic (anti-anxiety) medication. In addition to pharmacologic management, interventions such as the administration of oxygen, position changes, washcloth baths, massage, and music can increase comfort and at times, when culturally and medically appropriate, engage family members in the process of care.

Palliative interventions with the family also include treatment planning, counseling, and spiritual support to address their stress, emotional state, cultural and religious beliefs, and physical needs for privacy, rest, and reflection. Interventions with the family members are especially important in the ICU because of its unique culture and specialized technological environment, which is foreign to most families and friends. Families need support for their physical and emotional needs and may need assistance to learn to manage their energy and time at the hospital. Because most patients in the ICU cannot communicate their wishes or condition, ICU staff members rely heavily on family and friends for information, decision making, and support for the patient. Meeting with the family is a natural point of intervention for social workers, and the remainder of this chapter will be devoted to discussing this aspect of care.

Social workers engage families and friends in a variety of ways, including participation in family conferences with physicians, nurses, and chaplains; meetings with individual and small groups of family members; and telephone and e-mail contacts to distant family members. Social workers can employ a variety of interventions with family members. Intrapsychic counseling techniques can address the emotional responses of family members, reality and cognitive-based approaches can help clarify thinking and decision making related to the patient, and process-oriented approaches can help family members reflect on their loved one's life and the spiritual and cultural context of the family.

Interface of Social Work and Palliative Care in the Intensive Care Unit

Social work in the ICU has become a subspecialty of medical social work just as the ICUs themselves have become more specialized. In large hospitals, social workers are typically assigned to one ICU and can develop a specialty in a particular area of medicine. In smaller hospitals, the social worker may cover several ICUs, or there may be only one ICU with a variety of patients in it. These social workers often become generalists across a variety of medical specialties.

While hospitals have set up palliative care services in different ways, the Center for the Advancement of Palliative Care (CAPC, 2009) and the National Consensus Guidelines for Quality Palliative Care (National Consensus Project, 2009) affirm social work as part of the core palliative care team. Despite this understanding, funding limitations often prevent hospitals from assigning a dedicated social worker to a palliative care team. Where they are part of a team, palliative social workers may assess and intervene with patients and families in collaboration with primary providers and with unit social workers in a shared working relationship. In hospitals without a dedicated palliative social worker, the regularly assigned ICU social worker will interface with the palliative care team members.

Activities of Social Workers in Palliative Social Work

It may seem simplistic to highlight that the palliative social worker approaches patients and families differently than do doctors and nurses. Nevertheless, this difference is real and should not only be appreciated by social workers but also emphasized as we define the unique contribution that social workers provide to the care of patients, friends, and family. The classic ecological perspective of considering the client in his or her environment is especially evocative for a social worker in the ICU. The patient has been moved from his or her home and work environments to the foreign environment of the ICU. The family members and friends are caught between the ICU and home environments and are pulled by both. A social worker practicing an ecological approach can use crisis intervention techniques to assist families who are adapting to a new reality of having a family member or friend critically ill, with an uncertain prognosis and sometimes close to death. She or he can employ problem-solving skills, anticipatory guidance, and use cognitive interventions when families need assistance in making treatment decisions which may extend life or result in death. She or he can function as a liaison between patient and family and the medical staff, interpret medical language, and act as an advocate providing education and counseling services. From a task-oriented perspective, the social worker functions as a coordinator of services and as a broker for community services.

The narrative of Mrs. Amalu (See Box 6.1) illustrates several of these skills in a social work intervention that takes the family cultural background into consideration while clarifying the problem areas in the family members' decision making process.

Box 6.1
Patient/Family Narrative: Mrs. Amalu

Mrs. Amalu, a 73-year-old, married, Catholic, Hawaiian woman, was admitted to the Neurological ICU with end-stage liver disease and end-stage renal disease. Six months prior to this admission she had been hospitalized with bleeding in her brain from an aneurysm. After a period in the ICU and with very little recovery of cognitive and physical function, Mrs. Amalu was not able to wean from the ventilator. Rather than discontinue life-sustaining treatment, her husband agreed to have a tracheostomy placed to control her airway, ease the effort to breathe, and allow her to be taken off the ventilator. Following this procedure Mrs. Amalu was moved to a hospital floor and then transferred to a nursing home. Upon her readmission to the hospital, Mr. Amalu complained about the care his wife had received during her first admission and said he believed it may have led to her current condition, an attribution of blame that had not been expressed during the prior hospitalization.

Mrs. Amalu had remained minimally responsive for the entire 6 months and physicians wanted to discuss treatment options with the family. A conference was held to discuss the goals of care and a treatment plan. The participants included the patient's husband

---

and one adult son, the intensivist, the nephrologist, the ICU nurse, and the social worker. The intensivist summarized Mrs. Amalu's care and condition and said that it would be helpful to think together about what Mrs. Amalu would want done for her. He said the ventilator and dialysis treatments were keeping her alive and that if the ventilator was removed or dialysis was stopped, she would die very soon. The nephrologist said she had reached a decision to stop the dialysis because it was no longer helping and may actually be increasing Mrs. Amalu's suffering by causing pain during the procedure. Stopping dialysis would lead to her death within a short period of time as her kidneys failed. Mr. Amalu bargained for one additional dialysis treatment and said that he knew that his wife's death was a matter of when, not if. Despite this awareness he was not ready to make a decision to stop the ventilator.

At this point the social worker intervened to ask whether Mr. Amalu or his son had ever had a conversation with Mrs. Amalu about what she would want in this situation. Both men said they had not, because they did not expect things to worsen so quickly. Realizing that they were thinking about recent conversations, the social worker in an effort to help the family reflect on past values and articulated beliefs, suggested that such a conversation could have happened at any time in the past, and then provided the example of a person who might see a news item related to end-of-life care and then talk about how he or she would want his or her own end-of-life decisions to be made. Mr. Amalu then related a story about his wife's father, who had a living will which indicated that he did not want extraordinary care, and how Mrs. Amalu stayed with him as he died. The social worker commented on how brave she had been and the husband agreed, but he added that he did not seem to know what Mrs. Amalu would want at this time. He said he could not decide to discontinue treatments nor talk about death, adding that he feared a decision to stop the ventilator or dialysis would lead to her death. He asked for time to obtain input from many family members, which is traditional in the Hawaiian culture.

Mr. Amalu and his son agreed to call other family members to tell them they agreed with the nephrologist that the dialysis would be discontinued after the additional treatment, and to get the opinion of the family members before agreeing to the removal of the ventilator. The physicians said they would give Mrs. Amalu medication to control any pain or shortness of breath that might develop as the ventilator was removed. The team members agreed to give the family time to reach a decision and respect their cultural tradition. Mrs. Amalu remained on the ventilator for an additional 10 days before it was discontinued. During this time the social worker continued to meet with Mr. Amalu and the son to provide ongoing support and to continue discharge planning for a possible return to a skilled nursing facility. At the time it was unclear how long Mrs. Amalu would survive after dialysis was stopped and the ventilator was removed. A discharge to skilled nursing with hospice care might have been needed. She died in the hospital 2 days after the ventilator was removed.

An Ecological Approach to Family Decision Making

Decision making with the Amalu family was informed by several factors: *(a)* the husband's negative feelings about the hospital's care during her previous admission may have been a factor in his reluctance to remove the ventilator during the current admission; *(b)* Mrs. Amalu had not written an advance directive of her own and despite the care she provided for her father at the end of his life, the husband was doubtful about her wishes for herself; *(c)* the cultural belief among Hawaiians that they should not talk about death with a sick person and that doing so would hasten her death prompted Mr. Amalu to seek the counsel of his wider community; and *(d)* despite agreeing to only one additional dialysis treatment, the husband was reluctant to make a decision that would remove ongoing ventilator treatment because it would lead more directly to his wife's death.

The social worker's approach diverted from the medical presentations made by the two physicians. By leading the husband and son to prior conversations and retrospective review of values and beliefs, the social worker was acknowledging the value of informal discussions and family members' knowledge of Mrs. Amalu in determining her best interests and bringing her voice into the discussion. Comments that she may have made in the past could be used to inform the current decision making. This intervention to explore the past helped insulate the family members from the immediate pressure to make a decision and provided some time for them to consider their loved one at a time of less emotional intensity. This opening gave the husband the opportunity to relate the story of how the patient supported her father in his dying which provided all a glimpse into the life and values of the person who had become the ICU patient. As he was helped to move beyond the immediate task of decision making, he expressed family and cultural values that included the need to engage other family members in the decision, which is a common practice in many families and friend networks and is a reminder of the need for health care staff members to elicit cultural values and needs. Mr. Amalu was not able to make a decision to withdraw the ventilator during the conference. Although most ethicists agree there is no difference between withholding or withdrawing treatment, many patients and family members think there is a difference. Mr. Amalu felt more comfortable withholding treatment, in this case additional dialysis treatments, than withdrawing ongoing ventilator treatment. The palliative care team and unit social worker maintained contact with the husband and son in the days that followed the conference, and after several consultations with his family Mr. Amalu agreed to stop the ventilator treatment. In situations such as this one, social workers can also offer to set up a conference call with family members in distant locations to get their input on decision making.

Recent research has identified a number of activities engaged in by social workers working with families of patients who receive palliative care and die in the ICU (McCormick, Engelberg, & Curtis, 2007). In this study 20 social workers with no formal training in palliative care completed 133 questionnaires, which asked them to select from a list of 14 activities the ones they provided to families. These activities reflect a generalist ecological approach to practice,

Table 6.2. Palliative Care Activities of Social Workers in the ICU (n = 133)	
Total Activities per Family	Median (IQR)
Social Worker Activities Provided	6 (2, 10)
Social Worker–Identified Activities	Percent of Families
Talk about the family members' feelings	74
Support the family's decision about the patient's care	61
Talk about what the patient valued in life	54
Reminisce with the family about the patient	52
Talk about spiritual or religious needs	50
Discuss what the patient would have wanted	50
Locate a private space for the family	45
Take action to address spiritual needs	39
Assure the family that the patient would be kept comfortable	38
Tell the family what to expect in the family conference	32
Tell the family it is all right to talk to or touch their loved one	23
Talk about cultural needs	21
Take action to address cultural needs	19
Talk about a disagreement among family members	13

Source: Adapted from McCormick, A. J., Engelberg, R., & Curtis, J. R. (2007). Social workers in palliative care: Assessing activities and barriers in the intensive care unit. Journal of Palliative Medicine, 10, p. 933. Copyright 2007 by Mary Ann Liebert, Inc.

and the frequency with which each activity was provided reflects how this group of social workers allocated their time with families (Table 6.2). In over three-quarters of the families the social worker talked about the family members' feelings, and in nearly one-third the social worker supported the family member's decision about patient care. The activities of talking about the patient's past, his or her values, his or her spiritual or religious needs, and what the patient would have wanted were reported in half of the families. The social workers in this study demonstrated an understanding of the importance of addressing the wishes of the patient, in spite of the patient's inability to speak, as the primary source of information for enhanced work with the family. Social workers who reported providing more of these activities also scored significantly higher on their satisfaction that they had met the family's needs.

These activities were studied again after the social workers were trained in palliative care and an increase was noted in a number of reported activities (McCormick, Curtis, Stowell-Weiss, Toms, & Engelberg, 2010). Most notably social workers more frequently engaged families in talking about spiritual or religious needs, letting the family know it was all right to talk to or touch their loved one, talking with the family about a disagreement among the family members, and assuring the family the patient would be kept comfortable. The palliative care training had a positive effect on the activities chosen by social workers when they intervened with families. These activities that increased in frequency have a humanizing effect on the ICU experience for families and encourage them to stay involved with their family member's care.

In addition to the activities described in the survey and delineated in the narrative of Mrs. Amalu, social workers may also need to be active in locating a patient's legal next of kin or friend network, determining whether advance directives or durable power of attorney documents exist and getting the documents brought to the hospital, assisting in obtaining financial assistance to cover medical expenses, and setting up a family conference in person or by means of a speaker phone.

Palliative Care with Transition to Comfort Care and Death

Decisions to withhold or withdraw life-sustaining treatments are made in consultation with the patient's family members and in particular with the legal next of kin or appointed health care agent, who is most likely the spouse or adult children. Family members who find themselves as the surrogate decision maker have very different comfort levels with this taxing role. The family members of adult patients and the parents of children with chronic illness have often cared for their loved one for many years and are often quite expert in their care. They may be very comfortable caring for a very disabled person and have gone through many previous medical crises. They may also be very comfortable talking with physicians. In contrast the families of trauma patients are often in an unfamiliar environment, in a crisis, and in the unexpected role of having to make decisions in overwhelming circumstances.

Social workers can assist experienced families by making sure they have access to physicians and medical information that is provided in a manner that is respectful of their input and expertise while at the same time differentiating why this current medical crisis may be different from their prior experiences. Families who are overwhelmed require critical and skilled assessment and intervention. They may require more directive interventions helping them to identify preexisting supports and crisis management skills they have used in the past. During family conferences, social workers may have to take the lead in directing and interpreting questions and medical language, identifying cultural and spiritual influences, and assisting families to reorganize around the destabilizing reality of an ICU admission. Flexibility, critical thinking, and a varied skill set are required of social workers in assisting many different families with integrating and transitioning through the intensive care experience.

The narrative of Mr. Taylor (See Box 6.2) illustrates how a social worker can intervene with involved family members who know a patient's wishes and help them be sure they are communicated to physicians and carried out by the medical team.

Supporting a Family in Decision Making

The family members of Mr. Taylor were aware of the wishes of their father, but they were unfamiliar and uncomfortable with their role as surrogate decision makers. Their decision making was informed by the following factors: (a) they needed reassurance that they were doing the right thing, (b) they did not want their father to suffer during the process of stopping any interventions, (c) they were unfamiliar with the process of changing goals of care in response to the guidance provided to them by the advance directive, (d) they wanted to be supportive to their father at the end of his life, and (e) and they did not know how to negotiate the ICU experience so they might make their decision known to the physician.

The social worker met with the daughters to review the advance directive and explore their understanding of Mr. Taylor's wishes and the values that guided how he had lived his life. This process allowed the patient's voice to be brought into the discussion regardless of his ability to speak. Acting as a liaison for the family the social worker contacted the physician to inform her of the patient's wishes and the existence of the advance directive. During the family conference the social worker facilitated communication between the physician, nurse, and the daughters regarding the procedure for withdrawal of the ventilator and provision of comfort measures. Specific statements of support for the daughters' decision and an invitation to engage extended family, cultural, spiritual supports and ritual individualized this process and humanized the withdrawal of medical equipment not only for the patient and his daughters but also for the medical staff that participated. These are all important palliative care activities.

Changing Goals of Care

Curative care is all the care that can be provided to attempt to cure an illness or repair an injury. Oftentimes intensive, life-saving interventions do not provide a cure but rather remedy a crisis, improve health, and extend life. For many health care professionals, curative care is the primary goal of medicine. Cure has been the thrust of modern medical care and with the development of new techniques, technology, and medicines physicians can present a patient with an increasing number of options for treating disease. Once stabilized a

Box 6.2
Patient/Family Narrative: Mr. Taylor

Mr. Taylor was an 87-year-old, widowed, Protestant, Caucasian man who sustained a traumatic brain injury when he slipped and fell on the concrete steps leading to his front door. His injury was so severe that he was unable to breathe on his own or control his airway and he required the assistance of a ventilator. It was set to force oxygenated air into his lungs and was attached to an endotracheal tube, which was inserted into his mouth and down his throat to keep his airway open and make it easier for the nurse to suction secretions from his throat. He was given paralytic medications so that his body would remain quiet and he would not gag on the tube. Oxygen was being supplied to infuse his body and aid in healing his brain. He had leads from his body to a heart monitor, blood pressure monitor, intravenous fluids and medications, and an oximeter to monitor the oxygen level in his blood. He was not responsive but looked comfortable in bed. His prognosis was very poor. If he survived he would be severely disabled and dependent for long-term care in a nursing home setting.

Mr. Taylor's two adult daughters were in their 50s. They asked to meet with a social worker to talk about making decisions for their father because, as they put it, they were "unsure of how to do the right thing." They presented their father's signed living will, which said that if he was in a terminal condition or persistent coma, he would not want his death to be prolonged. Mr. Taylor had always been an active person and his daughters knew he would not want to live in a dependent condition, unable to participate in the things he enjoyed such as reading and talking with friends. They were also aware that the doctor might ask them whether their father would want a tracheostomy and a feeding tube, but their immediate concern was that he be kept out of pain. They requested a meeting with physicians to discuss Mr. Taylor's current condition, his prognosis for a meaningful recovery, options for his care, and his wishes as expressed in his advance directive.

The social worker conferred with the physician and nurse and scheduled a family conference. The social worker led the conference, introduced everyone, and advised the doctor of the content of the advance directive. Inviting the daughters to participate, he summarized their concerns, asking them to correct or amplify the summary. The attending physician acknowledged their thoughtfulness and validated their understanding of his prognosis, confirming that his condition did in fact meet the conditions set forth in his living will.

The treatment option agreed upon was to stop the interventions that were sustaining his body and let Mr. Taylor die as naturally as possible. The physician outlined the process of withdrawal, assuring the daughters that Mr. Taylor would be given medications to keep him comfortable the entire time. She let the daughters know that they could spend time in the room during the procedure, or if they wished, they could leave and return once withdrawal was completed. The nurse prepared the daughters for the change in environment, described the process of disconnecting all the monitors to both reduce the noise and create a physical setting in which it would be easier to be physically close to their father. The social worker asked that they consider whether additional family, including grandchildren, or friends might need to visit before or during the extubation (removal of the endotracheal tube). After this discussion the physician and daughters agreed on a time when the ventilator would be withdrawn.

The social worker supported the daughters in making this difficult decision and acknowledged that Mr. Taylor would likely have made the same choice as evidenced by his living will. He asked if there might be a cultural or spiritual ritual that would be helpful and offered the services of a spiritual care provider. He also let them know that they could have extended visitation hours and access to the conference room to spend some private time. In addition, the social worker explored concerns and questions related to grandchildren who had been aware of Mr. Taylor's serious condition and might need help as they integrated his death. He offered to speak with the grandchildren and to provide guidance and resources to assist the family with funeral arrangements and bereavement as they felt ready to do that.

patient may continue to live with a life-threatening or debilitating disease for many years. For the large group of chronically ill patients who will not be cured despite the best medical intervention, the medical team and family will confront the reality that continued intensive care might not achieve the intended benefit and hoped-for outcome. This realization can come to staff, patients, and family members at different times in the process. As this awareness increases it may compel changes in the goals of care and the need to revisit decisions in a process guided by advance directives, state-specific regulations, and the cultural and spiritual beliefs of the family.

The decision to change goals does not mean moving directly to stopping interventions which may improve health. Many patients continue treatment for progressive health conditions, and they will need continued palliative care provided in conjunction with curative or maintenance medical care. Those patients who survive a crisis in the ICU may have periods of stable health punctuated by exacerbations of their illness and future ICU admissions. Continued palliative care can not only provide relief for pain and other symptoms but also an opportunity to review treatment goals and clarify plans for handling the next crisis. This period between exacerbations of illness can be an excellent time for a palliative social worker to work with the patient and family to establish a future plan of care and work on legal documents such as a durable health care power of attorney, advance directive, and a will.

The profound decision to withdraw interventions or not to do so requires skilled communication. This is especially true in the ICU, where communication problems are consistently cited by family members as their most important concern (Levy & McBride, 2006). Good communication will include an ongoing, honest discussion of the progress of the patient and the work of weighing benefits against the burden of specific treatments. Such communication includes discussion of the recognition that an ICU admission with intubation and ventilator support may be traumatic for a patient and provide only temporary relief, without curing a chronic condition. A palliative social worker may test the readiness of the patient and family to make a decision for the future and agree to withhold life-sustaining treatment at the next crisis. This could mean withholding the ventilator and the breathing tube and continuing only palliative care with a goal of keeping the patient comfortable as death approaches.

Bioethical Considerations

The social work profession has made a strong, long-term commitment to client self-determination and this includes support for patients' rights to make their own decisions regarding their health care at the end of life. The bioethical corollary to self-determination is respect for autonomy. It is based on the philosophical concept of individual freedom to decide how one wants to live life. A decision made by a patient about his or her health care will be followed by physicians in almost all circumstances. The exception would be if the person did not have decisional capacity, which is the ability to understand information and the consequences of a decision. If a patient is mentally impaired in some way that prevents clear thinking and reflective decision making, then a surrogate family member or assigned agent may decide for the patient. In families where culture embraces a family decision-making process, the clinical and ethical task requires that clinicians insure that the patient is freely delegating this authority within the family.

The surrogate decision maker in the ICU has the same authority the patient would have, with the added responsibility of making the decision with an understanding of what the patient would want. In most states, this requirement is based on the concept of substituted judgment, which requires that the surrogate make the decision not as he or she wishes, but as the patient would choose. If the surrogate, in consultation with other family members and friends, is not able to determine what the patient would want, the surrogate is then expected to use a standard of decision making based on the best interests of the patient. This standard implies that the medical team and family members know what is best for the person. This can be difficult to determine at times, because the implication is that family, with the help of staff, have the ability to acknowledge their assumptive judgments about quality of life and move beyond them to review the values and past life choices of another person. While difficult, this process requires medical and prognostic information so that deducing best interest is set in the context of best medical input.

Social workers in their work with family members in the ICU have a role in assisting families in this decision-making process. As exemplified in the narrative of Mrs. Amalu, well-timed questions directed to family members can elicit important information that will aid them to reach a decision based on the patient's wishes and cultural variables and with which all parties may feel satisfied. The narrative of Mr. Taylor demonstrates the benefits of having written statements of the patient's wishes, information from family members based on prior conversations with the patient, and family members who are good advocates who can insure that a patient's wishes are carried out.

During this decision-making process, there are times when a family member might ask whether things can be speeded up a little, which often means the family member would like extra medications given to hasten death. There are some family members who confuse withdrawal or withholding of interventions with physician-assisted death, and they may either fear or request that a lethal dose of medication be given to a patient. At other times families fear that the withdrawal of interventions is "killing" rather than allowing the dying process to proceed. Families may infer that the intention of staff is to hasten the death. It is essential that inferences and innuendo about these issues be openly discussed so all participants are clear on the intent and goal of care. The inability to clarify these issues is a sign that continued work with the family is needed.

Social workers can often assist in clarifying the parameters and intent of a plan of care. For example, it is important to know that the assisted-suicide laws in the states of Oregon and Washington require that the patient self-administer the medication. An incompetent patient would not be able to accomplish that. Medications given to patients are intended for comfort rather than to intentionally hasten death. While some pain medications, such as morphine, can compromise breathing as a secondary effect, their primary use is to relieve pain and assist with shortness of breath. Many ethicists agree that the possibility of respiratory depression in an imminently dying patient is an accepted secondary effect when the intention is to provide pain relief and enhance the patient's comfort.

Proactive Palliative Care

Recent developments in ICU care have emphasized early intervention with families. This has been done successfully with an intensive communication intervention (Lilly et al., 2000), ethics consultation (Mularski et al., 2006), and proactive palliative care (Norton et al., 2007). These interventions have found that with early intervention families are more satisfied with care and patients have a shortened length of stay in the ICU. This kind of proactive approach can identify patients in need of palliative care earlier in their ICU stay, facilitate decision making, accelerate earlier withdrawal of interventions which are not beneficial to the patient, and shorten the time to death for those who are inevitably dying (Norton et al., 2007). Daily screening of the census and rounding with physicians and nurses are practices that will help a palliative social worker or a unit social worker collaborating with the team to identify patients for early intervention.

The social worker can initiate assessment and intervention early in the ICU stay and establish rapport in anticipation of a continued relationship if the patient transfers from the ICU to a hospital unit. If death occurs while the patient is in the ICU, the social worker will be well positioned to support the family with whom they have already established a relationship. All of the skills and intervention techniques discussed in this chapter are predicated on the quality of the relationship the social worker has with the patient and the family. Optimal palliative social work will begin at the time of admission to the ICU and carry through the initial rescue phase of treatment to hospital discharge or death of the patient in the hospital. A social worker on a palliative care team would be able to follow a patient through the hospital stay and provide good continuity of care, while a social worker assigned to the ICU would likely have to transfer the patient to a hospital unit social worker for discharge planning. In either scenario the ecological perspective of the social worker can have a humanizing effect on the ICU process and provide an important perspective to the health care team. It incorporates the values and culture of the patient, the home and community settings, the financial and social resources of the family, and plans for discharge from the hospital or for support to the family through death and bereavement. The need for a multifaceted approach to social work in the ICU provides a challenging opportunity for meaningful interventions for the palliative social worker.

LEARNING EXERCISES

- Jot down verbatim statements and questions from family members during several family conferences. Review them later, to ponder any symbolic meaning and to help prepare yourself and colleagues for future conferences.
- Patients in the ICU can seem to be ignored as staff members talk to the family. Upon entering a patient's room in the ICU, greet everyone and introduce yourself, then ask the patient or the family member if the patient is experiencing any pain. This practice will tune you into the patient and family needs at the beginning of your session. Imagine other ways that you might create a sense of the personhood of the patient despite the patient being attached to technology and unable to speak.
- Take on the role of leader of the family conference. Meet with the family before the conference to learn everyone's name and find out their concerns. Then lead the introductions at the start of the conference. Getting involved in the conference at the beginning can strengthen your role later in the session because it will be easier to speak having already broken the ice.

ADDITIONAL SUGGESTED READINGS

Beauchamp, T. L., & Childress, J. F. (2001). *Principles of biomedical ethics* (5th ed.). Oxford, England: Oxford University Press.

Curtis, J. R., & Rubenfeld, G. D. (Eds.). (2001). *Managing death in the intensive care unit: The transition from cure to comfort.* Oxford: Oxford University Press.

Field, M. J., & Behrman, R. E. (2003). *When children die: Improving palliative and end-of-life care for children and their families.* Washington, DC: Committee of Palliative and End-of-Life Care for Children and Their Families, Institute of Medicine.

Field, M. J., & Cassel, C. K. (1997). *Approaching death: Improving care at the end of life.* Washington, DC: Committee on Care at the End of Life, Institute of Medicine.

Gertais, M., Edgman-Levitan, S., Daley, J., & Delbanco, T. L. (1993). *Through the patient's eyes: Understanding and promoting patient-centered care.* San Francisco, CA: Jossey-Bass Publishers.

Lunney, J. R, Foley, K. M., Smith, T. J., & Gelband, H. (2003). *Describing death in America: What we need to know.* Washington, DC: National Cancer Policy Board and Division of Earth and Life Studies, Institute of Medicine.

Quill, T. E. (2001). *Caring for patients at the end of life: Facing an uncertain future together.* Oxford, England: Oxford University Press.

ADDITIONAL RESOURCES AND WEB SITES

Center to Advance Palliative Care: http://www.capc.org/ipal-icu This Web site is an excellent resource for a wide range of information about palliative care in the intensive care unit and includes sections on articles/publications, organizations, tools/toolkits, presentations and audio conferences, and books and videos. /

REFERENCES

Center to Advance Palliative Care (CAPC). (2009). *Building a palliative care program.* New York, NY: Author.

Curtis, J. R., & Rubenfeld, G. D. (2001). Introducing the concept of managing death in the ICU. In J. R. Curtis & G. D. Rubenfeld (Eds.), *Managing death in the intensive care unit: The transition from cure to comfort* (pp. 3–5). Oxford, England: Oxford University Press.

Field, M. J., & Behrman, R. E. (2003). *When children die: Improving palliative and end-of-life care for children and their families.* Washington, DC: Committee on Palliative and End-of-Life Care for Children and Their Families, Institute of Medicine.

Foley, K. M. (2001). Pain and symptom control in the dying ICU patient. In J. R. Curtis & G. D. Rubenfeld (Eds.), *Managing death in the ICU: The transition from cure to comfort* (pp. 103–125). Oxford, England: Oxford University Press.

Levy, M., & McBride, D. (2006). End-of-life care in the intensive care unit: State of the art in 2006. *Critical Care Medicine, 34*(11 Suppl.), S306–S308.

Lilly, C. M., DeMeo, D. L., Sonna, L. A., Haley, K. J., Massaro, A. F., Wallace, R. F., & Cody, S. (2000). An intensive communication intervention for the critically ill. *The American Journal of Medicine, 109*(6), 469–475.

Luce, J. M., & Prendergast, T. J. (2001). The changing nature of death in the ICU. In J. R. Curtis & G. D. Rubenfeld (Eds.), *Managing death in the intensive care unit* (pp. 19–29). Oxford, England: Oxford University Press.

McCormick, A. J., Curtis, J. R., Stowell-Weiss, P., Toms, C., & Engelberg, R. (2010). Improving social work in ICU palliative care: Results of a quality improvement intervention. *Journal of Palliative Medicine, 13*(3), 297–304.

McCormick, A. J., Engelberg, R., & Curtis, J. R. (2007). Social workers in palliative care: Assessing activities and barriers in the intensive care unit. *Journal of Palliative Medicine, 10*(4), 929–937.

Mularski, R., Curtis, J. R., Billings, J. A., Burt, R., Byock, I., Fuhrman, C., Mosenthal, A. C., Medina, J., Ray, D. E., Rubenfeld, G. D., Schneiderman, L. J., Treece, P. D., Truong, R. D., & Levy, M. M. (2006). Proposed quality measures for palliative care in the critically ill: A consensus from the Robert Wood Johnson Foundation Critical Care Workgroup. *Critical Care Medicine, 34*(11 Suppl.), S404–S411.

National Consensus Project for Quality Palliative Care. (2009). *Clinical practice guidelines for quality palliative care.* Pittsburg, PA: Author.

Nelson, J. E., & Nierman, D. M. (2001). Special concerns of the very old. In J. R. Curtis & G. D. Rubenfeld (Eds.), *Managing death in the ICU: The transition from cure to comfort* (pp. 349–367). Oxford, England: Oxford University Press.

Norton, S. A., Hogan, L. A., Holloway, R. G., Temkin-Greener, H., Buckley, M. J., & Quill, T. E. (2007). Proactive palliative care in the medical intensive care unit: Effects on length of stay for selected high-risk patients. *Critical Care Medicine, 35*(6), 1530–1535.

7 Robin Rudy Lawson

Palliative Social Work in the Emergency Department

A person doesn't die when he should but when he can.

—*Gabriel Garcia Marquez*

Key Concepts

- *Patients with serious illness and their families present to emergency departments (EDs) with symptom distress, caregiver distress, and for management of end-of-life issues.*
- *The palliative care needs of patients and families in the ED often revolve around pain and symptom management, clarification of advance directives (ADs), and death in the setting of the ED environment.*
- *Both ED and palliative social workers can improve the care that seriously ill patients receive in the ED by identifying unmet needs and providing specific palliative social work interventions.*

Introduction

The emergency department (ED) typically provides care for people with severe trauma or acute illness, and for those with minor acute problems that require rapid assessment. Increasing numbers of people with chronic diseases and those facing end of life are also being admitted to EDs (Chan, 2004; Tardy et al., 2002). Even though overall cancer deaths have decreased recently, ED visits for cancer-related emergencies are on the rise (Rondeau & Schmidt, 2009). Patients with serious illness and their caregivers arrive in the ED seeking assistance with distressing symptoms, caregiver distress, and for some patients and/or caregivers, fears about dying at home (Chan, 2004; Marco & Shears, 2006; Tardy et al., 2002;).

A burgeoning elderly population will only increase the number of people with significant life-limiting illnesses who present to the ED. The Centers for Disease Control and Prevention (CDC) (CDC & The Merck Company Foundation, 2007) estimate that by 2030, the number of Americans aged 65 and older will more than double and constitute 20% of the population. At nearly 10.2 million visits, people aged 75 and older had the second highest per-capita ED visit rate (CDC, 2008). Rapid triage and diagnosis can be difficult in older patients who may present with multiple diseases, numerous medications, and functional and cognitive impairments (Hwang & Morrison, 2007).

The relationship between palliative care and emergency medicine is in its infancy. There has been increasing interest among both emergency medicine and palliative medicine clinicians in improving the care that seriously ill patients receive in the ED while also moving palliative care consults upstream (Meier & Beresford, 2007). In 2006, the American Board of Emergency Medicine co-sponsored palliative medicine as a recognized subspecialty and the Education on Palliative and End of Life Care Project (EPEC) developed a new curriculum specifically for emergency medicine professionals.

Building relationships between palliative care and emergency medicine departments is dependent on many factors, including the goals of the institution, the availability of resources from the palliative care service, and a commitment by both departments to improve the care for seriously ill patients in the ED. Palliative social workers, and ED social workers with specific training, can play instrumental roles in fostering collaboration between departments, identifying patients/families with unmet palliative care needs, and providing specific interventions to improve the care of seriously ill patients in the ED.

Challenges in Providing Palliative Care in the Emergency Department

Modus Operandi

Lawson, Burge, McIntryre, Field, and Maxwell (2009) affirm that EDs can be chaotic, pressured environments where diagnosis and treatment for acute or traumatic events are the main goals. Patients are prioritized by the seriousness of their illness or injury, which produces an environment of persistent change and urgency (Chan, 2004). The most markedly ill or injured patient is given the most attention and care and is identified as the person who is at highest risk for an unforeseen or undesired death (Chan, 2004). Chan (2004) affirms that society's and community's standards for ED care include the assumption of consent for complete aggressive measures to prevent sudden death. Asking a patient/family to switch gears and consider palliative care or hospice can appear incongruous with these standards and requires clear conceptualization of the goals of care in the setting of extensive groundwork and collaboration among palliative care, emergency medicine, and primary care providers.

Environment of the Emergency Department

The physical environment of the ED is not conducive to providing palliative care. While the use of curtains rather than walls allows clinicians quick physical access to patients and increases visual and auditory awareness, it limits privacy for patients, families, and staff. These structural realities and the consequent lack of privacy, as in the intensive care unit (ICU), create a setting where family members are acutely aware that their own distress might agitate others (Lloyd-Williams, Morton, & Peters, 2009). As most EDs are on the ground floor of hospitals, they are typically windowless to protect patient privacy. Hwang and Morrison (2007) assert that this lack of natural light can be disorienting to both older patients with cognitive impairments as well as patients with a delirium or confusion. Finally, the constant noise from monitors that sound alarms, clinician discussions, and collective voices all in the same space contribute to communication difficulties for the hearing impaired (Hwang & Morrison, 2007); and for many patients and families, this creates a chaotic, noisy environment that is not ideal for care of seriously ill patients. Yet with skilled, vigilant, and collaborating clinicians there is an opportunity to intervene

effectively and focus on the palliative care needs of patients and their families.

Inadequate Information

Outside of their own clinical assessment, ED physicians and nurses have little information at hand to help guide decisions regarding patient care. Patient report and information from caregivers as well as the accompanying ambulance report are useful but limited and calls to the patient's primary physician/specialist may go unanswered or may only provide the necessary information to get the patient admitted to a floor. Many patients with life-limiting illnesses present to EDs in crisis, either from an acute illness event, severe symptom distress, or a psychosocial crisis. Emergent medical issues take priority and a comprehensive identification of palliative care issues such as advance directives (ADs) and prognosis are secondary to a busy staff who do not have the necessary time to spend with patients and families who look to them to act. Generally, staff are not familiar to patients and families and while crises can build rapport and trust and an immediate dependence, at other times these realities create a barrier and mitigate against the informed and emotional communication that is often at the basis of decision making in the setting of life-threatening illness. Finally, the nature of the emergency may mandate a discussion of ADs, goals of care, and resuscitation decisions concurrently with the provision of emergent medical interventions.

Compared to the emergency physician, the patient's primary doctor typically has the benefit of knowing the patient from time of diagnosis through end stage, has an understanding of the patient's life history, the strain of chronic suffering, the patient's prognosis, and the patient's wishes regarding life-prolonging therapy (Tardy et al., 2002). In Smith et al.'s (2009) study, emergency physicians reported that they typically had no documentation regarding the patient's conversation with their primary physician about goals of care. Discussing goals of care in the ED requires skillful communication focusing on the current reality and including inquiry about any discussions that may have already occurred with the patient's primary care team.

Palliative Care alongside Curative Care?

Some ED clinicians may have difficulty understanding why patients with life-limiting illnesses and their loved ones come to the ED for assistance. They may view an ED visit as negligence on the part of the patient or family in planning for disease progression or a collapse of caregiving coping skills (Rondeau & Schmidt, 2009). ED staff may also believe that it is the primary provider's fault for not foreseeing the patient's end-of-life needs (Rondeau & Schmidt, 2009).

When emergency clinicians (physicians, nurses, and social workers) were asked about patients with serious illness in the

Box 7.1
Patient/Family Narrative: Anne F.

3:35 p.m. *A 52-year-old Caucasian female, Anne F., arrives in the ED with severe shortness of breath. She has a history of lung cancer which has metastasized to her brain and liver, and she recently stopped chemotherapy and radiation treatment due to weakness, shortness of breath, and confusion. Her 80-year-old mother, Rosemary, is her primary caregiver and has accompanied her to the ED, where the patient and mother are assigned to an acute care bed because it has more space for life-saving equipment and affords more privacy.*

Upon arrival, the ED staff determines that she is actively dying and that her respiratory status is critical, and the emergency physician speaks to Rosemary about her daughter's wishes regarding resuscitation and intubation. Her mother begins to cry and says that she wants everything done for her daughter to save her life. When asked whether her daughter had previously expressed her wishes regarding end-of-life care, the mother responds that they never talked about it. The physician pages the ED social worker and calls Anne's oncologist.

4:00 p.m. *The ED social worker meets with Rosemary and provides support and comfort. The nurse assigned to the patient continues to check the patient's vital signs every 5 minutes, a routine behavior that increases the mother's anxiety as she is told that her daughter's condition is worsening. The social worker speaks with the nurse to determine whether checking vital signs every 5 minutes is essential. The nurse explains, "I just don't know what to do for them. I can't just stand there. I have to be doing something for the patient." As the patient's condition worsens, the ED staff contact the ICU regarding bed availability, and they inform the mother that they are prepared to intubate the patient when she stops breathing. Equipment for intubation is brought over to the patient's bed and, as the mother slowly integrates the meaning of this equipment, through her tears, she talks about "losing her baby." Anne's oncologist calls back and reports that he and Anne never talked specifically about resuscitation or intubation but that she had told him that she wanted to be as comfortable as possible at the end of life.*

5:00 p.m. *The ED staff page the palliative social worker (PSW), asking for assistance in talking with the mother about interventions that might only serve to prolong Anne's dying.*

Assessment

5:20 p.m. *During the PSW assessment, she learns that Anne, an only child, is unmarried, lives with her mother, and has no children. Prior to beginning chemotherapy and radiation treatment, she was an anthropologist at the local natural history museum and had a small, but close network of work friends. Her mother states that Anne was diagnosed with lung cancer 8 months ago and has had a rapid decline both physically and cognitively. She goes on to explain that both she and her daughter's attitude was that she would "beat it," even after they understood the prognostic significance of the metastasis. Anne's mother reports that Anne was spiritual but not religious and that she believes in a higher power.*

5:45 p.m. *When asked about her knowledge of her daughter's wishes, the mother states that Anne brought up dying once with*

her a few months ago and the mother immediately became upset and refused to continue the discussion. She feels guilty that she did not give Anne the opportunity to express her thoughts on death and is terribly frightened that she may have to make such decisions without this guidance. When asked whether Anne ever mentioned other people coming to the end of their lives, Rosemary recalls that Anne's mentor at work died of Alzheimer's disease a few years ago. She states that Anne was very upset after learning that he received very aggressive interventions before dying in the ICU; he was always adamant about wanting to die a natural death and had carefully specified his end-of-life preferences in a document that his children were unable to locate. Rosemary now remembers Anne stating that if she were "on her way out," she would want to go peacefully and "not be assaulted by people or equipment."

Interventions and Outcomes

6:15 p.m. *After a period of sitting silently, the PSW explains that although Anne is currently unable to communicate how she would want to die, her statements made in the past and in discussion about the death of her mentor provide guidance to Rosemary and the emergency medicine clinicians in how to respect her daughter's values and wishes. Rosemary understands but states she will not allow her daughter to die while she is alive and states that she will feel guilty if she does nothing to prevent her daughter's death. While it is possible that she will also feel guilty for not respecting Anne's values, the social worker chooses to remain silent about the potential conflict as the medical team provides additional information necessary for the consent process involved with intubation.*

6:30 p.m. *As the emergency physician discusses gently and directly the process of intubation, and the uncertainty regarding its outcome, as well as Anne's possible course in the ICU, Rosemary becomes quiet. She tells the social worker that if the intubation takes place, perhaps it might prolong the suffering that she believes her daughter is enduring from her disease. Rosemary goes back to her daughter's side, sits down, and weeps. Joined by the social worker, Rosemary explains that her daughter was very shy as a child and was teased for her quiet nature. She goes on to say that Anne "found her voice" as she got older and became more assertive and confident. In that context, the PSW reminds Rosemary that Anne's voice is not silent right now: Anne did provide specific guidance to her mother about how she would want her end of life to look by using descriptive words such as "peaceful" and "not being assaulted." Rosemary sits with this for a few minutes and tells the emergency physician that she does not want to intubate her daughter and asks what can be done so that her daughter might die peacefully.*

ED, they believed that fears about managing worsening symptoms such as pain and dyspnea contributed to families' decisions to come to the ED for care (Smith et al., 2009), which were acceptable reasons to the staff. Most emergency physicians and nurses have the training and experience to recognize patients with serious illness, but identifying the specific palliative care needs and how to intervene may require additional training or the expertise of a palliative care consultation team (Quest, Marco & Derse, 2009).

Role of the Emergency Department Social Worker

The ED social worker is a key player in identifying at-risk patients and families, providing crisis interventions, and assisting with "social admissions." Social admissions are non-medical admissions to the hospital, including elder abuse/neglect, psychosocial emergencies, and caregiver crises. A cost–benefit analysis of social work services in the EDs performed by Gordon (2001) found that large urban EDs would have a net benefit if they had a full-time social worker but only if the social worker could prevent social admissions and reduce the amount of time that doctors and nurses spend on the social needs of patients.

The ED social worker conducts psychosocial assessments, provides bereavement counseling for deaths in the ED (Wells, 1993), and may be heavily involved in the pediatric ED, intervening with pediatric psychiatric admissions, child abuse and neglect, and severely ill children. They provide emotional support to patients and families experiencing a crisis and provide counseling as needed (Wells, 1993). Due to their education and experience, ED social workers also serve as a resource for medical-legal (domestic violence, sexual assault) and guardianship issues (Bristow & Herrick, 2002). They are charged with making appropriate referrals to community resources and may assist with discharge planning, including setting up transportation and/or home care services (Bristow & Herrick, 2002).

Because of their extensive knowledge of ED processes and protocols and ability to rapidly identify patients and families in crisis, ED social workers are well positioned to identify patients and families with serious illness. With the proper tools, such as a comprehensive palliative care assessment and some targeted training, ED social workers can collaborate with the ED staff and palliative care clinicians to identify specific palliative care needs. With specialized training in palliative care principles and focused social work assessment and intervention skills, they can also intervene to guide and enhance a plan of care consistent with the stage of illness and the patient and family's goals and values.

Palliative Care Emergencies

Pain Management

Emergency clinicians assess a variety of pain syndromes, from patients with sickle cell disease who present in a pain crisis, to the head and neck oncology patient with esophageal mucositis, which causes severe pain, discomfort, and interferes with nutrition. Pain is the chief complaint for adult patients presenting to EDs (CDC, 2008), yet there are many barriers to effective pain management for this population. Todd et al. (2007) examined the current state of pain

management in 20 EDs in North America and found that 83% of patients had a pain assessment, but reassessments were not common. They also noted that after a median delay of 90 minutes, only 60% of patients who needed pain medication received an analgesic and 74% of patients were released in moderate to severe pain (Todd et al., 2007).

Other barriers to optimal pain management in the ED include well-documented ethnic and gender disparities. In a study looking at patients who presented with extremity fractures, white patients were significantly more likely than black patients to receive analgesics (74% versus 57%), even though pain complaints were similar in the medical record (Todd, Deaton, D'Adamo, & Goe, 1997). Black patients had a 66% greater chance than white patients of not receiving pain medication (Todd et al., 1997). In a study by Chen et al. (2007) looking at the administration of analgesia for acute abdominal pain, women were less likely than men to receive any analgesia (60% vs. 67%) even with similar pain scores, and they were 13% to 25% less likely to be given opioid analgesia than men.

Clinicians' concerns about the use of opioids in pain management either for patients with chronic pain or for patients with life-limiting illnesses persist in the ED. Fears of causing opioid addiction or that prescribing opioids encourages an already established addiction means that patients with chronic pain who present to the ED receive inadequate treatment from clinicians (Derse, 2006). Fears that clinicians will hasten death and cause respiratory depression in patients with cancer or other life-threatening conditions also prevents adequate pain management in palliative care patients (Derse, 2006).

Emergency nurses, as the clinicians who administer pain medications, may be particularly concerned about the use of opioids in the ED. Tanabe and Buschmann's (2000) study of emergency nurses knowledge of pain management principles identified significant deficits in two domains: comprehending and differentiating "addiction," "tolerance," and "dependence"; and education regarding various pharmacologic analgesic principles. Education and training in pain management with opioids and in patients with serious illness includes not only pharmacologic principles but also an understanding of ethical principles and legal parameters so that clinicians treat pain with confidence that they are making thoughtful and informed medical decisions.

Advance Directives

Patients with life-limiting illnesses who present to EDs at the end of life pose a unique challenge to emergency clinicians if treatment decisions are to be made without knowledge of the patient's wishes. It may be difficult for clinicians to evaluate a person's decision-making ability in the setting of stress or pain and without knowing the patient's baseline cognitive functioning (Rondeau & Schmidt, 2009).

For patients who do not have the capacity to make their own decisions, the responsibility of decision making in a crisis may be left to others who might very well be unaware of their loved ones wishes. Partners, life partners, or those in domestic unions who accompany loved ones to the ED may find that ED staff are unaware or confused about whether they can legally include them in decision making for cognitively impaired patients. Emergency clinicians may feel particularly helpless when a nursing home resident who is cognitively impaired comes to the ED without ADs. It may be impossible to find family and get in touch with the patient's primary physician in the timeframe available and can be particularly distressing if the patient is actively dying and decisions must be made.

In Smith et al.'s (2009) survey of emergency providers' experiences, beliefs, and attitudes with respect to palliative care, clinicians noted three problems with ADs: when available, they were too broad to be helpful; sometimes the AD conflicted with the wishes of the health care surrogate; and providers resuscitated patients with valid do not intubate (DNI) or do not resuscitate (DNR) orders. Advance directives may have limited usefulness for emergency clinicians because they may be unaware of the context in which these documents were completed and thus unaware of situation-specific wishes of the patient. For example, a patient may want intubation for shortness of breath or resuscitation when recovery to his or her current level of functioning is anticipated, but not if it is expected that he or she will be ventilator dependent. ED clinicians may not have the time nor the medical information needed to know whether the current medical reality fits the parameters of the AD and will err of the side of intervention, believing that the intervention can be withdrawn later, whereas allowing the death to occur is an irrevocable decision.

When the advance directive is in conflict with the health care surrogate's wishes and the patient is incapacitated, clinicians may be unsure as to how to handle this incongruity and default to providing life-prolonging care partly due to litigation fears (Smith et al, 2009). At the same time, there are ethical and legal issues for ED physicians who do not respect a patient's wishes or ADs. Derse (2006) states that emergency physicians typically use the maxim, "always err on the side of life" and assert that any dialogue regarding terminating these treatments can take place in the ICU after the treatment has begun. However, the legal consequences for not respecting a patient's wishes include "actions for battery, lack of consent, and medical malpractice" (Derse, 2006). As well as legal ramifications, the physical and emotional consequences of resuscitating patients who either had valid DNR/DNI orders or who had verbally requested DNR/DNI are complex and impact the patient and family well beyond the events in the ED. Choosing not to start a treatment (withholding treatment) is very different philosophically and emotionally for staff and family members than withdrawing a treatment that has been initiated (Derse, 2006).

Unique Challenges for Emergency Clinicians

In a survey conducted by Heaston, Beckstrang, Bond, and Palmer (2006), emergency room nurses perceived that the major challenges in providing end-of-life care in the ED were high caseloads, working with family members' emotions, the poor layout of the ED, lack of knowledge of the patient's wishes for treatments, and decisions to obviate the patient's known wishes because of a family member's desire to initiate or continue life-prolonging treatment and the inability of the staff to mediate this discrepancy.

As the ED is seen as a place of transition and triage, there may not be as much emphasis on the value of ADs. In addition, emergency clinicians whose goals are to stabilize the patient and get the patient admitted to a hospital unit or sent home may overlook valuable communication regarding the patient's wishes. Another challenging task is to determine whether the context of the current medical crises meets the context described in the AD. For example, a patient may choose not to be resuscitated if his cancer is the cause of his dying but may very well wish to have full support if he has pneumonia where treatment will allow return to a prior level of function. Where there are language differences, family members may be protective of patients who do not speak English or who, because of cultural, spiritual, or emotional reasons, may be unaware of their diagnosis and prognosis. Patients and family members may either have difficulty providing this information due to language differences or may withhold it out of fear that the information will be used to inadvertently harm the patient or deprive the patient of needed quality care. Home health aides or patient care attendants who care for patients at home and in the ED—providing personal care such as assistance with toileting and eating, helping with transfers within the hospital, and performing administrative tasks—spend a considerable time with patients and families and can be valuable resources for emergency clinicians seeking additional information about the patient and family.

Dying in the Emergency Department

Patients who are actively dying and are deemed unable to survive a transfer or hospitalization may remain in the ED instead of occupying an inpatient bed that could be used for someone with a reversible or treatable condition (Chan, 2004). Even the expected death of a patient who is at end of life is emotional and stressful for emergency clinicians. Charged with diagnosing and treating patients, emergency clinicians may feel helpless and uncomfortable with the adaptation required to move from emergency intervention to working with dying patients and the grief of family members. Fear of not knowing all the answers or being blamed and experiencing the emotions of patients and families are some of the perceived challenges in working with families in death notification and bereavement care in the ED (Chan, 2004; Olsen, Buenefe, & Falco, 1998). In some cases, clinicians may view the patient's death as preventable, prompting feelings of guilt, inadequacy, or failure among emergency clinicians (Olsen et al., 1998).

People who die abruptly and without warning in the ED, victims of violence or trauma, and those who commit suicide are potential cases for the medical examiner or coroner (Chan, 2004). The trauma room is regarded as a potential crime scene (Chan, 2004), and the person who died is "evidence," which can be depersonalizing for surviving family members who may also be interviewed by law enforcement and treated suspiciously. Emergency clinicians such as chaplains and social workers play a key role in the provision of emotional, spiritual, and cultural care pertaining to death and bereavement (Quest et al., 2009; Wells, 1993) and are specifically called upon for sudden, unexpected death. They can also assist to create a responsive environment where cultural or spiritual rituals are invited and respected in preparation for and at the time of death (Campbell & Zalenski, 2005).

Whereas common traditional practice used to be to separate the family from the patient during resuscitation and invasive procedures, there is mixed evidence in support for the presence of families at the patient's side (Boudreaux, Francis, & Loyacano, 2002). A critical review of the literature found that nurses may have a more approving opinion toward family presence during invasive procedures than physicians and that although family may want to be present and believe it is helpful, their presence may not actually reduce the patient's distress (Boudreaux et al., 2002). In Doyle et al.'s (1987) study of family presence during resuscitation attempts, 97% of families would witness it again, 76% believed their grieving was made easier, 67% thought their presence helped the patient, and 100% felt confident that everything had been done to save their loved one.

The death of a child in the ED is devastating. Allen (2009) describes the responsibility that a clinical nurse specialist can have in creating standards of practice for children who die in the ED, and these suggestions can be the shared work of interdisciplinary staff. She describes enlisting chaplain support, gathering community resources for families, providing mementos that represent contact with the child (pillow, etc.), educating staff on pediatric end-of-life care, supplying caregivers with support, and contacting families for bereavement follow-up (Allen, 2009). Truog, Christ, Browning, and Meyer (2006) highlight the importance of a formal debriefing session facilitated by a social worker so that staff can share feelings about the uncertainty, powerlessness, and hopelessness that often result from the sudden, traumatic death of a child. Knazik et al. (2003) also emphasize the importance of communicating with the child's "medical home" (providers that cared for the child prior to her death) and ensuring that critical incident stress management is available for ED staff.

Opportunities for Palliative Social Workers in the Emergency Department

Palliative social workers (PSW) can play an important role in introducing palliative care principles in the ED and, when death occurs, improving the end-of-life care provided to patients and families. By being able to identify patients and families with unmet palliative care needs, the PSW can serve as a liaison between the ED physician, nurses, and the palliative care team to ensure that these patients are seen by the palliative care team either during their hospitalization or as an outpatient if they are discharged from the ED to the community. Communication with the patient's primary physician is essential prior to any contact by the palliative care team to ensure that the patient's existing relationships are respected, to avoid duplication of service, and to reinforce the services of palliative care as complementary to primary clinicians. ED physicians who contact the primary physician while their patient is in the ED can convey needed clinical information and seek the primary physician's understanding of the patient, the patient's illness, and the patient's goals.

Palliative social workers who are introduced to the ED staff in a collaborative, respectful process can serve as the "face" of palliative care in the ED. They must be available and responsive because emergency clinicians want their patients to receive the best possible care and given the nature of the environment, responsiveness is a key to successful collaboration and excellence in care of patients and families. ED clinicians are, due to the nature of their work, open to other specialties (Chan, 2006), which means that there are opportunities for collaborative and reciprocal learning. This includes palliative care teams providing information and training to improve symptom management, care of actively dying patients, understanding of ADs, and death and bereavement practices. Reciprocally, ED staff can assist palliative clinicians to understand the culture, processes, and demands of the ED environment.

Clinical interventions that can be provided by palliative social workers in the ED emanate from a comprehensive palliative care assessment of patient, family, and caregiver, including their individual knowledge; awareness and concerns about diagnosis, prognosis, treatment, and side effects; specific religious or cultural values and expectations (Gwyther et al., 2005); and ethical and legal issues. By providing education and support to emergency clinicians and participating in goals of care or AD conversations, the palliative social worker serves as a resource and intervenes to help patients and families as they consider and integrate information and options for care. Palliative social workers can also provide individual and/or family counseling in the ED for specific palliative care concerns such as patient or caregiver distress, conflicts and clarification related to decision making, and need for caregiver support. Symptom management techniques such as relaxation exercises for anxiety, pain, or shortness of breath can be provided easily in the ED setting. Finally, crisis intervention counseling skills are essential to assist patients and caregivers whether in the setting of a new diagnosis, a medical crisis, or an actively dying patient.

Conclusion

Many patients with serious illness, their families, and caregivers present to the ED seeking assistance with symptom distress such as pain or shortness of breath, new or worsening functional impairment, and patient needs and demands that have grown to exceed the resources in place in the community. Because it is in the ED where a decision will be made about treatments and admission, there is a unique opportunity to intervene with patients and families who have life-limiting conditions. Both ED and palliative social work clinicians can play an active and pivotal role in identifying, assessing, and intervening with patients and families who present to EDs with unmet palliative care needs.

LEARNING EXERCISES

1. As the palliative social worker who has been called to the ED by the physician to assess for symptom management distress in Mr. L., a 45-year-old Cantonese-speaking male patient with head and neck cancer, you and an interpreter meet with him to assess need and levels of symptom distress. When you ask him if he has been sad at all in the past 2 weeks, he responds, "I think about killing myself all the time." How do you respond? How would you document a note in the ED chart for other clinicians to view? How might you view the cultural and gender aspects of this distress? What would be your recommendation to the physician?

2. An ED resident (physician in training) asks for your help in telling the 16-year-old son of a woman with advanced cancer that his mother is actively dying. How would you assist the ED resident? What steps might you take in preparation for this conversation? Do you need the patient's consent to have this conversation? What are you anticipating and preparing for to ensure the most supportive environment for this son? Do you agree to participate? Why or why not? How do you help the resident to think through and prepare for the possible outcomes of this discussion?

ADDITIONAL SUGGESTED READING

Coyle N., & Layman-Goldstein M. (2001). Pain assessment and management in palliative care. In M. L. Matzo & D. W. Sherman (Eds.), *Palliative care nursing: Quality care to the end of life* (pp. 363–486). New York, NY: Springer.

Meier, D. E., & Beresford, L. (2008). Social workers advocate for a seat at the palliative care table. *Journal of Palliative Medicine*, *11*(1), 10–14.

RESOURCES AND WEB SITES

American College of Emergency Physicians: http://www.acep.org
ACEP's mission is to promote the highest quality of emergency care, and it is the leading advocate for emergency physicians, their patients, and the public. See position statements on "Death of a Child in the ED," "Ethical Issues in Emergency Department Care at the End of Life," "Pain Management in the ED," and "Ethical Issues of Resuscitation."
The Education on Palliative and End-of-Life Care: http://www.epec.org
EPEC Project's mission is to educate all health care professionals on the essential clinical competencies in palliative care.
Emergency Nurses Association: http://www.ena.org
ENA's mission is to advocate for patient safety and excellence in emergency nursing practice. See position statements on "EOL Care in the ED" and "Resuscitative Decisions."

REFERENCES

Allen, M. (2009). A child dies in the emergency department: Development of a program to support bereaved families and staff. *Clinical Nurse Specialist*, *23*(3), 96.

Boudreaux, E. D., Francis, J. L., & Loyacano, T. (2002). Family presence during invasive procedures and resuscitation in the emergency department–a critical review and suggestions for future research. *Annals of Emergency Medicine*, *40*(2), 193–205.

Bristow, D. P., & Herrick, C. A. (2002). Emergency department case management: The dyad team of nurse case manager and social worker to improve discharge planning and patient and staff satisfaction while decreasing inappropriate admissions and costs: a literature review. *Lippincott's Case Management*, *7*(6), 243–251.

Campbell, M., & Zalenski, R. (2005). The emergency department. In B. R. Ferrell & N. Coyle (Eds.), *Textbook of palliative nursing* (pp. 861–869). New York, NY: Oxford University Press.

Centers for Disease Control and Prevention (CDC). (2008). National hospital ambulatory care survey: 2006 emergency department summary. Retrieved from http://www.cdc.gov/nchs/data/nhsr/nhsr2007.pdf

Centers for Disease Control and Prevention (CDC) & The Merck Company Foundation. (2007). *The state of aging and health in America 2007*. Retrieved from http://www.cdc.gov/aging

Chan, G. K. (2004). End-of-life models and emergency department care. *Academic Emergency Medicine*, *11*(1), 79–86.

Chan, G. K. (2006). End-of-life and palliative care in the emergency department: a call for research, education, policy and improved practice in this frontier area. *Journal of Emergency Nursing*, *32*(1), 101–103.

Chen, E. H., Shofer, F. S., Dean, A. J., Hollander, J. E., Baxt, W. G., Robey, J. L., ... Mills, A. M. (2008). Gender disparity in analgesic treatment of emergency department patients with acute abdominal pain. *Academic Emergency Medicine, 15*(5), 414–418.

Derse, A. R. (2006). Ethics and the law in emergency medicine. *Emergency Medicine Clinics of North America, 24*(3), 547–555.

Doyle C. J., Post H., Burney R. E., Maino, J., Keefe, M., & Rhee, K. (1987). Family participation during resuscitation: An option. *Annals of Emergency Medicine, 16*(6), 673–675.

Gordon, J. A. (2001). Cost-benefit analysis of social work services in the emergency department: A conceptual model. *Academic Emergency Medicine, 8*(1), 54–60.

Gwyther, L. P., Altilio, T., Blacker, S., Christ, G., Csikai, E. L., Hooyman, N., ... Howe, J. (2005). Social work competencies in palliative and end-of-life care. *Journal of Social Work in End-of-Life and Palliative Care, 1*(1), 87–120.

Heaston, S., Beckstrang R. L., Bond, A. E., & Palmer, S. P. (2006). Emergency nurses' perceptions of obstacles and supportive behaviors in end-of-life care. *Journal of Emergency Nursing, 32*(6), 477–485.

Hwang, U., & Morrison, S. (2007). The geriatric emergency department. *Journal of the American Geriatrics Society, 55*(11), 1873–1876.

Knazik, S. R., Gausche-Hill, M., Dietrich, A. M., Gold, C., Johnson, R. W., Mace, S. E., & Sochor, M. R. (2003). The death of a child in the emergency department. *Annals of Emergency Medicine, 42*(4), 519–529.

Lawson, B. J., Burge, F. I., McIntyre, P., Field, S., & Maxwell, D. (2009). Can the introduction of an integrated service model to an existing comprehensive palliative care service impact emergency department visits among enrolled patients? *Journal of Palliative Medicine, 12*(3), 245–252.

Lloyd-Williams, M., Morton, J., & Peters, S. (2009). The end-of-life care experiences of relatives of brain dead intensive care patients. *Journal of Pain and Symptom Management, 37*(4), 659–664.

Marco, C. A., & Schears, R. M. (2006). Death, dying, and last wishes. *Emergency Medicine Clinics of North America, 24*(4), 969–987.

Meier, D. E., & Beresford, L. (2007). Fast response is key to partnering with the emergency department. *Journal of Palliative Medicine, 10*(3), 641–645.

Olsen J. C., Buenefe, M. L., & Falco, W. E. (1998). Death in the emergency department. *Annals of Emergency Medicine, 31*(6), 758–765.

Quest, T. E., Marco, C. A., & Derse, A. R. (2009). Hospice and palliative medicine: New subspecialty, new opportunities. *Annals of Emergency Medicine, 54*(1), 94–102.

Rondeau, D. F., & Schmidt, T. A. (2009). Treating cancer patients who are near the end of life in the emergency department. *Emergency Medicine Clinics of North America, 27*(2), 341–354.

Smith, A. K., Fisher, J., Schonberg, M. A., Pallin, D. J., Block, S. D., Forrow, L.,... McCarthy, E. P. (2009). Am I doing the right thing? Provider perspectives on improving palliative care in the emergency department. *Annals of Emergency Medicine, 54*(1), 86–93.

Tanabe, P., & Buschmann, M. B. (2000). Emergency nurses' knowledge of pain management principles. *Journal of Emergency Nursing, 26*(4), 299–305.

Tardy, B., Venet, C., Zeni, F., Berthet, O., Viallon, A., Lemaire, F., & Bertrand, J. C. (2002). Death of terminally ill patients on a stretcher in the emergency department: A French specialty? *Intensive Care Medicine, 28*(11), 1625–1628.

Todd, K., Ducharme, J., Choiniere, M., Crandall, C., Fosnocht, D., Homel, P., & Tanabe, P. (2007). Pain in the emergency department: Results of the pain and emergency medicine initiative (PEMI) multicenter study. *The Journal of Pain, 8*(6), 460–466.

Todd, K., Deaton, C., D'Adamo, A., & Goe, L. (1997). Ethnicity and analgesic practice. *Annals of Emergency Medicine, 35*(1), 11–16.

Truog, R. D., Christ, G., Browning, D. M., & Meyer, E. C. (2006). Sudden traumatic death in children: "We did everything, your child didn't survive." *The Journal of the American Medical Association, 295*(22), 2646–2654.

Wells, P. J. (1993). Preparing for sudden death: Social work in the emergency room. *Social Work, 38*(3), 339–342.

8

Sherri Weisenfluh

Social Work and Palliative Care in Hospice

What do you mean? No one told me I was terminally ill.
—Lucille, hospice patient during the admission process

Key Concepts

- ◆ *Social workers play a key role by offering emotional and psychosocial care to patients and families.*
- ◆ *Despite efforts to standardize hospice services, variability in programs exists.*

Introduction

This chapter will provide a brief overview of hospice care, define the role of the social worker, and discuss a number of current challenges that impact hospice social work. Hospice is a philosophy of care aimed at relieving the suffering of the terminally ill and their families. In the United States, hospice can be traced back to the early 1970s, when the first program opened in Connecticut. U.S. programs differed from those in England, in that early programs in the United States were created as grassroots organizations, operated by dedicated volunteers, and unlike England, where care was provided in hospice units, the patient's home was thought to be the setting of preference. In 1982, Medicare Part A recipients became eligible for the Hospice Medicare Benefit, and hospice programs receiving Medicare revenues began to grow. The Hospice Medicare Benefit is provided for patients who have a terminal diagnosis, confirmed by two physicians, who anticipate and affirm that the patient has a prognosis of 6 months or less to live if the disease runs its normal course. The Centers for Medicare and Medicaid Services (CMS) certify hospice programs and through regulation create a level of standardization of services among hospice providers. Today, only 7% of hospice programs are not certified by Medicare (Conner, 2009).

Elements of Hospice Programs

Hospice philosophy can be characterized by the following components:

- *The patient and the family are the unit of care.* One premise of hospice care is that the patient is not the only one affected by a terminal diagnosis. This unique aspect differentiates hospice from many health care systems.
- *Care is provided in the home and in inpatient facilities.* Care for hospice patients can occur wherever the patient resides, providing the facility agrees.
- *Symptom management is a focus of treatment.* Patients who want to access the Hospice Medicare Benefit must

forego or have exhausted curative treatment to pursue hospice care.

- *Palliative care treats the whole person.* Terminal illness impacts patients physically, emotionally, and spiritually. Treating the whole person is a hallmark of hospice philosophy.
- *Services are available 24 hours a day.* Hospice care is provided when needed either through telephone guidance or in-person services. Hospice care is a 24 hour a day program.
- *Palliative care is interdisciplinary.* Patients can expect to receive care from a variety of disciplines that include the attending physician, a nurse, a social worker, a chaplain, a certified nursing assistant, and bereavement staff. Other disciplines such as physical or speech therapists, expressive arts therapists, or other integrative therapists may also be involved.
- *Palliative care is physician directed.* A hospice patient may maintain a relationship with his or her primary physician, but the patient may also receive care from a palliative trained hospice medical director.
- Volunteers are an integral part of hospice and an important aspect of the history of the hospice movement. They can provide a variety of patient and administrative services on behalf of hospice patients.
- *Hospice care is community based.* It is provided without regard to the ability to pay; a patient with no insurance is provided care.
- *Bereavement services are provided to families on the basis of need.* Patients and family members have access to bereavement services both prior to and after the patient's death (Conner, 2009).

Hospice programs that are certified by CMS must meet minimum regulations, which were created to protect the public and to prevent hospice providers from promising one set of services, only to deliver less care than promised. A number of factors influence the ability of a hospice program to go above and beyond the minimum regulatory standards. One of the primary factors is the size of the program. *Hospice and Palliative Care: The Essential Guide* (2nd ed.) (Conner, 2009) indicates that the majority of hospice programs are small with the median average daily census of 51 patients. A few programs serve over a 1000 patients per day, but the reader can easily see that size would make for vastly different types of programs. While size may not affect quality, size does correspond to the number of employees working in a hospice. Smaller programs may have one or two social workers but often do not employee a social work supervisor nor have enough staff to cover patient care while sending employees to state or national conferences.

A second factor that differentiates programs is the financial status of the program. Some hospices are for profit; other programs are 501c-3 organizations and have a not-for-profit status. Just as size does not directly correlate to quality of services, neither does for-profit versus not-for-profit status.

Hospice programs may also be parts of larger institutions, such as hospital-based hospice programs, or home health-hospice programs.

Rural versus urban service areas may also differentiate programs. Rural programs may cover vast geographic areas that require hospice staff to drive great distances between patients' homes. Medicare sets hospice reimbursement rates for rural programs lower than urban areas based on the premise that the wage index rate is lower in rural areas. For 2010 rural hospice programs are reimbursed for all levels of care at 82% of the set rate. Urban programs may receive as much as 150% of the set rate. Medicare reimbursement rates for rural programs are lower than urban programs, despite the fact that travel costs to provide care are often higher in rural settings. Rural providers also face the challenge of offering community programs such as memorial services or bereavement support groups to family members who also have large distances to travel. Hospice programs are constantly trying to find the best way to meet the needs of varying communities. Urban areas may also cover large geographical distances that may have vastly different ethnic composition. The growth of technology has created opportunities for creative programming that may bridge these geographic distances.

Reimbursement levels also affect variability of programs. When the Medicare Hospice benefit was created, CMS regulations required bereavement services to be provided to patients and families. Revenue to cover the cost of the services was considered a part of the daily rate paid to hospice providers. This daily rate is supposed to be enough to cover the cost of providing bereavement services, even though revenue stops once a patient dies. While regulation requires services, hospice providers are left the flexibility to create the form services will take. Some hospice programs may mail educational information to family members after a death or provide support groups with the use of volunteers. Other hospice providers have created extensive bereavement services, such as individual counseling, and support groups; they offer services to the community regardless of whether the family member was a hospice patient.

The Role of the Social Worker in Hospice Home Care

Hospice services can be provided in the patient's home, extended care facilities, assisted living facilities, group homes, inpatient units, residential programs, prison programs, or other environments of the patient's choice. This discussion will deal primarily with providing care in the patient's home because other chapters deal with palliative care in other settings.

Hospice care provided in the home setting can be both challenging and enriching. Entering a patient's home means you are a guest and initially a stranger. The ability to quickly put a patient and family member at ease, establish a level of rapport, and maintain a professional relationship is essential.

Working in the home environment allows social workers to get a glimpse of the patients' and families' life and a flavor for the atmosphere and relationships that can inform the assessment and plan of care. Social workers may be privileged to view cherished photos or collections and to see the patient in the setting that the patient and his or her family have created. Social workers can determine who lives in the home, whether there are neighbors who might be willing to help, or whether extended family members plan to visit. Working in the home environment provides an opportunity to assess the patient's environmental safety, including such issues as smoke alarms, grab bars, and medication storage. On the other end of the continuum is the dangerous home setting, which may include unrestrained aggressive pets, chaotic homes with violence or tenuous family relationships, meth labs, and evidence of active drug diversion. Abuse, neglect, and exploitation are also potential problems and can create dangerous and challenging situations for hospice staff.

The National Hospice and Palliative Care Organization (NHPCO) published *Social Work Guidelines* (*2008*) defined certain activities as within the scope of social work services. They recommend that every patient, family, and friend network have access to the following services:

- *Completion of an initial social work assessment.* Assessment is the foundation for all patient care. Each hospice program can determine the length, nature, and type of psychosocial assessment to be utilized. Regardless of the type of assessment, gathering relevant information is at the core of developing a care plan in collaboration with other team members.
- *Development of a plan of care that stems from the comprehensive social work assessment and is coordinated with the interdisciplinary team.* Social workers are required to use data gathered from the assessment to develop a plan in coordination with other team members to best meet the needs of the patient and family. The care plan reflects the goals that are important to the patient and family and is kept updated as the hospice patient's condition or environment change.
- *Provision of ongoing social work services.* Interventions are based on the assessment, reassessment, and availability of services. Interventions may include counseling, crisis intervention, patient and family education, resources and referrals, financial resource identification, discharge planning, advocacy, and bereavement care.
- *Frequency of visits.* Visits to the patient and family must be of a frequency that allows for adequate reassessment. Patient needs change, and social workers should reevaluate a patient and family's response to team interventions and thereby monitor outcomes. Visit schedules must be tailored to patient need, with some patients being seen daily, weekly, or less frequently based on assessment.

- *Social work interventions.* Ongoing social work interventions are focused on helping patients and family members reach their goals. Common interventions include education on advance care planning, discussions with the patient and family members on the benefits and burdens of palliative treatments, counseling to address anxiety and/or depression, assistance with accessing benefits and community resources, spiritual or philosophical discussions regarding the meaning of the illness experience, exploration and advocacy for management of pain and other symptoms, strengthening coping mechanisms, and development of a culturally and spiritually respectful plan to prepare the family for the patient's death.
- *Organization and provision of social work services and supervision.* Social workers should be involved in the development of agency policies and procedures. Examples include policies or procedures for reporting abuse and neglect, suicide assessment, crisis intervention, and social work supervision.
- *Social work participation in consultation, administration, education, and team meeting.* In addition to direct patient care, social workers have a role to play in developing educational material that might assist patients. Social workers, as part of the interdisciplinary team, attend team meetings to discuss patient/family response to interventions intended to help them meet their goals. Social workers may also have administrative duties, based on each agency's structure, and they may participate in ethics committees, safety committees, or quality assessment programs.
- *Advocacy within larger systems.* At times patients may require an advocate within their family system, within an acute care facility, or to obtain community resources. Social work advocacy, however, extends beyond the family to the macro level, which might involve working on a state or national level to change or improve laws dealing with palliative and end-of-life care.

CMS estimates over 7000 social workers are employed in hospice programs, and social workers are the primary providers of emotional and psychosocial support for the patient and family (Conner, 2009). A study conducted by Mary Raymer and Dona Reese (Project On Death In America, 2001) found that providing adequate social work services in conjunction with physical care significantly reduces overall hospice costs. Additional benefits included fewer hospitalizations for the patient, decreased nursing costs, and higher client satisfaction.

Donna Reese (2008) surveyed hospice directors and found that they view social workers as most qualified to address the following issues with patients and families:

- Financial counseling
- Referrals

- Counseling about suicide, denial, and anticipatory grief
- Facilitating social support
- Promoting cultural competence
- Providing community outreach
- Crisis intervention

The patient and family narrative and discussion will help illustrate the role of the hospice social worker (see Box 8.1).

Box 8.1
Patient/Family Narrative: Dean and Lydia

Dean speaks softly. Slowly he tells you he is 75 years old and has been married to his second wife, Lydia, for 15 years. "I'm having a rough day," he says. He has just gotten home from the hospital and is having trouble getting comfortable because of his pain. You ask where he would rank his pain on a scale of 0–10. He tells you the pain is around 5–6. He explains he has two daughters from his first marriage. One daughter lives in the same town and the younger daughter lives out of state. He moved to the area to be closer to his daughter and to find work. Both daughters have children and Dean has five grandchildren. He points to the pictures that cover the walls of his mobile home. His wife, Lydia, also has children from a previous marriage and her children all live out of state. He has more pictures to show you and talks lovingly about a recent visit from one of Lydia's sons and grandchildren.

Dean tells you he has lung cancer and over the last year he has completed several rounds of chemotherapy. He was diagnosed several years ago and experienced a period of remission, but a recent hospitalization confirmed the cancer has metastasized to other areas of his body. When asked what his doctor has told him about his prognosis he tells you, "The doctor said I don't have long to live." Lydia interrupts to say, "Doctors don't know everything." She also mentions that Dean got well before and he will get well again. Dean mentions his extended family, saying they are close but live out of state. He has three sisters and four brothers. He tells you he is the first in the family to have cancer.

When you look around, you see a neat, clean trailer with two small dogs sitting on the sofa next to Lydia. Dean is sitting in a recliner and says the recliner is more comfortable for him because of the pain. He asks how much longer the interview will take. Dean and Lydia say finances are tight and the only income is a combination of Social Security and a small amount from a part-time job Dean held until recently. Lydia is not working and seems confused regarding Dean's prognosis because she believes he will return to work as soon as he is better.

During the assessment, Dean wants to know what can be done for the pain he is experiencing as well as some shortness of breath. Dean mentions it would be nice to be able to sleep in a bed again. You offer to have a hospital bed sent out but Lydia adamantly refuses, saying there is no room and she does not want the living room disrupted. Dean does not disagree and drops the subject.

Dean agrees to elect the Hospice Medicare Benefit. You conclude the visit after explaining services and let Dean know to expect a visit from the nurse to help with the pain and shortness of breath.

Narrative Discussion

As the social worker, your first concern is the pain level Dean reported. You realize that Dean's pain and shortness of breath made it difficult to engage in conversation and is affecting his quality of life. Dean also is unable to sleep in his own bed and is having trouble getting comfortable. You contact the nurse immediately and discuss the information you gathered. You also share the information that you think a hospital bed would help and note Lydia's adamant refusal, the meaning of which is uncertain. The nurse agrees to make a visit later that day.

The following issues are identified for further assessment and possible intervention:

- *Finances.* Lydia is at risk for having decreased and ultimately little income as Dean physically declines. A conversation will be difficult because Lydia is acting as though she does not accept Dean's prognosis. With sensitivity, you can explore her responses, understand her unique process for integrating her reality, and help her hope for the best but plan for the worst.
- *Advance directive.* Dean's medical records show he has previously had a do not resuscitate order (DNR) while in the hospital. He has also been educated about advance directive documents but has made no decisions. A conversation that explores Dean's emotional and thought process that led to the previous DNR order will help you understand his wishes when he can no longer speak for himself. A phone call to the hospital oncology social worker might also be helpful in understanding the family dynamics, Lydia's previous responses and involvement in treatment decisions, and the process surrounding the previous DNR order. You also realize that conversations related to advance directive and resuscitation may be a difficult for Lydia and want to explore her views. You are also aware that it is not unusual for family members to call 911 before they call hospice. If Dean was to be admitted to a hospital, you cannot advocate for Dean without knowing his wishes.
- *Needs of the children and grandchildren.* You will want to meet as many members of Dean's family as possible to assess their needs. The daughter that lives in town visits often and you set up your next meeting to coincide with her visit. She has been bringing her daughters to see their grandfather, but they will be in school. You will want to ask Dean's daughter what she believes about her father's prognosis and what she shared with her daughters.
- *Equipment.* The nurse will be having a conversation about what equipment might be helpful for Dean, but you want to follow up with the wife to understand the meaning of having a hospital bed in her home. You realize it is important not to jump to conclusions about why Lydia is refusing equipment that might help Dean, because you know that equipment often has symbolic

significance for patients and family. You frequently encounter situations where there is disagreement within the family.

- *Safety needs.* A closer look at the home will help anticipate and identify safety concerns as Dean declines. You would be looking for the presence of smoke alarms, ability to move around the home without tripping on rugs, pets, and so on. Along with other team members you will want to watch for smoking, because oxygen will most likely be necessary. You will watch for decline because Dean will become too weak to attend to personal care. You know the more you can anticipate future changes, the easier it is to prevent problems, yet you balance this anticipatory guidance against Dean and Lydia's readiness to hear about future disease progression and potential symptoms.

- *Extended family.* You think it could be significant that Dean volunteered that he is the first member of his family to have cancer. He might have fears about his siblings, and he might be wondering, why me? This may be an area for exploration and intervention. There might be an opportunity to reach out and meet with his brothers and sisters.

- *Spiritual concerns.* You know from the referral that Dean and Lydia belong to a Baptist church, and you anticipate the team chaplain making a visit. You know patients often have spiritual questions at this point in their life and that sometimes patients with lung cancer who have smoked may experience a myriad of complex feelings. You will want to talk to the chaplain and work as part of a team to help address issues such as forgiveness, fears, or any feeling that Dean might have about burdening Lydia.

- *Blended family issues.* You may need to explore past relationships, as well as feelings and concerns surrounding divorce. Why did Dean move to be closer to one daughter and not the younger daughter? What is the nature of their relationship? What are their treasured moments, joys and sorrows, regrets, or misunderstandings?

- *Practical needs.* If finances are tight, there may be an immediate need to sensitively address unmet basic needs such as food and shelter. You realize that Dean's role as provider for Lydia may be an important part of his identity. As Dean's disease progresses and his inability to return to work becomes clear to all, you anticipate a financial crisis for the couple.

- *Bereavement needs.* As you work with the family, you will assess risk factors for complicated or prolonged grief responses (Prigerson, 2009). You will explore coping strengths, assess Lydia's ability to adapt to adversity, and explore any meaning Lydia might attach to Dean's illness (Neimeyer, 2005). You may want to give special attention to the potential for integrating the grandchildren into the evolving illness process.

- *Meaning making.* You will want to find out what has given Dean's life meaning. What has given him pleasure and a sense of pride? What does he want to pass on or be remembered by? There might be opportunities with Dean and his family to facilitate such discussions.

- *Educational and communication needs.* How do Dean and his family members integrate experiences in their lives? What educational material needs to be provided and what form should it take? Videos, teaching sheets, and pamphlets can all help educate Dean and Lydia and family about cancer, advance directives, caregiver stress, children's understanding of illness, and additional concerns. You will want to assess literacy level, any communication challenges, tools that can help, and their response to such intervention.

- *Cultural concerns.* You need to explore Dean's culture and the impact culture has on his values, beliefs, and attitudes. What does it mean to be sick? What does it mean to have cancer? Does his culture preclude open discussion of death and dying or impact the process of advance care planning? Are there family members that have differing views? How may cultural values and beliefs inform care planning?

- *Support systems and caregiver concerns.* What help will Lydia need? Who else in the family can provide care? If acceptable to Dean and Lydia, are there friends, family members, church members, or neighbors who might participate in care or provide respite for Lydia? How much stress is Lydia experiencing? What type of care can Lydia provide? How does the marital relationship impact the care Lydia may be able to provide and Dean may be able to receive? What can our team do to help Lydia feel more confident in providing care? Would it be helpful for Dean and Lydia to have a volunteer? Does Dean want to die at home and does Lydia agree with this plan? How can we help them to know how they can count on the hospice team if they decide to have Dean die at home? How can we help them prepare and know what steps to take? How can we validate Lydia and let her know she is giving Dean a precious gift?

This is not an exhaustive list of issues and concerns, but it can help convey some of the areas the social worker will assess over time, as he or she intervenes and works cooperatively with team members to create a care plan that responds to this family and illness experience. While two physicians have confirmed that Dean has a terminal diagnosis and a prognosis of 6 months or less to live, Dean may have much less than 6 months. Social workers must approach each patient with uncertainty as to when death will occur; when death is imminent, crisis intervention skills are often needed (Gardia & Raymer, 2005). Every death is unique and each plan of care individualized. Social workers may have to prioritize issues and concerns based on the patient's prognosis or length of stay in the hospice program.

Challenges and Opportunities

With the growth of hospice programs, a climate of dissatisfaction with health care, the evolution of health care reform, and the push to improve safety in health care, hospice has been under increased scrutiny by the Office of Inspector General, fiscal intermediaries of CMS, and Medicare Payment Advisory Commission (MedPac), a health care advisory group that reports to Congress. The increased scrutiny is welcomed by some hospice providers. Families that have had a poor experience with one hospice generalize the experience to all hospices and all other programs suffer. Knowing generalization occurs, the hospice industry cautions, "If you've seen one hospice program, you've only seen one hospice program." Despite efforts to enforce uniform care by Medicare, hospice care varies greatly in the United States. Scrutiny should improve services, and the public must be protected from hospice programs that fail to deliver the care they promised to provide.

In conjunction with closer scrutiny, hospice is now being expected to provide data to demonstrate outcomes. Hospice has been slow to embrace technology and has relied primarily on collecting data manually. If you are a hospice program with 50 or fewer patients a day, it is possible to manually collect quality assurance data. Larger programs may be drowning in data and often have multiple data collection systems that do not communicate with each other. Pharmacy records, patient financial information, human resources information, and patient records may all be tracked using separate software systems. The cost for hardware, software, and personnel has challenged many hospice providers. Hospice is under increased pressure to find electronic solutions so more systematic information can be collected to support the tracking of patient outcomes.

Given the drive to collect patient information on a national level, documentation is quickly changing in the hospice industry. Many programs are in the process of utilizing electronic medical records (EMRs) and software that may not have included the expert input of social work clinicians. Additionally, many hospice providers are requiring that documentation be done at the bedside of the patient, a practice referred to as point of service (POS). Initially some social workers are resistant to EMSs and POSs, believing both create a barrier to good communication (Cornwall, 2009). Many believe that the benefits of EMRs far outweigh the potential burden of laptops, and that EMRs will become commonplace in hospice in the near future (NHPCO, 2009).

In the past, most hospice programs assigned the task of creating a psychosocial assessment tool to social workers. It is a concern that in the past few years a number of programs have started to utilize electronic patient information systems that contain assessment tools that seem to have little input from hospice social workers. Assessment data are critical, because select data elements, such as the rating of a patient's pain level on admission, and on subsequent visits, will be used to demonstrate the effect of hospice services on a patient's quality of life. Data elements that capture and measure social work and spiritual care outcomes are in their infancy, and outcome research is desperately needed. In the meantime social workers can contribute to process improvement initiatives.

Social work has historically advocated for underserved populations. In recent years, hospice providers have made efforts to reach out to special populations such as minorities, prisons, and veterans programs (Bronstein & Wright, 2006; Edes, Shreve, & Casarett, 2007; Linder & Meyers, 2007; Washington, Bickel-Swenson, & Stephens, 2008; Winstron, 2004–2005). Social workers, in consultation with interdisciplinary colleagues, need to conduct research to understand barriers that prevent populations from utilizing hospice care and to shed light on the full range of attitudes toward death and end-of-life care.

Conclusion

Hospice care in the United States has existed for over 30 years. What started as a grassroots movement, with a small band of dedicated volunteers running hospice programs, has evolved into programs with professional staff, more physician input and oversight, and regulations designed to standardize services. Despite CMS efforts, variability remains a challenge in the hospice industry.

Social workers have a key role as members of the hospice interdisciplinary team and offer most of the emotional and psychosocial support provided to the patient and family. Assessment, interventions, and the creation of a care plan are the main responsibilities of the social worker in hospice. Specialized knowledge and skill are required to meet the needs of dying patients and their families, including the provision of bereavement services after the death of the patient. Responsibilities include patient education, administrative duties, and advocacy on micro and macro levels. In addition, many of the nationally recognized hospice programs viewed as innovative and award winning have been developed and are led by social workers.

Currently, there is a great deal of change confronting hospice providers and social workers. Electronic medical records and point-of-service models require social workers to alter their interaction with patients and families to accommodate electronic equipment. Higher levels of scrutiny are an opportunity to demonstrate positive outcomes for hospice patients and families. Finally, research is needed in multiple areas of psychosocial care, with immediate attention to measuring outcomes and to understanding the barriers that impact access to hospice for underserved populations.

Holistic, interdisciplinary care and consideration of the impact of disease on both the patient and the patient's family are the hallmarks of hospice philosophy. Health care in general could benefit from lessons learned in caring for the terminally ill and could create a new gold standard of care for all patients.

Hospice needs to continue to attract social workers to the field, mentor those currently working in end-of-life care, participate in succession planning to build leaders and insure a skilled workforce. The future of hospice depends on the next generation of social workers. Our patients and families and the systems within which we practice continue to need our voices.

LEARNING EXERCISES

Using the patient and family narrative about Dean and Lydia, explore the following questions:

1. What additional issues might arise?
2. How is religion different from spirituality? How comfortable are you with the patient asking you to pray with him or her? What do you do if you have a different belief system?
3. What are the physical signs to watch for that indicate a patient is close to dying?
4. Is denial a problem for dying patients, for family members? Why or why not?
5. Many phrases used by hospice social workers have not necessarily been researched, but they seem to provide comfort to family members, for example: "Maybe your loved one chose to die while you went to get coffee to spare you." Should social workers continue to use such phrases? What might be a potential positive outcome of these words; what might be a potential negative outcome for families?
6. How do we protect the rights of the dying/the bereaved while doing much needed research?
7. What types of information would you want to communicate with team members? What information would you as the social worker want communicated to you? What information do you consider confidential? Are there any limits to confidentiality?
8. What ethical dilemmas might arise when Dean can no longer speak for himself?
9. What age appropriate services might benefit Dean and Lydia's grandchildren?

ADDITIONAL RESOURCES AND WEB SITES

The Hastings Center. National Hospice Work Group. (2003). *Access to hospice care expanding boundaries, overcoming barriers*. Garrison, NY: The Hastings Center.

Huff, M., Weisenfluh, S., & Murphy, M. (2008). *End of life care: A manual for social work students and practitioners*. Alexandria, VA: National Hospice and Palliative Care Organization.

Munson, C. (2002). *Clinical social work supervision*. Binghamton, NY: Haworth Press Inc.

Parker-Oliver, D., Wiienberg-Lyles, E., Washington, K. T., & Seema, S. (2009). Social work role in hospice pain management: A national survey. *Journal of Social Work in End-of-Life & Palliative Care, 5*(E1-2), 61–74.

Rando, T. (1984). *Grief, dying and death, clinical interventions for caregivers*. Champaign, IL: Research Press.

Sharoff, K. (2004). *Coping skills manual for treating chronic and terminal illness*. New York, NY: Springer Publishing Company Inc.

WEB SITES

Centers for Medicare & Medicaid Services: http://www.cms.hhs.gov/CFCsAndCoPs/05_Hospice.asp#TopOfPage
Link to hospice conditions of participation.

National Association of Social Workers (NASW): http://www.socialworkers.org
Information on social work advance practice credential for hospice and palliative care and end-of-life online course.

National Council of Hospice and Palliative Care Organization: http://www.nhpco.org
Current statistical data on the member hospice and palliative care programs. The National Council of Hospice and Palliative Professionals, social work section provides resource materials to members (must be a member to access mynhpco, the social work list serv).

Respecting Choices: http://www.respectingchoices.org
Information on advance care planning. Offers online course work for becoming a trainer.

REFERENCES

Bronstein, L., & Wright, K. (2006). The impact of prison hospice: Collaboration among social workers and other professionals in the criminal justice setting that promotes care for the dying. *Journal of Social Work in End-of-Life and Palliative Care, 2*(4), 85–102.

Conner, S. (2009). *Hospice and palliative care: The essential guide (2nd ed.)*. New York, NY: Routledge Taylor and Francis Group.

Cornwall, J. (2009, Sept.). Point of care documentation: Perception versus reality. *Newsline*, p. 15–16.

Edes, T., Shreve, S., & Casarett, D. (2007). Increasing access and quality in Department of Veterans Affairs care at the end of life: A lesson in change. *Journal of American Geriatrics Society, 55*(10), 164–169.

Gardia, G., & Raymer, M. (2007). What social workers do. Alexandria, VA: National Hospice and Palliative Care Organization.

Linder, J., & Meyers, F. (2007). Palliative care for prison inmates: Don't let me die in prison. *Journal of American Medical Association, 298*, 894–901.

National Hospice and Palliative Care Organization (NHPCO). (2008). *National Hospice and Palliative Care Organization social work guidelines (rev. ed.)*. Alexandria, VA: Author.

Neimeyer, R. (2005). *Widowhood, grief and the quest for meaning: A narrative perspective on resilience, late life widowhood in the United States*. New York, NY: Springer.

Prigerson, H. G., Horowitz, M. J., Jacobs, S. C., Parkes, C. M., Aslan, M., Goodkin, K., … Maciejewski, P. K. (2009) Prolonged Grief Disorder: Psychometric Validation of Criteria Proposed for DSM-V and ICD-11. *PLoS Medicine, 6*(8), e1000121.

Project on Death in America. Open Society Institute. (2001, Dec.). A new social work study by social work leader Mary Raymer: Social work services save money (8th ed.). New York, NY: Open Society Institute.

Raymer, M., & Donna, M. (2004). Living with dying. In J. Berzoff & P. Silverman (Eds.), The history of social work in hospice (p. 150–160). New York, NY: Columbia University Press.

Reese, D. (2006). Interdisciplinary perceptions of the social work role in hospice. Paper presented at the Annual Program Meeting of the Council on Social Work Education, Chicago, IL.

Washington, K., Bickel-Swenson, D., & Stephens, N. (2008). Barriers to hospice use among African Americans: A systematic review. *Health and Social Work, 33*(4), 267–274.

Winstron, C., Leshner, P., Kramer, J., & Allen, G. (2005). Overcoming barriers to access and utilization of hospice and palliative care services in African-American communities. *Omega, 50*(2), 151–163.

9 *Stacy F. Orloff*

Pediatric Hospice and Palliative Care: The Invaluable Role of Social Work

The day our child was diagnosed, the world changed. Nothing looked the same; even the colors of the sky and grass looked different. Our family was shaken in a way we did not know was possible. I didn't think we'd survive.

—Parent of a child diagnosed with a life-limiting illness

Key Concepts

- ◆ *It is important to understand and identify the key skills utilized by the pediatric hospice or palliative social worker.*
- ◆ *Health care professionals desire to understand the unique pediatric social work role on the interdisciplinary team.*
- ◆ *Social workers learn to recognize the importance and influence of cultural factors in providing care to children and families.*
- ◆ *Biopsychosocial-spiritual assessments and interventions are much more successful when social workers recognize and understand the differences in providing care to infants, children, and adolescents.*

Introduction

This chapter will address the major roles of the hospital- and home-based hospice and palliative social worker, including assessment strategies and interventions when providing hospice and palliative care to children with life-limiting illnesses or conditions and their families. Consider narrative in Box 9.1A which provides an introduction to Maria and her family.

What might the hospital social worker ask first? Where to start? This chapter will help guide the reader in answering these and other questions. This narrative will be referenced throughout the chapter to reinforce major teaching points.

Key Concepts and Skills

Let's start at the beginning. Before discussing the role of the pediatric hospice and palliative social worker, it is important to agree upon key concepts and skills. While it is beyond the scope of this chapter to describe the core social work competencies in palliative and end-of-life care, a good review of these competencies can be found in Gwyther et al. (2005).

It is a standard tenet of pediatric and adult hospice and palliative care that all patients and their families benefit greatly from ongoing and seamlessly integrated care that focuses on the spiritual, emotional, social, and physical domains. Further, these efforts must be coordinated with all teams providing care to the child and family. This includes all hospital, home, and community-based providers (Heller & Solomon, 2005; Himelstein, Hilden, Boldt & Weissman, 2004).

Palliative care is based on relationships. Honest, caring, and sincere relationships between the child and his or her family with all health care providers are vital. Heller and Solomon (2005) interviewed 36 bereaved parents. Their research findings support the importance of these human relationships. The authors found that these relationships are a key element in how parents evaluated the continuity and quality of care their children received. Additionally, 78% of parents

---

Box 9.1A.
Patient/Family Narrative: Maria

Maria is a 12-year-old Latina female diagnosed with cystic fibrosis when she was a baby. Her mother, a single parent raising three additional children, was uncertain about how or when to share information about Maria's diagnosis. By the time Maria was 12, she had been hospitalized more than six times. She knew she had breathing problems that required her to take several different medications and breathing treatments. Because no one had ever really provided Maria with a developmentally appropriate explanation of her illness, she remained confused about what it really meant to have cystic fibrosis and when she would "outgrow" it.

Maria was recently hospitalized for an emergent breathing problem. She developed several complications, and her mother was quite worried. Maria's siblings (two younger, 7 years and 9 years; one older, 15 years) were scared. The younger siblings had little information about what was really wrong with Maria and what it meant. Maria's older brother understood much more about cystic fibrosis. Most of his information came from the Internet. He was afraid to ask his mother many questions because in the past she had made it clear she did not want to talk about it.

The hospital palliative social worker stopped in Maria's hospital room to say hello. Her older brother was visiting. Maria's younger siblings and mother were downstairs in the cafeteria. The social worker and Maria had developed a warm relationship based on time spent together during Maria's former hospitalizations. Although they had not talked in depth about Maria's illness and prognosis, Maria had talked about some of her other concerns such as missing school, her fears of being left out of her social group, and worry about her future.

Today Maria told the social worker she had some questions. Both Maria and her brother asked whether she had some time to talk privately with them. The social worker sat down on the side of Maria's bed and asked …

---

commented they had at least one or more staff who they could always "count on" to be involved in their child's care. Parental confidence in this consistent relationship relieved them of the burden they often felt having to coordinate all aspects of their child's care. In essence, parents felt access to a consistent caring member of the team ensured their child would receive excellent care. This level of confidence may also allow parents to leave the hospital setting at times to spend time with their other children, go home for a shower, or have a quiet respite. Pediatric social workers play an important role on the interdisciplinary team to ensure the team functions in this heightened capacity.

On the other hand, lack of consistency (whether from an individual or team) within the hospital environment intensified parental suffering and feelings of mistrust and anxiety. Parents also perceived that their child was more vulnerable and suffered. This lack of consistency may cause parents to be hypervigilant and attentive to every aspect of their child's care because they were less confident in the staff's ability to provide excellent care (Heller & Solomon, 2005). Team members, sensing parental discontent, may respond by withdrawing, blaming the parents for problems, and miscommunication or reacting defensively.

Social Work Skill Set

Social workers are qualified to build and maintain relationships of continuity because our education and training are based on relationships and values that foster client self-determination, empowerment, and social support (Jones, 2005; National Association of Social Workers [NASW], 2004). They are also trained in systems theory, family development, and counseling skills for children of different ages. Social workers learn cultural aspects of care in graduate school, although everyone must continue this training daily at one's workplace.

In 2004, the National Association of Social Workers (NASW) published a monograph entitled Standards for Social Work Practice in Palliative and End-of-Life Care. This important monograph contains 11 standards to guide social work practice. Additionally, in 2008, NASW and the National Hospice and Palliative Care Organization (NHPCO) jointly developed a certification for hospice and palliative social workers. Called the Advanced Hospice and Palliative Care Social Worker credential, it is one of the first official steps to recognize the specialized skill set of hospice and palliative social workers (National Association of Social Workers, 2008). Both the monograph and the credential reflect the "best of" skill set of palliative or hospice social workers.

A 2005 survey of the Association of Pediatric Oncology Social Workers (APOSW) by Jones yielded a response rate of 50% (N = 131). APOSW members ranked key services provided by pediatric social workers and identified the most important roles of the ideal pediatric oncology social worker. From this data Jones was able to collate six principal components of the ideal role. They are as follows:

- Advocate/educator
  - For control over treatment decisions
  - For family control
- Specialized pediatric palliative care service
  - Play therapy/expressive arts therapy
  - Access to complementary/alternative therapies
  - Timely discussion about transition from curative to palliative care
- Counselor for children
  - Supportive counseling for siblings
  - Supportive counseling for child
- Bereavement counselor
  - Bereavement support
- Provider of psychosocial assessment

- Individual psychosocial assessment of the family's needs
- Individual psychosocial assessment of the child's needs
- Confidant/companion
  - Listing to concerns, fears, hopes
  - Supportive counseling to parents (Jones, 2005, p. 46).

Social Work Assessments

Pediatric social workers assess the family as a unit and all members individually. Assessments include both the micro aspects obtained from the biopsychosocial-spiritual assessment and the macro view, including the greater community that interacts with the child and family unit, such as a faith community, school, and service groups. It is important to understand the developmental level of each person and the family as a unit in order to assess readiness to complete tasks, including those associated with normal development. The pediatric social worker's biopsychosocial-spiritual assessment focuses on the child and other family members' experiences of emotional, spiritual, social, and physical symptoms; the effectiveness and quality of the family's communication style; their decision-making process; and the need for case management assistance such as financial and social support (McSherry, Kehoe, Carroll, Kang, & Rourke, 2007; Meier & Beresford, 2008).

This comprehensive and ongoing assessment includes information about the family history, what is unique about their behavior, and how it is understood within the larger context. Training in systems theory enhances the social worker's understanding of the person in his or her environment. Cultural and spiritual practices are also an important component of the comprehensive assessment as well as identifying any mental health issues that could impact the family's ability to cope with the child's current illness and treatment (Sourkes et al., 2005).

Social workers assess for signs of anticipatory grief, beginning at the time of admission to the palliative care or hospice program and continuing throughout the treatment process until remission of disease or the child's death. A thorough assessment includes attention to the following:

- The nature of day-to-day losses over the course of the illness
- Assisting parents to stay connected to their ill child as well as their healthy children
- The unique nature of grief for the mother and the father (as well as other family members)
- Negotiating needed changes in the family routine and family communication, while maintaining healthy marital and parent–child relationships
- Ensuring effective communication between and among the family and health care provider

- Engaging in funeral preplanning as appropriate and as they may wish to do
- Recognizing manifestations of grief in the other children in the family, both during the illness and after the death
- Identifying and connecting with resources in the community for financial, emotional, and spiritual support (National Hospice and Palliative Care Organization [NHPCO], 2000).

For additional information on how social workers can assist in assessing spiritual concerns, see the Children's Project on Palliative/Hospice Services (ChiPPS) for a spiritual assessment that can used by a pediatric social worker (Davies, Brenner, Orloff, Sumner, & Worden, 2002). ChiPPS is an interdisciplinary pediatric workgroup organized under the auspices of the National Hospice and Palliative Care Organization (NHPCO). ChiPPS has its own Web page as part of the NHPCO website (http://www.nhpco.org/i4a/pages/index.cfm?pageid=3409).

Pediatric social workers provide education and support. We listen. We share. We intervene to guide the family along the path they are on. We do all this with as much presence and humanity as possible (Mellichamp, 2007).

So what did the hospital social worker do next when meeting with Maria and her brother? (See narrative in Box 9.1B.)

The hospital social worker has done a good job thus far recognizing some of the major cultural and family system issues related to communication with Maria's family. She was respectful of the mother and her role within the family. She understood the importance of letting Maria's mother know she responded to the children's request for a visit and did not initiate it herself. The social worker anticipated that the palliative care team might need some assistance in understanding Latino culture since most of Maria's health care providers are not Latino. As a member of the nondominant culture within the hospital setting, it is sometimes difficult for Maria's mother to ask questions and get her needs met. The social worker is also uncertain whether there are any linguistic concerns she or the other team members might be overlooking. Finally, she has learned much from Maria's mother about the different roles of family members in this Latino family, and she is eager to share these newfound insights with the team. The social worker understands that cultural beliefs and traditions play an important role in shaping attitudes, and they often affect behavioral responses related to diagnosis, treatment, symptoms, death, and bereavement (Knapp & Contro, 2009; Sourkes et al., 2005).

Additionally, Maria's mother was provided useful information about local community supports, which assisted with financial resources and helped her to reconnect with her local church. The social worker in this narrative understood that it can be difficult to assist a family with resolving emotional conflicts when their basic needs are not met. The social worker recognized that until Maria's mother's distress about her financial condition and lack of religious and spiritual

Box 9.1B.
Patient/Family Narrative: Maria (continued)

The hospital social worker asks whether it is okay to sit down on the side of Maria's bed. She tells Maria and her brother she is glad they invited her in for a visit. Knowing that it has only been a few months since her last hospitalization, and knowing that Maria's mother has struggled to provide her with developmentally relevant information about her disease, the social worker asks Maria whether there's something in particular she wants to discuss, The social worker is also aware that Maria's mother is worried about losing her job due to Maria's frequent hospitalizations. Their extended family does not live close by; however, the family is very involved with a local church. Based on previous short conversations the social worker has had with Maria, she wonders whether Maria is worried about her prognosis and how she might engage in conversation with her mother about this.

Based on her prior assessments and the veiled looks the social worker observes between Maria and her brother, the social worker asks the siblings whether they would like to do an art project to express their feelings. With permission from the children, the pictures are shared with their mother as a bridge to enhancing communication. She is careful to let the mother know that the children asked for the meeting and agreed to draw pictures of their feelings. The social worker shares the context in which the clinical work occurred to ensure that the mother understands that her role and family relationships have been respected and that her children created the opportunity for this clinical work. Maria's mother is shocked to see how much Maria and her brother comprehend both Maria's medical situation and the impact on the family emotionally, physically, financially, and spiritually. She goes into her daughter's hospital room and asks her whether she would like to talk about the picture. She also asks Maria whether she would like her brother to participate in the discussion. Maria says yes to both questions.

A few days later the social worker sees Maria's mother in a small day room on the hospital floor. After the social worker comments that she looks tired, Maria's mother shares her worry about paying her bills. The social worker is able to assist Maria's mother in obtaining some additional financial assistance as well as increased emotional support through her church.

connection were diminished, it would be difficult to invite her to focus on the emotional components of Maria's illness.

The palliative or hospice social worker provides care to all members of the family. Social work knowledge base includes information about child development, family life-cycle issues, parental needs, and extended family needs. The biopsychosocial-spiritual assessment is systems based and includes all key individuals and organizations. Assessment may also be thought of as an intervention because it has the potential to partialize experience and validate the child and family's perceptions. Key roles and tasks are similar regardless of whether the social worker is providing palliative care or hospice care. They are as follows:

- Ensure the team provides family-centered care
- Address the biopsychosocial-spiritual aspects of pain and symptom management

- Ensure access to community resources and assistance through case management
- Advocate for needs of patient and family within the community and the team
- Facilitate communication between the team and the family
- Balance family need for hope with open direct information
- Assist with advance care planning
- Provide psychosocial assistance that addresses needs of individual family members, including extended family such as grandparents
- Facilitate psychosocial care throughout the diagnostic, treatment, and final phases of illness (Kovacs, Bellin, & Fauri, 2006; Sourkes et al., 2005)

Parental Needs

Parents of ill children also have needs. They want health care providers who provide accurate and honest information. Parents appreciate the patience of the team in understanding that they may need to ask their questions repeatedly until they are able to comprehend and remember the answers. In a study by Brosig et al. (2007), bereaved parents whose infant children died ranked the following as the most important aspects of care:

- Honesty
  - Honest information, even if it meant receiving "bad news"
- Empowered decision making
  - Particularly regarding withdrawal of life support
- Parental care
  - Appreciated staff taking care of them also
- Environment
  - Hospital environment may be an issue for some parents; however, the people present at time of death are the most important
- Faith and trust in nursing care
  - Trust allowed parents to leave hospital for brief time
- Physician bearing witness
  - Particularly in hospital, important for physician to be present at time of death
- Support from other hospital care providers
  - Appreciated support from other hospital palliative care team members (Brosig, Pierucci, Kupst, & Leuthner, 2007, pp. 512–513).

Brosig et al.'s study (2007) also identified seven coping strategies bereaved parents used. Social workers regularly assist parents in utilizing these coping strategies when providing anticipatory grief and bereavement support. They are as follows:

- Providing support to the entire family unit (as defined by the family)
- Assisting in keeping the child's memory alive
- Providing spiritual and faith-based support
- Assisting the family to respond to their sense of altruism, to give back when they are ready
- Refocusing on life
- Validating decisions made by the family
- Providing information about bereavement support groups

Parents who felt they were part of all treatment decisions coped better during their bereavement and had a more positive perception about their child's end-of-life care regardless of how long the child lived. Conversely, parents who felt their decision to remove life support was not supported had more difficulty coping. A critical finding of Brosig et al.'s study is that the quality of relationships parents formed with providers was critically important in how they coped after their child's death. Ongoing contact with members of the health care team was important. Social workers' strength-based training is an important lens through which we assist parents in having the aforementioned needs met.

Social work is one of the few disciplines that may be involved with a child and his or her family throughout the illness, from diagnosis, treatment, final phase of care, and through bereavement. This unique role provides great opportunity and responsibility in providing patient/family-centered care and is critical in assisting parents in their bereavement. It also may help to reduce the sense of abandonment some families feel when they move from one health care setting to another (Sourkes et al., 2005). Social workers may serve as a companion and guide and thereby represent a continuity of relationship and a participation in the ongoing narrative of the ill child and family that may be reassuring and also have the potential to add a historical perspective to ongoing decision making. Social work training is helpful in identifying and understanding ethical dilemmas. Often a vocal member on the team, social workers encourage truth telling and honesty, frequently giving voice to the family's unique suffering and assisting the teams in understanding the effect of psychosocial and spiritual suffering (Jones, 2005).

Numerous studies describe the role of the social worker and palliative care/hospice teams in assisting families to maintain and reframe hope. Social workers frequently assist the family in redefining their goals from cure to remission; to comfort; to attending a significant event; to sharing stories and creating a living legacy (Keene, Reder, & Serwint, 2009). Many parents have difficulty coping with their child's illness and have been diagnosed with signs of posttraumatic stress disorder. Symptoms of posttraumatic stress include recurrent and distressing recollections of events, including intense feelings and thoughts that the particular event may continue to occur over and over. Further symptomlogy includes attempts to avoid any stimuli associated with the event. These feelings or behaviors seem to be mitigated when parents have access to honest, clear, and direct information. Parents also express a desire for privacy when death approaches so that they can hold their child (Gudmundsdottir, Elklit, & Gudmundsdottir, 2006; Knapp & Contro, 2009; Landolt, Vollrath, Ribi,Gnehm, & Sennhauser, 2003; Truog, Christ, Browning, & Meyer, 2006).

Developmental Assessments

Pediatric social workers understand child development and how the needs of a young child are different from those of an adolescent. They also consider the life-cycle needs of families. Biopsychosocial-spiritual assessments include an understanding of these multidimensional concerns, and interventions are chosen based on an integrated assessment.

In 2006, Jones surveyed social workers from the Association of Pediatric Oncology Social Workers (APOSW). Part of her query was to determine the psychosocial needs of children and adolescents with cancer. With a 50% response rate her quantitative results showed some distinct differences. APOSW social workers identified the following needs for younger children (0 to 14 years of age) at the end of life (in rank order):

- Communication and expression
  - Assistance with sharing concerns with parents and siblings
  - Choice of where to die
  - Ability to talk freely about fears and feelings
- Disease information and medical control
  - Medical information
  - Education about disease
  - Control over treatment decisions
- Normal activities
  - School interventions
  - Normal childhood activities
  - Assistance with talking to friends
- Counseling and support
  - Supportive counseling
  - Companionship
  - Structured conversations
- Consistent caregivers (Jones, 2006, p. 780)

Adolescent (ages 15 to 21 years) needs ranked slightly differently. They are as follows:

- Personal control
  - Education about disease
  - Medical information

- Structured conversations
- Spiritual support
- Assistance with funeral arrangements
- Normal activities
  - School interventions
  - Normal childhood activities
  - Assistance with talking to friends
- Communication and expression
  - Ability to talk freely about fears/feelings
  - Assistance with sharing concerns with parents and siblings
  - Creative expression
- Consistent caregivers and companionship
  - Consistent communication between caregivers
- Control over medical and treatment decisions
  - Pain control and symptom management
  - Choice of where to die (Jones, 2006, p. 781)

Parents often want to explore all options, regardless of how nonbeneficial they may seem to health care providers. For many, being a good parent means "leaving no stone unturned." Many parents are comforted by the belief they have explored all curative options for their child. Some bereaved parents will frequently remark that it is somewhat easier to cope with their child's death knowing that they considered all forms of treatment. The role of the social worker becomes even more important during these times of transition from hospital to home, from disease-modifying therapies to a primary focus on palliative interventions as described in Maria's evolving narrative (Box 9.1C). Oftentimes the social worker helps the hospice and/or palliative care team to understand how parents can balance the tension between hoping for the best, waiting for a miracle, and understanding their child's prognosis. This balance is typically more difficult for health care providers than it is for parents. The social worker is often the team member who serves as the common link in these discussions between the parents and the interdisciplinary team. Some team members may view uncertain prognosis as a threat; that is, they struggle when parents may not acknowledge a potential negative outcome, believing they must reinforce for the parents consistently and directly the outcome they are anticipating: the child's death. Parents, on the other hand, view this uncertainty as the continuing potential for a good outcome, however that may be defined by them (Keene Reder & Serwint, 2009). Social work training to meet the client where he or she "is" allows social workers to work more comfortably and confidently in this ambiguous and ambivalent area and to help the interdisciplinary team understand and accept this parental response. Their understanding of communication practices and the dynamics underlying behavior provides a context in which to work with the team to consider the thoughts and emotions that influence parents as they make treatment decisions

---

Box 9.1C.
Patient/Family Narrative: Maria (continued)

Eighteen months later, Maria is hospitalized yet again. This is her fourth hospitalization since she and her brother drew their pictures for the palliative social worker. It is very apparent to the hospital palliative care team that Maria's condition has worsened and that medically she meets the criteria for hospice care. The team meets to discuss this transition and decides, given the relationship the social worker has with Maria's mother, that she should initiate the discussion about hospice care.

The social worker guides Maria's mother in a conversation about her daughter's illness and treatment. They discuss the recurring hospitalizations, Maria's increasing weakness, and her difficulty breathing. The social worker also inquires about how the family is coping with all of these changes. Maria's mother is able to acknowledge the physical, emotional, social, and spiritual impact these changes have had on the family. The social worker shares information about hospice care and how closely the hospital palliative care team works with the home-based community hospice. She further explains that this close collaboration will ensure continuity in care for Maria and everyone else in the family. Maria's mother agrees to meet with the hospice pediatric team.

The palliative care team arranges for a pre-admission hospice consult at the hospital. The hospice pediatric nurse and social worker first meet with the palliative care team to learn about Maria's medical history and current status. The palliative social worker then brings them to meet with Maria's mother. After a conversation in which Maria's mother is able to ask questions, she agrees that home-based hospice care is the right choice for her daughter. Maria's mother brings the hospice pediatric nurse and social worker to meet Maria. After a brief introduction the hospital social worker leaves the room so that Maria can talk privately with her "new" team. The hospital palliative care team and hospice pediatric team collaborate on discharge planning and 2 days later Maria is discharged home with hospice care.

---

regarding their child's care (Bluebond-Langer, Bello Belasco, Goldman, & Belasco, 2007). Let's return to Maria and her family now that her care has transitioned to the pediatric hospice interdisciplinary team (see Box 9.1D).

Box 9.1D.
Patient/Family Narrative: Maria (continued)

Maria has been a hospice patient for 7 months. During those 7 months she has returned to the hospital twice. Her mother has talked with the hospice social worker and nurse about not sending Maria back to the hospital. The hospice pediatric team assures her they can provide the level of comfort care Maria will likely need in her final months and days. The pediatric hospice social worker understands the importance of helping Maria's mother and siblings maintain a sense of hope along with providing information that helps them to integrate the many signs of decline. The social worker understands that maintaining hope does not necessarily mean hoping for a cure; it is possible for families to balance hope with accepting the reality of a prognosis. What a family hopes for may

Box 9.1D *(Contd.)*

also change over time. For example, Maria's social worker helps the family to focus hope on Maria's ability to attend her younger sister's dance recital. They also hope to attend a social event at their church the following week. With assistance the family begins to consider immediate tangible events that Maria may be able to participate in. The hospice social worker maintains contact with her hospital palliative counterpart, alerting her to Maria's worsening condition.

The hospice pediatric social worker has been working closely with Maria's three siblings, utilizing many different interventions: play, art, music, and talking. Sometimes they meet all together and other times they prefer seeing the social worker individually. With the permission of Maria's mother, the social worker has provided developmentally appropriate information about Maria's condition and prognosis. In fact, Maria's mother most recently asked the social worker to assist her in telling the other children that Maria would be dying soon. The social worker has been a consistent presence in this family's life and Maria's mother has expressed gratitude that she no longer has to be hypervigilant in coordinating her daughter's care alone.

Today the hospice social worker meets privately with Maria, who wants to talk about her final wishes and her desire to leave a legacy to others. Together they talk about what that means. The social worker writes down Maria's individual thoughts to each of her siblings and her mother. Maria is able to sign her name. Maria also talks to the social worker about a gift she would like to give to each of her sibling and her mother. Maria has already given this a great deal of thought and she is ready to have this conversation. She asks the social worker to wrap the four personal items she has selected for each family member and they then place the personal note along with each item. While they are doing this, the social worker is able to guide Maria in life review. Maria thanks the social worker for assisting her in completing this important task and says she appreciates the social worker's comfort in having this conversation.

Maria later shares these items and her notes with each of her siblings and her mother privately. They cry and hug. Maria's mother told the social worker that she had never seen Maria so peaceful. Their priest comes to visit later that day. Two days later Maria dies. The hospice social worker, with permission from Maria' mother, alerts the hospital palliative care team. They all contact Maria's mother to express their sympathies and attend her funeral service.

The hospice social worker continues to meet regularly with Maria's family individually and together. Maria's siblings each attend a bereavement group at their respective schools that the hospice social worker facilitates. Maria's mother is considering attending a parental bereavement group. She is not sure whether she is ready and appreciates continuing to see the hospice social worker for her bereavement needs. The hospice social worker assures Maria's mother and her siblings that she will continue to provide bereavement support to them as long as they desire.

LEARNING EXERCISES

- Watch one or more of the following DVDs and review teaching guidelines or associated curriculum:
  - Lion in the House
    - http://www.pbs.org/independentlens/lioninthehouse/index.htm

- Initiative for Pediatric Palliative Care
  - http://www.ippcweb.org/
- Making Every Moment Count
  - http://www.fanlight.com/catalog/films/405_memc.php
- Review archived ChiPPS (Children's Project on Palliative/Hospice Services) newsletters at http://www.nhpco.org/i4a/pages/Index.cfm?pageID=4657
- Access the Initiative for Pediatric Palliative Care Web site and review the available curriculum at http://www.ippcweb.org/
- Seek out different mentors to assist in continuing professional development.
- Volunteer with an organization that provides pediatric palliative care or hospice care. Ensure the organization can also provide supervision and consultation to volunteers.

ADDITIONAL SUGGESTED READINGS

Armstrong-Dailey, A., & Zarbock-Goltzer, S. (Eds.). (2009). *Hospice care for children* (3rd ed.). New York, NY: Oxford University Press.

Carter, B. S., & Levetown, M. (Eds.). (2004). *Palliative care for infants, children, and adolescents: A practical handbook.* Baltimore, MD: The Johns Hopkins University Press.

Davies, B., Gudmundsdottir, M., Worden, B., Orloff, S., Sumner, L., & Brenner, P. (2004). Living in the dragon's shadow: Fathers's experiences of a child's life limiting illness. *Death Studies, 28,* 111–135.

Huff, S. & Orloff, S. (Eds.). (2004). *Interdisciplinary clinical manual for pediatric hospice and palliative care.* Arlington, VA: Children's Hospice International.

Journal of Social Work in End-of-Life and Palliative Care. (2007). *3*(3). A special thematic issue related to pediatric hospice and palliative care.

Orloff, S., & Huff, S. (Eds.). (2003). *Home care for seriously ill children: A manual for parents.* Arlington, VA: Children's Hospice International.

REFERENCES

Bluebond-Langer, M., Belasco, J. B., Goldman, A., & Belasco, C. (2007). Understanding parents' approaches to care and treatment of children with cancer when standard therapy has failed. *Journal of Clinical Oncology, 25*(27), 2414–2419.

Brosig, C. L., Pierucci, R. L., Kupst, M. J., & Leuthner, S. R. (2007). In fact end-of-life care: The parents perspective. *Journal of Perinatology, 27,* 510–516.

Browning, D. (2003). To show our humanness: Relational and communicative competence in pediatric palliative care. *Bioethics Forum, 18*(3/4), 23–38.

Davies, B., Brenner, P., Orloff, S., Sumner, L., & Worden, W. (2002). Addressing spirituality in pediatric hospice and palliative care. *Journal of Palliative Care, 18*(1), 59–67.

Gudmundsdottir, H., Elkilt, A., & Gudmundsdottir, D. (2006). PTSD and psychological distress in Icelandic parents of chronically ill children: Does social support have an effect on parental distress? *Scandinavian Journal of Psychology* 47(4), 303–312.

Gwyther, L., Altilio, T., Blacker, S., Christ, G., Csikai, E., Hooyman, N.,... & Howe, J. (2005). Social work competencies in palliative and end-of-life care. *Journal of Social Work in End-of-Life and Palliative Care, 1*(1), 87–120.

Heller, K., & Solomon, M. Z. (2005). Continuity of care and caring: What matters to parents of children with life-threatening conditions. *Journal of Pediatric Nursing, 20*(5), 335–346.

Himelstein, B., Hilden, J., Boldt, A., & Weissman, D. (2004). Pediatric palliative care. *New England Journal of Medicine,350*(17), 1752–1762.

Jones, B. (2005). Pediatric palliative and end-of-life care: The role of social work in pediatric oncology. *Journal of Social Work in End-of-Life and Palliative Care, 1*(4), 35–62.

Jones, B. (2006). Companionship, control, and compassion: A social work perspective on the needs of children with cancer and their families at the end of life. *Journal of Palliative Medicine, 9*(3), 774–788.

Keene Reder, E. A., & Serwint, J. R. (2009). Until the last breath: Exploring the concept of hope for parents and health care professionals during a child's serious illness. *Archives of Pediatric Adolescent Medicine, 163*(7), 653–657.

Knapp, C., & Contro, N. (2009). Family support services in pediatric palliative care. *American Journal of Hospice and Palliative Care Online First.* Published on October 16, 2009 as doi:10.1177/1049909109350205.

Kovacs, P., Bellin, M. H., & Fauri, D. (2006). Family-centered care: A resource for social work in end-of-life and palliative care. *Journal of Social Work in End-of-Life and Palliative Care, 2*(1), 13–27.

Landolt, M., Vollrath, M., Ribi, K., Gnehm, H., & Sennhauser, F. (2003). Incidence and associations of parental and child posttraumatic stress symptoms in pediatric patients. *Journal of Child Psychology and Psychiatry, 44*(8), 1199–1207.

McSherry, M., Kehoe, K., Carroll, J., Kang, T., & Rourke, M. (2007). Psychosocial and spiritual needs of children living with a life-limiting illness. *Pediatric Clinics of North America, 54,* 609–629.

Meier, D. E., & Beresford, L. (2008). Social workers advocate for a seat at palliative care table. *Journal of Palliative Medicine, 11*(1), 10–14.

Mellichamp, P. (2007). End-of-life care for infants. *Home Healthcare Nurse, 25*(1), 41–44.

National Association of Social Workers (NASW). (2004). Standards for social work practice in palliative and end of life care. Retrieved from http://www.naswdc.org/practice/bereavement/standards/default.asp

National Association of Social Workers. (2008). NHPCO and NASW announce the first advanced certified hospice and palliative care social worker credential [Press release]. Retrieved from http://www.nhpco.org/i4a/pages/index.cfm?pageid=5765

National Hospice and Palliative Care Organization (NHPCO). (2000). *Compendium of pediatric palliative care.* Alexandria, VA: Author.

Sourkes, B., Frankel, L., Brown, M., Contro, N., Benitz, W., Case, C.,... & Sunde, C. (2005). Food, toys, and love: Pediatric palliative care. *Current Problems in Pediatric Adolescent Health Care, 35,* 350–386.

Troug, R, Christ, G., Browing, D., & Meyer, E. (2006). Sudden traumatic death in children. *Journal of the American Medical Association, 295,* 2646–2654.

10

Elena Davis-Stenhouse, Kennan Moore, and Becky Niemeyer

Home-Based Palliative Care

[Having a home palliative care social worker] is like an angel dropping in on me. [The team] is like a family, always there for you. I've never had anything that makes me feel so good. [The home palliative program] makes all the difference in the world. If I'm scared about anything, I just call.

—Virginia Henriksen, 84-year-old patient with lung cancer

Key Concepts

- *Home palliative care is a type of specialty palliative care practice that includes a variety of different practice models, with and without social workers, designed to meet the needs of persons living at home with chronic, advanced, and, in some cases, terminal illnesses.*
- *Home palliative care is a relatively new, still evolving specialty practice that requires additional research to develop, maintain, and advance best social work practice standards.*
- *Palliative social workers are poised to impact the future of home palliative care with their unique approach to considering the "person in environment," sensitivity to safeguarding the needs of vulnerable and oppressed populations, and dedication to quality transdisciplinary care.*

Introduction

The creation of the Medicare Hospice Benefit in 1983 was crucial to the growth of the hospice movement in the United States and is discussed elsewhere in this textbook. While the Hospice Benefit created a funding stream for providing interdisciplinary palliative care to terminally ill patients, it also resulted in a difficult choice for patients and families. The Medicare Hospice Benefit "provides palliative care rather than traditional medical care and curative treatment" (Medicare and Medicaid Hospice Conditions of Participation, 2009). This either/or dichotomy has come to be known as "making the hospice choice." To some persons and families, this is a distressing dilemma. As medical interventions and treatments continue to prolong life and improve quality, the hospice capitated system is being challenged to adapt to an evolving health care system. Changes in health care policy and financing are ongoing, and social workers are actively involved in discussions and change efforts. Unmet needs are being identified in the evolving specialty of palliative care and, in some cases, are giving rise to the development of a continuum of palliative care program models.

In this chapter, we will describe the current research on home palliative care programs both in the United States and worldwide. Palliative care initially evolved in an acute care setting and has only recently expanded into the community. Over the last 10 years, various approaches to home palliative care have been piloted and new research models are being operationalized. We will discuss the various home palliative care programs and present a synopsis of three composite conceptual models and two practice variables. There are many diverse populations who are vulnerable to being underserved or missed entirely by home palliative care programs; this chapter will present several brief patient narratives that illustrate the role of the home palliative social worker as patient advocate and team educator. Navigating transitions of care is often a key challenge for home palliative care teams and presents opportunities for social workers to coordinate successful care transitions. This chapter will explore some of the care transitions that are unique to home palliative care.

Research: The United States and Beyond

A literature search on home palliative care programs yields a relatively small (as compared with hospice) but growing body of research. In the United States, while home hospice and other home health services covered under Medicare, or other insurances, have been available to people for many years, access to alternative models of palliative care such as home palliative care, which helps patients with pain and symptom management and maximizes quality of life, remains limited (Brumley et al., 2007). As many health care providers demand a strong evidence base before investing in new programs, additional scientifically rigorous research is needed to support implementing palliative care in the home setting. As such, social workers are needed to participate in research that supports wider access to palliative care for an increasingly diverse population; they are also needed to advocate, particularly for the role of palliative social workers in direct practice with all patients and families and in the continued development of palliative care policy (Kramer, Christ, Bern-Klug, & Francoeur, 2005).

Various models of home palliative care provide a wide array of services in alignment with the individual patient's goals and preferences, including pursuit of treatments that offer possibility of a cure or longer life expectancy, and interventions to manage pain and other distressing symptoms that impact overall quality of life (Brumley et al., 2007). In addition, the literature reveals a variety of team compositions in each model of home palliative care delivery—some models utilize an interdisciplinary team of physician, nurse, social worker, and chaplain, while others provide a physician and/or nurse as the primary care team with supplemental services of a social worker, chaplain, or physical therapist available upon request (Finlay et al., 2002). Finlay et al. conducted a systematic review of various palliative care models in different settings that included 22 studies that examined home palliative care models (2002). He commented that while most of these studies lacked strong comparative designs, there were nonetheless very positive outcomes for patients who received home palliative care from "multiprofessional teams" trained in palliative care, particularly increasing patient's satisfaction levels with pain and symptom management. This review also points to results that indicate that trained, multiprofessional teams help to deliver cost-effective care as well.

The effectiveness of home palliative care programs is the subject of ongoing research not just in the United States but worldwide. Researchers in Norway utilized a cluster randomized trial design to examine outcomes (location of death and amount of time during last month of life in nursing home or hospital) of a palliative care service that provided both inpatient and home palliative care (Jordhoy et al., 2000).

This model included a social worker as part of the inpatient consult team and for home support thereafter, but the doctor and nurse were considered the primary professional caregivers. The research team found that of the patients who died, more intervention patients died at home than those in control group ($p < .05$), and while hospital utilization was similar in both groups, the intervention patients did spend a shorter amount of time in nursing homes than did patients in the control group. A study in Sweden examined how a home palliative care service impacted perceptions of meaning for the family caregivers of cancer patients (Appelin, Broback, & Bertero, 2005). Italian researchers have offered insight into the experiences of palliative care patients, their family members, and the nurses providing care (Peruselli et al., 1999). In South Korea, researchers found that a model utilizing a palliative care nurse in the patient's home did positively impact patient quality of life, helped relieve pain and other symptoms, and increased family caregiver support (Hwang & Ryu, 2009). An English model offered home palliative care support to patients from a palliative care physician (Bush, Wearne, Reilly, Chacko, & Palmer, 2009). From Canada, Johnson, Abernathy, Howell, Brazil, and Scott (2009) looked at cost-related outcomes associated with utilization of acute and other health care for patients enrolled in an interdisciplinary home palliative care program. A study in Germany compared hospital and home palliative care (Jocham, 2006), while Kuhlen et al. (2009) provided results from a German pediatric home palliative care program. One care model in Australia provides a home palliative care nurse who delivers care to patients, and also offers palliative care education to other home health nurses (Arnaert & Wainwright, 2009).

In the United States, Kaiser Permanente has conducted significant research in home palliative care. A 2003 study by Brumley, Enguidanos, and Cherin, enrolled 558 patients (210 in the palliative care program and 338 in the usual care group receiving standard home health care) and evaluated whether a home palliative care service provided by an interdisciplinary team composed of a physician, nurse, and social worker demonstrated improved patient and family satisfaction. They also evaluated whether such care had an impact on utilization of other medical care services such as emergency room visits, hospitalizations, and skilled nursing facility admissions. The intervention group in this nonequivalent comparison group study was composed of patients with a prognosis of 1 year or less with a diagnosis of cancer, chronic obstructive pulmonary disease (COPD), or congestive heart failure (CHF), while the comparison group consisted of patients with a less-than 24-month prognosis and similar diagnoses but receiving more traditional home health services. Patients and caregivers in the intervention group were able to communicate with their palliative care teams about their treatment preferences and goals of care; based on individual goals, some patients received home palliative care concurrently with life-extending, curative treatment(s), while others preferred to receive home palliative care as part of a focus on "comfort care"—that is, care focused on relieving symptoms, enhancing quality of remaining life, and easing the dying process. Preferences and goals identified by the patients then guided specific interventions to regularly assess and manage pain and other symptoms, assist with medication management, offer psychosocial and spiritual support, and help with identification of resources to increase stability and safety at home as needed. Patients had access to the palliative care team 24 hours a day, 7 days a week via telephone, and after-hours home visits were available if needed. Patients in the comparison group were provided standard home health as regulated by Medicare guidelines and in response to acute care needs. The results of this study revealed that while being a comparison and not a randomized study, enrollment in this palliative care program did offer high-quality care defined as high patient satisfaction scores all while lowering costs and rates of access to acute care settings (Brumley et al., 2003). Brumley et al. suggest that a key to high levels of patient satisfaction is offering palliative care interventions while the patient is still seeking a cure and doing so as early as possible, thus reducing the need for trips to the emergency room, the hospital, or a skilled nursing facility.

In 2007, another Kaiser Permanente randomized controlled trial (N = 298) followed intervention and comparison group patients in California, Hawaii, and Colorado to examine whether palliative care provided at home by an interdisciplinary team of a physician, nurse, social worker, and chaplain would impact patient satisfaction, acute care utilization and costs, and the likelihood of dying at home (Brumley et al., 2007). Participating patients were able to continue with aggressive treatment concurrent with home palliative care enrollment. Patients with a diagnosis of cancer, COPD, or CHF and a life expectancy of 1 year or less received care from a team who developed care plans based on individual patient preferences and goals. While the study did not specifically report the preferences of study group patients, the results were significant: Patients in the intervention group reported higher satisfaction with care ($p < .05$), were less likely to access an emergency room ($p = .01$) or be admitted to a hospital ($p < .001$), and were more likely to die at home ($p < .001$). Intervention patients were asked to report satisfaction levels at 30 and 90 days, and as compared to the usual care group, they reported levels of satisfaction three times higher.

A 2009 study by the University of Chicago's Section of Geriatric and Palliative Medicine reported on the implementation of the Palliative Access Through Care At Home (PATCH) program, designed to offer support to "vulnerable" older adults and to help train clinicians to provide better care to this population and their caregivers (Holley, Gorawara-Bhat, Dale, Hemmerick, & Cox-Hayley, 2009). Study authors suggested that access to adequate medical and end-of-life care is often limited for older adults who are homebound, who have dementia, and/or who identify with particular racial or ethnic groups—all are generally less likely to access palliative or hospice care. The PATCH program staff consisted of a geriatrician, an advanced practice nurse, and a social worker. Specific supportive interventions provided by the team included pain and symptom assessments, coordination of care with other health professionals, arranging for durable medical equipment, patient education regarding medications, home safety evaluations, caregiver support, assistance with transitions from home to long-term care and/or from palliative care to hospice, as well as discussions around decision making, treatment preferences, and advance directives. Eighty-two percent of the study participants were African American, and more than half had a dementia diagnosis. While many people with dementia spend the last days of their lives in nursing homes, none of the PATCH patients who had a primary diagnosis of dementia died in a nursing home and, overall, the majority of PATCH patients died in their own homes. This study was limited by the homogeneity of the population and its small sample size, and the authors acknowledge that sustainability of such programs is always a concern. However, the authors reported that the PATCH program helped identify patient and caregiver needs and goals, such as remaining at home, while having access to specially trained social work palliative care "experts" and geriatricians who provided timely and meaningful interventions to achieve these goals.

Social Work Role in Home-Based Palliative Care

As mentioned previously, there is minimal research available on the social work role in home palliative care, as distinct from hospice social work. It might be tempting to suggest that documented outcomes relative to the social worker's role in hospice could be translated to that of palliative care; however, the scope of practice for palliative social worker involves caring for palliative care patients whose disease may or may not be at end stage and/or whose goals will likely shift and evolve over time (Lawson, 2007). Palliative social work may involve more case management tasks, participation in discussions about ethics, collaboration with additional providers outside of the palliative care team, as well as actively "experience[ing] the process that leads up to the hospice referral" (Lawson, 2007). Similar to home hospice, home palliative care focuses on the psychosocial, spiritual, and mental health aspects of the patient and family's experience—all while employing appropriate interventions relevant to patients who are pursuing disease-modifying, aggressive, curative, and life-prolonging treatment and/or are not emotionally aligned with a hospice comfort-only approach (Brumley et al., 2003; Brumley et al., 2007).

Anecdotally, many palliative social workers report coming to their role in palliative care with some level of experience working on hospice teams and reflect that while there is some overlap between the roles of hospice social worker and palliative social worker, there are also key differences. Some former hospice social workers have speculated that the differences in new palliative social work roles may increase their risk of emotional distress—especially for clinicians who are new to working with patients actively pursuing life-prolonging treatments. In the transition to working with a palliative care population, some hospice social workers report heightened emotional reactions and countertransference in working with home palliative care patients and families (N. Thompson, personal communication, November 2009). For example, new palliative social workers might presume that palliative care patients have a much longer life expectancy than typical hospice patients. The team may not feel prepared for the deaths of palliative care patients and therefore react with disbelief. They may believe that they ought to have noticed increased weakness or other warning signs and feel upset that they were not able to prepare the client, family members, and themselves for the death. The patient narrative in Box 10.1 illustrates an unexpected-death that caused considerable emotional distress for the palliative care team.

Patients such as Mrs. Carson are rarely considered eligible for or referred to hospice, even when their health is quite decompensated because, in general, determining heart failure prognosis has, until recently, been considered more variable than predicting the length of time until death from other diseases, such as cancer, which has a more established trajectory of decline. However, recent study of heart disease progression and prognosis, such as described in the Seattle Heart Failure Model (American Heart Association, 2007), can help teams prepare themselves as well as the families they serve. Similarly, understanding the trajectory of specific, individual chronic and progressive illnesses, such as amyotrophic lateral sclerosis or Parkinson's disease, can greatly assist teams, patients, and families in discussions and care planning. Understanding these diseases is specialized knowledge that requires ongoing study (Elman et al., 2007). In addition, there is some research to suggest that indicators of progressive

decline, like a declining palliative performance score (PPS), may increase palliative care teams' awareness about the nearness of death and assist the team to prepare the patient, family, and themselves proactively (Head, Ritchie, & Smoot, 2005). However, in the earlier narrative, Mrs. Carson did not show a clear decline in function, and the team was not cued to prepare for the patient's death. This narrative underscores the importance of being aware of the medical vulnerability of all palliative care patients, even those who may not have a clear prognosis.

Similarly, when home palliative care teams work with individual patients for extended periods of time, the increased duration of care may increase staff's development of strong emotional bonds to that patient and family. With an increased duration of the relationship, there is also an increased risk for strong grief reactions by palliative social workers and their teams at the time of death. As such, processing deaths of long-standing patients needs to be a subject for agency orientations and trainings, continuing education, and ongoing team support. In addition, it is vital that palliative care team members employ regular self-care strategies to address the emotional consequences of this challenging work. Seasoned palliative social workers are a valuable resource in highlighting this need for agencies in order to ensure staff's cumulative and/or complicated losses are being addressed and to support team sustainability and psychological health. The unique challenges of both hospice and palliative social work merit further study to understand both roles as well as to assist palliative care and hospice organizations to foster an environment of self-care for all staff.

The available literature on home palliative care programs underscores the need for further research and the boundless opportunities for social workers to participate in research design, direct practice, and research analysis of palliative social work practice. Social workers cannot depend on other disciplines alone to provide the evidence-based outcome measures; social work–led research is needed to demonstrate how the unique skills and perspectives brought by palliative social workers contribute to positive outcomes. In these changing economic and political climates, the role of social work risks being seen as supplemental, optional, or "as needed" rather than embraced as an integral part of the palliative care team. To ensure holistic, strengths-based, transdisciplinary home palliative care, social workers need to be actively involved in research that will motivate health care organizations to invest in new programs that honor the vital role of palliative social work, including working toward improved access to care for diverse populations impacted by health care disparities.

Home Palliative Care: A Model Quality Improvement Project in Canada

As in the United States, globally there exists much variety in the program models that provide home palliative care

---

Box 10.1
Patient/Family Narrative: Mrs. Carson

Mrs. Carson, a 52-year-old African American woman, was newly diagnosed with stage C heart failure. She and her spouse worked together to manage her many chronic conditions, but they experienced a great deal of stress given the demands of her care and her symptom burden. When the team first met them, Mrs. Carson was confined to her home most of the time. With close home management from the palliative care team to address medical, social, and emotional concerns, Mrs. Carson's quality of life and her heart failure gradually improved to the point that she was planning to resume care with her clinic physicians. Her other conditions— diabetes with poorly controlled blood sugar, neuropathic pain in her feet, stage 4 chronic kidney disease, and poorly controlled blood pressure would continue to need medical management. The social worker was developing a safety plan with Mr. and Mrs. Carson so that they could access the team quickly in the future when home palliative care was needed again. However, before the discharge could occur, Mrs. Carson had a sudden stroke and died at home while her husband was out at the gym.

services. Whether in the United States or abroad, home palliative care programs continue to face many organizational barriers and challenges, including providing sufficient access to services for patients desiring care, managing overall care coordination, and financial sustainability. Despite these challenges, the field of home palliative care has continued to grow and develop over the last decade and has resulted in a wide range of new and innovative programs.

In Canada, a quality improvement project for the care of persons diagnosed with cancer uses a *macro-meso-micro* sociological approach (Dudgeon et al., 2009) to demonstrate gains made coordinating palliative care across settings by standardizing training and use of two assessment tools. The project's development and implementation stages included palliative social workers at both the organizational management (*meso*) level and at the direct practice (*micro*) level as planners, subject matter experts, and as direct care providers. At the community (*macro*) level, two social workers were among the 19 individuals who served as members of the "working groups for the development of [three] generic Collaborative Care Plans"; two masters-level social workers helped identify and review the literature and develop the ongoing project plans. The project included 30 individual agency pilot sites throughout Ontario that participated in the project, without loss of autonomy. In addition, a social worker from one of the participating agencies was involved in reviewing the care plans and giving input prior to implementation of the pilot program.

At the *micro* level, as the program was implemented provincially over a 2-year time period, more social workers joined the project as direct care providers. A significant aspect of the pilot was to identify best practices and then to teach, implement, and evaluate these "interdisciplinary guides to practice [in order to]: 1) place the patient at the focal point of care; 2) promote continuity and coordination of care; and 3) promote communication among all disciplines" (Dudgeon et al., 2009, p. 487). One preliminary outcome of this project was the training of 800 providers to implement the Edmonton Symptom Assessment (ESAS) and Palliative Performance Scale (PPS) in their practices in order to provide standardized evaluations across multiple settings to improve the continuity of care. The overall aims and outcomes of this project are consistent with crucial aspects of palliative social work and provide a promising framework for addressing a fragmented health care system. Despite challenges related to the project's implementation and evaluation time table, direct care providers "reported that the [project] added value to their practice" as well as provided an opportunity for "continuous quality improvement activities" (Dudgeon et al., 2009, p. 489).

Home Palliative Care in the United States: Practice Themes

The development of new home palliative care programs and the implementation of ongoing quality improvement activities necessitates an understanding of existing home palliative care practice models. Some home palliative care programs in the United States replicate the hospice team model and provide for an interdisciplinary team, including a physician or overseeing medical director, nurse, social worker, chaplain, and additional team members such as a certified nurse assistant, pharmacist, and/or volunteer. Other home palliative care programs have evolved as *solo* practitioner models that provide primarily nursing and/or social work services. Given the essential nature of palliative care as a team intervention, these solo models represent care provided by a specialist professional.

The authors of this chapter have identified core themes in home palliative care practices and experiences through one-on-one discussions with social workers, nurses, and physicians in agencies across the United States. Participants in these discussions included palliative care professionals on the West coast, the intermountain West, the Midwest, and the East coast. The home palliative care programs involved were either established programs or pilot projects, with start-up dates ranging from 2001 to 2009. Through the course of these direct discussions, review of the current literature, professional involvement in the intervention phase of a home palliative care pilot study, experience with home palliative care program management and staff supervision, and the authors' direct work with patients in home palliative care, three basic social work practice themes have emerged: *(1)* direct interventions with patients and families; *(2)* collaborative transdisciplinary leadership opportunities; and *(3)* shaping the structure and delivery of home palliative care services through specific program models.

Direct Interventions with Patients and Families

The role of the social worker in home palliative care varies based on a number of factors, including the following: the relationships of agencies collaborating to provide care, regulatory requirements, contracts and limitations of practice settings, the client's medical and mental health needs, team/organization culture, and norms of the program environment (i.e., programs arising out of medical, community, or residential health care entities). In home palliative care, social workers and other advanced practice professionals typically provide billable services through their professional license and Medicare/Medicaid provider numbers. Home health regulations provide for billing federal and commercial insurances for necessary skilled care in the home. These billing mechanisms create various sanctions and limitations for the types of interventions. In addition, because program sustainability is largely based on financial reimbursement, programs tend to favor care provided by a professional in a single discipline, such as clinical social work, skilled nursing, or occupational therapy, rather than by an integrated team providing coordinated practice. In palliative care programs using the typical home health model, a specific skilled palliative care problem is identified and matched to the identified medical professional and a medical order is written. While traditional home health care needs are generally resolved over a relatively short period of time, home palliative care patients' needs may be more complex and last for an extended period of time, such as the duration of an end-stage illness.

The role of the palliative social worker in direct practice with patients and families includes assessment and interventions to address various psychosocial needs such as the following: reducing emotional and/or physical suffering and distress, management of preexisting or co-occurring mental health issues, interventions to reduce family conflicts, treating symptom-related anxiety, depression, and fears related to illness progression and thoughts of dying. Interventions are usually provided through a solution-focused, brief treatment modal and are typically focused around the patient's needs and desires. Interventions may also focus on family members' emotional distress, caregiver fatigue, caregiver support, and anticipatory grief. The single practitioner model provides a number of rewarding practice aspects for social workers, such as providing care to underserved or vulnerable populations, having a practice environment of relative independence, and having the opportunity to build practice skills in working with a wide range of medical and behavioral health challenges. The challenges may include managing large case loads and rapid care transitions, ensuring personal safety in unknown home environments, professional isolation, and fragmentation of care.

Additional roles for palliative social workers can include team leaders, peer educators, access specialists, care transitions coordinators, and program leaders and managers. Organizational leaders of home palliative care programs are usually physicians, registered nurses, or nurse practitioners. Social workers serve as program leaders or other administrators with much less frequency. While program, research, and policy leadership roles are still less numerous than direct care roles, palliative social workers can serve as mentors and role models—activities vital to forming the foundation for future professional leadership opportunities for palliative social workers.

Transdisciplinary Collaborative Leadership Opportunities

Collaborative team leadership roles and tasks vary across home palliative care programs, whether the program is a direct care, solo practitioner model or a transdisciplinary team model. Home palliative care programs structured under the home health benefit are multiplying in number, with skilled palliative care needs now being defined as appropriate for team interventions; each team member brings the skills of his or her unique discipline to the patient and creates an integrated team approach to care. Research by both Brumley et al. (2007) and Holley et al.(2009) demonstrates the value of interdisciplinary care in the home setting. The Clinical Practice Guidelines for Quality Palliative Care (National Consensus Project, 2009) also provides consensus on the importance of integrating all care domains for patients and families receiving palliative care services.

In many team-oriented home palliative care programs, team leadership, including the leadership role during interdisciplinary rounds, may be "entirely shared" or "based on the practice task at hand" (B. Mandel, personal communication, November 6, 2009). Practitioners who work in a transdisciplinary team model report that family meeting leadership is also not determined by discipline. Rather, the family meeting and other team leadership roles are more dependent upon matching the specific needs of the patient with the skill of the specific team member, or they are based upon the quality of the patient's relationship with individual clinicians rather than on the specific discipline of the individual team member. This open sharing of roles may be surprising to social workers who have long understood family meeting coordination and leadership to be the responsibility of the team social worker. The fluidity of roles in such teams suggests the development of transdisciplinary programs that operate in a truly collaborative team culture, made up of highly skilled professionals who are able to negotiate and share shifting roles in the best interests of the patient and family. The model of shared leadership and variable practice roles underscores the need for social workers to develop and maintain very high levels of group collaboration skills in addition to clinical intervention skills. Both skill sets are becoming core features for home palliative social work practice and are anticipated to continue as home palliative care models and best practices continue to evolve.

The staffing composition of large home palliative care programs reveals master's-level social workers in the role of clinical supervisor and/or program manager, creating additional opportunities to expand the range and depth of social work services and practice. Some programs employ master's-level licensed clinical social workers in program management and/or supervisory roles. Some employ bachelor's-level social workers assisting in managing case loads. Such programs capitalize on multiple tiers of social work training to effectively provide program services to patients and their families.

Shaping the Structure and Delivery of Home Palliative Care

Research, practice, and professional discussions concerning various models of home palliative care consistently demonstrate that each model has different effects and consequences for care of patients and families. In reviewing the similarities and differences of various home palliative care programs, three separate program models and two practice variables have emerged that illustrate the challenges of providing coordinated care for the patient and family in their environment.

The following section will describe these models in depth and provide analysis of each option. It is important for palliative social workers to understand the benefits and challenges of each practice setting—both for themselves professionally and for the patients and families served. Palliative social workers have an integral role as change agent in shaping the future delivery of home palliative care.

Home Palliative Care in the United States: Three Practice Models

The Single-Agency Program Model The single-agency program model is representative of home palliative care programs that are based on one single agency, usually a hospice, senior services residence, or other health care entity that does not contract out for any of its services (see Fig. 10.1). These single-agency entity programs are characterized by similar reimbursement mechanisms, and their sustainability is tied to the sustainability of the entire organization. Such organizations fund internal home palliative care programs (see Figures 10.1–10.3 for diagrammatic representation of the relationships) through one or more of the following funding sources:

a) Revenue brought in from core service (e.g., hospice or senior residential services) and allocated through the agency's internal budgets
b) Grant funding and/or fund raising
c) Billing Medicare, Medicaid, or commercial insurances for physician, nurse practitioner, licensed clinical social worker, home health aide, or chaplain services
d) Pediatric hospice waiver programs,
e) Contracts with hospitals or larger health systems to provide preventative or chronic care at home for persons with high urgent care or emergency department use patterns that yield low patient benefit and create a service burden to the contracting entity.

Some of these home palliative care programs also use cafeteria/private pay or fee-for-service billing mechanisms to finance services. One agency designed a monthly flat rate, fee-for-service billing structure as one of several income streams for their program. This program provides team-oriented service without any visit or service period limitations. The same agency also contracts with area hospitals to care for patients who frequently used emergency room care, although their needs were more often related to mental health disorders overlaying chronic medical conditions.

Persons receiving care in the single-agency model typically have chronic health conditions and high needs, have limited social support networks, need help navigating the health care system, and have limited financial resources. In addition, many are part of highly complex, discordant family systems. The patient narrative in Box 10.2 illustrates one example of an intervention by a single entity model home palliative care team.

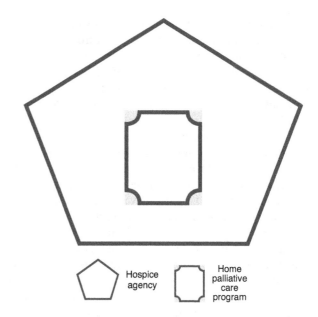

Figure 10.1. Single-Agency Program Model

The single-agency model often uses a solo practitioner approach that is common in traditional medical models or psychotherapeutic models of care. This model may or may not include interdisciplinary team meetings and/or standardized review and discharge practices such as those that are the norm in Medicare-regulated hospice practice. In a solo practitioner role, a key social work intervention can be conducting family meetings as well as coordinating patient and family needs with other medical providers to link an otherwise fragmented health care system. In senior residence home palliative care programs, the agency social worker may be responsible for the psychosocial needs of the residents but may not have prior training in palliative care, which raises the question as to the comprehensive nature of the palliative care services provided. Palliative social work interventions in this model often require a psychiatric diagnosis from the *Diagnostic and Statistical Manual of Mental Disorders* (*DSM IV-TR*) in order for billing to occur. This may lead to

---

Box 10.2
Patient/Family Narrative: Edward

Edward, a 68-year-old man, appeared at the hospital emergency room on multiple occasions complaining of acute health concerns. During the most recent visit, a thorough assessment concluded that the primary issues were anxiety and depression. The home palliative care team became involved to help manage the concurrent medical and psychological issues. The team social worker provided immediate psychotherapeutic interventions and helped Edward to discover and access ongoing mental health support services. The social worker also found additional resources to assist Edward with obtaining his prescriptions and helped him develop an individualized motivational program to increase the likelihood he would continue taking the medications recommended to relieve his psychological distress.

unnecessarily pathologizing of the patient's situation, rather than allowing the social worker to assess from a developmental or strengths perspective, which frames distress related to life-threatening illness and end of life as part of the normative journey along the human life span.

Because there are no universal standards for home palliative care programs, agencies that adopt the standards of the National Consensus Project's Clinical Practice Guidelines for Quality Palliative Care (2009) will provide some assurances to patients and families that they will receive the highest quality care. Social workers in all practice settings may at some time or another find themselves referring a client to a home palliative care program; as such, it is important to become familiar with these standards in order to be able to evaluate programs on the basis of quality indicators. At the time of this writing, when home palliative care programs are still in the early stages of development, there are not yet any standardized recertification periods or other standardization processes for individual palliative care programs.

In home palliative care programs that are provided by an individual hospice agency, there exists a potential bias for guiding the patient toward hospice enrollment with that agency versus allowing full choice of palliative care participation. This bias creates a concurrent responsibility to be transparent about the two program choices and their respective benefits to the patients and families. This complicates discussions with patients and family and necessitates a full evaluation of hospice enrollment practices to ensure ethical integrity. To effectively address this ethical concern, it is essential to elicit direct feedback and assess the needs of persons receiving care, establish clear goals, and openly address this issue with all program staff. That being said, home palliative care providers frequently report that clients express strong appreciation for the existence of palliative care programs, especially as an alternative to hospice enrollment. This is most often identified in cases where enrollment in hospice would have required a decision to stop seeking disease-modifying therapies. It is imperative that patients not feel pressured to make a transition to hospice care in order to receive comprehensive palliative services.

As individual agency programs choose their specific program model, it is important to understand that social work is not always considered a *standard* service for patients receiving home palliative care. In some program models, social work interventions may be ordered at the discretion of the physician or nurse practitioner. One social worker estimated that only about 30% of the patients in her home palliative care program are referred for social worker interventions by the nurse practitioner in a solo practitioner model. In another program, direct palliative social work services are provided to all patients through the use of both bachelor's- and master's-level clinicians. Because it is common for there to be an absence of clinical and/or administrative social worker professionals at the meso practice level, administrative supervision is typically provided to direct practice social workers by a physician, nurse, psychologist, or master's-level

public health practitioner. Most social workers who practice in this model rely on their social work peers and colleagues or other professional groups to provide for routine social work consultation, clinical supervision, and/or professional development activities.

Single Health System Program Model Large metropolitan, state-wide, regional, or multistate integrated health systems, especially not-for-profits systems, are able to provide a wide range of comprehensive health care services, including primary and specialty care, behavioral health care, home health care, hospice care, and hospital services (see Fig. 10.2). Sometimes called "all inclusive" or integrated care systems, internal funding mechanisms for the services provided are built in through governmental funding streams, regular health insurance premiums, and co-insurances and co-pays for covered services. These systems focus on monitoring service gaps because such gaps can lead to poor overall care outcomes, lower client and provider satisfaction, and higher overall health care costs both to consumers and the company. Some large health systems have developed home palliative care services to meet these identified gaps. Social workers who join these systems have the opportunity to become partners in addressing the moral imperative of providing genuinely individualized, quality health care in these highly complex systems (Otis-Green et al., 2009).

Single health systems may fund home palliative care programs out of their overall budget or provide palliative care services to specific at-risk patient populations for additional monthly or per-visit fees. Health systems may elect to provide palliative care for all their patients or to only offer the program for special populations or patients with unique needs. General fundraising and/or grants may provide

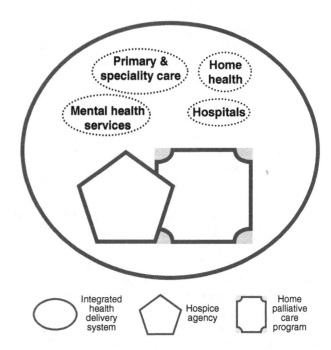

Figure 10.2. The Single Health System Program Model

a portion of the funding for palliative care programs. Some single health system programs may bill for individual visits under Medicare and have commercial contracts that reimburse for home health visits or even, in rare cases, for chaplain visits. However, the option of utilizing home health billing creates additional access problems, since patients receiving palliative care visits under this billing mechanism must be certified as home bound in order to receive services. The goal for many palliative care patients is to maximize function and engagement with life, which is in conflict with the billing criteria of "homebound." Providers must also ensure there are no other concurrent home health providers because this creates a duplication of services not allowed under Medicare rules. Despite their large overall budgets, some single health system models of care are challenged by a lack of adequate financial resources to support ongoing team involvement with patients. Some of these home palliative care services are thus designed as *consultative* services with an emphasis on short-term involvement.

Home palliative care programs provided by single health systems are typically comprised of interdisciplinary teams. The team's norms and practices may be either formal or informal, and they may or may not include regular care coordination and/or interdisciplinary team meetings during which topics are discussed, which may include staff coverage, patient symptom management or psychsocial/spiritual needs, shifting goals of care, and the need to consider discharge from the program or a transition to care in different settings and/or to different levels of care. One home palliative social worker described her team practice as nonhierarchical and collaborative, providing a culture in which clinical communication occurs between providers of all disciplines—nurses, physicians, and social workers alike. Most patients will require palliative social work interventions for a broad range of changing and evolving needs and wishes. Service in single health systems may become fragmented and, just as in any large complex systems, skilled palliative social workers help coordinate care, integrating home palliative care within a continuum of services and improving overall quality. Coordination with other social workers and nurses along the continuum is essential and guards against duplication of services, which are a significant waste of resources in the health care system. In one single-system home palliative care program, the team social worker coordinates with the home health social worker to maintain a consistent social work presence. The primary focus of the palliative social workers' interventions is to provide emotional support and counseling services; he helps with entitlements if requested, but this is not a primary function of his role. Whatever the length of care or type of services provided, when skilled transdisciplinary teams focus on quality individualized care for patients and their families there will be progress toward meeting their physical, emotional, spiritual, and pain and symptom management needs that will guide the future course of the patient's care plan in the health care system.

In discussing evolving care plans over time, palliative social workers have observed that patients enrolled in palliative care frequently will describe one or more philosophical or emotional barriers to accepting hospice care. Over time, the needs and goals of the same patients and families change as the illness progresses and function deteriorates. As palliative interventions become primary, hospice services become more coherent with the patient and family's needs and goals. While no research has been found to substantiate the commonly held belief among home palliative care providers, many in the field continue to assert that patients who receive home palliative care services enroll in hospice care *much earlier* than they otherwise would have, had they not received home palliative care services. Providers commonly believe that, as a result, patients and families may be able to experience more beneficial use of hospice services.

Community Partnership Model The community partnership model for home palliative care is created by the collaborative efforts of various health care entities such as hospitals, health plans or systems, home health agencies, cancer centers, hospices, and other health care providers (see Fig. 10.3). Funding for this collaborative model may include in-kind staffing, grants, support from general budgets, service development funds, and/or investment budgets. Home palliative care program models that arise out of a community partnership are praised by their advocates as having superior sustainability, since no one agency partner has to bear the entire financial burden of the program. This is especially helpful since most

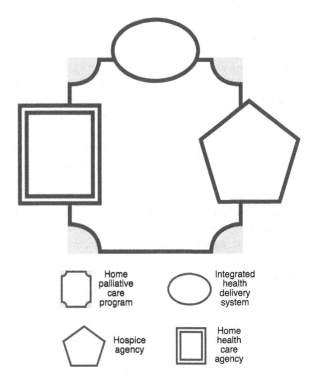

Figure 10.3. Community Partnership Models

home palliative care funding structures are not yet fully developed or consist of mainly grant funding or noninstitutional funds. On the other hand, these models sometimes face an even greater challenge than the single health system model in terms of coordination of patient care.

The setting for care in such models may be a hospital, home, or clinic. In one example of this continuum of care partnership model, the home palliative care service was the joint effort of a hospital, a cancer center, and a local home health hospice agency. The home palliative care service was comprised of physicians and nurse practitioners from the cancer center who made home visits and billed health insurances for their services. The social worker was available on an as-needed basis and provided by the community hospice partner.

Making the most of the potential for effective team practice and ensuring high patient satisfaction in a community partnership model is largely dependent upon social workers and other team members practicing alongside each other with high levels of skill and dedication to working together to provide care to clients and their families (Gardia, 2009; Johnson et al., 2009). Flexibility in team practice is a hallmark of this type of model, especially in younger programs. One direct care social worker in a palliative care pilot program created by a collaborative partnership described a fairly informal team meeting process in which staff routinely met to talk about successes and what was working well in their practices. The pilot phase of their program allowed for informal learning and case review rather than formal, structured team meetings at set intervals with a set leadership structure. The social worker interviewed identified the physician as the leader in conceptualizing and implementing the pilot project, with a nurse providing the day-to-day program management and all team members working together to develop best practices and work processes. Many models of collaborative agency care are small and able to provide a limited level of care to patients and families. From the perspective of a nurse in a partnership program, there is greater service flexibility and increased collaboration when working with multiple agency partners and community resources.

Direct care social workers in this practice model utilize their core skills to analyze systems and bring the resources of the whole community to bear in meeting the needs of the patient and family. In this collaborative model, however, there are generally fewer structural and institutional care processes that identify social workers as core members of the home palliative care team. Palliative social workers who demonstrate strong entrepreneurial, clinical, and leadership skills are needed to highlight the benefits social workers bring to the team and to patients and families. Leading through example, demonstration and advocacy will ensure that patients and their families will continue to receive the benefits of professional social worker involvement for the future. As palliative social workers commit to involvement in community collaborative home palliative care programs, gains in the quality of home palliative care through skilled social work interventions will continue to be woven into the fabric of community partnership home palliative care programs.

Bivariant Conceptualization of Program Models

The following diagram (Fig. 10.4) illustrates two variables that characterize individual home palliative care programs and the associated types of social work practice. The vertical (x) axis describes the Palliative Care Professional and Team Integration (micro-level practice). The horizontal (y) axis describes the Health Care Entity Collaborative Integration (meso-level practice). This conceptualization can be used as a guide for future social work research comparing service outcomes for programs with each service type and combination of variables. Such research will be essential in demonstrating the impact and value of core social work services for all palliative care clients as well as best practices in palliative care team and community practice.

Thematic Synthesis

The following are dynamic and interacting themes in home palliative care that have emerged during the first decade of the twenty-first century: (1) the role of the social worker, (2) collaborative team leadership, (3) emerging program models, (4) financial sustainability, and (5) the relationship of social work, team, and agency integration to create viable programs and best practices in transdisciplinary care. Early and evolving research in home palliative care, the dissemination of evidence-based program models, best practices, and policy development through consensus building have all added practice knowledge. We offer this thematic synthesis as the foundation for advancing home palliative care social work practice.

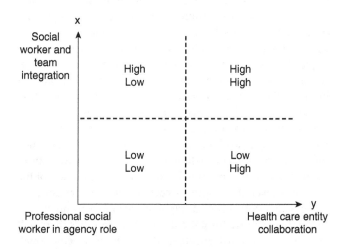

Figure 10.4. Bivariate model of home palliative care social work practice: aligning social work and team practice in collaborative organizations

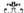

Adapting Home Palliative Care Services for Special Populations

Individual persons and families within unique populations, subgroups, and communities have their own distinct cultural needs that require individualized attention and care, and these populations are discussed elsewhere in this textbook. The following patient family narratives from our program research and patient interviews identify a small sampling of the wide variety of persons within special groups who have benefited from home palliative care interventions tailored to their unique situations.

Home Palliative Care with Native Americans

Native Americans have distinct spiritual practices and beliefs regarding healthcare that may be at odds with traditional western medicine. In addition, as an indigenous people with a history of persecution and mistreatment, Native American tribes and families may be mistrustful of the intentions and motives of medical personnel outside of their tribal background. The following narrative (see Box 10.3) describes the importance of nurturing relationships within Native American communities.

In working with such communities, it is imperative that social workers plan to spend a significant amount of time laying the foundational work of developing experiences of trust. This process can take many months or even years before a practitioner will be entrusted with the care of members of such a community.

Home Palliative Care with Persons Experiencing Homelessness

For a person experiencing homelessness, home palliative care visits may occur in a motel room, at a homeless shelter, under a bridge, or in a car. The patient's "home" may also change every day, every month, or may vary by the season.

For the home palliative care team, providing care to persons experiencing homelessness is an opportunity to truly embrace the metaphorical social work concept of *"meeting the client where they are"* (see Box 10.4).

Home Palliative Care with Lesbian, Gay, Bisexual, and Transgender Persons

Gay, lesbian, bisexual, and transgender (GLBT) individuals are a vulnerable population who may be fearful of discrimination and/or harassment from providers if their sexual orientation/gender identity is known. Thus, when working with patients in the home setting, it is essential to create an atmosphere of openness and acceptance that will allow GLBT persons to feel comfortable and supported as they receive care (see Box 10.5).

The initial assessment by the palliative social worker revealed Sara to be a gregarious, intelligent, confident, and assertive woman with a good sense of humor. Alexandra was polite but distant and did not seek to participate in conversations with any of the team members nor did she respond to the social worker's initial outreach efforts to engage her individually, to offer emotional support, or to begin an assessment of her needs as a family member and caregiver. The social worker continued to visit the home on a weekly basis, providing the opportunity for the relationship with both Sara and Alexandra to slowly develop, and creating a strong rapport within an atmosphere of trust. In this setting, the couple agreed to meet as a couple because both agreed to meet to address the underlying emotional conflicts in their relationship. Together, they were able to openly discuss Sara's terminal illness, to address the reports of verbal abuse, to explore the meaning of Alexandra's behaviors, and to understand the challenges to both in their marriage. Alexandra was helped to acknowledge her feelings of helplessness, inadequacy, and anger related to the Sara's decision to live as a woman, as well as to recognize the verbal abuse as destructive and unwarranted. Sara also learned new ways to handle her wife's anger, and both began to process their unexpressed

---

Box 10.3
Patient/Family Narrative: Native American Tribal Partnerships
A home palliative care program in the Midwest received a start-up grant to form partnerships with two area Native American tribes. (Detailed information on the specifics of this project is omitted out of respect for tribal sovereignty.) The individual social worker assigned to this project slowly developed partnerships and provided palliative care services within each unique tribal context. Initially, the social worker's contacts with the tribes were characterized by hesitancy and mistrust. Over time, as the social worker continued to spend time with families and various tribal subgroups, trust in the partnership with her program increased.

Box 10.4
Patient Narrative: Mr. Harrison
One home palliative social worker participated in a unique initiative to provide care to persons who were experiencing homelessness in the midst of advancing illness. Mr. Harrison had his home in a small area under a bridge; however, he was becoming increasingly bed-bound and concerned about meeting his daily needs as his terminal illness progressed. The palliative social worker had ongoing meetings with him at this location while she identified and mobilized resources to help meet his medical and shelter needs. She eventually helped Mr. Harrison accept palliative care in a setting where caregivers could attend to his safety, nutrition, and comfort through the end of his life.

Box 10.5
Patient/Family Narrative: Sara

Sara is a 64-year-old, married, male-to-female transgender patient who was referred to the home palliative care team by her primary care physician for help managing her end-stage congestive heart failure symptoms. She is a retired banker who lives in a well-cared-for trailer home with her spouse, Alexandra. There has been much conflict in their 20-year marriage related to Sara's decision to live her life as a woman. Alexandra refuses to call Sara by her chosen name and still calls her by her masculine birth name. Sara maintains that she told Alexandra of her gender issues when they met and so feels that Alexandra's anger is unwarranted. Upon enrollment in the home palliative care program, the team quickly became aware of several issues requiring intervention. First, one of the palliative care team providers reported to the team that she witnessed Alexandra verbally abusing Sara during the visit. Second, Sara was soon labeled by some members of the team as seeming "difficult to please" and "overly critical" of care providers; she was forthright in her demands for the best care possible from the palliative care providers. Lastly, the hospital-based palliative care team had noted in the patient's chart that she was expressing significant distress related to her transgender identity and numerous life regrets. The inpatient team felt that these concerns were increasing Sara's suffering and were having a negative effect on her ability to "come to peace" with her life-threatening illness and impending death.

---

feelings of sadness and anger related to Sara's rejection and estrangement by both sides of the family consequent to her transgender identity. As a result of the social worker's intervention, the couple was able to be kinder to one another and to handle conflicts in a more productive manner.

As Sara engaged in a full life review with the social worker, she incorporated her gender identity journey as part of her lifelong emotional growth process. Sara shared her feelings of alienation and marginalization as a transgender woman, as well as her underlying fears of mistreatment and discrimination. In the setting of an empathic relationship, the social worker assisted Sara to understand how these feelings and her fear of discrimination were manifesting in her ongoing assertions to the team that she should receive the best care possible. The social worker focused on Sara and Alexandra's courage and assertiveness in demanding the best care possible, while also linking the constant questioning of providers to fears that they would experience discrimination. After voicing and discussing these fears, Sara felt more assured that the team was fully accepting and committing to providing the best care and services possible. Once Sara was able to relax with this knowledge, interactions with other team members and providers became more collaborative, relaxed, and collegial. The social worker enhanced the sensitivity of the team by helping them to reframe Sara's "complaints" and "hostility" as simply assertive demands for the best care possible, given her history of marginalization and fears of discrimination. As a result of this explanation, the team was

also assisted to be more sensitive to these concerns when discussing treatment plans, specific care services, and limitations which for most patients did not engender fear and worry about discrimination. As a result of the social worker's skillful interventions and ability to create a strong therapeutic alliance, Sara was provided a venue to be able to process her life journey, including her regrets, accomplishments, and reflections about her life as a whole. Her emotional pain and suffering decreased and she expressed increased peace of mind and an open acceptance of her impending death.

The social worker was the team's leader in ensuring Sara was provided culturally sensitive care related to her transgender identity and that Alexandra's needs and distress were addressed as well. She led by example, consistently referring to the patient by her preferred pronoun and modeling respect and culturally sensitive care to the patient. At an interdisciplinary team meeting early on, a confused staff member referred to the patient as "gay" and the social worker seized the opportunity to educate the full team about the difference between sexual orientation and gender identity. (For additional information, please see Chapter 35.)

Transitions of Care

When a patient transitions from a home palliative care program to an alternate level of care, the needs and wishes of the patient and family must be given the highest priority. Quality, ethical standards of palliative care practice include focused attention to well-planned, smooth, and successful care transitions across multiple settings (National Consensus Project, 2009).

Transitioning to a Less Intensive Level of Care

There are four main reasons for a patient to be discharged from a home palliative care program to a less intensive level of care. First, when palliative care programs are structured as specific goal-directed care, discharge from the home palliative care program is appropriate as soon as all the care plan goals have been met. Second, a discharge is indicated if a patient's chronic medical illness (for which he or she was enrolled in the home palliative care program) stabilizes or if symptoms decrease to a level that the patient's needs are best met through the services of another program or agency. Third, when a program provides services for a patient who is concurrently pursuing disease-modifying treatments for an illness and the treatment results in a cure or remission, the patient may no longer need the services of the team. For example, in providing home palliative care to children diagnosed with cancer, "discharge is considered: when the disease goes into remission, symptoms and treatment side effects are managed easily, and the child is healthy enough to attend and stay in school" (K. Altieri, personal communication, November 11, 2009). In all instances requiring transition from home palliative care, the social worker and team should prepare the patient and family emotionally by acknowledging the complex emotions that may exist, including sadness at separation from the team, joyful celebration of a temporary or permanent cure from the disease, potential feelings of abandonment by the providers, and/or emptiness at the loss of the rigorous treatment schedule that might have become part of the person's life.

Transitioning to Home Hospice or a More Intensive Level of Care

In the single-agency palliative care model, aspects of ethical practice and standards for informed consent as well as Medicare guidelines provide structure for this care transition. When a patient enrolled in a home palliative care program becomes medically eligible to enroll in home hospice care, the patient and family need to be informed in a timely manner that hospice care is an option for them, including discussion of the benefits and costs to making such a change. In the process, it is important that the patient and family not feel coerced one way or the other and that information be provided in a clear manner that enhances the patient and family's understanding of the available options.

Palliative social workers need to be especially attentive to the psychological and physical vulnerability of the patient and family and their cognitive ability to process information, especially when in a heightened emotional state. During transition to hospice, the palliative social worker should serve as an advocate for the patient and family to ensure that related financial issues—both costs and benefits of the change—are fully disclosed and fully understood by the patient and family and that the choice of available hospice programs is discussed. In addition, every effort should be made to prevent actual or perceived abandonment by the team during and after the transition. As the care plan evolves, at each point in the decision-making process, medical factors and patient and family values and beliefs are essential components of an informed consent process. Ensuring that patients and families feel included and involved in care transitions will minimize potential feelings of abandonment and loss.

It is expected and essential that palliative social workers convey an attitude of respect for patient and family autonomy and for their personal decisions related to acute care and/or life-rescuing treatments, such as cardiopulmonary resuscitation (CPR) or long-term ventilator support. Informed decision making involves an understanding of the impact of these decisions, including the reality that some initial decisions produce a cascade of events. For example, a decision to be resuscitated requires that the patient leave his or her home setting for transfer to a hospital intensive care unit. Palliative social work skills include joining with medical colleagues to sensitively explore and process the multidimensional impacts of the treatment being considered

along with the patient and their family members to ensure that they make the best decisions that also uphold their personal values and wishes.

Death of the Home Palliative Care Patient

In addition to the tasks of active symptom management and spiritual and psychosocial support and interventions, home palliative care teams may be called upon to assist patients to plan for death in the home, when that is their preference. Most home palliative care programs develop educational handouts for their clients to provide information on what steps to take if the client dies and is not enrolled in a hospice program. It is crucial for families to know in advance how to handle the death of their family member because the county coroner or law enforcement officers may perceive a death without hospice involvement as "not expected" and thus require a formal investigation. The experience of treating the death as a possible crime scene can put the family and caregivers in a traumatic and vulnerable situation. Individuals may be required to explain the situation to law enforcement, coroners, and other officials who may react with suspicion and who are likely not trained in psychosocial care of grieving families. Preparation and prevention of distress at the time of death to prevent complicated bereavement is an essential element of home palliative care services and is an important role for the palliative social worker.

Conclusion

Palliative social workers play a vital role in ensuring the provision of quality, effective, culturally sensitive home palliative care services. As palliative care programs continue to grow and evolve over the next several decades, it will be imperative that social work professionals continue to emerge as leaders in research, direct practice, and program development to ensure that social work values and practices are built into the framework of home palliative care service delivery.

LEARNING EXERCISES

1. Identify and describe all of the following in your local practice area, with a focus on identifying, reducing, or eliminating home palliative care access gaps: *(a)* community consortium, *(b)* health entity partnerships, *(c)* government policy or legislative efforts, *(d)* research projects, *(e)* practice improvement projects, *(f)* community-based senior residences that offer any form of palliative care on site, and *(g)* educational programs. Choose one or more of these projects that has a unique or influential approach and arrange to

shadow or interview a key social worker in that service. Interview patients and families also if possible. Based on your results, write a journal article or create a presentation (e.g., breakout session, class presentation, or poster) for a local practice group, school of social work, or local or national conference.

2. Interview direct care social work professionals in home palliative care services. Consider questions that identify aspects of both (1) their individual practices (evidence base for their practice, practice theories used consistently with patients and their families, special populations, greatest practice challenges, collaboration with other professionals, identification of service disparities, leadership activities, research activities or opportunities) and (2) the characteristics of the program in which they practice (funding sources of the program, collaborations with other agencies or community groups, opportunities for advancement of social workers throughout their program and agency).

3. Perform a current literature search to determine whether there has been an increase in home palliative care research, both in general and per the specific role of the social worker, since the publication of this book.

4. Research current health policy in your local area, either where you live or practice. Consider what effect this policy may have on home palliative care and/or palliative social work at the provincial, state, national, and global levels. Does your policy search reveal any new home palliative care benefits under Medicare or Medicaid in the United States? What is your state's position on so-called right-to-die legislation or other controversial practices that may have an impact on home palliative care practices?

5. Identify and discuss some unique populations that would benefit from culturally sensitive palliative care. What role could the social worker play in each of these scenarios? What challenges and barriers exist for this population in accessing home palliative care? Consider whether home palliative care would be more or less acceptable, given this population's cultural and/or spiritual values and beliefs.

REFERENCES

American Heart Association. (2007). Prediction of mode of death in heart failure: The Seattle heart failure model. Boston, MA: Harvard Medical School and Harvard School of Public Health.

Appelin, G., Broback, G., & Bertero, C. (2005). A comprehensive picture of palliative care at home from the people involved. *European Journal of Oncology Nursing, 9,* 315–324.

Arnaert, A., & Wainwright, M. (2009). Providing care and sharing expertise: reflections of nurse-specialists in palliative home care. *Palliative and Supportive Care, 7,* 357–364.

Brumley, R. D., Enguidanos, S., & Cherin, D. A. (2003). Effectiveness of a home-based palliative care program for end-of-life. *Journal of Palliative Medicine, 6,* 715–724.

Brumley, R. D., Enguidano, S., Jamison, P., Seitz, R., Morgenstern, N., Saito, S., … Gonzalez, J. (2007). Increased satisfaction with care and lower costs: results of a randomized trial of non palliative care. *Journal of the American Geriatrics Society, 55,* 993–1000.

Bush, S. H., Wearne, H. J., Reilly, P. E., Chacko, R., & Palmer, J. L. (2009). Clinical findings and recommendations made during home visits by a palliative care specialist physician. *Palliative Medicine, 23,* 635–641.

Dudgeon, D. J., Knott, C., Chapman, C., Coulson, K., Jeffery, E., Preston, S., … Smith, A. (2009). Development, implementation and process evaluation of a regional palliative care quality improvement project. *Journal of Pain and Symptom Management, 38,* 483–495.

Elman, L. B., Houghton, D. J., Wu, G. F., Hurtig, H. I., Markowitz, C. E., & McCluskey, L. (2007). Palliative care in amyotrophic lateral sclerosis, Parkinson's disease, and multiple sclerosis. *Journal of Palliative Medicine, 10,* 433–457.

Finlay, I. G., Higginson, I. J., Goodwin, D. M., Cook, A. M., Edwards, A. G. K., Hood, K., … Norman, C. E. (2002). Palliative care in hospital, hospice, at home: results from a systematic review. *Annals of Oncology, 13*(4), 257–264.

Gardia, G. (2009). *The Interdisciplinary Team—Dysfunctional, barely functional or highly functional.* Tenth Clinical Team Conference. Conducted at the annual conference of The National Hospice and Palliative Care Organization, Denver, Colorado.

Head, B., Ritchie, C. S., & Smoot, T. M. (2005). Prognostication in hospice care: can the palliative performance scale help? *Journal of Palliative Medicine, 8,* 492–502.

Holley, A. P. H., Gorawara-Bhat, R., Dale, W., Hemmerick, J., & Cox-Hayley, D. (2009). Palliative access through care at home: Experiences with an urban, geriatric home palliative care program. *Journal American Geriatric Society, 57,* 1925–1931.

Hwang, M. S., & Ryu, H. S. (2009). Effects of a palliative care program based on home care nursing. *Journal of Korean Academy of Nursing, 39,* 528–538.

Jocham, H. R. (2006). Quality of life in palliative care: A comparison of hospital and home care. *Pflege Zeitschrift, 59,* 2–8.

Johnson, A. P, Abernathy, T., Howell, D., Brazil, K., & Scott, S. (2009). Resource utilization and costs of palliative care cancer care in an interdisciplinary health care model. *Palliative Medicine, 23,* 448–459.

Jordhoy, M. S., Fayers, P., Saltnes, T., Ahlner-Elmqvist, M., Janner, T., & Kassa, S. (2000). Apalliative-care intervention and death at home: a cluster randomized trial. *The Lancet, 356,* 888–893.

Kramer, B. J., Christ, G. H., Bern-Klug, M., & Francoeur, R. B. (2005). A national agenda for social work research and end-of-life care. *Journal of Palliative Medicine, 8,* 418–439.

Kuhlen, M., Balzer, S., Richter, U., Fritsche-Kansy, M., Friedland, C., Borkhardt, A., & Janssen, G. (2009). Development of a specialized pediatric palliative home care service. *Klinische Padiatrie, 221,* 186–192

Lawson, R. (2007). Home and hospital; hospice and palliative care: How the environment impacts the social work role. *Journal of Social Work in End of Life and Palliative Care, 3*(2), 3–17.

Medicare and Medicaid Hospice Conditions of Participation, Reg 42 C.F.R. § 418.100 (2009).

National Consensus Project for Quality Palliative Care. (2009). *Clinical practice guidelines for quality palliative care, second edition*. Retrieved from http://www.nationalconsensusproject. org/guideline.pdf

Otis-Green, S., Ferrell, B., Spolum, M., Uman, G., Mullan, P., Baird, P., & Grant, M. (2009). An overview of the ACE Project ~ Advocating for clinical excellence: Transdisciplinary palliative care education. *Journal of Cancer Education, 24*(2), 120–126.

Peruselli, C., Di Giulio, P., Toscani, F., Gallucci, M., Brunelli, C., Costantini, M., … Higginson, I. J. (1999). Home palliative care for terminal cancer patients: A survey on the final week of life. *Palliative Medicine, 13,* 233–241.

11 *Mercedes Bern-Klug and Kelsey Simons*

Palliative Care in Long-Term Care Facilities

We accepted that we are just passing through. We would accept a miracle, but we are not expecting one.

—Daughter of a nursing home resident

Key Concepts
- *Long-term care is care for persons with advanced chronic illness, persons who have had a debilitating accident, or persons with a serious developmental disability.*
- *Most people with long-term care needs live at home where they receive care from family members, friends, and community-based organizations.*
- *Most (90%) of persons who live in nursing homes are age 65 or older.*
- *The principles of palliative care are an excellent match for the needs of long-term nursing home residents.*

Introduction

Of all health care settings, it is the nursing home that stands to benefit the most from the philosophy and practice of palliative care. This is not an indictment of the staff. This is in recognition of the unique circumstances of contemporary nursing home living and dying. As is exemplified by Mrs. R's narrative in Box 11.1, nursing homes are settings serving people with advanced chronic illness, most of whom are also in advanced old age. Consequently, because people spend weeks, months, and years as nursing home residents, even modest improvements in nursing home care can enhance the lives of residents. The purpose of this chapter is to discuss the role of social workers in providing palliative care to residents and families in nursing homes. We begin by putting nursing home care into the context of long-term care. After briefly providing background information about nursing homes in general, we turn our attention to how the nursing home social worker can honor palliative care principles while involved in assessment, care planning, and group work with residents and family members. The chapter concludes with the bold assertion that if nursing homes were to fully embrace palliative care, the quality of care would increase and the stigma associated with nursing home living would diminish.

Palliative care is defined as care aimed at preventing and relieving pain and suffering in an effort to support the best possible quality of life for patients and families (National Consensus Project, 2009). The National Consensus Project for Quality Palliative Care's definition states that palliative care is appropriate for people of all ages who have a life-threatening or debilitating illness, including "persons living with progressive chronic conditions (such as peripheral vascular disease, malignancies, chronic renal failure, stroke with significant functional impairment, advanced heart disease, frailty, neurodegenerative disorders, and dementias)" (http://www.nationalconsensusproject.org/Guidelines_Download.asp). These health conditions are common among long-term care nursing home residents.

How the eight domains of the National Consensus Project's palliative care framework apply to the provision of

> **Box 11.1**
> **Resident/family narrative**
>
> *A nursing home resident (Mrs. R) with advanced lung disease and a weak heart was adamant that she did not want to be sent to the hospital as her health declined. She called a meeting between the administrator, the director of nursing, her two daughters, and herself. She reviewed—in front of everyone—that her wishes continue to be to remain in the nursing home and not be sent to the hospital as her health declined. After the meeting, I (as a researcher doing a study in the nursing home) talked with one of the daughters who was quite upset about the meeting. I asked the daughter to help me understand. She said, "They talked with her like she was going to die.... and that really upset me to have to hear that." The next day the social worker mentioned she thought Mrs. R was a good candidate for hospice but that she had to be careful how she would bring up the subject because the daughters may not be ready to hear it. (Bern-Klug, 2000-unpublished fieldnotes)*

psychosocial services in nursing homes is the focus of a recent book (Bern-Klug, 2010). In this chapter, the focus is on one of those eight domains, "social aspects of care."

As is true in all social movements, timing is important for success. The push toward incorporating palliative care principles into nursing homes is being facilitated by two other trends in the field, the person-centered care movement led by the Pioneer Network (http://www.pioneernetwork.net) and geriatrician and founder of the Eden Alternative and Green House movement, William Thomas (2003), as well as the movement to enhance the quality of life among nursing home residents, led in part by social work scholar Dr. Rosalie Kane (2003). All three of these movements—palliative care, person-centered care, and quality of life—have at their core the need to recognize and address the humanity of each resident by expanding the focus of care from physical care to also incorporate and indeed honor psychosocial and spiritual well-being.

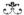

What is Long-Term Care?

Long-term care is care provided over months, years, and in some cases decades. Much of long-term care is in the form of assistance with activities of daily living (ADLs) such as help with personal care (e.g., bathing, dressing, using the toilet, or grooming) (Weiner, Hanley, Clark, & Van Nostrand, 1990). Some recipients of long-term care also receive assistance with instrumental activities of daily living (IADLs), which include help with grocery shopping, meal preparation, keeping track of finances, and using the phone.

The need for long-term care typically arises from a debilitating accident or as the result of advancing chronic illness. Most people with long-term care needs live in a private home, and they typically do so with the help of women—mothers, daughters, sisters, nieces, and neighbors. While

women are more likely to provide care, it must be said that men also play an important role in providing long-term care to family members and friends. Indeed, male caregivers face unique challenges because many have not been socialized to be caregivers (Kramer, 2000; Sanders, 2007). While often thought of as a concern of older adults, it is important to note that half of the people with long-term care needs in the United States are under the age of 65 (Feder, Komisar, & Niefeld, 2000). Most of the younger people with long-term care needs live in private residences. Although the *number* of people with long-term care needs who are under versus over age 65 is comparable, the *percentage* of older adults is much higher, because the likelihood of needing long-term care increases with age. Of the 1.4 million nursing home residents represented in the 2004 National Nursing Home Survey, 45% were age 85 or older (Jones, Dwyer, Bercovitz, & Strahan, 2009). Furthermore, the 85+ population, although small in number, is the fastest growing age group among persons age 65+ in the United States (Himes, 2002).

Long-term care can be contrasted with "acute" care, which is care in response to a need that appears rather suddenly or in the form of a sudden serious exacerbation of a chronic illness. Hospitals are designed to address acute care needs. Home—a house, apartment, condominium, or trailer—is where the vast majority of long-term care is provided. In some cases, only informal care from nonpaid caregivers is used, and in other cases formal community services such as adult day care services or home health augment the informal long-term care. Alternatively, the person who needs long-term care will move in with someone else, such as a sibling, daughter, or close friend, or move to an assisted living facility. Some communities have group homes or residential care facilities where 4–12 people with chronic care needs live together. Sometimes people move to nursing homes. This chapter is about the provision of palliative care to persons living in nursing homes. For information about receiving long-term care services outside of a nursing home, please refer to the National Clearinghouse for Long-Term Care Information (http://www.longtermcare.gov/LTC/Main_Site/index.aspx).

Nursing Homes in the United States

In the United States the federal government defines a nursing home as a setting with three or more beds that routinely provides nursing care services (Requirements for States and Long-Term Care Facilities, 2008). Nursing homes are charged with providing round-the-clock assistance to persons who cannot otherwise function in a private home due to their degree of physical and/or cognitive impairment and unmet need for support.

While a nursing home can have as few as three beds, most nursing homes have many more. Indeed, of the 16,000 certified nursing homes in the United States, about half (48%) have 100 beds or more; 1000 U.S. nursing homes have 200 or more beds (National Center for Health Statistics [NCHS], n. d., 2004–2006 data table 1). There are two opposing trends occurring in terms of nursing home size. On the one hand, some innovators are experimenting with "green houses" (small-scale nursing home–level care provided in group homes of 10 or 12 residents) (Kane, Lum, Cutler, Degenholtz, & Lu, 2007). On the other hand, there is a trend toward nursing homes with more beds. Twenty years ago, about one-third of nursing homes had 50 or fewer beds compared to less than 15% in 2004 (National Center for Health Statistics (NCHS) http://cdc.gov/nchs/nnhs/nnhschart.htm). If this latter trend continues, we can expect that most nursing home residents will live in facilities where their needs are balanced against the needs of a hundred or more other residents.

Today, most (two-thirds) of nursing homes are run as for-profit businesses and about one-third are nonprofit. About 6% of nursing homes are government owned (Jones et al., 2009, table 1). Nursing homes can be part of a continuing care retirement community, which include various levels of care, including independent and assisted living; part of a hospital system; or free standing.

Nursing homes are licensed at the state level. In addition to carrying a valid license, most nursing homes are certified to provide both long-term care *and* subacute care/rehab care. If certified, the nursing home can receive Medicare and/or Medicaid funding. Nursing home residents with Medicaid coverage are considered "long-term care" residents and typically have advanced organ failure, frailty, or neurological illnesses that are expected to eventually worsen and from which there is no recovery. In contrast, Medicare pays toward care in the nursing home but only under very narrow conditions. The care must be considered to be skilled subacute or rehab care (not long-term care) and must follow a hospitalization (for a discussion of nursing home payment options for palliative care, see Klug, 2010). Medicare pays for time-limited nursing home care—usually only weeks or months while the resident/patient receives skilled rehabilitation care after which time the patient can either return to his or her private home or remain in the nursing home but now as a "long-term care" resident. Medicare does not pay for long-term care in nursing homes; it pays only for time-limited skilled care in the nursing home. Long-term care in the nursing home is paid by Medicaid, private long-term care insurance, or out of pocket.

The Metlife Market Survey of Nursing Home and Home Health Care Costs reported that in 2009, the average annual cost of a semi-private room for a resident needing long-term care (also called custodial care) was $72,000 per year (about $198 per day), and for a private room, about $80,000 per year (or $219 per day) (http://www.metlife.com/assets/cao/mmi/publications/studies/mmi-market-survey-nursing-home-assisted-living.pdf). People pay these costs as long as their resources allow, with the hopes that Medicaid will deem them eligible to receive Medicaid assistance toward the nursing home bill thereafter. Once eligible, most nursing home residents continue to receive Medicaid assistance for the duration of their stay. which can be months, years, or decades.

Resident Characteristics

Despite the fact that nearly half (45.2%) of nursing home residents are aged 85 or older, it should be noted that 11% of residents are under the age of 65 (Jones et al., 2009). The majority of nursing home residents are women (which is why it can be hard to locate a masculine-looking lap robe in a nursing home—see narrative in Box 11.2). Moss and Moss (2007), in describing the perspectives of men who live in nursing homes, report the unique concerns that arise for the minority gender. Nursing homes need to be mindful to ensure that although most residents are older women, the setting must also meet the preferences and needs of younger people and of men. In nursing homes, as in other settings, in order for care to be good, it must be culturally responsive in terms of gender, age, ethnicity, religion, sexual orientation, and functional ability.

Nearly all residents require assistance with one or more activity of daily living (e.g., bathing, dressing, toileting, transferring, or eating) and indeed over half require assistance with five or more ADLs (Jones et al., 2009). Within the last several years, there has been a trend toward greater acuity among nursing home residents, as evidenced by a larger percentage of residents requiring help with multiple ADLs. This is due in part to the rise in less restrictive alternatives to nursing homes including assisted living and continuing care retirement communities. These alternatives can prevent or postpone the need for nursing home–level care. Furthermore, because states have adapted case-mix payment policies in which there is larger reimbursement when the nursing home provides care to residents with higher level of needs, there are incentives to admit residents with greater physical dependence (Feng, Grabowski, Intrator, & Mor, 2006). This increase in the complexity of care needs places greater demands on staff, including social workers. In addition, most nursing homes in the United States are considered to be "under-staffed" (Schnelle, Simmons, Harrington, Cadogan, Garcia , & Bates-Jensen , 2004).

While most people expect that nursing home residents require physical care, there is growing recognition of the enormous mental health needs of this population. For example, investigators with the National Nursing Home Survey (Jones et al., 2009) have documented that mental health disorders are the second most common diagnostic category in long-term care homes following circulatory disorders. The most common mental health issue is depression, which has been diagnosed in nearly *half to two-thirds of residents* (Bagley et al, 2000; McCurren, Dowe, Rattle, & Looney, 1999; Teresi, Abrams, Holmes, Ramirez, & Eimicke, 2001). Alzheimer's disease and other forms of dementia occur in half of all nursing home residents (Burns et al., 1993; Davis, 2005; Magaziner, Zimmerman, Fox, & Burns, 1998). Several researchers have noted the discrepancy between the need for mental health care in nursing homes and lack of access to such services (Borson, Loebel, Kitchell, Domoto, & Hyde, 1997; Castle & Shea, 1998; Linkins, Lucca, Housman, & Smith, 2006; Shea, Russo, & Smyer, 2000; Smyer, Shea, & Streit, 1994). In response to such concerns, the American Geriatrics Society and the American Association for Geriatric Psychiatry published a consensus statement (2003a) and policy statement (2003b) to encourage greater recognition of, and responsiveness to, the mental health care needs of nursing home residents. The statements underscore that psychosocial interventions should be part of the care plans for residents with mental health concerns. Social workers can address palliative psychosocial concerns by helping to ensure that nursing homes have good interdisciplinary systems for assessing and addressing depression and dementias. For a description of considerations in assessing cognitive and emotional problems among older adults, refer to McInnis-Dittrich (2005).

The complexity of providing excellent care in nursing homes goes beyond the higher acuity of physical needs and the growing recognition of the unmet mental health needs. Nursing homes are also settings where dying occurs frequently. Annually, about 20% of the nation's 2.4 million deaths occur in nursing homes. Among those ages 85+, nearly half (42%) of deaths occur in nursing homes (CDC/NCHS, 2004, table 309). Social work scholar Debra Parker Oliver and colleagues (2004) report that although death is common in nursing homes, there is a need for more empirical research geared toward how excellent end-of-life care can be provided.

Researchers have noted the challenges to providing palliative care in nursing homes. For example, Travis, Loving, McClanahan, and Bernard (2001) have suggested that the complexity of transitions between active, disease-modifying treatment options to palliative and end-of-life care contributes to confusion about treatment goals resulting in curative care as the default. Their hierarchy of obstacles to palliative and end-of-life care includes failing to recognize the futility of curative and restorative treatment, poor communication among decision makers, failure to agree on a course of care, and failure to implement a treatment plan (Travis et al., 2001).

There is a growing emphasis on the need for palliative care approaches in this setting given the complexity of bio-psychosocial-spiritual issues that the vast majority of people in nursing homes face. Indeed, for people with dementia, it has been suggested that palliative care should be part of the treatment protocol beginning at the time of nursing home admission, rather than, as is often the case, introducing it when a person experiences a precipitous decline in health (Powers & Watson, 2008). Engle (1998) goes further in saying that comfort-oriented care should be a goal for all permanently placed nursing home residents. Even when palliative

care–oriented goals dominate a nursing home resident's care plan, he or she should be free to augment palliative care with care aimed at modifying the disease or recovery. In other words, palliative care is always appropriate, whether in the presence or absence of care designed to modify the disease. In theory, palliative care geared toward aggressive comfort can coexist with care aimed at modifying the disease; in practice, it is not common to find palliative care and disease-modifying care goals coexisting in nursing homes.

To close this section, we recognize that nursing home staff members—including social workers—are increasingly called upon to juggle competing paradigms of care, including subacute, rehab, long-term, and end-of-life care. In all cases, attention to physical and psychosocial comfort is appropriate; palliative care can be thought of as an important aspect of best practice care.

As long as there is life there is hope. You don't bury a person before they are dead. If they still see breath on the mirror there is hope … I don't fight death but as long as I am living I want to be happy and well and not in pain … I'm ready to die when it is my time, but in the meantime I want to feel good. (95-year-old resident who has been living with a "terminal" brain tumor for 10 years; from Bern-Klug, 2000 field notes)

Nursing Home Social Work

Nursing homes certified to receive Medicare and/or Medicaid payments are held responsible for providing "medically-related social services to attain or maintain the highest practicable physical, mental and psychosocial well-being of each resident" (Nursing Home Reform Act [NHRA], 1987). Many—although not all—nursing homes meet this requirement by employing social work staff.

Social Work Staffing

While there is a great need for social workers in nursing homes, there are also barriers to the provision of effective social work services. Even though certified nursing homes are required to address the psychosocial needs of residents, current federal regulations require only nursing homes with more than 120 beds to employ one full-time social worker; furthermore, the regulations do not require that the social worker have a degree in social work (Code of Federal Regulations, 2010). A national study of nursing home social service directors documents that although most (over 90%) of nursing homes (even those with fewer than 120 beds) have at least one social services staff member, the majority (58%) have only one full- or part-time social service staff member (Bern-Klug et al., 2009). Furthermore, half the social service directors in the country have a social work degree. The other half is comprised of people with college degrees—but not in social work—as well as 14% who do not have a 4-year college degree (Bern-Klug et al., 2009).

A 2003 report by the Department of Health and Human Services (DHHS), Office of Inspector General identified issues in delivery of psychosocial service in Medicare skilled care units in nursing homes. They documented that 39% of nursing home residents with psychosocial needs had inadequate care plans to meet these needs, while 46% of residents with psycho-social care plans did not receive all planned services. The authors of the report later questioned "whether the present federal rule regarding social worker credentials is effective in achieving the desired level of psychosocial services for skilled nursing facility residents" (DHHS, OIG, 2003, p. 14).

Clearly, the current staffing situation for social workers presents challenges to adequately meeting residents' psycho-social needs, particularly for residents with more intensive needs, including those who are at the end of life. However, without data demonstrating the efficacy of excellent psycho-social care, it will be difficult to make changes. Toward this end, there is a pressing need for scholarship that investigates the outcomes of social work practice in nursing homes (Allen, Nelson, & Netting, 2007; Vourlekis, Zlotnik, & Simons, 2005).

In most nursing homes, because of their education and training, social workers are the only staff member with mental health expertise. They are likely to be the only staff members available to routinely participate in the meetings where care goals—including psychosocial care goals—are agreed upon. If palliative care needs are to be tailored to the needs of each client, palliative care–oriented discussions should be part of the care-planning discussions. Social workers have an important role in ensuring that palliative-oriented psychosocial concerns are identified and addressed.

The NASW *Standards for Social Work Services in Long-Term Care Facilities* (2003) provides a description of social worker roles and functions (pp. 13–15). In general, the scope of practice for nursing home social workers includes, but is not limited to, direct services to residents, families, and other individuals involved with residents' care; advocacy; care planning, discharge planning and documentation; participa-tion in policy and program planning; quality improvement; staff education pertaining to social services; liaison to the community; and consultation to other staff members (p. 13).

Social work is a discipline built on the core belief that a trusting, respectful relationship can be therapeutic and that how we work with clients is as important as completing tasks. In social work, process matters. This is illustrated in the nar-rative of Mr. A. (see Box 11.2) as the social worker listens attentively to the resident as he speaks about being in WWII; it is clear that the social worker is doing much more than providing factual information or a laprobe.

Notably, social work practice in a nursing home requires work within multiple system levels, including residents, family, members of the interprofessional team, facility administration, other providers (hospitals, hospices, etc.),

Box 11.2
Resident/Family Narrative: Mr. and Mrs. A

The social worker is paged to the subacute unit where a couple (Mr. and Mrs. A.) is waiting to speak with him. The wife tells the social worker that they are upset because the husband—who was admitted from the hospital 2 days ago to receive rehab for a broken hip—did not receive the assistance from the nursing staff that morning as expected. The first day of his stay his wife helped him to transfer from bed to chair and to the restroom. This morning, before the wife arrived, Mr. A. asked for help in transferring, and the nursing staff said he should do it on his own. That angered and humiliated him. He wanted to be as independent as possible, but he did not want to risk another fall. Mr. A. did not yet feel safe transferring without help. The past months have been a struggle for the couple. Mr. A. had been treated for prostate cancer and on his last day of radiation (his 37th treatment), he had a heart attack, and then needed bypass surgery (his fifth bypass surgery). When he finally got home from the surgery episode, he slipped off a breakfast stool and broke his hip—which is what led to the hospitalization, more surgery, and now this nursing home stay for rehab. It had been a long road of illness.

The social worker listens patiently and carefully. He apologizes on behalf of the staff and says that he will touch base with the nursing staff. The wife mentions that despite her husband's experience in serving in World War II, all the recent battles with health problems have really been a challenge for him. The social worker engages the husband in a detailed conversation about WWII and Mr. A. concludes with a story about how he was part of the effort to liberate the Philippines. The social worker takes a deep breath and, looking directly at Mr. A., says, "Mr. A., for all you have done for this country, and for me, and for everyone in my generation, I want to say 'thank you.'" Mr. A. smiles and looks down. Mrs. A. pipes up, "Honey—tell him about the nurse in the hospital." Mr. A. hesitates for a moment and then looks at the social worker and explains how embarrassing it had been for him to soil himself in the hospital and to have to ask a nurse to clean him up. He talks about how much he hated to bother the staff. One particular day he was apologizing to a nursing assistant as she changed his sheets and the nursing assistant said to him, "Oh you just forget about it. This is my chance to repay you for helping to liberate my country." The nurse was from the Philippines. Mrs. A. explains that the nurse's comment made it easier for her husband to accept help. The social worker thanks Mr. A. and his wife for sharing the story and then goes to fetch a lap robe for Mr. A. who had mentioned he was chilled. It takes a while for the social worker to return, "I'm sorry it took so long, I wanted to find a masculine lap robe—most of them around here are pink." The social worker hands the brown plaid lap robe to Mr. A. and assures the couple that he will speak with the nursing staff about helping with transfers. (Bern-Klug, 2000 unpublished field notes)

and the community as a whole. It is also one of the few health care settings where the possibility exists for long-term prac-titioner–client relationships, which draws some people to work in this setting.

Even the most qualified social worker depends on a realistic staffing ratio, an appropriate job description, auton-omy, support, and other team members in order to assure good resident outcomes. Interprofessional teamwork, as in other health care settings, is central to the process of providing good nursing home care. Nursing home teams are generally comprised of a nurse, physician (generally not on-site), rehabilitation specialists (e.g., physical, occupational, and speech therapists), dietician, pharmacist (generally not on-site), social worker, recreation therapist, resident, and family members. The exact composition of the care team should be determined by the needs of the resident and treatment goals under review. For example, speech therapists may play a lead in developing treatment goals and interventions for residents with swallowing difficulties, which are common among people recovering from strokes or living with other neurological conditions. Dieticians can address the consistency of food and nutritional needs of a person incapable of chewing and swallowing solid foods. Nurses and nursing assistants are responsible for ensuring that the resident is provided personal assistance at meal time as needed. In the best circumstances, residents are involved in the development of treatment goals. In situations where this is not possible (i.e., the resident lacks cognitive capacity), family members are called upon to serve as a voice for the resident. Staff members need to be turning to the family for information about the residents' preferences, hopes, and fears, and honoring the family's perspective.

Palliative Psychosocial Assessment and Care Planning

The Minimum Data Set (MDS) is a federally required comprehensive assessment tool that collects data about each nursing home resident in all certified nursing homes. The data are collected at admission and then on specified intervals thereafter (for long-term care residents, typically, every 90 days). The MDS is the driver of nursing home care. Goals related to care and also planned interventions are developed in relation to the clinical needs identified through the MDS. Along with physical health–related items, the MDS includes items that are psychosocial in nature, such as those related to mood, cognition, behavior, and preferences for routines and activities. Ideally, social workers are involved in conducting psychosocial assessments and completing psychosocial portions of the MDS, but in reality there are no regulations specifying which discipline should complete these sections. Federal regulations require that a registered nurse (RN) must sign off on the entire MDS document (Code of Federal Regulations). The new version, the MDS-3, is expected to be mandated as of fall 2010 (http://www.cms.hhs.gov/NursingHomeQualityInits/25_NHQ-IMDS30.asp) and includes questions on pain and the PHQ-9 (Brief Patient Health Questionnaire–Mood Scale) tool for screening depression and mood. Social workers who do not have the responsibility of completing the psychosocial sections of the MDS can still be effective catalysts for palliative psychosocial care by working with the MDS RN to record psychosocial issues and by including these aspects of the residents' experience in care plan discussion.

In addition to the MDS, social workers are involved in other forms of psychosocial assessment, such as the creation of psychosocial histories for residents and administration of standardized measures of mood and behavior as needed (Beaulieu, 2002; Sahlins, 2010). For example, although the MDS 3.0 includes an item intended to screen for suicidality, as part of a best practice approach, a social worker or other mental health professional should follow up with a standardized assessment tool in order to determine whether immediate intervention is required. Likewise, to the extent that MDS assessments rely on day shift observations, the social worker may team with evening or night shift staff in completing standardized assessment of residents with agitation and aggressive behaviors that could inform care planning and behavioral interventions. Clinical assessments in addition to the MDS will become part of the resident's record. The assessments can be administered on a routine basis to gauge changes in psychosocial status, thus creating a shared vigilance and accountability for this aspect of care. The National Consensus Guidelines for Quality Palliative Care call for a comprehensive interdisciplinary social assessment, including family structure and geographic location; relationships; lines of communication; existing social and cultural networks; social support; medical decision making; work settings; finances; sexuality; intimacy; caregiver availability; access to needed equipment; community resources; and legal issues (National Consensus Project, 2009). Morrison and colleagues (2005) documented that an intervention aimed at training nursing home social workers to identify and document resident medical care wishes increased the likelihood that the care received was consistent with resident wishes.

The National Consensus Guidelines emphasize the need for culturally sensitive care plans and openness to spiritual needs and desires. Nursing home social workers committed to infusing palliative care in their settings can begin by comparing current assessment forms with recommendations from the Clinical Practice Guidelines.

Once care needs are identified, nursing home team members should meet to develop appropriate treatment goals. These meetings are expected to take place at least quarterly and more often if there is a major change in a resident's condition or circumstance, such as readmittance from the hospital, which may trigger an immediate review of treatment goals and options. Goals of care can become confused between the hospital and the nursing home, and a meeting to ensure that everyone is on the same page can be helpful. Social workers often have a role in organizing and coordinating these meetings. For example, as liaisons to residents and family members, they are often involved in ensuring that family members are aware of the care plan meeting and have the opportunity to attend and provide input. Social workers may also be called upon to mediate family members' concerns relative to the care provided, including complaints made to administration. One study found that social workers were primarily responsible for resolving nearly half (43%) of all resident and staff conflicts (Vinton, Mazza, & Kim, 1998). In this case, nursing home social workers walk a fine line between being advocates for and with residents and families, while also serving as representatives of the facility and its concerns.

Palliative psychosocial care plan goals should be specific to the unique needs of residents. Often the goals and planned interventions are aimed at ameliorating psychological symptoms related to disease processes, adjusting to life within the facility, personalizing care based on the residents' personal preferences and previous life patterns, and accessing necessary mental health services, such as psychiatric consultation and/or counseling.

As in Mr. B.'s situation (see Box 11.3), the social worker can be instrumental in helping the family understand options for receiving care outside of the nursing home. Social workers honor residents' self-determination when they assist residents in leaving the nursing home if that is their desire; this holds for residents who are considered to be dying, like Mr. B., and residents who are not imminently dying. In the case of residents with end-of-life care needs, the social worker may be responsible for educating the family and resident on available care options, including hospice. Social workers can encourage residents and family members to discuss the option of hospice with their primary care provider. Hospice services can be provided to nursing home residents while they are in the nursing home, or they can be delivered in a hospice facility (if available in the community), or in a private home setting (under certain conditions). For a discussion about Medicare eligibility, coverage and financing, please consult the federal government's booklet, "Medicare and Hospice" (http://www.medicare.gov/Publications/Pubs/pdf/02154.pdf). For information about hospice eligibility, coverage, and financing specific to nursing home residents with Medicare and/or Medicaid, refer to Klug (2010). It has been documented that hospice involvement can improve end-of-life care by controlling pain and reducing the number of hospitalizations for nursing home residents (Miller, Williams, English, & Keyserling, 2002; Munn, Hanson, Zimmerman, Sloane, & Mitchell, 2006).

Experienced nursing home social workers have the knowledge and skills to facilitate discussions with residents, family members, staff, and the resident's physician regarding options for palliative and end-of-life care. Social workers are often responsible for discussing advance directives with residents and family members and for documenting the wishes so that all staff can access the information. When family members disagree on end-of-life treatment decisions, it may be the social worker that mediates these conflicts.

Group Work

Providing one-to-one counseling and mental health services to a large number of residents may not be feasible for most nursing home social workers given the typical level of resident-to-social worker staffing ratios. Instead, when the social workers' caseload precludes providing individual

Box 11.3
Resident/Family Narrative: Mr. B

The social worker mentioned that she felt badly for not getting to Mr. B.'s room before his wife left for the day, "I went in and she had already left." The social worker wanted to talk with the couple about home health care and hospice because they were thinking about bringing Mr. B. home for his last weeks and were confused about what Medicare would pay for and under what conditions. She said that her job was hectic and that no matter what she had planned to get done on any given day there were always interruptions and unexpected things that needed attention. She would try again tomorrow to meet with Mr. and Mrs. B. and talk through how the discharge to home could work. (Bern-Klug, 2000 unpublished field notes)

mental health services, the worker connects residents with other mental health professionals who are able to provide one-on-one services (Beaulieu, 2002).

Even when staffing ratios prohibit one-to-one counseling sessions, nursing home social workers can engage in group work with residents. Group work topics can address the desire to thrive, the challenges of suffering, and the need for meaningful social connections (Sahlins, 2010). Social workers facilitate educational and therapeutic groups with residents who share similar psychosocial needs. In the context of palliative care, social workers may work with a group of residents on strategies for self-management of pain as a complement to pharmacological interventions. Because of the many issues related to loss facing most nursing home residents, grief and bereavement groups are of benefit as well. There is also initial evidence to support the use of reminiscence and validation therapies to improve mood (Woods, Spector, Jones, Orrell, & Davies, 2005) and to reduce behavioral disturbances (Deponte & Missan, 2007) among people with dementia; more research in this area is needed. Social workers may also partner with recreation and expressive arts therapists to provide services and activities that are oriented toward meeting psychosocial needs.

Nursing home social workers are often the main contact between the nursing home and family regarding psychosocial issues. Solomon (1983) suggests that there are four events typically perceived as crises by families of nursing home residents, including the decision to admit to the nursing home; the actual admission process; the move to a more intensive level of care; and the death of the resident. Nursing home social workers can anticipate the high emotional content of these situations and devise methods to provide extra support to families around these events. Some of the support can come by way of a support group or psychoeducational sessions.

The nature or theme of the group is determined by the particular needs of family caregivers. For example, spousal caregivers of people with Alzheimer's disease and other dementias are often frequent visitors to the home and may struggle with grief, guilt, and their changed role as they adapt to both the nursing home admission and the functional changes experienced by their spouse. The nursing home social worker may organize and facilitate a support group to help caregivers cope and to build a support network of people who are sharing these same experiences. She or he may also organize, coordinate, or facilitate a caregiver support group through the local chapter of the Alzheimer's Association (http://www.alz.org/index.asp) and make information available on other types of support groups in the region and on the Internet. There are likely a number of groups that could be created. Drawing upon community resources to sponsor, coordinate, and facilitate such groups may also be necessary if social work staffing hours are limited, and it has a secondary benefit of connecting family to community supports. There is the potential for nursing home residents to use computers to join online support groups as well, especially if adaptive equipment is available.

Resident-Centered Care and Residents' Rights

Social workers can help the resident and his or her family members adjust to institutional living and can help the facility adjust to the resident. For example, it is typically the role of nursing home social workers to review the Residents' Rights information with each resident (or caregiver by proxy). By federal law, all homes must review and provide a physical copy of the Residents' Rights document (http://www.medicare.gov/Nursing/ResidentRights.asp; or http://www.nccnhr.org/sites/default/files/advocate/advocacy-groups/ResidentRights.pdf) before or during admission. At a basic level, Residents' Rights are meant to ensure the following:

- Residents are treated with dignity and respect (including freedom from abuse and neglect).
- Residents are provided written notice regarding the costs of services.
- Residents are given the right to manage their own money when they are at all capable of doing so.
- Residents are provided with privacy and have access to personal belongings.
- Residents are informed about their medical condition and given the right to refuse treatment.

An intention of Residents' Rights is that residents be encouraged to maintain previous lifestyles and preferences, including personalizing their daily schedule if they choose. It is here that the concept of "resident-centered care" has taken root. Resident-centered care has been described as embodying values that include "allowing older adults or those closest to the older adults to make decisions, promoting individualized care, knowing each older adult as a person, and putting the individual before the task" (Robinson & Rosher, 2006, p. 19). It is perhaps best articulated as part of the nursing home culture change movement, which began in the mid-1990s. Broadly defined, culture change is a quality of life

movement involving structural, attitudinal, and behavioral changes within the environment of care. The intention of these changes is to create a sense of community and to empower both frontline staff and residents in order to improve worklife satisfaction and decrease feelings of loneliness and depression among residents (Rahman & Schnelle, 2008). For example, culturally transformed facilities often redesign larger, hospital-like units into smaller "neighborhoods" with shared kitchens and living spaces. They also attempt to invert the organizational structure, so that those traditionally at the bottom (i.e., residents and frontline staff) have more power and greater decision-making capacity (Robinson & Rosher, 2006). The culture change and resident-centered care movements are a good fit with social work's professional mission and values, and they provide social workers with unique opportunities for leadership in culturally transforming facilities. They are also compatible with holistic approaches to care such as palliative care.

In addition to culture change, there is a small but growing movement for culturally responsive nursing home care. This includes the recognition that nursing homes are settings with ethnic and racial cultural diversity (not so much among the residents as *between* residents and staff) as well as, of course, age diversity. In addition, nursing homes—including the people who work, live, and visit there—like other societal institutions, are challenged by ageism, ableism, and heterosexism. Social workers can help enhance the cultural sensitivity of staff, residents, and families by providing training or arranging for others in the community to lead discussion and education sessions. Because nursing homes are home to residents, it is vitally important that the setting and the people within the setting aspire to cultural responsiveness. Excellent palliative care is culturally respectful care.

Practice Competencies for Social Work in Nursing Homes

Effective practice in nursing homes requires specific knowledge of the environment and its clientele as well as a unique skill set; however, it also shares much in common with other gerontological settings, particularly other residential and health care environments that serve elders. Building on the earlier work of the Council on Social Work Education's *Strengthening Aging and Gerontological Education in Social Work* to develop a set of competencies for gerontological social work practice (Rosen, Zlotnik, Curl, & Green, 2000), the Hartford Partnership Program for Aging Education developed a *Geriatric Social Work Competency Scale* intended to provide a self-assessment of skill in aging practice. The instrument has four conceptual domains: (1) values, ethics, and theoretical perspectives; (2) assessment; (3) intervention; and (4) aging service, programs, and policies. It can be found at: http://socialwork.nyam.org/nsw/competencies/competencies.php.

While general in nature, each of the scale items provides a description of skills that are necessary for effective practice in nursing homes as well as other gerontological settings. For example, items under "assessment" describe the use of sensitive interviewing skills; the adaptation of interviewing methods to meet sensory or cognitive imitations; the assessment of health status, psychosocial, and cognitive functioning (i.e., comprehensive bio-psychosocial-spiritual assessment); the assessment of caregivers' needs and stress levels; the use of standardized assessment tools; the development of service plans with measurable objectives; and the review and revision of service plans. Items under "intervention" describe establishing rapport with older adults and their family members; enhancing the mental health of elders through various therapeutic modalities; utilizing group interventions; mediating conflicts with elders and/or their family members; assisting caregivers to reduce stress and maintain well-being; providing case management services; using educational strategies related to wellness and disease management; advocating on behalf of elders to obtain needed services; and adhering to laws related to older adults (Damron-Rodriguez, 2006). Readers are encouraged to view and/or complete the scale themselves.

Beyond this broader set of competencies, nursing home social workers will require a working knowledge of Alzheimer's disease and other dementias as well as the range of chronic health conditions, including diabetes, heart disease, stroke, the most common forms of cancer, chronic pain conditions, and other neurological conditions such as Parkinson's disease and brain injury (Allegre, 2010). Although a social worker is not directly responsible for addressing the physical aspects of disease, she or he must be capable of identifying psychosocial consequences of the disease—or of the treatment of the disease—and creating and implementing appropriate interventions. For example, the federal government's interpretive guidelines indicate that nursing homes are responsible for ensuring that residents who are experiencing chronic or acute pain have access to medical social services (State Operations Manual, 2005). Furthermore, nursing home social workers must have knowledge of best practices in mental health with a frail elder population, including the assessment of depression because it is so prevalent in this environment. Serving the psychosocial needs of people with advanced dementia is particularly difficult because of communication challenges that impede conveying thoughts, feelings, and emotions. In this situation, observational assessment, which may include the use of standardized observational measures of depression and agitation, will be necessary. To thrive in the nursing home setting, as well as in other long-term care settings, social workers need educational opportunities to enhance their knowledge and skills related to the physical, mental, and emotional circumstances facing nursing home residents.

Beginning social workers and those fulfilling this role without a degree in social work will benefit from accessing clinical supervision from an experienced, licensed social worker.

When clinical supervision is not available at the facility, social workers may contact their local chapter of the National Association of Social Workers (NASW) to seek support in identifying a clinical supervisor. Nursing home social workers are also encouraged to become members of professional associations, such as the NASW (http://www.naswdc.org/), the Society for Social Work Leadership in Health Care (http://www.sswlhc.org/), and the Social Work Hospice and Palliative Care Network (http://www.swhpn.org/) as doing so will expand opportunities for networking and for accessing continuing education. The University of Iowa hosts a Web page for nursing home social workers and a listserv (http://www.uiowa.edu/~socialwk/NursingHomeResource/index.html). Networking is particularly important because many nursing homes have only one social worker, creating a situation that can lead to professional isolation.

Conclusion

This chapter discusses ways in which nursing home social workers can introduce and support palliative care. We believe that palliative care is good care. Furthermore, a nursing home may be more effective in providing palliative care to some residents if it is set up to provide palliative care to all residents (Bern-Klug, 2010). In other words, the entire nursing home environment should be organized to address bio-psychosocial-spiritual needs, rather than only conceptualizing palliative care as a type of care provided to certain residents. This is another example of how the movement toward person-centered care is clearing a way for palliative care. Person-centered care emphasizes improving the nursing home psychosocial and social environments. As nursing homes build a reputation for providing high-quality care that addresses both physical pain and psychosocial- spiritual suffering, the cloud of stigma currently shadowing nursing homes will likely lift.

Excellent palliative care will also require the scholarship necessary to document what are the best practices. This information can inform regulatory change. Scholarship is needed at multiple levels. Social workers have the opportunity to collect information about resident outcomes in relation to the palliative psychosocial services provided. For example, social workers can conduct pre- and postassessment of mood state among participants of support groups to determine whether mood improves as a result of the intervention. We need information that documents the amount of social worker time spent providing direct, clinical services to residents in relationship to nonclinical activities. We need the will to improve care, the vision, the education, and the resources to improve care. A philosophy of palliative care can be a guiding light.

If I ever go back to work again in a nursing home, and someday I might, I will have more feeling for the people

*there. I will keep my eyes open more for how I can help.
I like the people. I enjoy hearing the stories about their
life. After a while … they look forward to seeing you….
If I ever go back to that kind of work, when I look at a
person I will think, "this lady is somebody's momma—
like my momma was to me—I better treat her good."
(Daughter of a nursing home resident and former
certified nurse aide; Bern-Klug, 2000 field notes)*

LEARNING EXERCISES

1. Compare the "quality of care" provided by Medicare and/or Medicaid certified nursing homes in your zipcode by reviewing information posted by the federal government. Go to http://www.medicare.gov and then scroll down to "compare nursing homes" or use the Web site's search engine to locate. Compare at least three nursing homes. Discuss how the various measures of quality might affect resident psychosocial issues. How are addressing palliative care needs consistent with high overall quality of care? Also, how is palliative care related to quality of life?

2. Watch this DVD and discuss how a social work approach to palliative psychosocial care could be an asset to the family: http://www.forgetfulnotforgotten. com/the-film Also, using an ecological systems theory framework, identify four key psychosocial issues in a patient family narrative. Develop a case/care plan with specific, realistic treatment goals. What outcomes would you identify for each of these treatment goals as indicators of "success", and how would you measure these outcomes?

3. Learn about the TimeSlips training system for interactive storytelling with persons affected with moderate dementia. "TimeSlips is a group process that opens storytelling to people with cognitive challenges by replacing the pressure to remember with the encouragement to *imagine*." http://www.timeslips.org/ This activity can be organized by social workers, activities staff, and/or family members.

4. Consult http://www.medicare.gov to check current guidelines for Medicare Hospice coverage in the nursing home setting. Notice the "extra" benefits that hospice enrollees and their families get through hospice that are not otherwise available through Medicare.

ADDITIONAL RESOURCES/WEB SITES

Bern-Klug, (Ed). (2010). Transforming palliative care in nursing homes: The social work role. NY: Columbia University Press Available at: http://cup.columbia.edu/search?q=bern-klug&go. x=13&go.y=9

Henderson, M. L., Hanson, L. C., & Reynolds, K. S. (2003). *Improving nursing home care of the dying: A training manual for nursing home staff*. New York, NY: Spring Publishing Co. Available at: http://www.springerpub.com/ product/9780826119254

WEB SITES

Resource Page for Nursing Home Social Workers: http://www. uiowa.edu/~socialwk/NursingHomeResource/index.html Serves as a repository of information about nursing home social services and social work for people who work in nursing homes and people who conduct research about psychosocial care in nursing homes.

Toolkit of Instruments to Measure End-of-Life Care (TIME): http://www.chcr.brown.edu/pcoc/toolkit.htm Takes steps toward crossing this measurement barrier by creating patient-focused, family-centered survey instruments that address the needs and concerns of patients and their families, as defined by them.

REFERENCES

Allegre, A. (2010). Anticipating and managing common medical challenges encountered at the end of life. In M. Bern-Klug (Ed.), *Transforming palliative care in nursing homes: The social work role* (pp. 107–139). New York, NY: Columbia University Press.

Allen, P. D., Nelson, H. W., & Netting, F. E. (2007). Current practice and policy realities revisited: Undertrained nursing home social workers in U.S. *Social Work in Health Care, 45*(4), 1–22.

American Geriatrics Society (AGS) & American Association for Geriatric Psychiatry (AAGP). (2003a). Consensus statement on improving the quality of mental health care in U.S. nursing homes: Management of depression and behavioral symptoms associated with dementia. *Journal of the American Geriatrics Society, 51*, 1287–1298.

American Geriatrics Society (AGS) & American Association for Geriatric Psychiatry (AAGP). (2003b). The American Geriatrics Society and American Association for Geriatric Psychiatry recommendations for policies in support of quality mental health care in U.S. nursing homes. *Journal of the American Geriatrics Society, 51*, 1299–1304.

Bagley, H., Cordingley, L., Burns, A., Mozley, C. G., Sutcliffe, C., Challis, D., & Huxley, P. (2000). Recognition of depression by staff in nursing and residential homes. *Journal of Clinical Nursing, 9*(3), 445–450.

Beaulieu, E. (2002). *A guide for nursing home social workers*. New York, NY: Springer Publishing.

Bern-Klug, M. (Ed.). (2010). *Transforming palliative care in nursing homes: The social work role.* New York, NY: Columbia University Press.

Bern-Klug, M., Kramer, K. W. O., Chan, G., Kane, R., Dorfman, L. T., & Saunders, J. B. (2009). Characteristics of nursing home Social Services Directors: How common is a degree in Social Work? *Journal of the American Medical Directors Association, 10*(1), 36–44.

Borson, S., Loebel, J.P., Kitchell, M., Domoto, S., & Hyde, T. (1997). Psychiatric assessments of nursing home residents under OBRA-87: Should PASARR be reformed? *Journal of the American Geriatric Society, 45*(10), 1173–1181.

Burns, B. J., Wagner, H. R., Taube, J. E., Magaziner, J., Permutt, T., & Landerman, L. R. (1993). Mental health service use by the elderly in nursing homes. *American Journal of Public Health, 83,* 331–337.

Castle, N., & Shea, D. (1998). The effects of for-profit and not-for-profit facility status on the quality of care for nursing home residents with mental illnesses. *Research on Aging, 20*(2), 246–263.

Centers for Disease Control (CDC), National Center for Health Statistics (NCHS). (2006). *Worktable 309: Deaths by place of death, age, race, and sex: U.S., 2004.* Retrieved from http://www. cdc.gov/nchs/data/dvs/MortFinal2004_Worktable309.pdf

Code of Federal Regulations (2010). Title 42: Public Health, Part 483 Requirements for states and long term care facilities, sub-part B requirements for long term care facilities, Section 483:25 Quality of life. Washington DC; Government Printing Office: Accessed August 17, 2010: http://ecfr.gpoaccess.gov/ cgi/t/text/text-idx?c=ecfr&sid=baf734ca473c2a4a01abda2f738f d9b5&rgn=div8&view=text&node=42:5.0.1.1.2.7.6&idno=42

Damron-Rodriguez, J. (2006). Moving forward: Developing geriatric social work competencies. In B. Berkman (Eds.), *The Oxford handbook of social work in aging* (pp. 1051–1064). New York, NY: Oxford University Press.

Davis, J. A. (2005). Differences in the health care needs and service utilization of women in nursing homes: Comparison by race/ ethnicity. *Journal of Women and Aging, 17*(3), 57–71.

Department of Health and Human Services (DHHS), Office of Inspector General (OIG). (2003). *Psychosocial services in skilled nursing facilities.* Retrieved from http://oig.hhs.gov/oei/reports/ oei-02-01-00610.pdf

Deponte, A., & Missan, R. (2007). Effectiveness of validation therapy (VT) in group: Preliminary results. *Archives of Gerontology and Geriatrics, 44,* 113–117.

Engle, V. F. (1998). Care of the living, care of the dying: Reconceptualizing nursing home care. *Journal of the American Geriatrics Society, 46*(9), 1172–1174.

Feder, J., Komisar, H. L., & Niefeld, M. (2000). Long-term care in the United States: An overview. *Health Affairs, 19*(3), 40–56.

Feng, Z., Grabowski, D. C., Intrator, O., & Mor, V. (2006). The effect of state medicaid case-mix payment on nursing home resident acuity. *Health Services Research, 41*(4), 1317–1336.

Himes, C. L. (2002). Elderly Americans. *Population bulletin.* Retrieved from the Population Reference Bureau Web site: http://www.prb.org/Source/ACFD30.pdf

Jones, A. L., Dwyer, L. L., Bercovitz, A. R., & Strahan, G. W. (2009). *The national nursing home survey: 2004 overview.* U.S. Health and Human Services, Centers for Disease Control and Prevention. NCHS Publication Number (PHS) 2009-1738.

Kane, R. A. (2003). Definition, measurement, and correlates of quality of life in nursing homes: Toward a reasonable practice, research, and policy agenda. *The Gerontologist, 43*(2), 28–36.

Kane R. A., Lum, T. Y., Cutler, L. J., Degenholtz, H. B., & Yu, T. (2007). Resident outcomes in small-house nursing homes: A longitudinal evaluation of the initial green house program. *Journal of the American Geriatrics Society, 55*(6), 832–839.

Klug, M. (2010). Paying for advanced chronic illness and hospice care in America's nursing homes. In M. Bern-Klug (Ed.),

Transforming palliative care in nursing homes: The social work role (pp. 59–83). New York, NY: Columbia University Press.

Kramer, B. J. (2000). Husbands caring for wives with dementia: A longitudinal study of continuity and change. *Health and Social Work, 25*(2), 97–107.

Linkins, K. W., Lucca, A. M., Housman, M., & Smith, S. A. (2006). Use of PASRR programs to assess serious mental illness and service access in nursing homes. *Psychiatric Services, 57,* 325–332.

Magaziner, J., Zimmerman, S. I., Fox, K. M., & Burns, B. J. (1998). Dementia in United States nursing homes: Descriptive epidemiology and implications for long-term residential care. *Aging and Mental Health, 2*(1), 28–35.

McCurren, C., Dowe, D., Rattle, D., & Looney, S. (1999). Depression among nursing home elders: Testing an intervention strategy. *Applied Nursing Research, 12*(4), 185–195.

McInnes-Dittrich, K. (2009). Differential assessment and diagnosis of cognitive and emotional problems of older adults In *Social work with older adults: A biopsychosocial approach to assessment and intervention* (3rd ed., pp. 112–142). Boston, MA: Pearson, Allen & Bacon.

Miller, G. W., Williams, R. J., English, D. F., & Keyserling, J. (2002). *Delivering quality care and cost-effectiveness at the end of life: Building on the 20-year success of the Medicare hospice benefit.* Alexandria, VA: National Hospice and Palliative Care Organization.

Morrison, R. S., Chichin, E., Carter, J., Burack, O., Lantz, M., & Meier, D. (2005). The effect of a social work intervention to enhance advanced care planning documentation in the nursing home. *Journal of the American Geriatrics Society, 53*(2), 290–294.

Moss, S. Z., & Moss, M. S. (2007). Being a man in long-term care. *Journal of Aging Studies, 21*(1), 43–54.

Munn, J. C., Hanson, L. C., Zimmerman, S., Sloane, P. D., & Mitchell, C. M. (2006). Is hospice associated with improved end-of-life care in nursing homes and assisted living facilities? *Journal of the American Geriatrics Society, 54*(3), 490–495.

National Association of Social Workers (NASW). (2003). *Standards for social work services in long-term care facilities.* Washington, DC: Author.

National Center for Health Statistics (NCHS). (n. d.). *The national nursing home survey.* Retrieved from http://www.cdc.gov/nchs/ nnhs.htm

National Consensus Project for Quality Palliative Care. (2009). Clinical practice guidelines for quality palliative care. Retrieved from http://www.nationalconsensusproject.org/Guideline.pdf

Nursing Home Reform Act (NHRA) of 1987, Pub Law No. 100-203 § 4211, 101 Stat. 188 (1989).

Oliver, D. P., Porock, D., & Zweig, S. (2004). End-of-life care in nursing homes: A review of the evidence. *Journal of the American Medical Directors Association, 5*(3), 147–155.

Powers, B. A., & Watson, N. M. (2008). Meaning and practice of palliative care for nursing home residents with dementia at end of life. *American Journal of Alzheimer's Disease and Other Dementias, 23*(4), 319–325.

Rahman, A. N., & Schnelle, J. F. (2008). The nursing home culture-change movement: Recent past, present, and future directions for research. *The Gerontologist, 48*(2), 142–148.

Robinson, S. B., & Rosher, R. B. (2006). Tangling with the barriers to culture change creating a resident-centered nursing home environment. *Journal of Gerontological Nursing, 32*(10), 19–25.

Rosen, A. L., Zlotnik, J. L., Curl, A. L., & Green, R. G. (2000). *The CSWE SAGE-SW national aging competencies survey report.* Alexandria, VA: Council on Social Work Education.

Sahlins, J. (2010). *Social work practice in nursing homes: Creativity, leadership, and program development.* Chicago, IL: Lyceum Press.

Sanders, S. (2007). Experiences of rural male caregivers of older adults with their informal support networks. *Journal of Gerontological Social Work, 49*(4), 97–115.

Schnelle, J. F., Simmons, S. F., Harrington, C., Cadogan, M., Garcia, E., & Bates-Jensen, B. M. (2004). Relationship of nursing home staffing to quality of care. *Health Services Research, 39*(2), 225–250.

Shea, D. G., Russo, P. A., & Smyer, M. A. (2000). Use of mental health services by persons with a mental illness in nursing facilities: Initial impacts of OBRA 87. *Journal of Aging and Health, 12*(4), 560–578.

Smyer, M. A., Shea, D. G., & Streit, A. (1994). The provision and use of mental health services in nursing homes: Results from the national medical expenditure survey. *American Journal of Public Health, 84*(2), 284–286.

Solomon, R. (1983). Serving families of the institutionalized aged: The four crises. *Journal of Gerontological Social Work in Long-Term Care, 5,* 83–96.

State operations manual, appendix P, survey protocol for long-term care facilities. Retrieved from http://www.cms.hhs.gov/GuidanceforLawsAndRegulations/12_NHs.asp

Teresi, J., Abrams, R., Holmes, D., Ramirez, M., & Eimicke, J. (2001). Prevalence of depression and depression recognition in nursing homes. *Social Psychiatry and Psychiatric Epidemiology, 36*(12), 613–620.

Thomas, W. H., & Johansson C. (2003). Elderhood in Eden. *Topics in Geriatric Rehabilitation, 19*(4), 282–290.

Travis, S. S., Loving, G., McClanahan, L., & Bernard, M. (2001). Hospitalization patterns and palliation in the last year of life among residents in long-term care. *The Gerontologist, 41*(2), 153–160.

Vinton, L., Mazza, N., & Kim, Y. (1998). Intervening in family-staff conflicts in nursing homes. *Clinical Gerontologist, 19,* 45–67.

Vourlekis, B. S., Zlotnik, J. L., & Simons, K. (2005). *Evaluating social work services in nursing homes: Toward quality psychosocial care and its measurement. A report to the profession and blueprint for action.* Washington, DC: Institute for the Advancement of Social Work Research.

Weiner, J. M., Hanley, R. J., Clark, R., & Van Nostrand, J. F. (1990). *Measuring the activities of daily living: Comparisons across national surveys. ASPE-HHS Report.* Retrieved from the U.S. Department of Health & Human Services Web site: http://aspe.hhs.gov/daltcp/reports/meacmpes.htm

Woods, B., Spector, A. E., Jones, C. A., Orrell, M., & Davies, S. P. (2005). Reminiscence therapy for dementia. *Cochrane Database of Systematic Reviews, 2.* Art No. CD001120. doi: 10.1002/14651858.CD001120.pub2.

12 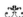 *Louisa Daratsos*

Palliative Care for Veterans

My dad always wanted a military funeral. I promised him that. Can you help me?
—The son of Mr. B, a 66-year-old Marine veteran
of the Vietnam War who was dying of lung cancer

Key Concepts

◆ *Veterans are a significant population receiving palliative and end-of-life care.*

◆ *Each war cohort has a set of central issues related to their era in the service that might influence how they experience life-threatening illness and end of life.*

◆ *The Department of Veterans Affairs (VA) and the respective state and local government agencies are the source of financial, educational, and health care benefits for veterans.*

◆ *The VA has a well-developed program and is a source of expertise and consultation for palliative and end-of-life care for veterans.*

◆ *The community at large and the VA serve veterans best when they collaborate on veterans' palliative and end-of-life issues on the federal, state, and local levels.*

Introduction

This chapter will discuss specific aspects of palliative care related to veterans who are living with life-threatening illness and those at end of life. Veterans of any country can be considered a special population because of their sacrifice and service to their nation, regardless of whether they served after volunteering or being drafted. This chapter, will, however, concentrate on veterans of the United States Armed Forces, and profile Vietnam Era veterans, who are the largest living veteran cohort. The history of the development of services for veterans sheds light on why, in the United States, there is much interest in quality palliative care for veterans. Veterans of the United States Armed Forces represent 8% of this country's population. The Department of Veterans Affairs (VA) is the federal agency responsible for the development and administration of a range of financial, educational, psychological, and health services for this population. The Veterans Health Administration (VHA) is the largest integrated health care system in the United States devoted almost exclusively to the physical and mental health of veterans. Nearly all veterans are entitled to receive benefits from the federal government, ranging from low-cost home loans, to educational benefits, to health care, to death benefits, which are based upon their military service. Therefore, this chapter will also discuss the benefits available to all veterans, with particular emphasis on services related to palliative care and end of life.

Need for Social Work Expertise in Veterans' End-of-Life Care

There have been various VA policy mandates to promote care that meets the needs and optimizes comforts for veterans who are coming to the end of their lives. The policy directive stems from the demographics of an older veteran population who are dying at the rate of 1800 per day according to VHA estimates as stated in the most recent VA Policy Directive, 2008-066. The VA has robust partnerships at the macro, mezzo, and micro level through the Veterans-Hospice

Partnership and with major organizations dedicated to promoting palliative care such as the National Hospice and Palliative Care Organization (NHPCO), the Center to Advance Palliative Care (CAP-C), and Joint Commission Accreditation Hospital Organizations (JCAHO), to name a few (Daratsos & Howe, 2007).

Social workers, together with physicians and nurses, have been core members of medical treatment teams as far back as the emergence of the profession of social work in the early twentieth century (Bartlett, 1975). Palliative care as both a social movement and as a treatment objective began on a micro level consequent to observations made by health care professionals at the bedsides of terminally ill individuals in the post–World War II era (Teno, 2004). Dame Cecily Saunders modernized the concept of hospice and influenced social workers worldwide to promote palliative care services in their communities. By talking to her patients, in particular a Holocaust survivor dying of cancer, Dame Cecily Saunders found that patients had a considerable agenda of wants, needs, and opinions about this phase of their lives. Dame Saunders began her career as a nurse, later to become a social worker and then a physician (Saunders, 2001). Along with Dame Saunders, another pioneer, a former chief of social work service at a VHA medical center, Zelda Foster, was influential in fostering the growth of palliative care in the United States when she was a relatively new social worker assigned to an inpatient hematology ward (Foster & Corless, 1999). It is interesting that these two innovators of the modern hospice and palliative care movement began their careers by working with patients affected by war. In contrast to Dame Saunders who acknowledged that her interest in palliative care was initiated by her patient who was a Holocaust survivor, Foster scarcely mentions the setting in which she works. Perhaps Foster intentionally chose not to highlight the veteran status of her patients so as to emphasize the universal condition of all dying people, where the "conspiracy of silence" generated a sense of powerlessness when it came to discussing end-of-life issues with the medical team and with their families in an era when a cancer diagnosis was almost always fatal (Foster, 1965).

Like Dame Saunders and Zelda Foster, medical social workers are particularly active and skilled in the area of end-of-life care (Hedlund & Clark, 2001; McCormick, Engelberg & Curtis, 2007). Beyond medical settings, social workers, wherever they are employed, are likely to encounter patients and clients affected either directly or indirectly by life-threatening illness, dying, and death. For this reason, social workers of all specialties need to have generalist competencies in the area of illness and end-of-life care for patients and their families (Gwyther et al., 2005; Howe & Daratsos, 2006). This competency extends beyond knowledge of disease trajectory, and it includes expertise that relates to every stage of the life span and incorporates a mastery of cultural diversity.

Historical Origins of Veterans as a Defined Population in American Society

The VA only became a cabinet-level division of the federal government in 1989. Yet its mission traces to the Plymouth Colony, when the settlers agreed to compensate any male colonist who was injured fighting against the Native Americans (Becerra & Damron-Rodriguez, 1995). Later, during the Revolutionary War, the Continental Congress was challenged to assemble and sustain an army. People were accustomed to defending their own land and property and that of their local surroundings, but the idea of becoming a part of a much larger political body was a difficult concept for some colonists to accept. By promising these individuals cheap or free land in exchange for enlisting in the military, the Continental Congress was able to form a moving army to fight the English and those who fought would be able to reestablish themselves and care for families at the war's conclusion. Even in the earliest days of the United States, it was recognized that men returning from military service were changed and needed societal assistance to cope with the physical and emotional effects of warfare and to readjust to civilian life (Resch, 1988).

Every major conflict during U.S. history includes a related story about how participation in that conflict affected members of the military and those close to them. In response to these observations, the government provided, created, or expanded services offered to veterans. For example, the VA's community living centers (CLCs) can be traced back to the period shortly before the Civil War, when the federal government established its first home for veterans who were undomiciled and in need of care. Again, after the Civil War, the precursor to today's VA granted an expanded package of benefits to veterans of the Union Army. Eventually, in 1958, benefits were extended to the single survivor of the Confederacy. The Hoover administration reorganized the various federal offices that had responsibility for veterans' issues into a new office known as the Veterans Administration. This action was a response to the needs of World War I veterans who not only suffered from the effects of the war but also were found to have particular economic difficulties as a result of the Great Depression (http://www4.va.gov/about_va/vahistory.asp). President Reagan expanded the agency and granted it cabinet status in 1988.

The VA's motto, taken from Lincoln's second inaugural address, is "To care for him who has borne the battle, his widow and his orphan." The phrase is striking for several reasons. It includes the veterans' families as being among the wounded in need of healing, with the associated suggestion that veterans are not isolated individuals. It looks across the life span and implies a responsibility to family after the veteran has died. The motto connotes a sense of values and ethics consistent with the profession of social work. Indeed, the agency is the largest employer and training site for master's level social workers in the nation, employing approximately 4000 social workers. Many Council on Social Work Education (CSWE) accredited schools of social work are affiliated with Veterans Heath Administration (VHA) facilities to provide internships in the social work specialties of gerontology, health care, rehabilitation, substance abuse, mental health, among others (http://www.socialwork.va.gov/). Several Veterans Integrated Service Networks (VISNs), the VHA term for districts, have Geriatric Research and Education Clinical Centers (GRECCs) that offer interdisciplinary fellowships in palliative care which are open to post-masters-level social work graduates. Specific information about these programs, their applications, and other details can be ascertained from the GRECC Web site (http://1va.gov/grecc).

The VA is now the third largest cabinet department. The VA has three divisions: the Veterans Benefits Administration (VBA), which manages veterans' financial and educational programs; the VHA, which operates the nation's largest health care system; and the National Cemetery Administration (NCA), which administers the VA cemetery system. The details regarding the gamut of VA benefits from the educational benefits to burial benefits can be found in the VA Handbook, which is updated yearly and readily accessible on the VA's Web site, which is available at: http://www.va.gov. In addition, states and local governments have their own agencies dedicated to veterans' affairs, and elected officials at every level have a staff person who is responsible for veterans' issues.

The Nature of the Veteran Identity

There are an estimated 70 million veterans in the United States who are eligible to use VA health and mental health services. Only 10% of this group are *enrolled veterans*, the term for veterans who use VA services. It has been reported that one factor in a veteran's decision to use VHA for health care is the degree to which he or she attaches to a self-definition as a veteran (Damron-Rodriguez, et al., 2004). While veterans are much discussed in the media and in the social sciences, until recently psychosocial research related to their experiences was confined to a relatively few interested scholars and clinicians who are mostly interested in the mental health research and interventions. This is increasingly problematic in light of current military actions in Iraq and Afghanistan, which are creating a new cohort of veterans and a demand for policy decisions regarding all manner of issues related to veteran status, including medical and mental health care. There are currently two related policy and practice imperatives, one which discusses the results of living with a traumatic injury caused during military service over the long term and a second which considers the aging of the World War II, Korean, and Vietnam era cohorts, especially those veterans at their end of life (Casarett et al., 2008).

A research question, yet unexplored, might involve understanding the process by which one transitions one's identity from "a member of the military" to "a veteran." Once someone has been discharged from military service, he or she is now called "a veteran." The word *veteran* always has been an iconic word, especially in today's society, generally depicting the notion of a "wounded warrior," who bears physical and emotional damage as the result of having been in war. The media, in particular, films, are full of images that promote stereotypical depictions of veterans and may influence their self-image and presentation to the medical team. However, in the process of psychosocial assessment of patients who are seriously ill, it is important to differentiate the nature of their experiences. For example, (1) not all members of a war cohort were in combat; (2) members of a war cohort not stationed in combat zones may have been exposed to traumatic situations; and (3) members of so-called peacetime cohorts may also have been exposed to traumatic situations.

To understand the veteran identity, one must first understand some basics of the military experience. The nature of a "veteran identity" stems from two concepts. As with all experiences that social work clinicians seek to understand, veterans are individuals and their military experiences and their related perceptions of their military lives are unique to them. Regardless of whether they enlisted or were drafted, a portion of their lives was detoured to serve the nation. It could be that the nature of the veteran identity does evolve from an individual's military history and his or her related perceptions of that experience, but there is a paucity of research that directly links one's military service time to later perceptions of life as a former military person. Yet the concept that one's identity as a veteran evolves from one's time in the service and is a self-defined concept seems to be a more informed way of viewing veterans as a population and as individuals.

Daley (1999) makes the case for the concept of the military identity and that each branch of the armed services has a particular culture. His descriptive chapter illustrates the structure of military life, which is rooted in the need to foster cohesion. Basic training is a full immersion into that culture and the new soldier soon learns to use an exclusive military vocabulary. Military communities, known as bases or posts, exist as self-sufficient entities, as Daley (1999) notes, with its own mega stores, the post exchanges (PXs), gas stations, restaurants, and recreational facilities. These communities serving as a source of uniformity and familiarity are designed to enhance group cohesion and stability as military personnel move from assignment to assignment. These full-service communities become preferred locations to conduct all manner of social and commercial discourse so that leaving the bases becomes unnecessary—a dynamic that serves to further the military culture's development (Daley, 1999).

In their literature review on cohesion, Griffith and Vaitkus (2000) relate cohesion to stress, strain, disintegration, and performance. Their meta-analysis of studies on military cohesion finds that the stressors of military life, including those events that put strains on the group's ability to maintain its identity and function, are antecedents to the development of social support within all branches of the military, especially in a small group context. It follows that this sense of belonging to the group may not vanish upon discharge from military service. Perhaps for some, the cohesion and expectation of support transfers to institutions closely related to the military experience such as veterans' service organizations, programs associated with the VA, and paramilitary activities.

The VA has sponsored a number of studies that attempt to collect, analyze, and disseminate data about the population of U.S. citizens who spent time in military service. Much of this research appears in two VA Web pages specifically dedicated to veteran data. In the first Web page, the VA offers demographic data in its simple, aggregated form (http://www1.va. gov/vetdata/). It contains data by geographic locations, race, gender, and service cohort. The intent of this Web site is to provide statistics on the veteran population within the United States for all who are interested in learning about veterans.

The Office of Academic Affiliations, the division of the VA that has responsibility of oversight for training clinicians, has an informative and easy-to-use learning tool called the Military Health History Pocket Card (http://www4.va.gov/oaa/pocket-card/default.asp). The Pocket Card is a two-sided, index card–sized document that directs clinical staff on how to obtain a military-specific health history that includes biopsychosocial issues common to the veteran population, such as inadequate housing, and issues specific to a war cohort, such as hepatitis C among veterans who were stationed in Vietnam.

The VA is invested in evidence-based practice guidelines and research as part of its continuing education curriculum for military-specific biopsychosocial issues driven both by its investment in palliative care and in the experience of the military related to the current conflicts in Afghanistan and Iraq. In fact, as early as the 1940s the VHA was planning for the aging of the World War II veteran population (Taylor & Siegal, 1948). Such planning proved to be fitting because the ability to prolong life had also advanced in the last half of the 1900s. Now a substantial majority of all deaths in the United States occur after a period of prolonged illness and dependence on health care settings such as intensive care units and nursing homes (Hallenback, 2003). Over 25% of all deaths in the nation, according to the NHPCO Veterans Hospice Resource page, are of men and women who are veterans of the armed forces (http://www.nhpco.org/i4a/pages/index. cfm?pageid=4390). Greater collaboration and research is needed between VHA social work providers as well as community social workers to better understand the needs of terminally ill veterans and their families of every war cohort.

Military Service as a Potential Risk Factor for Disease

Since the majority of veterans receive medical care outside the VHA system, palliative social workers practicing in the community will interface with veterans and their families and require skills in assessment and intervention with their unique veteran-related psychosocial and medical issues. Veterans with life-threatening illnesses may be eligible for financial support from the VA, known as service-connected compensation. Among the groups of affected veterans are sailors from World War II exposed to asbestos that was used throughout the construction of ships, Korean War veterans who developed frostbite serving during the harsh Korean winters, and Vietnam combat veterans who were exposed to the defoliant Agent Orange. Veterans of Operation Enduring Freedom/Operation Iraqi Freedom and the professionals who serve them should be aware of the VA's Office of Public Health and Environmental Hazards, which is responsible for disseminating research and information regarding potential physical and mental health issues related to these two combat theaters (http://www.publichealth.va.gov/exposures/oefoif/benefits.asp).

Since the 1980s former Vietnam-era combat soldiers who have one or more diagnoses that are deemed related to Agent Orange exposure are entitled not only to treatment for their disease but also compensation because the illness is assumed to be, at least in part, due to their exposure to the chemicals in the course of their combat status (http://www.va.gov/AgentOrange). The list includes several cancers and also contains diabetes and hepatitis C, among other illnesses. These data, coupled with the Department of Defense's current focus on posttraumatic stress prevention and early detection, infer that veterans have unique biopsychosocial issues across the disease continuum regardless of whether they use VHA as their health care provider.

There were 8.7 million soldiers in the military during the Vietnam era from 1964 to 1975. Of that number, 3.4 million soldiers were stationed in Southeast Asia. Currently, Vietnam Era veterans represent one-third of the veteran population in the United States (http://www1.va.gov/opa/fact/docs/amwars.pdf). As of 2007, 50% of this cohort is over the age of 65 and in addition to the diseases impacting the general population, this group is at additional risk. The Agent Orange Web site provides references regarding potential exposures to hazardous substances in areas outside Southeast Asia for a number of years well before the Vietnam Conflict.

Posttraumatic Stress Disorder and Its Role at the End of Life

Hymans, Wignall, and Roswell (1996) trace the etiology of what we now would broadly term PTSD from the Civil War to the Persian Gulf War. This group reports that every war era has an associated set of illnesses that contain a constellation of physical and psychological symptoms, the descriptions of which, whether offered by veterans or their clinicians, reflects the language of that era. For example, during World War I, a condition known as "war fatigue" was treated by giving affected soldiers a respite from the front lines and by providing opportunities for adequate rest and food.

According to the latest published VA data, approximately 350,000 veterans receive compensation for posttraumatic stress disorder (PTSD). Much of this section will focus on the Vietnam-era cohort where the rates of PTSD among those who were in combat are currently 15%. An estimated 31% of all combat veterans cohort are likely to have combat-related posttraumatic stress in their lifetimes according to Schlenger and colleagues (2007), who conducted the original National Vietnam Veterans Readjustment Study in 1983 and who continue to analyze the data. While there are hundreds of studies related to PTSD from the mental health professions, there are significant gaps in the research specific to veterans of any era who are living with life-threatening illness or who are at the end of their lives. The VA maintains a Web site, the National Center for Post Traumatic Stress, which is a central source of research regarding PTSD (http://www.ptsd.va.gov/index.asp).

Nye, Qualls, and Katzman (2006) reviewed the results of the trauma symptom inventory (TSI) on a sample of VHA using combat experienced veterans already having a diagnosis of PTSD and already known to the research team. A small subsample of veterans in their study rated themselves inconsistently more distressed than their actual symptom burden as documented in their medical records. This team concluded that these patients had certain commonalities among them; they endorsed higher levels of anxiety, anger, and substance abuse as compared to the rest of the sample. The researchers consider that the scores, though deemed inconsistent according to the comparisons between the survey instrument and their known mental health histories, is nevertheless the accurate representation of the level of distress for this group of veterans. They suggest that the research community continue to pursue improved ways of measuring long-term effects of traumatic experiences especially in the veteran population (Nye et al., 2006).

Some historians and sociologists, such as Modell and Haggerty (1991), state that because the Vietnam War was politically unpopular and that returning soldiers were not afforded the respect and social privileges given to World War II veterans, Vietnam-era veterans had and continue to have more difficulties adjusting to civilian life. The conclusions of their analysis underscore the basic assumptions about the Vietnam Conflict upon which so many of the social science research rests—that one's circumstances of having been in the military, more specifically to have been assigned to service in Vietnam, cause these veterans to have difficulties returning to civilian life and that these difficulties persist throughout the life course.

Kaylor, King, and King (1987) further illustrate these points through a meta-analysis of 67 studies published about the psychological status of Vietnam-era veterans. They noted the later studies in the meta-analysis had been impacted by the political and medical influences such as the inclusion of PTSD as a diagnosis in the *Diagnostic and Statistical Manual, third edition (DSM-III)* and the political and legal activities concerning the health effects Vietnam veterans associated with Agent Orange. Their analysis suggests that veterans who were in Vietnam did indeed develop a "Vietnam" effect, which they refer to as a psychological imprint of their experience. The Kaylor team found, however, that the imprint extended to those who did not actually fight, such as medical and allied health professionals working in field hospitals or those serving in the navy stationed on vessels in the Southeast Asian waters. The results of the meta-analysis are themselves limited by the fact that a similar examination has not been repeated to see whether the findings still have merit over time and as this wartime cohort ages.

Villa, Harada, Washington, and Damron-Rodriguez (2002) studied the differences among war cohorts from World War II to the Persian Gulf War with regard to socioeconomic status, mental health, and physical illness. The study is remarkable because of its findings specific to the Vietnam-era veterans. Even though logic and the passage of time would predict that the two oldest war cohorts, World War II and Korean War, would have the most biopsychosocial problems related to illness, the authors report that the oldest cohorts reported having the least amount of physical and mental health issues. It was the Vietnam-era cohort, however, who had the most mental health issues and the greatest difficulty with activities of daily living (ADLs) and independent activities of daily living (IADLs), when compared to the Korean War and Persian Gulf veterans. This finding remained even when the demographic variables of race and ethnicity were held constant.

Box 12.1
Patient/Family Narrative: Mr. A.

Mr. A. is a 75-year-old Korean War–era marine veteran with multiple medical problems, including advanced bladder cancer. He is in the medical intensive care unit and on a ventilator after having a stroke. In the family meeting with all the specialists involved in the veteran's care, including the social worker, one of his sons, John, is observed to be especially distressed at the news of the veteran's grave prognosis. Following the family meeting, several clinicians note that they smelled alcohol on John's breath. In a separate interview, the palliative social worker learns that this son is himself a combat veteran and the only other member of the family who was in the military. Their respective veteran status, coupled with the father's status as a former marine—a branch of the service with a reputation of surviving all manner of dangerous situations—has made the news of the father's expected death especially difficult for this adult child. In addition to the usual palliative social work interventions such as counseling related to coping with advanced disease and a long complicated hospital stay, the palliative social worker acknowledges the unique attachment to his father, educates the younger veteran son about services specific to his needs and military experience, such as the substance abuse program and assessment in the mental health clinic.

Veterans Health Administration Users Versus Veterans Who Seek Care in the Community

There is a concept among providers both within and without the VHA system that there is a set of characteristics attributable to VA users. While there are approximately 24 million veterans in the United States, only 10% of them use the VA as their health care providers (Zeber, Copeland, & Grazier, 2006). Research about the similarities and differences between VA-enrolled and non-VA-enrolled veterans is confined to very few studies. The current state of health care insurance in this nation has focused more awareness on the VA as a source of health care for eligible veterans, particularly those living with life-threatening illness. In addition, our veterans of the most recent conflicts in Afghanistan and Iraq will likely have physical and mental health needs unique to their wartime experiences and injuries, and therefore the descriptions of VA users and nonusers are likely to change in the future. Thus, social workers in clinical practice need to look at every veteran as an individual with his or her unique biopsychosocial and spiritual history and care needs. Research findings in clinical practice need to be coupled with comprehensive and compassionate assessment that individualizes the experience of each veteran and his or her family.

The current literature reports that African Americans were 3.7 times more likely to use the VHA for outpatient care than Caucasians and that Hispanics who separated from the military with a medical condition were 5.3 times more likely to use the VA (Villa, Harada, Washington, & Damron-Rodriguez, 2002). One predictor of whether a veteran enrolls and uses VHA services is the degree to which the individual identifies himself or herself as a veteran (Harada et al., 2002).

Damron-Rodriguez and colleagues (2004) examined the differences between veterans who use the VHA and those who do not. Their findings suggest that (1) veterans value having a particular status within society that provides them with a package of services and privileges; (2) veterans see themselves as deserving of these benefits, yet findings suggest respondents, both users and nonusers, express concern that veterans' services are somehow related to welfare and therefore stigmatizing; (3) among the VA users is the expectation that all VA employees treat them with courtesy and respect (Damron-Rodriguez et al., 2004). Harada, Valentine, Reifel, and Bayhylle (2005) examined veteran identity among Native Americans who served in the armed forces and their use of VA services. The study is notable because it validates common factors that this minority, which has made valuable contributions to the military history of this country, shares with other groups related to veteran identity. Perhaps because these veterans are getting care from the same institution to which they devoted their service and which demanded their best, veterans who use the VA expect the same culture of duty, honor, and respect from all its employees.

Citing a long list of variables found to be associated with VHA use, Long, Polsky, and Metlay (2005) reported on the results of their analysis comparing data from the 1992 and 2001 National Survey of Veterans. Long and his colleagues report that the 2001 survey indicates the VHA continues to service an overwhelmingly male population (94%) with a mean age of 58. Nearly 85% of the veterans served are Caucasian, almost 9% are African American, and less than 3% are Hispanic. About 75% are married and slightly less than 60% have education beyond high school. Nearly 28% have incomes less than $25,000 per year, about 26% have at least one problem with activities of daily living, and 10% have no other health insurance. A little more than 13% have a service-connected condition. These findings show that veterans who began to use the VHA during the 9 years between the two surveys are poorer, have no additional health insurance, and are older. Zeber, Copeland, and Grazier (2006) report that the VA expects that by 2010 the percentage of veterans over the age of 65 will rise to 51% of all veterans, and there will be about 1.3 million over the age of 85. The results underscore the need for all health care systems to prepare to provide comprehensive biopsychosocial care to this population.

Harada and Pourat (2004) found that membership in veteran service organizations (VSOs) also predicted whether veterans used the VHA and that having income less than $8200 was a predictor of veterans who do not use the VHA. Both of these variables may relate to how engaged an individual is in the community and how much access one has to information that could benefit eligible veterans financially or through access to mental and physical health services.

Psychosocial Care for Veterans

A central question that guides psychosocial care for persons with life-limiting disease revolves around understanding how clients' define the elements of their quality of life. Specifically, do team members caring for the veteran have objective evidence-informed data upon which to base their interventions? The absence of a comprehensive evidence base does not preclude the commitment to provide informed state-of-the-art biopsychosocial care to accompany the cutting-edge medical therapies that serve to extend lives. VA social workers have the benefit of their own practice wisdom, supervision, and VA-disseminated research to inform their assessment of the individualized experience of the veteran and the veteran's family. As this research becomes available, community social workers will also have access to this research to enhance the biopsychosocial-spiritual care provided to veterans and their families no matter where they chose to access care.

Sherwood, Shimel, Stolz, and Sherwood (2003) discuss the reemergence of trauma in the aging veteran population. This article is particularly valuable for non-VA social workers because through the use of case examples, the authors underscore the importance of an assessment that includes a complete military history. They explain the various ways in which older veterans have integrated the military trauma experience in their adult lives and in older age, when facing losses, such as poor health, the death of a spouse, or watching current events, the trauma reemerges. The authors describe effective interventions such as groups, cognitive behavioral therapy, and medication. They review obstacles to the treatment process, which include what the authors term "the sociocultural experiences of the WWII veteran." For instance, stoicism and societal views of that war as a "good war" inform the perception and belief that there should be no negative feelings associated with military service, especially so many years later (Sherwood, Shimel, Stolz, & Sherwood, 2003). In this context, any "negative feelings" of the veteran might be kept hidden and/or create a sense of being disenfranchised and isolated with complex and very private thoughts and feelings.

Another important contribution to the literature related to working with veterans at their end of life is *Peace at Last: Stories of Hope and Healing for Veterans and Their Families*, by VA Nurse Practitioner, Deborah Grassman (2009). Grassman's book recounts her growth as a clinician as she cares for veterans in her palliative care unit. In greater detail than the Sherwood article, she helps clinicians know what to do and say once a veteran has given his or her military history. She stresses the interdisciplinary nature of palliative care. Her interventions are drawn from many sources, including literature, history, art, music, religion, medicine, and psychology. She provides specific guidance about cultivating self-awareness, confronting stoicism by veteran patients, and seeking interventions and rituals that community agencies can incorporate to make their settings more hospitable to veterans.

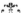

Enhancing Knowledge Related to Veterans and Their End-of-Life Care

There are a limited number of studies of terminally ill veterans, including the Vietnam Conflict, the war cohort that has visibly been affected by the long-term disease effects of wartime service. Additionally, the military and therefore the VA continue to be institutions where males represent the overwhelming majority of membership and studies to determine the longer term effects of military service on female veterans are now part of the VA's research agenda. As this research becomes public, social workers will be able to access the findings on the VA Web site for issues related to women veterans (http://www1.va.gov/womenvet/).

Furthering the knowledge base about veterans who are living with life-threatening illness, experiencing pain and suffering, and coming to the end of life can be the shared responsibility of clinicians within and beyond the VA.

Including the following essential variables in research studies would be a beginning: war cohort, combat/noncombat status, combat-related medical diagnoses, such as those under the Agent Orange grouping of diseases, and service-connected status for PTSD. Within the VA, research interest in palliative and end-of-life care for veterans has increased since the inception of the VA's Palliative Care Initiative of 2003 and the creation of the Veterans Hospice Partnership, a robust network poised to change and enrich the research landscape. We can look forward to new studies in the coming years that will more directly inform our practice.

Support of Studying Those Veterans with Terminal Illness

Hwang, Chang, Cogswell, Srinivas, and Kasimis (2003); Steinhauser and colleagues (2000); and Feldman and Periyakoil (2006) represent some of the VA research teams working in the area of veterans' end-of-life care. Steinhauser and her team (2000) employed focus groups of veteran patients enrolled in ambulatory care clinics to determine their preferences for end-of-life care. The themes developed by the veterans in this qualitative study placed great weight on pain and symptom relief and choice of place of death. Although the researchers note that their qualitative study used a small sample of well, elderly veteran patients, the responses are notable because the sample is representative of the demographics of VA users discussed in earlier sections of this chapter. In addition, their stated wishes are comparable to the work of Hwang et al., who extensively analyzed the symptom burden of dying patients in a large quantitative study of patients with terminal cancer (Hwang et al., 2003).

Feldman and Periyakoil (2006) are the first team of VA researchers to publish an article investigating the incidence of PTSD among VA users at the end of life. Their article discusses the incidence of PTSD within the VA population generally and describes clinical situations where inexperienced clinicians may mistake the behaviors of dying patients to be PTSD and treat it as such rather than the condition known as terminal restlessness. The article provides guidance to practicing clinicians to ensure that their interventions are based on critical thinking and differential diagnosis rather than assumptions.

Casarett and colleagues (2008) developed a survey instrument that assesses the end-of-life needs of veterans and their families. Their qualitative research consisted of 66 structured interviews of the identified next of kin of recently deceased veterans who received care in a VHA facility in the last month of life. In their preliminary research, the team has identified that many of the aspects of care for veterans are in fact the same as the majority of dying patients in the United States. On the other hand, they identify some domains of care that are unique to the VA system or that are complicated by the fact that many of the sickest veterans cycle through both the VHA and community health care institutions in their final months or weeks of life. Among the VA-specific concerns reported to be important to the veteran and his family, assessed through the eyes of the next of kin, are access to care issues, including long-term care and mental health services, and information about VA benefits such as burial and survivor benefits. Their findings about the positive and negative aspects of care in the last weeks of the lives of these veterans lend strong support to Harada et al.'s (2002) findings of a "veteran identity." Veterans and their families expect the best possible and most comprehensive care from the VA. The work of these and other researchers can further theory development to enrich the knowledge base specific to veterans and their families being cared for both within and beyond the VHA system, where most veterans appear currently to be coming to the end of their lives.

Conclusion

It is notable that both the Department of Defense and the VA are leaders in all forms of medical research that has extended life and improved medical outcomes (Sung et al., 2003). Consequent to the history of the VA, with its initial mission to care for veterans who could not care for themselves, VA clinicians may indeed become the palliative care experts for their population. The research and clinical work in which the VA is engaged both organizationally and in its collaborative relationships with the Veterans Hospice Veterans Partnership will continue to increase the knowledge base and skill sets necessary to understand and treat the veteran population. This is imperative so that the veterans' sacrifice in service to their nation is respected and acknowledged by offering the best biopsychosocial-spiritual care along the continuum of illness and at end of life.

ACKNOWLEDGMENT

The statements and opinions expressed in this chapter are those of the author and do not reflect those of the Department of Veterans Affairs.

LEARNING EXERCISES

1. Notice whether your practice setting includes a military history of all its adult clients. If it does not, discuss with your supervisor the possibility of incorporating a military history as part of your assessment of adults.
2. Visit a federal or state veterans' cemetery. For a list of locations, see http://www.cem.va.gov/cems/listcem.asp
3. Identify the names and the contact information for all public offices with jurisdiction or interest in veterans'

issues. In this exercise, note the level and branch of government of these individuals and their area of expertise, such as home loans, educational benefits, and so forth.

4. Invite a local public official or employee who is responsible for veterans issues to give a presentation to your class or agency to describe the essentials about what every social worker should know about the VA and its benefits and eligibility requirements. If possible, hold that presentation at the local VA office or clinic. For patient confidentiality reasons, you will not be permitted to tour patient care areas, but you can get a sense of what the VHA offers veterans and their families by visiting the public areas.

ADDITIONAL READINGS
AND RESOURCES

Beyond the list of references used for this chapter, there are many resources that inform us about the veteran experience. When evaluating these resources, especially with regard to artistic works, it is important to discern where the work reduces, expands, or otherwise departs from the real experience of being in the military or being a veteran.

The American Pain Foundation. The American Pain Foundation's Web site focuses on issues related to pain in the military and veteran population. Available at: http://www.painfoundation. org/learn/programs/military-veterans/

Department of Veterans Affairs. The Department of Veterans Affairs National Center for Post Traumatic Stress aims to help U.S. veterans and others through research, education, and training on trauma and posttraumatic stress. Available at: http://www.ptsd.va.gov/index.asp

Department of Veterans Affairs. Agent Orange Web site. Available at: http://www.publichealth.va.gov/exposures/agentorange/

Department of Veterans Affairs. Office of Public Health and Environmental Hazards Website. *OEF/OIF hazardous exposure benefits.* Available at: http://www.publichealth.va.gov/ exposures/oefoif/benefits.asp

Department of Veterans Affairs. VA social work Web site. Available at: http://www.socialwork.va.gov/

Department of Veterans Affairs, National Center for Veterans Analysis and Statistics. Veteran data and information. Available at: http://www1.va.gov/vetdata/

Department of Veterans Affairs. Center for women veterans Web site. Available at: http://www1.va.gov/womenvet/

Department of Veterans Affairs. (2003, June 20). *Directive 2003-034 National cancer strategy.* Available at: http://va.gov/ cancer/docs/NationalCancerDirective/doc

Department of Veterans Affairs. (2008, October 23). *Directive 2008-066 Palliative care consult teams.* Available at: http:// vaww1.va.gov/vhapublications/ViewPublication.asp?pub_ ID=1784

Department of Veterans Affairs Office of Academic Affiliations Web site. Available at: http://www.va.gov/OAA/pocketcard/ FactSheet.asp

Department of Veterans Affairs History Web site. Available at: http://www4.va.gov/about_va/vahistory.asp

Federal Benefits for Veterans, Dependents and Survivors, 2009 edition. Available at: http://www1.va.gov/opa/publications/benefits_book.asp

Grassman, D. (2009). *Peace at last: Stories of hope and healing for veterans and their families.* St Petersburg, FL: Vandamere Press.

Library of Congress Veterans History Project. The Veterans History Project of the American Folklife Center collects, preserves, and makes accessible the personal accounts by American war veterans so that future generations may hear directly from veterans and better understand the realities of war. Available at: http://www.loc.gov/vets/

Van Devanter, L., & Furey, J. (1991). *Visions of war, dreams of peace.* New York, NY: Warner Books.

REFERENCES

Bartlett, H. (1975). Ida M. Cannon: Pioneer in medical social work. *The Social Service Review, 49*(2), 208–229.

Becerra, R., & Damron-Rodriguez, J. (1995). Veterans and veterans' services. In R. Edwards (Ed.), *Encyclopedia of social work* (pp. 2431–2439). Washington, DC: NASW Press.

Casarett, D., Pickard, A., Bailey, A., Ritchie, C., Furman, C., Rosenfeld, K.,... Shea, J. (2008). Important aspects of end-of-life care among veterans: Implications for measurement and quality improvement. *Journal of Pain and Symptom Management, 35*(2), 115–125.

Daley, J. (1999). Understanding the military as an ethnic identity. In J. Daley (Ed.), *Social work practice in the military* (pp. 291–306). New York, NY: The Haworth Press.

Damron-Rodriguez, J., White-Kazemipour, W., Washington, D., Villa, V., Dhamani, S., & Harada, N. (2004). Accessibility and acceptability of the Department of Veterans Affairs health care: Diverse veterans' perspectives. *Military Medicine, 169*(3), 243–250.

Daratsos, L., & Howe, J. (2007). The development of palliative care programs in the Veterans Administration: Zelda Foster's legacy. *Journal of Social Work in End-of-Life and Palliative Care, 3*(1), 29–39.

Feldman, D., & Periyakoil, V. (2006) Posttraumatic stress disorder at the end of life. *Journal of Palliative Medicine, 9*(1), 213–218.

Foster, Z. (1965). How hospital social work can influence management of fatal illness. *Social Work, 10*(4), 118–127.

Foster, Z., & Corless, I. (1999). Origins: An American perspective. In Z. Foster & I. Corless (Eds.), *The hospice heritage: Celebrating our future* (pp. 9–14). Binghamton, NY: The Haworth Press.

Gwyther, L., Altilio, T., Blacker, S., Christ, G., Cskai, E., Hooyman, N., Kramer, B., Linton, J., Raymer, M., & Howe, J. (2005). Social work competencies in palliative and end-of-life care. *The Journal of Social Work in End-of-Life and Palliative Care, 1*(1), 87–120.

Grassman, D. (2009). *Peace at last: Stories of hope and healing for veterans and their families.* St Petersburg, FL: Vandamere Press.

Griffith, J., & Vaikus, M. (2000). Relating cohesion to stress, strain, disintegration, and performance: An organizing framework. *Military Psychology, 11*(1), 27–55.

Hallenback, J. (2003). *Palliative care perspectives.* New York, NY: Oxford University Press.

Harada, N., Damron-Rodriguez, J., Villa, V., Washington, D., Dhanani, S., Shon, H.,... Anderson, R. (2002). Veteran identity and race/ethnicity: Influences on VA outpatient care utilization. *Medical Care, 40*(Suppl. 1), 1117–1128.

Harada, N., & Pourat, N. (2004). Does membership in veterans' service organizations influence use. *Military Medicine, 169*(9), 735–740.

Harada, N., Valentine, V., Reifel N., & Bayhylle, R. (2005). Exploring veteran identity and health services use among Native American veterans. *Military Medicine, 170* (9), 782–786.

Hedlund, S., & Clark, E. (2001). End of life issues. In M. Lauria, E. Clark, J. Herman, & N. Stearns (Eds.), *Social work in oncology* (pp. 299–316). Atlanta, GA: American Cancer Society Health Content Products.

Howe, J., & Daratsos, L. (2006). The context of palliative and end of life care and the role of social work practice, In B. Berkman (Ed.), *Oxford handbook of social work in health and aging* (pp. 305–324). New York, NY: Oxford University Press.

Hwang, S., Chang, V., Cogswell, J., Srinivas, S., & Kasimis, B. (2003). Knowledge and attitudes toward end-of-life care in veterans with symptomatic metastatic cancer. *Palliative and Supportive Care, 1,* 221–230.

Hymans, K., Wignall, S., & Roswell, R. (1996). War syndromes and their evaluation: From the U.S. Civil War to the Persian Gulf War. *Annals of Internal Medicine, 125*(5), 398–405.

Kaylor, J., King, D., & King, L. (1987). Psychological effects of military service in Vietnam: A meta-analysis. *Psychological Bulletin, 102*(2), 257–271.

Long, J., Polsky, D., & Metlay, J. (2005). Changes in veterans' use of outpatient care from 1992 to 2000. *American Journal of Public Health, 95*(12), 2246–2251.

McCormick, A., Engelberg, R., & Curtis, J. (2007). Social workers in palliative care: Assessing activities and barriers in the intensive care unit. *Journal of Palliative Medicine, 10*(4), 929–937.

Modell, J., & Haggerty, T. (1991). The social impact of war. *Annual Review of Sociology, 17,* 205–224.

Nye, E., Qualls, C., & Katzman, J. (2006). The trauma symptom inventory: Factors associated with invalid profiles in a sample of veterans with post traumatic stress disorder. *Military Medicine, 171*(9), 857–860.

Resch, J. (1988). Politics and public culture: The Revolutionary War Pension Act of 1918. *Journal of the New Republic, 8*(2), 139–158.

Saunders, C. (2001). Social work and palliative care - The early history. *British Journal of Social Work, 31*(5), 791–799.

Schlenger, W., Kulka, R., Fairbank, J., Hough, R., Jordan, B., Marmar, C., & Weiss, D. (2007). The psychological risks of Vietnam: The NVVRS perspective. *Journal of Traumatic Stress, 20*(4), 467–479.

Sherwood, R., Shimel, H., Stolz, P., & Sherwood, D. (2003). The aging veteran: Re-emergence of trauma. *Journal of Gerontological Social Work, 40*(4), 73–86.

Steinhauser, K., Clipp, E., McNeilly, M., Christakis, N., McIntyre, L., & Tulsky, J. (2000). In search of a good death: Observations of patients, families, and providers. *Annals of Internal Medicine, 132*(10), 825–832.

Sung, N., Cowley, W., Genel, M., Salber, P., Sandy, L., Sherwood, L.,... Rimoin, D. (2003). Central challenges facing the national clinical research enterprise. *Journal of the American Medical Association*, 289(10), 1278–1287.

Taylor, M., & Siegal, I. (1948). Public expenditures for veterans. *Journal of Political Economy, 56*(6), 527–532.

Teno, J. (2004). Measuring end-of-life care outcomes retrospectively. *Journal of Palliative Medicine, 8*(Suppl. 1), S42–S49.

Villa, V., Harada, N., Washington, D., & Damron-Rodriguez, J. (2002). Health and functioning among four war eras of U.S. veterans examining the impact of war cohort membership, socioecomonic status, mental health and disease prevalence. *Military Medicine, 167*(9), 783–789.

Zeber, J., Copeland, L., & Grazier, K. (2006). Serious mental illness, aging and utilization patterns among veterans. *Military Medicine, 171*(7), 619–626.

13

Richard B. Francoeur, Susan A. Murty, and Bernice Sandowski

Special Considerations in Rural and Inner-City Areas

Courage is nine-tenths context. What is courageous in one setting can be foolhardy in another and even cowardly in a third.

—Joseph Epstein

Key Concepts

◆ *Access to services is a challenge in rural and inner-city communities.*

◆ *Continuity of care is difficult when patients are discharged to rural and inner-city communities where palliative care is not available.*

◆ *Community collaboration is necessary to improve palliative care in rural and inner-city communities.*

◆ *The financial viability of small hospices is threatened because they do not benefit from economies of scale and serve populations with low levels of health insurance coverage.*

◆ *Providing palliative care in inner-city and rural communities is challenging*

◆ *Access to medications to manage pain is problematic in some rural and inner-city communities.*

◆ *Palliative care for diverse and underserved populations in rural and inner-city communities requires sensitivity to health, cultural, and spiritual beliefs.*

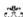

Introduction

Every chapter in this textbook contains information on palliative care that applies to patients and their families who live in inner-city or rural areas. The same principles apply and the same approaches are recommended for palliative social work wherever individuals and families are coping with serious and life-threatening illnesses. Why then were we asked to write about special considerations for palliative social work in inner-city and rural areas? The answer is that context matters. To use the approaches recommended in this textbook, and to ensure quality care in rural and inner-city areas, social workers must manage unique challenges related to delivering and integrating services into these unique communities. The capacity to take advantage of opportunities afforded by a particular local context requires insight, knowledge, and of course, courage. To be effective, social workers serving these areas must be innovative and develop partnerships with leaders and organizations in the local community. Effective programs serving inner-city and rural areas use creative strategies to deliver effective palliative care. Social workers are especially valuable in these programs because they have skills in community assessment, engaging stakeholders, and problem solving at individual, family, programmatic, community, interorganizational, and social policy levels.

It is a paradox that even though rural areas appear to be so different from urban areas, they have much in common. This paradox invites confusion when comparing the needs of rural and inner-city palliative care services and health services in general. The assumption that urban areas constitute a single type of community is very misleading because it does not distinguish the unique aspects of the inner city within metropolitan areas and separate them from suburbia. For example, on average, poverty rates are higher in rural than metropolitan areas; however, it would be quite misleading to say that poverty does not exist in urban communities. Poverty rates in urban areas within metropolitan areas are very high; between 2007 and 2008 urban poverty rose from 16.5% to 17.7%; suburban poverty also rose but only from 9.0% to 9.8% (Acs, 2009). It is important to carefully identify the geographical location and the characteristics of inner-city neighborhoods in order to understand their needs and challenges.

Many data are available for urban and metropolitan areas that describe the populations in general, often including the urbanized suburban communities associated with these cities. However, there is much less data available about *inner cities* within cities and metropolitan areas. It is generally agreed that inner cities are characterized by high proportions of low-income individuals and families and often by a high proportion of African American and other racial and ethnic minority groups. Latinos are highly represented in some of these communities. However, although a great deal has been written about inner cities, it is not easy to identify these areas precisely and obtain data describing them. Some research has attempted to do so by identifying census tracts or block groups with high proportions of residents living under the poverty line, high rates of unemployment, or high proportions of families with incomes below the median income level of the surrounding metropolitan area (Rankin & Quane, 2000). In certain metropolitan areas, inner-city neighborhoods have been defined (Committee on National Urban Policy, National Research Council, 1990). The Urban Institute, the Initiative for a Competitive Inner City, and other organizations have been active in promoting research on inner cities and have developed various ways to gather data. However, the lack of widely used standard definitions and methods to identify inner-city neighborhoods has limited the research on their characteristics and the challenges they face.

In contrast, rural areas have been the focus of a great deal of research and a variety of measures are used to locate geographical areas on the rural-to-urban continuum. The Economic Research Service of the U.S. Department of Agriculture has taken the lead in this work and provides guidance for researchers in defining rural areas and urban influence at the county and census tract level (Economic Research Service, 2008, 2000). There is a long tradition of research comparing rural and urban areas on a wide range of factors (Economic Research Service, 2009), including health status, insurance coverage, health care professional shortages, and poverty. As a result, there is a literature on rural services and rural health that can be very helpful in planning rural palliative care services. For example, lower levels of health care coverage (Bolin & Gamm, 2003) and higher rates of chronic illness (Dennis & Pallota, 2001) have been documented. There are also organizations that are active in formulating policies based on the data, such as the National Rural Health Association and the Office of Rural Health Policy. As a result, there is much more documentation of rural needs than inner-city needs. In this chapter, we note similarities between rural and inner-city environments and draw conclusions about approaches that may be successful in both locations, but we cannot draw on a comparable level of research publications concerning the inner city to support all our claims.

None of these generalizations is true of every rural or every inner-city area. In fact, it is especially important for palliative social workers to learn about the particular community and its residents, history, characteristics, and needs. Beginning with a community assessment is an important step in delivering effective palliative care in rural and inner-city areas. The social worker is uniquely qualified to initiate a community assessment and to engage the community in developing plans for effective services that will meet their needs and build on their strengths.

Innovative Approaches to Service Delivery

In this section, we will review particular challenges to delivering palliative care in inner-city and rural areas and suggest innovative approaches for effective service delivery. Some of the suggestions are based on approaches that have been used and documented; other suggestions seem promising and could be tested to determine their effectiveness.

Improving Transportation and Access

The most important barriers to palliative care in rural regions and inner cities are related to access. Barriers to access in rural communities have been documented (Van Vorst et al., 2006). Many rural areas are identified as "health professional shortage areas"; 68% of these shortage areas are located in rural regions (Health Resources and Services Administration [HRSA], 2009). Although inner cities may constitute many of the remaining shortage areas, the numbers are not reported for inner cities. We state this to support the general impression that there is much more documentation of rural needs than inner-city needs. In rural areas, the shortages of health care professionals are directly related to the low density of the population. The number of patients is too small to support full-service hospitals and clinics and even to sustain a primary care practice. Fewer rural and inner-city residents receive palliative care and fewer die receiving hospice care. Data on poor access to hospice in rural areas are well documented (Madigan, Wiencek, & Vander Schrier, 2009; Virnig, Ma, Hartman, Moscovice, & Carlin, 2006; Virnig, Moscovice, Durham, & Casey, 2004).

Rural residents tend to prefer local care rather than traveling long distances for care, and many rural residents cannot access services in metropolitan areas. As a result, individuals rely heavily on care by generalists, internists, and those in family practice who focus on acute and routine care. Seeking local services may still require that patients travel long distances (Jones, Parker, Ahearn, Mishra, & Variyam, 2009). For example, there may be a clinic in their county, but it may be located more than a 30-minute drive from their home (Chan, Hart, & Goodman, 2006). Patients who are suffering from chronic diseases may find it uncomfortable to travel for routine primary care, and their conditions may worsen without monitoring and attention. They may seek local care only when there is an emergency.

Rural areas rarely have professional providers trained in specialties such as palliative care (Kelley, 2007). Patients with severe chronic and life-threatening diseases are frequently transferred to regional health care centers for specialized care, often far away from their homes. Hospital-based palliative care may be available only at the regional health care centers where it is a specialty, whether as a separate hospital unit or as a hospital-wide consultation service. Therefore, rural patients are unlikely to benefit from palliative care until they are referred to a regional health center, and follow-up care with their primary care physician in their communities may not be adequate. Chan, Hart, and Goodman (2006) report that a quarter of those patients living in small and isolated rural areas who were seen for cancer (malignant neoplasm) had traveled nearly 1 hour one way to receive treatment, which was a great burden for these patients who were very sick. Rural patients must pay costs for travel (both financial and time costs) that urban residents do not have to pay (Jones et al., 2009). Because of shortages of palliative and hospice social workers serving rural and inner-city areas, new strategies are needed to attract students to practice in these settings, including grant and loan-forgiveness programs for bachelor's and master's education in social work (Hospice Association of America, 2005.

Home hospice might seem like the ideal alternative during the last 6 months of life so that rural patients can receive palliative care in their own homes. It is covered under the Medicare Hospice Benefit and many low-income rural elders are covered for this kind of palliative care. However, fewer patients receive hospice care in rural areas than in urban areas, and in many rural states, a large proportion of deaths occur in regions not served by a hospice (Virnig et al., 2006).

Other types of barriers to accessing palliative and hospice care exist in the inner city. Many patients and family members may not own a car, and as a result encounter barriers to traveling even moderate distances to the hospital or clinic. For instance, patients may endure cramped buses or subways with standing room only, and multiple bus or subway transfers can result in long, exhausting travel trajectories inappropriate for seriously ill patients. Staff travel to visit families at home involves transportation and safety problems that will be discussed later.

Telemedicine

One strategy for improving access to services for patients and families is telemedicine. Generally, telemedicine is used to supplement traditional face-to-face services rather than to replace them. Telephone contacts are frequently used to monitor and reassure patients and also to guide and support families struggling with the constant changes and the anxiety of caring for a palliative care patient. Videophone and computer-assisted communication can be used to enhance communication with families who live far from the hospital or the hospice office and when it is difficult for a nurse or social worker to travel to the home. There has been little research on the effectiveness of telemedicine. Some studies suggest that it is accepted by patients and families and could be helpful in improving quality of life (Bakitas et al., 2009; Demiris, Doorenbos, & Towle, 2009; Madigan et al., 2009). When there is resistance to using the new technologies, it may be more on the part of the service providers than the patients and families.

Obstacles to the use of telemedicine include limited equipment availability and the absence of telephone service in the home, which is sometimes limited in both rural and urban communities. Hearing impairment on the part of the patient or caregiver can be another hindrance (Whitten, Doolittle, & Mackert, 2004). An additional impediment is the reality that there is currently no reimbursement for home health or hospice service by telemedicine (Madigan et al., 2009). In addition, access to the Internet and high-speed Internet service providers is still limited in many rural regions (Carlton-LaNey, Murty, & Morris, 2005).

Although telemedicine has been recommended primarily to improve access to services in rural areas, its potential value in programs serving inner cities needs to be evaluated. Telemedicine precludes the travel and parking difficulties and provider safety concerns that may discourage routine home visits. A Hastings Center Report recommends research on improving access to hospice with

> ....telehospice demonstration projects, in which centrally located palliative care specialists may interact at a moment's notice both with family caregivers in private residences in a stratified selection of geographic settings, to include, urban, suburban, inner city, rural and wilderness areas, and with staff in nonhospice inpatient settings such as hospitals, nursing homes and assisted living facilities
> (Jennings, Ryndes, D'Onofrio, & Baily, 2003, p. 55)

Thus, telemedicine has the potential to be highly cost-effective as an innovation in the delivery of palliative and hospice care within rural and inner-city settings.

Improving Financial Viability of Palliative Care and Hospice Programs

Health care programs in both inner-city and rural areas face extreme financial burdens that put their viability at risk. Due to the concentration of poverty and the low levels of insurance coverage of the residents, providers that primarily serve these patients are likely to become impoverished themselves due to low levels of reimbursement for services provided. This phenomenon was documented in rural areas by Virnig et al. (2004):

In many rural areas, the number of patients is too small to support full-service hospitals and clinics and even to sustain a primary care practice. The unique challenges of delivering health services in rural areas have generally not been given sufficient attention

(Jones et al., 2009, p. 45).

Since many low-income patients may be eligible for Medicaid, policies to encourage Medicaid coverage for home health, hospice, and palliative care are recommended by the Hospice Foundation of America (2005).

One of the reasons that many rural regions are not served is that small hospices serve fewer patients and as a result they run into serious financial difficulties and many are unable to survive. Patients with high-cost needs in low-volume hospices can have a devastating effect; one patient who requires a high intensity of service or unusually expensive medications can bring about financial ruin in a system that is reimbursed at a daily rate. As a result, many small hospices are barely surviving financially. Casey et al. (2005) report that Medicare and insurance reimbursements were not sufficient to cover costs of the small rural hospices they studied. Some programs widen their patient base by combining home health and hospice programs in one organization; however, the financial risks remain high (Peterschmidt, 2006).

Some inner-city programs also encounter financial problems as a result of serving low-income, underinsured community populations; small size may contribute to problems of hospices in urban areas as well. Many inner-city patients and families do not seek hospice care because they do not see its value but rather view hospice care as second-rate or experimental care (Neubauer & Hamilton, 1990). The lack of a reliable family caregiver at home may characterize a greater proportion of inner-city patients, and this alone might exclude their acceptance by many hospice programs. Persons who live alone, are homeless, or live in environments with high drug addiction and drug dealing activity are generally excluded from hospice services (Colón & Lyke, 2003; Crawley et al., 2000; Rhymes, 1996). As a result, hospices in both geographic areas have the potential to experience financial difficulties, which can threaten their survival.

In addition to the risk that goes along with small size and low patient volume, rural hospices are under financial strain because they serve patients who are dispersed over a large geographic area. Providing staff and on-call coverage for a fluctuating census is challenging. The burden of travel costs and time is heavy. Distances between patients' homes and from the hospice home base make it difficult to respond quickly with a visit and create a burden on staff. Hospices serving inner cities may also encounter difficulties traveling to serve neighborhoods.

It is striking that instead of being compensated for their higher service delivery costs, rural hospices actually receive lower Medicare payments because the rates are based on lower wage rates in rural areas (Casey, Moscovice, Virnig, & Durham, 2005). The U.S. General Accounting Office (GAO) (2005) identified this problem and suggested that it might be appropriate to change these rules concerning payments to rural hospices. Financially strapped inner-city programs that serve primarily underinsured populations are also less able to afford sufficient qualified staff to deliver services. "Although costs for pharmaceutical and pharmacotherapy for symptom control and pain management have increased dramatically, the reimbursement system has not changed since its inception" (Hospice Foundation of America, 2008, p. 6). The Hospice Foundation of America (2008) recommends that the Centers for Medicare and Medicaid Services (CMS) should evaluate revision of the Medicare Hospice Benefit reimbursement system to make sure that it is adequate.

Availability of Medication for Pain Management

Adequate pain management is central to effective palliative care. The Hospice Foundation of America (2008) states that:

Inadequate pain management has been identified by experts in the field as a national public health issue. Terminally ill patients may require very high doses of pain medication to achieve effective pain control. Physicians and other health professionals often do not have adequate knowledge about pain control, and/or have fears of laws related to controlled substances. (p. 8)

The Hospice Foundation of America (2008) stresses that laws should be avoided that discourage or prohibit physicians from prescribing the controlled substances needed to manage pain across *all* stages of illness, and not just at the end of life.

Securing the medications to manage pain can be a challenge in rural regions (Dunham, Bolden, & Kvale, 2003) and in inner-city areas served by small or nonchain pharmacies with limited medication inventories or by pharmacies that do not stock opioids which are considered targets for theft (Morrison, Wallenstein, Natale, Senzel, & Huang, 2000). Health care providers serving these areas often find it especially difficult to obtain medications, often have to pay higher costs, and may struggle to ensure safe delivery of the medications palliative care patients need. Small hospices have difficulty obtaining medications at the lower bulk rates that higher volume hospices can obtain. These higher costs have been documented in small rural hospices (Virnig et al., 2004) but are likely to be an issue as well for small inner-city hospices. Forming a consortium of health institutions (including free-standing hospices, hospitals, and nursing homes) within an urban or rural area, or across an urban-suburban-rural region, may help them to negotiate collectively in purchasing medications at less expensive bulk rates (see Table 13.1).

Table 13.1.
Forming Consortia of Rural and Inner-City Health Providers to Negotiate Cost Savings from Bulk Medication Mail-Order Companies

Problems	Innovative Solution
1. Financial burden is a major barrier • Erodes financial viability of hospices, hospitals, nursing homes, and visiting nurse services that shoulder medication costs of inpatient, residential, or home care • Problem for uninsured, but also underinsured, patients and families through out-of-pocket costs, copayments, deductibles, and total reimbursement ceilings • Delays inpatient discharge • Prevents recently discharged inpatients, and clinic outpatients, from adhering to medication schedules • Unaffordable tamper- or abuse-resistant medications 2. Many inner-city providers belong to integrated health systems of hospitals, physicians, hospices, nursing homes, etc. These systems are in direct competition, which may discourage consortia.	1. Forming consortia of health institutions to negotiate cost savings from bulk medication mail-order companies • Small rural hospitals and affiliated health institutions, like nursing homes, have formed consortia. • Some regional hospitals and health systems are large enough to negotiate cost savings on their own. • Inner-city hospitals and affiliated institutions could form consortia. • Patient and family financial relief • Affordable tamper- or abuse-resistant medications 2. Competing health institutions/systems may still form a consortium due to shared self-interests in saving money. • Consider specific institutional cultures, local contexts • Inner-city, urban, suburban, and rural hospitals from the same, or even different regions, could form a consortium, just as small, unrelated employers pool risks that lower premiums in group health insurance. • Geography does not restrict the composition of consortia to negotiate via the Internet and to ship medications to hospital/community pharmacies, doctors offices, patient homes, and nursing homes.

A hidden, major cost to families and society may be the extent to which higher rates of hospitalization at the end of life stem from the lack of appropriate access to opioid medications (Cherny, Frager, & Ingham, 1995). Restrictions on physicians in prescribing medication, and on pharmacists in stocking them (Green, Ndao-Brumblay, West, & Washington, 2005; Morrison et al., 2000), exist where there are serious concerns over illegal drug trafficking and drug-related crime. Rural areas, as well as inner-city areas, have been experiencing growing problems with abuse and diversion of prescription medications. Some medications needed for treatment of symptoms may not be stocked by small pharmacies, and many rural areas do not have 24-hour pharmacy coverage (Dunham et al., 2003).

Because nursing homes operate much of the time without doctors or pharmacies on their premises, pain medications are delayed due to the mandate by the U.S. Drug Enforcement Agency (DEA) that pain medications be prescribed only after written signatures from physicians are faxed to off-site pharmacies (Johnson, 2009). Pain medication delays are especially lengthy for residents with pain exacerbation in the middle of the night or who are in transition from the hospital. These mandates are designed to lower the potential for drug theft and abuse by nursing home staff. New tamper- or abuse-resistant or deterrent formulations of opioids are designed to prevent prescription drug abuse (King, 2009).

In some common or repetitive circumstances, nursing homes could satisfy the intended purpose of the DEA mandate to prevent drug theft and abuse while avoiding delays in the administration of pain medications and needless patient suffering. In particular, limited supplies of tamper-/abuse-resistant or deterrent formulations of opioids, such as methadone/naloxine, could be stocked and closely monitored at the nursing home for circumstances when efforts to meet the DEA mandate are likely to result in prolonged episodes of untreated pain. Social workers and other health professionals should advocate in these circumstances for exceptions to the DEA mandate that pain medications be prescribed only after written signatures from physicians have been obtained and faxed to off-site pharmacies.

Patients with a history of addiction may experience lower tolerance for pain when measured experimentally (Compton, Charuvastra, & Ling, 2001), which may be related to the observation that the pain behaviors demonstrated by those with a history of addiction are sometimes assessed as out of proportion to injury. When this occurs, regardless of the factors responsible, it may predispose health providers to dismiss the pain and assume that the patient is drug seeking (Gureje, Simo, & Von Korff, 2001; Scimeca, Savage, Portenoy, & Lowinson, 2000). At the same time, patients addicted to drugs may manipulate their pain medications and secure nonprescribed, diverted medications to fuel their addiction

(King, 2009). Another risk is that family members or neighbors and acquaintances will steal, divert, or use the prescribed drugs, creating an unsafe environment for all.

Physicians monitor their prescribing practices in an effort to create a safe, effective treatment plan and/or in response to regulatory scrutiny. This may include state medical boards, and state and federal regulatory bodies such as the U.S. Drug Enforcement Agency (DEA), which is charged with investigating and prosecuting violation of the 1970 Controlled Substances Act (CSA). The CSA mandates that controlled substances be prescribed "for legitimate medical purpose by a practitioner acting in the usual course of his professional practice." (Joranson & Gilson, 2004; Tierney, 2007). At the same time, there is an ethical mandate to treat pain and suffering in patients, and the shared palliative care goal is to create a treatment plan that enhances the safety of patients, families, and prescribers. When these issues impact care, a structured plan of care can be created that includes frequent office visits or home visits, use of nonopioid medications, and inpatient admissions or residential care in the extreme circumstances where patient's symptoms cannot be managed in the home. Providing a lock box in the home is one suggestion for keeping all medications safely stored. Drug trafficking and abuse are serious problems in inner-city neighborhoods and growing problems in rural areas.

Home Visits: Challenges and Opportunities

Because of the impact of context on providing quality palliative care in rural and inner-city areas, home visits are strongly recommended. Social workers are skilled at assessments that will provide insight into the household situation, family dynamics, and the neighborhood and community context. Home visits provide excellent opportunities for palliative social workers to assess home conditions and to forge trusting bonds with the patient and family by engaging initially in task-oriented functions (Naleppa & Hash, 2001). Common task-oriented functions that are often highly valued by chronically ill patients and their families involve arrangements with formal home care services, housing, transportation, drug and alcohol counseling, financial and income support, service coordination among various providers, and illness education. Social workers in hospital, home, and community settings who understand the concept of family as the unit of care can advocate, in clinically appropriate situations, for the training of family caregivers to self-monitor their blood pressure using an analog blood pressure monitoring device, as one means of detecting whether strain may be reaching levels that threaten the caregiver's own health (Francoeur, 2010). Valued concrete services improve continuity of care and patient satisfaction (Pawling-Kaplan & O'Connor, 1989). Because family members may be present who might never be seen at a hospital or clinic visit, it is possible to convey respect for each of them and encourage their involvement in family problem solving. Once these

relationships have been established, other aspects of palliative social work (such as symptom assessment, work with grief, exploration of spiritual issues, support for caregivers, and resolution of family conflict) can be addressed in a deeper and more meaningful way.

Home hospice care offers the best opportunity for home assessment and intervention because it provides the social worker on the team ongoing opportunities to meet with the patient and family in the home environment. Unfortunately, not all palliative care patients are eligible for home hospice care. We recommend when possible that hospital palliative programs consider building in the potential for social workers to make home visits to gain a better understanding of the home and neighborhood context. When a patient is to be discharged from the hospital to home health care rather than hospice, continuity and transitions might be greatly enhanced if a palliative social worker and home health social worker can complete at least one joint home visit for assessment and consultation with the home health clinicians who will be entering the life of the patient and family. Hanley (2004) states that one-time consultations by hospice advance-practice nurses or physicians can be reimbursed through Medicare part B without an increment in cost to the home health care organization; it is not clear whether these consultations would include a palliative social worker. We advocate for systems to build support for home visits by palliative social workers for patients in inner-city and rural communities where a wide range of barriers to quality care are greatest. These visits will help to make the transition successful from inpatient to community providers.

Home visits, although they contribute to the quality of palliative care, are time consuming and involve some risks to palliative and hospice social workers. In rural areas the distances that must be travelled to visit families and the road and weather conditions are important considerations (Dunham et al., 2003). In inner-city areas, the time required for public transportation and lack of parking create special difficulties. Safety issues arise in home visits and high-crime neighborhoods that are not encountered in the hospital, clinic, or office (Naleppa & Hash, 2001). Social workers concerned about their safety in the home or neighborhood need to consult with their agency to create a plan to enhance their safety and ability to provide services. Some agencies have staff visiting in pairs or with escorts such as a trained volunteer (Pawling-Kaplan & O'Connor, 1989) or police officer. Social workers in hospices and palliative care programs can contribute to agency efforts to develop strategies that reduce barriers and increase safety when clinicians visit patients and families at home.

There are unique considerations related to home visits in both inner-city and rural areas. In rural areas, the most obvious concern relates to confidentiality. When a health care professional visits a home in a rural area, there is no way to keep the visit confidential from the community (Naleppa & Hash, 2001). Even if an agency vehicle is not used, the presence of an unknown vehicle at the home will be noted by neighbors and will raise questions. In most cases where palliative care is needed, the situation of the patient and family will already be known by the neighbors. Nevertheless, it is a good practice to discuss the situation with the family prior to the first visit and determine whether they have any concerns related to privacy or confidentiality. The distrust of outsiders is often pronounced and may make home visits a challenge in some inner-city and rural communities. Like other rural social workers, hospice and palliative social workers must be highly skilled in managing boundaries involved with home visits (Naleppa & Hash, 2001; Reamer, 2001). In inner-city neighborhoods where people are well acquainted with each other, similar issues related to confidentiality can arise and should be handled sensitively and openly discussed with patients and families.

Home visits can also be important because of the potential for abuse and diversion of drugs used for pain management. Access to these medications in the home is essential for good palliative care. Social workers need to balance an open and engaging disposition with good listening skills, and with vigilance and skilled assessment related to worries about abuse, addiction, or diversion. Families and patients may fear controlled substances or worry that any use equates with addiction. In families where individuals may be abusing or diverting prescribed medications, mutual dependency and protectiveness may draw family members to cover up evidence of these behaviors. Home visits provide social workers with a unique venue to detect whether families may be caught up in these protective strategies without assuming that they indicate bad intentions. There are opportunities for education, assessment, and the reframing of addiction as a disease needing expert evaluation and treatment. Social workers in consultation with their interdisciplinary teams develop expertise to assess and manage symptoms and create a treatment plan that structures care to enhance pain management, treatment of any addiction or substance abuse issues, and safety for patients, families, and prescribers.

In sections of inner cities, there are dwellings and specific neighborhoods that harbor pronounced violence, crime, drug use, rodent infestation, or seriously deteriorated and dangerous housing. Deteriorated, unsafe, and dangerous housing is also common in rural areas. It is important to consider that neighborhoods and dwellings that seem unacceptable to clinicians may have a very different history and meaning to patients and their families. Social workers, in consultation with patients and families, may create a care plan that includes collaboration with neighborhood groups and other organizations to advocate concerning the rights of patients and families with landlords and housing authorities. Frail, disabled, physically ill, and elderly individuals are at risk of self-imposed isolation due to deteriorated housing or from fear of crime, assault, and exploitation. Home assessments may also help uncover hidden issues such as physical, emotional, or financial abuse or neglect, including self-neglect that may occur in the struggle to accommodate to current conditions. Social workers, with

patient consent, may collaborate with others to work with the family, neighbors, and local groups to improve some of these conditions. However, at times social workers may also need to consult with their interdisciplinary health teams to work toward a plan of care that weighs options and impacts on patients, families, and staff, and which may include reporting situations to county or citywide Adult Protective Services. Deciding whether a situation should be reported requires deliberation guided by state regulations as well as the professional ethics of team members and individual clinicians (National Association of Social Workers [NASW], 2008). Whenever possible, Adult Protective Services seeks to retain patients at home and with family members by setting up support services.

Collaboration with Trusted Local Community Leaders and Organizations

To overcome the challenges of serving inner-city and rural populations, some programs are developing innovative strategies for service delivery that involve creating partnerships with community leaders and with local organizations. Many of these require collaboration with members of the community (Weil, 2005). Local churches and congregations are often very active in rural and inner-city communities (Cnaan, Boddie, & Yancey, 2005). Church members can be helpful in providing care to families struggling with serious chronic and life-threatening illnesses once they become informed and aware of the importance of palliative care and learn ways they can assist. Such care should be offered in a sensitive way and never be imposed on families who are uncomfortable with it. Many rural and inner-city patients and their families identify their congregation as an important source of social support.

Social workers are skilled at assessing communities, identifying their strengths as well as their needs (Murty, 2004). They can work to bring together stakeholders to plan programs to meet the needs of elders and disabled members of the community initially exploring the needs of the general community rather than focusing too narrowly on palliative care (Balaswamy & Dabelko, 2002). A capacity-building approach is an appropriate strategy for building community involvement and support. A local team is created of community members and providers who work together to initiate and develop and sustain the palliative care program. Although additional resources are necessary, it becomes an extension of the networks and relationships that are already in place in the community (Kelley, 2007).

Palliative care programs at regional specialized medical centers and university teaching hospitals can play an important role in improving palliative care for inner-city and rural populations by using a model of community collaboration to enhance local services and integrate them with palliative care services provided by the medical center. Better integration of care between these regional health centers and inner-city and rural communities needs to be an ongoing priority. When patients from inner-city and rural communities turn to these tertiary care centers for palliative care, much of it may not be reimbursed because they are uninsured or underinsured. It will be cost effective and improve quality of care for these medical centers to link patients to innovative, effective community programs for follow-up care and support that are developed by local teams, as described earlier. Social workers at regional health centers and university teaching hospital palliative care programs could work to create linkages with local partners and communities and develop collaborative planning for palliative care (Kelley, 2007; Weil, 2005).

An innovative strategy for bringing this about would be to assign social workers to develop relationships in particular communities, inner-city neighborhoods, or rural towns. It would be important to maintain continuity so that the same social worker travels to the community to represent the regional medical center (Murty, 2005). It might not be realistic to expect social workers to build these relationships in all the communities served by a regional medical center, but by dividing up the communities and gradually developing relationships, home care, outreach, discharge planning, and community partnerships could all be improved.

To overcome the challenges of serving inner-city and rural populations, some programs are developing partnerships with local organizations that are not necessarily specialized in palliative care but do intervene to reduce factors that precipitate or worsen illness conditions. For example, agencies and shelters that respond to domestic or gang violence might become important partners for sharing the care of palliative patients and their families, especially in the inner city. Victims of violence often suffer emotional trauma, physical injuries and symptoms, and disabilities and would benefit from palliative care as the uncertainty of their medical condition evolves. Schools may provide a network of support and counseling for children from families struggling with serious illness.

Another strategy is to work with home health care agencies that are able to provide services in the home, even though they are not as intensive as those provided by outpatient palliative care or hospice to meet some of the needs of patients facing serious and life-threatening diseases. Providers for this kind of home health program have often built the relationships and trust in the community that will enhance care. Some rural programs have been successful at developing home palliative care programs to supplement their hospice program by using creative approaches of billing a variety of sources. An example is a palliative care program provided by Hospice of Siouxland in Sioux City, Iowa (personal communication, Linda Todd, Director). Similar programs have been developed to serve inner-city areas. Some private insurers are beginning to provide outpatient and home palliative care for patients who are not eligible or do not choose to be cared for by a hospice program, for example, Wellmark in Iowa (Nuhn, 2009). However, fewer rural and inner-city patients have private health insurance, and many of these new programs will not be available to many of these patients. Coverage for these home palliative care programs under Medicaid would be helpful. (For more information on home based palliative care programs, please see Chapter 10).

Critical access hospitals (CAHs) have become common in rural areas and have saved many local rural hospitals from closing. These CAHs could play a role in improving palliative care in rural communities. They offer a limited set of services and are intended to provide critical care close to home for patients who live far from comprehensive and specialized medical care. Critical access hospitals are certified to receive cost-based reimbursement from Medicare rather than the standard payments based on disease-related groups (American Hospital Association, n.d.). This special arrangement with Medicare helps these small hospitals survive, even though they do not have the economies of scale that benefit larger hospitals. Effective integration of local care at a CAH with specialized palliative care programs at regional and teaching hospitals could be an important innovation. Continuity of care through short-term stays at CAHs could be incorporated into the discharge planning for palliative care patients along with follow-up care under home health and hospice programs. A similar status for hospitals serving populations of poor and underinsured patients could be explored in inner-city areas.

One of the organizations commonly found in rural communities and inner cities is the local nursing home. Those in rural areas are often small, but like those in the inner city, some have a long history in the community and maintain close ties with families and churches, especially those that are stand-alone, nonprofit organizations. Providing palliative care in nursing homes is a viable strategy for rural areas and inner cities and could be greatly expanded (Miller & Mor, 2004). Hospice in nursing homes is growing rapidly and has been shown to be effective at improving the quality of care for patients at the end of life (Stevenson & Bramson, 2009). Because administrators and staff at nursing homes often lack understanding and awareness of palliative care and hospice (Bern-Klug, 2010; Center to Advance Palliative Care [CAPC], 2008), palliative care programs and hospices need to provide outreach and education. In developing both the skill sets and relationships with nursing facilities, social workers from regional medical centers can expand options for discharge planning for palliative care patients who need skilled nursing. Policies are needed to encourage pilot projects and hospice/nursing home collaborations to enhance the care of patients who are not receiving adequate palliative and end-of-life care (Miller & Mor, 2004).

Religious institutions in inner cities have long traditions of outreach into their neighborhoods to provide sanctuary, hope, and uplift to seriously ill individuals who may not adopt their beliefs or practices. For instance, individuals who are homeless, struggle with addiction, or are diagnosed with HIV/AIDS may attend a church-operated soup kitchen or be visited at home by church members who offer social and material support. Francoeur, Payne, Raveis, and Shim (2007) point out that religious support networks appear to be dynamic, and not necessarily hierarchical, in how they operate. The process of outreach may operate in both directions since seriously ill individuals, family members, and friends may also be seeking connections to religious institutions at points in the illness trajectory that are especially difficult. Integration of these religious networks into palliative or hospice care is likely to depend upon the inclusion of program staff of the same ethnic, socioeconomic, and linguistic backgrounds as major populations in the community (Crawley et al., 2000; Krakauer, Crenner, & Fox, 2002). Volunteers and paraprofessionals can supplement professionally trained staff without these backgrounds and facilitate communication across these differences.

Religious leaders such as church pastors may serve uniquely influential roles as neighborhood "opinion leaders." Operating in conjunction with the Harlem Palliative Care Network (a grassroots network of community service providers who referred prospective patients for outpatient palliative care at North General Hospital), the Palliative Training and Education Program trained 130 local pastors and senior lay members from Harlem churches to provide bereavement ministries in their congregations with individuals, families, and support groups and to become better advocates for hospitalized church members (Canning & Payne, 2006). When clinically appropriate and if properly trained, pastors could also be called upon to explore spiritual beliefs and encourage patients and families to consider more adaptive coping beliefs to replace preoccupations that lack of faith is the cause of illness or that suffering is God's will. These preoccupations may cause delays in patients willingness to access health care. In a study of 146 inner-city African American and Latino outpatients from the Harlem Palliative Care Network, Francoeur and his colleagues (2007) revealed that among outpatients either identifying with a religion or affiliated with a religious institution, those who were uninsured reported *more hopeful* attitudes than other patients toward their pain and symptoms, while those who were covered only by Medicaid reported *less* hopeful attitudes. The authors suggest these findings may be related to evidence that referrals to palliative care are often delayed until late stages of the disease (i.e., Morita et al., 2005) and that uninsured populations may be at heightened risk. Consequently, "… exacerbated pain and symptoms may mean that full-blown conditions have become more difficult to control. Thus, more hopeful pain and symptom attitudes by uninsured patients anticipating Medicaid coverage could diminish over time once on Medicaid" (Francoeur et al., 2007, p. 426). These differences in health expectations between the uninsured and Medicaid groups suggest that clergy, church members, and neighborhood opinion leaders should give serious consideration about how to reach and refer uninsured (and underinsured) residents earlier in the disease course.

Clergy and church members may also be strong influences as neighborhood "opinion leaders" *within* inpatient palliative care settings and hospital hospice programs to personalize and uplift the institutional environments. An inpatient palliative care program serving inner-city African Americans in Birmingham, Alabama, The Balm of Gilead successfully tapped and directed neighborhood churches to visit patients, furnish their rooms, and host social events to overcome the depersonalized and institutional setting (Kvale, Williams, Bolden, Padgett, & Bailey, 2004). This Adapt-a-Room program resulted in high patient satisfaction with care, including high scores on the "transcendence/spiritual" domain of the Missoula VITAS scale, despite high illness severity and debilitation. Compared to outpatient and home-based models of care, this inpatient palliative care program was better able to meet the needs of this medically underserved population.

Influencing Community Perceptions of Palliative Care

Underserved inner-city and rural communities may be suspicious of palliative care, perceiving it as inferior or inadequate. This point of view may have been supported historically by hospice eligibility requirements that required patients to discontinue disease-modifying therapies, such as palliative chemotherapy or radiation treatment for cancer. In oncology, these types of palliative treatment can slow the advance or progression of cancer and the concomitant precipitation of new or intensified symptoms at later stages of the illness. These procedures can also provide satisfactory relief of pain. Fortunately, in some hospice programs *Open Access* policies have removed some of these restrictions (O'Mahony et al., 2008).

Many communities and practitioners are unaware that palliative care can be provided along the continuum of illness concurrently with disease-focused interventions. Palliative interventions provide holistic care, including relief of pain and symptoms throughout the illness continuum. When properly understood, palliative care may remain attractive to inner-city, minority, and rural populations as they continue to seek disease-modifying therapies. African Americans, for instance, are more apt to choose aggressive care when diagnosed with HIV (Mouton, Teno, Mor, & Piette, 1997) and agree to life support measures such as cardiopulmonary resuscitation, including residents of skilled nursing facilities (Braun, Beyth, Ford, & McCullough, 2008; Kwak & Haley, 2005; O'Brien et al.,1995). In addition to religious values, the limited options for health care available to lower socioeconomic and minority populations may also entrench preferences for aggressive care (Wolff, 2004). But these preferences can coexist with palliative care.

In some populations that have viewed hospice with suspicion, such as rural and inner-city African American communities, there might be greater receptivity to hospice if the patient and family received palliative care along the continuum of illness. Decisions about treatments should be based in an informed consent process and personal values and preferences and avoid suggesting that regulations, hospice philosophy, and financial limitations frame the options available. There is an important need for evidence to explore whether patients and families become more settled with coming to the end of life and receptivity to hospice, if they have engaged in a process that involved "prevailing against death" as long as they perceived any chance for survival.

Neighborhood "opinion leaders" knowledgeable about options for palliative and end-of-life care (Haas et al., 2007) may be critical messengers for broadcasting and marketing attractive program elements and overcoming misunderstanding about the options for care. The community reputation of the palliative care service may be reframed to one that integrates disease-modifying treatments along with palliative care. Moreover, the location of a palliative care service and an inpatient hospice within the same hospital, and educational outreach by opinion leaders about the roles and interface of both programs, may help build and maintain the viability of the hospice. In other settings, changing perceptions about the scope of palliative care requires an ongoing effort to differentiate palliative care from hospice programs. The assessment of the community in which one practices will determine the intervention most likely to enhance care and access to care for the populations requiring services.

The location of residential hospice programs within acute-care hospitals may help address fears by minority patients of lower quality care when hospice is received at home or in a separate hospice residence (Barrett, Hall, & Neuhaus, 1999; Barrett & Heller, 2001). An extended stay at a residential program within a hospital may also be a solution when potential for opioid diversion delays discharge home for a patient at the end of life. It should be recognized, however, that restricted Medicaid coverage or reimbursement rates in some states could limit their use unless private funding can be obtained. Recent legislation for federal health care reform raises Medicaid payments to doctors (Herszenhorn & Pear, 2010), which may be one variable that serves to enhance the feasibility of community hospices and residential hospices within acute care hospitals. Clearly, social work expertise and advocacy are important in assisting institutions to seek financial support for residences that provide care.

Hospice within skilled nursing facilities is often provided through a partnership with an outside, freestanding hospice organization (O'Mahony et al., 2008), but it may also be provided by the skilled nursing facility itself, who may choose to provide palliative and end-of-life care internally or have no access to a freestanding hospice. A critical constraint is that while hospice in skilled nursing facilities may be reimbursed through Medicare, some elderly residents cannot obtain Medicaid coverage for care in a skilled nursing facility (O'Mahony et al., 2008). Hospice housing/residence is another promising option that needs to be expanded in locations near inner-city or regional hospitals. In all options, provider teams reflecting the ethnic makeup of the community; outreach programs; trained volunteers and staff; and linkages with community programs are critical

components that improve viability (Born, Greiner, Butler, & Ahluwalia, 2004).

Outreach to Underserved and Minority Populations

In inner-city and rural areas, underserved and culturally diverse groups need special attention from palliative care and hospice service providers. Since each culture is unique, learning from the members of each group, building trust, and adapting the program to the community are essential for a culturally sensitive palliative care program.

Inner cities have had culturally diverse populations for many years. Although many rural communities have traditionally had little cultural diversity in the United States, some have Native American, African American, and Latino populations. Other rural communities have recently received immigrants and refugees representing a range of diverse cultures (Dalla, Villarruel, Cramer, & Gonzalez-Kruger, 2004). The immigrant population in inner cities has also increased; for example, Houston, Phoenix, Las Vegas, and Atlanta dramatically increased their Hispanic populations in the 1990s (RapidImmigration.com, n.d.). (See Table 13.2 for information on palliative care considerations that may be helpful in providing services for African Americans, Latinos and Native Americans in rural and inner city areas).

Many residents of rural areas share what may be considered rural culture. Typical values and attitudes are self-reliance; conservatism; work orientation; emphasis on family and religion; individualism; distrust of outsiders; and traditional gender roles (West Virginia University Center on Aging, Mountain State Geriatric Education Center, nd). Of course not all rural residents share in this culture, but it is helpful for service providers to be aware that they may encounter these values and attitudes, especially among older residents of rural communities.

Similarly, many residents of inner cities share what may be considered inner-city culture, which is also characterized by an emphasis on family, and in certain groups, religion and religious support networks, as well as traditional gender roles and distrust of outsiders. In some contexts or individuals, there may be attitudes and behaviors that reflect machismo and a "street smarts" sensibility, while in other contexts or individuals, there may be attitudes and behaviors of withdrawn invisibility. These strategies may be unconsciously adopted to protect individuals and their loved ones from violence, trauma, victimization, stigma, and unrelenting urban stress (Altman, 1995). Again, not all residents share in this culture, but service providers need to be aware that they may encounter these values and attitudes, which may restrict palliative social work assessments. For instance, mental illness concepts such as depression can be stigmatizing to inner-city and rural residents, suggesting a character defect, mental derangement, or weak masculinity. However, depression may exacerbate the experience of pain and other physical symptoms and increase the risk that regimens for care and

Table 13.2.
Issues Related to Palliative Care for Some Ethnicities in Rural and Inner-City Areas

Ethnicity	Inner City/Rural	Considerations	References
African Americans	Both in inner-city and rural areas; common in rural South	Hesitant to acknowledge dying Reluctant to complete advance directives May prefer to use all medical measures Distrust of professional medical care Religious beliefs that sufficient faith will cure serious illness Support of church community and family consensus important to many families Low hospice use but growth in enrollment over time	Bullock, 2006; Francoeur, Payne, Raveis, & Shim, 2007; Haas et al., 2007; National Hospice and Palliative Care Organization (NHPCO), 2003; Rosenfeld, Dennis, Hanen et al., 2007; Smith, 2004; Washington, Bickel-Swenson, & Stephens, 2008
Latinos	Both in inner-city and rural areas; recently many Latinos immigrate to rural communities to work in agriculture and meat packing (Henness, 2002)	Desire to return to home country to die and be buried Support of church community and family consensus important to many families Reliance on traditional medicine Language and cultural differences Many have no health care coverage and may be undocumented immigrants Low hospice use but growth in enrollment over time Believe death may occur prematurely from loss of hope when informed about dying	Barrett et al., 1999; Baxter, Bryant, Scarbro, & Shetterly, 2001; Dalla & Christensen, 2005; Diaz-Cabello, 2004; Gutheil & Heyman, 2006; Gouveia & Stull, 1997; National Hospice and Palliative Care Organization, 2003; Randall & Csikai, 2003; Rosenfeld, Dennis, Hanen et al., 2007; Smith, Sudore, & Pérez-Stable, 2009; Topoleski, 1997
Native Americans	Although Native American Nations are located primarily in rural areas, many Native Americans migrate to urban areas and may be found in inner-city areas.	Varied beliefs among different Native American nations May avoid acknowledging death is close Family tends to care for members who are ill and resists care from outsiders Language and cultural differences Traditional medicine Traditional culture and religion affect beliefs about medicine and death	Demiris, Doorenbos, & Towle, 2009; Finke, Bowannie, & Kitzes, 2004; Hobbs & Stoops, 2002; Lautenschlager & Smith, 2006

medication will not be followed. Ambivalent or missing responses to a single item screening for depression identified additional older minority men from Harlem who were at risk for hidden depression, and potential problems with care and impaired quality of life (Francoeur, 2006). Therefore, creative assessment screens should be incorporated into clinical assessment, especially short, standardized scales known as rapid assessment instruments (RAIs).

Homeless people are a unique group common in inner-city areas (Lee & Price-Spratlen, 2004). Homeless inner-city populations are described in Lashley (2006) and Kertesz, Hwang, Irwin, Ritchey, and LaGory (2009). Homelessness is also a problem in rural areas, even though it is less prevalent and more hidden (Rollinson & Pardeck, 2006). Providing palliative care and hospice to homeless individuals is especially challenging. Homeless shelters are often unable to manage health care demands for residents, and the lack of a primary care provider may limit access to hospice (O'Mahoney et al., 2008). They frequently have very limited financial resources and no health coverage, yet they commonly have serious chronic illnesses and would benefit from palliative care. Because homeless individuals are indigent, they tend to receive care from state-funded hospitals as the service provider of last resort, and their care can be quite expensive and unlikely to be reimbursed. End-of-life care is often received in the emergency room, where it is most expensive. Some development of hospital-based residential palliative care and homeless shelter-based hospice to serve the homeless population has occurred (Kushel & Miaskowski, 2006; Podymow, Turnbull, & Coyle, 2006). In addition, a hospice residence in the Bronx, established in 2005 and operated by the Jacob Perlow Hospice, admitted 38 homeless individuals out of 136 sequential total admissions (O'Mahony et al., 2008). Innovative approaches to reach homeless patients are needed so that they can be offered options and choose the kind of care they want, improving the quality of the end of their lives and perhaps also reducing public costs.

Continuity of Care throughout the Disease Course

An important strategy for improving palliative care in inner-city and rural areas is to work to establish continuity of care as patients' progress through various stages of a serious life-threatening disease. Regional health centers that deploy social workers in outreach programs to rural and inner-city communities can help maintain continuity of care and counter the shortages of social workers and other palliative care professionals that exist in these areas. Social workers have the skills to engage the interdisciplinary health team in identifying opportunities to work toward greater continuity and better coordination for patients who are cared for by various physicians and providers. We recognize that this may be challenging in many circumstances. Social workers in settings such as primary care, home health care, nursing homes, hospital, and hospice can integrate palliative care principles and assess needs, advocate and intervene from the time of diagnosis, and provide needed services at every phase of the disease rather than waiting until a hospice referral has been made (Jennings et al., 2003). The importance of coordination of care is highlighted by findings that many patients receive care from 10 or more physicians in the last 6 months of their life (Wennberg, 2008). Social workers can play a major role in building a relationship with the patient and family, which builds continuity of care among providers to ensure excellence and quality in ongoing care.

Conclusion

Social work can play a major role in improving palliative and hospice care in inner-city and rural areas. Although the challenges of providing services in these areas are daunting, the skills of social workers equip them well to engage in relationship building and problem solving to take on these challenges successfully. We have suggested a series of innovative strategies to consider for serving these underserved communities more effectively.

ACKNOWLEDGMENTS

The authors would like to acknowledge the generous assistance of colleagues with expertise in rural palliative social work (N. Joel Fry, Team Restoration Ministries, Johnston, IA; Sherri Weisenfluh, Hospice of the Bluegrass, Lexington, KY; and Marvin Fagerlind, Cedar Valley Hospice, Waterloo, IA) and pain medicine in the context of the disease of addiction (Russell Portenoy, MD, Department of Pain Medicine and Palliative Care, Beth Israel Medical Center, New York, NY).

LEARNING EXERCISE

Read Table 13.1 and answer the following questions:

1. Identify the integrated health care systems that serve inner-city and/or rural communities in your geographic region. Do you believe each health care system is large enough to negotiate successfully for significant cost savings from online bulk medication suppliers?
2. What smaller hospitals and health care affiliates might form a consortium? What may be some strategies for social work advocacy?

ADDITIONAL SUGGESTED READINGS AND RESOURCES

National Rural Health Association. (2005). *Providing hospice and palliative care in rural and frontier areas: A tool kit.* Kansas City, MO: Author.

O'Mahony, S., McHenry, J., Snow, D., Cassin, C., Schumacher, D., & Selwyn, P. A. (2008). A review of barriers to utilization of the Medicare hospice benefits in urban populations and strategies for enhanced access. *Journal of Urban Health, 85*(2), 281–290.

WEB SITES

American Medical Association. Health literacy videos: http://www.ama-assn.org/ama/no-index/about-ama/8035.shtml

The Dartmouth Atlas of Health Care: http://www.dartmouthatlas.org/

Economic Research Center, U.S. Dept. of Agriculture: http://www.ers.usda.gov/Briefing/Rurality/

Information on alternative ways to measure rurality

Health Resources and Services Administration (HRSA), U.S. Department of Health & Human Services: http://ers.hrsa.gov/ReportServer?/HGDW_Reports/BCD_HPSA/BCD_HPSA_SCR50_Smry&rs:Format=HTML3.2

Designated Health Professional Shortage Areas (HPSA) statistics.

Initiative for a Competitive Inner City: http://www.icic.org/

The National Association for Home Care and Hospice Vendor Mall: http://www.nahc.org/

Includes services for Internet Telemedicine.

National Association for Rural Mental Health: http://www.narmh.org/

National Council of Churches Health Task Force: http://www.health-ministries.org/

National Rural Health Association: http://www.ruralhealthweb.org/

National Rural Social Work Caucus: http://www.ruralsocialwork.org/

Office of Rural Health Policy (ORHP): http://ruralhealth.hrsa.gov/

Public Broadcasting Service (2006): http://www.pbs.org/wnet/religionandethics/episodes/november-24-2006/homeless-hospice/1793/

Homeless hospice (video on line, Religion and Ethics Newsweekly).

Rural Assistance Center: Health and Human Services for Rural America: http://www.raconline.org/

Rural Policy Research Institute: http://www.rupri.org/index.php

Telemedicine and e-Health (Electronic journal): http://www.liebertonline.com/loi/tmj

West Virginia University Center on Aging, Mountain State Geriatric Education Center

Rural Cultural Competence in Healthcare: http://www.hsc.wvu.edu/coa/msgec/RCC/RCCindex.asp

Urban Institute: http://www.urbaninstitute.org/

REFERENCES

Acs, G. (2009). *Poverty in the United States, 2008.* Washington, DC: Urban Institute. Retrieved from http://www.urban.org/UploadedPDF/901284_poverty_united_states.pdf

Altman, N. (1995). *The Analyst in the inner city: Race, class and culture through a psychoanalytic lens.* Hillsdale, NJ: The Analytic Press.

American Hospital Association. (n.d.) *Critical access hospitals.* Retrieved from http://www.aha.org/aha_app/issues/CAH/index.jsp

Bakitas, M., Lyons, K D., Hegel, M. T., Balan, S., Brokaw, F. C., Seville, J.,... Ahles, T. A. (2009). Effects of a palliative care intervention on clinical outcomes in patients with advanced cancer: The Project ENABLE II randomized controlled trial. *Journal of the American Medical Association, 302*(7), 741–748.

Balaswamy, S., & Dabelko, H. I. (2002). Using a stakeholder participatory model in a community-wide service needs assessment of elderly residents: A case study. *Journal of Community Practice, 10*(1), 55–70.

Barrett, R. K., Hall, A., & Neuhas, C. (1999). *U.S. minority health: A chart book.* New York, NY: The Commonwealth Fund.

Barrett, R. K., & Heller, K. S. (2001). Death and dying in the black experience: An interview with Ronald K. Barrett, PhD. *Innovations in End-of-Life Care, 3,* 5. Retrieved from http://www2.edc.org/lastacts/archives/archivesSept01/intlpersp.asp

Baxter, J., Bryant, L. L., Scarbro, S., Shetterly, S. M. (2001). Patterns of rural Hispanic and non-Hispanic White health care use: The San Luis Valley Health and Aging Study. *Research on Aging, 23,* 37–59.

Bern-Klug, M. (2010). The need to extend the reach of palliative psychosocial care to nursing home residents with advanced chronic illness. In M. Bern-Klug (Ed.), *Transforming palliative care in nursing homes* (pp. 6–30). New York, NY: Columbia University Press.

Bolin, J., & Gamm, L. (2003). Access to quality health care in rural areas—Insurance. In L. D. Gamm, L. L. Hutchison, D. J. Dabney, & A. M. Dorsey (Eds.), *Rural health people 2010* (pp. 19–24). College Station, TX: Texas A&M University System Health Science Center, School of Rural Public Health, Southwest Rural Health Research Center.

Born, W., Greiner, K. A., Butler, S. E., & Ahluwalia, J. S. (2004). Knowledge, attitudes, and beliefs about end-of-life care among inner city African Americans and Latinos. *Journal of Palliative Medicine, 7*(2), 247–256.

Braun, U. K., Beyth, R. J., Ford, M. E., & McCullough, L. B. (2008). Voices of African American, Caucasian, and Hispanic surrogates on the burdens of end-of-life decision making. *Journal of General Internal Medicine, 23*(3), 267–274.

Bullock, K. (2006). Promoting advance directives among African Americans: A faith-based model. *Journal of Palliative Medicine, 9*(1), 183–195.

Canning, E., & Payne, R. (2006). Harlem palliative care network. In B. Ferrell & N. Coyle (Eds.), *Textbook of palliative nursing* (pp. 1139–1146). New York, NY: Oxford University Press.

Carlton-LaNey, I., Murty, S. A., & Morris, L. C. (2005). Rural community practice: Organizing, planning, and development. In M. Weil (Ed.), *The handbook of community practice* (pp. 402–417). Thousand Oaks, CA: Sage.

Casey, M. M., Moscovice, I. S., Virnig, B. A., & Durham, S. B. (2005). Providing hospice care in rural areas: Challenges and strategies. *American Journal of Hospice and Palliative Care, 22*(5), 363–368.

Center to Advance Palliative Care (CAPC). (2008). Improving palliative care in nursing homes. New York, NY: Author.

Chan, L., Hart, L. G., & Goodman, D. C. (2006). Geographic access to health care for rural Medicare beneficiaries. *Journal of Rural Health, 22*(2), 140–146.

Cherny, N., Frager, G., & Ingham, J. (1995). Opioid pharmacotherapy in the management of cancer pain. *Cancer, 76*(7), 1283–1293.

Cnaan, R. A., Boddie, S. C., & Yancey, G. I. (2005). Rise up and build the cities: Faith-based community organizing. In M. Weil (Ed.), *Handbook of community practice* (pp. 372–386). Thousand Oaks, CA: Sage.

Colón, M., & Lyke, J. (2003) Comparison of hospice use and demographics among European Americans, African Americans and Latinos. *American Journal of Hospice and Palliative Care, 20*(3), 182–190.

Committee on National Urban Policy, National Research Council. (1990). *Inner-city poverty in the United States.* Washington, DC: National Academy.

Compton, P., Charuvastra, V. C., & Ling. W. (2001). Pain intolerance in opioid-maintained former opiate addicts: Effect of long-acting maintenance agent. *Drug and Alcohol Dependence, 63*(2), 139–146.

Crawley, L., Payne, R., Bolden, J., Payne, T., Washington, P., & Williams, S. (2000). Palliative and end-of-life care in the African American community. *Journal of the American Medical Association, 284*(19), 2518–2521.

Dalla, R. L., & Christensen, A. (2005). Latino immigrants describe residence in rural Midwestern meatpacking communities: A longitudinal assessment of social and economic change. *Hispanic Journal of Behavioral Sciences, 27*, 23–42.

Dalla, D. L., Villarruel, F., Cramer, S. C., & Gonzalez-Kruger, G. (2004). Examining strengths and challenges of rapid rural immigration. *Great Plains Research, 14*, 231–251.

Demiris, G., Doorenbos, A. Z., & Towle, C. (2009). Ethical considerations regarding the use of technology for older adults. The case of telehealth. *Research in Gerontological Nursing, 2*(2), 128–136.

Dennis, L. K., & Pallota, S. L. (2001). Chronic disease in rural health. In S. Loue & B. E. Quill (Eds.), *Handbook of rural health* (pp. 189–207). New York, NY: Kluwer Academic/ Plenum.

Diaz-Cabello, N. (2004). The Hispanic way of dying: Three families, three perspectives, three cultures. *Illness, Crisis & Loss, 12*(3), 239–255.

Dunham, W., Bolden, J., & Kvale, E. (2003). Obstacles to the delivery of acceptable standards of care in rural home hospices. *American Journal of Hospice and Palliative Care, 20*(4), 259–261.

Economic Research Service (2000). Measuring rurality: Rural-urban commuting area codes. Washington, DC: USDA. Retrieved from http://www.ers.usda.gov/briefing/Rurality/RuralUrbanCommutingAreas/

Economic Research Service. (2008). *Measuring rurality.* Washington, DC: USDA. Retrieved from http://www.ers.usda.gov/briefing/rurality/

Economic Research Service. (2009). *Rural America at a glance* (Economic Information Bulletin 59). Washington, DC: USDA. Retrieved from http://www.ers.usda.gov/Publications/EIB59/EIB59.pdf

Finke, B., Bowannie, T., & Kitzes, J. (2004). Palliative care in the Pueblo of Zuni. *Journal of Palliative Medicine, 7*(1), 135–143.

Francoeur, R. B. (2006). A flexible item to screen for depression in inner-city minorities during palliative care symptom assessment. *American Journal of Geriatric Psychiatry, 14*(3), 227–235.

Francoeur, R. B. (2010). Agency social workers could monitor hypertension in the community. *Social Work in Health Care, 49*, 424–443.

Francoeur, R. B., Payne, R., Raveis, V. H., & Shim, H. (2007). Palliative care in the inner-city: Patient religious affiliation, underinsurance, and symptom attitude. *Cancer, 109*(2 Suppl.), 425–434.

Gouveia, L., & Stull, D. D. (1997). Latino immigrants, meatpacking, and rural communities: A case study of Lexington, Nebraska (JSRI Research Report No. 26). East Lansing, MI: The Julian Samora Research Institute, Michigan State University.

Green, C., Ndao-Brumblay, S., West, B., & Washington, T. (2005). Differences in prescription opioid analgesic availability: Comparing minority and white pharmacies across Michigan. *The Journal of Pain, 6*(10), 689–699.

Gutheil, I. A., & Heyman, J. C. (2006). "They don't want to hear us": Hispanic elders and adult children speak about end-of-life planning. *Journal of Social Work in End-of-Life and Palliative Care, 2*(1), 55–70.

Gureje, O., Simo, G. E., & Von Korff, M. (2001). A cross-national study of the course of persistent pain in primary care. *Pain, 92*(1-2), 195–200.

Haas, J. S., Earle, C. C., Orav, J. E., Brawarsky, P., Neville, B. A., Acevedo-Garcia, D., & Williams, D. R. (2007). Lower use of hospice by cancer patients who live in minority versus white areas. *Journal of General Internal Medicine, 22*(3), 396–399.

Hanley, E. (2004). The role of homecare in palliative care services. *Care Management Journal, 5*(3), 151–157.

Health Resources and Services Administration (HRSA), U.S. Department of Health & Human Services. (2009). *Designated Health Professional Shortage Areas (HPSA) statistics.* Retrieved from http://ersrs.hrsa.gov/ReportServer?/HGDW_Reports/BCD_HPSA/BCD_HPSA_SCR50_Smry&rs:Format=HTML3.2

Henness, S. A. (2002). Latino immigration and meatpacking in the rural Midwest: An inventory of community impacts and responses. *Latinos in Missouri* (Occasional Paper Series, No. 2). Columbia, MO: Department of Rural Sociology, University of Missouri-Columbia.

Herszenhorn, D. M., & Pear, R. (2010, March 2). Obama offers to use some G. O. P. health proposals. *The New York Times.* Retrieved from http://www.nytimes.com/2010/03/03/health/policy/03health.html

Hobbs, F., & Stoops, N. (2002). *Demographic trends in the 20th Century* (Census 2000 Special Reports CENSR-4). Washington, DC: U.S. Census Bureau

Hospice Association of America. (2005). *Legislative blueprint for action.* Washington, DC: Author. Retrieved from http://www.nahc.org/NAHC/LegReg/05bp/2005_Leg_Blueprint.pdf

Hospice Association of America. (2008) *Legislative blueprint for action.* Washington, DC: Author. Retrieved from http://www.nahc.org/HAA/attachments/08_HAA_Leg_BP.pdf

Jennings, B., Ryndes, T., D'Onofrio, C., & Baily, M. A. (Eds.) (2003). *Access to hospice care: Expanding boundaries, overcoming barriers* (A special Supplement to the Hastings Center Report.) Garrison, NY: The Hastings Center. Retrieved from http://www.thehastingscenter.org/uploadedFiles/Publications/Special_Reports/access_hospice_care.pdf

Johnson, C. (2009, October 29). DEA crackdown hurts nursing home residents who need pain drugs. *The Washington Post*, p. A7

Jones, C. A., Parker, T. S., Ahearn, M., Mishra, A. K., & Variyam, J. N. (2009). *Health status and health care access of farm and rural populations* (EIB-57). Washington, DC: Economic Research Service, USDA. Retrieved from http://www.ers.usda. gov/Publications/EIB57/EIB57.pdf

Joranson, D. E., & Gilson, A. M. (1994) Controlled substances, medical practice and the law. In H. I. Schwartz (Ed.), *Psychiatric practice under fire: The influence of government, the media and special interests on somatic therapies* (pp. 173–194). Washington, DC: American Psychiatric Press, Inc.

Kelley, M. L. (2007). Developing rural communities' capacity for palliative care: A conceptual model. *Journal of Palliative Care, 23*(3), 143–153.

Kertesz, S., Hwang, S. W., Irwin, J., Ritchey, F. J., & LaGory, M. E. (2009). Rising inability to obtain needed health care among homeless persons in Birmingham, Alabama (1995–2005). *Journal of General Internal Medicine, 24*(7), 841–847.

King, S. A. (2009). Preventing prescription opioid abuse: New formulations—but who will benefit? *Psychiatric Times, 26*(2).

Krakauer, E. L., Crenner, C., & Fox, K. (2002). Barriers to optimum end-of-life care for minority patients. *Journal of the American Geriatric Society, 50*(1), 182–190.

Kushel, M. B., & Miaskowski, C. (2006). End-of-life care for homeless patients: "She says she is there to help me in any situation." *Journal of the American Medical Association, 296*(24), 2959–2966.

Kvale, E. A., Williams, B. R., Bolden, J. L., Padgett, C. G., & Bailey, F. A. (2004). The Balm of Gilead Project: A demonstration project on end-of-life care for safety-net populations. *Journal of Palliative Medicine, 7*, 486–493.

Kwak, J., & Haley, W. E. (2005). Current research findings on end-of-life decision making among racially or ethnically diverse groups. *The Gerontologist, 45*(5), 634–641.

Lashley, M. (2006). A targeted testing program for tuberculosis control and prevention among Baltimore City's homeless population. *Public Health Nursing, 24*(1), 34–39.

Lautenschlager, L., & Smith, C. (2006). Low-income American Indians' perceptions of diabetes. *Journal of Nutrition Education and Behavior, 38*(5), 307–315.

Lee, B. A., & Price-Spratlen, T. (2004). The geography of homelessness in American communities: Concentration or dispersion? *City and Community, 3*(1), 3–27.

Madigan, E. A., Wiencek, C. A., & Vander Schrier, A. L. (2009). Patterns of community-based end-of-life care in rural areas of the United States. *Policy, Politics, and Nursing Practice, 10*(1), 71–81.

Miller, S. C., & Mor, V. (2004). The opportunity for collaborative care provision: The presence of nursing home/hospice collaborations in the U.S. States. *Journal of Pain and Symptom Management, 28*(6), 537–547.

Morita, T., Akechi, T., Ikenaga, M., Kizawa, Y., Kohara, H., Mukaiyama, T.,… Uchitomi, Y. (2005). Late referrals to specialized palliative care service in Japan. *Journal of Clinical Oncology, 23*, 2637–2644.

Morrison, R. S., Wallenstein, S., Natale, D. K., Senzel, R. S., & Huang, L. (2000). "We don't carry that"—Failure of pharmacies in predominantly nonwhite neighborhoods to stock opioid analgesics. *The New England Journal of Medicine, 342*(14), 1023–1026.

Mouton, C., Teno, J. M., Mor, V., & Piette, J. (1997). Communication of preferences for care among human immunodeficiency virus—Infected patients. Barriers to informed decisions? *Archives of Family Medicine, 6*(4), 342–347.

Murty, S. (2004). Mapping community assets: The key to effective rural social work. In L. Scales & C. Streeter (Eds.), *Rural social work: Building assets to sustain rural communities* (pp. 278–289). Belmont, CA: Brooks/Cole/ Thomson Learning.

Murty, S. A. (2005). The future of rural social work. *Advances in Social Work, 6*(1), 132–144.

Naleppa, M. J., & Hash, K. M. (2001) Home-based practice with older adults. *Journal of Gerontological Social Work, 35*(1), 71–88.

National Association of Social Workers (NASW). (2008). *Code of ethics.* Washington, DC: Author.

National Hospice and Palliative Care Organization (NHPCO). (2003). *Facts and figures.* Retrieved from http://www. ccsnationwide.com/Facts_and_Figures.htm

Neubauer, B. J., & Hamilton, C. L. (1990). Racial differences in attitudes toward hospice care. *Hospice Journal, 6*, 37–48.

Nuhn, J. (2009, October 28). *Wellmark Blue Cross Blue Shield Palliative Care outpatient services.* Hospice and Palliative Care Organization of Iowa Fall Conference, Ames, Iowa. Retrieved from http://www.iowahospice.org/documents/filelibrary/ documents/pdf/2009_fall_conference/1B__Transparency_in_ Health_Plans__N_19FE20493800A.pdf

O'Brien, L. A., Grisso, J. A., Maislin, G., LaPann, K., Krotki, K. P., Greco, P. J.,… Evans. L. K. (1995). Nursing home residents' preferences for life-sustaining treatments. *Journal of the American Medical Association, 274*(22), 1775–1779.

O'Mahony, S., McHenry, J., Snow, D., Cassin, C., Schumacher, D., & Selwyn, P. A. (2008). A review of barriers to utilization of the Medicare hospice benefits in urban populations and strategies for enhanced access. *Journal of Urban Health, 85*(2), 281–290.

Pawling-Kaplan, M., & O'Connor, P. (1989). Hospice care for minorities: An analysis of a hospital-based inner city palliative care service. *American Journal of Hospice and Palliative Care, 6*(4), 13–21.

Peterschmidt, P. (2006). Home health and hospice in rural America. *Caring: National Association for Home Care Magazine, 25*(1), 26–32.

Podymow, T., Turnbull, J., & Coyle, D. (2006). Shelter-based palliative care for the homeless terminally ill. *Palliative Medicine, 20*(2), 81–86.

Randall, H., & Csikai, E. (2003) Issues affecting utilization of hospice services by rural Hispanics, *Journal of Ethnic And Cultural Diversity in Social Work, 12*(2), 79–94.

Rankin, B. H., & Quane, J. M. (2000). Neighborhood poverty and the social isolation of inner-city African American families. *Social Forces, 79*(1), 139–164.

RapidImmigration.com (n.d.) *US immigration facts.* Retrieved from http://www.rapidimmigration.com/usa/1_eng_ immigration_facts.html

Reamer, F. G. (2001). *Tangled relationships: Managing boundary issues in the human services.* New York, NY: Columbia University Press.

Rhymes, J. A. (1996). Barriers to palliative care. *Cancer Control, 3*, 230–223.

Rollinson, P. A., & Pardeck, J. T. (2006). *Homelessness in rural America: Policy and practice.* Binghamton, NY: Haworth.

Rosenfeld, P., Dennis, J., Hanen, S., Henriques, E., Schwarts, T. M., Correoso, L., Murtaugh, C. M., & Fleishman, A. (2007). Are there racial differences in attitudes toward hospice care?

A study of hospice-eligible patients at the Visiting Nurse Services of New York. *American Journal of Hospice and Palliative Medicine, 24*(5), 408–416.

Scimeca, M. M., Savage, S. R., Portenoy, R., & Lowinson, J. (2000). Treatment of pain in methadone-maintained patients. *The Mount Sinai Journal of Medicine, 67*(5/6), 412–422.

Smith, A. K., Sudore, R. L., & Pérez-Stable, E. J. (2009). Palliative care for Latino patients and their families: Whenever we prayed, she wept. *Journal of the American Medical Association, 301*(10), 1047–1057.

Smith, S. H. (2004). End-of-life care decision-making processes of African American families: Implications for culturally-sensitive social work practice. *Journal of Ethnic and Cultural Diversity in Social Work, 13*(2), 1–22.

Stevenson, D. G., & Bramson, J. S. (2009). Hospice care in the nursing home setting: A review of the literature. *Journal of Pain and Symptom Management, 38*(3), 440–451.

Tierney, J. (2007, March 27). Trafficker or healer? And who's the victim? *The New York Times.* Retrieved from http://www.nytimes.com/2007/03/27/science/27tier.html?_r=1

Topoleski, L. M. (1997). *An interpretive analysis of hospice underutilization by Mexican- Americans in Lansing, Michigan: En sus propias palabras (In their own words)* (JSRI Research Report #28). East Lansing, MI: The Julian Samora Research Institute, Michigan State University.

U.S. General Accounting Office (GAO). (2005). *Modifications to payment methodology may be warranted* (Report GAO-05-42). Washington, DC: Author.

Van Vorst, R. F., Crane, L. A., Barton, P. L., Kutner, J. S., Kallail, J., & Westfall, J. M. (2006). Barriers to quality care for dying patients in rural communities. *Journal of Rural Health, 22*(3), 248–253.

Virnig, B. A., Ma, H., Hartman, L. K., Moscovice, I., & Carlin, B. (2006). Access to home-based hospice care for rural populations: Identification of areas lacking service. *Journal of Palliative Medicine, 9*(6), 1292–1299.

Virnig, B. A., Moscovice, I. S., Durham, S. B., & Casey, M. M. (2004). Do rural elders have limited access to Medicare hospice services? *Journal of the American Geriatrics Society, 52*(5), 731–735.

Washington, K. T., Bickel-Swenson, D., & Stephens, N. (2008). Barriers to hospice use among African Americans: A systematic review. *Health and Social Work, 33*(4), 267–274.

Weil, M. (2005). Social planning with communities: Theory and practice. In M. Weil (Ed.), *The handbook of community practice* (pp. 215–243). Thousand Oaks, CA: Sage.

Wennberg, J. E. (2008). *Tracking the care of patients with severe chronic illness: The Dartmouth Atlas of Health Care 2008.* Lebanon, NH: Dartmouth Institute for Health Policy and Clinical Practice, Center for Health Policy Research, Dartmouth Medical School.

West Virginia University Center on Aging, Mountain State Geriatric Education Center. (n.d). *Rural cultural competence in health care.* Retrieved from http://www.hsc.wvu.edu/coa/msgec/RCC/RCCindex.asp

Whitten, P., Doolittle, G., & Mackert, M. (2004). Telehospice in Michigan: Use and patient acceptance. *American Journal of Hospice and Palliative Medicine, 21*(3), 191–195.

Wolff, S. H. (2004). Society's choice: The tradeoff between efficacy and equity and the lives at stake. *American Journal of Preventive Medicine, 27*(1), 49–56.

14 *Karlynn BrintzenhofeSzoc*

Clinical Trials and the Role of Social Work

Being a part of a clinical trial, even though I got standard of care, was the best decision I made. Not only did I have access to my doctor, but the research nurse was always there. If I had a problem and couldn't get in touch with the doctor, the research nurse was almost always available. The longest I had to wait was 1 hour for a return phone call. I know I would have gotten great care regardless, but I feel good about being able to help patients who come after me.

—61-year-old, white female, diagnosed with stage IV esophageal cancer

During the first visit with the oncologist—1 week after the initial diagnosis—he brought up the topic of clinical trials. I was so impressed and excited. To me this meant my sister would get the best care possible.

—Family member of patient above

Key Concepts

- *The five types of clinical trials focus on treatment, prevention, diagnostics, screening, and quality of life.*
- *Trial protocols must be approved by institutional review boards who ensure the ethical conduct of research that involves human participants.*
- *Barriers and misconceptions influence participation in clinical trials.*
- *Access to clinical trials is not equally available to all persons regardless of age, race, and socioeconomic class.*

Introduction

Clinical trials are the means by which improvements in medical treatments occur. They also increase the understanding of the etiology of a disease or condition, and they help assess the effectiveness of nonmedical treatments. The methodical process that is a clinical trial allows researchers to know more about how a treatment works, why it works with some people and not others, and what the next steps might be to improve the outcomes. Clinical trials are used in the study of almost every disease. They are not limited to biomedical treatments but include behavioral treatments as well. The manner in which clinical trials are planned and carried out is critical to moving the science from the bench to the bedside, to the clinic, to the primary health care providers, and eventually to influence policy decision makers.

Historically, clinical trials were typically conducted by those in the medical community to test treatments for illnesses—both acute and chronic—that have a relatively large number of people who either are at risk or live with the diseases. Over the past few years more attention has been paid and more funding has been designated for rare diseases (those diseases or conditions affecting fewer than 200,000 persons in the United States) and neglected diseases (such as malaria, which is common in developing countries where access to expensive treatments is limited). It is estimated that over 25 million people in the United States have one of the over 6800 rare disease with only 200 of them having a known effective treatment (National Institute of Health Office of the Director and Office of Rare Diseases Research [NIH OD & ORDR], 2009).

Clinical trials are usually organized in large research institutions and funded by federal government agencies such as the National Institutes of Health, the Department of Defense, the Department of Veterans Affairs, and private industry, including pharmaceutical and biotech companies, medical institutions, and foundations (CenterWatch, 2010). Being a part of a clinical trial usually does not increase the costs of care, because the cost of the actual treatment being tested is covered by the funder.

Given these conditions, one would expect current or future patients to be clamoring to participate. Unfortunately this is not the case. For example, only 3% of adults diagnosed with cancer enroll in a clinical trial. The reasons for the lack of participation are many and varied and are discussed later in this chapter under "Barriers to Participation." Some of the reasons include lack of awareness that clinical trials are available, not being asked to participate, fear of being treated like a guinea pig, not wanting to upset their physician, and simply fear.

The numbers are very different with children diagnosed with cancer, with over 60% participating in clinical trials (Education Network to Advance Cancer Clinical Trials [ENACCT] & Community-Campus Partnerships for Health [CCPH], 2008; Harnessing Science, 2004). The outcome of this high rate of enrollment is an improvement of survival of childhood cancers from about 55% survival at 5 years in the 1970s to a 70% survival at 5 years in 2002. The reasons that children have such a high proportion of participation include the following: parents are told about clinical trials and asked to enroll their child; clinical trials are the norm for children (which is not the case for adults); and often parents will do anything to increase the probability of survival for their children.

As social workers interested in palliative care, we need to understand how clinical trials work; how we can get involved to help recruit and retain patients into trials; how to ensure that all patients, especially people from minority groups, are aware of the possibility of clinical trials as a means of treatment; and how to be the conduit of clear communication about clinical trials between the research team, the patient's physician, and the patient and his or her family. Furthermore, being on the team that develops the trial will ensure that some of the well-documented barriers to enrollment are addressed and that the best psychosocial care is available to patients enrolled in the trials. It is my strong and long-standing belief that all social workers possess the exact skills needed to be an integral member of the clinical trial team. Having a social worker on the clinical trial team will improve recruitment, retention, and an understanding of the impact of trials on patients and families.

This chapter will describe the basics of clinical trials, including the history of protecting participants in clinical trials, the known barriers to enrollment in trials, and the role social workers can play in increasing the awareness of clinical trials with clients and patients so they can make informed treatment decisions. The potential ethical issues faced by social workers in this role will be presented as well. The chapter will end with an examination of the opportunities to increase skill and knowledge around clinical trials.

Clinical Trials

The purpose of clinical trials is to move basic scientific research from the laboratory into treatments for people. By evaluating the results of these trials, researchers can find better treatments and ways to prevent, detect, and treat diseases (ENACCT & CCPH, 2008). Sometimes clinical trials do not start as basic science but rather are used to determine whether a treatment that is effective in one disease has any efficacy with a different disease.

Types of Clinical Trials

There are five categories of clinical trials, each with a specific purpose:

- *Treatment trials* test experimental treatments, combinations of drugs, or new surgeries or radiation therapies.
- *Prevention trials* focus on finding new ways to prevent disease in people who do not have the disease or to keep a disease from recurring. The focus of these trials includes medicines, vaccines, supplements, and lifestyle or behavior modifications.
- *Diagnostic trials* have the objective of improving tests and procedures for detecting a disease or condition.
- *Screening trials* evaluate the most effective means to detect specific diseases or conditions.
- *Quality-of-life trials* (also known as supportive care trials) evaluate interventions to improve the comfort and quality of life of people diagnosed with a chronic illness.

The Stages and Phases of Clinical Trials

Years of work in the *preclinical stage* precede any treatment with humans. This is the work in the laboratory, testing the treatment's effectiveness in test tubes, petri dishes, and (in some cases) animals. Once there is evidence of biological activity and the safety of compounds, an application is filed with the U.S. Food and Drug Administration (FDA) to get approval to start trials with humans. This filing is called the investigational new drug (IND) application and is the shortest step in the process: If the FDA does not disapprove, the study can move into the *clinical stage* of trials. At this first stage, the FDA can take only one of two actions: It can disapprove the action, or it can "not disapprove," implying that the activity can proceed. Before a trial can recruit a human participant, the study must be approved by the institutional review board (IRB) of every institution where recruitment is planned (Pharmaceutical Research and Manufacturers of America [PhRMA], 2009). The role of the IRB is described in more detail under "Human Subject Protection."

The clinical stage of treatment development and testing is made up of three phases. Each phase has a specific purpose to answer specific questions, and each needs a progressively larger number of participants. The one purpose that is an important component of each phase is safety of the treatment. At the end of each phase the findings must be submitted to the FDA for approval to move to the next phase of testing. Once word is received from the FDA, the subsequent phase is considered a new study so the process of going through the IRB's of each institution to be involved in the study for human protection occurs again (PhRMA, 2009). Table 14.1 presents the purpose of each phase and the number of people needed to complete the trial. Of note is that in Phase I trials the first human participants are usually healthy volunteers, except in the cases of cancer and HIV/AIDS trails. In these two instances patients diagnosed with the type of cancer and the stage of HIV disease under study are the participants. This is because of the need to determine the interaction of the treatment and the disease process. A treatment might not have any side effects on a healthy person but when given to a person with the disease under study the interaction may have life-threatening side effects.

In Phase I trials, the documentation of toxicity of the treatment is to determine the parameters of safe dosage levels for future trials. The doses are increased incrementally to determine what the side effects are based on the dosage. This guides the decisions for the dosage used in Phase II trials. In Phase II trials the main question is, "Is the treatment effective?" Effectiveness is determined by an improvement in the disease or condition. For example, in a Phase II trial for lung cancer, the changes in the size of the tumor would be an indication of effectiveness. Safety information continues to be collected as well as information on side effects. Studies that have a quality-of-life component would also collect data on this issue. Unfortunately not all studies include any quality-of-life components. Phase III trials answer the question, "Does the new treatment work at least as well or better than the standard of care?" The standard of care is the current approved treatment for the disease under study. The number of patient volunteers needed for this phase range from 1000 to 5000 (PhRMA, 2009). The participants in Phase III trials are followed carefully to determine the effectiveness of the treatment under study on the progression of the disease and for side effects in comparison to the standard of care. It is in Phase III trials that the comparison may be a placebo if no standard treatment is available for the disease or condition. A placebo is an inactive substance or treatment that looks just like the substance or treatment under study (NCI, 2007). As Phase II and III trials need a much larger population, the clinical trials usually occur at many clinics and hospitals.

Table 14.1.
Phases of Clinical Stage of Clinical Trials

	No. of People Who Participate	Time to Completion
In Phase I trials, researchers test an experimental drug or treatment in a small group of people for the first time to evaluate its safety, determine a safe dosage range, identify means of administering the treatment, and identify side effects.	20–100 participants (in many trials healthy volunteers are the participants; in cancer clinical trials and HIV/AIDS trials, patients volunteers are the participants)	6 months to 1 year
In Phase II trials, the experimental study drug or treatment is given to a larger group of people to see whether it is effective and to further evaluate its safety.	100–300 (NCI) patient volunteers 100–500 (PhRMA)	6 months to 1 year
In Phase III trials, the experimental study drug or treatment is given to large groups of people (1000–3000) to confirm its effectiveness, monitor side effects, compare it to commonly used treatments, and collect information that will allow the experimental drug or treatment to be used safely.	From 100 to thousands of people (NCI) patient volunteers 1000 to 5000 (PhRMA)	1 to 4 years
In Phase IV trials, postmarketing studies delineate additional information, including the drug's long-term safety and effectiveness, risks, benefits, and optimal use.	Several hundred to several thousand people	Many years

Source: National Cancer Institute, 2007; PhRMA, 2009; TrialsCentral.org, n.d.

Phase III studies are those that include random assignment. As these trials are comparing the new treatment to the standard of care or placebo, participants are assigned to one arm or the other. In medicine a Phase III study has at least two arms: one arm is the group getting the study treatment, and the other arm is the standard of care. The outcome of random assignment is not known at the time of recruitment of a potential participant into a study. Random assignment gives every potential participant an equal chance of being in either arm. The goal of this procedure is to ensure that characteristics of the patients are likely to be spread equally across each group. Some of the characteristics include gender, race, genetic differences, potential differences in reactions to treatments, to name a few. This type of trial is called a randomized clinical trial and is considered the "gold standard" in medicine.

Each study has a specified list of inclusion criteria and exclusion criteria. These inclusion criteria usually address the age of the potential participants, the specific disease or condition, or the need for the participant to not be diagnosed with the disease under study (e.g., healthy participants), performance status, and types of treatments already received that are allowable. The exclusion criteria are those that the potential participant cannot have. These might include comorbidities such as diabetes or hypertension, current medications such as hormone replacement therapy, and having already received treatments for the disease or condition under study. The inclusion and exclusion criteria are sometimes seen as a barrier to access to clinical trials because some minority populations are more likely to have exclusionary conditions than those from the majority population.

Further, if newly diagnosed patients are not aware of the possibility of clinical trials as the first line of treatment, they may not have the opportunity if a specific treatment or procedure is one of the exclusions. An example of this situation is where a specific study is designed to investigate a treatment for patients who have not received any previous treatments for the condition. They are looking to see the effect of the treatment on a "virgin" disease. Another example would be if the procedure under study is a new type of surgery, and only those who have not had any surgery would be eligible to participate.

At the end of Phase III the results of the studies are written up and sent to the FDA for approval to offer in clinical practice. A report to the FDA can be up to 100,000 pages of information. The FDA can then take up to 2 years to give approval (PhRMA, 2009).

A treatment may be approved by the FDA with a request for postclinical trials. These are Phase IV trials and the goal is to determine long-term risks and benefits. As shown in Table 14.1 the process from preclinical to approval and availability to patients is a very long one, ranging from 10 to 15 years. Due to the large numbers of participants needed in Phase III trials and the low rate of accrual of patient volunteers, some of these trials are closed and the information gathered is not enough to warrant an application for approval to the FDA (NCI, 2007; PhRMA, 2009). Table 14.2 presents the drug discovery, development, and approval process. Each phase is described in term of the purpose of the phase, the number of participants, the average time for the phase to be completed, and the success rate of a drug. Two important

Table 14.2.
Drug Discovery, Development, and Approval Process

Stages	Preclinical Testing	Clinical Trials			FDA Approval	Postclinical Testing
Phases		Phase I	Phase II	Phase III		Phase IV
Purpose	Safety and biological activity in lab, animals, and xenografts (where tissues of one species are transplanted to another species)	Safety, how best administered, and dose-related toxicities	Effectiveness on disease or condition, identify side effects	Effectiveness as compared to standard of care or placebo if no standard of care available	File papers to FDA for review and approval	Efficacy and safety, larger group of people, does not include limitations of clinical trials with excluding comorbidities
Time	6.5 years	1.5 year	2 years	3.5 years	1.5 years	
Success rate	5000 compounds tested	5 enter trials			1 approved	

Source: NCI, 2007; PhRMA, 2009, p. 103.

messages in Table 14.2 are that the average time from beginning to study a drug to approval is 15 years, and 1 out of 5000 drugs make it to the marketplace.

Human Subjects Protection

As mentioned previously, before any participant can be recruited and enrolled in a clinical trial, the trial protocol must be approved by the IRB of each institution involved in the trial. The purpose of the IRB is to ensure the ethical conduct of any research that involves human participants taking place within an institution. The composition and work of an IRB is regulated by the U.S. Department of Health and Human Services (DHHS) under the Code of Federal Regulations (CFR) Title 45, Part 46, Subparts A through D (American Evaluation Association, 2005). An IRB must register with Office for Human Research Protections (OHRP) and have submitted an assurance of compliance to OHRP. The minimum requirements of an IRB is to have five members with a variety of backgrounds that will allow for the promotion of a complete and sufficient review of research activities and submitted protocols at the institution (OHRP, 2009). In "The IRB" section of this chapter, the various backgrounds of the members are presented, including the place for social work.

The protocol is the plan, much like a recipe or a blueprint, which will be followed for each study participant. There are specific guidelines that identify what must be included in the protocol: the purpose of the study; the number of participants; eligibility; how the study will be carried out; what information will be gathered about the participants (including demographic, psychosocial, and medical); and endpoints. This information also includes the amount of time required by the participant, the known risks and benefits of the study, and how the participants will be protected. The protocol is submitted for review to the IRB along with the informed consent form that each participant will need to read, understand, and sign before he or she can start the study. The NIH strongly suggests that the text of informed consent forms be written at the eighth grade reading level or lower as well as including graphics. Another suggestion to allow inclusion of participants who do not read English is to have multiple consent forms for each study. This means forms in different languages that are also culturally appropriate.

Approval of a clinical trial by an IRB is not guaranteed, and often the researchers must rewrite and resubmit the protocol and consent forms a number of times before final approval is received. Though this can be frustrating for the researcher, the important point is to protect the human participants in the research project (American Evaluation Association, 2009). The need for this protection arose due to the United States' disturbing history of taking advantage of participants and not putting the participants' safety and well-being first (ENACCT & CCPH, 2008; Frank, 2004; Perlman, 2004).

Table 14.3 presents a short history, starting with the Nuremburg Code, of the changes that have occurred at the legislative level (both international and national) to ensure protection of human participants in research. Some of the changes came about in response to specific abuses, while others were further development of standing policies and regulations.

The International Review Board

The makeup of the IRB is set forth in the Common Rule (OHRP, 2009). The IRB must have a minimum of five members who represent a cross-section of experience and expertise, diversity, and sensitivity to community attitudes, promoting respect and awareness of safeguarding the rights and welfare of study participants (Knowlton, 2003). Some of the specific guidelines are that no IRB shall be all men or all women or be made up of one profession; one of the five members must not be affiliated with the institution and is identified as the community representative. Another primary criterion for membership relates to the nonscientific aspects of the studies presented to the IRB, so one member is identified as a nonscientist. The remaining members need to be scientists who cover the range of topics presented for approval. Thus, if there are studies presented that include children, an expert in the area of pediatrics needs to be on the IRB (Knowlton, 2003, OHRP, 2009). The role of social work on the IRB could be as the nonscientist or as a scientist with expertise in the biopsychosocial-spiritual aspects of the potential participants and their families. Having social workers on IRBs might be one way to move toward more inclusion of quality-of-life indicators as a part of treatments.

Any researcher who presents a study for approval by an IRB must document that he or she has completed training in the protection of human participants. Some institutions have their own training, whereas others require the completion of the online training developed and offered by the NIH. For most clinical trials all study staff must complete the training, and the protocol includes current certificates as proof of completion. At this point in time some institutions require that the training be completed periodically, whereas others require completing the training once. There is a move toward requiring ongoing training and certification.

Barriers and Misconceptions Regarding Participation in Clinical Trials

There are many barriers to participation that are real and others that are perceptual. There are also a multitude of misconceptions about why people may not participate. An important aspect of understanding clinical trials is to know why people participate, what the concerns and fears are, and who helps people offered a trial to make the best decision for

Table 14.3.
History of Human Subjects Protection

Year	Event	Purpose	Event in Response to
1947	Nuremberg Code	Made explicit some of the following research concepts: the voluntary consent of the human subject is absolutely essential, minimization of risk and harm, a favorable risk/benefit ratio, qualified investigators using appropriate research designs, and freedom for the subject to withdraw at any time	Nazi Germany atrocities (see Fleischman, 2005)
1962	Senate adds the Kefauver-Harris Drug Amendments to the Food, Drug, and Cosmetic Act	Passed into law to ensure drug efficacy and greater drug safety, this was the first time drug companies had to prove to the FDA that a drug was effective	Thalidomide (see Rajkumar, 2004)
1964	Declaration of Helsinki: Recommendations Guiding Medical Doctors in Biomedical Research Involving Human Subjects	Adopted by the 18th World Medical Assembly	Nazi Germany atrocities (see Fleischman, 2005).
1966	NIH developed policies for the Protection of Human Subjects		
1971	Guidelines issued by the U.S. Department of Health, Education, and Welfare (DHEW) on Codes for the conduct of social and behavioral research		
1972	Establishment of the Office for Protection from Research Risks (OPPR), which reported to NIH		
1974, May	NIH policies raised to federal regulatory status	Established IRB as a means of protecting human subjects	
1974, July	National Research Act established the National Commission for the Protection of Human Subjects of Biomedical and Behavioral Research	Commission met from 1974 to 1978; its charge was to identify the basic ethical principles that should underlie the conduct of biomedical and behavioral research involving human subjects	In response to the Willowbrook School Study (1956–1971) (see Krugman, 1986), Tuskegee Syphilis Study (see Parker & Alvarez, 2003), Fernald State School (see D'Antonio, 2004) and Jewish Chronic Disease Hospital (see Lerner, 2004)
1975	Revised Helsinki Declaration adopted by the 41st World Medical Assembly		
1978, Sept.	The Belmont Report	The outcome of the Commissions work that started in July 1974	
1978, Nov	Additional protections for research involving fetuses, pregnant women, in vitro fertilization, and prisoners implemented		
1981	Department of Health and Human Services (DHHS) and the FDA regulations are codified in the Code of Federal Regulations: DHSS in Title 45 Part 46 FDA in Title 21 Parts 50 and 56	In response to the Belmont Report, changes focused on how the IRB was expected to accomplish its charge and specific procedures to follow	

Table 14.3. *(Contd.)*

Year	Event	Purpose	Event in Response to
1983	Title 45 Part 46 revisions made, which include additional protection for children involved in research		
1991	Title 45 Part 46 revision involved adoption of the Federal Policy for Protection of Human Subjects known as the "Common Rule"; Title 21 Parts 50 and 56 revised		
2000	OPPR changed to the Office for Human Research Participants; reports to the Assistant Secretary of Health	No longer reporting to the group it was to be overseeing	

FDA, Food and Drug Administration; IRB, institutional review board; NIH, National Institutes of Health.

Source: Penslar & Porter, 1993; Office of Research Integrity, n.d.; Perlman, 2004.

themselves with regard to participation. The following will address the literature on known barriers, misperceptions, as well as what has been reported about the public's beliefs about clinical trials.

Patient Barriers

The literature is replete with information about the distress that is experienced when being treated for chronic diseases (Ciechanowski, Katon, & Russo, 2000; Fortin et al., 2006; Johnson, 1989; Joshi, Kumar, & Avasthi, 2003; Zabora, BrintzenhofeSzoc, Curbow, Hooker, & Piantadosi. 2001). There is evidence that the rate of psychiatric disorders and distress increases as a patient moves toward the end of life. Crunkilton and Rubins (2009) in a review article report a range from 1% to 76% of patients at end of life who experience some form of psychological distress. Akechi et al. (2004) report ranges of psychological distress among cancer patients from 9% to 35%, rates of major depression from 8% to 26%, and rates of posttraumatic stress disorder (PTSD) from 3% to 35%. Akechi et al. also report on two studies among terminally ill patients with 34% to 43% and 28% to 80% experienced symptoms of PTSD. The role of psychiatric disorders, psychological distress, and PTSD play in the recruitment and retention of participants in clinical trials has not been formally investigated. Why might this be? The recruiter may believe the person is unable to give informed consent or that having the discussion about treatment participation will result in more distress or an exacerbation of psychiatric symptoms. Some perceive that these distressed patients will be less likely to comply with the rigors of the clinical trial.

Harris Interactive has conducted nationwide surveys to evaluate perceptions of clinical trials in the United States in 2001, 2003, 2004, and 2005 (http://www.harrisinteractive.

com). In the 2001 and 2003 surveys the respondents were asked if they would consider enrolling in a trial if asked, and the response went from 83% to 77%. This suggests that asking may be the first important step in increasing the rates of enrollments in clinical trials. The 2005 report shows that there is no real difference in the number of adults who report ever participating in a clinical trial by year (8%, 10%, 11%, and 10%). The number of adults who report ever being offered an invitation to participate in a clinical trial has changed some over time (13%, 16%, 19%, and 15%). These data suggest that, when offered the opportunity, a large percentage of individuals accept the invitation. Specifically, for the years 2001 and 2003 over 60% of the adults who had an opportunity to participate in a clinical trial, of any type, agreed to enroll in the trial.

The main reasons for consideration of a clinical trial were stable for 2004 and 2005, but they have changed since 2003. Table 14.4 presents comparative percentages of the reasons respondents considered for participating in a clinical trial if they were asked in 2003, 2004, and 2005. This information is helpful to social workers across the disease continuum because we can educate members of the health care team as to why patients agree to participate. Further, social workers could use this information to educate patients and family members around the issues that concern patients such as receiving a placebo rather than an active drug.

Family Barriers

Psychological distress is experienced by family members of those living with chronic illnesses (Holmes & Deb, 2003). As family members play a number of roles to assist an individual entering a clinical trial, it is important to understand the impact distress has on the family. A family that has negative perceptions and attitudes about clinical trials will likely not

Table 14.4.
Reasons Respondents Would Consider Participating in a Clinical Trial If Asked

	2003	2004	2005
If I had a terminal illness	48%	72%	72%
If I thought the drug might cure me	52%	71%	67%
If there were no other medical options available to me	39%	67%	66%
If I thought the drug/treatment would help me	n/a	71%	67%
The treatment was free of charge to me	66%	64%	53%
If my doctor recommended it	49%	54%	47%
If I received money for participating	63%	56%	46%
If I knew the risks associated with the treatment	72%	49%	45%
If it would benefit me or someone else (2003 question) If I thought the drug/treatment would help someone else in the future (2005 question)	71%	n/a	45%
If it were convenient for me	60%	54%	43%
If the location were convenient for me	n/a	54%	43%
If there were minimal side effects associated with the treatment	59%	48%	43%
If I knew that I would receive an active drug and not a sugar pill (placebo)	20%	37%	33%
If I had a condition other than a terminal illness	29%	36%	29%

Source: HarrisInteractive, 2003, p. 3; HarrisInteractive, 2005, p. 5.

support the individual's consideration of joining a trial (Frank, 2004).

Physician Barriers

As noted previously, clinical trial candidates depend on and follow the guidance given by their physician. So exploring some of the barriers for the physicians to be a champion of clinical trials is imperative for social workers who are interested in enhancing the opportunity for patients to consider enrollment into clinical trials. The information presented here can be used as a basis for understanding where the oncologists and internists stand in developing educational materials as well as advocating for changes in the process. A Web-based survey launched by Medscape was conducted to evaluate physician barriers to recruiting or referring patients to cancer clinical trials. The sample included oncologists and internists internationally. The responses to questions about what would motivate offering clinical trials to more patients revealed the top motivator to be a dedicated staff member to be responsible for the patients on trials (oncologists, 58%; internists, 39%). For oncologists this was followed by easier access to trials for their patient populations at 52%; better reimbursement and better patient-oriented educational information (both at 32%), and the final motivators, both at 26%, were trials that their patients would more likely accept, no randomization, and physician-oriented education

information about specific trials. For the internists 32% of the respondents would be motivated by easier access to trials and better physician-oriented education information about specific trials. These were followed by trials that did not include randomization (21%), and finally, better physician reimbursement (18%) (Markman & Grimm, 2009).

The top barriers the oncologists reported that kept cancer patients from enrolling in clinical trials were increased physician time to enroll, treat, and monitor patient on the trial (58%); complex consent forms (36%); lack of resources in the practice to enroll and monitor the patients (36%); and patients not meeting the eligibility criteria (26%). For the internists in the study the top barriers for patients were lack of resources in the practice to enroll and monitor the patients (54%); worries about side effects (50%); complex consent forms (42%); and increased physician time to enroll, treat, and monitor patient on trial (39%) (Markman & Grimm, 2009).

A study conducted by Simon et al. (2004) found that patients with a new breast cancer diagnosis were not offered a trial because physicians thought they would not be eligible (57%) or that there were no trials available for the stage of the disease (41%). Of note, black women were less likely to be offered a trial because the physician thought the patient would not be eligible (61.1%) as compared to white or other race patients (53.3%). Not being offered a trial due to no trial available for the stage of disease was lower for black women (33.3%) than for white or other race women (46.7%). Another potential barrier to offering cancer patients clinical trials is the proximity to American College of Surgeons (ACoS) approved hospital cancer programs and the number of American Society of Clinical Oncologist (ASCO) certified oncologists (Sateren et al., 2002). In other words, the physicians may not refer patients because they do not believe there are sites geographically close to their patients.

Somkin et al. (2005) report, based on a survey of 198 adult oncologists, that 94% agreed that enrollment in clinical trials improved patient care in general, 87% agreed that involvement in clinical trials results in a high quality of care for the participants, and 83% agreed that participation benefited the patient. Furthermore, research has shown that trial participants nearly always receive equivalent or better care than those receiving standard treatments, despite the experimental nature of these investigational treatments. The importance of these findings to social work is that we can help patients across the disease continuum to consider that clinical trials not only add to the knowledge base on moving toward better treatments but that there is a benefit to the patient. Patients often receive more attention from the health care team because every study has a core of research nurses. The quality of care is thought to be better because the procedures are monitored and followed by not only the principal investigator of the study but also overseen by the federal government.

Social Justice Issues

As noted previously, children with cancer are enrolled in clinical trials at a significantly higher rate than are adults. Sateran et al. (2002) reported that for children between the ages of 1 to 10 years, the accrual rate is over 50%, and there is no difference in rate of accrual between whites, African Americans, Asian Americans, and Hispanics. The comparability of accrual by race is similar up to the age of 29, while differences appear from the age of 30 and above. Specifically, African American men and Asian American and Hispanic men and women are enrolled in clinical trials at a lower rate than their white peers. The explanation of these differences is not known, although some posit that regardless of race or ethnicity parents will do everything possible for their children. The change that occurs over the age of 30 may be due to the previously mentioned barriers, including the fact that potential participants are just not asked. Simon et al. (2004), in a study of clinical trial accrual at one NCI Cancer Comprehensive Center in Detroit, MI, reported that five women were not offered the option of clinical trials due to the physician's perception that the women would likely be noncompliant. Of note is that all five women were black. Others have reported that patients from minority populations are not invited to participate in clinical trials (Greenlea, Murray, Bolden, & Wingo, 2000; Lara et al., 2001; Wendler, et al., 2006).

Wendler et al. (2006), in a review of 20 published studies with consent rates reported, found there were little to no differences in the rate of consent by race or ethnicity. In some cases, minority populations had a higher consent rate than the majority population. The problem identified was that there was a major difference in the number of racial and ethnic minorities *who were actually invited* to participate. Townsley et al. (2005) found a similar outcome when investigating the role of age in being invited to participate in a clinical trial; the older the patient, the less likely the discussion about clinical trials will take place. Finn (2000) reports that an increasing reason for physicians not starting the discussion about clinical trials with cancer patients is the perception that this will require taking more time with one particular patient than if no discussion is started. In other words, they would have less time for another patient who is not eligible for a clinical trial.

The end result of these barriers is that the most referred adult patients for clinical trials are white men and women; minorities and the elderly are underreferred. This leads to two problematic outcomes: (1) patients who are eligible for clinical trials are not referred, are thus not invited to participate, and trials end up being unable to recruit the numbers necessary to answer questions at all phases of clinical trials; and (2) those who end up in a clinical trial are not representative of the true population of people who are or might be diagnosed with the disease under study.

From the perspective of social work this is a social justice issue; access to clinical trials is not equally available to all persons regardless of age, race, and socioeconomic status. This is a core value of social work (NASW, 2008). ENACCT offers community trainings that include a component of "social justice to increase community literacy about cancer clinical trials" (2008, p. 11). In an editorial written by Otis Brawley, MD (2004), the issue of social justice comes up again. He suggests that equal and widespread access is less a matter of science than it is of social justice. After an effort by the National Cancer Institute (NCI) to address racial proportionality in clinical trials in the 1990s, there was an increase of 20% in the number of patients enrolled in clinical trials. Unfortunately, the rise has been in middle-class whites and not in any of the racial or ethnic minorities.

Role of Social Work

In August 2001 *Health & Social Work* published a series of short articles regarding the role of social workers in clinical trials, presented as a point–counterpoint. Sadler (2004) wrote the initial viewpoint article focusing on the inaugural collaborative effort between the NCI Cancer Clinical Trial Education Program (CCTEP) and the Association of Oncology Social Work (AOSW). The goal of the collaboration was to increase the number of social workers who would be knowledgeable about cancer clinical trials and be able to work in their communities to raise awareness of clinical trials, and to utilize their unique skills to improve recruitment into trials.

Her final argument was that the inclusion of social workers in the clinical trials process would likely result in a greater diversity of patients recruited into trials. As a member of the initial cohort of AOSW members who participated in this training, I left with the belief that all cancer clinical trial groups should include social workers. We bring the skill set that can improve the process, including the ability to educate patients and family members of the risks, benefits, and the availability of trials; ensure clear communication between the participants, family members, and the health care team; and the ability to assess for and address concerns and fears of patients and family members.

The three counterpoint articles (Freedman, 2001; Kadushin, 2001; Rankin, 2001) address questions of potential ethical issues if social workers are involved in the process of recruitment and retention of participants. The common ethical themes were the potential dual relationship between social workers and participants, the role social workers would have on the team, and the expectation of other team members about the outcomes the social worker would produce. Freedman makes the argument that a social worker in the role of recruiting participants in clinical trials is a dual relationship and the social worker should be available for education but not the actual recruitment. Kadushin and Rankin make very good points about the need for the social workers involved in the clinical trial process to be adequately trained, that all members of the clinical trials team have a clear understanding of the role of each team member, and that not all potential patients approached, whether by a social worker, research nurse, or physician, will be appropriate for enrollment.

The arguments made by these three authors are issues that most social workers face in all the varied places we are employed. It is not just in a setting where social workers are involved in clinical trials. Our Code of Ethics (NASW, 2008) provide specific guidelines for every social worker in providing ethical practice. The IRB process has been set up to ensure that the development of a trial is safe for the participants, and the regulations put forth by the OHRP provide further protection of participants. As long as social workers are aware of the potential ethical issues, know how to work through ethical dilemmas, and are adequately trained about clinical trials, their involvement will only improve the experience for patients and family members (Sadler, 2003).

Conclusion

This writer challenges social workers to continue to expand their knowledge about clinical trials, to develop collaborative relationships with the health care teams that offer clinical trials either in your institution or your community, and to include in your discussions with patients and families the potential of participating in clinical trials. This includes helping patients make fully informed decisions by engaging in an assessment of the benefits of the trial to the patient, the burdens, the role of the family, and how the patient might manage family differences of opinion and conflict. I believe this role can be undertaken by social workers who are focused primarily in either research or in clinical practice, as well as those who cross over into both arenas of health care. If you see yourself as an advocate for patients' access to treatments for whatever medical condition they may have, and if you advocate for patients to be able to make fully informed decisions about the care they receive, you must be able to engage in the clinical trials conversation with patients

LEARNING EXERCISES

1. Take the online tutorial offered by the NIH Office of Extramural Research entitled *Protecting Human Research Participants*, which is available at: http://phrp. nihtraining.com/index.php

2. *The SoCRA Source*, the journal of The Society of Clinical Research Associates, offers self-study articles with a quiz at the end of each. These self-study articles in the six issues from February 2003 through May 2004 are available at: http://www.socra.org/html/newslett. htm. Read each issue and take the quiz to improve your knowledge and understanding of how the Common Rule influences and guides clinical trials.

3. The NIH offers an online repository, ClinicalTrials.gov, of federally and privately sponsored clinical trials, both in the United States and internationally.

   a. Select a condition, disease, or disorder that you are interested in and locate a clinical trial using ClinicalTrials.gov, available at: http://www. clinicaltrials.gov/. After finding a trial, determine who would be eligible, the type of trial it is, what is required by the participants, what is the phase of the study, and where it is offered. Develop a script of how you would introduce this trial to a potential participant.

   b. Using the same online repository, put in the term *palliative care*. Determine whether there are any clinical trials currently being offered for patients, family members, or caregivers. After finding one, establish who is eligible, the type of trial, and what is required by the participants. Develop a script of how you would introduce this trial to a potential participant.

   c. For both of the above trials, identify ways in which you, as a social worker, could participate in the clinical trial. Develop a plan for how you would approach the principal investigator to offer your services to improve at least one of the following areas: recruitment, retention, or addressing barriers to enrollment.

ADDITIONAL SUGGESTED READINGS

EDICT (2008). *The EDICT Project: Policy recommendations to eliminate disparities in clinical trials.* Houston, TX: Baylor College of Medicine. Retrieved from http://www.bcm.edu/edict/PDF/EDICT_Project_Booklet.pdf

Education Network to Advance Cancer Clinical Trials (ENACCT) and Community-Campus

Partnerships for Health (CCPH). (2008). *Communities as partners in cancer clinical trials: Changing research, practice and policy.* Authors: Silver Spring, MD: Retrieved from http://www.communitiesaspartners.org

Wells, A. A., & Zebrack, B. (2009). Psychosocial barriers contributing to the under-representation of racial/ethnic minorities in cancer clinical trials. *Social Work in Health Care, 46*, 1–14.

WEB SITES

Education Network to Advance Cancer Clinical Trials; http://www.enacct.org
Includes CEU opportunities as well as the current state of community involvement in clinical trials.
Office for Human Research Protections (OHRP): http://www.hhs.gov/ohrp/
Includes access to regulations, information on special populations such as children, prisoners, and women, as well as educational information for health care teams, patients, and families.

REFERENCES

Akechi, T., Okuyama, T., Sugawara, Y., Nakano, T., Shima, Y., & Uchitomi, Y. (2004). Major depression, adjustment disorders, and post-traumatic stress disorder in terminally ill cancer patients: Associated and predictive factors. *Journal of Clinical Oncology, 22*, 1957–1965.

American Evaluation Association. (2005). The complexity of the IRB process: Some of the things you wanted to know about IRBs but were afraid to ask. *American Journal of Evaluation, 26*, 353–361.

Brawley, O. W. (2004). The study of accrual to clinical trials: Can we learn from studying who enters our studies? *Journal of Clinical Oncology, 22*, 2039–2040.

CenterWatch. (2010). Overview of clinical trials. Retrieved from http://www.centerwatch.com/clinical-trials/overview.aspx

Ciechanowski, P. S., Katon, W. J., & Russo, J. E. (2000). Depression and diabetes: Impact of depressive symptoms on adherence, function, and costs. *Archives Internal Medicine, 160*, 3278–3285.

Crunkilton, D. D., & Rubins, V. D. (2009). Psychological distress in end-of-life care: A review of issues in assessment and treatment. *Journal of Social Work in End-of-Life and Palliative Care, 5*, 75–93.

D'Antonio, M. (2004). *The state boys rebellion.* New York, NY: Simon & Schuster.

Education Network to Advance Cancer Clinical Trials. (2008). *2007-2008 annual report.* Silver Spring, MD: Author.

Education Network to Advance Cancer Clinical Trials (ENACCT) and Community-Campus Partnerships for Health (CCPH). (2008). *Communities as Partners in Cancer Clinical Trials: Changing Research, Practice and Policy.* Silver Spring, MD. Retrieved from http://www.enacct.org/sites/default/files/Communities%20Full%20Report_0.pdf

Finn, R. (2000). Oncologist's role critical to clinical trial enrollment. *Journal of the National Cancer Institute, 92*, 1632–1634.

Fleischman, A. R. (2005). Regulating research with human subjects—is the system broken? *Transactions of the American Clinical and Climatological Association, 116*, 91–102.

Fortin, M., Bravo, G., Hudon, C., Lapointe, L, Dubois, M., & José Almirall (2006). Psychological distress and multimorbidity in primary care. *Annals of Family Medicine, 4*, 417–422.

Frank, G. (2004, February). Current challenges in clinical trials patient recruitment and enrollment. *SoCRA SOURCE*, 30–38. Retrieved from http://www.socra.org/pdf/200402_Current_Challenges_Recruitment_Enrollment.pdf

Freedman, T. G. (2001). Clinical trials: A wider lens. *Health & Social Work, 26*, 201–203.

Greenlee, R. T., Murray, T., Bolden, S., & Wingo, P. A. (2000). Cancer statistics, 2000. *Cancer Journal for Clinical, 50*, 7–33.

Harnessing science: Advancing care by accelerating the rate of cancer clinical trial participation. Hearing before the Committee on Government Reform: U.S. House of Representatives. 108th Congress, Second Session (May 13, 2004). Serial No. 108-189. Retrieved from GPO Access Web site: http://www.gpoaccess.gov/congress/index.html; http://oversight.house.gov

HarrisInteractive. (2001, January 22). Misconceptions and lack of awareness greatly reduce recruitment for cancer clinical trials. *Health Care News, 1*(3). Retrieved from http://www.harrisinteractive.com/news/newsletters/healthnews/HI_HealthCareNews2001Vol1_iss3.pdf

HarrisInteractive. (2003, June 16). The many reasons why people do (and would) participate in clinical trials. *Health Care News, 3*(10). Retrieved from http://www.harrisinteractive.com/news/newsletters/healthnews/HI_HealthCareNews2003Vol3_Iss10.pdf

HarrisInteractive. (2004, June 11). Public awareness of clinical trials increases: New survey suggest those conducting trials are doing a better job of informing potential participants of opportunities. *Health Care News, 4*(10). Retrieved from http://www.harrisinteractive.com/news/newsletters/healthnews/HI_HealthCareNews2004Vol4_Iss10.pdf

HarrisInteractive (2005, June 27). New survey shows public perception of opportunities for participation in clinical trials has decreased slightly from last year. *Health Care News, 5*(6). Retrieved from http://www.harrisinteractive.com/news/newsletters/healthnews/HI_HealthCareNews2005Vol5_Iss06.pdf

Holmes, A. M., & Deb, P. (2003). The effect of chronic illness on the psychological health of family member. *The Journal of Mental Health Policy and Economics, 6*, 13–22.

Johnson, E. H. (1989). Psychiatric morbidity and health problems among black Americans: A national survey. *Journal of the National Medical Association, 81*, 1217–1223.

Joshi, K., Kumar, R., & Avasthi, A. (2003). Morbidity profile and its relationship with disability and psychological distress among elderly people in Northern India. *International Journal of Epidemiology, 32*, 978–987.

Kadushin, G. (2001). Clinical trials: A wider lens 2. *Health & Social Work, 26*, 203–206.

Knowlton, L. (2003, August). Self study: Title 45 Code of Federal Regulations Part 46 Protection of Human Subjects. *SoCRA SOURCE*, 8–15. Retrieved from http://www.socra.org/pdf/SelfStudy2003August.pdf

Krugman, S. (1986). The Willowbrook hepatitis studies revisited: Ethical aspects. *Reviews of Infectious Diseases, 8*, 157–162.

Lara, P. N., Higdon, R., Lim, N., Kwan, K., Tanaka, M., Lau, D. H. M., Wun, T.,… Lam, K. S. (2001). Prospective evaluation of cancer clinical trial accrual patterns: Identifying potential barriers to enrollment. *Journal of Clinical Oncology, 19*, 1728–1833.

Lerner, B. H. (2004). Sins of omission. *New England Journal of Medicine, 351*(7), 628–630.

Markman, M., & Grimm, M. (2009, October). Barriers to physician participation in cancer clinical trials: Results of a web-based survey of providers. *Medscape Hematology-Oncology*.

National Association of Social Workers (NASW). (2008). *Code of ethics*. Washington, DC: Author.

National Cancer Institute (NCI). (2007). *Taking part in cancer treatment research studies*. Retrieved from http://www.cancer.gov/clinicaltrials/Taking-Part-in-Cancer-Treatment-Research-Studies

National Institute of Health Office of the Director (NIH OD) and Office of Rare Diseases Research (ORDR). (2009, October 5). NIH announces expansion of rare diseases clinical research network. *NIH News Press Release*. Retrieved from http://www.nih.gov/news/health/oct2009/od-05.htm

Office for Human Research Protections (OHRP). (2009). *Code of Federal Regulations: Title 45 Public Welfare Department of Health and Human Services Part 46 Protection of Human Subjects*. Retrieved from http://www.hhs.gov/ohrp/humansubjects/guidance/45cfr46.htm#46.111

Office of Research Integrity – Human Subjects Research, University of Nevada, Las Vegas. (n.d.). *History of research ethics*. Retrieved from http://research.unlv.edu/ORI-HSR/history-ethics.htm

Parker, L. S., & Alvarez, H. K., (2003). The legacy of the Tuskegee Syphilis Study. In B. Jennings, J. Kahn, A. Mastroianni, & L, Parker (Eds), *Ethics and public health: Model curriculum* (pp. 35–74). Washington, DC: Association of Schools of Public Health.

Penslar, R. L. & Porter, J. P. (1993). *Institutional review board guidebook*. Retrieved from the Health and Human Services Office for Human Research Protections website: http://www.hhs.gov/ohrp/irb/irb_guidebook.htm

Perlman, D. (2004, May). Ethics in clinical research: A history of human subject protections and practical implementation of ethical standards. *SoCRA SOURCE*, 37–40. Retrieved from http://www.socra.org/pdf/200405_Ethics_Clinical_Research_History.pdf

Pharmaceutical Research and Manufacturers of America (PhRMA). (2009). *2009 report medicines in development for cancer*. Retrieved from http://www.phrma.org/files/attachments/meds_in_dev/09-046PhRMACancer09_0331.pdf

Rajkumar, S. V. (2004). Thalidomide: Tragic past and promising future. *Mayo Clinic Proceedings, 79*(7), 899–903.

Rankin, E. D. (2001). Clinical trials: Opportunities and responsibilities. *Health & Social Work, 26*, 206–208.

Sadler, G. R. (2001). A call to action: Patients' access to clinical trials. *Health & Social Work, 26*, 196–200.

Sadler, G. R. (2003). A call to action: Patients' access to clinical trials. *Health & Social Work, 28*, 79–80.

Sateren, W. B., Trimble, E. L., Abrams, J., Brawley, O., Breen, N., Ford, L.,… Christian, M. C. (2002). How sociodemographics, presence of oncology specialists, and hospital cancer programs affect accrual to cancer treatment trials. *Journal of Clinical Oncology, 20*, 2109–2117.

Simon, M. S., Du, W., Flaherty, L., Philip, P. A., Lorusso, P., Miree, C.,… Brown, D. R. (2004). Factors associated with breast cancer clinical trials participation and enrollment at a large academic medical center. *Journal of Clinical Oncology, 22*, 2041–2052.

Somkin, C. P., Altschuler, A., Ackerson, L., Geiger, A. M., Greene, S. M., Mouchawar, J.,… Wagner, E. (2005). Organizational barriers to physician participation in cancer clinical trials. *American Journal of Managed Care, 11*, 413–421.

Townsley, C., Pond, G. R., Peloza, B., Kok, J., Naidoo, K., Dale, D.,…Siu, L. L. (2005). Analysis of treatement practices for elderly cancer patients in Ontario, Canada. *Journal of Clinical Oncology, 16*, 3802–3810.

TrialsCentral.org (n.d.). *Phases of clinical trials*. Retrieved from http://www.trialscentral.org/clinical-trial-phases.html

Wendler, D., Kington, R., Madans, J., Van Wye, G., Christ-Schmidt, H., Pratt, L. A., Emanuel, E. (2006). Are racial and ethnic minorities less willing to participate in health research? *PLoS Medicine, 3*, e19.

Zabora, J. R., BrintzenhofeSzoc, K. M., Curbow, B., Hooker, C. & Piantadosi, S. (2001). The prevalence of psychological distress by cancer site. *Psycho-Oncology, 10*, 19–28.

15 John F. Linder and Sheila R. Enders

Key Roles for Palliative Social Work in Correctional Settings

More punishment is not going to make what the doctor says more clear, it's just more punishment. This is my body. I got only one. I put myself here and I'm gonna be here, but I don't feel my body parts should have to do time.

—Inmate, Central California Women's Facility

Key Concepts

♦ *Prison populations worldwide are growing in number, advancing in age, and composed primarily of the underprivileged in their respective societies.*

♦ *The incarcerated enter prison in poorer health, having received inferior health care compared to age-matched peers.*

♦ *Poor quality health care should not be part of the punishment imposed by society.*

♦ *Palliative care and hospice offer solutions to address the needs of aging and dying inmates.*

♦ *Interdisciplinary team care is the preferred model for end-of-life care, and social workers are integral to the success of that model, in prison and in the community.*

Introduction

The number of people held in prisons around the world has grown exponentially in the last 30 years, as have the rates of incarceration. Table 15.1 shows incarceration rates and prisoner totals for a variety of nations worldwide.

In the United States, the prison population has grown five-fold between 1980 and June 30, 2008, rising from 315,974 to 1,540,805 (Beck & Gilliard, 1995; Beck & Harrison, 2001; West & Sabol, 2008, 2009). According to 2008 year-end figures, the United States has the greatest number of prisoners and the highest incarceration rate in the world, 2.29 million and 756 per 100,000, respectively (Walmsley, 2009).

The disparity in these two figures for total number of prisoners in 2008 exposes one of the methodological issues to consider when discussing incarcerated populations. For clarity, reported figures should address whether *(a)* they include local as well as regional and national facilities (jails vs. prisons); *(b)* sentenced prisoners and pretrial detainees are combined or reported separately; and *(c)* special populations are included, for example, juveniles, detainees awaiting deportation, military prisoners, the criminally insane, political detainees and those on probation or parole, in work furlough, or in home detention. In the figures above, the 1.5 million figure is from the U.S. Department of Justice, Bureau of Justice Statistics (USDOJ-BJS) and includes only sentenced prisoners in state and federal prisons (West & Sabol, 2009). The 2.29 million figure is from the Kings College London International Centre for Prison Studies (Walmsley, 2009).

Another important methodological consideration arises specifically with respect to the aging of prison populations. The age categories have changed and the level of detail available has increased as older inmates have come to comprise a growing percentage of the prison population. A more extensive discussion of these methodological considerations can be found elsewhere (Linder & Meyers, 2009).

Table 15.1.
Incarcerated Populations by Rate, Total Number Incarcerated, and Percentage of Total Prison Population Who Are Women

Nation	Rate per 100,000 pop.	Total Incarcerated	% of Women Prisoners
United States	760	2,310,984	9.0
Russian Federation	622	880,671	7.9
Rwanda	593	59,311	2.6
Cuba	~531	~60,000	Not found
South Africa	330	163,479	2.2
Israel	325	22,734	2.3
Chile	320	54,365	8.2
Ukraine	314	144,380	6.1
Thailand	303	199,607	14.1
El Salvador	273	19,814	5.5
Brazil	242	469,546	6.5
Poland	225	85,598	3.1
Iran	222	158,351	3.7
Mexico	208	227,735	5.1
Libya	199	12,751	3.0
New Zealand	197	8509	5.8
Saudi Arabia	178	44,600	5.7
Spain	164	76,455	7.9
Columbia	163	74,718	6.3
Lebanon	159	5870	3.8
Turkey	157	113,493	3.6
United Kingdom	154	84,409	5.0
Argentina	132	52,475	5.5
Kuwait	130	~3500	14.9
Australia	129	27,615	7.1
Myanmar (Burma)	126	65,063	15
China	119	1,565,771	4.9
Canada	116	38,348	5.0
Zimbabwe	114	12,971	4.2
Greece	109	12,300	5.4
Philippines	108	91,530	7.9
Vietnam	107	92,153	11.2
Netherlands	100	16,416	8.7
Tanzania	100	41,613	3.3
Ethiopia	~98	~80,000	Not found
Italy	97	58,597	4.4
Korea (South)	97	47,097	5.3
France	96	59,665	3.7
Iraq	93	27,366	2.5
Uganda	91	29,000	3.1
Germany	90	73,592	5.3
Egypt	85	64,378	3.7

Nation	Rate per 100,000 pop.	Total Incarcerated	% of Women Prisoners
Table 15.1. *(Contd.)*			
Ireland (Republic)	85	3895	3.5
Switzerland	76	5780	5.8
Sweden	74	6853	5.5
Japan	63	80,523	7.0
Indonesia	58	136,017	4.7
Congo, Dem. Rep.	57	~30,000	3.2
Pakistan	55	90,000	1.5
Bangladesh	51	83,000	3.7
India	33	373,271	3.9

Note: The list includes the top 25 nations by total population, the top 25 nations by total prison population, all member nations of the G-20, and selected other nations.

Many factors have contributed to the increases in prison populations. One can argue about the extent to which the war on drugs (Sorensen & Stemen 2002; Thigpen & Hunter 1998), stricter sentencing and three-strikes legislation (Sorensen & Stemen, 2002; Thigpen & Hunter, 1998), and the deinstitutionalization of many of the mentally ill (Harcourt, 2006) have played a part in this escalation in the United States. Scraton and McCulloch argue that a succession of U.S. administrations consciously engaged in an orchestrated effort that "neglect(s) social disadvantage, the material reality of poverty and marginalization, and hit(s) offenders hard with harsher laws, zero-tolerance policing, and uncompromising prison regimens leading to bursting prisons, devastated cities and a violent crime rate still unmatched in the developed world" (Scraton & McCulloch, 2006, p.3). While the causes are numerous and interwoven, the result is the same: a mushrooming prison population.

Inmate Demographics and Health Status

Prison populations are aging (Harcourt 2006; Scraton & McCulloch 2006; Sorensen & Stemen 2002; Thigpen & Hunter 1998). As they age, the percentages of state and federal inmates who report a significant medical problem increase (Maruschak & Beck, 2001). It is anticipated that by the year 2030, more than one-third of U.S. prisoners will be over the age of 55 (Maruschak & Beck, 2001). Moreover, inmates have greater morbidity than do age-matched peers in the general population, as documented in official reports (Anno, 2004; Anno, Graham, Lawrence, & Shansky, 2004; Maruschak & Beck, 2001; Thigpen & Hunter, 1998) and the professional literature (Clear, Rose, & Ryder, 2001; Linder & Meyers, 2009; Sheu et al., 2002; Stephenson, Wohl, Kaplan,

Golin, Hsiao-Chuan, & Stewart, 2005). Inmates experience diseases commonly found in individuals 10 years their senior in free society (Aday, 1994; Linder & Meyers, 2007; National Hospice and Palliative Care Organization [NHPCO], 2008/2009). The risks to long-term health caused by incarceration, discontinuity of care, sexual violence, and discrimination are amplified for women (Clear et al., 2001; Sheu et al., 2002; Stephenson et al., 2005; van den Bergh, Gatherer, & Møller, 2009; Visher & Travis, 2003).

Inmates are threatened by aging and serious illness. Unlike the "free" community, prisons do not offer a choice of medical coverage or providers. As inmates age and health concerns increase, prison procedures and physical plants need to accommodate disabilities, including impaired mobility, sight, or hearing. Without accommodation, special needs inmates may fall victim to intimidation or violence and be unable to physically defend themselves.

The Socioeconomics of Incarcerated Populations

Across the globe, the incarcerated are drawn primarily from the socioeconomically disadvantaged as defined by the dominant population. Traditionally, this population has had decreased access to health care, has received less routine health care, and has experienced little if any continuity of care. Affordable medications are scarce. Both male and female inmates are equally likely to report having at least 1 of 6 developmental impairments that include learning, speech, hearing, vision, mobility, or mental health issues (Maruschak & Beck, 2001).

The lack of universal health care in developing nations and the United States means the uninsured and underinsured often have to forego medications to treat chronic conditions like diabetes or high blood pressure.

People of lower socioeconomic status (SES) often have less access to healthy, fresh food and many live in neighborhoods with increased risk of violence. The lack of sufficient food leads to starvation or chronic malnutrition, while an unhealthy diet can contribute to obesity and its many comorbidities, including diabetes, kidney failure, hypertension, and heart disease. Inadequate or nonexistent sanitation and/or an unsafe water supply increase the risk of typhoid, dysentery, and many other diseases. Many low-income individuals work more than one job, performing labor that takes a greater toll on physical well-being or may contain an elevated risk of on-the-job injury. Most are without employer-provided health care and lack the resources and time to make prevention, screening, and health promotion a routine part of their lives. Through advocacy and direct practice, social workers in many settings have opportunities to address these systemic problems, which will in turn have a positive effect on prison population and lessen the demand for prison palliative care.

Many of the crimes leading to incarceration also have an adverse impact on health. An estimated 60% of U.S. inmates have substance abuse histories (Prisons: Prisons for women—Problems and unmet needs in the contemporary women's prison, 2009). All forms of substance abuse have multiple adverse health consequences. Prostitution and bartering sex for drugs, shelter, or food likewise increase the risk of HIV, hepatitis C, and sexually transmitted diseases while increasing the risk of violence-related injury. Methamphetamines and crack cocaine have multiple adverse health consequences (National Institute of Health – National Institute on Drug Abuse [NIH-NIDA], 2008). Many male and female sex industry workers enter the correctional setting with HIV, human papilloma virus (HPV), or other sexually transmitted diseases. All of these illnesses result in higher levels of health care need once in the correctional system.

Violent crime itself sometimes results in permanent disability. In conflict zones, sexual and physical violence may be commonplace; in the worst cases these are instruments of control and punishment in prison settings.

Special Health Considerations of Female Inmates

The number of incarcerated women in the United States has grown at a faster rate than incarcerated men. Typical characteristics for female inmates include (a) a member of a racial or ethnic minority; (b) median age of mid-30s; (c) a history of drug abuse; (d) having experienced physical or sexual abuse with or without posttraumatic stress syndrome; (e) more than likely unmarried with at least one minor child; and (f) often homeless. Criminal acts by women are often the result of poverty or drug use and the need for financing their addiction (Baldwin & Jones, 2000). Social work interventions that strengthen the family, reduce substance abuse and lessen physical and sexual abuse can reduce women's exposure to the criminal justice system.

Although women historically represent a relatively small percentage of the overall prison population, their unique health care needs are not often met (Baldwin & Jones, 2000). Female inmates are ranked near the top of population subgroups for the seriousness of their health problems (Anderson, 2003; Maruschak & Beck, 2001). Lack of attention to the unique health care needs of incarcerated women will lead to future economic and social costs to society (Anderson, 2003).

Females are more than 1.5 times more likely to report two or more current medical problems than male inmates (Anderson, 2003). Nearly 95% of female prisoners are within the childbearing years, though this percentage will decline as the female prison population ages (Maruschak & Beck, 2001).

Box 15.1
Patient/Family Narrative: Marcy

For women, being able to access adequate health care in prison is a challenge. The availability and quality of health care from institution to institution varies widely. From first report of symptoms to diagnosis to treatment can take an inordinate amount of time—time that proves detrimental to the health of the inmate.

Marcy (a composite of several patients) is a multiracial 38-year-old single mother of two small children; Eva, age 6, and Kevin, age 4. They are living with their maternal grandmother and Marcy sees them infrequently. She is serving a sentence for selling drugs and prostitution. She has a history of injection drug use. Currently she is drug free and has been for a period of 18 months. Past medical history includes positive for Hepatitis B and C with no symptoms, and she has had multiple sexually transmitted diseases. Family medical history includes breast cancer in her mother, two maternal aunts, and a sister.

Years prior to incarceration, Marcy had been told that she had fibrocystic breast disease and that she was at high risk for breast cancer given her family history. Marcy did not have insurance coverage and did not follow up on her yearly exams and seldom did breast self-exams. Because of her younger sister being diagnosed with breast cancer, Marcy went to a clinic where she was able to obtain a mammogram at no charge. She did not go back to obtain her results, nor did she respond to the doctor's office calls. No follow-up care was done. She was arrested soon after that on drug charges and since this was a repeat offense, sentenced to prison.

She now has come to the prison physician because of a more pronounced lump in her left breast. The initial mammogram was done more than 2 years ago. On the current exam, the physician noted the lump, suggested they get the results of her previous mammogram for comparison, and ordered a new mammogram. She was to return to see the prison physician in 2 months for the results of her current study and a review of her past mammogram.

Marcy did not go back to see the doctor and her information and findings "slipped through the cracks." There was no follow-up by the physician or clinic staff. Only after she started experiencing pain under her arm did she make another appointment. More than a year had gone by. When the doctor repeated his examination and looked at the records and mammograms, he was stunned. The initial mammogram revealed a lump "suspicious" for "adenocarcinoma." The recommendation at that time was for fine needle aspiration or breast ultrasound. Neither was performed and Marcy was not given any results at that time.

Box 15.1 *(Contd.)*

Now, nearly 4 years later, not only does she have breast cancer, but it has spread into her lymph nodes under her arm. After lengthy discussion, Marcy elected to have a mastectomy with removal of her lymph nodes. She also underwent chemotherapy and radiation.

Marcy has kept her medical appointments and repeat mammograms. She received some bad news at her recent clinic visit. Although her most recent mammogram is negative, an X-ray taken of her spine because of recent onset of pain reveals several metastatic lesions related to her breast cancer.

Somewhere between 4% and 9% of women enter prison while pregnant (Prisons: Prisons for women—Problems and unmet needs in the contemporary women's prison, 2009). Little time is allowed for the new mother and child to bond. Social workers assist with the process of finding relatives, friends, or foster care for the child. According to the United Nations Office on Drugs and Crime ([UNODC], 2009), not only do prisoners feel the loss and separation of leaving their young children behind, but children separated from their mothers experience emotional and developmental difficulties. Psychological challenges for women becoming mothers in prison are many and extremely provocative emotionally. Receiving help

from social workers is essential if the inmate is going to adjust to separation from their infant and equally integral to success when families are being reunified upon the inmate's release.

The U.S. Department of Justice, Bureau of Justice Statistics reports that female inmates (11%) in state prisons are more likely to report having mental health issues than male inmates (6%). These percentages are both self-reported; official estimates are much higher (Anderson, 2003; Sentencing Project, 2007). Mental health issues occur more often and are more serious than those of their male counterparts. Dual diagnosis of substance abuse and mental illness is more prevalent among women in prison than men (Anderson, 2003).

Social workers, as mental health providers, work with prisoners to help them access treatment programs to move away from old habits and toward a more successful future.

Race and Ethnicity as Elements of Prison Demographics and Health Status

Incarceration rates disproportionately favor the host country's racial and ethnic minorities as well as the economically disadvantaged. For example, blacks and Hispanics are overrepresented in the United States (Golembeski & Fullilove, 2005), as Table 15.2 illustrates.

Table 15.2
Comparison of Census 2000 and Incarcerated Populations

	U.S. Census	State and Federal Inmates			
	2000[4a]	1980[1,4b]	1990[3,4b]	2000[4b]	2007[4b]
White	75.1% (211,460,626)	52.3% (165,400)	35.6%	37.0% (471,000)	36.6% (521,900)
Black	12.3% (34,658,190)	46.5% (146,900)	44.5%	47.9% (610,300)	41.1% (586,200)
Hispanic	12.5% (35,305,818)	— —	17.4%	17.0% (216,900)	22.3% (318,800)
Asian[2]	3.6% (10,242,998)	— —	— —	— —	— —
Native/ Indigenous[2]	0.9% (2,475,956)	— —	— —	— —	— —
Total	100% 281,421,906	100% 315,974		100% 1,273,469	100% 1,427,300

[1] White and black categories include an unreported percentage of individuals of Hispanic ethnicity, though the recalibration in 1990 suggests that most Hispanics were included as white in the 1980 data.

[2] These categories are not reported separately in the USDOJ-BJS annual reports on prisoners.

[3] Only reported as percentages (in the *Prisoners in 2000* narrative), based on inmates with sentences of more than 1 year.

[4] These columns do not add up to 100%. When they sum to >100% (4a), individuals are reported in more than one category. When the percentages and raw numbers sum to <100% (4b), other categories are not reported here

Source: Reprinted with permission from Meyers, F. & Linder, J. F. (2009). *Journal of Social Work in End-of-Life & Palliative Care, 5,* 7–33. Copyright Taylor & Francis Group, LLC.

Sources for data: Anonymous, 2002; Beck & Gilliard, 1995; Beck & Harrison, 2001; West & Sabol, 2008.

Whether there are genetic racial or ethnic predispositions to certain health conditions is a matter of ongoing debate (Kaufman, 2008; Latimer et al., 2007; O'Donnell & Kannel, 1998). It is difficult to establish a causal connection while successfully controlling for many of the other factors: SES, access to prevention, screening and routine health care, diet, living conditions, and occupation-associated risks. What can be said is that for some mixture of reasons, including inherited predisposition and acquired risk, blacks and Hispanics in the United States are at greater risk of developing diabetes, heart disease, high blood pressure, and its sequelae (stroke, kidney failure, vascular disease), and blacks and Asians worldwide are at elevated risk of sickle cell disorders. The overrepresentation of African American and Latino men and women in the U.S. prison system, in combination with the lower educational attainment and SES of the inmate population overall and the harmful synergies between mental health, substance abuse, and chronic illness experienced by many inmates yields a population who are sicker than their age-matched free peers (Tanne, 2009; Wilper et al., 2009)

Thinking of the inmate population as monolithic or static is erroneous. Despite longer sentences, the U.S. prison system's rate of turnover each year demonstrates that the inmate population is not static. Based on data from the Bureau of Justice Statistics *Prisoners in 2007* report (West & Sabol, 2008), almost half of all sentenced inmates are released each year (e.g., 45.4% in 2007 [725,402 of 1,598,316]). In the years from 2000 to 2007, between 57.2% and 62.3% of those admitted to state and federal prisons were new court commitments. This reinforces the importance of interventions to lessen poverty, increase educational and occupational opportunity, and strengthen families among marginalized populations, all within the province of the social work profession.

Inmates' Right to Health Care

In most instances, the imprisoning entity is responsible for addressing the health care needs of its detainees. U.S. and international agencies have clearly stated that poor-quality health care should not be part of the punishment.

In the United States, several key legal decisions have framed the responsibilities of prison administrators, established the principle that inmates are entitled to adequate health care, and defined what constitutes adequate health care. Health care comparable to the free community is the standard set in the United States. In Estelle v. Gamble (1976), the Supreme Court held that "deliberate indifference to serious medical needs of prisoners constitutes the unnecessary and wanton infliction of pain, proscribed by the Eighth Amendment" (of the United States Constitution, which prohibits cruel and unusual punishment). The decision went on to state that "denial of medical care is surely not part of the punishment which civilized nations may impose for crime." The decision in Ramos v. Lamm (1980) held that either

"repeated examples of negligent acts which disclose a pattern of conduct by the prison medical staff" or "proving there are such systemic and gross deficiencies in staffing, facilities, equipment, or procedures that the inmate population is effectively denied access to adequate medical care" was sufficient to demonstrate "deliberate indifference."

In Wellman v. Faulkner (1983), the Federal 7th Circuit Court reinforced this precept, stating that

> When a state imposes imprisonment as a punishment for crime, it accepts the obligation to provide persons in its custody with a medical care system that meets minimal standards of adequacy. This obligation is enforceable in federal court, since inadequate medical care for prisoners violates the Eighth Amendment.

U.S. federal courts have also held that mental health falls under the rubric of overall health care. In Gates v. Cook (2004), the court sided with death row inmates in determining that providing insufficient mental health care is also a violation of the Eighth Amendment.

Hospice and Palliative Care for Incarcerated Individuals

I have a terminal illness. I just wish you could step into my head for a minute and see what I'm feeling. Then you could understand the helplessness I feel.
—*Inmate, Central California Women's Facility*

Hospice is the accepted community standard for end-of-life care in the United States and in many nations worldwide. While hospice care is delivered in private homes, in designated hospice residences, and increasingly, in the United States, in a variety of other congregate living facilities, including convalescent or skilled nursing facilities, adapting prisons to deliver hospice care requires innovation and a shift in thinking.

The Quality Guidelines for Hospice and End-of-Life Care in Correctional Settings, published by NHPCO in 2008, provide the most up-to-date and complete guide available (NHPCO, 2008). Security is the primary task for prisons; maintaining security at times adversely impacts the housing and care of infirm inmates. Guards and other prison personnel often think inmates do not deserve the compassionate treatment integral to hospice and palliative care. Most prison physical plants are not easily adaptable to the hospice model of care. Consequently, the integration of hospice and palliative care into prisons has proceeded slowly.

The exact number of prison hospices in the United States is not known; as of 2008 the National Hospice and Palliative Care Organization (NHPCO) put the number at about 75 (NHPCO, 2008/2009). A US-Canadian survey conducted in 2001 found that 25 of the 49 jurisdictions that responded from the United States, Canada, and U.S. territories had hospices (Anno et al., 2004). Many prison hospices (22/25) are operated as part of prison infirmaries. Free-standing hospice units are the exception (5/25) (Anno et al., 2004; Linder, Knauf, Enders, & Meyers, 2002; Lum, 2005). Descriptions of some prison hospice programs are available elsewhere (Anno et al., 2004; Bauersmith & Gent, 2002; Boyle, 2002; Dawes, 2002; Evans, Herzog, & Tillman, 2002; Ratcliff, 2000).

Inmates are free to identify themselves (or not) as having a medical condition needing attention. Being treated for a serious condition often means being transferred, either within a facility or between facilities, which in turn may lead to separation from one's prison family. This can serve as a disincentive to step forward as needing medical attention until symptoms become unmanageable, and it can cause inmates to underreport pain or declining functional status.

Hospice Inmate Volunteers

Many prison hospice programs use inmate volunteers who provide companionship, may help inmates with basic activities of daily living, and sit vigil with the dying. Dying behind bars is widely viewed as the ultimate failure (Bolger, 2005), and the fear of dying alone in prison is nearly universal. Terminally ill inmates take solace knowing someone will sit with them around the clock, and they often state that inmate-volunteers understand them and can connect in ways no free staff or volunteers can.

Prison staff employ stringent guidelines when screening inmates to be hospice volunteers. Prospective volunteers need to have records free of disciplinary action for 1 or more years, committal offenses unrelated to substance abuse, and lower security classifications. Initially, many of the volunteers had conditions such as HIV/AIDS, likely to lead to their demise; among the motivations for volunteering was the hope that when their turn to be the dying patient came, someone else would care for them.

Traits like vulnerability and compassion are not conducive to survival in prison. Add to this the troubled backgrounds of most inmates, and the need for training volunteers is obvious. Hospice inmate volunteers receive training in communication skills, problem solving, tolerance for alternative values and ideologies, and coping strategies for identifying and dealing constructively with strong emotions.

One unintended outcome of hospice inmate volunteer programs is the redemptive aspect to this work (Barnard, 1999; Head, 2005; Lampman, 2000). In the words of one Angola (Louisiana) prison hospice volunteer: "I did a lot of wrong and hurt a lot of people out there. When I heard about hospice, it was in my heart to join because this would be my way of giving back to society" (Barens, 1998).

As part of the hospice team, social workers may assist in the selection and training of inmate volunteers, provide ongoing direction and support, including bereavement support, and help volunteers be effective advocates for the patients they serve. Sometimes the social worker can bring a concern from a volunteer to the treatment team more effectively and credibly than can the volunteer. As new programs are contemplated, planned, and implemented, social workers can advocate for inmate participation, not only as volunteers but in the creation of the program itself. This will help programs address the needs as perceived by the consumers, ill inmates, while decreasing suspicion and increasing a sense of ownership of the program among inmates.

Many terminally ill prisoners and their inmate volunteers become family to one another. Addressing the bereavement needs of inmate family, including volunteers, is also a key element of comprehensive care, and social workers are well-suited to this task.

Volunteer Training: A Sample Exercise

For this and all training exercises with inmate volunteers, ground rules for the group are essential, as is a basic level of trust between participants. A professional (ideally a social worker) should be leading the exercises and monitoring closely for any adverse reactions.

Using simple outline pictures of common objects (e.g., a car, a house, a flower, a coffee cup, a chair, a table) have inmate volunteers sit in pairs, back to back. One inmate is given the drawing, the other a blank pad and a writing instrument. The participant with the drawing must describe the object without using any words that would give away the object (e.g., a window, a door, wheels, petals, legs) but rather only descriptive guidance ("Draw a 3-inch square in the middle of the page. Next draw four lines, each one 3 inches long, one at each corner of the square, all pointing to the bottom of the page" as a description of the top and legs of a table). Participants quickly learn how many assumptions are made when communicating, how people rely on nonverbal information, how easily miscommunication can occur, and how to manage frustration. After several minutes, the one doing the drawing shows the product to their partner. Usually both get a good laugh while learning many valuable lessons they can apply when communicating with the patients to whom they will be assigned.

Family Relationships

Many inmates have two families: a biological family and their inmate family. Inmates often hide or deny symptoms or illness out of fear of being transferred away from their biological or prison families. This is a fear particularly for incarcerated women. There are fewer women's institutions. Facilities that can handle long-term or life-limiting illness can be hundreds of miles from family, whether biological or prison family.

Being seriously ill, alone, and in unfamiliar surroundings increases feelings of abandonment and the intensity of fear. Palliative care programs within the institutions with social workers experienced in end-of-life care and bereavement play an important role in mitigating these circumstances.

Relations with biological families are often strained and sometimes irreparably damaged, but most inmates maintain some contact with family outside the walls. Confinement results in missed opportunities to participate in important family events, including the deaths and funerals of relatives. Many inmates are unprepared for receiving bad news; notification of the death of a family member or loved one is often delivered impersonally, posing additional bereavement risks for inmates. Prison social workers can facilitate communication between inmates and family members. Details of the loved one's death and funeral arrangements can be communicated to the inmate. If the inmate is dying, the social workers engage in the process of exchanging information with the inmate's family. Providing detailed answers to the family's questions helps them in the process of grieving.

Community social workers in hospitals, long-term care settings, or hospice programs may work with patients whose loved ones are in prison. Both parties can suffer greatly—the dying patient aching to see the incarcerated family member before he or she dies, and the inmate feeling frustration and shame at being unable to see the dying loved one. Community social workers can draw on their creativity and resourcefulness to provide a greater sense of connection and participation in the dying process. The patient and caregivers outside could journal or write letters chronicling the dying process. Sometimes an intermediary can facilitate more direct communication; prison chaplains and social workers might be able to arrange for special phone calls or viewing a DVD or video made by the patient and caregivers outside. The community social worker might facilitate a conversation between the patient's physician or other care team members and the inmate or a prison physician who could then explain the patient's condition to the inmate.

Imprisonment adversely affects postrelease employment, educational attainment, marital stability, school performance for inmates' children, and mental and physical health for inmates and their families (Arditti, Lambert-Shute, & Joest, 2003; Clear, 2005; King, 1993; La Vigne, Naser, Brooks, & Castro, 2005; London & Myers, 2006; Massoglia, 2008). As a result, social workers inside and outside of the institution will have opportunities to intervene. When an inmate is dying inside the walls, helping families arrange for transportation and housing to visit the inmate during his or her final days and hours draws upon social work's trademark ingenuity and resourcefulness. When an inmate is to be released to die in the community, social workers can help with placement, continuity of care, expedited access to resources, and overcoming resistance from facilities and communities (Wood, 2007). Social workers can also lead efforts at familial reconciliation and healing.

Resuscitation Status, Do Not Resuscitate Orders, and Advance Directives

Many of the legal decisions regarding inmate health care in the United States arose out of a pattern of "deliberate indifference." Inmates' experience of the health care system prior to incarceration and incidents like the Tuskegee experiment (Freimuth et al., 2001; Jones, 1993; Roy, 1995) serve to further lower expectations and raise suspicion of the medical community's ethics. The health care experience of people of lower SES, which includes many communities of color, has done little to disabuse anyone of these suspicions. The literature on pain control likewise demonstrates that communities of color, women, and the elderly routinely experience undertreatment of pain (Anderson et al., 2000; Bonham, 2001; Cleeland et al., 1994; McNeill, Sherwood, & Starck 2004; McNeill, Sherwood, Starck, & Nieto, 2001; Todd, Samaroo, & Hoffman, 1993). Doubts about health providers' beneficence are widespread among the incarcerated.

The issue of resuscitation status can be particularly problematic. Patient-inmates have a fundamental right to make their own health care and treatment decisions, including whether to take medications, consent to surgical procedures, and request or refuse life-support interventions. Clinical staff are responsible for initiating appropriate discussions about end-of-life decision making and the goals of care. Most prison hospice programs do not require inmates to have a do not resuscitate (DNR) order, though both advance directives (71%) and DNR orders (86%) (Anno et al., 2004) are available. For most of the terminally ill, arriving at a decision to implement a DNR order is a process of acknowledging approaching death; for inmates the decision may symbolize the loss of opportunity for forgiveness and repair of relationships at the same time one is asked to face the fear of dying in prison.

Inmate-patients should be educated about their rights and be able to specify their end-of-life preferences. Inmate literacy is an important consideration. Limited health literacy and overall literacy can impede inmates' ability to understand and weigh alternatives and express preferences. Innovative approaches (Enders, 2004a; Enders, Paterniti, & Meyers 2005) can help overcome the barrier of limited literacy.

Learning Exercise: The Go Wish Game

GO WISH (CodaAlliance, 2009; Steinhauser et al., 2000; a product of CODA–http://www.codaalliance.org) gives individuals an easy way to think and talk about how they would want to be treated should they become seriously ill. The game can make it easier for prison staff to follow an inmate's wishes when the time comes.

The GO WISH cards describe things that people often say are important when they are very sick or dying. The cards use value statements like "To be free from pain" or "To have my family prepared for my death" to describe how people want to be treated, who they want near them, and what matters to them. The cards are simply worded so they present few literacy barriers. One card is a "wild" card. An individual can use this card to stand for something he or she wants that is not on any of the other cards. Using a deck of 36 cards, each participant sorts and prioritizes, finally arriving at the 10 value statements most important to them. This can then be shared with hospice staff, discussed with the doctor, or used to inform choices for an advance directive.

Social workers in prison settings could use these cards with patients to help them determine what is most important to them as they live with life-threatening illness and come to the end of life. They can also be used with hospice inmate volunteers to increase their understanding of the many aspects of living with illness as they explore the sick inmates' wishes and or their own desires if faced with terminal illness.

Symptom Control

Primary responsibility for pain management and symptom control rests with the doctors and nursing staff in prison hospices. Strategies and guidelines for addressing pain and other symptoms for these professionals are available elsewhere (Bick, 2002; Lin & Mathew, 2005) as are broader professional guidelines for inmate health care and palliative care (American Board of Hospice and Palliative Medicine [ABHPM], 2007; Byock, Twohig, Merriman, & Collins, 2006; Centers for Disease Control and Prevention [CDC], 2007; Ferrell & Grant 2009; National Commission on Correctional Health Care [NCCHC], 2003; Puisis, 2006) including the EPEC (Education in Palliative and End-of-life Care) project (http://www.epec.net/EPEC/Webpages/index.cfm).

Because many inmates have a history of substance abuse, several issues arise affecting the clinical and nonclinical management of pain. Substance abuse has many roots: simple addiction, undiagnosed or untreated chronic pain or mental illness, as a numbing agent for deadening or escaping the feelings associated with physical or sexual abuse or irremediable poverty, and many more.

Inmates' responses to pain are likewise varied. For some in recovery, accepting opioid pain medicine violates their commitment to be drug free; for others, a chance/risk to legitimately return to their addiction, blurring the line between symptom management and substance abuse. Religious or cultural beliefs can exert powerful influence over the interpretation of pain's meaning. Some will see the pain of their terminal condition as fitting retribution, divine or otherwise, for their misdeeds, or as a vehicle for atonement.

Pain management issues could come to the attention of a social worker in a number of ways. Medical staff are not immune to bias toward inmate pain; social workers who are knowledgeable about pain and addiction can advocate for

patients and can help others understand the patient's reactions. The mechanisms for distributing pain medications may break down or prevent adequate continuous pain relief; creative problem solving is integral to social work practice. Medical staff may seek help from social workers in discriminating between "real" pain and attempts to obtain analgesics for recreational use or as contraband to barter. Inmate volunteers may believe a patient's pain is being undertreated, yet be powerless themselves to act as advocates. Social workers, in consultation with medical and nursing staff, can insure that a comprehensive pain assessment focuses on the physical, emotional, cognitive, and spiritual aspects of the inmate's pain experience. They can also advocate on the patient's behalf and can help the inmate volunteer appreciate his or her role in bringing the patient's suffering to light in the first place and empathize with the feelings of powerlessness. Maggie Bolger eloquently states that "prisons are environments of enduring loss" (Bolger, 2005, p. 619). Social workers can ease some of that sense of loss by helping volunteers truly appreciate their contribution, by being a consistent voice for justice and compassion, thereby extending the healing work of the inmate volunteers.

Social workers also have a variety of integrative pain management techniques to offer sick prisoners and inmate volunteers: various forms of distraction or diversion, including reading, being read to, playing games, watching television or movies, as well as techniques like praying, controlled breathing, relaxation exercises, meditation, and the use of guided imagery.

When an inmate makes choices that run contrary to others' values or cause additional suffering for themselves or staff and volunteers, social workers can also assist volunteers and medical staff to manage their own anxiety. An example would be an inmate who chooses to forego pain relief for spiritual or philosophical reasons and who consequently is visibly suffering.

Interdisciplinary Palliative Care

Most prisons are hierarchic and rigid; the interdisciplinary hospice team model stands in sharp contrast yet must operate within the overall organization. Social workers fulfill critical functions on interdisciplinary teams: developing and maintaining team cohesion, identifying and countering efforts to split the team, working on behalf of inmates to facilitate family visits, and, when possible, facilitating a smooth transition to a community setting. Social workers must also be aware that we can feel any of the same prejudices as our professional counterparts, and we should seek counsel and supervision accordingly.

Medical Parole or Compassionate Release

Releasing terminally ill inmates into the community for their care at first seems an obvious choice. Freed inmates will not die behind the walls, and prisons are relieved of these very sick detainees who are a significant drain on medical personnel and resources. Aging inmate-patients with a chronic condition or serious illness become the costliest patients in the system. This higher intensity of care includes tests, procedures, treatments, and hospitalizations. Within the prison system, added costs include transportation to outside contract hospitals and 24-hour guarding. If medical parole is broadly implemented, institutions have less need for specialized services and facilities that are difficult to create and maintain in aging physical plants. Wardens do not have to face staff who cannot reconcile the compassion of palliative care with their population of miscreants.

Despite these favorable arguments, the first mission of any department of corrections or public safety is maintenance of that public safety and preservation of the separation between inmates and free society. Correctional facilities are most reluctant to take any action that risks failure in their prime directive: public safety. Prisons are highly risk averse, and medical parole procedures reflect this.

For example, although 43 of the 49 jurisdictions surveyed in 2001 (Anno et al., 2004) offered some procedure to release the terminally ill from their confinement, in many jurisdictions the process to secure an inmate's release cannot begin until the patient is bedbound and no longer represents any threat to society (Bolger, 2005). Those charged with making the final decision often respond to political pressures rather than compassionate impulses. Inmates and their families are not the most vocal or powerful of constituencies. The advocacy skills of the social work professional can be put to good use in these instances. Currently, most inmates die before the request makes it all the way through the process.

Additional impediments include the scarcity of placements for individuals being released under these circumstances and in some instances the funding mechanisms for medical care, shelter, and food. If families are unavailable or unwilling to provide care, residential placement is often the only other option, and community resistance can be powerful (Wood, 2007).

Social Work and End-of-Life Care with Inmates

There is an ethical imperative as well as the legal mandate to provide quality health care to inmates in correctional settings (Cohn, 1999; Dubler, 1998; Watson, Stimpson, & Hostick, 2004), including terminally ill prisoners (Byock, 2002). For social workers, involvement in this endeavor is an extension of the profession's international code of ethics (International Federation of Social Workers & International Association of Schools of Social Work, 2004; National Association of Social Workers [NASW], 2008) and the codes of ethics of various national organizations (Association of Social Workers in Turkey, 2005; Australian Association of Social Workers, 2002; British Association of Social Workers, 2002; Blake, Kim, & Bong, 2004; Canadian Association of

Social Workers, 2005; Irish Association of Social Workers, 2006; NASW, 2008; Union of Social Workers [USW], 2007). Key social work values are embodied into these codes, such as social justice, the dignity and worth of each individual, advocacy for the disadvantaged and marginalized, autonomy, as well as a belief in the individual's ability to change.

The practice of social work within the prison setting, particularly in a palliative care or hospice program, offers opportunities to provide these services to one of the most vulnerable and disenfranchised populations. Social workers must learn to work within the context of security first, needs of the prisoner second. Mutual understanding of each others' viewpoints—social workers trained in dealing with psychosocial issues, and custody working with security issues—is essential for everyone's goals to be met. End-of-life care in the prison setting offers a wide range of experiences and can provide social workers opportunities to apply traditional social work theory and practice in a nontraditional setting (Enders, 2004a).

Developing palliative care and hospice programs in prison requires specific education and training of staff and medical providers. Although security must be first and foremost, traditional hospice care does have a place in the prison setting. Attention to prison policies and procedures must be maintained, but attention to pain control, symptom management, emotional needs, and spiritual needs cannot be excluded (Enders, 2004a).

LEARNING EXERCISES

Consider Marcy's narrative in Box 15.1
1. What can the social worker do for her? Her children and other family members?
2. How could the social worker be integrated into the health care team?
3. What social work interventions might dispel some of Marcy's anxiety, anger, or depression?
4. When might palliative care be introduced?
5. What custody issues might arise due to her change in health condition?
6. If she was to be released soon, what would need to happen to assure continuity of health care, and should a social worker be involved in that process? If so, in what capacity and to what end?
7. If she is not eligible for release and her prognosis is 6 months or less to live, what resources might the social worker employ?

ADDITIONAL RESOURCES AND WEB SITES

Academy of Correctional Health Professionals: http://www.correctionalhealth.org/index.asp
The Academy of Correctional Health Professionals connects clinicians with peers from across the country through publications, educational activities, and special events.
American Correctional Association: http://www.aca.org

The American Correctional Association serves all disciplines within the corrections profession and is broadly focused. Areas of interest include professional development and certification, standards and accreditation, networking, consulting, research, publications, and technology.

American Correctional Health Services Association: http://www.achsa.org

The American Correctional Health Services Association's mission is to be the voice of the correctional health care profession and to serve as a forum for addressing current issues and needs confronting correctional health care. The association holds annual multidisciplinary conferences designed to provide education on the latest developments in correctional health care.

American Jail Association: http://www.corrections.com/aja/

The American Jail Association (AJA) is a national, nonprofit organization dedicated to supporting those who work in and operate our nation's jails.

End of Life Care Standards of Practice for Inmates in Correctional Settings (Original) :

http://www2.edc.org/lastacts/archives/archivesMayoo/standards.asp

Standards of Practice were developed by the GRACE (Guiding Responsive Action for Corrections in End of life) Project, a Robert Wood Johnson Foundation Promoting Excellence in End of Life Care initiative, administered by Volunteers of America. Included in *Innovations in End of Life Care*, an international journal of leaders in end of life care.

The GRACE (Guiding Responsive Action for Corrections in the End of Life) Project: http://www.dyingwell.org/grace2001.htm

This foreword for *A Handbook for End of Life Care in Corrections Facilities* summarizes the issues challenging health care and hospice in the corrections system and includes valuable links related to prison hospice.

Health in Prisons Project, World Health Organization: http://www.euro.who.int/prisons

The WHO Health in Prisons Project (HIPP) arose in recognition of the gap between public health and prison health. HIPP's main purpose is to support Member States in improving public health by addressing health and health care in prisons, and to facilitate the links between prison health and public health systems at both national and international levels.

Health through Walls: http://www.healththroughwalls.org/

Health through Walls (HtW) is a nonprofit volunteer organization composed of doctors, nurses, and technicians primarily specializing in prison health care services, as well as laypersons in the United States working to assist jail and prison programs in developing countries to provide sustainable health care.

International Community Corrections Association: http://www.iccaweb.org/index.html

The International Community Corrections Association is a private, nonprofit, membership organization that acts as the representative voice for residential and other community corrections programs. ICCA requires of its members the professional background, research, and expertise necessary to ensure performance of effective quality services delivered with integrity and competence. ICCA affirms that its primary goal is the successful reintegration of the client into the community.

International Corrections and Prisons Association: http://www.icpa.ca/

The ICPA was formed to operate as an Association for corrections and prison professionals, dedicated to improving global understanding and professionalism in corrections. Improving the professionalism and competence of correctional officers through the respectful exchange of ideas, technology, and best practices in the profession of corrections is likely to have a positive impact on prison conditions and the humane treatment of prisoners.

The Journal of Correctional Health Care: http://jcx.sagepub.com/

The Official Journal of the National Commission on Correctional Health Care. *The Journal of Correctional Health Care* is the only U.S. peer-reviewed scientific journal devoted to correctional health care topics.

National Commission on Correctional Health Care: http://www.ncchc.org

The National Commission on Correctional Health Care's mission is to improve the quality of health care in jails, prisons, and juvenile confinement facilities.

National Hospice and Palliative Care Organization: http://www.nhpco.org/i4a/pages/index.cfm?pageid=5371

Quality Guidelines for Hospice and End-of-Life Care in Correctional Settings (Revised End-of-Life Care Standards of Practice for Inmates in Correctional Settings). This revision of the End of Life Care Standards of Practice for Inmates in Correctional Settings was completed in 2008 by a panel of experts under the direction of the National Hospice and Palliative Care Organization.

National Institute of Corrections: http://www.nicic.org

The National Institute of Corrections is an agency within the U.S. Department of Justice, Federal Bureau of Prisons. The agency provides training, technical assistance, information services, and policy and program development assistance to federal, state, and local corrections agencies.

National Prison Hospice Association: http://www.npha.org

The National Prison Hospice Association promotes hospice care for terminally-ill prisoners. Its purpose is to assist corrections and hospice professionals in their continuing efforts to develop high quality patient care procedures and management programs. It also provides a network for the exchange of information between corrections facilities, community hospices, and other concerned agencies about existing programs, best practices, and new developments in the prison hospice field.

REFERENCES

Aday, R. H. (1994). Aging in prison: A case study of new elderly offenders. *International Journal of Offender Therapy and Comparative Criminology, 38,* 79–91.

American Board of Hospice and Palliative Medicine (ABHPM). (2007). Physician board certification in hospice and palliative medicine, American Board of Hospice and Palliative Medicine. Retrieved from http://www.aahpm.org/certification/index.html

Anderson, K., Mendoza, T., Valero, V., Richman, S., Russell, C., Hurley, J., DeLeon, C., Washington, P., Palos, G., Payne, R., & Cleeland, C.S. (2000). Minority cancer patients and their providers. *Cancer, 88*(8), 1929–1938.

Anderson, T. (2003). Issues in the availability of health care for women prisoners. In S. F. Sharp & R. Muraskin (Eds.), *The incarcerated woman: Rehabilitative programming in women's prisons* (pp. 49–61). Upper Saddle River, NJ: Prentice Hall.

Anno, B. (2004). Prison health services: An overview. *Journal of Correctional Health Care, 10,* 287–301.

Anno, B., Graham, C., Lawrence, J., & Shansky, R. (2004). *Addressing the needs of elderly, chronically ill and terminally ill inmates.* Middletown, CT: Criminal Justice Institute, Inc. for National Institute of Corrections, U.S. Department of Justice.

Arditti, J. A., Lambert-Shute, J., & Joest, K. (2003). Saturday morning at the jail: Implications of incarceration for families and children. *Family Relations, 52*(3), 195.

Association of Social Workers in Turkey (ASWT). (2005). *Ethical principles and responsibilities of social workers.* Retrieved from http://www.ifsw.org/p38000300.html.

Australian Association of Social Workers (AASW). (2002). *AASW code of ethics.* Retrived from http://www.aasw.asn.au/document/item/92

Baldwin, K., & Jones, J. (2000). *Health issues specific to incarcerated women: Information for state maternal and child health programs.* Baltimore, MD: U.S. Department of Health and Human Services, Women's and Children's Health Policy Center, Johns Hopkins University, School of Public Health.

Barens, E. (Writer). (1998). Angola Prison Hospice, Opening the Door. In Center on Crime, Communities and Culture & The Prioject on Death in America (Producers). *The Open Society Institute (Producer).* New York, NY: Open Society Institute.

Barnard, J. (1999, August 1). Convicted murderers relearn compassion in prison hospice Oregon: With the spread of tough sentencing laws and HIV, more inmates are dying behind bars. When other prisoners volunteer to ease their last days, everyone benefits. *Associated Press.* Retrieved from http://www.aegis.com/news/ap/1999/ap990801.html

Bauersmith, J., & Gent, R. (2002). The Broward County Jails Hospice Program: Hospice in the jail. *Journal of Palliative Medicine, 5*(5), 667–670.

Beck, A., & Gilliard, D. (1995). *Prisoners in 1994.* Washington, DC: U.S. Department of Justice, Bureau of Justice Statistics.

Beck, A., & Harrison, P. (2001). *Prisoners in 2000* (Bulletin No. NCJ 188207). Washington, DC: United States Department of Justice, Bureau of Justice Statistics.

Bick, J. (2002). Managing pain and end-of-life care for inmate patients: The California medical facility experience. *Journal of Correctional Health Care, 9,* 131–147.

Blake, M., Kim, N., & Bong, B. (2004). *SASW code of professional ethics.* Singapore: Singapore Association of Social Workers.

Bolger, M. (2005). Dying in prison: Providing palliative care in challenging environments. *International Journal of Palliative Nursing, 11*(12), 619–621.

Bonham, V. (2001). Race, ethnicity, and pain treatment: Striving to understand the causes and solutions to the disparities in pain treatment. *The Journal of Law, Medicine and Ethics, 29*(1), 52–68.

Boyle, B. A. (2002). The Maryland Division of Correction Hospice Program. *Journal of Palliative Medicine, 5*(5), 671–675.

British Association of Social Workers (BASW). (2002). *The code of ethics for social work.* Brighton, England: Author.

Byock, I. (2002). Dying well in corrections: Why should we care? *Journal of Correctional Health Care, 9,* 107–117.

Byock, I., Twohig, J., Merriman, M., & Collins, K. (2006). Promoting excellence in end-of-life care: A report on innovative models of palliative care. *Journal of Palliative Medicine, 9*(1), 137–146.

Canadian Association of Social Workers/Association Canadienne des Travailleuses et Travailleurs Sociaux (CASW/ACTS). (2005). *Code of ethics.* Ottawa, Canada: Author.

Centers for Disease Control and Prevention (CDC). (2007, February 6, 2007). *Correctional Health.* Retrieved from http://www.cdc.gov/nchstp/od/cccwg/health_issues.htm

Clear, T. R. (2005). Imprisoning America: The social effects of mass incarceration. *American Journal of Sociology, 111*(3), 923–925.

Clear, T. R., Rose, D. R., & Ryder, J. A. (2001). Incarceration and the community: The problem of removing and returning offenders. *Crime Delinquency, 47*(3), 335–351.

Cleeland, C. S., Gonin, R., Hatfield, A. K., Edmonson, J. H., Blum, R. H., Stewart, J. A., & Pandya, K. J. (1994). Pain and its treatment in outpatients with metastatic cancer. *New England Journal of Medicine, 330*(9), 592–596.

CodaAlliance. (2009). The Go Wish Game: Values sort cards. Retrieved from http://www.codaalliance.org/gowishcards.html

Cohn, F. (1999). The ethics of end-of-life care for prison inmates. *Journal of Law, Medicine and Ethics, 27*(3), 252–259.

Commerce USDo. U.S. Summary: 2000. Census 2000 Profile. In: US Dept of Commerce, ed: U.S. Government Printing Office; 2002:6

Dawes, J. (2002). Dying with dignity: prisoners and terminal illness. *Illness, Crisis and Loss, 10*(3), 188.

Dubler, N. (1998). The collision of confinement and care: End-of-life care in prisons and jails. *Journal of Law, Medicine and Ethics, 26*(2), 149–156.

Enders, S. (2004a). End-of-life care in the prison system: Implications for social work. In J. Berzoff & P. Silverman (Eds.), *Living with dying: A handbook for end-of-life health practitioners* (pp. 609–627). New York, NY: Columbia University Press.

Enders, S. (2004b). *Simple answers to difficult healthcare questions: Choice.* Carmichael, CA: Autumn Indigo Books.

Enders, S. R., Paterniti, D. A., & Meyers, F. J. (2005). An approach to develop effective health care decision making for women in prison. *Journal of Palliative Medicine, 8*(2), 432–439.

Estelle v. Gamble, 429 U.S. 97, No. 75-929 (1976).

Evans, C., Herzog, R., & Tillman, T. (2002). The Louisiana State Penitentiary: Angola Prison Hospice. *Journal of Palliative Medicine, 5*(4), 553–558.

Ferrell, B., & Grant, M. (2009, May 2009). *ELNEC: End-of-Life Nursing Education Consortium.* Retrieved from http://www.aacn.nche.edu/ELNEC/factsheet.htm

Freimuth, V., Quinn, S., Thomas, S., Cole, G., Zook, E., & Duncan, T. (2001). African Americans' views on research and the Tuskegee Syphilis Study. *Social Science and Medicine, 52*(5), 797–808.

Gates v. Cook, 376 F.3d 323, (US 5th Circ. 2004).

Golembeski, C., & Fullilove, R. (2005). Criminal (in)justice in the city and its associated health consequences. *American Journal of Public Health, 95*(10), 1701–1706.

Harcourt, B. (2006). From the asylum to the prison: Rethinking the incarceration revolution. *Texas Law Review, 84*(7), 1751–1786.

Head, B. (2005). The transforming power of prison hospice. *Journal of Hospice and Palliative Nursing, 7*(6), 354–359.

International Federation of Social Workers (IFSW) & International Association of Schools of Social Work (IASSW). (2004). *Ethics in social work, statement of principles.* Bern, Switzerland: Author.

Irish Association of Social Workers (IASW). (2006). *Irish Association of Social Workers' code of ethics*. Dublin, Ireland: Author.

Jones, J. H. (1993). *Bad blood: the Tuskegee syphilis experiment*. New York, NY: Free Press.

Kaufman, J. S. (2008). Epidemiologic analysis of racial/ethnic disparities: Some fundamental issues and a cautionary example. *Social Science and Medicine, 66*(8), 1659–1669.

King, A. (1993). The impact of incarceration on African American families: Implications for practice. *Families in Society-the Journal of Contemporary Human Services, 74*(3), 145–153.

Lampman, J. (2000). Caring for sick, prisoners learn compassion. *Christian Science Monitor, 92*(168), 1.

La Vigne, N. G., Naser, R. L., Brooks, L. E., & Castro, J. L. (2005). Examining the effect of incarceration and in-prison family contact on prisoners' family relationships, *Journal of Contemporary Criminal Justice, 21*(4), 314–335. doi:10.1177/1043986205281727.

Latimer, W. W., Moleko, A-G., Melnikov, A., Mitchell, M., Severtson, S. G., von Thomsen, S., Graham, C., Alama, D., Floyd, L. (2007). Prevalence and correlates of hepatitis A among adult drug users: The significance of incarceration and race/ethnicity. *Vaccine, 25*(41), 7125–7131.

Lin, J. T., & Mathew, P. (2005). Cancer pain management in prisons: A survey of primary care practitioners and inmates. *Journal of Pain Symptoms Management, 29*(5), 466–473.

Linder, J., & Meyers, F. (2007). Palliative care for prison inmates: "Don't let me die in prison." *Journal of the American Medical Association, 298*(8), 894–901.

Linder, J., & Meyers, F. (2009). End-of-life care in correctional settings. *Journal of Social Work in End-of-Life and Palliative Care, 5*(1-2), 27.

Linder, J. F., Knauf, K., Enders, S. R., & Meyers, F. J. (2002). Prison hospice and pastoral care services in California. *Journal of Palliative Medicine, 5*(6), 903–908.

London, A. S., & Myers, N. A. (2006). Race, incarceration, and health: A life-course approach. *Research on Aging, 28*(3), 409–422.

Lum, K. (2005). Palliative care in a New Zealand prison. *International Journal of Palliative Nursing, 11*(12), 619–621.

Maruschak, L., & Beck, A. (2001). *Medical problems of inmates, 1997* (Special Report No. NCJ 181644). Washington, DC: United States Department of Justice.

Massoglia, M. (2008). Incarceration, health, and racial disparities in health. *Law and Society Review, 42*(2), 275–306.

McNeill, J., Sherwood, G., & Starck, P. (2004). The hidden error of mismanaged pain: A systems approach. *Journal of Pain and Symptom Management, 28*(1), 47–58.

McNeill, J., Sherwood, G., Starck, P., & Nieto, B. (2001). Pain management outcomes for hospitalized Hispanic patients. *Pain Management Nursing, 2*(1), 25–36.

National Association of Social Workers (NASW). (2008). *Code of ethics of the National Association of Social Workers*. Retrieved from http://www.socialworkers.org/pubs/code/code.asp

National Commission on Correctional Health Care (NCCHC). (2003). *Standards for health services in prisons*. Chicago, IL: Author.

National Hospice and Palliative Care Organization (NHPCO). (2008). *Quality guidelines for hospice and end-of-life care in correctional settings* (guidelines for care). Alexandria, VA: Author.

National Hospice and Palliative Care Organization (NHPCO). (2008/2009). *End of life care in corrections: The facts*. Retrieved from http://www.nhpco.org/files/public/access/corrections/Corrections_The_Facts.pdf

National Institute of Health, National Institute on Drug Abuse (NIH-NIDA). (2008). *NIDA InfoFacts: Methamphetamine*. Retrieved from http://www.nida.nih.gov/pdf/infofacts/Methamphetamine08.pdf

O'Donnell, C. J., & Kannel, W. B. (1998). Is there a racial predisposition to hypertension? *Hypertension, 32*, 817–819.

Prisons: Prisons for women - Problems and unmet needs in the contemporary women's prison. (2009). Retrieved from http://law.jrank.org/pages/1805/Prisons-Prisons-Women-Problems-unmet-needs-in-contemporary-women-s-prison.html

Puisis, M. (Ed.). (2006). *Clinical practice in correctional medicine* (2nd ed.). Philadelphia, PA: Mosby Elsevier.

Ramos v. Lamm, 639 F.2d 559; 485 F. Supp. 122 (US 10th Circ. 1980).

Ratcliff, M. (2000). Dying inside the walls. *Journal of Palliative Medicine, 3*(4), 509.

Roy, B. (1995). The Tuskegee syphilis experiment: Medical ethics, constitutionalism, and property in the body. *Harvard Journal of Minority Public Health, 1*(1), 11–15.

Scraton, P., & McCulloch, J. (2006). Introduction: Deaths in custody and detention. *Social Justice, 33*(4), 1–14.

The Sentencing Project. (2007, May 2007). Women in the criminal justice system: Briefing sheets. Retrieved from http://www.sentencingproject.org/doc/publications/womenincj_total.pdf

Sheu, M., Hogan, J., Allsworth, J., Stein, M., Vlahov, D., Schoenbaum, E. E., Schuman, P., Gardner, L., & Flanigan, T. (2002). Continuity of medical care and risk of incarceration in HIV-positive and high-risk HIV-negative women. *Journal of Women's Health, 11*(8), 743.

Sorensen, J., & Stemen, D. (2002). The effect of state sentencing policies on incarceration rates. *Crime and Delinquency, 48*(3), 456.

Stephenson, B. L., Wohl, D. A., Kaplan, A. H., Golin, C. E., Hsiao-Chuan, T., & Stewart, P. (2005). Effect of release from prison and re-incarceration on the viral loads of HIV-infected individuals. *Public Health Reports, 120*(1), 84–88.

Steinhauser, K. E., Christakis, N. A., Clipp, E. C., McNeilly, M., McIntyre, L., & Tulsky, J. A. (2000). Factors considered important at the end of life by patients, family, physicians, and other care providers. *Journal of the American Medical Association, 284*(19), 2476–2482.

Tanne, J. H. (2009). US prisoners are much sicker than average Americans. *BMJ: British Medical Journal, 338*(7688), 197–197.

Thigpen, M., & Hunter, S. (1998). *Hospice and palliative care in prisons*. Longmont, CO: U.S. Department of Justice, National Institute of Corrections Information Center.

Todd, K., Samaroo, N., & Hoffman, J. (1993). Ethnicity as a risk factor for inadequate emergency department analgesia. *Journal of the American Medical Association, 269*(12), 1537–1539.

United Nations Office on Drugs and Crime (UNODC). (2009). *Women's health in prison: correcting gender inequity in prison health*. Copenhagen, Denmark: United Nations Office on Drugs and Crime, World Health Organization.

Union of Social Workers (USW). (2007). *Code of professional ethics of the social workers in Israel*. Tel Aviv, Israel: The Association for the Advancement of Social Work.

van den Bergh, B. J., Gatherer, A., & Møller, L. F. (2009). Women's health in prison: Urgent need for improvement in gender equity and social justice. *Bulletin of the World Health Organization, 87*, 406–406.

Visher, C. A., & Travis, J. (2003). Transitions from prison to community: Understanding individual pathways. *Annual Review of Sociology, 29*(1), 89–113.

Walmsley, R. (2009). *World prison population list* (8th ed.). London, England: Kings College London, International Centre for Prison Studies.

Watson, R., Stimpson, A., & Hostick, T. (2004). Prison health care: A review of the literature. *International Journal of Nursing Studies, 41,* 119–128.

Wellman v. Faulkner, 715 F.2d 269, Nos. 81-3060, 81-3061 (US 7th Circ. 1983).

West, H., & Sabol, W. (2008). *Prisoners in 2007.* Washington, DC: U.S. Department of Justice, Bureau of Justice Statistics.

West, H., & Sabol, W. (2009). *Prison and jail inmates at midyear 2008 - Statistical tables.* Washington, DC: U.S. Department of Justice, Bureau of Justice Statistics.

Wilper, A. P., Woolhandler, S., Boyd, J. W., Lasser, K. E., McCormick, D., Bor, D. H., & Himmelstein, D. U. (2009). The health and health care of US prisoners: Results of a nationwide survey. *American Journal of Public Health, 99*(4), 666–672.

Wood, F. J. (2007). The challenge of providing palliative care to terminally ill prison inmates in the UK. *International Journal of Palliative Nursing, 13*(3), 131–135.

III

Social Work Practice: Screening, Assessment, and Intervention

"It's never the same thing every day. What is unique about each patient and family along with the commonalities they share in coping with illness can drive innovation in our work. Psychosocial interventions can't be "cookbooked."

Sue Stephens LCSW, ACSW
Social Worker, Pediatric Hematology/Oncology
Cancer Institute of New Jersey

"To engage in life to its fullest is to live simultaneously in the experience of mastery and surrender; surrender demands the capacity to simply allow everything to be while mastery entails the ability to know when to act and how."

Glenn Meuche MSW, MA, LCSW
Senior Program Coordinator for Bereavement Services
CancerCare of New Jersey

*"Learning to be
at home with liminality free of outcomes
a privileged and mindful presence
a spacious listener in the heart of silence."*

Jose San-Pedro MA, MLS, MSW/RSW
Palliative Care Social Worker
St. Joseph's Health Centre
Toronto, Ontario, Canada

16 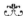 *James R. Zabora*

Screening, Assessment, and a Problem-Solving Intervention for Distress

You were the first person to ask questions about me and how I was doing. Everyone else wants to talk about my tumor and my treatments.
  —From a newly diagnosed cancer patient after completion of a psychosocial screening instrument

Key Concepts

♦ *The term* screening *is not interchangeable with* assessment.

♦ *Screening identifies patients that need to take priority for assessment.*

♦ *Assessment should be based on the needs and concerns of patients as documented in the relevant biopsychosocial-spiritual literature.*

♦ *Evidence-based interventions, such as problem-solving education, can benefit both patients and family caregivers in terms of management of distress and symptoms related to disease.*

Introduction

Rationale for the Early Detection of Distress

In terms of social work approaches and models of palliative care, the development and application of screening, assessment, and interventions are critical to clearly delineate how patients and family members are responding to life-threatening diagnoses, illnesses, and the prospect of end of life. While cancer serves as the basis for much of this chapter, these concepts and models can be applied to patients with end-stage renal disease, chronic obstructive pulmonary disease (COPD), and HIV/AIDS (Institute of Medicine, 2007). Given the significant variations that exist in each patient's and family's attempts to adapt and manage life-threatening diagnoses and end-of-life issues, models are necessary that apply brief and effective methods of psychosocial screening followed by evidence-based assessments and interventions. Estimates suggest that more than 10 million Americans live with some form of cancer with a lifetime risk to develop cancer of 1 in 2 for men, and 1 in 3 for women (American Cancer Society, 2009). Furthermore, nearly 100 million Americans live with some form of chronic medical conditions that may be managed with the assistance of palliative care clinicians and potentially referred for hospice (Zabora, 2009). Medical costs related to all of these chronic conditions are staggering, but the psychological and social consequences are also great.

Even with a disease such as cancer, which has a large literature attesting to psychosocial and spiritual sequelae, and despite the development of Distress Management Guidelines by the National Comprehensive Cancer Network (NCCN) in 1999, availability and access to formalized and structured psychosocial screening and intervention programs for patients and families are severely lacking (NCCN, 2010). In the United States only a few comprehensive cancer centers designated by the National Cancer Institute provide comprehensive palliative and hospice services. Frequently, the high-quality psychosocial programs tend to be located in comprehensive cancer centers where the overwhelming majority of cancer patients and survivors will not be seen. In reality, nearly 85% of all cancer patients receive treatment in a range of community-based programs and settings (Institute of Medicine, 2008).

The diagnosis of a life-threatening illness and the transitions over time related to illness progression generate a sense of vulnerability for virtually every patient and family (Weisman, 1976). These transition points engender fear, produce uncertainty, and create significant demands for any patient and family. However, significant evidence indicates that the majority of newly diagnosed cancer patients, patients with recurrent disease, or even a terminal diagnosis gradually adapt to these crises (Zabora et al., 1997). Weisman, Worden, and Sobel and others (Holland, 1992; Weisman, Worden & Sobel, 1980; Zabora, Loscalzo, & Smith, 2000) have described in detail the adaptive process that patients experience. Adaptation begins when patients manage to incorporate the diagnosis or the new transition into their daily lives and effectively address problems or concerns created by their changed health status.

Based on the early work of Holland and others (Holland & Rowland, 1989; Mishel, Hostetter, King, & Graham, 1984), the study of psychological responses to cancer and other chronic illnesses such as chronic obstructive pulmonary disease (Blinderman, Homel, Billings, Tennstedt, & Portenoy, 2009) and congestive heart failure (Blinderman, Homel, Billings. Portenoy, & Tennstedt, 2008) and appropriate interventions has expanded to include time points beyond the initial diagnosis. With the diagnosis of cancer, as patients move through the early reactions, patients gain experience as survivors. Survivorship is said to begin on the day of diagnosis as cancer patients begin to redefine all aspects of their lives (Insitute of Medicine & National Research Council, 2006). Three primary points exist in the psychosocial care of cancer patients. First, patients experience an "existential plight" (Weisman, 1976) during the first 3 months following their diagnosis. While many patients strive to regain a sense of normalcy, many experience intense feelings of distress exacerbated for many by the physical trauma associated with cancer therapies. For the most part, patients are forced to acknowledge that their lives will never again be the same. Second, if a recurrence occurs, patients learn to live with the return of their cancer (Wordon, 1989). Patients incorporate disruptions of daily life into their day-to-day routines. Third, the fear of significantly advanced disease and transition to end-of-life care further complicates the psychosocial course for each patient. While many health care providers assume patients may experience end of life as the point of highest distress, this is sometimes not the case. Patients and families gain critical information and knowledge concerning their disease and treatments across the entire disease continuum beginning at diagnosis. Over the course of illness, patients have formed supportive relationships with members of the health care team, as well as with other patients and families. Knowledge and support from the team enable patients to anticipate and understand their course of treatment following recurrence as well as the problems associated with the end-of-life phase (Zabora & Loscalzo, 1998).

Consequently, using cancer as a model and given these three critical points in time, screening for distress followed by an evidence-based assessment provides an optimal opportunity to identify patients with the highest level of psychosocial risk.

Definition and Measurement of Distress

At the core of any patient's ability to adapt to these types of stressors is the concept of psychological distress that has been defined as:

> ...an unpleasant emotional experience of a psychological, social, and/or spiritual nature that interferes with the ability to cope effectively with cancer and its treatments. Distress extends along a continuum, ranging from common normal feelings of vulnerability and sadness to problems that can be disabling, such as depression, anxiety, and social isolation. (NCCN, 2010)

Distress was chosen by the NCCN as the foundation for their national guidelines because it was a term that was more acceptable to patients as well as less embarrassing and stigmatizing. All patients experience some level of distress as they attempt to normalize their early reactions to a cancer diagnosis, a recurrence, or the anticipation of death. For social workers, distress has been correlated with many concepts that are of importance to their clinical practice. For example, studies have found that the higher the social support (Baker, Zabora, Jodrey, Polland, & Marcellus, 1995), the lower the distress. Or in the case of spirituality, the higher the level of spirituality the lower the distress (Smith et al., 1993). Similar correlations can be found between distress and performance status, family functioning, problem-solving skills, symptoms, and quality of life.

Of primary importance, distress can be measured with a high level of reliability and validity. Of all of the measures of distress in psychosocial oncology, the Brief Symptom Inventory (BSI) has been used more frequently to measure distress than any other instrument (Gotay & Stern, 1995). Please see Table 16.1. Furthermore, investigators developed cancer norms for the Brief Symptom Inventory-18 (BSI-18) in order to use this shorter form of the BSI as a screening instrument to identify patients at elevated risk for significant distress. As a screening instrument, the BSI-18 performs with higher levels of sensitivity (to correctly identify positive cases or high-distress patients) and specificity (to correctly identify negative or low-distress patients) than other measures such as the Distress Thermometer (DT) or the Hospital Anxiety and Depression Scale (HADS). Given the growing popularity of the DT as a screening tool, it should be emphasized that the level of sensitivity and specificity for the DT are as low as .77 and .68 versus .91 and .92 for the BSI-18 (Zabora et al.,

2001b). It should be noted that a lower level of specificity of .68 will result in a higher number of false positives, that is, the identification of patients as high distress that in fact possess a lower level of distress. However, the salient point here is that it is critical to screen for distress with any of these measures so that patients with higher levels of vulnerability can be targeted for immediate interventions. Even though screening identifies high-risk patients, higher levels of distress are associated with cancer diagnoses such as lung, pancreatic, and brain due to the prognosis often associated with these tumor sites (Zabora, BrintzenhofeSzoc, Curbow, Hooker, & Piantadosi, 2001a). However, the effect of psychosocial interventions such as psychoeducation, cognitive-behavioral therapy, skill-building groups, short-term therapy, and problem solving remain the same (Bucher et al., 2001: Fawzy, Fawzy, Arndt, & Pasnau, 1995; Houts, Nezu, Nezu, & Bucher, 1996).

Comparison of Screening Tools

Patients who cannot adapt to their clinical circumstances challenge the interdisciplinary team to respond to a multitude of psychological and social problems. Often, the vulnerability associated with these problems generates significant distress that may not become manifest to the clinical team until the patient reaches an observable crisis event. Frequently, referrals to psychosocial providers occur when the patient is severely depressed or anxious, experiencing significant conflicts within the family, or is suicidal (Rainey, Wellisch, & Fawzy, 1983). In addition, studies indicate that oncologists and oncology nurses often do not identify patients with elevated levels of anxiety and depression in a timely manner. On the other hand, screening and early detection of vulnerability can enable social workers or other psychosocial clinicians to provide prospective and appropriate interventions responsive to the identified problems.

Finally, while many methodologies have been used to screen patients for distress, technology must be integrated in order to efficiently screen large numbers of patients. One of the most promising applications is SupportScreen as developed by Loscalzo and colleagues at the City of Hope in Duarte, CA. This system uses PC tablets with touchscreen technology so that patients can easily record their responses to screening questions. At the conclusion of the screen, data are transmitted to a database while messages are transmitted to members of the health care team related to the patient's specific concerns and problems. In this way, numerous critical tasks are completed simultaneously (Clark, Bardwell, Arsenault, DeTeresa, & Loscalzo, 2009).

Theoretical Foundations for Psychosocial Screening

Given the issues defined earlier, an appropriate theoretical model must be used to guide the development of instruments to identify chronically ill patients who are at risk to experience significantly elevated levels of distress. Stress model theory (SMT) suggests that any individual experiences a series of cognitive appraisals related to any crisis event such as a diagnosis of a life-limiting illness or news that disease-modifying therapies have been unsuccessful (Lazarus & Folkman, 1984). In other words, before one can act and respond to a crisis in order to reduce the distress associated with it, the person must develop a personal meaning of the specific crisis or event. Primary appraisal describes this process as defining what the crisis event means to the person at this point in his life. To define the crisis event, people use all of their available resources. Stress model theory postulates that each person possesses a number of internal and external resources. Examples of internal resources include personality, level of optimism, ability to solve problems, and spirituality. Numerous studies have demonstrated the relationships between distress and resources such as spirituality (Smith et al., 1993),

---

Table 16.1.
The PS/PSE Model for Patients and Family Caregivers

- BSI-18 and Patient Problem Checklist to identify the level of distress as high or low.

- *For high-distress patients*, a 90-minute educational session to begin to learn the COPE model in the *Home Care Guide for Cancer* (*HCG*) and apply same to disease-related problems identified on the Problem Checklist.

- Sixty-minute educational session 1 week after initial session: applying COPE to patient/caregiver identified problems.

- Sixty-minute education session 2 weeks after initial session: applying COPE to patient/caregiver-identified problems.

- Monthly telephone support and reinforcement for both patient and caregiver for 4 months following the intervention with the potential for booster sessions.

- *Low-distress patients* should receive a 90-minute session, the *HCG*, and telephone follow-up intervention.

PS, problem-solving; PSE, problem solving education.

problem-solving skills (Bucher et al., 2001), and social support such as the family (Baker et al., 1995). Therefore, distress is an "appropriate marker" for the identification of high-risk patients, and if a resource such as effective problem solving is lacking, then it would be a critical internal resource to strengthen. Identification of distress leads clinicians to those patients who are in need of assessment as soon as possible.

External resources often consist of social supports such as the family and valued friends. If the social supports are adequate and available, there is a greater likelihood that the individual will define this event in a positive, rather than negative, manner. These internal and external resources not only influence the definition of crisis but also promote the development of a secondary appraisal related to effective strategies to respond to any specific crisis event (Lazarus, 1991). Failure to respond to the demands of a crisis event and to solve related complex problems may result in significant levels of emotional distress. Emotional distress may cause disruptions in daily functioning. However, most people attempt to conceal their distress from their families and those around them (Houts et al., 1996).

Most often, newly diagnosed cancer patients with limited resources experience significant distress at the time of their diagnosis (Weisman et al., 1980). As might be anticipated with other diagnoses, if this distress could be detected much earlier in time, psychosocial interventions could be offered at a more appropriate time in the course of care such as at the time of diagnosis. If emotional distress is undetected and untreated at any point on the disease continuum, unhealthy behaviors can occur, satisfaction with life decreases, and inappropriate use of health care resources may increase (Allison et al., 1995; Zabora, Loscalzo, & Weber, 2003).

Specifically, undetected and untreated distress may lead to a significant increase in somatic complaints such as fatigue, pain, or nausea which may be unrelated to their actual diagnosis or status of their disease (Allison et al., 1995). In turn, health care providers may respond by ordering unnecessary evaluations, tests, medications, and treatments. As a result, patients who experience higher levels of distress can generate higher rates of health care utilization, and therefore health care costs associated with these patients can also be significantly higher. In a critical study of 381 coronary artery disease patients, "high-distress patients" were 12 times more likely to be rehospitalized and 10 times more likely to have a second cardiac event. Further, when rehospitalized, high-distress patients "cost" on the average $7000 more than low-distress patients (Allison et al., 1995).

Evidence-Based Psychosocial Assessments

The introduction of palliative care into the treatment of patients may occur early in the illness, at crises points or during periods of uncertainty. This process may be seamless and as simple as the integration of another medical consult team or may come at a time of high distress when all or some

components of social integration—family, work, finances, and friendships—as well as patient's psychological status, faith, and spiritual beliefs are challenged. Over the extended course of the illness, physical changes due to advanced disease and evolving symptoms create multiple and complex problems and demands for the patient and family. These problems and demands, in conjunction with significant financial assaults, generate a negative synergy, which may be overlooked as palliative care services are introduced into the plan of care. An integrated model of psychosocial screening can identify patients with higher levels of distress that would benefit from evidence-based interventions which might include problem-solving education, pharmacology, and family intervention and such. If this occurred at the time of the initial meeting with palliative care clinicians or the hospice team, screening and early intervention could produce a significant benefit to numbers of patients and their families.

While screening seeks to identify patients with greater levels of psychosocial vulnerability, a comprehensive biopsychosocial-spiritual assessment needs to focus on issues that are amenable to change and that promote dignity. While dignity can be defined as the state of feeling worthy or esteemed, researchers have identified specific factors that promote dignity among patients with advanced disease. Pain, intimate dependency, hopelessness versus worthlessness, depression, informal social support, formal social support, and quality of life contribute to or diminish a patient's sense of dignity at a time when treatment options may be limited. If these concepts form the basis for assessment, then methods could be employed that address depression, foster hope, and enhance functional independence (Hack et al., 2004). In the setting of a referral to hospice, the transition from treatment-focused care can be rapid and brief. The National Hospice and Palliative Care Organization (NHPCO) reports that median length of service in 2008 was 21.3 days, which was an increase from 1.3 days from 2007. In essence, this indicates that half of all hospice patients received care for less than 3 weeks (NHPCO, 2009). This timeframe challenges hospice social workers to quickly screen, assess, and develop a timely and effective intervention. The BSI-18 and the Problem Checklist (PCL) offer the foundation for assessments by providing the social worker with an overall distress score, a depression score, an anxiety score, a somatization score (distress caused by physical symptoms), and the PCL presents a series of the most common problems that are specifically relevant to the patient. In addition, a number of psychosocial programs add pain and fatigue to the PCL, but display these symptoms on 10-point Likert scales. If additional time is available, Table 16.2 details items for a more comprehensive assessment.

Domains and Elements of a Psychosocial Assessment

Given the growing research related to the importance of spirituality (for additional information, see Chapter 19,) and

Table 16.2.
Critical Domains and Elements of a Psychosocial Assessment

DOMAIN	Physical	Psychological	Social	Financial	Legal	Spiritual	Existential
	Performance status	Level of distress	External resources	Insurance status	Will	See HOPE assessment	Meaning of life
	Mental status Symptoms	Internal resources	Adequacy of support	Level of income	Estate planning		Value of my life
	Physical limitations	Problem-solving skills	Availability of support	Access to other financial resources			Helplessness vs. worthlessness
	Sexuality (see PLISSIT assessment)	Quality of life	Employment history	Debts			Life review
	Advance directive		Family functioning				

sexuality (see Chapter 24) to patients with various chronic illnesses, these issues are also important to patients living with life-threatening illness. Consequently, there are well-designed methodologies for social workers to assess these salient issues. Research indicates that spirituality or religious involvement acts as a protective factor evidenced by the finding that patients with high involvement experiencing lower rates of cardiovascular disease, hypertension, depression, anxiety, stress hormones, social isolation with corresponding higher rates of immune functioning, hope, optimism, and social support (Koenig, 2001). Spirituality can be defined as "... the search for meaning, purpose, and connection with self, others, the universe, and the ultimate, however one understands it. This may or may not be expressed through religious forms or institutions" (Sheridan, 2009). The HOPE Approach to Spiritual Assessment (Anandarajah & Hight, 2001) provides clear guidance to assess this domain and begin to formulate interventions. The following framework offers examples of specific questions:

H: Sources of hope, meaning, strength, peace, love, and connection
  What in your life makes you feel strong inside?
  What sustains you and keeps you going?
O: Organized religion
  Do you consider yourself to be part of an organized religion?
  What parts of your religion do you find helpful? Not helpful?
P: Personal spirituality and practices
  Do you have personal spiritual beliefs that are not part of your religion?
  Do you have any spiritual practices such as prayer or mediation that you find helpful?
E: Effects on medical care and end-of-life issues
  Has being ill interfered with your spiritual or religious practices?
  Are there any spiritual beliefs and practices that you would want the health care team to know?

As for sexuality, there are a number of obstacles that prevent social workers from actively addressing issues related to sexuality and intimacy in palliative care and hospice settings. First, sexuality and death are two highly emotional and sensitive topics, and while these issues should be addressed in any type of comprehensive psychosocial assessment, little education and research are available to guide social workers. Second, there is a question of whose responsibility it is to explore sexuality and intimacy with a patient and family. While a strong rationale can be made for the social work here, other disciplines within the health care team may lay claim to this role as well. In addition, psychologists and nurses may have a higher level of training and assume this responsibility. Third, social workers may tend to avoid these issues altogether given their own discomfort and lack of knowledge in terms of assessment and intervention. Studies have indicated that as many as 63% of hospice care providers

that include social workers lack the skills to address sexuality and intimacy with their patients and their family members (Kutner, Kassner, & Nowels, 2001).

Cagle and Bolte (2009) attempted to address these issues for social workers with their review of the pertinent literature, discussion of clinical skills, strategies for assessment, and intervention based on defined categories of problems such as body image and self-concept, sexual functioning and desire, relational concerns, and systemic barriers. While the implications of the first three categories should be clear, the final issue of systemic barriers requires clarification. This category refers to institutional policies and government regulations that may create obstacles to an open and honest discussion of concerns and problems related to sexuality and intimacy. Examples here include advocating for "privacy please" signs and hospital beds that accommodate more than one person in order to allow patients and their significant others to enjoy intimate moments without fear of an abrupt interruption.

These authors also present concise definitions of the concepts of sexuality and intimacy within the context of palliative care as well as three models for assessment and intervention. Based on studies of palliative care patients, sexuality becomes a sense of emotional and physical closeness that does not necessarily involve sexual intercourse. To quote these authors, "sexuality is whatever it means to patients," and intimacy is a critical part of expression of sexuality.

Models for assessment and intervention include the ALARM model, the BETTER model, and the PLISSIT model. While each model has strengths, the PLISSIT model provides a flexible framework for social work clinicians in palliative care and hospice settings.

- *Permission (P).* Communication of a willingness to openly discuss concerns about intimacy and sex
- *Limited information (LI).* Provision of brief education concerning potential sexual problems related to a specific diagnosis or treatment regimen
- *Specific suggestions (SS).* Provision of concrete strategies to enable the patient who prefers to include a partner to address specific problems associated with sexual functioning and/or intimacy
- *Intensive therapy (IT).* Thirty percent (30%) of patients will probably require short-term therapy related to the first three levels or, in the case of more severe problems, a referral for sex therapy (Anon, 1976).

Finally, given the sensitivity of these areas, providers must focus on the issue of cultural diversity. As our society and others continue to become more multicultural, health care providers' individual experiences with diverse cultures and groups vary in depth and scope. Consequently, issues such as sexuality and spirituality need to be explored with recognition of cultural diversity, sensitivity, awareness, and competence. To be effective with assessment, providers seek information about the patient's expectations of care, cultural practices or taboos, and other data that results in an understanding of the patient's attitudes and beliefs about his or her illness and how it impacts the patient's life. Awareness and recognition of diversity leads to a greater level of knowledge of cultural differences, which in turn, influences clinician sensitivity during the assessment phase. These concepts as a whole create the opportunity for the achievement of cultural competence (Doorebos, Schim, Benkert, & Borse, 2005).

Necessity for the Inclusion of the Family

The effects of cancer reverberate throughout the family (Loscalzo & Zabora, 1998). Families can exhibit significant variation in their ability to adapt and respond to the overall cancer experience (Zabora et al., 2000). But, in many ways, this is also true of other chronic illnesses. While a variation in family response exists, family members can experience increased anxiety and depression, disruptions in social roles, and diminished physical health with an escalation of somatic complaints. Cancer generates demands that impose severe levels of stress that challenge even the most well-functioning family (Zabora, Fetting, Shanley, Seddon, & Enterline, 1989). These struggles occur as families attempt to serve as the primary source of support for the patient, a buffer against stress, and a facilitator for effective decision making and problem solving (Bucher et al., 2001).

When family caregivers are incapacitated by their reactions to a life-threatening diagnosis and treatment, the health care team loses a significant resource in the overall care of the patient. Distress in the family undermines decision-making and problem-solving skills (Zabora, & Smith, 1991). Family members' capacity to be effective caregivers is related to family functioning along the dimensions of adaptability and cohesion. The level of family functioning may simply be inadequate to meet the caregiving expectations of the health care team. Nearly all families experience difficulties and problems if the role of caregiving is prolonged over time (Houts et al., 1996; Zabora et al., 1989). Consequently, an imperative in palliative care has emerged to develop effective interventions to assist family caregivers as they provide care to patients over the continuum of illness. (For additional information, please see Chapter 21.)

Based on the aforementioned material, screening methodologies can also be employed with family caregivers. Olsen and colleagues developed the Circumplex Model of Family Functioning (1983) that provides the basis for screening individual family caregivers or the family unit as a whole. Family caregivers could be screened via the BSI-18 for their own individual level of distress, but additional insights could be generated through the use of the Family Adaptability Cohesion Evaluation Scale (FACES) as developed by Olsen and colleagues. This brief 20-item instrument examines adaptability and cohesion and allows the clinician to place the family in one of 16 family types. Some types experience significant difficulty in managing the multiple and complex

problems associated with palliative care. If possible, this instrument is completed from the patient's perspective, but all family members may complete it to provide broader information to the clinician prior to assessment. Families that fall on the extremes of the adaptability and cohesion subscales may exhibit difficult behaviors that truly challenge the health care team (Zabora et al., 1989). Finally, clinicians could also use the Family APGAR scale, which is a brief instrument of only five items that elicits a patient's view of his or her level of satisfaction with each item. The acronym APGAR stands for adaptation, friendship, growth, affection, and resolve; each item is scored 0 to 2 to quickly screen a family on a range of 0 to 10, similar to an infant APGAR score. Families who score 6 or below may be experiencing significant internal difficulties (Smilkstein, 1978).

Although there are many potentially appropriate interventions that may be useful for managing patient and family distress, COPE is a social problem-solving model that can be taught to patients and family caregivers and has been defined as "the metacognitive process by which patients and family members understand the nature of problems in living and direct their coping efforts at altering the difficult nature of the situations themselves, the patients' reactions to them or both (Nezu, 1983)" With this conceptual model, problems are defined as specific life circumstances that demand responses for adaptive functioning. Persons confronted with these circumstances do not meet them with effective coping responses because of the presence of a variety of obstacles, which may include ambiguity, uncertainty, conflicting demands, and lack of resources, novelty, or all of these (D'Zurilla & Nezu, 1999).

The Evidence for the Problem-Solving Education Intervention: COPE

According to this theoretical model, successful problem solving requires five component processes, each of which contributes directly to effective problem resolution (Nezu, Nezu, Felgoise, McClure, & Houts, 2003). The five components are as follows: *(1)* problem orientation, definition, and formulation; *(2)* generation of alternatives; *(3)* decision making; *(4)* solution implementation; and *(5)* verification. Problem orientation involves a motivational process; the other components consist of specific skills and abilities that enable a person to effectively solve a particular problem. Because problem solving is a set of skills, this approach lends itself to being provided in an educational format.

Problem-solving theory has led to the development of problem-solving education that adapts the five components for use with the special needs of chronically ill patients and their family caregivers. . The acronym COPE summarizes the four essential elements of the motivational approach: *creativity, optimism, planning, and expert information.* These four elements are essential in the development and implementation of a course of action that results in control, direction, and hope for patients and family caregivers (Houts et al., 1996).

The basic notion underlying the relevance of problem solving for patients and family caregivers lies in the moderating role that problem solving serves to enhance coping in the general stress–distress relationship (Houts et al., 1996). The more effective people are in resolving or coping with stressful problems, the more probable it is that they will experience a higher level of quality of life (QOL) as compared with those persons facing similar problems who have difficulty in coping. Families require guidance and support in how to manage the multiple problems associated with cancer, treatments, adverse reactions, and palliative care. Following the diagnosis of a life-threatening illness, families need to have honest, intelligible, and timely information while being reassured that competent and caring health care professionals are caring for their family member.

Houts et al. (1996) proposed a new conceptual model that adapts problem-solving counseling and applies these principles in an educational format for cancer patients and family caregivers. Each of the four components of COPE is defined as follows:

The *Creativity* component of the problem-solving educational model is related to overcoming obstacles in caregiving, and managing the emotional and interpersonal problems that result from a chronic illness. Creativity enables caregivers to see problems in new ways, as well as the potential solutions.

The *Optimism* component of the model addresses the attitudes and expectations that the patient and family caregiver have regarding the problem-solving process. Chronically ill patients and family caregivers need realistic optimism that recognizes the seriousness of problems, and that new solutions are possible.

The *Planning* component is the central activity of problem solving. Patients and families must develop plans to implement medical instructions, and to address the accompanying psychosocial concerns associated with aggressive therapies, advanced disease, and multiple symptoms.

The *Expert* information component is essential for solving complex medical problems. Guidance from health care professionals on how to manage physical and emotional problems due to a chronic illness and related treatments is a salient part of the problem-solving process. Expert information engenders autonomy and control by enabling patients and family caregivers to develop effective and responsible medical caregiving plans.

Based on data analyses from the author's study funded by the Project on Death in America (Bucher et al., 2001), a refined intervention emerged that consists of one 90-minute session followed by two 60-minute sessions and monthly follow-up or weekly monitoring for up to 12 months for the most distressed patients. The first 90-minute session opens with the acknowledgment that all people have some problem-solving abilities. Also, an opening discussion that focuses on the specific illness and the need for solving a series of ongoing and complex problems is provided in the context of palliative care. This preliminary discussion attempts to enable the patient and the family member to support one another while attempting to maintain a sense of normalcy as each adapts to evolving illness over time. Both the patient and the family member are encouraged to acknowledge the problems associated with transitions and adaptations. In addition, the patient and the family member may never have experienced any problem this severe or complex, and with as many negative implications for their dreams and aspirations. Patients and family members are then oriented to the negative influences that emotions can have on the overall problem-solving process. Behaviors and symptoms such as anxiety, depression, cognitive distortions, demoralization, confusion, anger, and fear may inhibit the ability to provide support to one another. Under these conditions, even the best problem solver can benefit from the knowledge and skills necessary to effectively manage the problems associated with life-threatening illness.

As a result, the social worker as educator can inquire about how the patient and family member have solved problems in the past. Next, the patient and family member are also encouraged to identify a specific problem that generates sadness or distress that is still of concern to them so that the problem-solving training can be directly related to this situation. Typical problems (identified in the study funded by Project on Death in America) include the following: how to balance time between simultaneously coming in for treatment and completing household responsibilities; how to best use financial resources; how to provide emotional support and to manage sadness and depression; how to engage a doctor who is consistently unhelpful; how to cope with the reality that life will never be the same again; how to advocate for adequate pain relief; how to prepare for the after effects of treatment; how to find additional help and resources; how to monitor the progress of a child's school work; and how to control complex unpleasant physical symptoms, such as fatigue (Bucher et al., 2001). These identified problems become the focal points for high-distress patients in the two follow-up sessions and the monthly telephone contacts.

Table 16.1 summarizes the psychoeducational intervention.

Table 16.3 summarizes the specific content of the problem-solving psychoeducational sessions. All teaching visits can be conducted in the outpatient clinic or at home with patients and family caregivers participating and the protocol can be adapted for those who are medically fragile. Please note that high-distress patients should receive at least three problem-solving education (PSE) sessions while low-distress patients will benefit from one session. This single session for low-distress patients parallels Session #1 for high-distress patients.

Table 16.3.
Examples of Content Outline of the PS/PSE Intervention for High-Distress Patients

SR/PSE Session	Content	Time
Session #1	• General introduction about the purpose of PSE	5 min
	• Elicit patient's willingness to participate in teaching	5 min
	• Provide teaching about problem-solving strategies—participants told to look at problems in a new way	10 min
	• Patients and caregivers are educated as to the value of expert and accurate information	20 min
	• The focus of the remaining problem-solving session will be communication skills.	
	• Give copy of Home Care Guide for Cancer to each participant	
	• The COPE education skills are reinforced through a brief analysis of the problem using the appropriate chapter in the book.	20 min
	• Family caregivers and patients are then guided through the problem-solving process and develop a plan that they commit to using. Family is reminded that at the beginning of the session, the focus was on a problem and at the end of each session, the focus is on a specific resolution and plan of action.	25 min
	• Participants are praised for their use of the problem-solving principles and encouraged to continue using the COPE model, followed by a discussion of how families can follow the same problem-solving procedures for issues they will face during the evolving process of illness.	5 min
Session #2 and Session #3	• Elicit patient's willingness to continue participating	5 min
	• Review PSE training and answer questions about problem solving	10 min
	• Provide teaching about effective problem solving, review terms used in book, role-play solving by caregiver and patient of one problem identified as the most troublesome at that time	25 min
	• Develop skills to assess and communicate these QOL problems	10 min
	• Discuss weekly telephone support that will be offered for both patient and caregiver	10 min
	• Session #3 only: Conclude intervention, elicit patient's desire to continue participating	(see above)
Monthly telephone support for patients and caregivers for 4 months	• The social worker contacts each caregiver and patient monthly to discuss problems, problem solving, and family dynamics	15–30 min
	• The social worker will encourage problem solving and the use of the Home Care Guide	
	• The social worker will praise the problem-solving efforts, discuss strategies to manage family dynamics that inhibit problem solving, and guide the development of new caregiving plans. The social worker refrains from giving specific advice. If new problems are identified during these calls, the patient or family caregiver is urged to contact the patient's primary physician as soon as possible.	
	• If during the follow-up calls there is an indication the COPE problem-solving approach is not being used, the social worker will attempt to discover why, and develop an appropriate plan to move the family forward.	
	• Thank patient and family caregivers for participating in the SR/PSE program and review the next steps in participating in the program.	

PS, problem solving; PSE, problem-solving education.

Patient Family Narratives: Integrating Screening and Care Planning

The following narratives exemplify the potential integration of screening, assessment and care planning.

Box 16.1
Patient/Family Narrative: Ms. A.

Ms. A. is a 54-year-old African-America woman who has avoided screening mammography for the past 5 years due to financial concerns and a lack of insurance coverage. A computed tomography (CT) scan suggested multiple positive nodes, so a mastectomy was recommended. Upon biopsy, 14 of 17 nodes were positive. Needless to say, her reaction to this news was one of devastation. Ms. A. works as an administrative assistant in a small business in East Baltimore that does not provide any type of health care insurance. She has been divorced for the past 10 years, and she has one daughter who is attending college in Atlanta, GA. Ms. A. has a distant relationship with her church and appears to have limited friendships.

On the BSI-18, Ms. A. scores as high distress with a total score of 15 with many of the depression items scoring at 3 or above. The PCL indicates that her primary problems to be addressed are more effective communication with her physician, how to discuss all of these developments with her daughter, the potential for pain due to the upcoming surgery, and the desire to reconnect with members in her church.

If a comprehensive assessment were employed, Additional items might be identified. However the PSE intervention could be applied immediately following a prioritization of the problems identified on the PCL. In all probability, communication with her physician and insurance issues might be the best point for focus in the context of her advanced diagnosis and pending surgery.

Box 16.2
Patient/Family Narrative: Mr. Z.

Mr. Z. is an 82-year-old male diagnosed with stage IIB lung cancer who underwent resection of nodules 3 years ago followed by participation in a Phase II clinical trial. Mr. Z. is married with two adult sons and worked as a steelworker for nearly 50 years. His level of education is limited, and he normally needs a family member present to examine the complex information presented. Currently, he had been experiencing an intense cough and blood in his sputum. A magnetic resonance image (MRI) reveals a severe relapse with multiple new nodes present in both lungs.

Mr. Z scores 16 on the BSI-18 with a number of physical concerns generating elevated levels of distress. On the PCL, Mr. Z. described his extreme level of fatigue and the

potential for pain. In addition, he stated that he worried about being a burden on his family with a particular concern for the costs of his future care. As in the first narrative, the PSE intervention could immediately focus on potential interventions for fatigue. Once this concern began to be addressed, attention would be directed to his sense of burden on his family and perceived or actual financial issues.

LEARNING EXERCISES

- To understand the patient's perspective in terms of psychosocial screening, it might be helpful to acquire a set of these instruments such as the BSI-18, the PCL, and a QOL measure and complete them yourself. If you choose to do this, pay careful attention to each item, the response pattern on each instrument, and so forth. After completion, what is your reaction?
- Most often, clinical social workers do not maintain their familiarity with the relevant social work literature in their field of practice. Select one domain or element from Table 16.2 that truly interests you. Set time to do a MEDLINE search on domain or element, such as spirituality, AND palliative care. Then, review each of the abstracts from the articles that interest you the most. From the abstracts, select no more than five articles to read. If possible, read each of the articles twice. From these articles, can you construct 1–3 new questions that you believe would be valuable to add to your psychosocial assessment?
- Make an attempt to test the PSE intervention in a role play with a social work colleague. Ask your colleague to construct a case scenario without divulging the content to you. Have your colleague complete the PCL based on the case scenario and ask you to review the PCL. Then, begin your interview and attempt to deliver the PSE intervention within this role play. It is critical to remember that this is a psychoeducational intervention, and not a clinical one. Therefore, you should maintain the role of an educator rather than a clinician. The goal is for the educator to enable your colleague as the patient to solve the identified problem, rather than solving the problem for the patient.

ADDITIONAL RESOURCES AND WEB SITES

American College of Physicians Home Care Guide for Advanced Cancer Advanced Cancer: http://www.acponline.org/patients_families/end_of_life_issues/cancer/
American Psychosocial Oncology Society: http://www.apos-society.org
Association of Oncology Social Work: http://www.aosw.org

City of Hope Professional Resource Center: http://prc.coh.org

National Catholic School of Social Service, Center for the Promotion of Health and Mental Health: e-mail: zabora@cua.edu

National Center for the Advancement of Palliative Care: http://www.capc.org

National Comprehensive Cancer Network: http://www.nccn.org

REFERENCES

Allison, T. G., Williams, D. E., Miller, T. D., Patten, C. A., Bailey, K. R., Squires, R. W., & Gau, G. T. (1995). Medical and economic costs of psychologic distress in patients with coronary artery disease. *Mayo Clinic Proceedings, 70,* 734–742.

American Cancer Society. (2009). *Cancer facts and figures, 2009.* Atlanta, GA: The American Cancer Society, Inc.

Anandarajah, G., & Hight, E. (2001). Spirituality and medical practice: Using the HOPE questions as a practical tool for spiritual assessment. *American Family Physician, 63*(1), 81–99.

Anon, J. (1976). The PLISSIT Model: A proposed conceptual scheme for the behavioural treatment of sexual problems. *Journal of Sexual Education Theory, 2*(1), 1–15.

Baker, F., Zabora, J., Jodrey, D., Polland, A., & Marcellus, D. (1995). Quality of life and social support of patients being evaluated for bone marrow transplantation. *Journal of Clinical Psychology in Medical Settings, 2*(4), 357–372.

Blinderman, C. D., Homel, P., Billings, J. A., Portenoy, R. K., & Tennstedt, S. L. (2008). Symptom distress and quality of life in patients with advanced congestive heart failure. *Journal of Pain and Symptom Management, 35*(6), 594–603.

Blinderman, C. D., Homel, P., Billings, J. A., Tennstedt, S., & Portenoy, R. K. (2009). Symptom distress and quality of life in patients with advanced chronic obstructive pulmonary disease. *Journal of Pain and Symptom Management. 38*(1), 115–123.

Bucher, J. A., Loscalzo, M. J., Zabora, J. R., Houts, P. S., Hooker, C., & BrintzenhofeSzoc, K. (2001). Problem-solving cancer care education for patients and caregivers. *Cancer Practice, 9,* 66–70.

Cagle, J.G. & Bolte, S. (2009). Sexuality and life-threatening illness: Implications for social work and palliative care. *Health and Social Work, 34*(3), 223–233.

Clark, K., Bardwell, W. A., Arsenault, T., DeTeresa, R., & Loscalzo, M. (2009). Implementing touch-screen technology to enhance recognition of distress. *Psycho-Oncology, 18*(8), 822–830.

Doorebos, A. Z., Schim, S. M., Benkert, R., & Borse, N. N. (2005). Psychometric evaluation of the cultural competence assessment instrument among healthcare providers. *Nursing Research, 54*(5), 324–331.

D'Zurilla, T. J., & Nezu, A. M. (1999). *Problem-solving therapy: A social competence approach to clinical intervention.* New York, NY: Springer-Verlag.

Fawzy, F., Fawzy, N., Arndt, L. A., & Pasnau, R. O. (1995). Critical review of psychosocial interventions in cancer care. *Archives of General Psychiatry, 52,* 100–113.

Gotay, C. C., & Stern, J. D. (1995). Assessment of psychological functioning in cancer patients. *Journal of Psychosocial Oncology, 13*(1/2), 123–160.

Hack, T. F., Chochinov, H. M., Hassard, T., Kristjanson, L. J., McClement, S., & Harlos, M. (2004). Defining dignity in terminally ill cancer patients: A factor-analytic approach. *Psycho-Oncology, 13,* 700–708.

Holland, J. C. (1992). Psycho-oncology: overview, obstacles, and opportunities. *Psycho-Oncology., 1*(1), 1–13.

Holland, J. C., & Rowland, J. (Eds.) (1989). *Handbook of psycho-oncology: Psychological care of the patient with cancer.* New York, NY: Oxford University Press.

Houts, P. S., Nezu, A. M., Nezu, C. M., & Bucher, J. A. (1996). The prepared family caregiver: A problem-solving approach to family caregiver education. *Patient Education and Counseling, 27,* 63–73.

Institute of Medicine. (2007). *Cancer care for the whole patient: Meeting psychosocial health needs.* Washington, DC: National Academies Press.

Institute of Medicine & National Research Council. (2006). *From cancer patient to cancer survivor: Lost in transition.* Washington, DC: National Academies Press.

Koenig, H. G. (2001). Religion, spirituality, and medicine: How are they related and what does it mean? *Mayo Clinic Proceedings, 76*(12), 1189–1191.

Kutner, J. S., Kassner, C. T., & Nowels, D. E. (2001). Symptom burden at the end of life: Hospice providers' perceptions. *Journal of Pain and Symptom Management, 21,* 473–480.

Lazarus, R. S. (1991). *Emotion and adaptation.* New York, NY: Oxford University Press.

Lazarus, R. S., & Folkman, S. (1984). *Stress, appraisal and coping.* New York, NY: Springer Publishing Co.

Loscalzo, M. J., & Zabora, J. R. (1998). Care of the cancer patient: Response of family and staff. In E. Bruera & R. K. Portenoy, (Eds.), *Topics in palliative care* (pp. 209–245). New York, NY: Oxford University.

Mishel, M., Hostetter, T., King, B., & Graham, B. (1984). Predictors of psychosocial adjustment in patients newly diagnosed with gynecological cancer. *Cancer Nursing, 7*(4), 291–299.

National Comprehensive Cancer Network (NCCN). (2010). *NCCN clinical practice guidelines in oncology: Distress management.* Ft. Washington, PA: NCCN Clinical Practice Guidelines.

National Hospice and Palliative Care Organization (NHPCO). (2009). *NHPCO facts & figures: Hospice care in America.* Alexandria, VA: Author.

Nezu, A. M., Nezu, C. M., Felgoise, S. H., McClure, K. S., & Houts, P. S. (2003). Project genesis: Assessing the efficacy of problem-solving therapy for distressed adult cancer patients. *Journal of Consulting and Clinical Psychology, 71*(6), 1036–1048.

Nezu, A. (1987). A problem-solving formulation of depression: A literature review and proposal of a pluralistic model. *Clinical Psychology Review, 7*(2), 121–144.

Olsen, D. McCubbin, W. I., Barnes, H., Larsen, A., Muxen, M., & Wilson, M. (1983). *Families: What makes them work?* Beverly Hills, CA: Sage Publications.

Rainey, L. C., Wellisch, D. K., & Fawzy, F. I. (1983). Training health care professionals in psychosocial aspects of cancer: A continuing education model. *Journal of Psychosocial Oncology, 1*(1), 41–60.

Sheridan, M. J. (2009). Spiritually-sensitive social work practice in healthcare. *Department of Social Work Grand Rounds.* New York, NY: The Mt. Sinai Hospital (November 18th).

Smilkstein, G. (1978). The family APGAR: A proposal for a family function test and its use by physicians. *Journal of Family Practice, 6*(6), 1231–1239.

Smith, E. D., Stefanek, M. E., Joseph, M. V., Verdieck, M. J., Zabora, J. R., & Fetting, J. H. (1993). Spiritual awareness, personal perspective on death, and psychological distress among cancer patients: An initial investigation. *Journal of Psychosocial Oncology, 11*(3), 90–103.

Weisman, A. D. (1976). The existential plight in cancer: Significance of the first 100 days. *International Journal of Psychiatry in Medicine, 7*(1), 1–15.

Weisman, A. D., Worden, J. W., & Sobel, H. J. (1980). *Psychosocial screening and intervention with cancer patients: A research report.* Boston, MA: Harvard Medical School.

Worden, J. W. (1989). The experience of recurrent cancer. *CA: A Cancer Journal for Clinicians, 39*(5), 305–310.

Zabora, J. R. (March 26, 2009). *A white paper on health care reform in the United States: The need to integrate mental health services into health care delivery.* Washington, DC: The Catholic University of America.

Zabora, J. R., Blanchard, C. G., Smith, E. D., Roberts, C. S., Glajchen, M., Sharp., J.W., … Hedlund, S. C. (1997). Prevalence of psychological distress among cancer patients across the disease continuum. *Journal of Psychosocial Oncology, 15*(2), 73–87.

Zabora, J. BrintzenhofeSzoc, K., Curbow, B., Hooker, C., & Piantadosi, S. (2001a). The prevalence of psychological distress by cancer site. *Psycho-Oncology, 10,* 19–28.

Zabora, J., BrintzenhofeSzoc, K., Jacobsen, P., Curbow, B., Piantadosi, S., Hooker, C., Owens, A., & Derogatis, L. (2001b). A new psychosocial screening instrument for use with cancer patients. *Psychosomatics, 42*(3), 241–246.

Zabora, J. R., Fetting, J. H., Shanley, V. B., Seddon, C. F., & Enterline, J. F. (1989). Predicting conflict with staff among families of cancer patients during prolonged hospitalizations. *Journal of Psychosocial Oncology, 7*(3), 103–111.

Zabora, J. R., & Loscalzo, M. J. (1998). Psychosocial consequences of advanced cancer. In A. M. Berger, J. L. Shuster, & J. H. Von Roenn (Eds), *Principles and practice of palliative care and supportive oncology* (pp. 531–545). Philadelphia, PA: Lippincott-Raven Publishers.

Zabora, J. R., Loscalzo, M. J., & Weber, J. (2003). Managing complications in cancer: Identifying and responding to the patient's perspective. *Seminars in Oncology Nursing, 19* (4 Suppl. 2), 1–9.

Zabora, J. R., Loscalzo, M. L., & Smith, E. D. (2000). Psychosocial rehabilitation. In M. D. Abeloff, J. O. Armitage, A. S. Lichter, et al. (Eds), *Clinical oncology,* (2nd ed., pp. 2845–2865). New York, NY: Churchill Livingstone.

Zabora, J. R., & Smith, E. D. (1991). Family dysfunction and the cancer patient: Early recognition and intervention. *Oncology, 5*(12), 31–35.

17 *Katherine Walsh and Susan Hedlund*

Mental Health Risk in Palliative Care: The Social Work Role

In times of difficulty, take refuge in compassion and truth.

— *Jack Kornfield*

Key Concepts
- *Social workers are essential members of the interdisciplinary team performing the functions of assessing and addressing psychosocial distress across the continuum of care.*
- *Differential diagnosis of mental health disorders is a requisite skill for social workers in palliative care, as accurate assessment will determine the effectiveness of the treatment plan.*
- *Cognitive/behavioral interventions can be helpful for patients experiencing anxiety and depression as well as other symptoms of distress such as sleep disturbance and lack of hope.*
- *Treatment plans to address mental health risk involve interdisciplinary collaboration and include both medication and psychosocial interventions*

Introduction

This chapter discusses the roles and functions of social workers in addressing mental health risk in patients requiring palliative care. Relevant *DSM-IV* diagnoses and other mental health issues such as demoralization and despair are reviewed and treatment approaches discussed through an illustrative narrative of a complex patient and family treated in a semi-rural medical setting.

Social Work Role and Functions

In the past decade, much has been written about the social work roles and functions in palliative and end-of-life care (Berzoff & Silverman, 2004; Gwyther et al., 2005; Hedlund & Clark, 2001; Miller, Hedlund, & Murphy, 1998; Taylor-Brown, Altilio, Blacker, Christ, & Walsh-Burke, 2001), and in 2004 the National Association of Social Workers (NASW) published Standards for Social Work Practice in Palliative and End of Life Care (NASW, 2010. More recently, however, the expanding development of both inpatient and outpatient palliative care programs that are antecedent to, integrated into, or independent of end-of-life care has resulted in evolving roles and research in social work in this specialized area, some of which has been published in the relatively new *Journal of Social Work in End of Life and Palliative Care* (Otis-Greene, Lucas, Spolum, & Ferrell, 2009). Yet there is still relatively little literature published about the roles and functions of social work members of the interdisciplinary team in addressing psychosocial distress in patients in the wide variety of settings in which palliative care is delivered. The evolution of palliative care as a specialty is partly due to postponement of hospice services in the pursuit of disease-modifying treatment and medical advances that have extended life expectancy for those with life-limiting or chronic illnesses. In this context, providers and insurers have recognized that patients and families with serious acute and chronic illness and injuries may live for long periods of time with debilitating symptoms, side effects, and psychosocial distress. The Institute of Medicine Report on Improving Palliative Care and Cancer (2001) underscored the importance of addressing both physical and psychosocial symptoms and has been influential in the development and utilization of best practice guidelines and standards. These standards require expert assessment and intervention by an interdisciplinary team in order to develop and implement comprehensive treatment plans that address the complex factors that contribute to physical and psychosocial distress (Meier & Beresford, 2008).

The complexity of assessment and treatment is underscored in the National Framework and Preferred Practices for Palliative and Hospice Care report endorsed by the National Quality Forum in 2006 (Hultman, Keene Reder, & Dahlin, 2008; National Quality Forum, 2008; National Quality Forum, 2006; http://www.qualityforum.org/Publications/2006/12/A_National_Framework_and_Preferred_Practices_for_Palliative_and_Hospice_Care_Quality.aspx). The document includes 38 preferred practices, three of which refer directly to the mandate to identify and manage mental health concerns:

- Measure and document anxiety, depression, delirium, behavioral disturbances, and other common psychological symptoms using available standardized scales
- Manage anxiety, depression, delirium, behavioral disturbances, and other common psychological symptoms in a timely, safe, and effective manner to a level that is acceptable to the patient and family
- Assess and manage the psychological reactions of patients and families (including stress, anticipatory grief, and coping) in a regular, ongoing fashion in order to address emotional and functional impairment and loss (National Quality Forum, 2006; http://www.qualityforum.org/Publications/2006/12/A_National_Framework_and_Preferred_Practices_for_Palliative_and_Hospice_Care_Quality.aspx)

These practices may be carried out differently depending on the delivery model and practice venue; for instance, a dedicated inpatient or outpatient palliative care program versus other medical units, hospice, or home care programs.

Diane Meier, physician, national leader, and director of the Center to Advance Palliative Care (CAPC), notes that various palliative care programs compose their teams differently, but in the *Journal of Palliative Medicine*, she and colleague Larry Beresford have advocated for social workers as an essential member of the interdisciplinary team noting,

Social workers are trained in counseling, family systems, community resources, and patient and family psychosocial assessment; skills with obvious relevance to the needs of patients with serious illness and their family caregivers. Ideally, each team includes a

dedicated palliative care social worker, dedicated full or part time to the team. (Meier & Beresford, 2008, p. 19)

This is not only because social workers are equipped to assess clinical disorders such as major depression, generalized anxiety disorder, acute stress disorder, and posttraumatic stress disorder but also because "... quality clinical social work care attends to a range of biological, psychological and social issues that patients, families and children [dealing with serious illness] regularly face" (Berzoff & Silverman, 2004, p. 266).

The narrative in Box 17.1 illustrates both the complex array of symptoms contributing to mental health risk in patients and families requiring palliative care as well as the strengths that can be maximized as social workers assess and intervene to mitigate distress and maximize quality of life.

Box 17.1
Patient/Family Narrative: Nuala

Nuala, a 39-year-old Irish American bank clerk, had initially been seen by the oncology social worker at her semi-rural community hospital cancer clinic after the diagnosis with breast cancer during the eighth month of her first pregnancy. The diagnosis had come as a shock because the 3 months of symptoms had initially been attributed to the pregnancy. She insisted on waiting until after the healthy birth of her only, and long awaited, daughter Kristini before undergoing a recommended mastectomy and chemotherapy for estrogen receptor positive cancer. She and husband Richard, age 55, had been married for 8 years, 4 years after they had met in a 12-step program. Both were in stable recoveries until the pregnancy when Richard began drinking secretively almost immediately following Nuala's cancer diagnosis and Nuala resumed "occasional" alcohol consumption. She had a history of early childhood sexual abuse that had contributed to her parents' divorce, and although she had never been treated for posttraumatic stress disorder or received therapy for resulting emotional distress, she acknowledged that the experience had a significant influence on her and contributed to a strong need for control over her environment.

She was extremely labile in the weeks following her diagnosis, weeping openly in the oncology clinic, and although she was enormously invested in her daughter, she reported that the combination of cancer-related anxiety, insomnia, fatigue, and sadness were making it difficult for her to attend as fully to her daughter as she had imagined she would, and she struggled to adhere to the recommended treatment regime. She had given up her job, as planned, following Kristini's birth but expected financial stress was exacerbated by unexpected medical expenses, and Richard began working longer hours, traveling out of town more frequently to earn more money at his job as a sales rep for a local manufacturing firm. Nuala's oncologist prescribed ativan as needed (prn) for anxiety and a trial of antidepressant medication was initiated shortly after her first chemotherapy treatment. The clinic's oncology social worker completed an initial family assessment followed by biweekly sessions coordinated with her clinic visits to address Nuala's feelings of fear, anger, and sadness about the impact of her illness. She was also referred to community

Box 17.1 (Contd.)

financial and child care supports. When Nuala continued to wrestle with questions about continuing treatment, the social worker referred her to a community therapist who specialized in serious illness. Weekly psychotherapy sessions with an ego supportive and cognitive behavioral focus were initiated with goals of developing strategies and supports to reduce depression and anxiety, find constructive outlets for anger, and identify internal and external resources to make treatment more manageable. One of these resources was the 12-step program Nuala had found helpful in her previous effort to attain and maintain sobriety. Nuala also urged Richard to reengage with a 12-step program, and although he did resume work with a previous therapist, he attended sessions only sporadically and did not utilize the 12-step program. His continued use of alcohol caused additional anxiety for Nuala.

Nuala's own sense of self-efficacy increased and not long after her breast reconstruction and intensive chemotherapy were completed the psychotherapy sessions were reduced to every other week, and then to once a month with successful reduction of anxiety and depression and improved sleep. Fourteen months later, Nuala was reveling in parenthood, bringing Kristini to follow-up medical appointments and proudly citing each new developmental milestone. She felt she no longer needed psychotropic medication and had just decided to seek part-time employment and extend Kristini's day care hours when back pain began to impede her mobility. She initially attributed this to the increasing weight and pressure of lifting her daughter, but 1 month later a workup revealed bone metastasis to her spine. Initially Nuala hoped that resumption of chemotherapy and local radiation would "reverse it," but as pain increased and additional metastatic sites were identified, she was plunged into alternate periods of hope and determination countered with despair. Her level of distress fluctuated in accordance with her pain and she wept during most clinic and therapy sessions, stating repeatedly, "I can't die, I want to see Kristini graduate from high school." She was reluctant to use opioids for pain due to her addiction history and her worry that Richard, who was by this time drinking heavily again, might abuse available medication. The breathing exercises and guided imagery she had been taught in her cognitive behavioral therapy were reinitiated and, in consultation with her oncologist, a plan was developed that included the use of adjuvant pain medication, including steroids and a bisphosphonate infusion to treat her bone pain. Within days she was hospitalized through the emergency room on a weekend, after she "hadn't slept for a week," and, according to Richard, she was "crying out so continuously" that Richard understood that he could not care for her at home and that her expressions of pain and suffering were causing enormous distress for their young daughter.

During the 5-day hospitalization on a medical floor that did not have a designated palliative care team or specialist, a patient controlled analgesia pump (PCA) was started with an infusion of morphine which Nuala agreed to try in the safe setting of the hospital. She complained of feeling "out of it," a side effect which impaired her ability to be mentally clear for her daughter's visits. During one visit, when she was in acute distress, she took the hands of both her therapist and her husband and said, "This is so bad that I'm thinking of ending it all and, trust me I wouldn't do it, but sometimes I even think of taking Kristini with me."

When her thoughts and feelings were explored further, she affirmed that she wanted to live and that Kristini was the reason she was willing to endure pain and treatment side effects. Her concern that Richard's drinking impaired his ability to parent effectively served as further motivation to live. In addition to partializing the aspects of her suffering, the clinical team viewed her pain as an emergency, rotating opioids and adding adjuvant medications to achieve a better level of pain relief without the intolerable side effects that disturbed Nuala and impacted her ability to be with Kristini.

She and Richard recommitted themselves to a comprehensive treatment plan that included combined antidepressant medication and individual weekly psychotherapy therapy sessions interspersed with couples counseling and a new oral pain medication regimen. This regimen was overseen by her oncologist and included opioids, which were prescribed within a very structured treatment agreement to attempt to ensure safety, minimize chance of relapse and control of the medications. Richard joined a caregiver support group and Nuala added massage therapy and increased child care assistance for Kristini to her treatment plan. During joint counseling sessions, advance directives were completed with Nuala taking the lead, using the Five Wishes document as a guide. A psychiatric consultation was obtained and Social Security disability payments were secured, which reduced financial strain. Money raised by Richard's coworkers was used by the family to attend a young breast cancer survivor's conference at a distant city; this provided respite and renewal as well as reinforced the couple's sense of self-efficacy. While her pain still caused limited mobility and psychosocial distress, these combined efforts did lead to some improved pain management and quality family time for the next 4 months preceding Nuala's death.

Patient Family/Narrative: Themes and Concepts

This family narrative illustrates several key "themes" that infuse the experiences of those who live with uncertain and debilitating illness such as advanced cancers, diabetes, and pulmonary and heart diseases. This particular example illuminates the complexities of mood and anxiety symptoms, suicidal thinking, uncontrolled pain, suffering, and substance abuse in the context of palliative care along with the closely related feelings of grief, hopelessness, despair, and demoralization. This young woman and her family suffered numerous losses in quick succession, including loss of health, work, and income; loss of the anticipated dream of the first year with her infant daughter; and loss of hope for the future. In addition to a disrupted sense of self, her family equilibrium was disrupted by the illness and treatment side effects, the relapse, and the threat to financial and physical security. After a period of stability, her disease recurred and she anticipated additional losses, including the dream of seeing her daughter into adulthood and loss of connection with her husband. Anxiety and depression, along with feelings of fear, despair, and demoralization prevailed until a combination of therapy and medication, integrative treatments, caregiver support, and financial help decreased her depression and increased her sense of self-efficacy. This narrative also illustrates how histories of addiction can further complicate the overall clinical picture. Richard resumed alcohol use in an attempt to numb his own distress and complex feelings related to his wife's diagnosis and disease progression. For Nuala, her history of addiction and her worry about her husband's potential opioid abuse, combined with a desire for mental clarity, made her reluctant to accept opioid treatment for her pain from metastatic disease. Her concern that Richard's drinking impaired his ability to care for their daughter served not only as a motivation to live but also incentive to complete advance directives that addressed her own and her daughter's future care.

All of these dynamics are compelling and the focus of both oncology and palliative care. It is essential that social workers assisting patients and families in palliative care be aware of, and clinically skilled in working with these dynamics. Psychosocial distress is a common presentation in chronic and life-limiting illness and can be manifested as mood and anxiety disorders (included in the *Diagnostic and Statistical Manual of Mental Disorders* by the American Psychiatric Association [APA], 2000) as well as hopelessness, despair, and demoralization (World Health Organization [WHO], 2004). Accurate identification and assessment and effective treatment planning are key social work functions. In the following section each of these manifestations of mental health risk will be discussed.

Hopelessness

People diagnosed with "incurable" illnesses may report feelings of hopelessness and despair. (Clark, 1997a). Many report they have lost their dreams of long and healthy lives, and they struggle through the day-to-day demands of dealing with symptoms, treatment, and management of diseases that create uncertainty about longevity and suffering. Hopelessness has been described as having no expectation of good or success. Alternatively, "hope" has been described as having an expectation of future good or success: it is something that really matters (Groopman, 2004). Many people like Nuala, who live in the context of a serious illness, experience periods of disillusionment and hopelessness alternating with periods of hopefulness when treatment appears to be helping. For many the task is to establish an internal equilibrium in the setting of an evolving and changing disease course. Hope, in the context of illness, can be derived from many sources. Social workers can explore with patients, family, and caregivers, sources of meaning that may help the person regain some degree of hope within the experience and beyond the medical framework. For Nuala, there could be hope for a day with fewer treatment side effects, hope that a new pain management program would be effective; or hope for spending meaningful time with her child. Fostering

hope and meaning may also involve life review and identification of previous challenges that were met in a way that reinforce the individual's or family's self-efficacy. Interventions may involve both reconnecting the client to strategies or coping methods that have previously been effective or teaching new strategies such as those based on the mindfulness work of Jon Kabot-Zinn (2003). These as well as integrative therapy approaches such as acupressure and self-hypnosis can increase the sense of empowerment that may be threatened by the illness progression, treatment, or symptoms. Utilizing techniques such as meditation and guided imagery offers patients and family members the opportunity to make choices, and this often enhances their sense of control and self-advocacy. While evidence-informed literature is in its early stages of development, there exists evidence that a sense of efficacy, choice, and control, may help patients to cope more effectively. (Holland & Lewis, 2000). Clients may be energized by hope to move forward in a positive way and to take active steps that contribute to their well-being (Clark, 1997a). Sources of hope for persons living with life-threatening illness include family, spiritual beliefs, friends, inner strength, employment, health care providers, and activities that bring meaning to life. Health care professionals contribute to a patient's hope by listening empathically, giving accurate information in a compassionate manner, and demonstrating caring behaviors (Hedlund, 2006). In addition to strengths-based empowerment strategies, psychotherapeutic interventions such as cognitive-behavioral therapy targeting pessimistic cognitions or spirituality based interventions to address existential issues such as loss of meaning may decrease hopelessness (Rousseau, 2009; Spiegel,1995). Chochinov has developed a dignity therapy model specifically to foster meaning and hope in patients with life-limiting illness. Social workers may find the Dignity Psychotherapy Question Protocol developed by Chochinov (2004) useful in implementing dignity therapy. The protocol contains questions such as "Can you tell me about your life, and what was most important?" and "What would you like your family to remember?" that are intended to help the patient achieve a sense of dignity, meaning, and hope despite the patient's circumstances. They also serve as a general guide for eliciting information from clients about what is meaningful in their lives.

"Despair" is described as "losing all hope or confidence" (Farron, Herth, & Popovich, 1995). The patient may lose hope that the disease can be cured, lose confidence in doctors or other health care providers, or in their own ability to cope with the demands of advanced disease and its treatment. All of these concerns can be challenging not only for the patient but also for their caregivers and the clinical team. As noted, strategies utilized by social workers and other health care providers can be structured to identify global and more immediate threats to hope and intervene accordingly.

"Cure" and other hopes may need to be refocused in some ways. Along the continuum of illness and in life experience, hopes are often adapted and reframed and mediated by emerging realities. Identifying and redefining the *"possible"* can kindle the spark of hope by extending its frame beyond the restrictive focus of illness and cure to a broader vision of hope. Careful use of language by professionals can alleviate or circumvent despair. For example, instead of phrases like *"there is nothing more we can do,"* language can reinforce patient's options and the commitment of the health care team to provide care rather than the implication of abandonment and helplessness at a time when patients and families need to know *the care that will be provided* in the setting of progressing disease. Consider the impact of an alternative statement such as "we will continue to provide the best treatment for the symptoms and support you and your family" (Altilio & Walsh-Burke, 2002, p. 48). Much of what the patient or family perceives about the hope or hopelessness of their situation contributes to their suffering and can be modified through use of language that instills confidence and reinforces a shared commitment to problem solving. Actions by the team that address the physical and psychological distress that patients experience further instill a sense of hope, capacity, and trust.

Eric Cassell (1982) notes a distinction between physical distress and suffering:

> *Suffering is experienced by persons, not merely by bodies, and has its source in challenges that threaten the intactness of the person as a complex social and psychological entity. Suffering can include physical pain but is by no means limited to it. (p. 640)*

Cassell goes on to state that relief of suffering and the cure of disease are twin obligations of a medical profession that is truly dedicated to the care of the sick. This mandate to relieve suffering extends beyond the medical profession to social workers who must strive to identify the kaleidoscope that frames the unique experience of suffering and work with the patient and family to relieve that which can be relieved and to be quietly present with that which cannot.

Demoralization

The concept of demoralization has received increasing attention in the psychiatric and medical literature, since it is often encountered in individuals with serious illness. Frank (1974) believed that demoralization left one feeling impotent, isolated, and in despair, and he linked it to depression and anxiety. Subsequent literature has identified demoralization as distinct from depression and having two states: distress and a sense of incompetence that results in not knowing which direction to go in (Jaycobson, Maytal, & Stern, 2007). "Demoralized patients may suffer from disturbances in sleep, appetite or energy and their thinking can be pessimistic or even suicidal" (Jacobson, Maytal, & Stern, 2007, p. 141). Kissane et al. (2004) have identified five relatively distinct dimensions of demoralization in a study with 100 cancer patients: loss of meaning, dysphoria, disheartenment,

helplessness, and a sense of failure. Depression is distinct from demoralization in that it is a clinically described experience that may have symptoms of helplessness, hopelessness, worthlessness, guilt, and inability to experience pleasure (Holland & Lewis, 2000).

Some of these troubling feelings are illustrated in Nuala's narrative. There is expressed helplessness related to the management of her pain, disheartenment at the progression of her disease, a sense of failure as she became less able to parent her daughter and a loss of meaning as she anticipated the complete loss of her ability to parent and the reality that she would not see her daughter into adulthood. These feelings were so powerful that she articulated suicidal ideation, which included a thought of ending her daughter's life, thereby warding off the ultimate separation. However, her desire to parent her daughter as long as possible gave her a sense of purpose and became the source of her strength and determination to exercise some sense of agency and to create a legacy. Jacobson, Maytal, and Stern (2007) note the following:

> *Confusion, isolation, despair, helplessness, cowardice, and resentment make a patient more vulnerable to demoralization. By contrast, coherence, communion, hope, agency, purpose, courage and gratitude characterize and facilitate resilience ... help for the demoralized patient targets relief from suffering and the mobilization of his or her resilience. (p. 141)*

Suicidal Ideation

Rugh Van Loon (1999) considers "desire to die" statements from three perspectives: the expression of suffering, of suicidal intent, or coping. Careful evaluation can help the social worker, the patient, and caregivers understand the meaning of a particular statement and address the contributing factors. While every effort is made to safeguard the well-being of both the despondent patient, and the patient's significant others, it is critical for palliative social workers to assess either "suicidal" or "desire to die" statements for their meaning and their intent, to discuss their assessment with their team, create a shared treatment plan, and refer for additional assistance if appropriate. Through careful assessment, the social worker can distinguish whether the patient is depressed, suicidal, or suffering from a lack of hope and identify if the patient is using these statements as a way of coping. As Eychmueller (2009) notes:

> *The wish to die may symbolize more the acceptance that life comes to an end instead of reflecting a depressive or anxiety disorder. Communication about concrete preparation for death, life completion discussions, expressing religious struggle and giving back a sense of coherence seem to be promising non-pharmacological strategies and may lead to improved social function and better management of physical symptoms. (p. 187)*

It is incumbent upon social workers and the health care team to differentiate meaning and to identify and target the cause of distress and suffering, and this requires accurate assessment that leads to differential diagnosis. Some patients' distress will begin to be relieved through this process of assessment and attention to targeting the causes of despair, hopelessness, and demoralization. Others' distress may be a manifestation of a mental disorder that requires additional or different intervention. These are discussed next.

✿ *DSM-IV* Disorders

The following section will consider assessment of mental disorders that are most commonly seen in the palliative care setting, including differential diagnosis of *DSM-IV* disorders. Accurate assessment is essential for development of effective components of a comprehensive treatment plan.

Gender, age, and culture can influence attitudes toward disclosure of psychiatric symptoms and diagnoses, medication, psychosocial distress, and mental health treatment. Cultural inquiry and sensitivity, a requisite aspect of social work training, enhances social work's contribution to the team when it comes to understanding symptom expression, mental health risk assessment, intervention, and response to treatment.

We will review below the *DSM-IV* Axis I diagnoses that are most commonly the targets of treatments in the context of palliative care and some of the evidence-informed interventions that social workers offer to address these.

Medical Conditions that are Associated with Psychosocial Distress

In the assessment of all Axis I disorders, it is essential to consider medical conditions and treatment side effects that may contribution to, or cause, symptoms such as depressed mood or panic episodes. Many steroids, for example, used in the management of symptoms such as pain or swelling, can cause mood changes that may appear to fit the diagnostic criteria for a unipolar or bipolar depression. Skilled assessment by a social worker who is well versed in medical conditions and treatment effects as well as the *DSM-IV* will enable the team, the patient, and family, to accurately target interventions, including psychoeducation and medication modification or cognitive-behavioral therapy approaches, depending on the etiology of the problem.

Palliative care is implicitly directed at physiological conditions or symptoms that require medical management such as pain, dyspnea, anorexia, and fatigue. Much of the psychological or emotional distress social workers are called upon to address is directly related to physical symptoms and illness progression. If depression or anxiety is evidenced in the presence of untreated pain and/or dyspnea, *these somatic symptoms must be addressed* immediately. Not only can adequate management of these symptoms prevent or alleviate depression and anxiety, but inadequate management can contribute to unnecessary suffering (Emanuel, 2005; Miller et al., 1998). It is therefore essential that social workers be active advocates to ensure that these physiological symptoms are thoroughly assessed and effectively treated before a diagnosis of a mental disorder is made (Walsh-Burke, 2004).

Once medical conditions are identified (Axis 3 of the *DSM-IV* Multiaxial Assessment) and are being responded to, psychosocial and spiritual distress can also be targeted for assessment and intervention. Symptoms such as pain, anxiety, and depression need to be evaluated separately but concurrently, particularly since pain and physical and spiritual suffering can contribute to depression. And while they are often treated separately, there are some interventions that can provide relief from both. Some antidepressant medication, for example, can have a beneficial effect on pain from medical conditions and are considered adjuvant medications used for pain even in the absence of depression (University of Chicago, 2010). Sometimes when treatments such as this are offered to address physical symptoms, they are more palatable to patients and families who may be biased and have preconceived fears about opioid medications. Patient and family education can reduce resistance to medications that can alleviate different forms of distress.

Depression

The case of Nuala is illustrative of the blurred boundaries between a mental disorder diagnosis such as major depression (*DSM-IV-TR* code 296.2x–single episode) and demoralization. Sometimes these are caused by similar influences and amenable to similar treatment approaches. As Rayner et al. (2009) note,

> The ability to detect cases of depressive disorder may be less important than the ability to detect depressive symptoms remediable to treatment … Evidence-based guidelines on the detection and management of depression in palliative care are needed to help standardize practice and improve patient outcomes. (p. 58)

Accurate assessment of contributory factors (physiological, psychological, cultural, social, and spiritual) is a shared responsibility of the interdisciplinary team, since effective treatment will depend on identifying and ameliorating causative factors. When depressed mood is caused by the physiological effects of illness or treatment, a diagnosis of depression related to a medical condition (*DSM-IV-TR* code 293.83) is made.

> Consideration should be given to obtaining laboratory data to assist in detection of electrolyte or endocrine imbalances or the presence of nutritional deficiencies.

Clinical experience suggests that pharmacotherapy is more advantageous than psychotherapy alone in the treatment of depression that is caused by medical factors, particularly if the dosages of the causative agent(s), i.e., steroids, antibiotics, or other medications, cannot be decreased or discontinued. (The National Cancer Institute Fact Sheet on Depression and Cancer, 2010 p. 4)

These important differentiations illustrate the essential need for critical thinking and interdisciplinary team collaboration in both the assessment and treatment planning for palliative care patients. In addition to the physiologic factors, the emotional weight of a chronic and progressive disease such as metastatic cancer or COPD, can impact an individual's and family's motivation, energy, and sense of emotional control and result in symptoms that meet the diagnostic criteria for depression (Breitbart, Bosenfeld, Pessin, et al., 2000). Patients who are receiving palliative care for cancer may have frequent feelings of depression and anxiety, leading to a much lower quality of life. Patients suffering from depression report being more troubled about their physical symptoms, relationships, and beliefs about life (http://www.cancer.gov/cancertopics/pdq/supportivecare/depression/Patient/page2).

Axtell (2008) notes that many life-threatening illnesses cause depression. Along with targeted treatment for the illness, additional interventions may include the following:

- Medications
- Individual, group, and/or family therapy
- Hypnotherapy
- Meditation
- Existential therapy (related to the meaning of life)
- Complementary and alternative [integrative] medicine

The multifactorial and fluctuating nature of symptoms was represented by Nuala, who was alternately listless and labile when her pain was not under control, but who was able to regain a sense of self-efficacy and hope in her role as parent as she experienced the active, committed response of the interdisciplinary team to her pain and existential crises. Her disclosure of suicidal thoughts was indicative of her depressed affect, which was connected to a loss of hope. Accurate identification of the factors contributing to depressed mood can lead to a comprehensive discussion and joint decisions to implement an evidence-informed treatment plan. For Nuala, this included identifying sources of meaning to increase her motivation to utilize a combination of antidepressant medication, a new pain management program, individual and couples therapy, pastoral counseling, and integrative approaches.

Anxiety

Emerging data regarding anxiety and depression suggest a strong link to neurotransmitter dysregulation when these disorders are physiologically based, and some combination of psychotropic medication is often most effective in decreasing symptoms of anxiety and panic. However, like depression, anxiety is an expected psychoemotional reaction to an illness accompanied by the threat of death, chronic physical pain, and other disabling symptoms (Cambridge and Huntingdon Palliative Care Group, 2009). Differentiating when manifestations of anxiety are related to illness-related functional disturbance (such as thyroid or pituitary dysfunction), a medication response (steroids), a manifestation of a preexisting anxiety disorder (such as Generalized Anxiety Disorder (300.02), or a reaction to diagnosis or treatment (Adjustment Disorder with Anxiety (309.24) is essential in determining a treatment plan. Similar to depression, if the physiological causes are managed medically, the social work focus is on advocacy and referral for proper pharmacological treatment in addition to assisting the patient and family to understand and manage the symptoms through psychosocial interventions.

Support groups, individual or family counseling with a cognitive-behavioral focus, and teaching stress management techniques such as progressive muscle relaxation and guided imagery are useful in the treatment of anxiety, just as they are in depression (WHO, 2004). In particular, cognitive reframing can help to lessen the anxiety generated by negative or catastrophic thoughts associated with the diagnosis or treatment that often cause the patient to believe the experience is unmanageable, thus increasing anxiety. Thought-stopping techniques that involve learning to identify, explore, and dismiss negative, intrusive thoughts are often used in conjunction with diaphragmatic breathing and can significantly reduce anxiety that interferes with daytime activities and improve sleep at night (Bourne, 2000). Patients and families can be helped as anxiety symptoms are normalized and they experience increasing self-efficacy that comes from using these strategies alone or in combination with anti-anxiety medication.

Posttraumatic Stress Disorder

Posttraumatic stress disorder (PTSD, *DSM-IV-TR* code 309.81) is caused by experiencing or witnessing an unusually traumatic event that involved actual threatened death or serious physical injury to the person or to others. Individuals who have experienced childhood abuse (as Nuala did), rape, or domestic violence, and veterans and military personnel who have experienced combat, may all exhibit the symptoms that fit the diagnostic criteria for PTSD. The U.S. Veteran's Administration fact sheet for primary health providers discusses why it is important for health care providers as well as mental health professionals to be knowledgeable about PTSD:

Fifty to ninety percent of all adults and children are exposed to a psychologically traumatic event (such as a life-threatening assault or accident, human-caused or natural disaster, or war) at some point in their lives. As many as 67% of trauma survivors experience lasting psychosocial impairment, including posttraumatic stress disorder (PTSD); panic, phobic, or generalized anxiety disorders; depression; or substance abuse. Symptoms of PTSD include the persistent, involuntary re-experiencing of traumatic distress, emotional numbing and detachment from other people, and hyper-arousal (e.g., irritability, insomnia, fearfulness, and nervous agitation). (Retrieved from http://ncptsd. va.gov/ncmain/ncdocs/fact_shts/fs_primary_care.html)

When individuals have experienced prior trauma, both the PTSD symptoms and the psychosocial distress due to illness may be exacerbated, particularly if they feel a loss of control due to the illness and/or treatments. Guilt, shame, anger, and sadness, all normal reactions to losses associated with serious illness, may be intensified if a patient or family member has PTSD, and these symptoms may interfere with their ability to comply with invasive diagnostic or treatment procedures or to manage progressive dependence and potential feelings of vulnerability. In the course of psychosocial assessment, social workers may learn about an early trauma and can identify the symptoms of PTSD. Some patients will come into the palliative care setting without symptoms and distress ever having been assessed within a trauma framework. In identifying the cause (the traumatic experience) and the effect (PTSD symptoms such as flashbacks and hyperarousal), the social worker can contribute significantly to the patient, family, and team's understanding of both the patient's distress, its relationship to the past and the present, and their therapeutic needs.

Psychotherapy that includes cognitive-behavioral interventions is recommended for survivors of PTSD, and social workers in palliative care can assess need and either provide the interventions directly or make effective mental health referrals. According to the National Institute of Mental Health, psychotherapy for PTSD can help in the following ways:

- Teach about trauma and its effects
- Use relaxation and anger control skills
- Provide tips for better sleep, diet, and exercise habits
- Help people identify and deal with guilt, shame, and other feelings about the event
- Focus on changing how people react to their PTSD symptoms (Retrieved from http://www.nimh.nih.gov/ health/publications/post-traumatic-stress-disorder-ptsd/psychotherapy.shtml)

In addition to these interventions for the patient and family, it is important to educate the interdisciplinary team about the impact of trauma and the need to minimize traumatizing aspects of medical care and the medical environment. Invasive procedures as well as exposure to others' distress in the hospital or clinic setting may serve as triggers or additional traumatic stimuli to those with PTSD as well as everyone else who is experiencing life-threatening or chronic

illness. Much can be done to lessen risk of trauma or retraumatization when care is delivered with sensitivity within a comforting environment. Social workers can be instrumental in sensitizing other providers to these aspects of care.

Substance Abuse and Dependence

It is estimated that between 6% and 15% of the U.S. population has a substance use disorder that may involve the use of illicit drugs or misuse of prescription medications (Collier & Kopstein, 1991; Groerer & Brodsky, 1992; Zachny et al., 2003). Some of the medications used in the management of chronic pain and in palliative care are controlled substances which may be preferred drugs of abuse for those with a history of substance dependence or abuse. As illustrated by Nuala's narrative, patients and family caregivers with histories of substance abuse may be vulnerable to relapse under the stressors of a diagnosis of a chronic or life-limiting illness. Of equal concern is the reluctance of those who have successfully "recovered" from addictions to accept treatment for pain and other symptoms for fear of relapse or dependency, or concern about family members' abuse of the patient's prescribed medication. These concerns also impact patients and families where there is no history of abuse but confusion and worry about the potential for addiction with certain classes of medications such as opioids and benzodiazepines.

Palliative social workers need to understand these issues so they can debunk myths and misunderstandings; educate patients, family, and staff; and frame addiction as a medical diagnosis that requires assessment to establish a diagnosis such as alcohol dependence (303.90) and other preexisting substance-related disorders. Navigating the multidimensional issues that pervade this concern requires an informed assessment of history, risk, and worry as well as a knowledge of interventions. These may include structured and frequent visits to clinicians and treatment agreements that enhance the possibility of safely prescribing medications to patients who may suffer from coexisting conditions of a life-threatening illness and a substance use disorder. Differential diagnosis is essential because treatment for substance dependence will need to be included in the treatment plan.

Dementia of the Alzheimer's Type

Palliative care is increasingly integrated into the care of patients with Alzheimer's disease (290.0) and other forms of dementia. These diagnoses bring with them multiple impairments and heavy demands on caregivers, who may be at risk for depression and anxiety or demoralization. Patients with other chronic physical conditions may evidence cognitive impairment that mimic or resemble those of Alzheimer's disease. While a physician will make the differential diagnosis of this and other physiological conditions, social workers have unique listening and observational skills and may notice changes in patients' speech or thinking that will contribute to diagnoses such as dementia or delirium. These changes not only impact the patient's self-concept and function but they also shatter the equilibrium of the family system and cause enormous distress in family and caregivers who may misinterpret behaviors. In addition, social workers with their environmental perspective may be the members of the team most likely to assess caregivers' stress and mental health and then to intervene to create an interdisciplinary plan of care. This is essential whether the social worker is in a hospice and palliative care setting, acute or rehabilitation setting, or in a community service setting where patients and their families are either receiving or require palliative care. Since fewer family caregivers may be aware of palliative care options for persons with dementia, social workers in these settings can be key community and caregiver educators about the needs and services for this vulnerable population. (For additional information please see Chapters 11, 34, and 37.)

Conclusion

This focused description of the process of assessing mental health risk, making a differential diagnosis, and selecting appropriate treatments illustrates the very complex nature of this essential aspect of palliative care. Since social workers provide palliative care in multiple settings, a high level of training and skill is needed, not only in mental health in the context of medical illness but also in interdisciplinary collaboration. Comprehensive psychosocial-spiritual assessment, an essential social work contribution to the interdisciplinary team in every setting, enables social workers to identify mental health disturbance as well as risk and address the specific factors influencing patient and family coping. Through accurate assessment, treatment planning, and implementation, the psychosocial distress that emanates from untreated mental health symptoms can be ameliorated in patients and families requiring palliative care.

REFERENCES

Altilio, T., & Walsh-Burke, K. (2002). The words we choose and the messages they convey. *Oncology Issues, 17*(1), 48.

American Psychiatric Association (APA). (2000). *Diagnostic and statistical manual of mental disorders* (4th ed., text rev.). Arlington, VA: Author.

Axtell, A. (2008) Depression in palliative care. *Journal of Palliative Medicine, 11*(3), 30.

Berzoff, J., & Silverman, P. (2004). *Living with dying: A handbook for end-of-life care health professionals.* New York, NY: Columbia University Press.

Bourne, E. (2000). *The anxiety and phobia workbook.* (3rd ed.) Oakland, CA: New Harbinger Publications.

Breitbart, W., Bosenfeld, B., Pessin, H., Kaim, M., Funesti-Exh, J., Gallieta, M., . . Brescia, R. (2000). Depression, hopelessness, and desire for hastened death in terminally ill patients with cancer. *Journal of the American Medical Association, 284*(22), 2907-2911.

Cambridge and Huntingdon Palliative Care Group. (2009). Fact sheet 15 on anxiety, depression and palliative care. Retrieved from http://www.arthurrankhouse.nhs.uk/documents/FACTSHEET_15.pdf

Cassell, E. J. (1982). The nature of suffering and the goals of medicine. *New England Journal of Medicine, 306,* 639-645.

Chochinov, H. V. (2004). Dignity is in the eye of the beholder. *Journal of Clinical Oncology, 22*(7), 1336-1340.

Clark, E. J. (1997a). *You have the right to be hopeful* (2nd ed.). Silver Spring, MD: National Coalition of Cancer Survivorship.

Collier, J. D., & Kopstein, A. N. (1991). Trends in cocaine abuse reflected in emergency room episodes reported to DASW. *Public Health Report, 106,* 59-68.

Emanuel, E. J. (2005). Depression, euthanasia and improving end-of-life care. *Journal of Clinical Oncology, 23*(27), 6456-6458.

Eychmueller, S. (2009). Management of depression in the last month of life. *Current Opinion In Supportive And Palliative Care, 3*(3), 186-189.

Farron, C., Herth, K., & Popovich, J. (1995). *Hope and hopelessness. Critical clinical constructs.* Thousand Oaks, CA: Sage Publications.

Frank, J. D. (1974). Psychotherapy: The restoration of morale. *American Journal of Psychiatry, 131,* 271-274.

Groerer, J., & Brodsky, M. (1992). The incidence of illicit substance abuse in the United States, 1962-1989. *British Journal of Addiction, 87,* 1345.

Gwyther, L. P., Altilio, T., Blacker, S., Christ, G., Csikai, E. L., Hooyman, N.,.Howe, J. (2005). Social work competencies in palliative and end of-life care. *Journal of Social Work and End Life and Palliative Care, 1*(1), 87-120.

Hedlund, S., & Clark, E. J. (2001). End of life issues. In M. Lauria, E. Clark, J. Hermann, & N. Stearns (Eds.), *Social work in oncology: Supporting survivors, families, and caregivers* (pp.299-310). American Cancer Society.

Hedlund, S. C. (2006). Hope and communication in cancer care: What patients tell us. In P. Angelos (Ed.), *Ethical issues in cancer patient care* (pp. 65-77).

Holland, J. C., & Lewis, S. (2000). *The human side of cancer; Living with hope, coping with uncertainty.* New York, NY: Harper/Collins.

Hultman, T., Keene Reder, E. A., & Dahlin, M. (2008). Improving psychological and psychiatric aspects of palliative care: The National Consensus Project and the National Quality Forum preferred practices for palliative and hospice care. *Omega: The Journal of Death and Dying, 57*(4), 323-339.

Institute of Medicine. (2001). *Improving palliative care for cancer.* Retrieved from http://www.iom.edu/Reports/2003/Improving-Palliative-Care-for-Cancer-Summary-and-Recommendations.aspx

Jacobson, J., Maytal, G., & Stern, T. (2007). Demoralization in medical practice. Primary care companion. *Journal of Clinical Psychiatry, 9*(2), 139-143.

Katcheressian, J., Cassell, J. B., Lyckholm, L., Coyne, P., Hagenmueller, A., & Smith, T. (2005). Improving palliative and supportive care in cancer patients. *Oncology, 19*(10), 1365-1376.

Kabot-Zinn, J. (2003). *Full catastrophe living: Using the wisdom of your body and mind to face stress, pain and illness. Fifteenth anniversary* edition. New York, NY: Delta Press.

Kissane, D. W., Wein, S., Love, A., Lee, X. Q., Kee, P. L., Clarke, D. M. (2004) The Demoralization Scale: a preliminary report of its development and validation. *Journal of Palliative Care*, *20*(4), 269–276.

Meier, D. E., & Beresford, L. (2008). Social workers advocate for a seat at the palliative care table. *Journal of Palliative Medicine*, *11*(1), 10–14. doi:10.1089/jpm.2008.9996.

Miller, P. J., Hedlund, S. C., & Murphy, K. A. (1998). Social work assessment at the end of life: Practice guidelines for suicide and the terminally ill. *Social Work in Health Care*, *26*(4), 23–36.

National Association of Social Workers. (2010). Standards for Social Work Practice in Palliative and End of Life Care. Retrieved from http://www.naswdc.org/practice/ bereavement/standards/default.asp

National Cancer Institute. (2010). Depression (PDQ). Retrieved from http://www.cancer.gov/cancertopics/pdq/supportivecare/ depression/Patient/page2

National Consensus Project for Quality Palliative Care. (2009) *Clinical practice guidelines for quality palliative care, second edition*. Retrieved from http://www.nationalconsensusproject. org/Guideline.pdf

National Institute of Mental Health (2010) Post Traumatic Stress Disorder Retrieved from http://www.nimh.nih.gov/health/ publications/post-traumatic-stress-disorder-ptsd/ psychotherapy.shtml)

National Quality Forum. (2006). *A national framework and preferred practices for palliative and hospice care quality: A consensus report*. Retrieved from http://qualityforum.org/ Publications/2006/12/Executive_Summary_for_Hospice_ Report.aspx

National Quality Forum. (2008). *National framework and preferred practices for palliative and hospice care quality: A national quality forum consensus report*. New York, NY: Retrieved from http://www.qualityforum.org/Publications/2006/12/A_

National_Framework_and_Preferred_Practices_for_Palliative_ and_Hospice_Care_Quality.aspx

Otis-Greene, S., Lucas, S., Spolum, M. & Ferrell, B. (2009). Promoting excellence in pain management and palliative care in social workers. *Journal of Social Work in End-of-Life and Palliative Care*, *4*(2), 120–134.

Rousseau, P. (2009). Spirituality and the dying patient. *Journal of Clinical Oncology*, *18*, 2000–2002.

Spiegel, D. (1995). Essentials of psychotherapy interventions for cancer patients. *Supportive Care in Cancer*, *3*(4), 252–256.

Taylor-Brown, S., Altilio, T., Blacker, S., Christ, G., & Walsh-Burke, K. (2001). *Best practices in end of life care*. Philadelphia, PA:Work and Health Care.

University of Chicago. (2010). Anti-depressants (as pain relievers). Retrieved from http://millercenter.uchicago.edu/learnaboutpn/ treatment/pain_med/antidepressants/index.shtml

United States Department of Veterans Affairs. (2010) FactPTSD Fact Sheet Retrieved from Fhttp://ncptsd.va.gov/ncmain/ ncdocs/fact_shts/fs_primary_care.html

Van Loon, R. A. (1999). Desire to die in terminally ill people: a framework for assessment and intervention. *Health and Social Work*, *24*(4), 260–268.

Walsh-Burke, K. (2004). Mental health risk assessment. In J. Berzoff & P. Silverman (Eds.), *Living with dying: A handbook for end-of-life health care practitioners*. New York, NY: Columbia University Press.

World Health Organization (WHO). (2004). *Palliative care: Symptom management and end-of-life care: Integrated management of adolescent and adult care*. Geneva, Switzerland: Author.

Zachny, J., Bigelow, G., Compton, P., Foley, K., Iguchi, M., & Sannerud, C. (2003). College on problems of drug dependence taskforce on prescription opioid non-medical use and abuse: Position Statement, *Drug and Alcohol Dependence*, *69*(3), 215–232.

18

Lissa Parsonnet and Carrie Lethborg

Addressing Suffering in Palliative Care: Two Psychotherapeutic Models

Every morning I wake up and I'm generally not feeling the best. I don't sleep so well these days and never wake feeling refreshed and various things ache and I sigh and think, "OK girl, pull yourself together, today's another day." You muster up whatever you have inside you to get you going again and then you face another day, and often you even enjoy that day!

—*Jacinta, a young single mother with recurrent breast cancer 1 month before she died (names and details changed to ensure anonymity)*

Key Concepts

- *Interventions in the setting of palliative care require a range of therapeutic models to respond to the individual lived experience of patients.*
- *Social work practice is informed by a variety of theoretical constructs that assist practitioners in making sense of adjustment issues and meeting the complex needs of those facing life-threatening illness and the end of their life.*
- *Meaning-based and schema therapy are two broad models used in the setting of palliative care, both suggesting ways to view and work with the process of adjustment.*

Introduction

Faced with the major life challenge of serious life-threatening illness, individuals vary in the way they view both the threat and the resources available to them. Similarly, from a psychotherapeutic perspective, social workers vary in the models, skills, and conceptualizations they use to help patients negotiate their illness journey.

This chapter will offer two broad models for psychotherapy found to be useful and adaptable to many palliative settings: meaning-based therapy and schema therapy. Each model is predicated on the belief that every patient is a social person existing within a system of others—a person of strength who brings resilience to the challenges he or she faces; a person with a past that informs his or her view of the present and contributes to the way the patient copes with challenge; and a person with a history, who is a member of a culture with specific values, roles, and practices to be understood and respected within any therapeutic setting. Each model suggests a different way of viewing personal challenges and offers different therapeutic methods. These therapeutic approaches, which have utility in both medical and mental health settings and in short- and long-term relationships, were developed to help people at different junctures of their lives meet their core human needs in healthy, adaptive, and effective ways.

A Meaning-Based Model for Psychotherapy in the Palliative Setting

Part of the clinical complexity of social work in the palliative setting is that life-limiting illness can be experienced simultaneously as suffering and as a trigger to seek meaning in the experience (Lethborg, Aranda, Bloch, & Kissane, 2006). While suffering may be an expected component of the illness experience, the role of meaning may be less apparent. Recent research suggests, however, that meaning may well have a significant role in the adjustment process of living with a life-threatening illness (Breitbart et al., 2010; Lee, 2008; Lethborg, Aranda, & Kissane, 2007; Park, Edmondson, Fenster, & Blank, 2008). This section aims to discuss the role of meaning in the setting of palliative care from the perspective of the illness experience of the patient and the clinical perspective of the social worker.

"Meaning" in this context refers to the process of making sense of life situations and deriving purpose from existence (Speck, Higginson, & Addington-Hall, 2004, p. 124). The term thus has a cognitive and an existential component; "making sense" relates to how the person *understands* his or her current circumstances and "deriving purpose" relates to the aspects of a person's life that are most *significant* to that person.

Making Sense of Life Circumstances

The cognitive perspective of meaning focuses on the thought processes individuals use in their life. Central to making sense of a situation is the way a person views the world and his or her place in it. This view becomes the lens through which appraisal of situations occurs. Thus, the set of assumptions a person holds about the world forms the background from which the cognitive aspect of meaning originates. This individual's worldview is pertinent in that he or she approaches life challenges such as a serious illness with a preconceived viewpoint about how events are regulated and where their energies should be directed.

A person's worldview also provides them with a sense of equilibrium in the way he or she processes experiences. As such, it incorporates a degree of "illusion of invulnerability," a sense that bad things will not happen (Janoff-Bulman, 1989, p. 116). When a traumatic event occurs, this illusion is often stripped away, leaving the person with the reality of mortality and ultimate aloneness. A life event such as a serious illness may then challenge this sense of stability and threaten beliefs and values. In particular, a person's assumptions that life has meaning, that the world is safe, and that he or she has worth may be tested in the face of trauma and suffering, prompting a need to regain a sense of equilibrium by searching for a coherence in the experience that stabilizes the self (Antonovsky, 1987). The need for stability in the way a person views the world and understands the events that occur thus forms a motivation or drive to find meaning. Hence, a central task in living with serious illness may involve an effort to integrate the severity of the situation with the way the person's world is understood (Frankl, 1963; Puchalski, 1999).

Deriving Purpose from Existence

The existential component of meaning is associated with fulfilment in life and the drive to live a life that has purpose.

Frankl (1963) described the "will to meaning" as an innate drive to find value in personal existence, especially in the face of suffering (Frankl, 1963, p. 98). For some, this motivation to find meaning emanates from the belief that life is a gift, and that the goal is to live it with meaning and authenticity (Hartman & Zimberoff, 2003). The tendency toward acquisition of meaning then is driven by the need to have a depth to life beyond merely existing (Yalom, 1980).

Sources of meaning vary in response to each person's worldview; they can be found by feeling a connectedness with God or a higher being (Benzein & Saveman, 1998; Halstead & Mickley, 1997), through the arts, family, work, money, or other people (Dyson, Cobb, & Forman, 1997; Oldnall, 1996).

While living with a life-threatening illness does not necessarily mean that one accepts death as an inevitable outcome, it commonly brings to the fore notions of existence, purpose, and meaning. In this setting, the reality of death is difficult to avoid, and it is more likely to become a focus as one searches for true meaning and purpose. "The sacred nature of life finds an unequalled focus in its conclusion," Cobb (2001) states, "which is why, for many people, dying and death are holy ground because of the intensity they bring to what is precious and meaningful" (p. 49).

Loss of Meaning

An inability to find meaning in the experience of living with illness can result in profound despair, loss of joy, and disconnection with life. Neimeyer (2000) suggests; "For those who seek meaning and find none, the loss can be excruciating, and data suggest that they report intense suffering on a variety of outcome measures" (p. 349). Indeed, loss of meaning in life has been found to be a factor in suicide, especially in the elderly (MacKinlay, 1997). As Frankl (1985) suggested, "Man is not destroyed by suffering, but by suffering without meaning" (p. 133).

Meaning in the Palliative Setting

Meaning as a concept is thus important when working with patients and their families. Gaining an understanding of how to view life circumstances (cognitive meaning) and balancing suffering and loss with significant relationships and experiences (existential meaning) are important goals for patients and families in this context. Nietzsche's (1844–1900) famous quote, "He who has a why to live can bear almost any how" (as quoted in Frankl, 1985, p. 97) offers a summary of the power of meaning in adjustment. Finding meaning in suffering can involve a period of intense growth, even self-transformation. People living with life-threatening illness may talk about reprioritization of goals, changed lifestyles and values, increased appreciation for nature and others, and spiritual development (Lutha & Cicchetti, 2000). The life review prompted by suffering often accounts for a positive reframing of what is significant in life. Anne Frank (1953) in the moving diaried account of her Holocaust experience talked about realizing the simple things, such as the sky, walking outside, fresh air, that we take for granted. It is often the meaning attached to life, rather than to the length of time remaining, that becomes important (Nuland, 1994). Indeed, finding fulfilment in life regardless of the experience of illness has been found to have a buffering effect, protecting against depression and hopelessness in those facing the end of life (Breitbart et al., 2000; Nelson, 2002).

Meaning-Based Psychotherapy

The complexity around meaning in the palliative setting calls for a range of therapeutic modalities when intervening with a meaning focus. Six main principles inform this approach (see Table 18.1).

From these principles, meaning-based psychotherapy focuses on the need people have for meaning and purpose, connection with others, to make sense of their situation, to have purpose and authenticity in their lives, and to "take a break" from suffering.

Overview of Meaning-Based Interventions

Understanding that the context of meaning is specific to the individual, meaning-based psychotherapy begins with the patient's narrative. The clinician draws out the patient's unique experience of illness as it relates to his or her view of the world. Balancing the need to debrief and understand suffering with the need to find meaning and purpose, the therapist uses cognitive and existential strategies. Narrative processes are used to elicit the expression of existential pain and suffering, the

processing of a life that has been disrupted, and to enhance dignity by enabling the patient to share who he or she is as a unique person. Meaning-based cognitive therapeutic interventions are used to amplify a sense of coherence (through the use of positive reappraisal), to increase the appreciation of and gratitude for what is meaningful in life (through finding benefit in their experiences), and promoting self-efficacy, acceptance of external support and care, and the aim of living life fully (through revising beliefs and goals). Though the acknowledgement of suffering is an important aspect of this work, meaning-based therapeutic techniques are used to shift attention away from this suffering to something meaningful in the person's life and to a greater concentration on meaning in life as a whole. Concurrently, the clinician listens for opportunities to strengthen interpersonal connections by exploring how individuals view themselves, their significance, and their goals in relation to others.

This narrative focus runs throughout meaning-based psychotherapy as the patient's unique story forms the basis of each session. Narrative therapy centers people as the experts in their own lives (Morgan, 2000). People have stories that include the events of their life, family, relationships, culture, work, achievements, losses, regrets, and so on. The narrative of a person's life is the thread that draws these stories together. Meanings are attributed based on the person's own interpretation, and this individualized focus serves as the context that frames the person's unique worldview.

Understanding the way in which people view their lives and the events that occur is the landscape within which clinicians identify and validate the natural use of positive reappraisal, and the process of finding benefit and revising beliefs and goals (Park & Folkman, 1997) that people often describe in their narratives. Where a person offers a positive view of an event, for example, the clinician highlights this view and feeds back the fact that the person has *chosen* a way of considering his or her experiences that encourages adjustment. In addition, the therapist makes suggestions of alternative views, goals, and beliefs for patients to consider.

Table 18.1.
Principles to Guide Meaning-Based Psychotherapy

Principles to Guide Meaning-Based Psychotherapy	References
Human beings have a propensity toward meaning—a will to meaning.	(Frankl, 1963)
We are driven to find fulfilment and significance in life.	(Davis et al., 1998)
In a stressful situation, making sense assists in the process of coping.	(Antonovsky, 1987)
The way a person makes sense of his or her world is generally prejudiced by the need for stability in life and an optimistic bias.	(Janoff-Bulman, 1989)
We are social beings who need to feel significance and a sense of belonging.	(Suchman & Matthews, 1988)
Those who lose meaning or are unable to find meaning in suffering can experience profound despair.	(Kissane, Clarke, & Street, 2001)

Meaning-Based Psychotherapy in Practice

The overall goal of meaning-based psychotherapy is to assist patients to access the meaning in their lives and to empower them to focus on meaning in spite of suffering. Meaning-based psychotherapy is thus a directive therapy in that the therapist actively works with the patient to direct attention toward meaning and purpose. The use of questions is important to guide an individualized exploration of the patient's unique meaning. The therapist might start by explaining the concepts of meaning and purpose. For example:

> When we talk about "meaning" we are referring to the things, people, and experiences that are significant or important to you in your life. "Purpose" refers to the intention of your life, the things you have aimed for, your goals, and the reasons why you have done the things you have done in your life.

The therapist may also ask:

> I am interested in your story, how your illness has impacted on your life, and how your life has changed since your diagnosis.

Within this discussion, questions are asked to discover how the patient experiences the world, his or her place in it, the people important to the patient, and whether the patient's illness has created a discontinuity and fracture in his or her life story. Individual *sources* of meaning are helpful to explore. The clinician is both guided by the participant's narrative and may also ask about specific themes to guide the unfolding of the patient's unique story.

Other questions that may be used to explore meaning and purpose include the following:

> What is meaningful in your life?
> What gives you the greatest joy?
> What ordinary moments do you treasure?
> What gets you out of bed in the morning?

When specific areas of meaning are identified, questions can again be used to focus further on those areas deemed significant to the patient, such as:

> It sounds like these are the things that are important to you and enrich your life? Would you agree? Can you tell me more about that?
> I am interested in what aspects of your life you would like to increase or encourage in order to enhance meaning and purpose.

One of the challenging and rich aspects of meaning-based therapy is that the unique nature of meaning makes the work with each patient so varied. The two patient narratives illustrate this uniqueness (see Box 18.1 and Box 18.2).

Box 18.1
Patient/Family Narrative: Anna

Anna, age 39, was a young mother of a 4-year-old boy, happily married and in the middle of renovating her home when she was diagnosed with advanced breast cancer. Treatment did not contain the cancer's growth. Anna asked to see the social worker for counselling and wanted to pursue the process of "finishing up." Meaning-based interventions were used to undertake life review and to draw out the specific areas of her life of most significance, using these as the focus for goal setting. Anna was remarkably at peace with the inevitability of her premature death but felt strongly that she "did it well" in that she "made the most of her life, however long." In drawing a focus on the relationships most important in her life, she noted that she had never had a family portrait done. She also wanted a portrait of herself—something she had always dreamed of. A weekend at her family's farm with a photographer friend created a forum to celebrate the closeness of her relationships and produced the legacy she desired: a book of photographs for those she would eventually leave behind.

Meaning-based therapy in the palliative setting is not about putting a positive spin on the suffering of life-limiting illness; rather, it provides an alternative focus to balance suffering and meaning and to illuminate those aspects of a person's life deemed to be central to the person's sense of significance and purpose.

Box 18.2
Patient/Family Narrative: Ed

Ed, a 73-year-old high court judge was struggling with the inevitability of his retirement as his lymphoma progressed. During his interview with the social worker, he was agitated and stated that he would rather die than have to focus on life as a sick person. The social worker persevered with questions about Ed's life, achievements, and interests. Ed shared that while he had achieved career and financial success, he had never felt the sense of authenticity that comes with being able to "be yourself." He regretted being absent from his children's early lives and found it hard to know what to do with himself now that his work was gone. He shared a number of stories about time spent at the family's beach house—as a child and then while raising his own children. As he spoke about this house, the coast, the beach, and in particular sailing, he had a different energy in his voice and was more alert and animated in his body. When the social worker pointed this out, Ed admitted that his "secret desire" was to be a boat builder and that this would have been preposterous to his father if he had ever mentioned it. After two sessions exploring this love of the ocean and sailing and life choices Ed had made to please others, he decided to move to the beach house and build a boat. Not a grand sailing ship, but a fine boat all the same, and he wanted to have "the hands of all the people he loved" involved in the making of this boat.

A Schema Therapy Model of Psychotherapy in the Palliative Setting

An individual's means of coping with pain, suffering, and loss is perhaps best predicted by the person's ways of coping with previous loss and pain. While nothing fully prepares an individual to face life-threatening illness, certain constructs may help determine how a person is likely to appraise and cope with this challenge. Schema therapy developed by Jeffrey Young, PhD, as an outgrowth of cognitive therapy offers a unified model of psychotherapy incorporating elements of Gestalt therapy, object relations and attachment theory, self-psychology, and interpersonal neurobiology. This model provides a framework for understanding an

individual's and family's response to pain, suffering, and impending loss, while also guiding a psychotherapeutic response to both psychological/psychiatric symptomatology and coping efforts.

Early Maladaptive Schemas

In the language of psychotherapy, a schema can be understood as an organizing principle for understanding one's life and life experience. Often these schemas are constructed early in life and may be elaborated upon over time. Schemas when adaptive can be useful ways of organizing and understanding one's view of oneself, one's world, and one's future. When maladaptive, however, they can become anachronistic or distorted constructs that are no longer relevant, and they may confound effective coping and undermine effective behavior. Schema therapy explores and intervenes with *early maladaptive schemas* (Young, Klosko, & Weishaar, 2003), which are understood as "self-defeating emotional and cognitive patterns that begin early in our development and repeat throughout life." An early maladaptive schema can be understood as follows:

- A broad, pervasive theme or pattern
- Comprised of memories, emotions, cognitions, and bodily sensations
- Regarding oneself and one's relationships with others
- Developed during childhood or adolescence
- Elaborated throughout one's lifetime
- Dysfunctional to a significant degree (Young et al., 2003)

Maladaptive behaviors are viewed as responses to these schemas.

Schemas form in childhood or adolescence as reality-driven representations of a child's experiences and environment. They are frequently accurate and useful constructs that help the child make order of his or her life and develop a sense of stability and predictability in a functional way. These schemas lead to a set of behavioral responses that may be extremely adaptive to the child, but when applied to adult life, mature relationships, and different demands may become highly dysfunctional, contributing to depression and anxiety as well as to the development of personality disorders, including borderline and narcissistic personality disorders. Maladaptive schemas can also lead to difficulty accurately understanding a stressful environment.

Development of Early Maladaptive Schemas

According to Dr. Young, early maladaptive schemas develop in response to unmet core emotional needs in childhood.

Table 18.2.
Schemas Organized by Domains

Schema Domain	Early Maladaptive Schema
Disconnection and rejection	Abandonment/instability
	Mistrust/abuse
	Emotional deprivation
	Defectiveness/shame
	Social isolation/alienation
Impaired autonomy and performance	Dependence/incompetence
	Vulnerability to harm or illness
	Enmeshment/undeveloped self
	Failure
Impaired limits	Entitlement/grandiosity
	Insufficient self-control/self-discipline
Other-directedness	Subjugation
	Self-sacrifice
	Approval-seeking/recognition-seeking
Overvigilance and inhibition	Negativity/pessimism
	Emotional inhibition
	Unrelenting standards/hypercriticalness
	Punitiveness

Source: Table adapted with information from Young et al., 2003.

Schema therapy delineates five core emotional needs, which correspond to "schema domains":

- Secure attachments to others (includes safety, stability, nurturance, and acceptance)
- Autonomy, competence, and a sense of identity
- Freedom to express valid needs and emotions
- Spontaneity and play
- Realistic limits and self-control

Early maladaptive schemas develop when these core emotional needs are not met in a consistent, reliable way. Innate temperament and childhood environment are believed to converge to either gratify or frustrate these basic universal needs. Schema therapy focuses on helping people find adaptive ways to meet core needs that were not adequately met in childhood. In the face of life-threatening illness, these core emotional needs may assume a more poignant and immediate importance.

Early Maladaptive Schemas and Schema Domains

This model identifies 18 early maladaptive schemas, which are organized into five "schema domains," each of which relates to a set of core unmet childhood emotional needs (Young et al., 2003). The 18 schemas, organized by the five domains, are shown in Table 18.2.

For the purposes of this chapter those schemas will be highlighted that most often impact patients and families as they integrate and adapt to life-threatening illness.

The Process and Practice of Schema Therapy

The overarching goal of schema therapy is to help patients find adaptive and effective ways to meet their core emotional needs. To achieve this, the clinician helps the patient to promote psychological awareness of the memories, emotions, body sensations, cognitions, and coping styles that comprise the patient's schemas. This understanding promotes the ability to control or modify behavior, create healthy environments, increase conscious control over schemas, and weaken the power of the memories, thoughts, feelings, and behavior that emerge when a schema is evoked. Schema therapists believe that the way(s) people respond to their schemas actually *prevents* them from meeting these core needs, thus reinforcing the distorted perception that embodies the schema. In daily life, and particularly in acute situations (including life-threatening illness), schemas can be either *perpetuated*, that is, reinforced; or *healed*, meaning that *maladaptive coping styles*, cognitive, affective, and behavioral, are weakened and replaced with healthy, adaptive, and effective ways of coping with stressors and "triggers." Traditionally schema therapy proceeds from an assessment and education phase to a change phase.

Assessment and Education Phase

In this phase patients are educated about the concept of schemas and helped to understand how these schemas have and/or can interfere with their functioning, relationships, and general well-being. Once an assessment has been completed, a schema conceptualization is formulated and schema-focused goals are established. In the palliative care setting social workers may meet patients early in their illness, and fully assess schemas, or meet them later in the disease process in which assessment is abbreviated and specifically targeted to identify schema activation and responses which are elicited by the illness, symptoms, and/or end-of-life issues. These interventions become relevant in so far as schemas interfere with immediate issues such as treatment, decision making, or coping with related psychosocial stresses.

Change Phase

In the change phase of treatment the clinician incorporates cognitive, experiential, behavioral, and interpersonal strategies to heal schemas and promote healthy and adaptive efforts to help the patient meet his or core needs.

Cognitive techniques much like those used in traditional cognitive therapy include the use of Socratic questioning. Schema validity will be tested rationally, looking for alternative or more likely explanations for the past experiences explained by the schema. Patients are helped to understand how and why the schema developed and to appreciate how its past utility and accuracy may no longer be relevant. Schema flashcards are among the tools that may be used to reinforce new cognitive understanding.

Experiential techniques, including imagery, dialogues, and writing, encourage the patient to address and battle schemas from a more emotion-activated state. Through dialogues patients' "rational" sides may debate the schema side. In imagery patients may reexperience the traumatic experiences that contributed to the development of the schema and come to a more accurate, less distorted comprehension of the traumatic event. In imagery the therapist and patient may battle with the schema or engage with the person who promoted the patient's distorted self-appraisal.

Behavioral pattern-breaking offers patients the opportunity to achieve different results and reactions in their lives as they experiment with new, more adaptive behaviors instead of repeating the maladaptive behaviors they have come to rely upon. This may involve different partner selection or life choices, different ways of responding to perceived rejection or criticism, or asserting one's wants, needs, and preferences (to name a few).

The therapist–patient relationship is a fundamental component of the change process. The relationship itself may serve to combat some schema-driven beliefs. The use of *limited reparenting*, providing the patient with what he or she did not receive from his or her parents in childhood (*within the appropriate bounds of the therapeutic relationship*) helps heal schemas.

Empathic confrontation in which the therapist shows compassion and empathy for patient's schemas when they arise in reaction to the therapist, while identifying ways that the patient's responses are distorted or dysfunctional is a prominent tool in schema therapy.

Schema Therapy in Palliative Care

Life-threatening illness, pain, suffering, and confrontation with mortality are likely to activate schemas that may be a regular part of a patient's experience or may have been dormant until the trauma of this life event elicits their expression. Because patients in the palliative care context need to rely on others, including family, friends, physicians, nurses, and social workers, to receive the care they need, patients with schemas in the domain of disconnection and rejection could be "triggered" by their illness and the reliance it creates.

A patient with abandonment/instability schema assumes:
> *instability or unreliability of those available for support and connection (Young et al., 2003)*

These patients may have particular difficulty adapting to a teaching hospital in which physicians and medical teams "rotate" the care of a patient. Similarly the transition from disease-modifying interventions to hospice care, and the movement from one health care team to another, may be particularly difficult for patients with this schema. Confrontation with mortality is a challenge for patients facing life-threatening illness, but for the patient with abandonment/instability schema the ability to sustain relationships in the setting of anticipated separation and potential abandonments may be particularly difficult. An understanding of this schema and ways of coping with it may enable the health care team as well as the family to heighten efforts to provide a stable schedule of care, with as much consistency of personnel as possible.

Patients with mistrust abuse schema expect:
> *that others will hurt, abuse, humiliate, cheat, lie, manipulate or take advantage ... usually involves the perception that the harm is intentional or the result of unjustified and extreme negligence (Young et al., 2003, p. 14)*

These patients are likely to have difficulty relying upon the health care team and their family. These patients may have difficulty trusting that they are getting the "right" care and may become nonadherent, abrasive, or accusatory when provoked by symptoms that do not abate as quickly or readily as they expect. If it is understood that these patients are not being "difficult," but that they are reacting to a set of learned, albeit distorted, assumptions about what they can expect from others, the health care team may have an easier time tolerating the mistrust and providing additional information and reassurance to help these patients feel safe. Patients who are able to come to understand the reasons for their global mistrust may be able to separate past abuses from the current efforts of others to truly be helpful.

Patients with an emotional deprivation schema expect:
> *that one's desire for a normal degree of emotional support: nurturing, empathy and protection will not be adequately met by others (Young et al., 2003, p. 14)*

These patients may experience an *intense* sense of loneliness and isolation. While it may be common for patients to feel alone in their suffering, or abandoned and helpless when disease-modifying treatments are discontinued, these feelings may be heightened in people with emotional deprivation schema. They may withdraw or isolate in response to these beliefs/feelings. Neither the health care team nor the well-meaning family and friends may understand this, and consequently they may respond to the patient's withdrawal by "respecting their boundaries" and distancing from the patient rather than seeking ways to provide the emotional care that the patient yearns for but believes he or she can never receive.

Patients with defectiveness/shame schema feel:
> *defective, bad, unwanted, inferior, or invalid in important respects, or that one would be unlovable to significant others if exposed (Young et al., 2003, p. 14)*

These patients may experience a diagnosis of cancer or HIV as validation of the feeling that there is something *within them* that is "bad," "defective," or "malignant" for which they have reason to be ashamed. They may be more prone to depression, helplessness, and withdrawal if their shame over their illness and condition eclipses other experiences and beliefs. These patients may be misunderstood, potentially by themselves and others, and described as "melodramatic," self-indulgent, or "having a pity-party," all of which further reinforces their feelings of shame and defectiveness and perhaps triggering a response to an emotional deprivation schema. Helpful interventions include cognitive reframing, education about illness, and imagery with the vulnerable child part of themselves that was "taught" that they were "defective."

From the domain of other-directedness,

Patients with self-sacrifice schema maintain:
> *excessive focus on voluntarily meeting the needs of others in daily situations at the expense of one's own gratification ... to avoid guilt from feeling selfish or to maintain the connection with others perceived as needy (Young et al., 2003, p. 16)*

Patients with subjugation schema experience:
excessive surrendering of control to others, feeling
coerced and submitting in order to avoid anger,
retaliation or abandonment (Young et al., 2003, p. 16)

These patients may find it exceedingly difficult to rely on others for care. This difficulty may result in nonadherence with treatment, unsafe or help-rejecting behaviors, or impaired judgment or decision making. Helping patients accept a healthy sense of entitlement to and comfort with *receiving* good care from family, friends, and the health care team is essential to safe and effective medical care. Patients in this situation can be helped by cognitive, behavioral, and experiential interventions as well as by the corrective emotional experience of limited reparenting.

Patients with schemas in the domain of impaired
autonomy or performance may present with a
dependence/incompetence schema and believe:
that one is unable to handle one's everyday responsibilities
in a competent manner, without considerable help from
others. ... (Young et al., 2003, p. 15)

Often presenting as helplessness, these individual are challenged by treatment decisions, medical/nursing instruction and have difficulty adhering to self-care regimens. It is important for the treatment team to understand this behavior as a lack of confidence, skill, or experience to make decisions or accept responsibility in a normal way. They may require additional time, guidance, and support from the treatment team.

Persons with vulnerability to harm or illness schema
have:
exaggerated fear that imminent catastrophe will strike
at any time and that one will be unable to prevent it
(Young et al., 2003, p. 15)

Consequently the diagnosis of a life-threatening illness may seem to confirm the validity of the schema-driven cognitive distortion. These patients may be particularly fearful, negative, and difficult to reassure. Their exaggerated fear may result in alarm, apprehension, and sensitivity to treatment side effects and complications. They may misinterpret normal sensations and effects as serious threats to their health and well-being, and respond with frequent anxious calls to the treatment team and visits to the emergency room. They are helped by very available and consistent support and education that is repeated and reinforced over time.

In the palliative care setting, the needs of patients and families may be acute, intense, and highly emotionally charged. The schema therapy framework for understanding and intervening with people's needs, pain, and suffering offers social workers across settings a rapid way to understand patients'/families' responses to their situation and to assist team members to depersonalize their reactions and respond therapeutically. It provides clear and targeted ways to effectively help people at this vulnerable time to receive care that is not only medically/socially effective but also helps them to meet the core needs reawakened or intensified by pain, suffering, and life-threatening illness.

Conclusion

I am about to take my last voyage, a great leap in the dark.
— *Thomas Hobbes, 1679*

Working in the palliative care setting offers professionals the opportunity to affect people's voyage into a world that is unfamiliar; a world that includes fear and suffering but may also include comfort, clarity, and meaning. Viewed this way it is imperative that skilled and competent clinicians approach this population in a way that systematically identifies needs and provides an avenue toward meeting these needs with compassion and understanding.

LEARNING EXERCISE
FOR MEANING-BASED THERAPY

Meaning-based interventions do not focus on the illness as such but rather on the things that are meaningful and significant in the person's life. The next time you are talking with a patient about their lived experience, ask questions such as:

- When are you most fulfilled/happy/authentic?
- What is it about that time that makes you feel that way?
- Is there a way you can have more of those times?

Focus on who the person is aside from the illness—telling the person directly that it can be helpful to put the illness aside for the moment because he or she is more than the illness. You may also like to ask yourself these questions and see whether you are able to create more meaningful times in your own life. It can be an important aspect of sustaining yourself.

LEARNING EXERCISES
IN SCHEMATHERAPY

1. Imagine that you have an emotional deprivation schema and believe with all of your being that no one can or will ever meet your needs for understanding, support, guidance, and nurturing. Picture yourself moving through your "normal" day—going to work, meeting friends or family, having a meal, running some errands. How do you see your emotional deprivation schema being triggered by these routine activities? How do you imagine you may respond to the schema as it arises?

2. Imagine that you have a defectiveness/shame schema that informs you that there is something inherently wrong with you, defective, not good enough, unlovable. Speak for that schema-driven part of yourself. Now get into a different chair and speak for your "healthy adult self," which does not believe the distortions of the schema. Let that healthy part tell the schema why it is wrong, that you are not unlovable—use examples of people who do/have loved you. Refute the argument of the schema through examples of times you were "good enough" and achieved goals or were well-regarded by yourself or others. Return to the "schema chair" and argue the schema side—continue debate until the schema part surrenders—How defective/shameful do you feel in this moment? Is your belief in the schema in any way shaken?

ADDITIONAL RESOURCES AND WEB SITES

BOOKS

Arntz, A., & Van Genderen, H. (2009). *Schema therapy for borderline personality disorder.* West Sussex, England: Wiley-Blackwell.

Behary, W. T. (2008). *Disarming the narcissist: Surviving and thriving with the self-absorbed.* Oakland, CA: New Harbinger Publications.

Young, J. E. (1990, 1999). *Cognitive therapy for personality disorders: A schema-focused approach.* (rev. ed.). Sarasota, FL: Professional Resource Press.

> *This is the original book describing schema therapy. It includes the basic rationale, theory, intervention strategies, and an extended case study based on schema therapy. The book is very succinct and nontechnical, and provides the underlying basis for the entire approach.*

Young, J. E., & Klosko, J. S. (1993, 1994). *Reinventing your life.* New York: Plume Books.

> *This popular self-help book based on Young's schema approach is essential reading for both the practitioner and client. The book includes detailed descriptions of the 11 most common life traps (schemas), including specific treatment techniques, the most common childhood origins, partner choices, self-defeating behavior patterns, self-help exercises, and extensive case vignettes. Written in easy-to-understand language, this book serves as an ideal client's guide to schema therapy.*

JOURNAL ARTICLES

Giesen-Bloo, J., van Dyck, R., Spinhoven, P., van Tilburg, W., Dirksen, C., van Asselt, T ... Arntz, A. (2006). Outpatient psychotherapy for borderline personality disorder: Randomized trial of schema-focused therapy vs. transference-focused psychotherapy. *Archives of General Psychiatry, 63,* 649–658.

WEB SITES

Center for Schema Therapy: http://www.schematherapy.com
International Society of Schema Therapy: http://isst-online.com/

REFERENCES

Antonovsky, A. (1987). *Unravelling the mystery of health: How people manage stress and stay well* San Fransisco, CA: Jossey-Bass.

Benzein, E., & Saveman, B. (1998). One step towards the understanding of hope: A concept analysis. *International Journal of Nursing Studies, 35*(6), 322–329.

Breitbart, W., Rosenfeld, B., Gibson, C., Pessin, H., Poppito, S., Nelson, C.,... Olden, M. (2010). Meaning-centered group psychotherapy for patients with advanced cancer: A pilot randomized controlled trial. *Psycho-Oncology, 19,* 21–28.

Breitbart, W., Rosenfeld, B., Pessin, H., Kaim, M., Funesti-Esch, J., Galietta, M.,... Brescia, R. (2000). Depression, hopelessness, and desire for hastened death in terminally ill patients with cancer. *Journal of the American Medical Association, 284*(22), 2907–2911.

Cobb, M. (2001). *The dying soul - Spiritual care at the end of life.* Buckingham, Philadelphia: Open University Press.

Davis, C. G., Nolen-Hoeksema, S., & Larson, J. (1998). Making sense of loss and benefiting from the experience: Two construals of meaning. *Journal of Personality and Social Psychology, 75*(2), 561–574.

Dyson, J., Cobb, M., & Forman, D. (1997). The meaning of spirituality: A literature review. *Journal of Advanced Nursing, 26*(6), 1183–1188.

Frank, A. (1953). *The diary of a young girl.* New York, NY: Pocket Books.

Frankl, V. (1985). *Man's search for meaning.* New York, NY: Washington Square Press.

Frankl, V. E. (1963). *Man's search for meaning: An introduction to logotherapy.* (Originally published in 1946 as Ein Psycholog erlebt das Konzentrationslager). New York, NY: Washington Square Press.

Halstead, M. T., & Mickley, J. R. (1997). Attempting to fathom the unfathomable: Descriptive views of spirituality. *Seminars in Oncology Nursing, 13,* 225–230.

Hartman, D., & Zimberoff, M. A. (2003). The existential approach in heart-centred therapies. *Journal of Heart-Centred Therapies, 6*(1), 3–46.

Janoff-Bulman, R. (1989). Assumptive worlds and the stress of traumatic events: Applications of the schema construct (Special Issue). *Social Cognition. 7*(2), 113–136.

Kissane, D., Clarke, D. M., & Street, A. F. (2001). Demoralization syndrome—a relevant psychiatric diagnosis for palliative care. *Journal of Palliative Care, 17,* 12–21.

Lee, V. (2008). The existential plight of cancer: Meaning making as a concrete approach to the intangible search for meaning. *Supportive Cancer Care, 16*(7), 779–785.

Lethborg, C., Aranda, S., Bloch, S., & Kissane, D. (2006). The role of meaning in advanced cancer- integrating the constructs of assumptive world, sense-of-coherence and meaning based coping. *Journal of Psychosocial Oncology, 24*(1), 27–42.

Lethborg, C., Aranda, S., & Kissane, D. (2007). To what extent does meaning mediate adaptation to cancer?—The relationship between physical suffering, meaning in life and connection to others in adjustment to cancer. *Palliative and Supportive Care*, 5(4), 377–388.

Lutha, S. S., & Cicchetti, D. (2000). The construct of resilience: Implications for interventions and social policies. *Development and Psychopathology*, 12(4), 857–885.

MacKinlay, E. (1997). Ageing, spirituality and the nursing role. In S. Ronaldson (Ed.), *Spirituality: The heart of nursing* (pp. 99–118). Melbourne, Australia: Ausmed Publications.

Morgan, A. (2000). *What is narrative therapy? An easy to read introduction*. Adelaide, Australia: Dulwich Centre Publications.

Neimeyer, R. A. (2000). Searching for the meaning of meaning: Grief therapy and the process of reconstruction. *Death Studies*, 24, 541–558.

Nelson, C., Rosenfeld, B., Breitbart, W., & Galietta, M. (2002). Spirituality, religion and depression in the terminally ill. *Psychosomatics*, 43, 213–220.

Nuland, S. (1994). *How we die: Reflections on life's final chapter*. New York, NY: Alfred A Knopf.

Oldnall, A. (1996). A critical analysis of nursing: Meeting the spiritual needs of patients. *Journal of Advanced Nursing*, 23, 138–144.

Park, C., Edmondson, D., Fenster, J., & Blank, T. (2008). Meaning making and psychological adjustment following cancer: The mediating roles of growth, life meaning, and restored just-world beliefs. *Journal of Consulting and Clinical Psychology*, 76(5), 863–875.

Park, C., & Folkman, S. (1997). Meaning in the context of stress and coping. *Review of General Psychology*, 1(2), 115–144.

Puchalski, C. M. (1999). Touching the spirit: The essence of healing. *Spiritual Life*, (Fall), 155–159.

Speck, P., Higginson, I., & Addington-Hall, J. (2004). Spiritual Needs in Health Care. *British Medical Journal*, 329, 123–124.

Suchman, A., & Matthews, D. (1988). What makes the patient-doctor relationship therapeutic? Exploring the connexional dimension of medical care. *Annals of Internal Medicine*, 108, 125–130.

Yalom, I. (1980). *Existential psychotherapy*. New York, NY: Basic Books.

Young, J. E., Klosko, J. S., & Weishaar, M. (2003). *Schema therapy: A practitioner's guide*. New York, NY: Guilford Publications.

19 *Dona J. Reese*

Spirituality and Social Work Practice in Palliative Care

Why would God do this to me?

Key Concepts

- *Spirituality is the most important way of coping for many patients, families, and their intimate network.*
- *Confrontation with a life-threatening illness can spur spiritual growth in patients, families, their intimate network, and the staff who work with them.*
- *Palliative social workers have an important role in addressing spirituality with clients.*
- *Spirituality can be defined in two dimensions: (1) philosophy of life, which is an intellectual dimension that includes philosophical, religious, nonreligious, and existential perspectives; and (2) unity consciousness, which is an experiential dimension that includes direct spiritual experience.*
- *Transpersonal social work, Jungian theory, the biopsychosocial-spiritual model of care, along with deep ecology, can provide frameworks for interventions.*

Introduction

Spirituality has always been an important aspect of the palliative care movement in the United States. In the past two decades, spirituality has been recognized as an important area for intervention in social work practice. What is spirituality? What are the spiritual concerns that arise for patients and families in palliative care, and what are models for addressing it? How does a social worker know when to address a spiritual concern and when to refer to a spiritual caregiver on the palliative care team? This chapter provides guidance for this important area of practice.

From the beginning of the hospice and palliative care movement in the United States, its leaders have advocated for a holistic approach that addresses biopsychosocial-spiritual needs. Medicare regulations for hospice certification require an interdisciplinary team that includes a spiritual caregiver. The National Consensus Project for Quality Palliative Care (2009) has espoused eight domains of palliative care, one of which is spiritual, religious, and existential aspects of care. In 2009, an interdisciplinary Consensus Conference developed guidelines for spiritual care and recommended that all members of the palliative care team be trained in spiritual care and that a board-certified chaplain be included on the team (Puchalski et al., 2009). These guidelines call for evidence-based practice, including the following:

- Documented assessment and periodic reevaluation using standardized instruments
- Addressing needs in a manner consistent with patient and family cultural and religious values, including facilitating practices as desired by the patient and family
- Facilitating contacts with religious leaders and communities desired by patient and family
- Documentation of the impact of spiritual interventions; services provided by professionals trained in pastoral care and spiritual issues that arise in life-threatening illness
- Referrals to professionals with specialized knowledge when appropriate (Puchalski et al., 2009, p. 887; see Table 19.1)

This requirement to address spirituality is justified by its importance as a way of coping for patients, families, friends,

Table 19.1.
Consensus Conference Guidelines for Spiritual Care within Palliative Care
Guideline 5.1 Spiritual and existential dimensions are assessed and responded to based upon the best available evidence, which is skillfully and systematically applied. Criteria: • The interdisciplinary team includes professionals with skill in assessment of and response to the spiritual and existential issues common to both pediatric and adult patients with life-threatening illnesses and conditions, and their families. These professionals should have education and appropriate training in pastoral care and the spiritual issues evoked by patients and families faced with life-threatening illness. • The regular assessment of spiritual and existential concerns is documented. This includes, but is not limited to, life review, assessment of hopes and fears, meaning, purpose, beliefs about afterlife, guilt, forgiveness, and life completion tasks. • Whenever possible a standardized instrument should be used to assess and identify religious or spiritual existential background, preferences, and related beliefs, rituals, and practices of the patient and family. • Periodic reevaluation of the impact of spiritual existential interventions and patient-family preferences should occur with regularity and be documented. Spiritual-existential care needs, goals, and concerns are addressed and documented, and support is offered for issues of life completion in a manner consistent with the individual's and family's cultural and religious values. • Pastoral care and other palliative care professionals facilitate contacts with spiritual religious communities, groups, or individuals, as desired by the patient and/or family. Of primary importance is that patients have access to clergy in their own religious traditions. • Professional and institutional use of religious-spiritual symbols is sensitive to cultural and religious diversity. • The patient and family are encouraged to display their own religious, spiritual, or cultural symbols. • The palliative care service facilitates religious or spiritual rituals or practices as desired by patient and family, especially at the time of death. • Referrals to professionals with specialized knowledge or skills in spiritual and existential issues are made when appropriate (Puchalski et al., 2009, p. 887)

or intimate networks and professional staff when a patient is facing life-threatening illness (Sessanna, 2008). In addition, the end of life may be seen as an additional life stage with spiritual developmental tasks, characterized by the potential for great spiritual growth for all, including the staffs who work with patients and their families (Seccareccia & Brown, 2009). There is also evidence that much of what patients and families want to discuss has to do with spirituality (Sheehan, 2003).

The National Hospice Social Work Survey conducted by Reese and Raymer found that 58% of a sample of 65 social workers in 65 hospices said they addressed spirituality with their interdisciplinary teams (Reese, 2001). Twenty-three percent of the social workers reported addressing spiritual issues directly with patients; but a chart review revealed that 62% of the social workers actually had addressed spiritual issues in counseling sessions with clients. In other words, the social workers were addressing spirituality without knowing it- they were unable to identify issues being discussed as spiritual in nature and reported a lack of training in spirituality in their social work education. This underscores the importance of training for social workers in addressing spirituality in practice. This chapter will help to address that need.

What Is Spirituality?

Definitions of spirituality within the social work literature usually reflect one or both of two dimensions. The *philosophy of life* dimension is intellectual in nature and has to do with worldview, values, and belief systems about the meaning and purpose of life and suffering. Both religious beliefs and non-religious worldviews, including existential perspectives, fit into this dimension. Philosophy of life becomes transcendent when it is focused on the welfare of all rather than one's own self-interest.

The *unity consciousness* dimension is transrational and experiential, referring to direct spiritual experience and a sense of relatedness to an Ultimate Reality. This dimension may be described as a feeling of unity with the totality of the universe, a sense of oneness with God, others, nature, and so forth, communication with the spiritual dimension, peace of mind, a sense of compassion, or a sense of awareness of one's higher or spiritual self. Unity consciousness is inherently transcendent, since it has to do with an awareness of existence beyond one's separate identity.

Canda (1990) defined spirituality as "the person's search for a sense of meaning and morally fulfilling relationships between oneself, other people, the encompassing universe, and the ontological ground of existence" (p. 13). The 2009 Consensus Conference developed the following definition:

> *Spirituality is the aspect of humanity that refers to the way individuals seek and express meaning and purpose and the way they experience their connectedness to the moment, to self, to others, to nature, and to the significant or sacred. (Puchalski et al., 2009, p. 3)*

Theoretical Frameworks

Transpersonal Social Work

Transpersonal social work encompasses spirituality as a universal aspect of human development, client strength, and an important area of attention in social work practice. Wilber (1996) described three stages of consciousness within spiritual development: (1) pre-egoic, in which a young child has no clear sense of a separate ego or identity; (2) egoic, in which a mature adult has a clear identity and role in society; and (3) transegoic, in which individuals are able to move beyond a focus on concerns of the separate ego and develop a holistic sense of union between the "ultimate" and the "ordinary." According to transpersonal social work, the transegoic stage of consciousness promotes an ability to cope with life-threatening illness, through the perspective that one's identity is more than one's separate body and ego.

Elizabeth Smith (1995) developed a model of therapy, the *transegoic model*, based on transpersonal theory. This model uses interventions designed to help clients develop an awareness of an identity that is broader than social roles and physical abilities. She discussed a patient and family narrative of a young woman dying of cancer. Through social work intervention, the woman was able to profoundly identify with nature and to learn to view her identity as connected to all, rather than limited to her physical body and its abilities (Smith, 1995). In addition to awareness of a transpersonal identity, transpersonal theory proposes that transpersonal experiences become more common for individuals who have reached the transegoic stage of development. Rather than being viewed necessarily as psychopathology, transpersonal theory explains these experiences as crucial to the self-fulfillment, healing, and transformation of individuals at the transegoic stage of spiritual development (Robbins, Canda, & Chatterjee, 1998). When facing life-threatening illness, patients experience spiritual growth and commonly report transpersonal experiences (Gibbs & Achterberg-Lawlis, 1978; Pflaum & Kelley, 1986). (See Box 19.1.)

In this example, evidence of transpersonal growth can be seen in both dimensions of spirituality, along with characteristics of the transpersonal stage of development. Within the philosophy of life dimension, a change can be seen from a lack of concern for others (not living a very moral life) to a more transcendent life purpose and belief system focused on the welfare of all (he now "prayed for everybody"). A change can also be seen within the unity consciousness dimension—the patient now had frequent direct spiritual experiences, receiving guidance from "the Lord."

For other patients and families, transpersonal experiences may not be an issue. A common Jewish perspective, for example, is to place primary importance on the life the patient has lived on this earth, without focus on an afterlife or a transpersonal dimension. In this spiritual view, the patient can find an equal degree of peace through appreciation of the meaning of a life well lived. The focus of spirituality from this perspective, then, may be more rooted in the philosophy of life dimension of spirituality. Theoretical perspectives and models other than transpersonal theory might be more appropriate for use with these patients and families—theory developed by Carl Jung, for example, which is discussed next.

Jungian Theory

Carl Jung described the psyche as a *personal* and *collective conscious* and *unconscious* (Jung, 1960). The collective conscious explains the concept of spiritual connection. Jung's *principle of opposites* describes humans as peaceful and warlike, loving and hating. The *conscious ego* represents much of what a person knows of himself or herself. The *persona* is the socialized presentation of the conscious self to the world. The *shadow*, a part of the unconscious, is where one hides the things one wishes to avoid in consciousness: fears, thoughts, and desires perceived as immoral. Becoming aware of unconscious content allows a patient to integrate the polarities and resolve *polarization* (Jung, 1960; Woodruff & Reese, 2005).

Goelitz (2001a, 2001b) has used a dream work model individually and in groups to help patients access unconscious thoughts and feelings that they might normally avoid acknowledging. The elements represented in patients' dreams have included healing as well as anxiety and vulnerability. The clinician trained in this approach guides the investigation into the personal meaning of the dream images, using Jung's technique of amplification. Amplification asks the patient to reexperience and reenact the dream using all the senses. This approach promotes access to the unconscious, through which healing then takes place. Goelitz (2001a) does caution that patients often reveal intimate content earlier than they normally would through the use of this approach. In some cases this could occur before a group has developed a strong sense of cohesion. The social worker should screen patients before using this model in a group setting, keeping this concern in mind.

Biopsychosocial-Spiritual Model of Care

The interdisciplinary Consensus Conference (Puchalski et al., 2009) developed a theoretical framework for spiritual

---

Box 19.1
Patient/Family Narrative: Jerry

Jerry died of chronic heart disease. His wife relates the following:
    Jerry died of a heart attack, and went through a black tunnel with a tiny light at the end. He saw Jesus Christ in the tunnel, handing him a note. Jerry had not lived a very moral life, and was afraid to look, because he was afraid the note would say he was going to Hell. He finally looked at the note, which said, "Follow me, I will show you the way." The note was signed, "Jesus Christ." At this point, Jerry spontaneously resuscitated, and was filled with the Holy Spirit. The bed was shaking; Jerry was shouting. Jerry was "saved" and "born again" after that day. The Lord gave him scriptures he should read in church. He was a different person; he prayed for everybody. He saw Jesus at the foot of the bed again that night, and knew everything would be O.K. He kept saying to his wife Shirley, "Can't you see him?" (Reese, 2001).

care, based on the work of Engel (1977), White and colleagues (1996), Jonas (2001), and Sulmasy (2006). This model is holistic, reflective of a systems perspective, focusing on the relational nature of life. The relationship between humans and themselves, others, nature, and the significant or sacred is considered spiritual. Illness is viewed as a disturbance in these relationships. The biopsychosocial-spiritual model looks at the spiritual history of a patient, whether religious or not, to add shape to his or her holistic identity. Illness strikes the whole person; interventions therefore focus on the biological, psychological, social, and spiritual dimensions. The Consensus Conference recommended a number of intervention techniques, which will be discussed later in this chapter. Deep ecology, discussed in the next section, is a similar articulation to the biopsychosocial-spiritual model.

Deep Ecology

Fred Besthorn (2001) applied deep ecology to social work practice. This theory is an expansion of systems theory to include the natural world and the spiritual dimension and naturally leads to a call for activism. On the micro level of practice, deep ecology can be used as a framework for expressing the pain caused by the split between humans and nature and the healing that is possible when synergy is again created. Through this approach, clients can use the transpersonal properties of nature to realize the transpersonal self, and to discover deeper purpose, meaning, and connection in their lives. Examples of intervention approaches include pet therapy, equine therapy, wilderness practice—which includes experiences with wild and pristine places as well as simple encounters with nature—and environmental meditation (Delaney & Barrere, 2009).

Addressing Spirituality in Palliative Care

Two patient/family narratives drawn from this author's experience as a hospice social worker illustrate how different the experience of life-threatening illness can be for different people. In the first example, *an elderly African American woman, Joan, felt at peace, her little dog resting on the bed with her, her church choir singing softly around her bed. Joan often mentioned God and I asked her once, "Do you feel the presence of God?" and she answered, "Oh, yes, all the time!"* In the second example, *a young white state policeman, Ed, who was extremely fearful of dying, asked his doctor to continue treatments to extend his life, but the doctor said he had already received everything available, and sent him to hospice, promising to call him if a new experimental treatment was developed. Ed became combative, punching the hospice staff if they came near, and died yelling, "Code 13! Code 13," which means "officer in distress!"*

Why was one person so peaceful, and one so anxious? What makes the difference and how can we help them? These two examples are quite distinct. Joan expressed a sense of the presence of God, which implies a sense of spirituality in the unity consciousness dimension. Ed, on the other hand, was younger, with a higher likelihood of some spiritual concerns, such as unfinished business and questions about the meaning and lack of justice exemplified by his terminal illness. Research indicates that spirituality reduces anxiety about death and life-threatening illness (Broderick, Birbilis, & Steger, 2008). To further delineate factors that may have influenced Joan and Ed's end of life, the following section will discuss aspects of experience that inform spirituality within palliative social work practice, including personal preparation, philosophy of practice, spiritual assessment, intervention with spirituality in palliative care, utilizing the spiritual dimension therapeutically, and cultural diversity considerations.

Personal Preparation

The 2009 Consensus Conference emphasized the importance of personal preparation. To prepare for effective work in this area, social workers must reflect upon their own perspectives and experiences within the two dimensions of spirituality: philosophy of life and unity consciousness. Self-awareness is a prerequisite to spiritually sensitive practice that honors diverse religious and nonreligious worldviews (Puchalski, 2002). One must examine one's own spiritual concerns, negative reactions, and stereotypes related to other perspectives; one's ability to support self-determination; and one's personal tendency to proselytize. In addition, knowledge of spiritual leaders, mentors, and resources in the community is invaluable.

Philosophy of Practice

Spiritual intervention in palliative social work starts with a philosophy of practice that views the patient and family members as sacred beings, a concept very similar to the social work value of dignity and worth of the person (National Association of Social Workers [NASW], 2008), and the foundation for a spiritually sensitive relationship. Some therapists suggest taking a moment just before a client session to "create a sacred space" (Lord, 2008), in which the social worker engages in a brief meditation and a belief statement: "I intend to perceive this client as a unique sacred being." Within this philosophy, patients and families are viewed as having unconditional worth and unlimited possibilities for growth, a perspective that creates an environment of attention and intention, no matter what the focus of intervention. Crises are seen as opportunity for growth; problems are understood within an awareness of and support for the possibility of spiritual development. The Consensus Conference asserts that transformation occurs within both the health care professional and the patient, and it emanates from the quality of the relationship, the spiritual self-awareness of the clinician, and the ability to learn the practice of "compassionate presence" with patients (Puchalski et al., 2009).

This spiritually sensitive relationship is characterized by a perspective that honors diversity and the ability to relate across belief systems. It includes skills in cooperating with diverse religious and nonreligious spiritual support systems. Similar to our approach to culture, spiritually sensitive practice respects differing worldviews, understands that the social worker's own perspective is only one of many in a very diverse world, and operates with the purpose of helping the patient and family to clarify their own views rather than imposing one's own belief system.

Spiritual Assessment

Assessment of spirituality is necessary in order to respond in a manner that is appropriate to the needs and belief system of the patient. Clinicians evolve an understanding of the client perspective in a variety of ways. Often patients and families tell stories that express spiritual experiences, beliefs, or concerns through metaphor or symbolic terms. An example may be a patient who expressed to the social worker that he was having dreams at night of leaping flames. The social worker explored this with the patient, wondering whether this reflected the religious concept of hell, and whether he had concerns related to punishment by God. She found that the patient was only comfortable discussing the symbols, not the possible meaning of these symbols. A spiritually sensitive social worker could recognize this as an expression of spiritual issues and possibly use the dreamwork approach discussed earlier if the patient expressed a desire to further his understanding of this dream.

In addition to exploring statements and thoughts raised spontaneously by the patient and family, the Consensus Conference recommended using validated scales to assess spirituality, including the following:

- FICA (adapted from Puchalski, 2006; Puchalski & Romer, 2000; See Table 19.2)
- SPIRIT (Ambuel, 2000; See Table 19.3)
- HOPE—*H* (sources of hope and meaning), *O* (organized religion), *P* (personal spirituality and practices, *E* (effects of medical care and end-of-life decisions) (Anandarajah & Hight, 2001)
- Domains of Spirituality, which was developed by leaders in the field of spirituality in social work (Nelson-Becker, Nakashima, & Canda, 2006)

The Social Work Assessment Tool (SWAT) is based on social work research, and it can be used to measure spiritual adjustment along with major psychosocial issues found to be predictive of hospice social work outcomes (Reese et al., 2006).

Finally, Hodge (2001) has developed a Framework for Spiritual Assessment that uses interview questions to explore *(1)* an initial narrative framework focusing on spiritual experiences throughout life, and *(2)* an interpretive anthropological framework discussing with the client the relationship between spirituality and affect, spiritual behavior, cognition (religious/spiritual beliefs), communion (relationship to the Ultimate), conscience (values, guilt, and forgiveness), and intuition.

In summary, important areas to address in a spiritual assessment include the belief system of the patient and family, spiritual issues and concerns, functional and dysfunctional use of religion, and spiritual development. These aspects will be discussed next.

Belief system. Knowledge of the belief system of the patient and family allows the social worker to gear interventions toward the patient and family's point of view. This inquiry might include spiritual, religious, or existential background; preferences, rituals, and practices that might be integrated into care; and spiritual leaders and supports within the community that the patient and family would like to involve.

Spiritual issues and concerns. Major issues within the philosophy of life dimension of spirituality include meaning of life and suffering, unfinished business, and belief systems.

Table 19.2.
The FICA spirituality assessment scale.

F—Faith, Belief, Meaning

"Do you consider yourself spiritual or religious?" or "Do you have spiritual beliefs that help you cope with stress?" If the patient responds, "No," the health care provider might ask, "What gives your life meaning?" Sometimes patients respond with answers such as family, career, or nature.

I—Importance and Influence

"What importance does your faith or belief have in your life? Have your beliefs influenced how you take care of yourself in this illness? What role do your beliefs play in influencing your health care decisions?"

C—Community

"Are you part of a spiritual or religious community? Is this of support to you and how? Is there a group of people you really love or who are important to you?" Communities such as churches, temples, and mosques, or a group of like-minded friends can serve as strong support systems for some patients.

A—Address/Action in Care

"How would you like me, your health care provider, to address these issues in your health care?"

Source: FICA (Puchalski, 2006; Puchalski & Romer, 2000).

Table 19.3.
The SPIRIT spirituality assessment scale.

S- Spiritual belief system

- Do you have a spiritual life that is important to you?

- What is your clearest sense of the meaning of your life at this time?

P- Personal spirituality

- In what ways is your spirituality/religion meaningful for you?

I- Integration with a spiritual community

- Do you belong to any religious or spiritual groups or communities?

- What types of support and help does or could this group provide for you in dealing with health issues?

R- Ritualized practice and restrictions

- What specific practices do you carry out as part of your religious and spiritual life (e.g.,prayer, meditation, service, etc.)?

I- Implications for medical care

- What aspects of your religion/spirituality would you like to keep in mind as I care for you?

- Would you like to discuss religious or spiritual implications of health care?

T- Terminal event planning

- Are there particular aspects of medical care that you wish to forgo or have withheld because of your religion/spirituality?

- Are there religious or spiritual practices or rituals that you would like to have available in the hospital or at home?

- Are there religious or spiritual practices that you wish to plan for at the time of death, or following death?

- From what sources do you draw strength in order to cope with this illness?

Source: SPIRIT (Ambuel, 2000).

Issues within the Unity Consciousness dimension include relationship with the "Ultimate," connectedness to others, and transpersonal experiences (Reese, 2001). How one defines and experiences the "Ultimate" is a highly personal matter and depends upon one's belief system. This concept might refer to God, the divine self (Bullis, 1996), or the general experience of union with all described by transpersonal or deep ecology theorists. Connectedness to others refers to human relationships and a sense of support and closeness.

Functional and dysfunctional use of religion. Understanding that religion may serve as a source of resiliency (Nakashima, 2007; Peckham, 2009), but in other cases may be used as a rationale for unresolved psychosocial issues (York, 1989), allows social workers to better respond to patient and families' spiritual needs. An example of this is described later in this chapter in the narrative of Sister Frances, where her son David expresses belief in a miracle, a belief that is often included in traditional African American cultures. The concern is whether the belief was in the service of denial of the seriousness of his mother's condition and created an aura of blame, isolation, and judgment of his mother and her acceptance of death.

A word of caution is necessary here, however. Whether the use of religion is functional or dysfunctional could be in the eyes of the beholder. It is too easy to judge a religious perspective that differs from one's own. A concern that religious beliefs may be masking psychosocial problems or creating an environment of distress is only valid if the psychosocial problems result in interference with daily functioning, safety of the patient and family, legal concerns, or great emotional distress. Even then, the intervention should be centered on asking questions, clarifying values, and helping the patient and family to discuss and consider alternative conceptualizations always in an atmosphere of acceptance and respect for the patient and family's beliefs.

Spiritual development. One technique for gathering information about spiritual development is to use a genogram that includes information on religious background and how family members coped with death and illness (Cascio, 1998). Bullis (1996) also describes the use of a timeline to illustrate significant events, persons, and experiences that have had a formative effect on the patients' spiritual development throughout their childhood, adolescence, and adulthood (Bullis, 1996). Such a timeline can also be therapeutic in exploring and discovering meaning in difficult life experiences.

Intervention with Spirituality in Palliative Care

Despite our awareness of the potential for spiritual distress, the social work value of self-determination leads us to wait for the patient and family to determine the direction of the discussion and whether these issues will be addressed. Some patients and families may choose not to engage in any discussion of spiritual concerns, or they may choose others with whom they explore these aspects of their life. Social work interventions may focus on the myriad of other needs that a patient and family may identify, and in fact meeting these needs may metaphorically bring meaning and purpose to their life and relationships. The following section will discuss social work intervention approaches with spiritual issues in palliative care.

Philosophy of Life Dimension of Spirituality

Meaning of life and suffering. Reminiscing or life review is often used to help patients reflect on the meaning of their lives (Reese, 2001). Social workers can help patients see crisis as an opportunity for transpersonal growth (Robbins et al., 1998), to come to terms with painful events in their lives, and to discover one's transpersonal mission (Smith & Gray, 1995), thus providing a sense of meaning to what has happened. A powerful approach to life review is Bullis's (1996) spiritual genogram or timeline exercise, which may help a patient see positive impacts that peak events, whether joyful or painful, have had on his or her spiritual development. Other methods are journaling (Vaughn & Swanson, 2006), discussion of dreams and drawings (Early, 1998; Goelitz, 2001a, 2001b), and meaning-based group psychotherapy (Breitbart & Heller, 2003). Dignity therapy enhances a sense of meaning and purpose and a will to live in palliative care patients by recording and transcribing patients' discussion of aspects of their lives that have been most meaningful (Chochinov, Hack, McClement, Harlos, & Kristjanson, 2002). Patients and families may also find meaning by using their own situation as an opportunity for helping others (Trombetti, 2006). An example is a 10-year-old girl born with sirenomelia (fused legs), who inspired other children with chronic illness and disabilities through television, news articles, Facebook, and other Web sites (Associated Press, 2009). Other examples are patients who volunteer for research, participate in clinical trials, donate organs, or contribute money to serve others.

Unfinished business. Several authors suggest planning for the use of remaining time with the aim of completing "unfinished business" (Early, 1998). Unfinished business may include resolution of prior grief (Smith & Gray, 1995), accomplishing final goals (Reese, 2001), or resolving concerns related to sin or guilt and the need for forgiveness of self and others (Canda & Furman, 2010; Puchalski, 2002; Puchalski et al., 2009). There may always be unfinished business in life and family, and part of social work intervention may be to help patients come to terms with this (Goelitz, 2001b). With others, it may be possible to support them in accomplishing final goals or taking care of unresolved issues. Examples include going on a cruise, finishing a novel, or sharing a written or recorded legacy. Several groups exist, such as Make a Wish Foundation, which help both children and adults with serious health problems plan an experience they have always wanted.

The following narratives are examples of patients struggling with anxiety or guilt over past actions:

Robert, a palliative care patient, struggled with guilt over killing enemy soldiers during World War II. Within the social work relationship, he ventilated his feelings and expressed remorse about these events. This expression, though not directly to the persons who were harmed or to their loved ones, helped him to forgive himself. He did not feel the need or express the desire to ask for God's forgiveness; thus, this was not part of the intervention.

Barbara, a Catholic patient, agonized over a past abortion, which she viewed as a sin. She believed that God had stricken her with cancer as a punishment. The social worker at first tried values clarification by exploring the question of whether God would punish someone in this way. Barbara was unwavering in her belief, and she agreed to speak with a spiritual caregiver from her own faith. The social worker contacted a Catholic priest from the interdisciplinary team, who met with Barbara and performed the Catholic ritual of reconciliation, helping to resolve her conflict in this area.

The Consensus Conference identified two issues in this area: the first related to guilt and shame—"the feeling that one has done something wrong or evil"—and the second related to the need for reconciliation—"I need to be forgiven for what I did." Wade, Worthington, and Haake (2009) outline techniques that may promote mutual forgiveness within troubled relationships, including owning one's hurtful actions, eschewing future hurtfulness, forgiving the partner for past hurts, perhaps atonement for hurting the partner, and sacrifice for each partner.

Belief system. The life crisis inherent in life-threatening disease can challenge a patient and family's belief system. Comments that allude to abandonment by God, religious or spiritual struggle, or an inability to engage in a previously comforting ritual such as prayer or reading scripture invite exploration to determine whether a person's faith or belief system has been challenged. In addition, clarification and development of a belief system may lessen aspects of death anxiety (Reese, 2001) and enhance the ability to integrate and adapt to the uncertainty implicit in the experience of living with serious illness. Interventions include joining in an exploration of the patient and family's beliefs (Reese, 2001), reading religious materials (Bullis, 1996), journaling about beliefs (Vaughn & Swanson, 2006) and exploring poetry and narrative.

With a Filled Silk Sail

Down by the sound of the green roaring sea
Wet sand lies white and the salt wind blows free.
Beneath a pale wreathe of light from the moon
Wild boiling waves leap and ride the lagoon.
Rough sand in my hand glows golden and white.
Low music booms from the breakers tonight.
To be kissed with the mist from wet lipped foam
Makes my heart ache for the sea as my home.
I stand in wet sand washed clean by the tide.
I gaze at a sea that always has sighed
To roar in at shore with fury and sound,
While washing the beach with ripple and bound.
Soft sigh in the cry of sea gulls to me
Is but a faint call that drifts from the sea.

I harked, I embarked. I sailed long ago
On waves of the sea to smell its winds blow.
Although I am slow and bent by my years,
To live with the sea holds for me no fears.
I'll ride by the side of a filled silk sail
In a soft summer breeze or a howling gale.
And if breath of that death blows to me on ship
Then I may sleep sound with salt on my lip.

Don Reese, 1987
(used with permission)

Unity Consciousness Dimension of Spirituality

Accessing the unity consciousness dimension can reduce stress and promote resilience, physical comfort, and healing. Interventions to address issues in this dimension are experiential rather than cognitive and do not require use of the term *spirituality*. They include all kinds of traditional religious and spiritual practices, including guided imagery, breathing techniques, healing imagery, art and music therapies, deep relaxation exercises, among many others. Such exercises may promote an altered state of consciousness. Some therapists caution that they should not be used with patients and family members with psychotic disorders for this reason. In addition, some recommend obtaining consent before using interventions that promote altered states of consciousness.

It is essential that the social worker be trained and competent in using these interventions. Training in spirituality, although becoming more common and now required by the Council on Social Work Education for accreditation, is still lacking in social work education, however (Barker, 2007). Social workers must therefore make an effort to include workshops on this topic when planning for continuing education. The Society for Spirituality and Social Work, founded by Edward Canda in 1990, is the leading professional organization specifically focused on this topic. This organization holds an annual conference and is an important source of information; its Web site can be accessed at http://ssw.asu.edu/portal/research/spirituality. Spiritual issues within the unity consciousness dimension of spirituality, along with suggested intervention approaches, are discussed next.

Relationship with the "Ultimate." The Consensus Conference identified spiritual concerns related to relationship with a deity and with God as the most frequently discussed issue regardless of discipline in a Midwestern chart review with 37 patients in one hospice (Reese & Brown, 1997). After gaining an understanding of the patient's unique history and perspective, it may be helpful to assure a patient and family of the normalcy of anger toward God during life-threatening illness or life crises. Ventilating anger within a relationship of safety and acceptance can sometimes help to lessen distress. Joseph (1988) also discusses the impact of the childhood relationship with one's father on one's view of God, especially if the nature of God is seen as masculine, and the relationship with one's father was difficult. The social worker may be able to help the patient separate feelings about God from significant others, assist the patient in clarifying his or her own individuated view of God, and focus counseling on unresolved developmental issues as a way to address problems in the patient's or family member's relationship with God and possibly in other relationships as well. Meditation, prayer techniques, art depicting one's conceptualization of God (Smith, 1993), and guided imagery can also be used as "a means of communicating and communing with God, a transcendent reality, or the divine self" (Bullis, 1996, p. 62). Canda and Furman (2010) note the impact of mutually beneficial human–nature relationships in experiencing a profound sense of connection. Another experiential approach that promotes a sense of connection is music therapy (Hilliard, 2005).

Connectedness to others. A number of factors can interfere with a patient's sense of connection to others. The Consensus Conference framed the issue as abandonment by others, which includes lack of love, loneliness, and not being remembered—"No one comes by anymore." The authors also note the impact of isolation, including separation from one's religious community or other sources of spiritual and social support—"Since moving to the assisted living I am not able to go to my church anymore" (Puchalski et al., 2009, p. 894).

Social workers may be helpful in assisting the patient to restore close relationships, build new ones, and resolve conflicts with others. Helpful approaches include exploring ways to maintain intimacy, stressing the importance of sharing thoughts and feelings as a way to connect and cope, helping to engage the family in the illness experience (Reese, 2001), and arranging meetings between loved ones wanting to share meaningful time, play, and possibly, when appropriate and necessary, work on reconciliation. A hospice or palliative care program itself may serve as a cohesive community that promotes a sense of belonging, and the clinical relationship can lead to an increased awareness of one's commonality with the rest of humanity (Reese, 2001). Cultural and gender differences inform these efforts. In some cultural traditions, such as traditional African American and Chinese cultures, there may be a taboo about discussion of death. In China, family members may perform end-of-life rituals that symbolically indicate that they are aware of the patient's condition, rather than directly discussing terminality (Chan, Epstein, Reese, & Chan, 2008; Reese, Ahern, Nair, O'Faire, & Warren, 1999). These differences do not preclude the important clinical task of encouraging patients and families to share meaningful time, creating memories, valuing each day, all of which do not require an acceptance or direct acknowledgement of an expected death.

Transpersonal experiences. It is not uncommon for patients nearing end of life to have visual and auditory experiences that others do not (Kelley & Callanan, 1992). They are often calm and accepting of their experiences, expressing relief at the opportunity to discuss them without judgment or rejection (Gibbs & Achterberg-Lawlis, 1978; Pflaum & Kelley, 1986). Such experiences are considered healthy and a source of resilience, may provide comfort to the patient, and may offer the opportunity for spiritual growth (Cowley, 1993; Nakashima, 2007).

Approaches with patients and families include normalizing the experience and exploring the meaning or symbolism without imposing any value or belief system (Pflaum & Kelley, 1986). Grof (1988) suggests that we support the experiential process with full trust in its healing nature, without trying to change it, even without full understanding of its meaning. Gibbs and Achterberg-Lawlis recommend reducing an intellectualizing atmosphere (1978) in discussing these issues and replacing it with an approach of active listening and acceptance.

It is important to note that the meaning of transpersonal experiences varies by culture. In some families, visions of deceased family members may be comforting if the patient interprets them as evidence of a benevolent afterlife and that the deceased loved one has come to be an escort to heaven. In other families, (such as in Hong Kong), such a vision may be quite frightening, as it would traditionally be interpreted as a sign of a "hungry ghost," who cannot reincarnate until it seeks revenge for a wrongful or early death (Reese, Chan, Chan, & Wiersgalla, 2009). In still other religious or cultural traditions, visions such as these may be interpreted as evidence of witchcraft. As in all clinical care, it is important for the social worker to be respectful and supportive of the client's world view and consult with his or her religious or spiritual leader for further guidance.

Guidelines for Referral to a Spiritual Caregiver

Interdisciplinary team collaboration in the fields of hospice and palliative care has been challenged by turf battles and lack of consensus regarding which discipline should address which aspect of care. Some of the reasons for this include lack of knowledge of the expertise of other professions, role blurring, conflicts arising from differences between professions in values and theoretical base, negative team norms, client stereotyping, and administrative barriers (Reese & Sontag, 2001). Egan and Labyak (2001) expanded the concept of the *transdisciplinary* team, in which the team transcends these turf issues by providing core training for all disciplines regarding primary biopsychosocial-spiritual needs, with patient and family values guiding all interventions. Similarly, the Consensus Conference (Puchalski et al., 2009) recommends that all health care professionals develop core skills to enable a culturally sensitive spiritual screening to identify spiritual distress. Palliative care professionals (including social workers) are encouraged to develop a more comprehensive skill set to aid them in the provision of basic spiritual support. All professionals need to be mindful of the limits of their training and scope of practice so that they can make timely and appropriate referrals to spiritual care specialists such as board-certified chaplains. This author concurs that professionals providing assessment and spiritual intervention should have the training and skills to do so. Research has repeatedly demonstrated that social workers are frequently addressing spirituality despite a lack of attention to this area in their formal social work education. As with any aspect of palliative care, if social workers face needs that they are not prepared to address, they refer to a member of the team with the needed skills; in this instance perhaps a board-certified chaplain or community spiritual care provider.

At the same time, since spirituality is of such primary importance for palliative care patients and their families and often raised with other disciplines, social workers cannot ignore the importance of obtaining continuing education in this area. If social workers do possess this knowledge and skill based on the recognized body of knowledge of their profession, this author's view is that they address the patient and family's needs when they arise, to the degree they are responsibly capable. The first time this author was faced with a hospice patient's question, "Why would God do this to me?" she answered, "Let me refer you to the hospice chaplain." The sad fact that led her on this course of study was that the patient died before the chaplain could get there, the question remaining unexplored.

Another point to keep in mind is that for some diverse cultural groups, such as African Americans, the patient's own pastor is traditionally the one sought out for guidance in life-threatening illness and end-of-life care (Bullock, 2006). In the Jewish faith it may be the community rabbi who is the trusted spiritual provider with whom profound questions are explored. Collaboration within a high-functioning team requires coordinated intervention to insure that needs and concerns are approached in a consistent way, without repeating interventions and with the inclusion of the patient and family's personal spiritual caregiver, or a caregiver of their religion, to explore specific religious questions.

Analysis of Patient/Family Narrative: Sister Frances and Family

The following are elements of addressing spirituality in palliative care that can be seen in the patient and family narrative in Box 19.2.

Philosophy of life dimension of spirituality. In the attempt to understand why his mother was dying of cancer—*the meaning of her suffering*—David developed the explanation that she was dying because she had a lack of faith and a lack of will. If only she would believe, God would perform a miracle. This is a common traditional belief among African Americans (Reese et al., 1999), but at some point the prayers for a miracle can change to accepting God's will that Sister Frances would die. In this patient/family narrative, David was having difficulty in making that transition because of his

Box 19.2
Patient/Family Narrative: Sister Frances and Family

This narrative of an African American family receiving hospice care may demonstrate how cultural and spiritual beliefs are identified, understood, and addressed.

Sister Frances was a 50-year-old African American woman who was dying of cancer. Her husband had died several years earlier in the care of hospice, and the patient preferred hospice care for herself. Her family was very active in their Southern Baptist church; Sister Frances sang in the choir, and her 30-year-old son David, a single child, was a lay minister in the church. David believed that his mother was dying because she did not have enough faith; he thought she was giving up rather than believing that God would perform a miracle. He was frustrated with her acceptance of her death and her desire for hospice care. He thought she just wanted to go to heaven to be with her husband, choosing therefore to leave her living son rather than fighting to survive.

On a home visit, the social worker observed Sister Frances tossing back and forth on her bed, appearing in great agitation and distress. She had a look in her eyes often described as "seeing but not seeing," meaning that she was not comatose, she had her eyes open, looking somewhere beyond, but her focus was not in this world. The social worker used a guided imagery exercise to promote relaxation and calm in spite of her lack of responsiveness, trusting the widely articulated perspective that the patient could hear, even if she could not respond. She then walked into the living room, where son David was watching television and the patient's sister, Aunt Laura, was sitting on the couch. The social worker asked a question that called for values clarification—"Is it the patient's fault if they are dying?" Aunt Laura replied, "No, and no one here would think that." David remained silent. After the social worker left, David went into his mother's room and saw her looking at the foot of the bed and shaking her head "no." David believed Sister Frances was seeing an angel who had come to take her to heaven and she was refusing to go. David said, "It's O.K., mom, you can go," and Sister Frances died 20 minutes later.

David and Aunt Laura invited the social worker to attend the funeral, which David conducted as a lay minister. The church bulletins were titled, "Homecoming Celebration for Sister Frances," and David sang in a beautiful voice the traditional hymn, "In the Sweet Bye and Bye, when we meet on that beautiful shore…" The choir members sang as they filed by Sister Frances' open coffin, each kissing her on the cheek. David asked the social worker to stand and speak. David preached, "We loved you, but God loved you more." At the end of the service, they invited the social worker to a wonderful church lunch in celebration of Sister Frances' homecoming.

his mother for a lack of faith in God's power to perform a miracle. The social worker's question, *"Is it the patient's fault if they are dying?"* created cognitive dissonance and invited David to reconsider the messages and meaning implicit in his response. Perhaps his giving of permission reflected his transition to a perspective that it was God's will that his mother die; a perspective that he was able to express at her funeral. The outcome of a peaceful environment and a funeral which engaged the social worker and was congruous with patient and son's values may serve to assist David in his grief and bereavement.

Unity consciousness dimension of spirituality. (1) *Connectedness.* The social worker was able to help Sister Frances and David reconnect by helping David resolve his anger at his mother for accepting her death, understanding that she was not choosing to leave him. (2) *Transpersonal experience.* David believed that his mother saw an angel at the foot of her bed, who had come to accompany her to heaven. The worker was able to respect that belief without interpretation or judgment.

Cultural diversity considerations. A key element in this patient/family narrative was a conflict between traditional African American religious beliefs and acceptance of death. David believed that God would perform a miracle, if only his mother had enough faith. Meanwhile, his mother accepted her death and had chosen hospice care rather than disease-modifying treatments. Despite the fact that the possibility of miracle is a traditional belief for many African American people, David was using this belief in the service of a psychosocial problem, which included a denial of his mother's expected death and an assumption that her will and faith could obviate the outcome, which many would identify as an example of *dysfunctional use of religion.* It was necessary for the social worker to understand and respect David's beliefs, while at the same time inviting him to reflect on the implications of those beliefs as well as to understand his mother's perspective. The message of acceptance and the quiet challenge and comfort this provided was attested to by the social worker's invitation to the funeral. The social worker's attendance and participation in the funeral demonstrated respect and furthered a community connection that would be important in the continued utilization of hospice by the African American community.

Conclusion

Social workers address spirituality with patients and families, but they are unlikely to have requisite training and may be less likely to recognize the many ways spiritual concerns are expressed. Social workers are unlikely to have conducted a spiritual assessment and have produced few evaluation studies of the effectiveness of their spiritual interventions. Further development of models of practice is needed, as is

own personal pain in losing both of his parents. The question asked by the social worker, "Is it the patient's fault if they are dying?" helped him to objectify his behaviors, clarify his beliefs, and change his focus from blaming his mother for a lack of faith and will to accepting the will of God, which for this family meant the acceptance of death. At the funeral, the explanation was expressed, "We loved you, but God loved you more." The funeral was experienced as a homecoming celebration, in which belief in an afterlife was a comfort in grief. *Unfinished business* was represented in David's anger at publication of models that are being used in practice but have not been disseminated to the profession as a whole. Further research is needed, subsequently, to test these practice models for effectiveness.

Training is needed to develop skills in defining spirituality, identifying issues, and the use of intervention techniques. Canda (1991) suggests that conventional and transpersonal theories be placed together in the curriculum to provide breadth and diversity of perspectives. In addition, social work education should especially address the following:

- The importance of spirituality to low-income and diverse populations
- The hesitation and ambivalence on the part of social workers to address spirituality, usually based on a fear of proselytizing, failure to understand spirituality and religion as separate concepts, and turf battles between spiritual caregivers and social workers on the interdisciplinary team
- Personal issues of the social worker that inhibit intervention in this area
- Proper documentation of spiritual interventions in patient charts

A number of hospice and palliative care policy issues need to be addressed in order to permit adequate spiritual care. Research shows that budgeting for increased social work and spiritual caregiver services increases intervention with spiritual issues (Reese, 2001). Turf issues between social workers and chaplains need to be resolved, perhaps by interdisciplinary training (Otis-Green et al., 2009). Finally, the short length of stay in hospice needs to be addressed at a programmatic and national level. Medicare regulations need to be reviewed for barriers to referral, and transitional programs, including both palliative care and hospice, need to be developed. Palliative social workers practicing in hospitals, clinics, extended care facilities, and in the community have opportunities to intervene with spiritual aspects of care early in the continuum of illness through the end of life.

In the end, the chronically ill and dying will teach us much more than we will teach them. The experience of facing one's own mortality propels many people into a transegoic perspective, entailing enhanced spiritual development according to transpersonal theory. It is then that they become our teachers, allowing us to experience with them their connection to a transcendent reality.

The most beautiful people we have known are those who have known defeat, known suffering, known struggle, known loss, and have found their way out of the depths. These persons have an appreciation, sensitivity and an understanding of life that fills them with compassion, gentleness, and a deep loving concern. Beautiful people do not just happen. (Elisabeth Kubler-Ross, retrieved from the Elisabeth Kubler-Ross Foundation Web site at:) http://www.ekrfoundation. org/quotes

LEARNING EXERCISES

Forgiveness exercise

- The purpose of this exercise is to assist clients in forgiving past hurts, even in situations where face-to-face contact between the client and the one he or she needs to forgive is impossible.
- The client imagines an umbilical cord connecting him or her to the person he or she needs to forgive. The client imagines a filter on this connection so that only positive energy, not negative, may flow through. Next the client imagines positive spiritual energy flowing through himself or herself, through the umbilical cord, and through the other person, so that all are washed clean of negative energy. If necessary, the connection may be cut altogether and the other person allowed to go his or her own way (from Bruce Swett, M.Div., M.S.W., Counseling Associates, Salisbury, MD [cited by Reese, 2001]).

ADDITIONAL SUGGESTED READINGS

Berzoff, J., & Silverman, P. (Eds.). (2004). *Living with dying: A comprehensive resource for end-of-life care.* New York, NY: Columbia University Press.

Furman, L., & Bushfield, S. (2000). Clerics and social workers: Collaborators or competitors? *ARETE, Journal of University of South Carolina School of Social Work, 24*(1), 30–39.

Hodge, D. (2003). Value differences between social workers and members of the working and middle classes. *Social Work, 48*(1), 107–119.

Kubler-Ross, E., & Kessler, D. (2001). *Life lessons.* Llandeilo, Wales: Cygnus Books.

Puchalski, C., & Ferrell, B. (2010). *Making health care whole: Integrating spirituality into patient care.* West Conshohocken, PA: Templeton Press.

Raboteau, A. (1978). *Slave religion: The "invisible institution" in the antebellum South.* New York, NY: Oxford University Press.

ADDITIONAL RESOURCES AND WEB SITES

City of Hope Professional Resource Center: http://prc.coh.org
Edward Canda's Web site: http://www.socwel.ku.edu/canda/
The George Washington Institute: http://www.gwumc.edu/gwish/ soerce
Global Alliance for a Deep Ecological Social Work, Fred Besthorn: http://www.ecosocialwork.org/
Society for Spirituality and Social Work: http://ssw.asu.edu/portal/ research/spirituality
Physician Education Resource Center www.eperc.mcw.edu.

REFERENCES

Ambuel, B. (2000). *Fast facts and concepts #19: Taking a spiritual history*. Retrieved from the End of Life Physician Education Resource Center Web site: http://www.eperc.mcw.edu/fastFact/ff_19.htm

Anandarajah, G., & Hight, E. (2001). Spirituality and medical practice: Using the HOPE questions as a practical tool for spiritual assessment. *American Family Physician, 63*, 81–89.

Assagioli, R. (1993). *Psychosynthesis: A manual of principles and techniques*. London: Aquarian/Thomsons.

Associated Press. (2009, October 25). *Maine girl with "mermaid syndrome" dies at 10. Southern Illinoisan*, retrieved from http://www.thesouthern.com/news/.

Barker, S. L. (2007). The integration of spirituality and religion content in social work education: Where we've been, where we're going. *Social Work and Christianity, 34*(2), 146–166.

Besthorn, F. H. (2001). Transpersonal psychology and deep ecological philosophy: Exploring linkages and applications for social work. *Social Thought, 20*(1/2), 23–44.

Breitbart, W., & Heller, K. S. (2003). Reframing hope: Meaning centered care for patients near the end of life. *Journal of Palliative Medicine, 6*, 979–988.

Broderick, D. J., Birbilis, J. M., & Steger, M. F. (2008). Lesbians grieving the death of a partner: Recommendations for practice. *Journal of Lesbian Studies, 12*(2-3), 225–235.

Bullis, R. (1996). *Spirituality in social work practice*. Washington, DC: Taylor & Francis.

Bullock, K. (2006). Promoting advance directives among African Americans: A faith-based model. *Journal of Palliative Medicine, 9*(1), 183–195.

Canda, E. R. (1990). An holistic approach to prayer for social work practice. *Social Thought, 16*(3), 3–13.

Canda, E. (1991). East/West philosophical synthesis in transpersonal theory. *Journal of Sociology and Social Welfare, 18*(4), 137–152.

Canda, E., & Furman, L. (2010). *Spiritual diversity in social work practice: The heart of helping*. New York, NY: Oxford University Press.

Cascio, T. (1998). Incorporating spirituality into social work practice: A review of what to do. *Families in Society, 79*(5), 523–532.

Chan, W. C. H., Epstein, I., Reese, D., & Chan, C. L.W. (2008). Family predictors of psychosocial outcomes among Hong Kong Chinese cancer patients in palliative care: Living and dying with the "support paradox". *Social Work in Health Care, 48*(5), 519–532.

Chochinov, H. M., Hack, T., McClement, S., Harlos, M., & Kristjanson, L. (2002). Dignity in the terminally ill: An empirical model. *Social Science Medicine, 54*, 433–443.

Cowley, A-D. S. (1993). Transpersonal social work: A theory for the 1990s. *Social Work, 38*(5), 527–534.

Delaney, C., & Barrere, C. (2009). Ecospirituality: The experience of environmental meditation in patients with cardiovascular disease. *Holistic Nursing Practice, 23*(6), 361–369.

Early, B. (1998). Between two worlds: The psychospiritual crisis of a dying adolescent. *Social Thought: Journal of Religion in the Social Services, 18*(2), 67–80.

Egan, K. A., & Labyak, M. J. (2001). Hospice care: A model for quality end-of-life care. In B. R. Ferrell & N. Coyle (Eds.), *Textbook of palliative nursing* (pp. 7–26). New York, NY: Oxford University Press.

Engel, G. L. (1977). The need for a new medical model: A challenge for biomedicine. *Science, 196*, 129–136.

Gibbs, H., & Achterberg-Lawlis, J. (1978). Spiritual values and death anxiety: Implications for counseling with terminal cancer patients. *Journal of Counseling Psychology, 25*, 563–569.

Goelitz, A. (2001a). Dreaming their way into life: A group experience with oncology patients. *Social Work With Groups, 24*(1), 53–67.

Goelitz, A. (2001b). Nurturing life with dreams: Therapeutic dream work with cancer patients. *Clinical Social Work Journal, 29*(4), 375–385.

Grof, S. (1988). *The adventure of self-discovery*. Albany, NY: State University of New York Press.

Hilliard, R. E. (2005). Music therapy in hospice and palliative care: A review of the empirical data. *Evidence-Based Complementary and Alternative Medicine, 2*(2), 173–178.

Hodge, D. R. (2001). Spiritual assessment: A review of major qualitative methods and a new framework for assessing spirituality. *Social Work, 46*(3), 203–214.

Jonas, H. (2001). *The phenomenon of life: Towards a philosophical biology*. Evanston, IL: Northwestern University Press.

Joseph, M. V. (1988). Religion and social work practice. *Social Casework, 69*, 443–452.

Jung, C. G. (1960). The structure and dynamics of the psyche. In H. Read, M. Fordham, & G. Adler (Eds.), *The collected works of C. G. Jung* (Bollingen Series, Vol. 8) (R.F.C. Hull, Trans.) New York, NY: Pantheon Books. (Original works published 1929 to 1944).

Kelley, P., & Callanan, M. (1992). *Final gifts: Understanding the special awareness, needs, and communications of the dying*. New York, NY: Bantam Books.

Kubler-Ross, E. (n.d.). Elisabeth Kubler-Ross Foundation. Retrieved from http://www.ekrfoundation.org/quotes

Lord, S. (2008). Therapeutic work with trauma: Revictimization and perpetration: Bearing witness, offering hope, embracing despair. *Psychoanalytic Social work, 15*(2), 110–131.

Nakashima, M. (2007). Positive dying in later life: Spiritual resiliency among sixteen hospice patients. *Journal of Religion, Spirituality and Aging, 19*(2), 43–66.

National Association of Social Workers (NASW). (2008). *Code of ethics*. Retrieved from http://www.socialworkers.org/pubs/code/code.asp

National Consensus Project for Quality Palliative Care. (2009) *Clinical practice guidelines for quality palliative care, second edition*. Retrieved from http://www.nationalconsensus project.org/

Nelson-Becker, H., Nakashima, M., & Canda, E. R. (2006). Spirituality in professional helping interventions. In B. Berkman & S. D'Ambruoso (Eds.), *Oxford handbook of social work, health, and aging* (pp. 797–807). New York: Oxford Press.

Otis-Green, S., Ferrell, B., Spolum, M., Uman, G., Mullan, P., Baird, P., & Grant, M. (2009). *An overview of the ACE project ~ Advocating for clinical excellence: Transdisciplinary palliative care education. Journal of Cancer Education, 24*(2), 120–126.

Peckham, M. (2009). Street-involved youths' constructs of God. *Relational Child and Youth Care Practice, 22*(2), 44–54.

Pflaum, M., & Kelley, P. (1986). Understanding the final messages of the dying. *Nursing, 16*(60), 26–29.

Puchalski, C. M. (2002). Spirituality and end-of-life care: A time for listening and caring. *Journal of Palliative Medicine, 5*(2), 289–294.

Puchalski, C. M. (2006). Spiritual assessment in clinical practice. *Psychiatric Annals, 36*, 150.

Puchalski, C., Ferrell, B., Virani, R., Otis-Green, S., Baird, P., Bull, J.,… Sulmasy, D. (2009). Improving the quality of spiritual care as a dimension of palliative care: The report of the Consensus Conference. *Journal of Palliative Medicine, 12*(10), 885–904.

Puchalski, C., & Romer, A. L. (2000). Taking a spiritual history allows clinicians to understand patients more fully. *Journal of Palliative Medicine, 3*, 129–137.

Reed, P. (1987). Spirituality and wellbeing in terminally ill hospitalized adults. *Research in Nursing and Health, 10*(5), 335–344.

Reese, D. J. (2001). Addressing spirituality in hospice: Current practices and a proposed role for transpersonal social work. *Social Thought: Journal of Religion in the Social Services, 20*(1-2), 135–161.

Reese, D. J., Ahern, R., Nair, S., O'Faire, J., & Warren, C. (1999). Hospice access and utilization by African Americans: Addressing cultural and institutional barriers through participatory action research. *Social Work, 44*(6), 549–559.

Reese, D. J., & Brown, D. (1997). Psychosocial and spiritual care in hospice: Differences between nursing, social work, and clergy. *The Hospice Journal, 12*(1), 29–41.

Reese, D. J., Chan, C. L. W., Chan, W. C. H., & Wiersgalla, D. (in press). A cross-national comparison of Hong Kong and U.S. student beliefs and preferences in end-of-life care: Implications for social work education and practice. *Journal of Social Work in End-of-Life and Palliative Care).*

Reese, D. J., Raymer, M., Orloff, S., Gerbino, S., Valade, R., Dawson, S.,… Huber, R. (2006). The Social Work Assessment Tool (SWAT). *Journal of Social Work in End-of-Life and Palliative Care, 2*(2), 65–95.

Reese, D. J., & Sontag, M-A. (2001). Barriers and solutions for successful inter-professional collaboration on the hospice team. *Health and Social Work, 26*, (3), 167–175.

Robbins, S. P., Canda, E. R., & Chatterjee, P. (1998). *Contemporary human behavior theory: A critical perspective for social work.* Boston, MA: Allyn & Bacon.

Seccareccia, D., & Brown, J. B. (2009). Impact of spirituality on palliative care physicians: Personally and professionally. *Journal of Palliative Medicine, 12*(9), 805–809.

Sessanna, L. (2008). The role of spirituality in advance directive decision making among independent community dwelling older adults. *Journal of Religion and Health, 47*(1), 32–44.

Sheehan, M. N. (2003). Spirituality and medicine. *Journal of Palliative Medicine, 6*(3), 429–431.

Smith, D. (1993). Exploring the religious-spiritual needs of the dying. *Counseling and Values, 37*, 71–77.

Smith, E. (1995). Addressing the psychospiritual distress of death as reality: A transpersonal approach. *Social Work, 40*(3), 402–412.

Smith, E., & Gray, C. (1995). Integrating and transcending divorce: A transpersonal model. *Social Thought, 18*(1), 57–74.

Sulmasy, D. (2006). The rebirth of the clinic: An introduction to spirituality in healthcare. Washington, DC: Georgetown University Press.

Trombetti, I. A. (2006). Meanings in the lives of older adults: In their own voices. *Dissertation Abstracts International: Section B: The Sciences and Engineering, 66*(9-B), 5130.

Vaughn, M., & Swanson, K. (2006). Any life can be fascinating: Using spiritual autobiography as an adjunct to therapy. In K. B. Helmeke & C. F. Sori (Eds.), *The therapist's notebook for integrating spirituality in counseling: Homework, handouts and activities for use in psychotherapy* (pp. 211–219). New York, NY: Haworth Press.

Wade, N. J., Worthington, E. L., Jr., & Haake, S. (2009). Comparison of explicit forgiveness interventions with an alternative treatment: A randomized clinical trial. *Journal of Counseling and Development, 87*(2), 143–151.

White, K. L., Williams, T. F., & Greenberg, B. G. (1996). The ecology of medical care. *Academy of Medicine, 73*, 187–205.

Wilber, K. (1996). *A brief history of everything.* Boston, MA: Shambhala.

Woodruff, L., & Reese, D. (2005, July) *God, guns, & gays: A Jungian analysis of the United States as global power.* Paper presented at the Inter-University Consortium for International Social Development's Biennial Symposium, Recife, Brazil.

York, G. (1989). Strategies for managing the religious-based denial of rural clients. *Human Services in the Rural Environment, 13*(2), 16–22.

20 *Susan Cadell, Sheryl Shermak, and Meaghen Johnston*

Discovering Strengths and Growth in Palliative Care

… the strengths perspective is about the revolutionary possibility of hope
—*Saleebey (2002, p. 18)*

Key Concepts

- *Palliative social workers have an important role to play in identifying strengths and positive outcomes in patients and family members.*
- *Practicing palliative social work with a strengths perspective acknowledges that, along with negatives, positive changes can take place for patients, families, and for professionals.*
- *Of the various models that focus on positive aspects of the negative situations, the strengths perspective and posttraumatic growth are the most applicable in palliative care.*
- *Posttraumatic growth includes the five domains of: new possibilities, relating to others, personal strength, appreciation of life, and spiritual change.*
- *Strengths and growth can emerge at any time along the illness continuum.*
- *Social workers are encouraged to be open to strengths as little is known about facilitating positive aspects.*
- *Positive aspects of stressful life circumstances do not replace the negative aspects: positive and negative states coexist.*

Introduction

The focus of this chapter is on discovering strengths and positive outcomes in palliative care. As palliative social workers, providing support through a strengths perspective lens means acknowledging that along with the negatives that come with a diagnosis of a life-threatening illness, there may also be experiences of positive changes and growth. In palliative social work, we work with people because of a diagnosis of a life-threatening illness, either of the person or of a family member. Despite this, indeed sometimes because of this, there are strengths awaiting discovery in every situation.

CONSIDER THE FOLLOWING PATIENT/
FAMILY NARRATIVE EXAMPLES[1]:
Rosemary is 41 years old with two daughters: Amanda, 19, and Christine, 17 (Cadell, Janzen, & Fletcher, 2004, November). Christine was diagnosed with a brain tumor in January. The next month she began treatment, but the tumor did not respond. It is now October and Christine has just died. Rosemary's husband left her 9 months before the diagnosis and has not been helpful throughout this year. Rosemary has some support from her extended family but has been Christine's primary caregiver. Some time later, Rosemary comments: "I think, you know, I have had an amazing life. … I didn't wish for [Christine] to die, but good things [have happened] … It is really hard…"

Amanda is a 21-year-old woman whose mother was first diagnosed with breast cancer 5 years ago (Puterman & Cadell, 2008). Her mother went through treatment and then her cancer recurred when Amanda was 20. Amanda has struggled a great deal to come to terms with her mother's illness at a time in her own life when, as a young adult, she is naturally beginning to separate from her family. Now, however, she wonders if she should stay close because her

---

1 All scenarios are based on people who have participated in research projects. Identifying information has been changed to protect their anonymity. Quotes are accurate.

mother is ill. Amanda has come to refocus her awareness in the present time; she explains a positive aspect:

> I think it just sort of makes you appreciate living more. I mean obviously I have days where I lose that perspective, but yeah, it makes you appreciate the small things in life, just like … the uncertainty of life for everybody, really. I mean, you never really know what's going to happen. You're not invincible. You're not here forever. (Puterman & Cadell, 2008, p.111)

Joseph is a 50-year-old man who has been HIV-positive for more than 10 years (Cadell, Janzen, & Haubrich, 2007). Joseph has transformed the French equivalent of HIV to be his own personal motto. HIV in French is VIH which for him meant "Vivre Intensément l'Humain" or in English to "Live Humanity Intensely." Joseph considered that instead of it being a death sentence, HIV was an opportunity for him to live his life to the fullest. Joseph credited this interpretation of HIV with allowing him to survive and thrive for so long.

The diagnosis and death of a friend or family member, of any relation, in a short timeframe such as Rosemary experienced has the potential to be traumatizing. The young age of Amanda could lead some professionals to assume that she would not be able to fully engage with her mother's illness, care, and potential death or that the impact of her mother's illness may have long-term negative effects on her development. Joseph could have been depressed by the realities of living with HIV. Instead he engaged with his disease and lived his life more intensely and fully. Indeed, many aspects of these scenarios have the potential to lead to depression and complicated grief.

As social workers, many of us have not been prepared to assess strengths and anticipate the possibility of growth, especially in situations that involve the potential for or the reality of the end of life. While some social workers might pathologize any of the aforementioned situations, we advocate for a strengths approach to social work practice in order to facilitate or initiate the possibility for growth. We believe that affirming the strengths in individuals and families is essential in the service of their future. By focusing on areas of strength and growth we are supporting a process of developing the skills and wisdom to cope with various life challenges, however long or short the future might be.

In this chapter we seek to achieve three aims. First, we provide an overview of the various concepts of positive approaches and processes. Second, to illustrate strengths and growth in the voices of those experiencing it, we present pilot research data concerning growth in bereaved parents whose child died of a life-threatening illness. Finally, based on approaches and processes, we will review implications for social work practice in palliative care.

An Overview of Positive Approaches

First, what is needed is an overview of concepts. There are a number of models that focus on positive aspects of negative situations. While all may be generalizable to palliative social work, some have more applicability than others.

Resilience is defined as the ability to adapt to and bounce back from adverse circumstances (Masten, Best, & Garmezy, 1990; Scannapieco & Jackson, 1996). The study of resilience grew out of developmental psychology and a concern for identifying risk factors for children of developing psychiatric disorders in adulthood (Garmezy, 1971). The emphasis shifted from risk to resilience when a large longitudinal study of children in Kauai, Hawaii, found that across all risk factors, there were always some children who became competent adults despite the life stressors they faced (Werner & Smith, 1982). Resilience as a concept is most often applied to children and youth, but some studies have examined resilience in families (McCubbin & McCubbin, 1988) and in adults (Aldwin & Sutton, 1998). Despite the years of research, the concept of resilience is still somewhat elusive and is coming under scrutiny due to the subjective nature of its use. Indeed, Ungar (2004) suggests that resilience should be conceptualized as a socially constructed phenomenon.

The transactional model of stress and coping was developed by Lazarus and Folkman (1984). The original model only allowed for the possibility of positive emotions if there was a favorable resolution to the stressor. Following longitudinal research on gay men caring for a partner with AIDS, Folkman (1997) reworked the model to involve positive emotions when the outcome was not favorable or there was no resolution of the stressful situation, which was clearly the case in the context of the AIDS epidemic. Along with positive emotions, the new model includes the process of meaning making. In essence, the model is designed to indicate that positive and negative psychological states co-occur.

The strengths perspective in social work was first articulated by Weick and colleagues (Weick, Rapp, Sullivan, & Kisthardt, 1989) and then advanced by Dennis Saleebey in his series of books on the strengths perspective in social work practice (Saleebey, 1992, 1997, 2002, 2006). The strengths perspective is not limited to social work: Psychology has also begun the process of understanding strengths though the positive psychology movement (Joseph & Linley, 2008). Saleebey (2002) states:

> *The strengths perspective is about the revolutionary possibility of hope; hope realized through the strengthened sinew of social relationships in family, neighborhood, community, culture, and country. That contextual sinew is fortified by the expression of the individual and communal capacities of all. (p. 18)*

The strengths perspective is not a theory or a method, but a way of understanding human concerns that provides a fuller appreciation of both assets and problems. It is based on a number of principles, the first of which is that all individuals, groups, families, and communities have strengths. Therefore, a social work practice grounded in a strengths perspective can lead the practitioner to consider the varied resources in many different types of situations. Other foundational principles are that professionals ought not to underestimate upper limits of growth and change and that we best serve clients through collaboration. It is not an approach that advocates neglecting problems; instead it is about assessing and building upon strengths in order to better approach issues in people's lives.

Posttraumatic growth refers to the idea that individuals can experience positive life changes as they attempt to cope with a traumatic event or life crisis (Helgeson, Reynolds, & Tomich, 2006; Hogan & Schmidt, 2002; Tedeschi & Kilmer, 2005; Tedeschi, Park, & Calhoun, 1998). Other terms commonly used to describe this concept are personal growth, stress-related growth, adversarial growth, benefit finding, and perceived growth. The term *posttraumatic growth* was coined by the psychologists Tedeschi and Calhoun (1995) who had noticed that the widows with whom they worked were expressing positive aspects of the negative experience of bereavement. Posttraumatic growth consists of five domains: new possibilities, relating to others, personal strength, appreciation of life, and spiritual change (Tedeschi & Calhoun, 1996).

We believe none of the models described capture the complexity of the occurrence of positive and negative human experiences coexisting completely, although each highlights or illustrates an important aspect to understand. For the most part, the models theorize that the occurrence of a highly stressful or traumatic event results in a violation of one's personal beliefs about the world and themselves. Consequently, a person will engage in various forms of meaning making or cognitive processing in an attempt to rebuild his or her goals and beliefs and that growth can be an outcome (Park & Helgeson, 2006). The process of growth is presented as co-occurring alongside the negative aspects that are traditionally given prominence when considering the outcome of trauma, stress, or grief (Calhoun & Tedeschi, 2006).

Of all of these, the concept of resilience may be the least applicable to palliative social work. Resilience signifies becoming strengthened in order to meet new hardships. When considering individuals who are facing the end of life, the idea of preparing for the next challenge is less salient than the concept of strengths and growth. As well, family and friends who are also impacted by the illness of the person and the potential impact of his or her death may perceive the notion of building resilience as something that should not be explored or talked about. The models of growth and strengths seem more congruent with palliative care: that people surpass their pretrauma or prediagnosis state through facing death, be it their own or that of others. These concepts are borne out through anecdotal and research evidence.

The following results from a pilot study will help illustrate the strength and growth that can occur.

Posttraumatic Growth in Palliative Care: A Study of Bereaved Parents

To better understand posttraumatic growth in a population of bereaved parents, we (Cadell, Janzen, & Fletcher, 2004) undertook a qualitative study. While in the study there were data from a wide range of causes of death, only the data from the parents whose children died of life-threatening illnesses are reported on here. In this subsample are five mothers and one father whose children received palliative care. Although parents were recruited, the sample was mostly comprised of mothers. More attention needs to be paid to purposely recruiting fathers (Macdonald, Chilibeck, Affleck, & Cadell, 2009).

Ethical approval from all the institutions involved was obtained. The data were collected through face-to-face interviews, which were audio-taped and transcribed. Open-ended questions were used to explore the changes in the parents' life experience subsequent to the child's death. The parents were interviewed at least 1 year after the death of their child. Data were analyzed using the constant comparative method to identify themes.

All of the parents involved in the study responded to a request for participants to address positive aspects of the bereavement experience. Because so little research attention has been paid to positive aspects of negative experiences, this sample was purposively sought in order to better understand the positive aspects. The data of the bereaved parents were organized into five categories according to the domains of posttraumatic growth. In the quotes that follow you will hear evidence of these individuals finding new possibilities, a new way of relating to others, an increase in personal strength, and greater appreciation of life as well as the experience of spiritual change (Tedeschi & Calhoun, 1996).

New Possibilities

All of the parents identified at least one new possibility that they had found in life after the death of their child. Some of these were new ways of coping that were learned from other parents and often took the form of giving of service to others. One mother highlighted the growth involved in learning to accept contradictions in life:

I think it is an acceptance, and I think the best thing that parents can do for themselves is just to stop trying to change everyone and change themselves in the sense of learning to accept the impossible, learning to accept [that you] will never accept it, that you can never change it, that this is it, this is the way it is, and start a new life. You have to start a new life.

Relating to Others: Family

We broke the idea of relating to others into three subcategories: family, friends, and the deceased child. All of the parents experienced positive aspects in how they related to others. Some of the mothers learned to accept that their spouses mourned differently than they. In families with surviving children, many discovered a new appreciation for the relationships that they had with their other children. One mother commented:

> [My surviving son][2] certainly is not replacing [my son who died] because it is a different feeling that mother feeling, but I am just so much more aware of [my surviving son]. I consider that the best gift. I may have lost a son but I gained one too. I know that sounds kind of funny.

Relating to Others: Friends

All of the parents expressed the need to have someone in their life with whom they could be completely honest in talking about their bereavement and deceased child. These relationships are ones where they could talk in depth about the bereavement experience without worry of burdening the other person. For some this entailed new relationships that were forged during the illness or after the death; for others this meant the deepening of relationships that already existed. One mother provided an example of how she behaved in a new way in an old relationship:

> [my one close friend and I] have had our ups and downs, again because she's never been through it, she doesn't get it, she doesn't understand and we have had a few little set-tos ... it was on the anniversary of [my son's] passing and she didn't call, which really set me off and I told her exactly, exactly how I felt and I find most times people are more than willing to take it because it actually helps them understand where I live and where I come from. So they're better able to talk or say things thereafter.

Relating to Others: The Deceased Child

All parents reported a close and strong relationship with their deceased child. For some this meant having conversations with that child; others felt the child's presence often. The relationship was also nurtured by discussing the deceased child with their other children. One mother said:

> [My son] sits on my shoulder everyday and has since the day he died. I view him as my guardian angel, my mentor, someone who is looking out for me and hopefully his dad and his brother, and I am sure he is.

Personal Strength

The theme of personal strength was well-developed among participants and derived from wrestling with the adversity of loss. The parents reported that they felt they had more strength than they did prior to their child's death; and also that they had more of a capacity to deal with hardships than they thought they did. One mother talked about being too young to be bereaved but said, "I am getting through this. I'm putting one foot in front of the other. I'm learning how to live a life again without that child."

Another mother described one of the possible contradictions between recognizing the need to be strong and fully believing that one is capable of strength in the midst of loss: "… I kept saying in my mind, you know, you're a strong person and a hard worker. But I didn't believe it, but I found out that I am a strong person."

Appreciation of Life

Over time the parents came to appreciate life in new ways. This theme often included a new way of relating to one's own mortality. One mother said:

> I used to be afraid to die, of course because my greatest fear would be saying good-bye to my children, and I had to do that didn't I, so I guess I was forced to, to face that fear. The way I look at it now is when I die I will be going to [my son who died], I will be sad to be leaving [my remaining child], but I will be going to [my son who died] so it is a fifty-fifty split. So I am not afraid anymore…

Spiritual Change

Many parents talked about how their spirituality or religion sustained them throughout the process of loss. For some this meant change through a deepening of their spiritual or religious beliefs. One mother commented:

> The night she passed away it stopped raining … [we] went outside … it was a full moon, clouds in the sky, but they had broken, cause it rained pretty much the day on, and then the next morning it was beautiful and I never forgot. That's how I believe there is somebody out there, because man could not have made that, it was just too beautiful for anybody to make.

Searching for meaning was viewed as a chance to learn more about themselves, their views of life and death, and their relationship with religion or spirituality. One mother said:

> I believe there is something after death. I believe in God, I believe in Jesus, I do not go to church but I don't believe you have to. I believe there is a stronger being somewhere. I do believe that there is something after death, because basically it's just one big cruel joke if not. I believe this is a

---

2 Identifying information has been removed and explanatory words replace it in square brackets

place of learning your lesson; I'm not sure if it was [my son] who had to learn the lesson or whether it was me who had to learn the lesson through [my son's] death.

In summary, we chose to include the data from this research project to provide evidence of growth within one of the most challenging life experiences, the death of a child. The voices of these parents are a profound expression of the possibility of growth in the face of enormous pain and suffering. These words remind us that grief is not about detaching from the person who died; instead, it is about forming new bonds (Klass, Silverman, & Nickman, 1996). When we consider all that was shared in the interviews, it is clear that the forming of new bonds extends not just from the bereaved to the deceased but also a new bond formed with oneself, with one's spirituality, and with many other relationships within the context of the bereaved person's life. Through these new bonds and by other means, the bereaved can grow. Strengths and growth exist not only in bereavement experiences but in other palliative care contexts as well. A notable example is patients and families across the spectrum of illness from diagnosis to death. So how do practitioners broach this topic with families in a sensitive and helpful manner? A discussion of the questions and issues surrounding positive approaches in palliative care will serve to further elucidate the question of who grows as well as other implications for social work practice, assessment and intervention.

Implications for Social Work of Strengths and Growth in Palliative Care

What is a strengths approach to social work practice in palliative care? It requires that we as professionals, critically and constructively challenge the medical culture in which many of us work. We need to challenge because the overarching paradigm of the medical model, which tends to guide or at least influence our work, is at odds with the strengths perspective, as envisioned by Dennis Saleebey (2006). As with general social work practice, honoring and supporting the resources of our palliative patients is vital for healing. As professionals in palliative practice, we know that the healing work does not end with a palliative diagnosis but continues as our patients, whether the individual diagnosed or their loved one(s), engage with the new challenges in their lives. In contrast to pathologizing or medicalizing the issues and experiences of our patients, a strengths approach is "driven by the search for, the definition, and employment of peoples' resources in helping them walk, however hesitatingly, in the direction of their hopes and dreams" (Saleebey, 2000, p. 127).

In social work palliative practice, we believe it is valuable to consider the three life elements that Saleebey (2006) argues are central to the strengths perspective. Saleebey presents his CPR of strengths as a triangle, showing the interconnectedness of core life elements, and he argues all must be part of

holistic helping. The letter "C" represents *competencies, capabilities, courage,* and *character.* In palliative social work, we need to remember the strengths, such as character, that our patients bring with them to the palliative context. The "P" of CPR signifies *promise, purpose, possibility,* and *positive expectations.* In thinking about the concept "possibility," a key element within strengths-based practice is hope for the future (Saleebey, 2006). In our work with bereaved parents, we have come to learn that the nature of what is hoped for might change, but embracing new possibilities is still important for growth. Finally, R stands for *resources, resilience, relationships, resourcefulness, resolve,* and *reserves.* Relationships are particularly important for holistic palliative care. Hawthorrne and Yurkovich (2004) argue relationships are of particular value for those facing issues of life-threatening illness, in part because connecting with others is a way to restore a sense of humanity during a challenging time. However, Hawthorne and Yurkovich also argue that relationships tend to be a dynamic of palliative care that is neglected. A strengths perspective provides a possible solution, with the goals of honoring the world of relationships within which the patient exists as well as the potential implicit in the collaborative partnerships established with professionals. Overall, reflection on all the CPR strengths can encourage new possibilities in social work palliative practice. Consideration of this model can serve to prompt exploration of aspects of the individual's life experience that might otherwise go unexplored, and it reminds us to envision all aspects of the individual's situation, past, present and future. Importantly, as we embrace the strengths perspective in palliative care, assessing strengths may be just the beginning. Consider now the possibility of facilitating growth: how do we as social work practitioners work to discover strengths and encourage growth?

Discovering Strengths and Facilitating Growth

A great deal of the growth that is documented in the literature has occurred spontaneously, rather than having been facilitated by a professional of any sort. If we as professionals have a better idea of the concepts and the possibilities, perhaps there is potential to create an environment to facilitate more growth than what is occurring spontaneously. Time and further research are required in order to determine the nature and amount of growth that may occur when it is facilitated. Nonetheless, there are many skills that social workers and other health care professionals have and can acquire with the goal to facilitate growth in patients, families, and fellow health care professionals in a palliative care context. Weick et al. (1989) suggest that one way to facilitate growth is to understand strengths:

Continuing growth occurs through the recognition and development of strengths. The interplay between being and becoming and between what a person is in totality and what may develop into greater fullness mark the essential dynamic of growth. But an emphasis on the positive aspects of human capability serves as a stimulus for new growth. (p. 353)

Cowger, Anderson, and Snively (2006) offer suggestions for assessing strengths with questions to uncover possibilities, such as "Are there any critical moments or turning points in your life that helped you?" (p. 108). Saleebey (2006) suggests that we listen to people's stories instead of trying to follow an assessment protocol. Cowger et al. further suggest documenting the story as told by the person or people themselves, in order to value their language and create a vehicle for mutual discovery. Such narratives often reveal people's interests and hopes. To see and understand strengths is often a matter of changing the frame of practice (Blundo, 2006) such as a pathological worldview (Grant & Cadell, 2009). This serves to narrow the divide between professional and client as we accept the view that social workers are not different from clients: We are all human. If we are to embrace a strengths-based practice, we need to understand to whom it applies and when.

Timing of Positive Processes and Who Grows in Palliative Care?

The question of who grows and when is not fully understood (Cadell & Sullivan, 2006). The bereaved parents discussed here and other bereaved caregivers (Cadell, Regehr, & Hemsworth, 2003) all demonstrated growth that comes not from the negative experience itself, but with the person's "struggle to survive and come to terms with what has happened" (Calhoun & Tedeschi, 1999, p. 67). The timing of this struggle to make meaning is still not clear in relation to illness, caregiving, and bereavement experiences. For instance, when someone is very ill or busy caregiving, is it possible to have the energy to wrestle and ruminate in order to come to terms with illness?

There is concern that the process of growth can be hampered by well-meaning professionals who wish to help: The risk of proposing the possibility of growth too early can serve to minimize pain and suffering, hampering the growth that can occur (Calhoun & Tedeschi, 1999). Rather it is suggested that social workers and others make room for growth (Berger, 2008). This entails not seeking to solve problems, but listening for positive aspects from the people we work with rather than suggesting them (Calhoun & Tedeschi, 1999).

The literature abounds with anecdotes of growth in patients at the end of life (Byock, 1997; de Hennezel, 1997), but very little research has sought to understand that growth in those who are approaching death. Nelson-Becker (2006) examined strengths and resilience in older adults at the end of life. This qualitative study found themes of self, spirituality, social investment, and independence. Growth was nurtured through continuity of care and the ability of professionals to be fully present with the older adults. Nelson-Becker recommends listening carefully to the narratives of older adults and using creativity in the linking of patients to resources. In a study of advanced cancer patients in Greece, posttraumatic growth was measured and found to have a positive relationship with posttraumatic stress disorder: the more traumatized the person, the more likely the person was to report growth (Mystakidou et al., 2007). More research that examines, qualitatively and quantitatively, the growth that can occur along the continuum of illness and at the end of life, needs to be undertaken.

There is a notion that the demand on family caregivers' time and energy is so high that it is not possible for them to realize growth during the caregiving experience while the care recipient is still alive: that growth does not occur until after death. However, a recent project (Cadell et al., 2007) has been gathering evidence that parents who are actively caring for a child with a life-limiting illness are demonstrating growth, as measured by the posttraumatic growth inventory (Tedeschi & Calhoun, 1996). In palliative care, it cannot be assumed that the death of someone is traumatic. If the negative aspects can occur well before the death, then the resulting struggle to survive and come to terms with the stress may begin before the death as well. Certainly, for the patients that struggle must come before they themselves die.

Dying people and their families are not the only ones who may experience growth in palliative care. Calhoun and Tedeschi (1999) discuss the possibility of vicarious posttraumatic growth in professionals who can also experience benefit from working with people who are emerging changed in meaningful ways from adverse experiences. In addition, they have numerous suggestions and strategies for self-care, such as ensuring proper nutrition and regular exercise, accessing nature, and the thoughtful use of humor. Meaghen worked as a palliative social worker for more than a decade. She reflects on her work:

When I put myself in a place to really "think" about the lessons I have learned through my work with families, I find myself in a space that is wallpapered with the stories and experiences of many families. Some of the images are positive and others make me feel uncomfortable and sad. I cannot, however, see one without the other and I think this is important ... there is going to be both ... there has to be both ... we just need to learn how to "see" both without looking away from one or the other. There are times in life when we are inclined to see the glass as either half empty or half full; however, the reality is that it doesn't have to be one or the other, it is in fact, both.

Meaghen's experience demonstrates both growth from her own experience and the notion that wisdom engenders the ability to tolerate contradiction. Indeed, Calhoun and Tedeschi (1999) state:

... individuals who experience posttraumatic growth appear to show an increase in life wisdom.... Wisdom can be characterized as the ability to balance reflection

and action, weigh the knowns and unknowns of life, be
better able to accept some of the paradoxes of life, and
to more openly and satisfactorily address the
fundamental questions of human existence. ... life is
changed both for better and for worse; existential
questions are more salient, yet answers may be less
satisfying; the individual is more vulnerable, yet
stronger. (p. 21–22)

One of the paradoxes of growth is that the positive aspects do not replace the negative.

Positive and Negative Aspects Coexist

Of the models of positive processes and outcomes presented in the first section, most of them underline the coexistence of the negative and the positive. The strengths perspective reminds us as professionals that to promote change, we need to assess the assets of people along with the problems (Saleebey, 2006). The model of stress and coping reworked by Folkman (1997) is designed to illustrate the co-occurrence of positive and negative emotions. As noted earlier, the ultimate outcome of posttraumatic growth is wisdom and a tolerance of paradox (Calhoun & Tedeschi, 1999).

As social work practitioners in palliative care, we are aware of the need to question dichotomies. The essence of our work is to enhance living while dying; therefore, life and death are not diametrically opposed to one another. Indeed, the notions of the strengths perspective invite us to question the client-practitioner or us-them dichotomy (Grant & Cadell, 2009): We are not different from the people we work with and indeed we too will face the end of life. Similarly, we need to understand that the pain and suffering coexists with strengths and growth; the positive does not replace the negative.

Conclusion

Positive processes and outcomes of difficult or traumatic experiences are possible for people in palliative care, be they patients, family caregivers, or professionals. Little is known about positive outcomes, as research has only recently begun to include positive aspects as possible results of adverse circumstances. The notion that growth follows adversity is an ancient one, but it has only recently been understood in the context of social work practice.

Social work has long been noted for its person-in-context approach; this fits well with the philosophy and values of palliative care. This holistic perspective brings an important aspect to interprofessional teams working in palliative care, as well as adding to patient and family care. Palliative social work entails an acknowledgement of the stresses along the continuum of illness for patients and families. One of the hallmarks of the profession is its ability to discover the strengths and positive outcomes that also occur.

LEARNING EXERCISES

1. What is your experience with these various positive lenses? Are you familiar with them, by these names or any other related concept?

2. As palliative social workers we are encouraged to develop reflective practice. How would you assess any of the situations of the people mentioned in this chapter? In your practice, are you inclined to look for the possibility of both positive and negative outcomes? Are you surprised to know of the positive aspects of their various situations?

3. Reflect on a story in which you or someone you know experienced posttraumatic growth following a negative event.

4. How might individuals and families in palliative care benefit when assessment takes a strengths-based perspective as opposed to a deficit-based perspective? Are there any disadvantages to this?

5. In the context of your own professional practice, reflect on how you and your colleagues already implement these positive lenses or not. Can you identify any similarities or differences between your practice and the various professions you work with? What are some ways in which you can enhance your use of the strengths-based perspective within your own practice, as well as promote it among colleagues?

6. Think of a situation in which you have found it challenging to identify an individual's or a family's strengths. How did that affect your relationship?

7. How do we engage people in conversations about growth and strengths while respecting adversity? Reflect on some examples of questions we might ask.

REFERENCES

Aldwin, C. M., & Sutton, K. J. (1998). A developmental perspective on posttraumatic growth. In R. G. Tedeschi, C. L. Park, & L. G. Calhoun (Eds.), *Posttraumatic growth: Positive changes in the aftermath of crises* (pp. 43–63). Mahwah, NJ: Lawrence Erlbaum.

Berger, R. (2008). Fostering post-traumatic growth in adolescent immigrants. In L. Liebenberg & M. Ungar (Eds.), *Resilience in action* (pp. 87–110). Toronto, ON: University of Toronto Press.

Blundo, R. (2006). Shifting our habits of mind: Learning to practice from a strengths perspective. In D. Saleebey (Ed.), *The strengths perspective in social work practice* (4th ed., pp. 25–45). Boston MA: Allyn & Bacon.

Byock, I. (1997). *Dying well: Peace and possibilities at the end of life.* New York, NY: The Berkley Publishing Group.

Cadell, S., Davies, B., Siden, H., Steele, R., Straatman, L., Hemsworth, D., & Liben, S. (2007). Caregiving parents of children with life-limiting illnesses: Beyond stress and coping to growth. *Journal of Palliative Care, 23*(3), 227.

Cadell, S., Janzen, L., & Fletcher, M. (2004, November). *Parents finding meaning: Examining the post traumatic growth and the role of support with two bereavement programs.* Paper presented at the National Hospice Palliative Care Organization's First Pediatric Palliative Care Conference, Dearborn, MI.

Cadell, S., Janzen, L., & Haubrich, D. J. (2007). Engaging with spirituality: A qualitative study of grief and HIV/AIDS. In J. Coates, J. Graham, & B. Swartzentruber with B. Ouellette (Eds.), *Spirituality and social work: Select Canadian readings* (pp. 175–190). Toronto, ON: Canadian Scholars Press.

Cadell, S., Regehr, C., & Hemsworth, D. (2003). Factors contributing to post-traumatic growth: A proposed structural equation model. *American Journal of Orthopsychiatry, 73*(3), 279–287.

Cadell, S., & Sullivan, R. (2006). Posttraumatic growth in bereaved HIV caregivers: Where does it start and when does it end? *Traumatology, 3*(12), 45–59.

Calhoun, L. G., & Tedeschi, R.G. (1999). Facilitating posttraumatic growth: A clinician's guide. Mahwah, NJ: Lawrence Erlbaum Associates Publishers.

Calhoun, L. G., & Tedeschi, R.G. (2006). The foundations of posttraumatic growth: An expanded framework. In L. G. Calhoun & R. G. Tedeschi (Eds.), *Handbook of posttraumatic growth: Research and practice* (pp. 3–23). Mahwah, NJ: Lawrence Erlbaum Associates Publishers.

Cowger, C. D., Anderson, K. M., & Snively, C. A. (2006). Assessing strengths: The political context of individual, family, and community empowerment. In D. Saleebey (Ed.), *The strengths perspective in social work practice* (4th ed., pp. 93–115). Boston, MA: Allyn & Bacon.

De Hennezel, M. (1997). *Intimate death: How the dying teach us how to live.* (C. Brown Janeway, Trans.). New York, NY: Knopf.

Folkman, S. (1997). Positive psychological states and coping with severe stress. *Social Science and Medicine, 45*(8), 1207–1221.

Garmezy, N. (1971). Vulnerability research and issue of primary prevention. *American Journal of Orthopsychiatry, 41*(1), 101–116.

Grant, J., & Cadell, S. (2009). Power, pathological worldviews and the strengths perspective in social work. *Families in Society, 90*(4), 425–430.

Hawthorne, D. L., & Yurkovich, N. J. (2004). Hope at the end of life: Making a case for hospice. *Palliative & Supportive Care, 2*(4), 415–417.

Helgeson, V., Reynolds, K., & Tomich, P. (2006). A meta-analytic review of benefit finding and growth. *Journal of Consulting and Clinical Psychology, 74*, 797–816.

Hogan, N., & Schmidt, L. (2002). Testing the grief to personal growth model using structural equation modeling. *Death Studies, 26*, 615–634.

Joseph, S., & Linley, P. A. (Eds.). (2008). *Trauma, recovery, and growth: Positive psychological perspectives on posttraumatic stress.* Hoboken, NJ: John Wiley & Sons, Inc.

Klass, D., Silverman, P. R., & Nickman, S. L. (1996). *Continuing bonds: New understandings of grief.* Philadelphia, PA: Taylor & Francis.

Lazarus, R. S., & Folkman, S. (1984). *Stress, appraisal, and coping.* New York, NY: Springer Publishing Company.

Macdonald, M. E., Chilibeck, G., Affleck, W., & Cadell, S. (2009). Gender imbalance in pediatric palliative care research samples. *Palliative Medicine.* doi: 0269216309354396v1.

Masten, A. S., Best, K. M., & Garmezy, N. (1991). Resilience and development: Contributions from the study of children who overcome adversity. *Development and Psychopathology, 2*, 425–444.

McCubbin, H. I., & McCubbin, M. A. (1988). Typologies of resilient families: Emerging roles of social class and ethnicity. *Family Relations, 37*, (3) 247–254.

Mystakidou, K., Parpa, E., Tsilika, E., Pathiaki, M., Galanos, A., & Vlahos, L. (2007). Traumatic distress and positive changes in advanced cancer patients. *American Journal of Hospice and Palliative Medicine, 24*(4), 270–276.

Nelson-Becker, H. (2006). Voices of resilience: Older adults in hospice care. *Journal of Social Work in End-of-Life and Palliative Care, 2*(3), 87–106.

Park, C., & Helgeson, V. (2006). Introduction to the special section: Growth following highly stressful life events–Current status and future directions. *Journal of Counseling and Clinical Psychology, 74*, 791–796.

Puterman, J., & Cadell, S. (2008). Timing is everything: The experience of parental cancer for young adult daughters–A pilot study. *Journal of Psychosocial Oncology, 26*(2), 103–121.

Scannapieco, M., & Jackson, S. (1996). Kinship care: The African American response to family preservation. *Social Work, 41*(2), 190–196.

Saleebey, D. (1992). *The strengths perspective in social work practice.* New York, NY: Longman.

Saleebey, D. (1997). *The strengths perspective in social work practice* (2nd ed.). New York, NY: Longman.

Saleebey, D. (2000). Power in the people: Strengths and hope. *Advances in Social Work, 1*(2), 127–136.

Saleebey, D. (2002). *The strengths perspective in social work practice* (3rd ed.). Boston, MA: Allyn & Bacon.

Saleebey, D. (2006). *The strengths perspective in social work practice* (4th ed.). Boston, MA: Allyn & Bacon.

Tedeschi, R. G., & Calhoun, L. G. (1995). *Trauma and transformation: Growing in the aftermath of suffering.* Thousand Oaks, CA: Sage Publications.

Tedeschi, R. G., & Calhoun, L. G. (1996). The posttraumatic growth inventory: Measuring the positive legacy of trauma. *Journal of Traumatic Stress, 9*(3), 455–471.

Tedeschi, R., & Kilmer, R. (2005). Assessing strengths, resilience, and growth to guide clinical interventions. *Professional Psychology: Research and Practice, 36*(3), 230–237.

Tedeschi, R. G., Park, C. L., & Calhoun, L. G. (1998) Posttraumatic growth: Conceptual issues. In R. Tedeschi & L. Calhoun (Eds.), *Posttraumatic growth: Positive changes in the aftermath of crisis* (pp. 1–22). Mahwah, NJ: Lawrence Erlbaum Associates.

Ungar, M. (2004). A constructionist discourse on resilience: Multiple contexts, multiple realities among at-risk children and youth. *Youth and Society, 35*(3), 341–365.

Weick, A., Rapp, C., Sullivan, W. P., & Kisthardt, W. (1989). A strengths perspective for social work practice. *Social Work, 34*(2), 350–354.

Werner, E., & Smith, R. (1982). *Vulnerable, but invincible: A longitudinal study of resilient children and youth.* New York, NY: McGraw-Hill.

21 *Myra Glajchen*

Caregivers in Palliative Care: Roles and Responsibilities

This is not a good ending. I feel like we are just watching her die. It's heartbreaking to see my mother like this, unable to eat or speak.
        —62-year-old son of Mrs. B., a week before she died in the palliative care unit

Key Concepts
- ◆ *Definitions of palliative care embrace the patient and family as the unit of care.*
- ◆ *Involvement of family caregivers is essential for optimal treatment of the patient with advanced medical illness.*
- ◆ *Family caregivers carry out a wide range of support tasks that span the entire trajectory of disease and include unique physical, psychosocial, and spiritual domains.*
- ◆ *Caregivers have their own emotional responses to the patients' diagnosis and prognosis, and they require interventions targeted toward their specific needs.*
- ◆ *The multifaceted role of family caregivers is demanding, posing significant challenges for the palliative care team.*

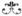
Introduction

Family caregivers play a major role in providing care to sick or disabled relatives in the United States. The actual numbers are difficult to estimate because many caregivers do not self-identify as such. However, the most recent survey estimates there are 44.4 million American caregivers, or 21% of the adult population. Most caregivers are women, the average age is 45 years, and most are providing care for women over 50. The amount of time devoted to caregiving is substantial, at least 40 hours of care each week for an average of 4.3 years (National Alliance for Caregiving and American Association of Retired Persons [AARP], 2004).

As people have enjoyed the benefits of early detection, aggressive treatment protocols, outpatient care, and longer survival times for many serious illnesses, so have family caregivers assumed more responsibilities that used to be performed by health care professionals (Schumacher et al., 2008). The goal of this chapter is to elucidate the wide range of roles and tasks performed by family caregivers, increase awareness of caregivers' emotional responses and unmet needs, and develop specific treatment recommendations for the palliative social worker.

Caregivers in Palliative Care

Definitions of palliative care embrace the patient and family as the unit of care. In particular, the National Consensus Project places the family caregiver in a central role during discussions about ongoing care and decision making (Altilio, Otis-Green, & Dahlin, 2008). The hallmarks of palliative care that relate to caregivers include an interdisciplinary focus, concern for quality of life in both patients and family caregivers, and involvement of caregivers in symptom management, communication, and medical decision making (Morrison & Meier, 2004). Ideally, the family caregiver should be treated as an integral part of the unit of care, at diagnosis, in the emergency room, through active treatment and beyond. The focus of this chapter will be to embrace caregivers as part of the unit of care, acknowledge their contribution, and recognize their needs along the continuum of patient illness including end of life care.

Hospital palliative care programs have been shown to improve caregiver well-being and family satisfaction, improve physical and psychological symptom management, and reduce hospital costs. In a retrospective study involving 524 caregivers, palliative care consultation prior to death was associated with higher scores in nine caregiver-related domains of care during the last month of life. These differences were attributable primarily to improvements in communication and emotional support (Casarett et al., 2008).

Caregivers derive benefit from the improved patient outcomes associated with inpatient palliative care consultations. These include identifying and treating new symptoms, addressing unmet needs, improving pain relief, documenting goals of care, and lowering the likelihood of an intensive care unit death (Higginson et al., 2003; Manfredi et al., 2000; Morrison et al., 2008; Norton et al., 2007; Penrod et al., 2006). The literature suggests that earlier consultations may be more valuable for patients and caregivers who need these services. This is probably because team effectiveness depends on a close rapport with patients and families, which takes time to develop (Rosenfeld & Rasmussen, 2003).

Definitions of family caregivers are many and varied. As early as possible, a social work inquiry about who the patient considers "family" and who has been providing the most care will lead to identification of caregivers. The team's inquiry and interest acknowledges the family's history of dealing with the disease and their familiarity with the patient's needs and wishes (Levine, 2003). Because many acute care hospitals have a policy of "Don't ask, don't tell" when it comes to caregivers, it often falls to the palliative social worker to recognize the contribution of the family caregiver and make it explicit. For Mrs. B.'s distressed son who is described in the opening quote, the social worker can respond to the helplessness and frustration of "just watching her die", explore what he would consider a "good ending," provide him with support, and identify meaningful tasks he can still perform. They can also discuss approaches for enriching the environment to reflect her history and the special relationship shared by mother and son.

Family Caregivers' Roles and Tasks

The U. S. health care system has shifted to shorter hospital stays and an increase in outpatient and home care for many advanced diseases. This has resulted in patients going home "quicker and sicker," and it has loaded caregivers with higher expectations for complex medical and nursing tasks that used to be done in the hospital. For example, family caregivers play a major role in pain and symptom management, which includes assessment and reporting of symptoms, dispensing medication, managing side effects, refilling prescriptions, and changing patches, dressings, tubing and other medical equipment. In this way, modern-day caregivers have replaced the role of skilled health care workers but often without training or explicit informed consent (McCorkle & Pasacreta, 2001).

In palliative care, the caregiver's role will shift along with the needs of the patient. During diagnosis and treatment, the caregiver is expected to integrate medical information and play an active role in decision making. This may involve unfamiliar terminology, new treatment settings, and frightening procedures or medications. During active treatment, caregivers may have to juggle competing demands by trying to provide emotional and tangible support to the patient while meeting ongoing obligations of home, work, and family. The demands of transportation, hospital visits, home care, and dealing with insurers can be exhausting. The palliative social worker is ideally positioned to address caregivers' physical and emotional needs, analyze family dynamics, and advocate on behalf of caregivers as needed.

At the time of a new diagnosis, change in diagnosis, or change in disease status, family caregivers have to integrate new medical information with prognostic significance, while also adjusting to functional limitations and emotional responses in the patient. If the patient is hospitalized, the caregiver is expected to work with professional staff to facilitate the transition to the home, hospice, or long-term care facility. For patients receiving home care, caregivers have to adjust to having health care professionals in the home, learn to manage them, deal with medical emergencies, and interact with insurance companies. In addition, for those patients at end of life, the caregiver's daily responsibilities are compounded by the anticipated death and its aftermath.

Family caregivers play a major role in home-based palliative care and hospice programs where they may have to assume the role of primary caregiver (Singer, Bachner, Shvartzman, & Carmel, 2005; Stajduhar & Davies, 1998). In the home setting, caregivers may master skills related to physical symptom and comfort management, nutrition, personal hygiene, positioning, technical equipment, 24-hour support, and emergency measures. Some studies suggest that caregivers providing care at home experience technical difficulties with medication management and more emotional strain in comparison to caregivers of hospital inpatients (Singer, Bachner, Shvartzman & Carmel, 2005). Anxiety related to ineffective symptom control and fear of administering medication seem to be the most prevalent concerns expressed by caregivers across many palliative home care studies (Armes & Addington-Hall, 2003; Hudson, Aranda, & McMurray, 2002; Oldham & Kristjanson, 2004; Wong et al., 2002).

In addition to the more obvious tasks just outlined, caregivers also provide valuable but less-defined contributions such as companionship, listening, physical comfort, and distraction. Caregivers also take on roles as patient advocates and as communicators between patients and medical providers

(Glajchen, 2010).Whatever specific roles the caregiver is performing, it is helpful for the social worker to acknowledge the work so the caregiver not only feels validated, but also invited to share the varied and complex emotions elicited by this role.

The Infusion of Culture

Palliative care teams confront cross-cultural influences on a daily basis. In immigrant families, traditional patterns of caregiving may conflict with professional expectations. It generally falls to the social worker to identify salient cultural variables and assist the team to integrate their significance and potential impact on the plan of care. In a recent meta-analysis of 116 empirical studies, Asian American caregivers were found to provide more caregiving hours than white, black, and Hispanic caregivers; to use lower levels of formal support services; and to have fewer financial resources, lower educational levels, and higher levels of depression than the other subgroups (Pinquart & Sorensen, 2005). These findings can inform the work of the palliative care team who may explore the unique reasons for refusing home care and assess for depression in caregivers over time. In a study involving unmet needs and service barriers among Asian caregivers, the reasons for refusing outside help included "too proud to accept it" or "didn't want outsiders coming in." Other reported barriers included "bureaucracy too complex" or "couldn't find qualified providers." Access to care may also be compromised by a reluctance to discuss the disease or death within the family. For example, "among the Chinese, it is bad luck to speak of death or dying, and doing so even for discussing prognosis or for informed consent purposes may offend or elicit fear and uneasiness" (Pinquart & Sorensen, 2005). Keeping a life-threatening diagnosis secret from the patient, and avoiding discussions of disease progression in light of increasing pain or weakness, further add to the caregivers' sense of burden, isolation, and responsibility.

These are only a few of the aspects of culture that infuse and enrich palliative care. Language is always an important consideration, although culture really transcends language. Often the role of translator is assigned to a family member by default, and this role may go to the person most fluent in the language or most compliant with the request. When chronic illness is involved, and family members have to take on the dual role of caregiver and translator, the potential for conflict becomes more likely (Levine, Glajchen, & Cournos, 2004). Generally speaking, the use of medical interpreters is associated with errors in imparting accurate medical information (Pham, Thornton, & Engleberg, 2008) and in providing less medical information and emotional support to family members (Thornton, Pham, Engelberg, Jackson, & Curtis, 2009). In a comprehensive social work assessment, cultural beliefs about such aspects of life as illness, caregiving, truth telling, role expectations, pain and symptoms, and death are identified and infused into the plan of care.

Caregivers' Emotional Responses and Unmet Needs

Extensive research has been conducted to identify the needs of caregivers and to characterize those that are unmet. Most of these studies have focused on cancer and dementia. In cancer, the patient's stage of illness and goals of care have been shown to impact the burden of caregiving with the physical and emotional demands reaching their peak as the disease progresses to the terminal phase. Caregivers of patients receiving palliative care report significantly lower quality of life and physical health scores than caregivers of patients in active, curative treatment (Weitzner, Jacobsen, Wagner, & Friedland, 1999). In addition to assuming many of the patients' prior domestic responsibilities, family caregivers may have to sacrifice social activities and work duties, leaving them isolated, financially vulnerable, and insecure. Caregivers providing end-of-life care have been shown to experience increased emotional distress, regardless of the amount of care provided, when limited in their ability to participate in valued activities and interests (Cameron, Franche, Cheung, & Stewart, 2002).

Caregivers of patients with advanced medical illness frequently report unmet needs in physical, psychosocial, economic, and concrete domains. In comprehensive reviews, researchers have found that 60% to 90% of caregivers of cancer patients reported a need for assistance in adjustment to illness, psychosocial support, transportation, financial assistance, home care nursing, personal care for the ill person, and medical information (Shelby, Taylor, Kerner, Coleman, & Blum, 2002). In a 2000 study involving terminally ill patients, 87% reported unmet needs for transportation, homemaking services, nursing care, and personal care, yet most patients relied completely on family and friends to provide the assistance they needed; only 15% relied on paid assistance (Emanuel, Fairclough, Slutsman, & Emanuel, 2000). All of these needs are within the range of social work skills either through direct clinical interventions, advocacy, or resource finding.

Unrelieved psychological symptoms of seriously ill patients may predispose their surviving caregivers to long-term psychological and physical morbidity (Valdimarsdottir, Helgason, Fürst, Adolfsson, & Steineck, 2002). In their landmark caregiver health effects study, Schultz and Beach found that caregiver strain increased mortality risk by 63% within 5 years. After adjusting for sociodemographic factors, and underlying caregiver disease, older spousal caregivers who were providing care and experiencing strain had mortality risks that were 63% higher than noncaregiving controls (Schultz & Beach, 1999). In a recent study of family caregivers of dying cancer patients, caregivers scored higher on levels of anxiety and depression than the general population. Routine screening of anxiety and depression in family caregivers appears warranted based on the results of this study (Gough & Hudson, 2009).

While the emotional needs of caregivers have been extensively researched, their practical needs have received far less attention. Family caregivers of home-based palliative care patients report the need for coaching in acquiring practical nursing skills and more access to professional advice to increase their self-confidence and ability to perform the practical aspects of home-based care (Bee, Barnes, & Luker, 2008). In a study involving caregivers and patients with early-stage lung cancer, the caregivers' sense of competence in pain and symptom management showed beneficial effects for patients and caregivers alike. Specifically, caregiver self-efficacy for managing pain, symptoms, and function promoted better adjustment and resilience among patients and lower levels of strain and psychological distress among caregivers (Porter, Keefe, Garst, McBride, & Baucom, 2008).

Caregiving has been shown to impact quality of life. The more time spent assisting the patient, the more disrupted are the caregiver's schedule and emotional well-being. Family members confronting serious illness experience as much, if not more, distress as the person with the illness. This distress arises from the caregiver role itself as well as witnessing the patient's suffering (Miaskowski, Kragness, Dibble, & Wallhagen, 1997). A meta-analysis of psychological distress among cancer patients and family caregivers found that both members of the dyad experienced similar levels of distress (Hodges, Humphris, & MacFarlane, 2005.) Accepting the responsibility of caregiving may lead to depression. Caregivers who have no outside help are more depressed than those who receive help from formal resources.

Caregivers report that their informational needs are largely unmet, and they highlight problems in the content, delivery, and timing of that information (Grbich, Parker, & Maddocks, 2001; Hudson et al., 2002; Singer et al., 2005; Wilkes, White, & O'Riordan, 2000). In response to direct inquiry, family caregivers express a firm preference for receiving information in person, as early as possible, and in written format. In a study that looked at pain education for caregivers of cancer patients, caregivers reported concerns related to lack of knowledge of pain medications, lack of information about comfort therapies, and difficulty remembering pain management strategies such as subcutaneous drug administrations (Oldham & Kristjanson, 2004). Lack of confidence in one aspect of caregiving, such as pain, tends to have a spillover effect and can result in broad feelings of inadequacy for caregivers (Broback & Bertero, 2003) and helplessness for patients (Porter et al., 2008).

Finally, the social worker should consider the costs of caregiving in terms of money, resources, and time away from usual activities. Included in these costs are time spent traveling to and from care, waiting for patient appointments, lost work time, preparation for surgery and medical procedures, hospitalization, and time away from other relationships (Yabroff et al., 2007). Caregivers also spend time managing the patient's recovery time at home, addressing insurance issues, and providing companionship, emotional support, conversation, and other forms of support.

Caregiver Assessment

The palliative social worker is trained in individual and family assessment. Assessment is key to identifying those caregivers at risk for future distress, family problems, and greater need for psychosocial services (Alderfer et al., 2009). There are many caregiver assessment tools available, some of which are accessible through the websites and resources listed at the end of this chapter.

To be effective, any assessment should take into account not only what the patient requires but also what the caregiver is able and willing to provide. For example, gender stereotyping may lead the palliative care team to assume that women are more able and willing to perform such tasks as wound dressing, feeding, bathing, and wheelchair manipulation, but this is not always the case (Levine, 2008). If the patient's daughter-in-law comes to the hospital to visit daily, the team cannot presume that the daughter-in-law does not work, is available to be a caregiver, or that she and the patient get along. Nor can it be assumed that the dynamics within a family support a plan of care which includes any family member becoming a caregiver to another member who has suddenly become a patient. These details should be assessed through a comprehensive patient family assessment that respects the unique history of each family.

Caregiving may be influenced by gender and the customary roles that family members have adopted within their particular family unit. In their meta-analysis of 84 studies of caregiver burden, Pinquart and Sorensen found that spousal caregivers were more distressed than other caregivers, and women were more distressed than men. Generally speaking, spouses who are caregivers provide four times the amount of care provided by nonspousal family caregivers (Tennstedt, McKinlay, & Sullivan, 1989); and they report a lack of social roles and activities outside the home, which might act as buffers against caregiver stress (Barber & Pasley, 1995). In terms of gender, women tend to demonstrate greater psychological distress than men because they provide more personal care tasks, they are more likely to assume the primary caregiver role, less likely to obtain formal help, and may experience cultural and social pressure to become caregivers (Miller & Cafasso, 1992; Yee & Schulz, 2000). In a study of spouses providing care for a terminally ill husband or wife, women provided more toileting-related tasks and reported higher levels of caregiver strain, but they also had lower odds of receiving support from family and friends than did male caregivers (Brazil, Thabane, Foster, & Bédard, 2009).

In looking at caregiver age, older caregivers are more likely to report higher levels of depression and lower levels of self-efficacy than younger caregivers. Older caregivers may have their own health problems and have access to fewer psychological, physical, and financial resources (Baltes & Mayer, 1999). Older caregivers may have fewer outside roles in the workplace (Barber & Pasley, 1995) and be less comfortable with formal support services (Hooker, Monahan, Bowman, Frazier, & Shifren, 1998).

Spiritual well-being may provide a stress-buffering effect for caregivers. Research has shown that higher levels of spirituality are associated with lower psychological distress and improved well-being for caregivers (Kim, Wellisch, Spillers, & Crammer, 2007). In addition, maintaining faith and finding meaning have been shown to buffer the adverse effect of caregiving stress on mental health (Colgrove, Kim, & Thompson, 2007). Spirituality can act to fortify against hopelessness, help caregivers to derive meaning, and provide an existential perspective on hope and suffering (Ward, Berry, & Misiewicz, 1996). The social worker can explore the spiritual or religious values that inform a person's response to caregiving.

Caregiver burden is commonly used to describe multiple dimensions of distress arising from an imbalance between care demands and resources to meet those demands. Caregiver burden is profoundly affected by the patient's symptom burden, stage of disease, and quality of care received (Teno et al., 2004). More physical demands for the family caregiver may result in social isolation and impairment in other quality-of-life domains (Weitzner et al., 1999). As the patient deteriorates, caregiver quality of life worsens, with burden reaching its peak during the terminal phase. This is probably related to increased physical demands plus alterations in role functioning as progressing disease forces changes in family structure, with caregivers taking on additional responsibilities in anticipation of the patient's death (McCorkle et al., 1998).

Studies suggest that the psychosocial status of caregivers may fluctuate over time, so frequent reassessment is essential. In addition, the involvement of palliative, hospice, and home care teams most likely will identify psychosocial problems among caregivers that might otherwise be missed.

Social Work Interventions

Despite the fact that caregiver burden and distress have been studied since the early 1980s, few documented intervention studies have been published to show which interventions produce specific outcomes. The lack of standardization in type of caregiver intervention, method of service delivery, and outcome variables present major challenges. Interventions for caregivers have focused on increasing knowledge through education and information; reducing anxiety and depression through counseling and psychotherapy; providing medical care and emotional comfort through palliative and hospice home care; and increasing confidence through problem solving and skill building (Glajchen, 2004; McCorkle & Pasacreta, 2001). Recent studies suggest that patient and caregiver self-efficacy for managing pain, other symptoms, and function may be important factors affecting adjustment, and that couple-based interventions aimed at increasing

self-efficacy and improving communication skills may be effective (Porter, Keefe, Garst, McBride, & Baucom, 2008; Porter, Keefe, Wellington, & de Williams, 2008). The palliative social worker, based on the social work assessment, is poised to select appropriate interventions or to refer caregivers to appropriate resources.

Social work clinicians generally agree upon the value of *providing information* to caregivers. Information provides caregivers with guidance for implementing care, and may reduce caregiver stress and the associated feelings of inadequacy and helplessness arising from ambiguity (Given, Given, & Kozachik, 2001). Information about the disease trajectory, the anticipated course, and the range of emotions experienced by families helps normalize the experience and enhances the sense of control so often missing in advanced illness. In addition, caregivers derive benefit and support from the time spent with the professional. Giving information is a process that bears repeating because anxiety often interferes with learning, and caregivers' information needs change over time (Wong et al., 2002). Although several descriptive investigations have reported on the value of educational programs for caregivers, outcome data are scarce.

Counseling, support, and psychotherapy are typically designed to enhance caregivers' morale, self-esteem, coping, and sense of control, while reducing anxiety and depression. Individual counseling provides caregivers with support, education, and problem-solving or coping skills. In this way, counseling can reduce caregiver distress by helping caregivers adjust psychologically to the demands of caregiving (Given, Given, & Kozachik, 2001; Kozachik et al., 2001). There have been few reports of the effectiveness of individual counseling in the literature. Available data suggest that individual counseling is effective in reducing caregiver burden, helping caregivers to challenge negative thoughts, effectively manage psychological issues (Harding & Higginson, 2003; Porter, Keefe, Garst, McBride, & Baucom, 2008), and provide guidance about role overload and time management (Honea et al., 2008). The palliative social worker can provide this counseling or refer to a therapist or support group. In addition, the social worker can give the caregiver permission to pursue relaxation and social activities. Many new forms of social support now exist for patients and their caregivers, including online support groups and social networking sites. However, outcome data on these techniques are still in their infancy.

Psychoeducational interventions involve structured programs with a combination of education and support. The setting and format may vary from home visits, phone calls, guidebooks, and audiotapes (Hudson, Aranda, & Hayman-White, 2005) to specialized home care (McCorkle et al., 1998). A recent synthesis of caregiver interventions found that caregiver burden and strain were more likely to be reduced through multiple psychoeducational interventions, which involved coping and problem-solving skills, as well as a symptom management component (Honea et al., 2008; McMillan et al, 2006; Porter, Keefe, Garst, McBride, &

Baucom, 2008). These programs seem to work best for caregivers with high rates of burden.

Numerous studies have investigated the impact of hospice care on caregivers. The results present a mixed picture, with some reports that involvement in a hospice home care program did not influence caregiver burden or adjustment (Haley et al., 2001; McMillan et al., 2006; Meyers & Gray, 2001), and others finding the positive impact of earlier hospice referrals and less aggressive care on the quality of life and adjustment of bereaved caregivers. In a well-designed, multisite, prospective, longitudinal cohort study of 332 patient–caregiver dyads, end-of-life discussions and hospice enrollment for patients with advanced cancer led to less caregiver regret, improved physical and mental health, as well as better overall quality of life for caregivers more than 6 months after the patient's death (Wright et al., 2008). Clearly, caregivers benefit from hospice participation. The potential for hospice home care to ameliorate caregiver burden is a ripe area for further study.

Skill training for caregivers has proven effective in improving caregiver quality of life, reducing the burden associated with symptom management, and strengthening caregiving competence. Such programs are effective for caregivers of patients at all stages of the disease process, including those at end of life (Hodges et al., 2005.) The most effective programs tend to combine guidance and support, as well as home visits, during which hands-on symptom management can be taught (McCorkle & Pasacreta, 2001). Successful nurse-led transition coaching programs help prepare patient and caregiver for what to expect, coach them on communicating with the doctor, and provide tools such as the personal health records and medication lists. In such programs, a nurse provides continuity of care through a single point of contact (Naylor, 2006). Such transition programs have shown promise in alleviating caregiver burden, increasing knowledge, confidence, morale, and new problem-solving skills for caregivers (Grbich et al., 2001; Kaasalainen, Craig, & Wells, 2000; Pasacreta, Barg, Nuamah, & McCorkle, 2000).

The *family meeting,* often a routine intervention in palliative care, is seen as a valuable clinical tool with many potential goals, including communicating medical information, delineating the goals of care, and facilitating decision making. The palliative social worker can take the lead in organizing and structuring the meeting, ensuring that the caregivers' needs for information and support are met, and encouraging a safe setting where caregivers may ask questions, process emotions, and receive validation for their contribution and concerns. Outcome studies confirming the effectiveness of the family meeting are just now beginning to emerge, especially from the intensive care unit literature. The family meeting is an ideal forum for eliciting caregiver concerns, providing clear information about treatment, facilitating end-of-life care decisions, and avoiding inappropriate and burdensome life-sustaining therapies. In addition, caregivers can receive reassurance that symptoms will be adequately managed and patient preferences will be respected (Boyle,

Miller, & Forbes-Thompson, 2005; Gueguen, Bylund, Brown, Levin, & Kissane, 2009; Radwany et al., 2009).

Expanding the Role of Palliative Social Work for Caregivers

Despite the rapid increase in the prevalence of inpatient palliative consultation teams, evidence about their effectiveness is still in its infancy. Future research is needed to better understand the mechanisms and processes of care that contribute to consultations' effectiveness (Casarett et al., 2008). Social workers can take the lead in this venture.

Focus groups conducted with doctors, nurses, social workers, home health aides, and administrators suggest that there is no uniform system for providing advice to caregivers in the home care setting (Grbich et al., 2001). This leaves family members susceptible to the weaknesses inherent in ad hoc communications (Adam, 2000). The palliative social worker can systematize the information given to caregivers, taking into consideration literacy, preferred language, and learning style. Working with the interdisciplinary team, the social worker can create a plan for follow-up and continuity of care. The social worker is ideally situated }at the interface between home-based and in-hospital services to enhance transitions so they are seamless and supportive of patients, families, and caregivers. The social worker can help caregivers by meeting their practical needs, raising awareness, improving communication, and ensuring that needs for information and skills training are met (Bee, Barnes, & Luker, 2008) as well as providing psychological support as they manage stress and the emotional sequelae of caregiving.

Caregivers assume caregiving for a variety of reasons, including a sense of familial obligation and loyalty, caring, cultural expectations, and out of necessity. Some caregivers assume the role because of the lack of resources to pay for care and lack of insurance coverage for services. Some report benefits such as personal growth, improved sense of self-worth, and increased personal satisfaction from caregiving. The positive aspects of caregiving are noteworthy and should be reinforced (Balducci et al., 2008; Kim, Schulz, & Carver, 2007). Caregiver assessment can include exploration of the positive aspects in addition to inquiry about the attributed meaning of this role in their lives

Many palliative care teams are uncertain about the specific needs of the caregivers they encounter. Good communication includes clear, reliable information tailored to caregivers' specific needs. These may be informational needs, emotional and support needs, or skill-based training. In an ideal world, such communication is best heard as part of a trusting relationship that has been built over time, is tailored to caregivers' needs and uncertainty, and allows time for them to process the information and complete important tasks (Hebert, Schulz, Copeland, & Arnold, 2008).

Emanuel and colleagues found that caregiver burden and distress were significantly reduced by physicians who practiced active listening. If the treating physician listened to their needs and opinions, caregivers felt validated in their role, and supported in their caregiving activities (Emanuel, Fairclough, Slutsman, Alpert, & Emanuel, 1999). There are interventions that social workers can encourage which involve the active, focused, and personal presence of the physician. A recent position paper of the American College of Physicians promotes recognition of the value of the caregiver role, suggesting that validation of the caregiver role may contribute to a positive caregiving experience and decreased rates of hospitalization and institutionalization (Mitnick, Leffler, & Hood, 2010). In addition, the American Medical Association advocates the use of the Caregiver Self-Assessment Questionnaire to improve communication and enhance the physician–family caregiver health partnership (http://www.ama-assn.org/ama/upload/mm/36/caregivertooleng.pdf).

Caregivers often derive benefit and satisfaction from information and clear communication regarding the prognoses of patients, even if the prognosis is poor (The SUPPORT Principal Investigators, 1995). These conversations are enhanced by the presence of a social worker because they often bring out caregivers' concerns, explore related cultural values, and set the stage for important adjustments and adaptations such as redefining expectations about care, accepting the patient's diminished capacities, struggling with ambivalence, searching for meaning, and ultimately, preparing for death (Levine, 2003).

Supporting the caregiver through the bereavement process may be one of palliative care's most important challenges. Caregivers who have been involved in full-time caregiving may have a difficult time reengaging in regular life once the patient has died. Many caregivers miss the familiar routines and social support from the palliative care team. Meeting with bereaved caregivers may be beyond the scope of practice for most palliative care teams, but it can help enormously with closure and help create meaningful memories of the person's dying and death (Levine, 2003). While bereavement is implicit in hospice care, palliative care teams may not provide bereavement services but rather refer within the community.

The palliative social worker can provide caregivers with resources for physical care, home health aides, respite programs, counseling, support groups, financial assistance programs, and other information (Travis et al., 2007). The social worker can advocate and provide direct guidance in negotiating the health care system, which may become overwhelming for overburdened and fatigued caregivers. Social workers can make a meaningful contribution to the assessment and treatment of caregivers in palliative care through their excellent communication skills, expertise in family systems, training in psychosocial aspects of well-being, psychological interventions, cultural awareness, and thorough knowledge about community resources.

In sum, members of the health care team should include caregivers in treatment planning explicitly and continuously. Such conscious involvement of family caregivers can do much to reduce stress, monitor caregivers' physical health, acknowledge their vital role, and, most important, fulfill our clinical responsibility to provide services reflective of our commitment to patient and family as the "unit of care."

LEARNING EXERCISE

Read the patient/family case narrative in Box 21.1. As the social worker on the team, what would be your first priority? Do you think the family can interpret Mrs. L.'s wishes, even though they never discussed these issues when she was well? How would you help them? How do you understand the family's responses in the family meeting? How will you work with the caregivers' reluctance to discuss advance directives? How will you think about the request that "everything be done?" Do you think this response represents a form of denial or cultural values and beliefs that are different than those reflected in the concept of advance directives? During the meeting, you may feel torn between the physician's focus on decision making and the family's need for emotional support and answers to specific questions. Do you see these as competing agendas and, if so, how

---

Box 21.1
Patient/Family Narrative: Mrs. L.

Mrs. L. is a 47-year-old Caucasian woman who is sightseeing with her husband and adult daughters in New York City. During dinner at a restaurant, Mrs. L. suffers a massive heart attack and is found unconscious on the floor of the restaurant bathroom. She is revived in the emergency department of the nearest hospital and admitted to the medical intensive care unit (MICU). When it becomes clear that she has sustained severe brain damage with little hope of neurologic recovery, the palliative care team is called. Mrs. L. has no oral or written advance directives, and her family asks that "everything be done" to keep Mrs. L. alive and restore her to her previous level of functioning. In the meantime, she shows significant medical decline, which includes lack of kidney function, a high fever, cardiac insufficiency, and bowel obstruction. She is completely dependent on a ventilator for respiratory support.

The palliative care attending convenes a family meeting to let the family know the severity of Mrs. L.'s medical condition, prognosis, and the likely course over the coming weeks. He asks the palliative care social worker and the MICU doctor to attend the meeting. To the surprise of the physicians, the L. family members divert the focus from the complex medical condition and discussion of decision making to their major concern, which is that Mrs. L.'s personal hygiene and dignity as a person be preserved by the staff. They request assurance that she is not experiencing pain, hunger, thirst, or any other kind of suffering, and they seek an estimate of how much longer she "has left."

will you negotiate them? If the patient is maintained on a ventilator, is it important for the family to know how long she might live as a ventilator-dependent person? How will you balance allowing the family the time that they need to process this tragedy and respect the institutional pressures to makes decisions and discharge patients? Do you believe that Mrs. L. is experiencing hunger and thirst? What is your understanding about suffering, and is this the same definition as the L. family's?

LEARNING EXERCISE

Consider the patient/family narrative presented in Box 21.2. Research the law that guides institutions in the use of medical interpreters. What are the clinical, family, and legal issues implicit in using young family members as interpreters of medical information? What might be the emotional and cognitive factors involved for a 15-year-old girl who is asked to deliver serious life-threatening medical information while simultaneously absorbing its meaning? What cultural and family rules may be violated by this request, which places the daughter in a leading role, while her mother and older brothers are passed over because of their poor English abilities? How would you advise the cardiologist from a family systems/legal and liability perspective? Would you be comfortable functioning as the intermediary between the family and the cardiologist, giving them the choice between using an interpreter and preserving the role of the daughter, or allowing her to translate if that is their cultural preference? If the family refuses a trained medical interpreter, what is the risk involved for the clinicians who will have no way of knowing what the daughter is saying to her family? Last, but not least, can you see any value in the daughter assuming this role for her immigrant family (Levine et al., 2004)?

Box 21.2
Patient/Family Narrative: Mr. C.

Mr. C. is a 58-year-old Chinese immigrant admitted to a major medical center with chest and arm pain. After a cardiac workup, he is diagnosed with end-stage heart disease. His prognosis is poor and his life span is limited. The C. family does not have a regular physician, so it falls to Dr. M., the attending cardiologist on call, to present Mr. C. with the extent of his heart disease and a range of treatment options, some of which are risky and complicated. Upon learning that no Cantonese interpreter is available until Monday morning, Dr. M. looks at the family members who visit Mr. C. on a daily basis, his wife and three children. Dr. M. decides to use the C. family's 15-year-old daughter, May, as the interpreter because her English is fluent and she seems smart enough to handle the task at hand.

ADDITIONAL RESOURCES
AND WEB SITES

American College of Physicians: http://www.acponline.org/ running_practice/ethics/issues/policy/caregivers.pdf

Position paper on Ethics, Professionalism, and Human Rights Committee Family caregivers, patients, and physicians: ethical guidance to optimize relationships. The paper consists of directives to physicians regarding accessibility, communication, advance care planning, and validation of the family caregiver's role in chronic and serious illness.

Center to Advance Palliative Care (CAPC): http://www.capc.org

A national organization that provides health care professionals with tools, training, guidelines, clinical resources, and technical assistance for starting a palliative care program in hospitals and other health care settings.

National Cancer Institute (NCI): http://www.cancer.gov/ cancertopics/pdq/supportivecare/caregivers/healthprofessional

The PDQ Caregiver Summary, *Family Caregivers in Cancer: Roles and Challenges*, provides a comprehensive evidence based overview about the roles, challenges and helpful interventions for caregivers of cancer patients. In addition, readers are encouraged to review the specific instruments for evaluating caregiver burdens included in the section on caregiver assessment.

The Family Caregiver Alliance: http://www.caregiver.org

Addresses the needs of caregivers providing long-term care at home. Its National Center on Caregiving serves as a central source of information on caregiving and long-term care issues for policy makers, service providers, media, and funders. The Web site provides useful information on caregiver research, publications, information, resources, technical assistance, training, and public policy initiatives.

The National Family Caregivers Association: http://www. thefamilycaregiver.org

Educates, supports, and advocates for caregivers who care for loved ones with a chronic illness or disability or the frailties of old age.

Net of Care: http://www.NetofCare.org

This interactive Web site is a community resource network for caregivers of the medically ill. The site is designed to put caregivers in touch with local and national resources searchable by type of illness, service need, and zip code; provide education on health topics such as communicating with health care professionals, managing medical emergencies, and self-care; and better educate caregivers of the medically ill to participate in informed decision making.

Next Step in Care: http://www.nextstepincare.org

This interactive Web site, designed by the United Hospital Fund, helps caregivers with transitions among different care settings, through tools and guides geared toward planning, communication, and coordination.

American Medical Association (AMA). (2009). Caregiver self-assessment questionnaire. Retrieved from http://www. ama-assn.org/ama/upload/mm/36/caregivertooleng.pdf

Andrews, S. (2001). Caregiver burden and symptom distress in people with cancer receiving hospice care. *Oncology Nursing Forum, 28,* 1469–1474.

Davis, C., Darby, K., Likes, W., & Bell, J. (2009). Social workers as patient navigators for breast cancer survivors: What do

African-American medically underserved women think of this idea? *Social Work in Health Care, 48*(6), 561–578.

Docherty, A., Owens, A., Asadi-Lari, M., Petchey, R., Williams, J., & Carter, Y. H. (2008). Knowledge and information needs of informal caregivers in palliative care: A qualitative systematic review. *Palliative Medicine, 22,*153–171.

Haley, W. E., LaMonde, L. A., Han, B., Narramore, S., & Schonwetter, R. (2001). Family caregiving in hospice: Effects on psychological and health functioning among spousal caregivers of hospice patients with lung cancer or dementia. *Hospital Journal, 15*(4), 1–18.

Hebert, R. S., Schulz, R., Copeland, V. C., & Arnold, R. M. (2009). Preparing family caregivers for death and bereavement: Insights from caregivers of terminally ill patients. *Journal of Pain and Symptom Management, 37*(1), 3–12.

Hudson, P., Thomas, T., Quinn, K., & Aranda S. (2009). Family meetings in palliative care: Are they effective? *Palliative Medicine, 23*(2),150–157.

Kramer, B. J., Christ, G. H., Bern-Klug, M., & Francoeur, R. B. (2005). A national agenda for social work research in palliative and end-of-life care. *Journal of Palliative Medicine, 8*(2), 418–431.

Kurtz, M. E., Kurtz, J. C., Given, C. W., & Given, B. A. (2004). Depression and physical health among family caregivers of geriatric patients with cancer—a longitudinal view. *Medical Science Monitor, 10*, CR447–456.

McCorkle, R., Robinson, L., Nuamah, I., Lev, E., & Benoliel, J. Q. (1998). The effects of home nursing care for patients during terminal illness on the bereaved's psychological distress. *Nursing Research, 47*(1), 2–10.

Tennstedt, S. L., McKinlay, J. B., & Sullivan, L. M. (1989). Informal care for frail elders: The role of secondary caregivers. *Gerontologist, 29*(5), 677–683.

Weitzner, M., McMillan, S. C., & Jacobsen, P. (1999). Family caregiver quality of life: Differences between curative and palliative cancer treatment settings. *Journal of Pain and Symptom Management, 17*, 418–428.

REFERENCES

Adam, J. (2000). Discharge planning of terminally ill patients home from an acute hospital. *International Journal of Palliative Nursing, 6*, 338–345.

Alderfer, M. A., Mougianis, I., Barakat, L. P., Beele, D., DiTaranto, S., Hwang, W. T., & Kazak, A. E. (2009). Family psychosocial risk, distress, and service utilization in pediatric cancer: Predictive validity of the Psychosocial Assessment Tool. *Cancer, 115*(18 Suppl), 4339–4349.

Altilio, T., Otis-Green, S., & Dahlin, C. M. (2008). Applying the National Quality Forum Preferred Practices for Palliative and Hospice Care: A social work perspective. *Journal of Social Work in End of Life and Palliative Care, 4*(1), 3–16.

Armes, P., & Addington-Hall, J. (2003). Perspectives on symptom control in patients receiving community palliative care. *Palliative Medicine, 17*, 608–615.

Balducci, C., Mnich, E., McKee, K.J., Lamura, G., Beckmann, A., Krevers, B., … Oberg, B. (2008). Negative impact and positive value in caregiving: Validation of the COPE index in a six-country sample of carers. *Gerontologist, 48*(3), 276–286.

Baltes, P. B., & Mayer, K. U. (1999). *The Berlin Aging Study: Aging from 70 to 100.* New York, NY: Cambridge University Press.

Barber, C., & Pasley, K. (1995). Family care of Alzheimer's patients: The role of gender and generational relationship on caregiver outcomes. *Journal of Applied Gerontology, 14*, 172–192.

Bee, P. E., Barnes, P., & Luker, K. A. (2008). A systematic review of informal caregivers' needs in providing home-based end-of-life care to people with cancer. *Journal of Clinical Nursing, 18*, 1379–1393.

Boyle, D. K., Miller, P. A., & Forbes-Thompson, S. A. (2005). Communication and end-of-life care in the intensive care unit: Patient, family, and clinician outcomes. *Critical Care in Nursing Quarterly, 28*(4), 302–316.

Brazil, K., Thabane, L., Foster, G., & Bédard, M. (2009). Gender differences among Canadian spousal caregivers at the end of life. *Health Social Care in the Community, 17*(2), 159–166.

Broback, G., & Bertero, C. (2003). How next of kin experience palliative care of relatives at home. *European Journal of Cancer Care, 12*, 339–346.

Cameron, J. I., Franche, R. L., Cheung, A., M., & Stewart, D. E. (2002). Lifestyle interference and emotional distress in family caregivers of advanced cancer patients. *Cancer, 94*(2), 521–527.

Casarett, D., Pickard, A., Bailey, A., Ritchie, C., Furman, C., Rosenfeld, K., … Shea, J. A. (2008). Do palliative consultations improve patient outcomes? *Journal of the American Geriatric Society, 56*(4), 593–599.

Colgrove, L. A. A., Kim, Y., & Thompson, N. (2007). The effect of spirituality and gender on the quality of life of spousal caregivers of cancer survivors. *Behavioral Medicine, 33*(1), 90–98.

Emanuel, E. J., Fairclough, D. L., Slutsman, J., Alpert, H., & Emanuel, L. L. (1999). Assistance from family members, friends, paid care givers, and volunteers in the care of terminally ill patients. *The New England Journal of Medicine, 341*, 956–963.

Emanuel, E. J., Fairclough, D. L., Slutsman, J., & Emanuel, L. L. (2000). Understanding economic and other burdens of terminal illness: The experience of patients and their caregivers. *Annals of Internal Medicine, 132*, 451–459.

Given, B. A., Given, C. W., & Kozachik, S. (2001). Family support in advanced cancer. *CA A Cancer Journal for Clinicians, 51*(4), 213–231.

Glajchen, M. (2004). Emerging role of caregivers in cancer care. *Journal of Supportive Oncology, 2*, 145–155.

Glajchen, M., Kornblith, A.B., Homel, P., Fraidin, L., Mauskop, A., & Portenoy, R.K. (2005). Development of a brief assessment scale for caregivers of the medically ill. *Journal of Pain and Symptom Management, 29*, 245–254.

Glajchen, M. (2010). Family Caregivers in Cancer: Roles and Challenges, National Cancer Institute, Rockville: MD. http://www.cancer.gov/cancertopics/pdq/supportivecare/caregivers/healthprofessional

Gough, K., & Hudson, P. (2009). Psychometric properties of the Hospital Anxiety and Depression Scale in family caregivers of palliative care patients. *Journal of Pain and Symptom Management, 37*(5), 797–806.

Grbich, C., Parker, D., & Maddocks, I. (2001). The emotions and coping strategies of caregivers of family members with a terminal cancer. *Journal of Palliative Care, 17*(1), 30–36.

Gueguen, J. A., Bylund, C. L., Brown, R. F., Levin, T. T., & Kissane, D. W. (2009). Conducting family meetings in palliative care: Themes, techniques, and preliminary evaluation of a communication skills module. *Palliative Support Care, 7*(2), 171–179.

Harding, R., & Higginson, I. J. (2003). What is the best way to help caregivers in cancer and palliative care? A systematic review of interventions and their effectiveness. *Palliative Medicine, 17,* 63–74.

Hebert, R. S., Schulz, R., Copeland, V., & Arnold, R. M. (2008). What questions do family caregivers want to discuss with health care providers in order to prepare for the death of a loved one? An ethnographic study of caregivers of patients at end of life. *Journal of Palliative Medicine,11*(3), 476–483.

Higginson, I. J., Finlay, I. G., Goodwin, D. M., Hood, K., Edwards, A. G. K., Cook, A., … Normand, C. E. (2003). Is there evidence that palliative care teams alter end-of-life experiences of patients and their caregivers? *Journal of Pain and Symptom Management, 25*(2), 150–168.

Hodges, L. J., Humphris, G. M., & MacFarlane, G. (2005). A meta-analytic investigation of the relationship between the psychological distress of cancer patient and their caregivers. *Social Science in Medicine, 60,* 1–12.

Honea, N. J., Brintnall, R., Given, B., Sherwood, P., Colao, D. B., Somers, S. C., & Northouse, L. L. (2008). Putting evidence into practice: Nursing assessment and interventions to reduce family caregiver strain and burden. *Clinical Journal of Oncology Nursing, 12*(3), 507–516.

Hooker, K., Monahan, D. J., Bowman, S. R., Frazier, L. D., & Shifren, K. (1998). Personality counts for a lot: Predictors of mental and physical health of spouse caregivers in two disease groups. *Journal of Gerontolgy and Behavioral Psychology Social Sciences, 53*(2), 73–85.

Hudson, P. L., Aranda, A., & Hayman-White, K. (2005). A psychoeducational intervention for family caregivers of patients receiving palliative care: A randomized controlled trial. *Journal of Pain and Symptom Management, 30*(4), 329–341.

Hudson, P., Aranda, S., & McMurray, N. (2002). Intervention development for enhanced lay palliative caregiver support—the use of focus groups. *European Journal of Cancer Care, 11,* 262–270.

Juarez, G., & Ferrell, B. R. (1996). Family and caregiver involvement in pain management. *Clinical Geriatric Medicine, 12,* 531–547.

Kaasalainen, S., Craig, D., & Wells, D. (2000). Impact of the caring for aging relatives group program: An evaluation. *Public Health Nursing, 17*(3), 169–177.

Kim, Y., Schulz, R., & Carver, C. S. (2007). Benefit-finding in the cancer caregiving experience. *Psychosomatic Medicine, 69,* 283–291.

Kim, Y., Wellisch, D. K., Spillers, R. L., & Crammer, C. (2007). Psychological distress of female cancer caregivers: Effects of type of cancer and caregivers' spirituality. *Support Care Cancer, 15* (12), 1367–1374.

Kozachik, S. L., Given, C. W., Given, B. A., Pierce, S. J., Azzouz, F., Rawl, S. M., & Champion, V. L. (2001). Improving depressive symptoms among caregivers of patients with cancer: Results of a randomized clinical trial. *Oncology Nursing Forum, 28*(7), 1149–1157.

Levine, C. (2003). Family caregivers: Burdens and opportunities. In R. S. Morrison & D. Meier (Eds.), *Geriatric palliative care* (pp.376-85). New York, NY: Oxford University Press.

Levine, C. (2008). Supporting family caregivers: Needed: Nursing and social work leadership. *American Journal of Nursing, 108*(9 Suppl.), 13–15.

Levine, C., Glajchen, M., & Cournos, F. (2004). Case study: A fifteen year-old translator. *Hastings Center Report, 34,* 10–12.

Manfredi, P. L., Morrison, R. S., Morris J., Goldhirsh, S. L., Carter, J. M., & Meier, D. E. (2000). Palliative care consultations: How do they impact the care of hospitalized patients? *Journal of Pain and Symptom Management, 20,* 166–173.

McCorkle, R., & Pasacreta, J. V. (2001). Enhancing caregiver outcomes in palliative care. *Cancer Control, 8,* 36–45.

McMillan, S. C., Small, B. J., Weitzner, M., Schonwetter, R., Tittle, M., Moody, L., & Haley, W. E. (2006). Impact of coping skills intervention with family caregivers of hospice patients with cancer. *Cancer, 106,* 214–222.

Meyers, J. L., & Gray, L. N. (2001). The relationships between family primary caregiver characteristics and satisfaction with hospice care, quality of life, and burden. *Oncology Nursing Forum, 28*(1), 73–82.

Miaskowski, C., Kragness, L., Dibble, S., & Wallhagen, M. (1997). Differences in mood states, health status and caregiver strain between family caregivers of oncology patients with and without cancer-related pain. *Journal of Pain and Symptom Management, 13,* 138–147.

Mitnick, S., Leffler, C., Hood, V. L., & American College of Physicians Ethics and Human Rights Committee. (2010). Family caregivers, patients and physicians: Ethical guidance to optimize relationships. *Journal of General Internal Medicine, 25,* 255–260. doi:10.1007/s11606-009-1206-3.

Miller, B., & Cafasso, L. (1992). Gender differences in caregiving: Fact or artifact? *Gerontologist, 32*(4), 498–507.

Morrison, R. S., & Meier, D. E. (2004). Clinical practice: Palliative care. *New England Journal of Medicine, 350*(25), 2582–2590.

Morrison, R. S., Penrod, J. D., Cassel, J. B., Caust-Ellenbogen, M., Litke, A., Spragens, L., & Meier, D. E. (2008). Cost savings associated with US hospital palliative care consultation programs. *Archives of Internal Medicine, 68*(16), 1783–1790.

National Alliance for Caregiving and American Association of Retired Persons (AARP). (2004). *Caregiving in the US.* Retrieved from http://www.caregiving.org/data/04finalreport.pdf

Naylor, M. D. (2006). Transitional care: A critical dimension of the home healthcare quality agenda. *Journal of Healthcare Quality, 28,* 48–54.

Norton, S. A., Hogan, L. A., Holloway, R. G., Temkin-Greener, H., Buckley, M., & Quill, T. E. (2007). Proactive palliative care in the medical intensive care unit: Effects on length of stay for selected high-risk patients. *Critical Care in Medicine, 35,* 1530–1535.

Oldham, L., & Kristjanson, L. (2004). Development of a pain management programme for family careers of advanced cancer patients. *International Journal of Palliative Nursing, 10,* 91–99.

Pasacreta, J. V., Barg, F., Nuamah, I., & McCorkle, R. (2000). Participant characteristics before and 4 months after attendance at a family caregiver cancer education program. *Cancer Nursing, 23*(4), 295–303.

Penrod, J. D., Deb, P., Luhrs, C., Dellenbaugh, C., Zhu, C. W., Hochman, T., … Morrison, R. S. (2006). Cost and utilization outcomes of patients receiving hospital-based palliative care consultation. *Journal of Palliative Medicine, 9,* 855–860.

Pham, K., Thornton, J. D., & Engleberg, R. A. (2008). Alterations during medical interpretation of ICU family conferences that interfere with or enhance communication. *Chest, 134,* 109–116.

Pinquart, M., & Sorensen, S. (2005). Ethnic differences in stressors, resources, and psychological outcomes of family caregiving; a meta-analysis. *Gerontologist, 45,* 90–106.

Porter, L. S., Keefe, F. J., Garst, J., McBride, C. M., & Baucom, D. (2008). Self-efficacy for managing pain, symptoms, and function in patients with lung cancer and their informal caregivers: Associations with symptoms and distress. *Pain, 137*(2), 306–315.

Porter, L. S., Keefe, F. J., Wellington, C., & de Williams, A. (2008). Pain communication in the context of osteoarthritis: Patient and partner self-efficacy for pain communication and holding back from discussion of pain and arthritis-related concerns. *Clinical Journal of Pain, 24,* 662–668.

Radwany, S., Albanese, T., Clough, L., Sims, L., Mason, H., & Jahangiri, S. (2009). End-of-life decision making and emotional burden: Placing family meetings in context. *American Journal of Hospice and Palliative Care, 26*(5), 376–383.

Rosenfeld, K., & Rasmussen, J. (2003). Palliative care management: A Veterans Administration demonstration project. *Journal of Palliative Medicine, 6,* 831–839.

Schulz, R., & Beach, S. R. (1999). Caregiving as a risk factor for mortality: The caregiver health effects study. *Journal of the American Medical Association, 282,* 2215–2219.

Schumacher, K. L., Stewart, B. J., Archbold, P. G., Caparro, M., Mutale, F., & Agrawal, S. (2008). Effects of caregiving demand, mutuality, and preparedness on family caregiver outcomes during cancer treatment. *Oncology Nursing Forum, 35,* 49–56.

Shelby, R. A., Taylor, K. L., Kerner, J. F., Coleman, E., & Blum, D. (2002). The role of community-based and philanthropic organizations in meeting cancer patient and caregiver needs. *CA A Cancer Journal for Clinicians, 52,* 229–246.

Singer, Y., Bachner, Y., Shvartzman, P., & Carmel, S. (2005). Home death–the caregivers' experiences. *Journal of Pain and Symptom Management, 30,* 70–74.

Stajduhar, K., & Davies, B. (1998). Death at home: Challenges for families and directions for the future. *Journal of Palliative Care, 3,* 8–14.

The SUPPORT Principal Investigators. (1995). A controlled trial to improve care for seriously ill hospitalized patients. The study to understand prognoses and preferences for outcomes and risks of treatments (SUPPORT). *Journal of the American Medical Association, 274,* 1591–1598.

Teno, J. M., Clarridge, B. R., Casey, V., Welch, L. C., Wetle, T., Shield, R., & Mor, V. (2004). Family perspectives on end-of-life care at the last place of care. *Journal of the American Medical Association, 291*(1), 88–93.

Thornton, J. D., Pham, K., Engelberg, R. A., Jackson, C., & Curtis, J. R. (2009). Families with limited English proficiency receive less information and support in interpreted intensive care unit family conferences. *Critical Care in Medicine, 37*(1), 89–95.

Travis, S. S., McAuley, W. J., Dmochowski, J., Bernard, M. A., Kao, H. F. S., & Greene, R. (2007). Factors associated with medication hassles experienced by family caregivers of older adults. *Patient Education and Counseling, 66,* 51–57.

Valdimarsdóttir, U., Helgason, A. R., Fürst, C. J., Adolfsson, J., & Steineck, G. (2002). The unrecognised cost of cancer patients' unrelieved symptoms: A nationwide follow-up of their surviving partners. *British Journal of Cancer, 86*(10), 1540–1545.

Ward, S. E., Berry, P. E., & Misiewicz, H. (1996). Concerns about analgesics among patients and family caregivers in a hospice setting. *Research in Nursing and Health, 19,* 205–211.

Weitzner, M. A., Jacobsen, P. B., Wagner, H., & Friedland, J. (1999). The Caregiver Quality of Life Index–Cancer (CQOLC) scale: Development and validation of an instrument to measure quality of life of the family caregiver of patients with cancer. *Quality of Life Research, 8,* 55–63.

Wilkes, L., White, K., & O'Riordan, L. (2000). Empowerment through information: Supporting rural families of oncology patients in palliative care. *Australian Journal of Rural Health, 8*(1), 41–46.

Wong, R., Franssen, E., Szumacher, E., Connolly, R., Evans, M., Page, B., & Danjoux, C. (2002). What do patients living with advanced cancer and their carers want to know? A needs assessment. *Supportive Care in Cancer, 10,* 408–415.

Wright, A. A., Zhang B., Ray A., Mack, J. W., Trice, E., Balboni, T., … Prigerson, H.G. (2008). Associations between end-of-life discussions, patient mental health, medical care near death, and caregiver bereavement adjustment. *Journal of the American Medical Association, 300*(14), 1665–1673.

Yabroff, K. R., Davis, W. W., Lamont, E. B., Fahey, A., Topor, M., Brown, M. L., & Warren, J. L. (2007). Patient time costs associated with cancer care. *Journal of the National Cancer Institute, 99,* 14–23.

Yee, J. L., & Schulz, R. (2000). Gender differences in psychiatric morbidity among family caregivers: A review and analysis. *Gerontologist, 40*(2), 147–164.

22

 Iris Cohen Fineberg and Amy Bauer

Families and Family Conferencing

You know, all families should be able to do this [have a family conference]. I feel sorry for the other families that aren't able to do that, to participate in that way. It's just sort of a source of strength of a family coming together at times like this. We all come together and face this together.

—Anonymous patient

Key Concepts

- The family is the central social system in which people experience serious illness and face end of life, regardless of how involved or absent the family is in people's lives.
- Palliative care recognizes the family, including the patient, as the unit of care. This requires a systemic perspective that integrates individual- and family-oriented approaches to palliative social work assessment, intervention, and overall practice. Designation of who constitutes "family" should be based on the patient's guidance.
- Social workers are uniquely educated and positioned to provide expertise and leadership within the palliative care team regarding family care. Their background in family systems, family and group dynamics, and family therapy provides strong theoretical grounding for professional practice.
- Communication in the setting of palliative care has a tremendous impact on the patient and family experience of what is a momentous life process. Family conferences are a powerful clinical tool for family and team communication and represent an ideal forum for social work leadership in palliative care.

Introduction

Families are a central part of people's lives. They are the immediate social system that shapes who people are and the lives they lead. The importance of family becomes magnified at times of serious illness, when people must grapple not only with the illness experience but also with facing end of life. During times of illness, and certainly in the context of palliative care, families often become important sources of support and practical assistance (Ell, 1996; Harris et al., 2009). They may help with transportation, child care, finances, physical care, and emotional support. Yet they may also be tremendous sources of distress, by their absence, their inner turmoil, and their conflicting needs. The importance of family remains central whether the family is traditional or nontraditional, intact or disjointed, present or absent. In fact, the lack of a family presence or involvement is in itself a powerful family force. In some cases, it may leave patients particularly vulnerable.

Health care providers are in a privileged social position that sanctions their entrée into the intimate lives of families because they deal with illness and impending death. Social workers' respect for this position should include a conviction that they have valuable knowledge, skills, and perspectives to offer in their care to families (Gwyther et al., 2005). The roles of families become highlighted at times of illness, and it is therefore essential that social workers working with seriously ill patients and providing palliative care have an inclusive and thorough understanding of the family, including the patient, as the recipient of care (Kristjanson & Aoun, 2004). Core clinical social work values and skills (O'Hare, 2009), such as relationship and trust building, are central to creating a care environment that fosters empathic, effective communication about the family's situation, needs, and wishes. This chapter will discuss the concept of family, family assessment, and common challenges for families in the palliative care context. Information about caring for families, and especially conducting family conferences, will be presented. Social work practice in the context of palliative care, either within or outside of a palliative care team, can provide expertise and leadership in the area of excellent family-oriented care.

Defining and Conceptualizing the Family

Defining the Family

Formal study of the concept of family is a long-standing topic in social work, sociology, anthropology, and other social sciences. While theoretical debate is outside the scope of this chapter, it is important to define family for the purposes of discussion. In the setting of palliative care provision, "family" is defined as whomever the patient designates as family (National Consensus Project for Quality Palliative Care, 2009). The patient is a member of the family and not external to it. Written language discussing palliative care often refers to the "patient and the family," which may unintentionally lead readers to forget that the patient too is a family member. He or she is part of the family group, a person with family roles, a participant in the family history, and someone integral to the family dynamics.

Family members may be related by biology (or blood, as some would state). These include parents, children, siblings, grandparents, aunts/uncles, and cousins of varying degrees. Other family members are related by legal or structural relationships, such as spouses, civil partners, in-laws, stepparents, and stepchildren. Furthermore, there are "chosen" family members who are close friends who have a significant social role in the life of the patient such that the patient defines them as family members (Beder, 2009). People have a mix of family members, with the balance of the different types varying from person to person. Definitions of family are both individually and culturally constructed, and as a result, patients' definition of their family will be influenced both by their individual perspective of who constitutes their family and by the broader culture or cultures from which they come (Kaslow, Celano, & Dreelin, 1995).

Exploring patients' views of their families is essential to avoid assumptions, incorrect attributions of family status, and the overlooking of important information about individual and cultural family norms. Cultures vary in how families are organized and function, with some emphasizing the individual patient as central in the family during a period of illness, while others emphasize the family unit as taking priority and having authority over the patient's process of care. Since behaviors may have different meanings in different cultures, it is important to explore and understand the significance of a particular family's behavior rather than assuming that the behavior has the same meaning in all families. For families with complex histories of tragedy, trauma, or loss, social work attention and understanding of family definitions and configurations may be especially critical for providing the best care for the family.

The Family in Palliative Care

Regardless of whether family definitions are explicit in specific documents, the importance of family in palliative care is clearly recognized in palliative care literature and policy documents (Department of Health, 2008; World Health Organization, 2007). Illness and end of life are understood to be periods of life when the involvement of those related and/or close to the patient have a magnified role. Furthermore, the contemporary conceptual model of palliative care defines the scope of care as continuing into the realm of bereavement care, acknowledging that the illness and death of the patient is an experience that impacts family members well after the moment of death (Milberg, Olsson, Jakobsson, Olsson, & Friedrichsen, 2008; Zaider & Kissane, 2009). Interactions with the patient and family during the illness process culminating in the end of life will have tremendous impact on how surviving family members recall, integrate, and endure their memories of the experience. While palliative care maintains the patient at the center of the process, it views the family as the unit for whom excellent care is also provided.

Family Systems

Social work has long applied family systems theory to clinical practice and brings the strength of this perspective to palliative social work. A key characteristic of a system is that change in any one part of the system influences the rest of the system (Mehta, Cohen, & Chan, 2009). The event of a life-threatening diagnosis in one family member, together with the subsequent changes that occur with the experience of illness, has a tremendous impact on the rest of the family system (King & Quill, 2006; Monroe & Oliviere, 2009). Conversely, behaviors and events in the family affect the patient family-member, including their experience of illness, coping, and decision making. The family systems conceptual framework offers a broad-view lens through which to consider potential factors influencing the behaviors and choices of patients and other family members. Thus, attempts to understand a patient's reaction to news about treatment would include exploration and consideration of other family events and dynamics that may be affecting the patient in non-obvious ways. Social workers using family systems theory are thus well equipped to offer insights to the care team about the patient and family, providing expert knowledge and subtly educating team members from a perspective less common to other health care professions.

Assessment of Families

Conducting a comprehensive biopsychosocial-spiritual assessment is central to the work of the palliative social worker (Gehlert & Browne, 2006; National Association of Social Workers [NASW], 2004; Puchalski et al., 2009; Sulmasy, 2002). Integral to the palliative care approach to understanding an individual facing life-threatening illness is to understand this family context (Zaider & Kissane, 2009). This assessment, which includes family characteristics and dynamics, is the basis for interventions aimed at assisting the family unit to adjust to the emotional, psychological, and social changes inherent to accommodation to illness in the family (Blacker & Jordan, 2004).

Family assessment often begins with gathering structural information identifying members of the "immediate" family, usually focused on those with biological and legal relations to the patient. The assessment explores the nature of the internal family relationships, determining the patient's conceptualization of family, and identifying key members of the family according to the patient. Particularly supportive or stressful relationships are helpful to identify. The assessment attempts to capture an overall "picture" to understand family roles, supports, and stressors that are relevant to the particular family and patient. Changes in family roles, such as who becomes the primary earner or caregiver, are common and profound for many families. The assessment explores cultural issues and their potential as sources of strain or strength for the patient within the context of illness and the health care system. Geographic distribution of the family is determined, especially as it relates to support for the patient and planning for optimal communication (Mitnick, Leffler, & Hood, 2010).

Specific attention is focused on a sensitive exploration of family history as it relates to illness and death, traumas, and other notable family experiences. The family's experience with mental and/or physical disabilities is assessed, as well as previous experiences with caregiving. Social workers need to consider difficult topics such as emotional, physical, and sexual abuse, as well as substance abuse. As information unfolds in the assessment process, so does a thoughtful exploration of significant social experiences as they are identified. Attention to such topics as poverty, immigration, refugee status, or exposure to violence and war may be appropriate with some families and not others.

Family Resilience

Resilience, "the ability to withstand and rebound from adversity" (Walsh, 2002, p. 130), has become an important concept in our understanding of healthy family functioning (Monroe & Oliviere, 2007). Although some families are shattered by crisis or chronic stressors, many families emerge strengthened and more resourceful (Walsh, 2003). A family systems approach suggests that crisis and adversity have an impact on the family as a unit, resulting in derailment of functioning, with a ripple effect to all members and relationships. In turn, key processes of the family mediate the recovery of all members within the unit. It is these processes that enable the family to rally in times of crisis, buffer stress, reduce dysfunction, and support adaptation to change (Walsh, 2003). More than managing stressful situations or surviving an ordeal, resilience involves the potential for personal and relational transformation that can occur as a result of adaptation to adversity.

In a holistic assessment that evaluates resilience, family characteristics such as effective family responses and adaptive relationships will inform clinicians. Key processes in family resilience include *(1)* belief systems, *(2)* organizational patterns, and *(3)* communication/problem solving (Walsh, 2002). It is valuable to explore how families respond in their proactive stance, immediate responses to stress, and long-term survival strategies. Interventions are then tailored to the particular situations that can overwhelm the system and capitalize on processes that strengthen the family system. This can have both short-term and long-term effects as families in palliative care traverse their bereavement experience (Monroe & Oliviere, 2006). (For more information on resilience, see Chapter 20)

Common Challenges for Families

Family life is inherently filled with challenges, from the pressures of everyday life to the debates and uncertainties of major life decisions. The challenges are not necessarily negative and may have positive sequelae, but nevertheless they may create stress and distress. The same issues that challenge families when life is "usual" may become more significant, magnified, and overwhelming when a family member is facing life-threatening illness and end of life (Rolland, 2005). This section, while not exhaustive, will review several types of challenges. Challenges will vary depending on when in family development the illness process occurs. Difficult family histories, including experiences of abuse or trauma may create difficult family dynamics that are especially problematic if they involve secrets. Practical challenges such as financial strains can be significant sources of distress. Because each family will have a unique set of circumstances, the social work assessment and subsequent family contacts needs to sensitively create opportunities for families to share their individual stories, circumstances, and concerns (Fineberg, 2010).

Developmental and Life Course Issues

The impact of serious illness will vary depending upon the life course phase of the family (Veach & Nicholas, 1998). Families go through various periods of development, when the focus of family life shifts depending on the age and needs of the family members, as well as the amount of time the family has been together. Young couples or newly formed families may face difficulties of a brief shared history, little experience of coping together with difficult situations, and many unknowns about how the family members manage challenges. They may be in the process of developing their own organizational and decision-making patterns, defining roles and boundaries, and struggling with dynamics of extended family influence. At the same time, they may bring stores of energy and optimism to dealing with difficulties, perhaps more so than some families fatigued by endurance of past difficulties. There may also be a network of other young families that can support and assist. Families with young children and adolescents may be balancing child care needs with care needs of the patient, navigating sensitive age-appropriate conversations and decisions with the children, anticipating future plans for the children's care, and struggling with the knowledge and preparation for the profound loss that the children may face (Turner et al., 2007). Clinical support to families in these early points of development can assist in building shared decision making and effective communication (Veach, Nicholas, & Barton, 2002) and integrating skills needed to live with uncertainty.

For families in a later stage of their development, challenges may center around relationships within the couple, with adult children, and the impact of the illness and death on the future of the surviving adults and grandchildren. Adults in mid life may be more established in their careers or jobs, focusing on creating and maintaining stability and financial security. Members of an older family, at or beyond retirement age, may have fewer competing demands on their time but may be physically limited in their ability to provide care to ill spouses or partners. Even aging parents, who have their adult children in close proximity, may find that the demands of employment make the availability of their children limited. This may create not only a practical but an emotional vacuum in the aging family.

Some families face the challenge of balancing multigenerational needs such as caring for children, older family members, and the midlife adults in the family. Such configurations may be especially difficult as the likelihood of competing needs and high-intensity care requirements may burden and stretch the family's emotional, psychological, spiritual, social, physical, and financial resources.

In conjunction with developmental issues related to age and time together, variations in family configurations, and sequential family constellations may add additional layers of complexity to communication and decision making. For example, families may include stepparents and stepchildren and couples who have shifted from heterosexual to same-sex relationships or vice versa, and married or unmarried cohabiting couples. Complex configurations may call for managing communication among large numbers of family members or family members who have strained or hostile relationships (Holst, Lundgren, Olsen, & Ishoy, 2009). Individual family members may require private time with the patient, and separate visitation schedules may make visitation more comfortable for all concerned. Differences in family members' status and power within the family may influence communication and decision making regarding the care and treatment of the patient. Social workers' attention to family configurations, including use of family genograms when helpful, can be essential for effectively assisting families (McGoldrick,

Gerson, & Petri, 2008). Such assistance will usually focus on facilitating functioning related to the illness situation, but in some rare instances family therapy aimed at long-term change in functional patterns may be pursued.

In the narrative in Box 22.1, an older couple that has been together for many years faces the end of life with other members of the family. Together they face the challenges of geographically distant adult children with competing

---

Box 22.1
Patient/Family Narrative: Dr. Anna Worthing

Dr. Anna Worthing is a 69-year-old retired Jewish woman diagnosed with chronic leukemia (CML) 5 years ago. She had emigrated from Eastern Europe to the United States, where she met her husband. She worked in the garment industry and later earned her doctoral degree in anthropology after she already had children. She enjoyed many years of teaching at the local university before her retirement. Always grateful for the opportunities that life allowed her, she volunteered in her local community, Jewish charities, and a nearby nursing home. She had just begun chemotherapy a few weeks ago and was tolerating it well until she collapsed at home and required hospitalization at the community hospital. She was diagnosed with pneumonia and transferred to the intensive care unit (ICU), where she was placed on a ventilator. Her husband of 40 years remains by her side, and her two adult children have arrived from around the country. Dr. Worthing's only sibling lives in England and is unable to visit due to poor health but remains informed and available by telephone.

The family has maintained a constant presence with the patient, bringing in music and pictures of the grandchildren to enrich the environment as well as to help the staff to view Dr. Worthing as a person as well as a patient. Mr. Worthing is retired, and both adult children are married with young children and full-time careers. The children are juggling their family and work situations. One has come from across the country with a baby and finds sporadic and temporary child care that enables her to be in the hospital for a few hours each day; the other lives in a neighboring state and has driven back and forth a few times to handle family and work responsibilities.

Several specialists have been involved with Dr. Worthing's situation, each coming in from the community at different times and providing their impressions and recommendations for treatment. The patient's oncologist, the only professional previously familiar with the family, visits the patient but does not direct immediate care. After 2 weeks of intensive treatment, the pneumonia improved and staff attempted to remove the ventilator support. A poor response to this attempt led to tests that revealed Dr. Worthing had had a profound stroke while on the ventilator.

The family was approached at this point to make a decision about maintaining or removing ventilator support for Dr. Worthing. Several years ago, Dr. Worthing had completed an advance directive, discussed her priorities regarding end of life with her family, and had appointed her husband and daughter as her agents. Over a number of days, the family considered the available information about the potential for Dr. Worthing's recovery and quality of life and determined that she would not have wanted to be kept alive under the current conditions, which would include permanent dependence on a ventilator and a low likelihood of being able to communicate or function.

Box 22.1 *(Contd.)*

The social worker assisted the family and team in coordinating a care plan that allowed time for additional family members to come from far distances before ventilator support would be discontinued. The family was assisted in exploring approaches to engage and assist the grandchildren, ages 7 months to 13 years and the older grandchildren were given the opportunity to see their grandmother and tell her whatever they wished.

Dr. Worthing's husband and two children were with her when the ventilator support was stopped, holding her hands, caressing her brow, reassuring her with their words and tone of voice. The respiratory therapist overseeing the ventilator removal thoughtfully explained to the family what was being done and what to anticipate. Dr. Worthing ceased to breathe within a few minutes of the ventilator being turned off. Her family remained with her for the coming hour, staying in the room together and then allowing each other individual private time in the room before leaving.

responsibilities, young grandchildren, and painful decisions to make.

The Worthing family's decisions were guided by their clarity regarding commitment to supporting each other, their attention to the patient's preferences and values, and their recognition of the importance of enabling each family member to participate. Questions to consider include the following: *(a)* What did staff do that was especially helpful to the family? *(b)* What could staff have done better to assist the family? and *(c)* How did Dr Worthing's character, personal history, and culture impact her care at the end of her life?

Family History and Current Relations

Family discord. Existing family conflict may have a tremendous impact on how a family behaves and adjusts as they integrate the experience of life-threatening illness and end of life. The underlying causes of the conflict do not magically disappear because a family member becomes ill. More often, discord leads to difficulties in the family's ability to support the patient, adjust to the illness, and participate positively in care (Holst et al., 2009). Exploration and discussion of the psychosocial issues underlying conflict will assist families to function more effectively as they have to negotiate treatment options and decision making.

Substance abuse. Abuse of alcohol, illicit drugs, or prescription medications has a profound impact on families (Otis-Green & Rutland, 2004). Long-term substance abuse by a family member will have influenced the family dynamics and functioning over time, with potential consequences such as anger, resentment, blame, guilt, shame, and reduced cohesion within the family (Lorber et al., 2007). The management of chemical dependency in a patient with advanced illness is a major endeavor for the patient, family, and health care team (Passik & Theobald, 2000). Assessment of frequently associated mental health difficulties, especially depression

and anxiety, is critical. The deleterious impact of untreated substance abuse extends to the patient's family. Patients and families may have fears of threatening recovery or perpetuating or triggering addiction that surface when addressing the management of pain and other symptoms (Altilio, Otis-Green, Hedlund, & Fineberg, 2006). They may fear use of controlled substances or the potential of inadequate pain management due to the withholding of pain medications. Social workers' can provide crucial psychoeducational support and advocacy both with the family and the health care team. Social work interventions help people to separate facts from myths and fears, promote a treatment approach focused on patient/family care rather than stereotypes and labels (such as "addict"), and advocate for appropriate pain and symptom management and a structured, informed plan of care that centers on the patient's well-being. (For additional information, see Chapter 25)

Abuse within the family. Current or past abuse, often kept secret by the involved individuals and/or family members aware of the abuse, may create tumultuous undercurrents in the family dynamics. When assessing physical, sexual, and emotional abuse by family or nonfamily members, it is critical to recognize that the patient may be a victim, perpetrator, or witness of the abuse. Patients who are elderly, isolated, and dependent on caregivers are especially at risk (Kahan & Paris, 2003). Palliative and hospice care providers are in an ideal position to identify and potentially prevent abuse in this vulnerable group of patients (Jayawardena & Liao, 2006). Feelings of vulnerability, guilt, fear, shame, blame, and anger are extremely powerful in influencing individual and family adjustment during illness and end of life. Social workers assess abuse concerns explicitly and with sensitivity, knowing that they may be denied or hidden (Fisher, 2003). Awareness of verbal and nonverbal cues from the patient or other family members and creation of opportunities for private conversation are important if abuse is suspected. If the patient is a victim, his or her sense of vulnerability due to life-threatening illness may be magnified because the illness experience and health care setting involve decreased sense of control, increased dependence, frequent physical touch by strangers, and usually, the need for direct caregiving by family members, potentially from the abusive family member. Social workers who communicate in a clear but nonthreatening manner demonstrate a willingness to listen and invite discussion of these difficult topics. Communication of the sensitive information to the rest of the health care team must be carefully discussed with the patient (or family member) to protect confidentiality, if it is requested, while facilitating situation-appropriate care by team members (Macpherson, 2009). Maximizing opportunities for patient control over interactions and care decisions, no matter how small, enhances abuse victims' sense of safety.

Family experience with illness and death. A family's past experience with illness and death will influence members' reactions to a current situation of life-threatening illness. Social workers explore not only the existence but also the timing of such experiences. Exposure to death not only from illness, but from suicide, homicide, accident, violence, or war, must also be considered. Family members may have memory of painful illness and inadequate treatment, regret their own behaviors, retain anger at the deceased, or have not fully faced or adjusted to their loss. By contrast, family members may have histories of well-handled, peaceful processes of illness and death which they feel led to personal growth and family strengthening. Social work assessments of past experiences do not assume positive or negative consequences but rather explore the nature and perceived outcomes of those situations, especially as they relate to the current illness in the family.

Social Forces

The social environment outside of the family is a source of both support and challenge as families navigate through the process of illness and end of life. These ecological issues influence the internal psychosocial functioning of the family system and thus must be considered in order to holistically assess, understand, and care for families.

Immigration, acculturation, and assimilation. For families who are living in a country different than their country of origin, social workers need to be aware of unique challenges. A professional interpreter, rather than a family member or friend, is essential to facilitate communication with patients and families whose primary language is different than that of the health care providers (Pham, Thornton, Engelberg, Jackson, & Curtis, 2008; Rosenberg, Seller, & Leanza, 2008; Schapira et al., 2008). In settings where clinicians choose not to use professional interpreters and rely on family members, they access the emotional or factual content as it is filtered through the family, creating uncertainty as to what is being expressed and understood. Recent immigration is often accompanied by language differences, lack of familiarity with cultural norms and expectations in the new place of residence, lack of knowledge about health care and civic systems, and limited social support. For families who have been in the "new" country for a longer period of time and have had children in the new country, intrafamily differences in the level of family members' acculturation and assimilation to the current setting may cause family tensions as differing value systems and expectations are applied in the illness and treatment context (DeSanto-Madeya et al., 2009). Social workers can assist families to recognize the source of such tensions, identify the core concerns related to the illness and treatment setting, help families identify similarities in views and priorities, and facilitate communication and understanding regarding differences (McGrath, Vun, & McLeod, 2001).

Culture, language, and the health care system. Families who have immigrated may need particular attention to cultural and language issues, and this is an important consideration for all families (Thomas, 1998). All people have a cultural background, whether it is that of the dominant culture in a society or a minority culture. Culture can be defined as a "set of distinctive spiritual, material, intellectual, and emotional features of society or a social group that encompass, in addition to art and literature, lifestyles, ways of living together, value systems, traditions and beliefs" (Goh, 2009, p. 51). In the context of working with families who are facing illness and end of life, awareness of culture is extremely important (Crawley, Marshall, Lo, & Koenig, 2002). Perspectives and attitudes about illness and death, views on autonomy and decision making, and expectations about the role of family are specifically explored because they will greatly influence the process of treatment and care. Health care professionals need to be sensitive to situations in which cultural perspectives of the family differ from that of the health care system in which care is taking place (Crawley, 2005).

Western and non-Western cultures hold divergent views of autonomy, highly influencing the ways in which patients and families will approach decision making and care (Volker, 2005). Western-minded families may prioritize individuality and autonomy, focusing on self-determination. Non-Western cultures, in contrast, often value interdependence over independence, resulting in very different perspectives on decision making and expectations. It is important for the health care team not to make assumptions based upon people's ethnic grouping but rather openly explore the role and expression of culture in patients' and families' perspectives (Green, Betancourt, & Carrillo, 2002). As noted earlier, levels of acculturation and assimilation will strongly influence individuals as they integrate their culture of origin with their current culture over time. Social workers offer an open, respectful, and collaborative approach that helps to emphasize similarities and negotiate differences that arise between the families and the system in which they are receiving care.

Financial and employment strains. The complex financial issues associated with advanced illness are often hidden as families struggle to preserve routine functioning while facing new roles, patterns, and strains. Financial difficulty associated with cancer is severe and may not be solely associated with the cost of treatment, but to related changes such as lost income and/or increased expenses (Grunfeld et al., 2004). Common sources of financial pressures focus on employment changes and treatment-related costs (Pawlecki, 2010). Challenges for patients include loss of income and loss of employment, and for family members, assuming caregiving roles may lead to the same changes (Yun et al., 2005). For family members who may have been working part time or not at all, the context of illness and end of life may require them to enter the paid workforce and/or take on the role of primary income earner. The strain of treatment-related costs are multilevel, including direct costs of the treatment and care as well as peripheral costs. For those who have the benefit of insurance or government health plans, medical equipment, medications, hospitalization, and medical care are expenses that are covered to greatly varying degrees (Hogan, Lunney, Gabel, & Lynn, 2001). Hiring private nursing or caregiving professionals to assist in the home or paying for residential options such as assisted living, nursing home, or inpatient hospice care can be very expensive. Peripheral costs such as transportation to and from health care facilities for treatment or visitation, lodging and food costs related to being away from home, and additional child care costs add to the overall financial burden of illness.

Family caregiving. Changes in family infrastructure and gender roles have influenced how available family members are to provide care and who becomes the designated and assumed caregiver. Historically, women have provided the majority of the caregiving to ill family members (Fredriksen, 1996, 1999; Navaie-Waliser et al., 2002). However, social changes have affected the availability of female family members to provide the hands-on attention so often necessary in palliative care. Variations in family structures and movement between them, such as divorce, marital separation, serial marriage, stepparenting, single parenting, and cohabitation of same-sex and heterosexual couples, have become common (Casper & Bianchi, 2002). These social shifts, together with increases in women's involvement with work out of the home and greater geographic mobility, further challenge the availability of female caregiving. At the same time, changes in health care delivery have resulted in a shift from inpatient hospital care to ambulatory and home settings, leading to a demand for increased family involvement in the day-to-day care of the person with advanced illness (Grunfeld et al., 2004; Waldrop, 2006). Thus, alterations in social systems and social patterns have added tensions to the already challenging circumstances of providing family caregiving to patients.

Research reflects that caregivers are at higher risk for depression and health problems and increased mortality rates (McMillan et al., 2006). Monitoring the well-being of caregivers is part of ongoing family assessment. Family members providing care may themselves have medical conditions, especially if they are older adults, as well as concurrent responsibilities to others (Waldrop, 2008). The physical, psychological, emotional, spiritual, and social impact of care provision can be tremendous and quite subtle and require ongoing assessment at the time of caregiving initiation and throughout the illness course and into the bereavement period. The goal of this proactive vigilance is to ensure the well-being of both patients and caregivers (Kinsella, Cooper, Picton, & Murtagh, 2000; Siegel, Raveis, Mor, & Houts, 1991) and may mitigate the patient's worry that their care needs are a burden and harming those that they depend on. At the same time, it is important to recognize that for some people, the experience of caregiving is positive and informed with meaning, providing an enduring sense of contribution, worth, and peace (Haley, 2003). (For additional information, please see Chapter 21)

Facilitating Family Care

Social Work and Family Care

When an individual is diagnosed with a serious illness, the entire family system is impacted. Each family is in a different state of well-being, with some more than others able to endure, grow, and adapt positively to the new situation. The needs of families vary widely, and not all families need specialized intervention (Kissane et al., 2003). Differences in culture and family style will influence the variations that families demonstrate in their desire and acceptance of professional support, and their capacity to cope with challenges and change will determine their need for support, regardless of whether accepted (Bowman, 2000).

Core social work skills for working with individuals and families are the foundation for social work practice in palliative and end-of-life care (Kovacs, Bellin, & Fauri, 2006). Assessing families' circumstances and needs, building trust and therapeutic alliances, providing ongoing psychotherapeutic and practical support, and intervening appropriately are integral components of social workers' roles with families. Coordination and optimization of complex discharge planning is often also necessary and calls for an inclusive approach with patients, their families, and caregivers. The addition of home health care services and durable medical equipment is often symbolically meaningful to patients and their families and requires the attention of skilled clinicians who explore the emotional responses and attributed meaning. For example, the need for medical equipment changes the physical environment and may be a very obvious and public reminder of progressing illness and disability.

There is frequent need for decision making over the course of illness, and social workers are often essential facilitators of the communication and processes that support informed decision making (Gwyther et al., 2005; Parsons, 1991). This expertise in facilitating communication focuses both within families as well as between families and their health care providers. Such facilitation takes place in individual discussions, family discussions, team conversations, whether in person, on the telephone, or through electronic media. In palliative care, however, the family conference, discussed in the next section, is a format for communication that offers powerful opportunities for family care.

In working with families along the continuum of illness and palliative care, an underlying and essential theme is to convey to patients and families that their care providers, including the social worker, will not abandon them as the process of illness and end of life becomes more difficult and imminent (West, Engelberg, Wenrich, & Curtis, 2005). Vigilance to this principle is often lost as the care of patients and families is transitioned between teams and programs such as when patients enroll in hospice programs or are moved to extended care facilities. This message is conveyed in language and behaviors and, while crucial for all patients and families, is especially important for those whose history includes abandonment and trauma that has created a pervasive sense of mistrust and vulnerability.

Bereavement

The palliative care model clearly and importantly includes bereavement care, reinforcing the concept that health care providers will not abandon families during the processes of care (National Consensus Project for Quality Palliative Care, 2009). Realistically in the current health care system, the degree to which social workers provide bereavement care will vary depending on their work setting, the structure of services in that setting, the expected scope of practice, the team's relationship with the family, and the family's needs. Often times, priorities in health care settings do not allow sufficient time for bereavement work. However, some form of bereavement follow-up is an integral part of care, whether that involves sympathy cards, written support materials, provision of information about support options, or phone calls (National Consensus Project for Quality Palliative Care, 2009).

Most important, the groundwork for bereavement begins before the death of the patient (Rolland, 1990). Family members' experiences of illness, treatment, and care will influence their adjustment to the death and loss of the patient (Lynn et al., 1997). For families whose emotional and family process, culture, and values allow for open discussion of the anticipated death, social workers can explore concerns and feelings and intervene clinically, while providing anticipatory psychoeducation related to grief and bereavement. Social workers can encourage families to tolerate members' individual differences in expression of feelings, reactions to the anticipated and actual death, as well as tolerating different styles and expressions of grief (Walsh & McGoldrick, 1991). While for most family members the death of the patient will provoke sadness and emotional pain, positive memories and feelings may also accompany the loss, and for some there is a prevailing sense of relief or vindication. The complexity of the families and their histories as described in prior sections of this chapter are reflected in the complexity of the feelings that attach to the death of a family member. Furthermore, adaptation following bereavement is marked with personal growth for many. It is important to remember this aspect of family need because the potential to influence the grief process exists along the continuum of illness and is impacted by the clinical assessment and interventions chosen to enhance the quality of care and assist patients and families as they negotiate the illness experience. (For more information on this subject, see Chapter 29)

Family Conferences

Family conferences, sometimes called family meetings, are vehicles for communicating with families in the setting of palliative care (Fineberg, 2010; Lautrette, Ciroldi, Ksibi, & Azoulay, 2006). They have the potential to optimize interdisciplinary collaboration among health care providers, create a climate of inclusion and empowerment for families, promote communication, and contribute to families' experience of care (Hudson, Thomas, Quinn, & Aranda, 2009). Like other clinical skills, leadership and conduct of family conferences need to be learned and practiced (Fineberg, 2005). For the purposes of this discussion, a family conference will be defined as a one-time meeting including the patient (when possible), family members of the patient, and relevant health care staff to discuss a topic related to the health and care of the patient and family. While family conferences may occur on multiple occasions, each meeting is usually viewed as a discrete event focused on a particular topic or aspect of care. In contrast to family therapy sessions, family conferences are not intended to facilitate fundamental or long-term changes in family functioning, although such consequences may occur as a secondary benefit (Kushner & Meyer, 1989; Meyer, Schneid, & Craigie, 1989).

Conference Functions
Family conferences serve many functions. They are a place for information exchange, clarification of information, correction of misinformation, and creation of shared understanding. They are settings for the expression of emotions, consideration of choices, decision making, conflict illumination, conflict negotiation, and consensus building (Hansen, Cornish, & Kayser, 1998; McDonagh et al., 2004; Radwany et al., 2009; Yennurajalingam et al., 2008). They are often used at times of crisis and decision making. In fact, they can be of substantial assistance to families as they struggle to make difficult decisions (Joling et al., 2008; Lautrette et al., 2007). Topics of family conferences often include delivery of diagnoses and prognoses, updates on illness and treatment status, discussion of treatment options and decisions, discussion of discharge plans, and advance care planning (Hollingsworth & Sokol, 1978; Miller, Krech, & Walsh, 1991). All too often, conferences are used later than would be ideal, when emotions and decision-making pressures are high (Fineberg, Asch, & Golden, 2007).

Conference Participants
Who attends a family conference usually depends on the topic to be discussed, who requests the conference, and logistical practicalities. Conference organizers consider the balance of number of providers to patient/family participants, realizing that power dynamics will impact the conference. Ideally, the patient's input assists clinicians in their decisions about who is invited to the meeting, especially with regard to family members. Advocacy for such inclusion of patient preference is warranted when appropriate, but it is common for health care staff to make such decisions (Hudson, Quinn, O'Hanlon, & Aranda, 2008). Staff participants often include health care providers who are immediately involved with the patient and/or those who have cared for the patient over a

lengthy period of time. When test results or care plans are discussed, specialists or consultants who have expertise or are essential to the care plan may be appropriate to include. For example, a family conference about results of a cardiac evaluation includes the consulting cardiologist, while a discussion of discharge to a care facility may include staff from the receiving facility to enhance continuity for the patient and family.

Family participants are often those most involved in the patient's life and care and may attend, depending on the patient's preferences, cultural issues, and conference topics. For patients who want to be part of the conference, all efforts are made to make that possible. This may involve holding the conference around the bedside, holding medications so that patients are more alert for the discussion, or timing the meeting to optimize attendance by the patient and family members. In some instances, the conference includes an interpreter to ensure that language and cultural issues do not prevent the patient or family members from participation and to insure that the health care staff has access to an interpreter whose communication is not impacted by the complex cognitive and emotional response of family members. Involvement of children and adolescents in family conferences is a consideration that reflects the family's values and a clinical assessment of the benefits and risks. Similarly, family members who may be viewed as "vulnerable" for reasons such as mental health issues or developmental disabilities require the same consideration. A decision to involve a child, adolescent, or vulnerable person requires that they be prepared for the experience and that the setting, process, and content of the conference be respectful of their needs. This includes preparation of the health care staff whose language and behaviors may need to be modified and adapted to the participants' cognitive level of development.

Conducting Family Conferences
There is no one model for family conferences, but several components are frequently noted in the literature (Altilio, Otis-Green, & Dahlin, 2008; Curtis et al., 2001; Hudson et al., 2008). A common-sense progression exists for some of the components, but others may vary in inclusion and order.

- *Preparation for the conference.* Before the conference begins, consideration needs to be given to the meeting space that will be used, the number and composition of participants, and any special circumstances for which preparation is needed, such as the inclusion of interpreters or participants with special needs whose presence may require scheduling additional conference time. Preparing for the conference includes identifying and inviting the desired participants, taking into account not only who is necessary but who would be valuable to include both to optimize the conference experience and outcome and to be respectful of the power dynamics that exist when health care

professionals meet with those receiving care. Proper preparation ensures that that relevant written materials or test results are available. Having preparatory discussions with the interdisciplinary care team to agree upon an agenda and conference leadership will optimize staff interactions in the conference and enhance the flow of the meeting. Conferences are often led by social workers, physicians, or collaboration between the two depending on the team members as well as the topic and goals of the meeting.

- *Introductions.* It is essential that introductions take place at the beginning of the family conference so that all participants are aware of who is present and what their relationship is to the patient. While this may seem like a basic step, it is frequently overlooked.

- *Agenda setting.* A brief but clear overview of the agenda and goals for the conference will create clarity and provide opportunity for participants to indicate additional or alternate agenda items. Alternately, it is possible to begin by inviting the patient/family to express their wishes for the meeting or their understanding of why the conference was organized.

- *Facilitation of discussion.* The conference discussion will be structured according to the goal and topic of the meeting. A number of social work skills are invaluable for conference facilitation. These include ongoing assessment and understanding of group dynamics, observation of family dynamics, and careful listening. Strengths in communication and advocacy are especially useful as complex and emotional discussions and decisions are navigated. It is helpful to begin conferences by exploring what the patient/family knows and understands about the conference topic. In some cases, discussions focus on staff providing new information or presenting a situation, medical, ethical, or psychosocial, that requires guidance or decision making. At other times, the discussion may begin with a set of questions between the family and staff. For example, family members may present their understanding of the patient's condition and ask questions about why palliative care is being introduced at this point in time into the plan of care of the patient who continues to receive care in the intensive care unit in the setting of uncertain outcome. Another scenario may be that family members are anticipating the patient coming home and thus have many questions about what to do in the event that various needs or situations arise in the house.

- *Soliciting patient and family reactions.* When new information is provided, patient and family are invited to articulate their reactions, questions, and concerns. When decisions need to be made, staff elicits patient/family perspectives, questions, and concerns including the cultural and spiritual values that inform their decision-making processes. Clear options are reviewed and considered with conference leaders encouraging open discussion, clarifying that respectful disagreement and debate are welcome. Consensus about decisions will not always be possible, but this may be acceptable to participants if they feel the process of decision making has been thoughtful and respectful. In some situations, a decision may be made to try a particular course of action with a designated time limit for reviewing whether it has worked. In conflict situations, lack of agreement may require that additional or senior staff people be included in the discussion, patient representatives be invited, or that consultation is sought from a clinical ethics committee.

- *Summary and conclusion.* In most instances, the conference ends with a summary of what was discussed and agreed upon as well as the outstanding issues that are unresolved. The summary reviews next steps that will be taken, by whom, and in what time frame. Social workers reinforce their valuable participation by having contact with the patient and family after the conference, creating a sense of continuity and connection. A summary of the family conference is documented in the medical record, noting participants, key topics, outcomes, and plans for follow-up.

Family conferences are flexible forms of communication that may be structured to meet the needs of the topic and participants. They are powerful forums that offer family care in an integrated, active, and inclusive format (see Box 22.2).

Box 22.2
Patient/Family Narrative: Mr. Carlos Santiago

Mr. Carlos Santiago is a 55-year-old Mexican American man with end-stage renal disease (ESRD). His condition has declined quickly, and he has decided to pursue comfort-focused treatment. Mr. Santiago lives alone, has never been married, and has no children. His five siblings are geographically dispersed, with two living within an hour of him. He was working until recently as a restaurant manager but has been hospitalized for 2 weeks. He is closely involved with his local Catholic church and has welcomed spiritual care providers in the hospital. Mr. Santiago was independent at home before his hospitalization but now faces difficult decisions related to his discharge plan.

With the patient's permission, the social worker arranged a family conference to discuss discharge and care plans. Mr. Santiago had invited all his siblings to the conference and seemed sad that only one could attend due to distance and work/family commitments. Efforts to have family members participate via speaker phones were unsuccessful, but the plan was made for the social worker to provide feedback after the meeting. The meeting focused on Mr. Santiago's decision to forgo further invasive interventions and his preference to spend the rest of his time, estimated as a few months, at home. Mr. Santiago's sister, Maria, expressed disbelief of the prognosis, expressing her belief that God will heal him. Nonetheless, she invites Mr. Santiago to move in with her family until he becomes stronger. She is uncertain of her

ability and that of her husband to provide appropriate care due to lack of experience. Both she and the patient express concerns about finances.

Staff members at the conference introduce the idea of hospice care in the home. Mr. Santiago and Maria have never heard of this service, and the explanation is met with the patient sitting quietly and the sister saying that she does not see that hospice is relevant for her brother since God will heal him. Staff offer support and respect of the family's spiritual perspective, and there is no attempt to dissuade Maria of her beliefs; rather, the discussion is framed with a focus on her brother's immediate needs, wishes, and priorities. Further discussion of alternative care options concludes with an agreement to try the hospice service and review the outcome within a week's time. Negotiating time limits for such care plans is an important clinical intervention. Providers encourage Mr. Santiago and his sister to maintain close contact with their church communities, and the pastoral care provider offers to call their community priest. A separate meeting is arranged with the social worker to assist the patient and his sister with concerns about the transition to home, including the practical, financial, psychological, and emotional issues involved for both the patient and family. A verbal and written summary of the conference includes who will arrange the hospice referral and partializes the steps that need to be taken to achieve a seamless transition. All staff ensure that both they and the patient and sister have mutual contact information before leaving the meeting.

Conclusion

Before people become patients or recipients of medical care, they are people with established lives, embedded in social systems. People are born into a family of origin, a biological family, to which they then add members by legal connection and close personal association. Families are often the centers of people's lives, whether they realize it or not. It is therefore logical that at times of serious illness and end of life when people are in palliative and hospice settings, care extends beyond the patient alone to encompass the family. Social workers working in palliative and end-of-life care contexts bring knowledge, skills, and perspectives that are particularly valuable for the care of families. As health care team members, social workers must articulate, model, and apply their clinical expertise to optimize the care and experiences of families.

LEARNING EXERCISES

- (For readers or for instructors to use with students) Create a genogram of your families, illustrating your biological/legal family, including as far as grandparents, aunts/uncles, and first cousins. This would include any adopted and stepfamily members, as well as people married/partnered into the family.

Think about and then circle who you would like to have closely involved if you were seriously ill. Then, separately make a list of "chosen" family members, not related by biology or legal connections.

As you look at your genograms and list, think about what it is about those people and relationships that you have circled that leads you to choose them. Think about how your cultural background (ethnic, national, urban/rural, group affiliation, etc.) is influencing your choices. Think about other factors that might be influencing your choices.

For instructors: Give students approximately 10 minutes to individually do this exercise. Then ask them to partner with someone to discuss for 5–10 minutes what they learned about how and who they might choose. Make it clear to students that they are invited to disclose only information that they are comfortable sharing. Finally, bring the class together and facilitate a discussion about the various considerations that we all make in how we think of family, the influences that cause people to define and include family in different ways, and how those definitions and influences matter when facing serious illness.

- (For readers or for instructors to use with students) Think about a family, other than your own, who you know well through your student placement, your professional practice, or your everyday life. Imagine that you are working with this family in the context of a member who is facing end of life. Try to determine some of the following aspects of the situation:

  - How does the ill person approach decision making in terms of individuality and collectivity? Does the ill person value individuality and personal choice, does he or she focus more on family and collective choices, or does the person have a blended approach to decision making? How does his or her approach match or conflict with the approach of the larger family? How does his or her approach match or conflict with that of the health care system?

  - What type of communication does the ill person seem to value? For example, is there a preference for open communication, metaphoric communication, or for gathering cues from the context of the situation? Does the person prefer individual or group discussions about illness/care, or some combination of the two?

  - What explanatory model does the patient have about how he or she understands the causes and progression of the illness, as well as his or her impending death? How does this explanatory model relate to the model of other family members? How does this explanatory model match or conflict with the model used by the staff in the facility caring for the patient?

For instructors: If using this with a class, divide the class into three groups. Provide all the students with a copy of the exercise, but assign one bulleted set of questions to each group. Within each group, have each student *(a)* describe a family and *(b)* describe how he or she would answer the questions about that family. Encourage each group to then discuss similarities and differences across families. At the end, ask each group to report to the whole class some of the main ideas they learned from the group's discussion.

- (For instructors) Present the students with the following scenario: A 50-year-old Eastern European woman has been diagnosed with advanced cancer for which there is no curative treatment. She is being treated at a large medical center in the United States, although she has lived in the area for only 2 years. The family members have made it clear to staff that they do not want the patient informed of her diagnosis and that they, the family members, will be making decisions on her behalf. The staff are trying to determine how to proceed with communication with this patient and family.

  Divide the students into two groups and ask each group to conduct a role played family conference that includes 2–3 family members and 2–3 staff members. Each group can determine whom they want their family members and staff members to be, including whether they want the patient involved. Each group conducts a 10-minute role play after which they report their experience to the entire class, including who they included in the conference and why, what they thought were the key issues in the interaction, and how it felt to actually engage in the role play. Be sure to leave time at the end for student group "debriefing" to make sure that no students leave unduly distressed by the exercise.

ADDITIONAL SUGGESTED READINGS

Berzoff, J., & Silverman, P. R. (Eds.), (2004). *Living with dying: A handbook for end-of-life healthcare practitioners.* New York: Columbia University Press.

Fadiman, A. (1997). *The spirit catches you and you fall down.* New York: Noonday Press.

Oliviere, D., & Monroe, B. (Eds.), (2004). *Death, dying, and social differences.* Oxford, UK: Oxford University Press.

Patterson, J. M. (2002). Integrating family resilience and family stress theory. *Journal of Marriage and the Family, 64*(2), 349–360.

RESOURCES AND WEB SITES

African Palliative Care Association: http://www.apca.org.ug/
APCA Web site with information to promote and support affordable and culturally appropriate palliative care throughout Africa.
American Psychosocial Oncology Society (APOS): http://www.apos-society.org/
APOS is a multidisciplinary professional organization in the United States dedicated to the psychosocial aspects of cancer

treatment and advancing the science and practice of psychosocial care for people with cancer.

Association of Oncology Social Work (AOSW): http://www.aosw.org/

AOSW is a nonprofit, international organization dedicated to the enhancement of psychosocial services to people with cancer and their families.

British Psychosocial Oncology Society (BPOS): http://www.bpos.org/

BPOS is a multidisciplinary organization founded in 1983. Its aims are to advance education and research in psychosocial oncology and to promote increased knowledge of this subject within oncology.

Canadian Hospice Palliative Care Association (CHPCA): http://www.chpca.net/

CHPCA is the national voice for Hospice Palliative Care in Canada. Advancing and advocating for quality end-of-life/hospice palliative care in Canada, its work includes public policy, public education, and awareness.

Center to Advance Palliative Care (CAPC): http://www.capc.org/

CAPC provides health care professionals with the tools, training, and technical assistance necessary to start and sustain successful palliative care programs in hospitals and other health care settings. CAPC is a national organization dedicated to increasing the availability of quality palliative care services for people facing serious illness.

European Association for Palliative Care: http://www.eapcnet.org/

The aim of the EAPC is to promote palliative care in Europe and to act as a focus for all of those who work, or have an interest, in the field of palliative care at the scientific, clinical, and social levels.

Family Caregiver Alliance: http://www.caregiver.org/

FCA was the first community-based nonprofit organization in the country to address the needs of families and friends providing long-term care at home. It now offers programs at national, state, and local levels to support and sustain caregivers.

International Psycho-Oncology Society: http://www.ipos-society.org/

IPOS was created to foster international multidisciplinary communication about clinical, educational, and research issues that relate to the subspecialty of psycho-oncology and two primary psychosocial dimensions of cancer: *(1)* response of patients, families, and staff to cancer and its treatment at all stages; *(2)* psychological, social, and behavioral factors that influence tumor progression and survival.

National Hospice and Palliative Care Organization: http://www.nhpco.org/

NHPCO is a nonprofit membership organization representing hospice and palliative care programs and professionals in the United States. The organization is committed to improving end-of-life care and expanding access to hospice care with the goal of profoundly enhancing quality of life for people dying in America and their loved ones.

Palliative Care Australia: http://www.palliativecare.org.au/

PCA is the peak national organization representing the interests and aspirations of all who share the ideal of quality care at the end of life for all. It is an incorporated body whose members are the eight state and territory palliative care associations and the Australian and New Zealand Society of Palliative Medicine. The membership of these associations includes palliative care service providers, clinicians, allied health professionals,

academics, consumers, and members of the general community.

Social Work Hospice and Palliative Care Network: http://www.swhpn.org/

SWHPN was created to bridge the gaps in social work's access to information, knowledge, education, training, and research in hospice and palliative care.

REFERENCES

Altilio, T., Otis-Green, S., & Dahlin, C. M. (2008). Applying the National Quality Forum Preferred Practices for Palliative and Hospice Care: A social work perspective *Journal of Social Work in End-of-Life and Palliative Care, 4*(1), 3–16.

Altilio, T., Otis-Green, S., Hedlund, S., & Fineberg, I. C. (2006). Pain management and palliative care. In S. Gehlert & T. A. Browne (Eds.), *Handbook of health social work* (pp. 635–672). Hoboken, NJ: John Wiley & Sons.

Beder, J. (2009). It's about family: The death of a close family friend. *Families in Society, 90*(2), 227–230.

Blacker, S., & Jordan, A. R. (2004). Working with families facing life-threatening illness in the medical setting. In J. Berzoff & P. R. Silverman (Eds.), *Living with dying: A handbook for end-of-life healthcare practitioners* (pp. 548–570). New York, NY: Columbia University Press.

Bowman, K. W. (2000). Communication, negotiation, and mediation: Dealing with conflict in end-of-life decisions. *Journal of Palliative Care, 16*(Suppl.), S17–23.

Casper, L. M., & Bianchi, S. M. (2002). *Continuity and change in the American family.* Thousand Oaks, CA: Sage Publications.

Crawley, L. M. (2005). Racial, cultural, and ethnic factors influencing end-of-life care. *Journal of Palliative Medicine, 8*(Suppl. 1), S58–69.

Crawley, L. M., Marshall, P. A., Lo, B., & Koenig, B. A. (2002). Strategies for culturally effective end-of-life care. *Annals of Internal Medicine, 136*(9), 673–679.

Curtis, J. R., Patrick, D. L., Shannon, S. E., Treece, P. D., Engelberg, R. A., & Rubenfeld, G. D. (2001). The family conference as a focus to improve communication about end-of-life care in the intensive care unit: Opportunities for improvement. *Critical Care Medicine, 29*(2), N26–33.

Department of Health. (2008). *End of life care strategy—Promoting high quality care for all adults at the end of life.* London, England: Author.

DeSanto-Madeya, S., Nilsson, M., Loggers, E. T., Paulk, E., Stieglitz, H., Kupersztoch, Y. M., & Prigerson, H. G. (2009). Associations between United States acculturation and the end-of-life experience of caregivers of patients with advanced cancer. *Journal of Palliative Medicine, 12*(12), 1143–1149.

Ell, K. (1996). Social networks, social support and coping with serious illness: The family connection. *Social Science & Medicine, 42*(2), 173–183.

Fineberg, I., Asch, S., & Golden, J. (2007). A research-based model for family conferences in palliative care. *Psycho-Oncology, 16*(S1), S67–S67.

Fineberg, I. C. (2005). Preparing professionals for family conferences in palliative care: Evaluation results of an interdisciplinary approach. *Journal of Palliative Medicine, 8*(4), 857–866.

Fineberg, I. C. (2010). Social work perspectives on family communication and family conferences in palliative care. *Progress in Palliative Care, 18*(4), 213–220.

Fisher, C. (2003). The invisible dimension: Abuse in palliative care families. *Journal of Palliative Medicine, 6*(2), 257–264.

Fredriksen, K. I. (1996). Gender differences in employment and the informal care of adults. *Journal of Women and Aging, 8*(2), 35–53.

Fredriksen, K. I. (1999). Family caregiving responsibilities among lesbians and gay men. *Social Work, 44*(2), 142–155.

Gehlert, S., & Browne, T. A. (Eds.), (2006). *Handbook of health social work.* Hoboken, NJ: John Wiley & Sons.

Goh, C. (2009). Culture, ethnicity, and illness. In D. Walsh, C. T. Augusto, R. Fainsinger, K. Foley, P. Glare, C. Goh, M. Lloyd-Williams, J. N. Olarte, & L. Radbruch (Eds.), *Palliative medicine* (pp. 51–55). Philadelphia, PA: Saunders Elsevier.

Green, A. R., Betancourt, J. R., & Carrillo, J. E. (2002). Integrating social factors into cross-cultural medical education. *Academic Medicine, 77*(3), 193–197.

Grunfeld, E., Coyle, D., Whelan, T., Clinch, J., Reyno, L., Earle, C. C., … Glossop, R. (2004). Family caregiver burden: Results of a longitudinal study of breast cancer patients and their principal caregivers. *Canadian Medical Association Journal, 170*(12), 1795–1801.

Gwyther, L. P., Altilio, T., Blacker, S., Christ, G., Csikai, E. L., Hooyman, N., … Howe, J. (2005). Social work competencies in palliative and end-of-life care. *Journal of Social Work and End of Life in Palliative Care, 1*(1), 87–120.

Haley, W. E. (2003). The costs of family caregiving: Implications for geriatric oncology. *Critical Reviews in Oncology/Hematology, 48*(2), 151–158.

Hansen, P., Cornish, P., & Kayser, K. (1998). Family conferences as forums for decision making in hospital settings. *Social Work in Health Care, 27*(3), 57–74.

Harris, J., Bowen, D. J., Badr, H., Hannon, P., Hay, J., & Sterba, K. R. (2009). Family communication during the cancer experience. *Journal of Health Communication, 14*, 76–84.

Hogan, C., Lunney, J., Gabel, J., & Lynn, J. (2001). Medicare beneficiaries' costs of care in the last year of life. *Health Affairs, 20*(4), 188–195.

Hollingsworth, C. E., & Sokol, B. (1978). Predischarge family conference. *Journal of the American Medical Association, 239*(8), 740–741.

Holst, L., Lundgren, M., Olsen, L., & Ishoy, T. (2009). Dire deadlines: Coping with dysfunctional family dynamics in an end-of-life care setting. *International Journal of Palliative Nursing, 15*(1), 34–41.

Hudson, P., Quinn, K., O'Hanlon, B., & Aranda, S. (2008). Family meetings in palliative care: Multidisciplinary clinical practice guidelines. *BMC Palliative Care, 7*, 12.

Hudson, P., Thomas, T., Quinn, K., & Aranda, S. (2009). Family meetings in palliative care: Are they effective? *Palliative Medicine, 23*(2), 150–157.

Jayawardena, K. M., & Liao, S. (2006). Elder abuse at end of life. *Journal of Palliative Medicine, 9*(1), 127–136.

Joling, K. J., van Hout, H. P., Scheltens, P., Vernooij-Dassen, M., van den Berg, B., Bosmans, J., … van Marwijk, H. (2008). (Cost)-effectiveness of family meetings on indicated prevention of anxiety and depressive symptoms and disorders of primary

family caregivers of patients with dementia: Design of a randomized controlled trial. *BMC Geriatrics, 8*, 2.

Kahan, F. S., & Paris, B. B. (2003). Why elder abuse continues to elude the health care system. *Mount Sinai Journal of Medicine, 70*(1), 62–68.

Kaslow, N. J., Celano, M., & Dreelin, E. D. (1995). A cultural-perspective on family theory and therapy. *Psychiatric Clinics of North America, 18*(3), 621–633.

King, D. A., & Quill, T. (2006). Working with families in palliative care: One size does not fit all. *Journal of Palliative Medicine, 9*(3), 704–715.

Kinsella, G., Cooper, B., Picton, C., & Murtagh, D. (2000). Factors influencing outcomes for family caregivers of persons receiving palliative care: Toward an integrated model. *Journal of Palliative Care, 16*(3), 46–54.

Kissane, D. W., McKenzie, M., McKenzie, D. P., Forbes, A., O'Neill, I., & Bloch, S. (2003). Psychosocial morbidity associated with patterns of family functioning in palliative care: Baseline data from the Family Focused Grief Therapy controlled trial. *Palliative Medicine, 17*(6), 527–537.

Kovacs, P. J., Bellin, M. H., & Fauri, D. P. (2006). Family-centered care: A resource for social work in end-of-life and palliative care. *Journal of Social Work and End-of-Life Palliative Care, 2*(1), 13–27.

Kristjanson, L. J., & Aoun, S. (2004). Palliative care for families: Remembering the hidden patients. *Canadian Journal of Psychiatry, 49*(6), 359–365.

Kushner, K., & Meyer, D. (1989). Family physicians' perceptions of the family conference. *Journal of Family Practice, 28*(1), 65–68.

Lautrette, A., Ciroldi, M., Ksibi, H., & Azoulay, E. (2006). End-of-life family conferences: Rooted in the evidence. *Critical Care Medicine, 34*(11), S364–372.

Lautrette, A., Darmon, M., Megarbane, B., Joly, L.M., Chevret, S., Adrie, C., … Azoulay, E. (2007). A communication strategy and brochure for relatives of patients dying in the ICU. *New England Journal of Medicine, 356*, 469–478.

Lorber, W., Morgan, D. Y., Eisen, M. L., Barak, T., Perez, C., & Crosbie-Burnett, M. (2007). Patterns of cohesion in the families of offspring of addicted parents: Examining a nonclinical sample of college students. *Psychological Reports, 101*(3 Pt 1), 881–895.

Lynn, J., Teno, J. M., Phillips, R. S., Wu, A. W., Desbiens, N., Harrold, J., … Connors, A. F., Jr. (1997). Perceptions by family members of the dying experience of older and seriously ill patients. SUPPORT investigators. Study to Understand Prognoses and Preferences for Outcomes and Risks of Treatments. *Annals of Internal Medicine, 126*(2), 97–106.

Macpherson, C. (2009). Childhood abuse uncovered in a palliative care audit. *Palliative and Supportive Care, 7*(4), 481–486.

McDonagh, J. R., Elliott, T. B., Engelberg, R. A., Treece, P. D., Shannon, S. E., Rubenfeld, G. D., Patrick, D. L., & Curtis, J. R. (2004). Family satisfaction with family conferences about end-of-life care in the intensive care unit: Increased proportion of family speech is associated with increased satisfaction. *Critical Care Medicine, 32*(7), 1484–1488.

McGoldrick, M., Gerson, R., & Petri, S. (2008). *Genograms: Assessment and intervention* (3rd ed.). New York, NY: W. W. Norton & Company.

McGrath, P., Vun, M., & McLeod, L. (2001). Needs and experiences of non-English-speaking hospice patients and families in an English-speaking country. *American Journal of Hospice and Palliative Care, 18*(5), 305–312.

McMillan, S. C., Small, B. J., Weitzner, M., Schonwetter, R., Tittle, M., Moody, L., & Haley, W. E. (2006). Impact of coping skills intervention with family caregivers of hospice patients with cancer: A randomized clinical trial. *Cancer, 106*(1), 214–222.

Mehta, A., Cohen, S. R., & Chan, L. S. (2009). Palliative care: a need for a family systems approach. *Palliative and Supportive Care, 7*(2), 235–243.

Meyer, D. L., Schneid, J. A., & Craigie, F. C., Jr. (1989). Family conferences: Reasons, levels of involvement and perceived usefulness. *Journal of Family Practice, 29*(4), 401–405.

Milberg, A., Olsson, E. C., Jakobsson, M., Olsson, M., & Friedrichsen, M. (2008). Family members' perceived needs for bereavement follow-up. *Journal of Pain and Symptom Management, 35*(1), 58–69.

Miller, R. D., Krech, R., & Walsh, T. D. (1991). The role of a palliative care service family conference in the management of the patient with advanced cancer. *Palliative Medicine, 5*, 34–39.

Mitnick, S., Leffler, C., & Hood, V. L. (2010). Family caregivers, patients and physicians: Ethical guidance to optimize relationships. *Journal of General Internal Medicine, 25*(3), 255–260.

Monroe, B., & Oliviere, D. (2006). Resilience in palliative care. *European Journal of Palliative Care, 13*(1), 22–25.

Monroe, B., & Oliviere, D. (Eds.), (2007). *Resilience in palliative care: Achievement in adversity*. New York, NY: Oxford University Press.

Monroe, B., & Oliviere, D. (2009). Communicating with family carers. In P. Hudson & S. Payne (Eds.), *Family carers in palliative care* (pp. 1–20). Oxford, England: Oxford University Press.

National Association of Social Workers (NASW). (2004). *NASW standards for social work practice in palliative and end of life care*. Washington, DC: Author.

National Consensus Project for Quality Palliative Care. (2009). *Clinical practice guidelines for quality palliative care, second edition*. Retrieved from http://nationalconsensusproject.org/guideline.pdf

Navaie-Waliser, M., Feldman, P. H., Gould, D. A., Levine, C. L., Kuerbis A. N., & Donelan, K. (2002). When the caregiver needs care: The plight of vulnerable caregivers. *American Journal of Public Health, 92*(3), 409–413.

O'Hare, T. (2009). *Essential skills of social work practice: Assessment, intervention, evaluation*. Chicago, IL: Lyceum Books.

Otis-Green, S., & Rutland, C. B. (2004). Marginalization at the end of life. In J.

Berzoff & P. R. Silverman (Eds.), *Living with dying: A handbook for end-of-life healthcare practitioners* (pp. 462–481). New York, NY: Columbia University Press.

Parsons, R. J. (1991). The mediator role in social work practice. *Social Work, 36*(6), 483–487.

Passik, S. D., & Theobald, D. E. (2000). Managing addiction in advanced cancer patients: Why bother? *Journal of Pain and Symptom Management, 19*(3), 229–234.

Pawlecki, J. B. (2010). End of life: A workplace issue. *Health Affairs, 29*(1), 141–146.

Pham, K., Thornton, J. D., Engelberg, R. A., Jackson, J. C., & Curtis, J. R. (2008). Alterations during medical interpretation of ICU family conferences that interfere with or enhance communication. *Chest, 134*(1), 109–116.

Puchalski, C., Ferrell, B., Virani, R., Otis-Green, S., Baird, P., Bull, J., … Sulmasy, D. (2009). Improving the quality of spiritual care as a dimension of palliative care: The report of the Consensus Conference. *Journal of Palliative Medicine, 12*(10), 885–904.

Radwany, S., Albanese, T., Clough, L., Sims, L., Mason, H., & Jahangiri, S. (2009). End-of-life decision making and emotional burden: Placing family meetings in context. *American Journal of Hospice and Palliative Care, 26*(5), 376–383.

Rolland, J. S. (1990). Anticipatory loss: A family systems developmental framework. *Family Process, 29*(3), 229–244.

Rolland, J. S. (2005). Cancer and the family: An integrative model. *Cancer, 104*(11 Suppl.), 2584–2595.

Rosenberg, E., Seller, R., & Leanza, Y. (2008). Through interpreters' eyes: Comparing roles of professional and family interpreters. *Patient Education and Counseling, 70*(1), 87–93.

Schapira, L., Vargas, E., Hidalgo, R., Brier, M., Sanchez, L., Hobrecker, K., Lynch, T., & Chabner, B. (2008). Lost in translation: Integrating medical interpreters into the multidisciplinary team. *Oncologist, 13*(5), 586–592.

Siegel, K., Raveis, V. H., Mor, V., & Houts, P. (1991). The relationship of spousal caregiver burden to patient disease and treatment-related conditions. *Annals of Oncology, 2*(7), 511–516.

Sulmasy, D. P. (2002). A biopsychosocial-spiritual model for the care of patients at the end of life. *Gerontologist, 42*(Suppl. 3), 24–33.

Thomas, A. J. (1998). Understanding culture and worldview in family systems: Use of the multicultural genogram. *The Family Journal, 6*(1), 24–32.

Turner, J., Clavarino, A., Yates, P., Hargraves, M., Connors, V., & Hausmann, S. (2007). Development of a resource for parents with advanced cancer: What do parents want? *Palliative and Supportive Care, 5*(2), 135–145.

Veach, T. A., & Nicholas, D. R. (1998). Understanding families of adults with cancer: Combining the clinical course of cancer and stages of family development. *Journal of Counseling and Development, 76*(2), 144–156.

Veach, T. A., Nicholas, D. R., & Barton, M. A. (2002). Cancer and the family lifecycle: A practitioner's guide. New York, NY: Brunner-Routledge.

Volker, D. L. (2005). Control and end-of-life care: Does ethnicity matter? *American Journal of Hospice and Palliative Care, 22*(6), 442–446.

Waldrop, D. P. (2006). Caregiving systems at the end of life: How informal caregivers and formal providers collaborate. *Families in Society, 87*(3), 427–437.

Waldrop, D. P. (2008). Treatment at the end of life. *Journal of Gerontological Social Work, 50*(Suppl. 1), 267–292.

Walsh, F. (2002). A family resilience framework: Innovative practice applications. *Family Relations, 51*(2), 130–137.

Walsh, F. (2003). Family resilience: A framework for clinical practice. *Family Process, 42*(1), 1–18.

Walsh, F., & McGoldrick, M. (Eds.). (1991). *Living beyond loss: Death in the family*. New York, NY: W. W. Norton & Co.

West, H. F., Engelberg, R. A., Wenrich, M. D., & Curtis, J. R. (2005). Expressions of nonabandonment during the intensive care unit family conference. *Journal of Palliative Medicine, 8*(4), 797–807.

World Health Organization (WHO). (2007). *Cancer control: Knowledge into action. WHO guide for effective programmes: Palliative care*. Geneva, Switzerland: Author.

Yennurajalingam, S., Dev, R., Lockey, M., Pace, E., Zhang, T., Palmer, J. L., & Bruera, E. (2008). Characteristics of family conferences in a palliative care unit at a comprehensive cancer center. *Journal of Palliative Medicine, 11*(9), 1208–1211.

Yun, Y. H., Rhee, Y. S., Kang, I. O., Lee, J. S., Bang, S. M., Lee, W. S., … Hong, Y. S. (2005). Economic burdens and quality of life of family caregivers of cancer patients. *Oncology, 68*(2-3), 107–114.

Zaider, T., & Kissane, D. (2009). The assessment and management of family distress during palliative care. *Current Opinion in Supportive and Palliative Care, 3*(1), 67–71.

23 *Lucia McBee*

The Doctor within: Integrative Medicine, Social Work, and Palliative Care

This group makes me feel at peace with the world. It helps my whole body and spirit. I forgot all my troubles.

—*Wellness group member*

Key Concepts

◆ *Use of integrative medicine and complementary and alternative medicine (CAM) has increased.*

◆ *Seventy-four percent of U.S. health care consumers use CAM already (National Center for Complementary and Alternative Medicine-NCCAM, 2002).*

◆ *Integrative medicine and CAM are currently offered in most health care settings, studied and published in major peer-reviewed journals, taught in medical settings, and are responsible for an increased expenditure of health care dollars.*

◆ *Integrative medicine, CAM, social work, and palliative care share similar values and approaches toward care.*

Introduction

What is health care, and what do we want in a health care system? In many ways, health care has come full circle, returning to its traditional roots of healing and holistic well-being. In the interim, Western medicine is responsible for tremendous progress in diagnosing and treating acute disease. Consequently, we are living longer, but with more chronic pain and illness (Centers for Disease Control and Prevention [CDC], 2009). When we broaden our vision of health care from curing to include healing, we encompass the domains of palliative care and integrative, complementary, and alternative medicine.

In *A Place of Healing*, Michael Kearney (2000) recalls Hippocrates forgotten colleague Asklepios. The foundation of Western health care was built on the teachings of Hippocrates in ancient Greece. The Hippocratic system embodied all that conventional Western medicine values: rational, evidence-based practice provided by an external expert. But when the Greeks suffered from chronic or incurable illness, they sought help from Asklepios, the Greek god of healing. Asklepian practice used dream work, rituals, and holistic approaches that honored each individual's unique ability to find internal balance and to heal himself or herself.

Integrative medicine and complementary and alternative medicine (CAM) mark a natural evolution and expansion of Asklepian healing, encompassing healing modalities from a range of traditions and cultures. In the same way that Greeks used both the rational Hippocratic and the subjective Asklepian approaches to healing, integrative medicine, social work, and palliative care overlap and complement each other in a variety of ways. This chapter will present an overview of this synergy; review integrative therapies as a whole; and describe examples of specific modalities and their applications to social work and palliative care. It is not intended to be an all-inclusive survey of integrative therapies. It is intended to describe the general reasons that integrative medicine might be effective in palliative care and illustrate selected specific treatments, applications, and recommendations. Illustrative therapies will be those most appropriate to social work rather than those that require advanced training, such as acupuncture. The reader also will be given exercises, so that the therapies can be experienced. The application of these modalities for professional and family caregivers is equally important. Caregivers are often the primary contact for palliative care patients. If the caregiver is distressed, the patient will be distressed. Integrative therapies offer a means to heal and support both caregiver and care receiver.

Some Definitions

The National Institute of Health's Center for Complementary and Alternative Medicine (NCCAM) defines conventional medicine as the medicine practiced by most Western medical doctors and doctors of osteopathy and allied professionals. Complementary medicine is practiced *with* conventional medicine, and alternative medicine is practiced *in place of* conventional medicine. Integrative medicine is defined as practice using well-researched combinations of CAM and conventional medicine (NCCAM, 2009). This chapter will use integrative medicine or therapies in deference to their integration with conventional medicine and the social worker's role in considering all aspects of treatment and patient choice.

The National Consensus Project for Quality Palliative Care defines best practices for palliative care that include the relief of suffering, patient choice, and a holistic approach (2009). The integrative approach often targets symptom management, embraces diverse cultures, and is holistic, aligning with the principles of palliative care. Evidence for efficacy of integrative modalities is mounting, although the effects of holistic treatments are often preventative, diffuse, and subtle, and therefore harder to measure. While not following Western research standards, 3000 years or more of practice and application (as in Ayurveda, yoga, meditation, acupuncture, shamanistic practices, bodywork, creative therapies) may also be considered as evidence of efficacy. In addition, the increasing trend of consumers to use integrative therapies points to the consumer's personal experience of efficacy. A 2007 study released by the NCCAM found that 4 out of 10 U.S. adults used at least one form of CAM in the previous 12 months (Barnes, Bloom, & Nahin, 2008). Integrative approaches are generally low risk and low cost, and they appeal to culturally diverse populations. These interventions tend to be holistic, not only addressing the physical dimensions of disease but also the emotional and spiritual. These modalities often view illness as systemic, a view supported by increasing scientific evidence (see the NCCAM Web site for research studies). They also may identify and strengthen spiritual resources, especially important for those facing illness, loss, and death.

CAM and integrative modalities include over 100 therapies, practices, and systems (Institute of Medicine, 2005). NCCAM defines the following categories of CAM:

- Alternative medical systems
- Mind/body interventions
- Biologically based therapies
- Manipulative and body-based methods
- Energy therapies

Alternative medical systems fundamentally differ from the *diagnose-and-treat* model of Western medicine. Alternative systems include Ayurveda (the ancient and holistic medical system of India), traditional Chinese medicine, and homeopathy. *Mind/body interventions* are based on the assumption that the mind, body, and emotions are linked, and they incorporate meditation, prayer, and cognitive and creative therapies. *Biologically based therapies* use herbs, vitamins, and food. *Manipulative therapies* comprise massage and chiropractic medicine. *Energy therapies* offer healing by using the patient's energy fields and include Reiki, chi gong, and magnetic fields (NCCAM, 2009). Categories overlap at times, pointing to the holistic, fluid nature of these interventions. Yoga, for example, is considered a mind–body modality, and yet it is also part of the Ayurvedic medical system. While often viewed as an adjunct, these modalities are best viewed as an integral part of good practice.

A study performed by NCCAM and AARP (2009) found that the large majority of adults over 50 used CAM, but 69% did not report this usage to their physicians. While most CAM interventions are mild and offer symptomatic relief, some are more aggressive and advertise cures. Coffee enemas and alternative diets, for example, have been proposed to cure cancer, with little or no scientific evidence on their safety and effectiveness. The herbal remedies of kava kava, ginkgo biloba, and St. John's Wort have all been found to have contraindications with certain medical conditions and medications. Since patients may be experimenting with these treatments, it would be important for their medical teams to be aware of this. It is also important not to automatically dismiss unproven treatments. Radiation treatment for cancer was considered radical at one time, and many pharmaceuticals are based on herbs many of which have been used by traditional healers for centuries.

Social workers will find integrative approaches to health and healing to be an important aspect of palliative care. As advocates for patients and families, social workers are obliged to be knowledgeable regarding the modalities used by their populations. For social workers functioning in diverse cultural environments, knowledge of the relevant approaches to healing is an important beginning. For example, if working with an Afro-Caribbean population, familiarity with the use of sarsaparilla, catnip, lemongrass, and other herbs for medicinal purposes (Thomas-Stevenson, 1991) and Santeria, an Afro-Caribbean religion with roots in Africa and Roman Catholicism (Lefever, 1996), would be essential.

In addition, mind–body modalities, especially aligned with social work, have benefited from new technologies able to scientifically describe and measure their effectiveness. Garland and Howard (2009) summarize the increasing evidence describing the brain's ability to change and the connection to the biopsychosocial perspective. Brain imaging and the measurement of immune responses also provide information on the links between emotions, stress, and illness. For example, Gouin, Hantsoo, and Kiecolt-Glaser (2008) found evidence to suggest that high stress may lead to accelerated cellular aging in caregivers. Davidson et al. (2003) demonstrated that those who participated in a stress reduction program were more resistant to infection and evidenced increased brain activity in areas associated with positive affect. Lazar et al. (2005) found evidence to suggest that meditation might be associated with changes in the brain's structure, including the offsetting of age-related cortical thinning. Social workers trained to teach relaxation techniques can expand their skills to include additional therapies designed to reduce stress, including breathing exercises, meditation, and guided imagery.

Palliative Social Work and Integrative Medicine: Common Themes

Palliative care, integrative medicine, and social work share both values and approaches toward health care. In general, the philosophies of palliative care, social work, and integrative medicine are similar in their holistic approach, generally viewing care of the individual disease in the context of the whole person and his or her environment. Approaches to healing include not only physical conditions but also spiritual, emotional, cultural, and psychosocial issues. Integrative modalities are not identical, but they tend to share common principles. Key elements of integrative medicine, palliative care, and social work include the following:

- Expanding curing to include healing
- Approaching health holistically
- Encouraging individual choice
- Focusing on strengths, not illness
- Including diverse cultures

Expanding Curing to Include Healing

I feel more alive in spite of the pain.

—Wellness group member

Conventional Western medicine's focus on curing disease has led to great progress in eliminating many life-threatening ailments and in preventing others. As life expectancy has been extended, the number of those living with chronic illness has increased. Professionals and patients are now considering *quality* of life, as well as *quantity* of life, in measuring successful treatment. Expanding the narrowly focused goal of "curing," the goals of palliative care, social work, and integrative medicine include "healing." Healing modalities address relief from pain and suffering, in body, mind,

---

> **Box 23.1**
> **Patient Narrative: Ms. R.**
>
> *Ms. R. is a 62-year-old African American nursing home resident with complaints of chronic pain. She was admitted to the nursing home following a motor vehicle accident that killed her husband. She suffered multiple fractures and traumatic injuries, ultimately resulting in bilateral below-the-knee amputations. Her adjustment to these losses and nursing home placement was very difficult. She developed complications related to congestive heart failure and diabetes mellitus and began to have tingling, burning sensations in the hands, and phantom limb pain. She began to isolate herself in her room, refusing to get out of bed. As a result of incontinence and being bed bound, she developed decubitus ulcers. In addition, staff reported that Ms. R. was becoming increasingly tearful and withdrawn. Offered pharmacological treatment for her pain and depression, she declined higher doses, stating that the medications made her feel nauseous and sleepy. Her social worker began meeting with Ms. R. weekly to offer a variety of CAM modalities, including breathing exercises, guided imagery and meditation, gentle stretches, and aromatherapy, and the social worker also provided her with tapes to listen to guided imagery. Ms. R. particularly responded to a guided imagery that included visualizing a beach, and she used breath work to release and soften pain. Over time, Ms. R. reported that she was able to use these interventions to help in alleviating her pain and distress. She also found that this process helped to give a greater sense of control over her symptoms and her life.*

and spirit. While quantity of life has standard measurements, quality of life is individually defined and culturally relevant. Quality of life may mean reducing physical symptoms; addressing emotional or spiritual crises related to health, prognoses, or symptoms; or finding meaning in the remaining time left. It may also mean coming to terms with difficult life circumstances as the vignette in Box 23.1 illustrates.

In the narrative (see Box 23.1), the social worker used a variety of mind–body, manipulative, and biologically based CAM interventions. The successful interventions were selected by the patient and the practitioner together based on experimentation and in response to the patient's ability and environment. The goals were not to change Ms. R.'s conditions or the tragic circumstances that led to them, but to ease her suffering in her current circumstances and to help her find meaning in her life as it currently existed.

FOR NOW
Dropping down
Lower and lower.
The quiet grows within.
Doing nothing
My wanting mind stills.
In the silence
In the space

What
I have been seeking
Is found.
It is nothing
Less than everything
and
More than anything.
Being here
For now
Now.

(Elana Rosenbaum, 2005)

Approaching Health Holistically

I feel uplifted. I realize we all have pain. We talk about how we are getting along. It is important to be with other people.

—*Wellness group member*

Conventional Western medicine is characterized by a deep and narrow focus. Health care specializations have allowed in-depth discoveries and yet, at times, do not include the broader, more inclusive perspective. Social work biopsychosocial-spiritual assessment and intervention is based on the person in his or her environment. Increasingly, health care professionals are promoting this holistic approach. In the conclusion of the 2009 Summit of the International Organization of Medicine Summary, Johns states:

> *The care must pay attention to the body, the mind, and the soul and treat the individual as a full and equal partner in care decisions. Integrative health is not merely piling a series of new practitioner tools onto conventional medicine, but a whole new orientation toward person-centered care. (IOM, 2009, p. 155)*

Psychosocial support or the lack of it can be a crucial aspect of health care. Environmental conditions cannot be separated from the healing process. The mind–body connection is well established, as is the importance of social systems (CDC, 2005; Cohen & Wills, 1985; Da Costa et al., 1999). Palliative care, social work, and integrative therapies view healing in a biopsychosocial, spiritual, and cultural context. The patient is also viewed in the context of his or her support system and environment. The relationship between physical symptoms and emotional, spiritual, and mental aspects of the person's experience are considered. Interventions may target one aspect, but they are understood to have ramifications beyond the targeted point of entry.

The use of integrative therapies at the end of life may be especially well received. At this time, patients and families may feel as though treatment has been limited or withdrawn; these therapies may offer healing and hope of continued quality of life. One simple application, easy to use and appreciated by most, is aromatherapy (a biologically based therapy) at the bedside. Lavender oil is the most all-purpose scent, shown to decrease agitation and increase relaxation and sleep (Ballard, O'Brien, Reichelt, & Perry, 2002; Holmes et al., 2002; Wolfe & Herzberg, 1996). Families and patients may also enjoy selecting their own essential oil. Social workers may find this a readily accessible intervention to share with both caregivers and care receivers. Sold online or in health food stores, pure essential oils are those in dark bottles with the Latin name on the bottle. There are many application methods, including placing a few drops of the essential oil on a cotton ball to have nearby the patient, or putting a little in the bath water. For further information on aromatherapy, see the Additional Resources section at the end of this chapter.

TRY THIS

Find a health food store or an aromatherapy boutique. Make sure the essential oils are pure. Sample a variety and see which appeals to you. Take some home to try. You can put a few drops in your bath or lotion. Put some on a cotton ball next to your pillow or a drop or two on the lamp bulb. If you are not sure what to try, start with lavender, the all-purpose essential oil.

Encouraging Individual Choice

Social workers seek to enhance the capacity of people to address their own needs.

—*Preamble, NASW Code of Ethics, 2009*

Integrative medicine, palliative care, and social work all consider the inclusion of the patient and their families in both the assessment and treatment phase. Healing is individualistic and may mean different things to each of us. Professional CAM practitioners are trained to engage the patient and family, present alternatives, receive feedback, and encourage choice. In conventional Western medicine, the health care professional is considered the expert, and the patient may not be encouraged to provide feedback or participate in treatment choices. More recently, health care consumers have been unwilling to accept this role, partially due to increased educational levels and access to information over the Internet and other media. In palliative conditions, symptoms can be complex and intractable, frustrating both the professional and the patient. Often the patient may feel disempowered, perhaps leading to depression or hopelessness. In conventional medicine, the shift to inclusion of the patient is well illustrated by changes in pain assessment. Previously, patients were not asked to rate their own pain; now they are. Integrative modalities have offered a route to self-care and empowerment as the following vignette illustrates:

Two weeks before I left work, I offered Ms. S., a 102-year-old woman, a hand massage. She rarely speaks and is usually hunched over in her wheel chair with a cup of black coffee and a plate of cookies by her side. She is probably the only centenarian that I have met who actually does look her age. When I offer her something, be it cake or coffee, she insists that I have some too. When I decline, she says, "Why not?" and breaks off a piece of whatever treat I have given her. I usually explain that I have already eaten a box full of cookies and that I could not possibly eat anymore. She seems satisfied with this answer. What happened, then, when I offered her a hand massage? I was holding her hands, and she said, "Let me give you one." I accepted. She bent each joint in each finger and what ensued was a 20-minute conversation—the most I have ever seen her talk in nearly 3 years. "There is always hope that things will get better," she told me. And more, "It is good to have strong hands. If you have strong hands, you have something. Strong hands is a start, you must keep your hands strong." I asked her if she felt strong, and she told me she did. I felt her hands and told her that they felt strong to me; she agreed and said that she must keep them strong because it gives her hope. I am constantly reminded that I must never underestimate a person. (M. Levine, personal correspondence, October 9, 2009)

Chronically ill or disabled persons often acutely feel the loss of role. For many, disempowerment and dependency increases their suffering, and they yearn to give back. In this case, the use of a manipulative therapy, a gentle hand massage, allowed this elder to connect and give back both physically and by sharing her wisdom.

Each patient carries his own doctor inside him. They [patients] come to us not knowing that truth. We [doctors] are at our best when we give the doctor who resides within each patient a chance to go to work. (Albert Schweitzer, MD, from Cousins, 2005, p. 78)

Focusing on Strengths, Not Illness

Social workers respect the inherent dignity and worth of the person.
—NASW (2009)

Social work practice, CAM, and palliative care all emphasize the strengths of the client and patient. The focus is on ability, not disability. This focus itself can lend hope to the hopeless and remind those whose time is short that quality may be as important as quantity of time. In the following narrative, a woman with a terminal diagnosis was treated by an experienced practitioner of energy work. The patient lived 1 year beyond the doctor's prognosis and also reported that the energy work enabled her to experience quality time with her family. In biofield energy work, the practitioner works with the energy fields that exist within and without the body. This intervention can include touching the body, passing hands around the body, and both:

Cathy was a 40-year-old white woman with five children ages 10–19 years. Her children's father had divorced her, and their relationship was adversarial. She remarried a supportive man and, within a few months, she was diagnosed with brain cancer and given the prognosis of a 6-month survival. Cathy started visiting an energy-medicine practitioner biweekly. She was also receiving radiation treatments and would often schedule appointments for energy sessions after these treatments. These sessions would begin with a discussion and assessment of her emotional status and for energy levels in the body. The energy work focused on body balance, increasing energy levels, and opening up blockages. Following the radiation treatments, the energy sessions would also work on "clearing the debris from the radiation." Cathy was an active participant in the work, providing feedback before, during, and after the healing. The intention of this practice was palliative, to ground Cathy in this world and to allow total relaxation throughout the healing. During the period of her illness, Cathy's current husband died of a heart attack, and her ex-husband filed for parental rights of the five children, stating that Cathy would be unable to care for them. Despite this, Cathy lived 1 year beyond the doctor's prognosis, and she also observed an increased ability to enjoy the time with her children and to cope with the multiple challenges of her life. (K. Mitcheom, personal communication, October 25, 2009)

While the connection of the energy work to Cathy's life extension is not scientifically proven, the evidence of her quality of life was clear. This hands-on healing worked with Cathy's energy consciousness system to create physical, emotional, mental, and spiritual health, while conventional medicine fought her cancer. Energy healing has been practiced throughout history via shamans and traditional native healers and is now the subject of research (Pierce, 2007; vanderVaart, Gijsen, de Wildt, & Koren, 2009). This energy worker was a nurse practitioner trained in the style of Barbara Brennan, but social workers are also trained in energy work. Also congruent with the underpinnings of palliative care and social work: "The biofield energy therapists share a common energetic world view, wherein they must surrender to a universal energy while simultaneously creating a therapeutic alliance with the client who is also an active agent in healing process" (Warber, Cornelio, Straughn, & Kile, 2004).

TRY THIS

Sit quietly, close your eyes, and center yourself by focusing on your breath. When you feel ready, bring your hands in front of your chest, palms open and facing each other, about a foot apart. Very slowly and attentively, bring your hands toward each other. At some point, you may notice a change in sensation, as though you are feeling a subtle energy field. When you feel this sensation, stop bringing your hands toward each other and, instead, gently explore this field with your palms.

Including Diverse Cultures

Many CAM practices have originated or are traditional in cultures and countries outside the United States and were brought here by immigrating racial and ethnic minority populations. In the new homeland, these CAM practices may have been modified over time, making them all the more interesting to study and to compare with practices in their countries of origin. There the particular system of healing may well constitute the routine system of health care for the majority of citizens (NCCAM, 2009).

Most integrative modalities are descended from ancient healing practices and are based on centuries of experiential practice and viewed in the cultural, holistic, spiritual context. In traditional cultures, creativity was also integrated into holistic healing. Music, art, and dance were often included in spiritual practices, such as worship and healing rituals. Many cultures continue to integrate the practices used for generations, whereas others are rediscovering the practices of their ancestors. Recognizing the importance of identifying and researching diverse healing modalities and interventions, NCCAM has introduced the Office of International Health Research to study these practices in their place of origin and to study their adaptations after relocation (NCCAM, 2009).

While anecdotal reports and personal experiences may demonstrate to many the efficacy of creative therapies in healing, a recent study has demonstrated their impact on health. Cohen et al. (2006) showed that elders who participated in creative groups visited their doctor less often than a similar population who did not participate in such groups. Some call music the universal language. Recently, drum circles have been offered in a variety of settings, providing an opportunity for connection, communication, and expression. One nursing home in New York City, initiated a weekly, ritual drum circle to connect and heal staff, families, and residents.

DRUM CIRCLE EXERCISE

The drum circle has grown to be a tradition and provided expected and unexpected benefits for residents, staff, and families. The residents no longer need to be reminded when Monday at 3 p.m. arrives. One 99-year-old resident will excuse herself from family visits at drum circle time. The staff also looks forward to this time. Ms. B., a certified nursing assistant in the community, traditionally improvises a costume from a shower curtain skirt and shower ring earrings. During the drum circle,

community is built, not discussed. Staff, families, and residents see each other in new ways, no longer patient and professional. Ms. B. is no longer just a caregiver, she is an amazing dancer. One resident, who frequently was seen as demanding, brought eight of her family members of all ages to the drum circle. As the children danced and drummed, the staff admired her beautiful, involved family. Sometimes the group will share music traditions from their culture of origin. The group forged new relationships and new avenues of communication. One 103-year-old member was disconnected from the community due to vision impairment. Through the drum circle, she was able to connect and communicate. (P. Padial, personal communication, November 12, 2009)

This drum circle provides nursing home residents and their families improved quality of life, focusing on creative expression in a format where all are equal and connected.

Why Social Work and Integrative Medicine? Starting with Ourselves

Social work core values include the following:

- Service
- Social justice
- Dignity and worth of the person
- Importance of human relationships
- Integrity
- Competence (NASW, 2009)

Social work and palliative care practice may promote a variety of interventions and practices, but more important, they promote an approach to care informed by underlying values and ethics. Cultivating these values and making treatment choices based on them can be challenging when immersed in a medical system that seems antithetical at times, and when faced with the most exigent circumstances. Our medical system has externalized and reinforced our internal belief and delusion that all illness can be cured and death can be defeated. Consider the Five Remembrances in the next section.

The Five Remembrances

I am sure to grow old; I cannot avoid aging.

I am sure to become ill; I cannot avoid illness.

I am sure to die; I cannot avoid death.

I must be separated from all that is dear and beloved to me.

I am the owner of my actions. Whatever actions I do, good or bad, of these I shall become their heir.

(Nyanaponika & Bodhi, 1999, p. 135)

Countertransference and Mindfulness

Social workers are asked to recognize, understand, and acknowledge their feelings, responses, wishes, and actions arising from interactions with clients (countertransference). Therapeutic training and practice experience teach us that unrecognized and unresolved countertransference will damage therapeutic relationships and the clinical work. Examining potential countertransferential issues when working in palliative care would include examining universal feelings that arise when facing loss, illness, and death. While this internal work may conceptually make sense, it may also prove challenging. Kabat-Zinn describes mindfulness as "paying attention, in a particular way: on purpose, in the present moment, and nonjudgmentally" (1994, p. 4). Practicing mindfulness over time cultivates increased awareness of and comfort in staying with difficult emotions and life circumstances. In turn, mindfulness practice may increase the therapist's ability to identify and utilize the universal wisdom identified in the Five Remembrances.

TRY THIS

Find a quiet space where you will not be interrupted for the next few minutes. Sit or lie comfortably in a position that you can hold without moving. Also make sure you can breathe comfortably. Make sure your chest and belly are open, and if your clothing is tight around the waist, loosen it. Close your eyes if it is comfortable for you; otherwise find a spot on the floor, wall, or ceiling to gaze at. Keep this gaze soft and steady, focusing internally. Notice your breath. Is it fast or slow, even or ragged, deep or shallow? Stay with each breath. In and out, notice the pauses between the in and the out, the exhalation and the inhalation. Do this exercise for 1–3 minutes. Has your mind wandered? At times, our mind may pull us away to events in the past or the future. At times, physical sensations may distract us, or emotions may arise. When this happens, and you become aware of it, simply take note and return your attention to your breath (McBee, 2008, p. 17.)

Mindfulness and meditation have been practiced for thousands of years and found by many to offer equanimity. More recent research has confirmed the results of mind-body practices in changing unhelpful, fear-based patterns in our brain (Begley, 2007; Garland & Howard, 2009). Mind-body practices may also prevent compassion fatigue by supporting self-care in caregivers (McCracken & Yang, 2008; Singh et al., 2004).

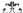

Conclusion

The holistic approaches of integrative medicine have the potential to bring relief from both chronic physical suffering and also from spiritual distress. The core principles of integrative medicine align with both social work and palliative care principles. It is important for social workers to be versed in CAM given its increasing usage among clients. Many patients may not discuss their use of CAM with their medical team, and yet these modalities have implications for treatment, and at times, contraindications. Social workers, whatever their personal beliefs regarding the effectiveness of integrative medicine, can best advocate for their clients by obtaining education about CAM and remaining nonjudgmental. By supporting our patients' choices and assuring they are fully informed, we increase their control in situations that often make them feel out of control. At the least, social workers with sufficient knowledge are able to explore integrative modalities with their palliative care patients and refer them to practitioners trained and certified in their specialty.

Most social workers who utilize integrative modalities in their professional practice begin with a personal usage of the modality. When social workers find that meditation, for example, decreases their reactivity and increases their attentive awareness and self-compassion, they often want to bring this practice to their clients. Many of the CAM therapies described earlier require additional training beyond social work. Integrative therapies may enhance and complement social work practice, especially in palliative care. As social workers learn more about integrative medicine and, perhaps, incorporate these practices into our own lives, we may also be able to offer another avenue of support and healing to our patients and clients. The most important intervention social workers bring to their clients is their presence, embodying respect, hope, strength, and authenticity. Faced with multiple challenges, it may be difficult to embody these qualities. Consider what nurtures you and cultivate it!

ACKNOWLEDGMENT

The author wishes to gratefully acknowledge Victoria Weill-Hagai for her editorial assistance.

ADDITIONAL RESOURCES

BOOKS

Baer, R. A. (Ed.). (2006) *Mindfulness based treatment approaches: Clinician's guide to evidence base and applications* Amsterdam, The Netherlands: Academic Press.

Brennan, B. A. (1988) *Hands of light: A guide to healing through the human energy field.* New York, NY: A Bantam Book.

Cappy, P. (2006). *Yoga for all of us: A modified series of traditional poses for any age and ability.* New York, NY: St. Martin's Press.

Dass, R. (2000). *Still here.* New York, NY: Riverhead Books.

Farhi, D. (1996). *The breathing book: Good health and vitality through essential breath work.* New York, NY: Henry Holt and Company.

Kabat-Zinn, J. (1990). *Full catastrophe living: Using the wisdom of your body and mind to face stress, pain and illness.* New York, NY: Dell Publishing.

Levine, S. (1987). *Healing into life and death.* New York, NY: Anchor Books.

Mackenzie, E. R., & Rakel, B. (Eds.). (2006). *Complementary and alternative medicine for older adults.* New York, NY: Springer Publishing Company.

Naperstek, B. (1994). *Staying well with guided imagery.* New York, NY: Warner Books.

Mindell, A. (1989). *Coma: The dreambody near death.* London, England: Penguin Books.

Price, S., & Price, L. (1999). *Aromatherapy for health professionals.* Edinburgh, U. K. Churchill and Livingstone.

Remen, R. N. (1996). *Kitchen table wisdom.* New York, NY: Riverhead Books.

Reynolds, R. A. (1995). *Bring me the ocean.* Acton, MA: VanderWyk & Burnham.

Santorelli, S. (1999). *Heal thy self.* New York, NY: Bell Tower.

Sapolsky, R. (2004). *Why zebras don't get ulcers.* New York, NY: Owl Books.

Worwood, V. A. (1991). *The complete book of essential oils and aromatherapy.* Novato, CA: New World Library.

WEB SITES

Belleruth Naparstek's guided imagery CDs: http://www.healthjourneys.com/

CDs and tapes from a variety of spiritual and healing traditions: http://www.soundstrue.com

Mindfulness-Based Elder Care: http://www.luciamcbee.com

Resource section contains a manual describing the use of aromatherapy in a nursing home. Mindfulness-Based Elder Care focuses on quality of life and is for those who are elders and who care for elders. Mindfulness-Based Elder Care adapts practices such as meditation, mindfulness, yoga, creative therapies, aromatherapy, massage, and other holistic modalities.

The National Association for Holistic Aromatherapy (NAHA): http://www.naha.org/

The NAHA is an educational, nonprofit organization dedicated to enhancing public awareness of the benefits of true aromatherapy. NAHA is involved with promoting and elevating academic standards in aromatherapy education and practice for the profession.

The National Institute of Health: Complementary and Alternative Medicine (NCCAM): http://nccam.nih.gov/

NCCAM is the U.S. federal government's lead agency for scientific research on the diverse medical and health care systems, practices, and products that are not generally considered part of conventional medicine.

The Touch Research Institute: http://www6.miami.edu/touch-research/

The Touch Research Institute studies the effects of touch therapy. The Institute has researched the effects of massage therapy at all states of life, from newborns to senior citizens.

Basic safety information and links for MSDS sheets on essential oils: http://www.mountainroseherbs.com/newsletter/essential_oils_handle_with_care.php

POETRY

Poetry can provide another voice for healing. Poems are about paying attention and seeing things in new ways. Below are listed a few poetry books. One easy way to discover and enjoy new poems is to listen to the Writer's Almanac on National Public Radio. If you sign up to receive it on your e-mail at http://writersalmanac.publicradio.org/, you will receive a poem each day.

PRACTITIONER RESOURCES

Alliances of International Aromatherapies (AIA) : http://www.alliancearomatherapists.org/Aromatherapy_schools.htm

This nonprofit organization was formed as the result of the vision and devotion of a Denver, Colorado, group of aromatherapists.

Barbara Brennan School of Healing: http://barbarabrennan.com/welcome/introduction.html

"M" massage technique and aromatherapy: http://www.rjbuckle.com

Practitioners and training in from R. J. Buckle in gentle massage and aromatherapy.

Mindfulness-Based Stress Reduction: http://www.umassmed.edu/cfm/

The Center for Mindfulness in Medicine, Health Care and Society; information and training resources.

REFERENCES

Ballard, C. G., O'Brien, J., Reichelt, K., & Perry, E. (2002). Aromatherapy as a safe and effective treatment for the management of agitation in severe dementia: The results of a double blind, placebo controlled trial. *Journal of Clinical Psychiatry, 63*(7), 553–558.

Barnes, P. M., Bloom, B., & Nahin, R. (2008). *CDC National Health Statistics Report #12. Complementary and Alternative Medicine Use Among Adults and Children: United States, 2007.* Retrieved from http://www.cdc.gov/nchs/data/nhsr/nhsr012.pdf

Begley, S. (2007). *Train your mind change your brain: How a new science reveals our extraordinary potential to transform ourselves.* New York, NY: Ballantine Books.

Centers for Disease Control and Prevention (CDC). (2005). *Social support and health related quality of life among older adults–Missouri, 2000. Morbidity and Mortality Weekly Report.* Retrieved from http://www.cdc.gov/mmwr/preview/mmwrhtml/mm5417a4.htm

Centers for Disease Control and Prevention (CDC). (2009). *Chronic disease and health promotion.* Retrieved from http://www.cdc.gov/nccdphp/overview.htm.

Cohen, G. D., Perlstein, S., Chapline, J., Kelly, J., Firth, K. M., & Simmens, S. (2006). The impact of professionally conducted cultural programs on the physical health, mental health and social functioning of older adults. *The Gerontologist, 46*(6), 726–734.

Cohen, S., & Wills, T. A. (1985). Stress, social support, and the buffering hypothesis. *Psychological Bulletin, 98*(2), 310–357.

Cousins, N. (2005). *Anatomy of an illness.* New York, NY: W. W. Norton and Company.

Da Costa, D., Clarke, A. E., Dobkin, P. L., Senecal, J.-L., Fortin, P. R., Danoff, D. S., & Esdaile, J. M. (1999). The relationship between health status, social support and satisfaction with medical care among patients with systemic lupus erythematosus. *International Journal for Quality in Health Care, 11*, 201–207.

Davidson, R. J., Kabat-Zinn, J., Schumacher, J., Rosenkranz, M., Daniel Muller, D., Santorelli, S. F., … Sheridan, J. F. (2003). Alterations in brain and immune function produced by mindfulness meditation psychosomatic medicine. *Psychosomatic Medicine, 65*, 564–570.

Garland, E. L., & Howard, M. O. (2009). Neuroplasticity, psychosocial genomics, and the biopsychosocial paradigm, the 21st century. *Health and Social Work, 34*(3), 191–199.

Gouin, J. P., Hantsoo, L., & Kiecolt-Glaser, J. K. (2008). Immune dysregulation and chronic stress among older adults: A review. *Neuroimmunomodulation, 15*(4-6), 251–259.

Holmes, C., Hopkins, V., Hensford, C., MacLaughlin, V., Wilkinson, D., & Rosenvinge, H. (2002). Lavender oil as a treatment for agitated behaviour in severe dementia: A placebo controlled study. *International Journal of Geriatric Psychiatry, 17*(4), 305–308.

Institute of Medicine(IOM). (2009). *Integrative Medicine and the Health of the Public: A summary of the February 2009 summit.* Retrieved from http://www.nap.edu/catalog/12668.html

Institute of Medicine of the National Academies. (2005). *Complementary and alternative medicine in the United States.* Washington, DC: National Academies Press.

Kabat-Zinn, J. (1994). *Wherever you go, there you are: Mindfulness meditation in everyday life.* New York, NY: Hyperion.

Kearney, M. (2000). A place of healing: Working with suffering in living and dying. Oxford, England: Oxford University Press.

Lazar, S. W., Kerr, C., Wasserman, R. H., Gray, J. R., Greve, D., Treadway, M. T., … Fischl, B. (2005). Meditation experience is associated with increased cortical thickness. *Neurology Report, 16*(17), 1893–1897.

Lefever, H. (1996). When the saints go riding in. *Journal for the Scientific Study of Religion, 35*(3), 318–330.

McBee, L. (2008). *Mindfulness-based elder care.* New York, NY: Springer.

McCracken, L. M., & Yang, S. Y. (2008). A contextual cognitive-behavioral analysis of rehabilitation workers health and well-being: Influences of acceptance, mindfulness, and values-based action. *Rehabilitation Psychology, 53*(4), 479–485.

National Association of Social Workers (NASW). (2009). Code of ethics. Retrieved from http://socialworkers.org/pubs/code/code.asp

National Center for Complementary and Alternative Medicine (NCCAM). (2009). Retrieved from http://nccam.nih.gov/health/whatiscam/overview.htm#integ

National Center for Complementary and Alternative Medicine (NCCAM). (2009). Retrieved from http://nccam.nih.gov/news/2007/011807.htm

National Consensus Project for Quality Palliative Care. (2009). *Clinical practice guidelines for quality palliative care.* Retrieved from http://www.nationalconsensusproject.org/AboutGuidelines.asp

Nyanaponika, T., & Bhikkhu, B. (1999). *Numerical discourses of the Buddha: An anthology of suttas from the Anguttara Nikaya.* Walnut Creek, CA: Altamira Press.

Pierce, B. (2007). The use of biofield therapies in cancer care. *Clinical Journal of Oncological Nursing, 11*(2), 253–258.

Rosenbaum, E. (2005). *Here for now: Living well with cancer through mindfulness.* Hardwick, MA: Satya House Publications.

Singh, N. N., Lancioni, G. E., Winton, A. S., Wahler, R. G., Singh, J., & Sage, M. (2004). Mindful caregiving increases happiness among individuals with profound multiple disabilities. *Research in Developmental Disabilities, 25*(2), 207–218.

Thomas-Stevenson, B. (1991). *Ozarkian and Haitian folk medicine.* (2009) Retrieved from http://www.webster.edu/~corbetre/haiti/misctopic/medicine/ozark.htm

VanderVaart, S., Gijsen, V. M., de Wildt, S. N., & Koren, G. (2009). A systematic review of the therapeutic effects of Reiki. *Journal of Alternative and Complementary Medicine, 15*(11), 1157–1169.

Warber, S. L., Cornelio, D., Straughn, J., & Kile, G. J. (2004). Biofield energy healing from the inside. *Alternative and Complementary Medicine, 10*(6), 1107–1113.

Wolfe, N., & Herzberg, J. (1996) Can aromatherapy oils promote sleep in severely demented patients? *International Journal of Geriatric Psychiatry, 11*, 926–927.

24 *Les Gallo-Silver*

Sexuality, Sensuality, and Intimacy in Palliative Care

I am still alive and I still want to give to my man. Time's wasting and I want loving too—as much as I can handle.
    —*Esther, 46-year-old African American woman with recurrent ovarian cancer*

Key Concepts

- *Sexuality is a key aspect of a person's quality of life and is consistent with the goals of palliative care.*
- *Patients are too often seen as asexual beings with sexual activity being a part of their past but not their future.*
- *Patients can project their rejection of their own bodies onto their partners, believing they will be rejected by them as well.*
- *Partners become desexualized by their anxiety, sadness, and caregiver fatigue.*
- *Helping patients and partners problem solve issues of sexuality can result in increased physical closeness.*

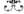

Introduction

Physical touch as an aspect of comfort, support, and affection is a basic human need and as crucial to an infant as is food and warmth. Freud described sex as one of the key primitive urges in people (Freud, 1922). Other theorists point out that our helplessness as infants drives us toward connection with others. This drive is not only in the form of urges as described in Freud's writings but for a sense of human companionship and affection as developed by Fairbairn (1954). Zoldbrod conceptualized milestones of sexual development that begins with the experience of love and touch in infancy. (For a more complete description of the milestones, see Zoldbrod, 2003.) Human sexuality is immersed in the sensation of touch; of touching; and being touched (Gallo-Silver, 2006; Zoldbrod, 2003). Human sexuality can therefore be conceived as the need for physical connection and proximity as well as a desire for specific types of physical contact. In viewing human sexuality in its broadest terms, it takes its rightful place as a universal element of being human rather than owned by people of specific ages, physical abilities, or health statuses. Sexuality is a key aspect of a person's quality of life and is consistent with the goals of palliative care (Howlett, Swain, Fitzmaurice, Mountford, & Love, 1997; Lemieux, Kaiser, Periera, & Meadows, 2004; Shell, 2008; Wilmoth, 2007; Woodhouse & Baldwin, 2008).

This chapter will use the concepts of sexuality, sensuality, and physical intimacy to expand and liberate the human repertoire of loving connection for people receiving palliative care, as well as for the people who love them.

The Touch Continuum

Touch is the primary vehicle for mammals to express comfort, support, and caring to each other. What we as humans call love is often referred to as gentling or being gentled for other mammals. Without sufficient positive physical contact with a caretaker, people are unable to develop crucial adaptive behaviors and coping abilities (Kroll & Klein, 2001).

For infants, parental love is communicated primarily by touch. It is later enhanced by sound/timbre recognition of the parent's voice and further embellished by face and expression recognition (Gallo-Silver, 2006). Parental reinforcement of the infant's smiles and laughing encourages the infant to repeat these behaviors. Parental reinforcement is frequently in the form of touching, whether through holding, kissing, hugging, or touching the infant's face, hands, or feet (Zoldbrod, 2003). This also becomes the foundation of the development of trust because the parent's touch is consistently pleasurable to the infant in a sensual manner (Maltz, 2001). We learn about our bodies through physical affection, bathing, diapering, and eating. For instance, the parent's gentle sponging of the infant's body followed by the drying process, which is often accompanied by hugging and comments of how nice the infant smells, is one way the infant learns about his or her body. The physicality of the diapering process and the accompanying soothing—soothing is a combination of holding, rocking, and kissing—and the parent's embrace while feeding the infant either by breast or bottle, usually accompanied by kisses, give the infant her or his first conceptions of "the pleasures of having a body" (Zolbrod, 2003).

As the descriptions of touch indicate, the various types of touch fall on a continuum of sensations. There are several ways of conceptualizing a touch continuum. Maltz's touch continuum portrays the progression from soothing touch, to sensual touch, and then to sexual touch (Maltz, 2001, 2003). Maltz's continuum begins with the holding and rocking of soothing touch and then progresses to playful contact (i.e., tickling), hugging, kissing, and stroking of sensual touch. The continuum ends with massaging and pleasuring of sexual touch (Maltz, 2001, 2003).

Serious illness can cause distress and the ill person may regress to earlier levels of adaptation and coping in response to his or her distress (Holland & Lewis, 1999; Latona & Stricklin, 1999). Within the realm of touching, this regression presents as a return to earlier parts of the touch continuum. As sexual touch is at the end of the continuum, this regression leaves the patient both less available and less interested in sexual contact (McCabe & Taleporos, 2003). As demonstrated in the narrative of Rita and Carmen in Box 24.1, pain and fatigue are the physical factors that in addition can cause this withdrawal from one's own sexuality. Yet Rita allowed herself to be open to the sensuous touch of Carmen's physical care. This then demonstrates where Rita fell on the touch continuum. This also becomes the benchmark for the palliative social worker to assist the patient and partner to progress further, if that is their goal.

Assessment and Treatment

Health care professionals, particularly nurses, have offered the field of medicine four basic models of assessing sexual

---

Box 24.1
Patient/Family Narrative: Rita

Rita, age 54, was paralyzed from the waist down due to her spinal cord injuries from a car accident. She and Carmen (age 52) became partners many years after her injury. She is currently receiving palliative care due to multiple urinary tract infections and progressive skin breakdown on her buttock from "bed sores." It became Carmen's job to assist with managing the bed sores and general bathing. Carmen also took over the job of inserting a straight catheter to help Rita urinate more frequently and efficiently. Rita had always been in charge of this part of her care but now weakened by infections and pain she needed more help. As Carmen provided this care, Rita refused to engage Carmen in any way including conversation. Carmen was hurt by Rita's behavior, thinking that she would rather have a stranger care for her than her own partner. Carmen presented her sadness and asked for help (see Post, Bloemen, & DeWitte, 2005 for more on caregiver burden). The palliative social worker asked Carmen to make a list of what she enjoyed about taking care of Rita's physical needs. After several tries, Carmen felt comfortable enough to talk about her sensations when touching Rita during the care process, how she relaxed as she felt the natural warmth of Rita's skin, how the softness of her skin pleased her, and how she wanted to kiss Rita. Carmen gradually introduced her feelings into Rita's care activities. At first Rita cried and asked Carmen to stop sharing. Yet Carmen persisted and Rita allowed herself to feel Carmen's touch. Rita's commented to the palliative social worker, "I feel I have so little to give her, the least I can do is be open to what she wants to give me. ... Now I find I enjoy the feel of her hands and I want to touch her, too" (see Cort, Munroe, & Oliviere, 2004; Frohlick & Meston, 2005; for more on responsiveness to touch).

Carmen's need to touch Rita is also the wish to be touched in return. This would be considered an expression of her sexuality. The actual sensation that Rita and Carmen feel can be described as sensuality. Sensuality is a series of pleasurable physical feelings that can be felt by any part of the body. Many people find eating chocolate a highly pleasurable activity in terms of the sensations experienced by the tongue and mouth. It is considered highly sensual but not explicitly sexual (see Small, Zatorre, Dagher, Evans, & Jones-Gotman, 2001 for more on this study). Some people enjoy having their hair washed by someone else. Often you do not know that person very well or at all. The sensation can be very pleasurable, but there is rarely any sexual attraction to the hair-washer and little thought about the person's gender or appearance. Therefore, while sensuality makes a considerable contribution to us in terms of our sexuality, it exists independent of our sexuality (see Gallo-Silver, 2006 for more on sensuality). For Rita and Carmen, their ability to enjoy their sensuality provides both relief and respite from Rita's mounting medical difficulties (see Bowden & Bliss 2009 for more on secondary obstacles to intimacy).

Physical intimacy is the concrete physical contact that is comforting, supportive, affectionate, sensual, and/or erotic. Physical intimacy does not necessarily involve our body's culturally selected and identified erogenous zones (see Kaplan 1974; Katzin 1990 for more information on body sensitivity). Caring for a person's wounds is in of itself a physically intimate act. When accomplished by a health care professional, it would trend toward being supportive and comforting. In Rita's instance, her partner

Box 24.1 (Contd.)

provided her with wound care. Carmen could choose to follow the process used by the health care professional who taught her this skill. She could be as supportive and comforting to Rita as the professional. Yet as her partner she also has the option of moving the care process toward being more affectionate. The affection could be demonstrated by Carmen kissing an unaffected part of Rita's body. This may seem to be a very simplistic progression, yet without instruction and permission the likelihood of Carmen trending Rita's wound care toward affectionate physical intimacy was not likely to occur.

issues for patients. While these models have been used with patients with a variety of medical conditions, they have most frequently been used with cancer patients (Cagle & Bolte, 2009). As a way of helping one to remember the pattern of each model, acronyms were developed. These acronyms then became the name for that specific model. The oldest and most frequently used of these is the original PLISSIT model and the updated version, EX-PLISSIT (Annon, 1976; Cagle & Bolte, 2009; Gallo-Silver, 2006). The PLISSIT model uses a gradual progression of inquiry that enables the health care professional to pace the process to suit the patient's needs. The PLISSIT acronym is based on the following: *P*, providing *p*ermission to discuss sexual concerns often using generalizing and normalizing techniques; *LI*, educating the patient and partner using *l*imited *i*nformation that shares the basic parameters of the functional obstacles to sexual expression experienced by patients with similar conditions; *SS*, making *s*pecific *s*uggestions is the introduction of recommendations to address specific problems and also to explore the patient's (and partner's) general level of sexual adaptation before the illness; and *IT*, addressing the potential referral to specialists in the field of sexual rehabilitation to obtain *i*ntensive *t*herapy (Annon, 1976; Cagle & Bolte, 2009). The *EX*-PLISSIT model widens the reach of the original PLISSIT by *ex*tending the model in two key ways. The permission phase is enlarged to include acceptance of the patient and by the patient as a sexual person. This issue is then carried through to the other phases as well. In addition, EX-PLISSIT includes a review and reflection upon what has been discussed and shared by the patient, the partner, and the professional (Cagle & Bolte, 2009; Taylor & Davies, 2006).

PLISSIT and Ex-PLISSIT have been used by social workers in health care settings, including those who specialize in palliative care (Cagle & Bolte, 2009; Taylor & Davies, 2006). There could be a potential weakness of the model if there is an assumption that it is an isolated topic of inquiry or an item within the history and physical rather than a way to address a clinical need. The palliative social worker focuses on several areas of clinical need involving the social, interpersonal, psychological, and economic domains. Discussions about sexual issues and concerns can be a natural part of the social work counseling relationship (Gallo-Silver, 2006). The

intimacy that the counseling relationship provides enables patients and partners to be open about their concerns with a palliative social worker who presents as accessible and able to address sexuality, sensuality, and physical intimacy. An assessment and intervention tool that emphasizes counseling as the foundation of intervention for sexual issues could be helpful to the palliative social worker. Another option is the adoption of a palliative social work–focused method of assessment and intervention identified with the acronym of CARESS. The word *caress* often means an affectionate touch, embrace, and gentle stroking/touching, thus reinforcing the importance of touch in the restoration of physical intimacy. It captures the cycle of human sexual response initially developed to address female sexuality so poorly served by the tradition linear phasic schema of desire, excitement, and orgasm (Kaplan, 1983; Masters & Johnson, 1966). The cyclical schema begins with emotional intimacy and ends with emotional intimacy more closely mirroring Fairbairn's theories (Fairbairn, 1946). Following the initial emotional intimacy, this cycle continues on to incentives, receptivity, sexual stimulation, subjective arousal, objective arousal, responsive desire, orgasm, resolution, and then a return to emotional intimacy (Basson, 2001). As sexual expression for palliative care patients often takes place within the relationship with the care partner, the cyclical schema grounded in emotional intimacy addresses the interpersonal dynamics of palliative care (Hazan & Shaver, 1987; McCabe, 1994).

The CARESS acronym stands for the following:

> *C*-Counseling is based on rapport, trust, and shared goals focused on the patient's quality of life. The palliative social worker's counseling addresses the patient's and partner's recognition that day-to-day routines, activities, and relationships change, which is validation of the disruption caused by the illness itself. The counseling co-occurs with the need to aggressively manage symptoms, treatment side effects, and pain within the context of palliative care. The social worker is presented with people in crisis attempting to find a new equilibrium to live by. The counseling relationship also becomes the platform for the palliative social worker to assist with sexual concerns as an integrated part of the counseling process (Gallo-Silver, 2006).
>
> *A*-Assessment: As the initial problem is solved interpersonally (the patient, the social worker, and family working together) as well as practically, the palliative social worker can begin to explore the levels of emotional intimacy between the patient and their partner. Key areas of inquiry are as follows (Andrews, 2000; Cagle & Bolte, 2009; Gallo-Silver, 2006; Lemieux et al., 2004):
>
> 1. Prior to the illness what did the couple do together for recreation or leisure?
> 2. How did the couple meet?

3. How and why did the couple decide to become partners?
4. Can they identify one time in their lives as a couple that was enjoyable; if so, what was taking place and what were they sharing together?
5. What were the sleeping arrangements prior to the illness?
6. Does the couple at times use the bathroom together?
7. Was there a physical relationship shared by the partners prior to the illness?
8. Do the individual members of the couple enjoy affection?
9. How does each member of the couple define affection?
10. What level of personal care does the partner provide to the patient at this time?

These areas of inquiry are suggestions based on the therapeutic use of reminiscing that would typically be addressed in couples counseling (Maltz, 2001). Notice that there were no frank questions about sex and that a gentle euphemism was used to refer to sex as a "physical relationship." It is important to be clear in helping patients and partners with sexual issues, but it is also best to learn the couple's language and words. The clinical decision to use more direct or explicit language is often based on the safe relationship the social worker has established with the patient/partner by using their words at first. This establishes a sense of comfort and safety that may lead to the use of more explicit terminology. It is important to establish the level of emotional intimacy the couple shared prior to the illness to establish a baseline for further clinical work. This type of assessment by its very nature nurtures emotional intimacy in couples who self-identify as "close" (Bowden & Bliss, 2009). The less "close" in terms of sharing, intermingling, and having a history of intimate living together (double bed, enjoying affection, co-use of bathroom, providing personal care, etc.), the less likely the possibility of successfully restoring physical intimacy on some medically appropriate level. Depending on the stated wishes of the couple, the social worker would need to help the partners develop emotional intimacy within their preferred context through couples counseling. The fact that the couple that is historically less close is willing to proceed with counseling on this basis is a good prognostic sign of their potential and interest in deepening their physical relationship.

R-Research by the social worker: The palliative social worker becomes knowledgeable over time about the limitations set by specific illnesses. Nonetheless, the individuality of how medical illnesses manifest in different patients requires the social worker to do research before proceeding further into the realm of restoration of physical intimacy. Issues of risk of bone fractures, high blood pressure, low blood pressure, blood counts (includes red, white, and platelet cells), oxygenation, exercise tolerance, residual treatment

radioactivity, diabetes, paralysis, and skin's integrity are some but not all of the medical issues that the palliative social workers need to consider (Gallo-Silver, 2006). This is a collaborative process that involves nursing, the physicians (from multiple areas of specialty depending on the patient's treatment plan), allied health professionals (dieticians, nutritionists, physical therapists, occupational therapists, speech therapists, respiratory therapists, etc.) and clergy. Faith-based and cultural issues for many people are closely intertwined with the expression of physical intimacy. The palliative social worker is obligated to know the "rules" of the patient's faith (if observant) and ethnic culture. Rules, taboos, and special permissions relating to culture and/or faith-based ideals can be varied, unfamiliar, and unexpected by the social worker or other members of the palliative care team. The palliative social worker often has the responsibility to research these issues to benefit the patient as well as the health care team. In addition, research includes identifying specialized resources to enable appropriate referrals to experts in the field of sexual rehabilitation.

E-Education for the social worker and the patient/partner: The palliative social worker self-educates by reviewing the outcome of the aforementioned research and the information obtained through collateral discussions with others. Once prepared, the palliative social worker, within the counseling relationship, begins to educate the couple about how the medical condition impacts on both physical and emotional intimacy. Education must be a paced process. The palliative care social worker needs to be reasonably comfortable that the couple is integrating information before going on to a new topic. New, previously undisclosed, or briefly described medical information should first be presented by either the patient's nurse or physician.

S-Strategies for problem solving including appropriate referrals: Helping a couple put into practice an idea that they have been thinking about or have created is a typical palliative social work function. Giving permission to the couple to experiment with their own ideas similar to the narrative about Lily and Herman (see Box 24.2) is within this same scope of practice (Esmail, Yashima, & Munro 2002; McInnes, 2003). Recommendations and suggestions may focus on communication, responses to new physically intimate activities, and the results of the social worker's research. Sex therapy is often out of the scope of practice for the palliative social worker because it uses a specific skill set that requires additional training and in many states licensure. Referrals to a certified sex therapist, counselor, or educator involve a professional who can identify specific sexual rehabilitation exercises, help the health care team manage and modify medical obstacles, and act as a resource to the team and patient/partner concerning the impact of illness progression. If professionals in this specialty are not available, contact the America Society of Sex Educators, Counselors, and Therapists (ASSECT) to locate a professional accessible to the patient and partner. Palliative social workers are eligible to enroll in training courses sponsored or certified by ASSECT (see Additional Resources section).

S-Sustaining gains in the couple's emotional intimacy: Many patients receiving palliative care may have chronic deteriorating conditions. The palliative social worker needs to be able to anticipate to the extent possible (through communication with the nurses/physicians) changes in the patient's physical condition. This would ultimately help the couple make adjustments in their pattern of physical intimacy. Even in the most integrated and communicative health care teams, patient information may not be exchanged in a timely way. The palliative social worker may learn of a change in the patient's condition either from the patient himself/herself or the partner, which is a signal to return to the Research phase to gain a better understanding of the patient's evolving situation. The goal is to help the couple retain emotional intimacy in the face of further losses and intense emotions (see Boxes 24.3 and 24.4). Sustaining strategies include identifying a couple's strengths, encouragement, normalization, confirmation, and validation interventions. Modifications in physical intimacy can be introduced gradually as the palliative social worker returns to the Strategies phase.

Sexual Reenfranchisement

The medically ill are too often seen as asexual beings with sexual activity being a part of their past but not their future (Gallo-Silver, 2006; Katzin, 1990; Kaufman, Silverberg, & Odette 2007.) Yet it is important to keep in mind the obvious: that pain, shortness of breath, seizures, and edema among other symptoms of serious illness, diminish a person's responsiveness to sexual feelings. One of the key missing pieces is that while the aggressive symptom management of palliative care ameliorates the severity of these symptoms, there is little thought given to the possibility that a person's needs as a sexual person would return (Schover, 2000). The intellectual interest may return in the form of reminiscing about the feelings of sexual activity rather than in a specific request for help with concrete questions about changes in sexual functioning (Kroll & Klein, 2001; McCabe, 1994).

Sometimes it is important for the patient to address the issue of physical intimacy. The partner is often depleted by the anxiety, sadness, and physical tiredness of being

---

Box 24.2
Patient/Family Narrative: Lily

Lily is a 46-year-old Korean woman with congestive heart failure (CHF). She is married to her husband, Herman (55), who is also Korean. Lily has been in and out of the hospital four times in the last 6 months and had met the palliative social worker at Lily's bedside numerous times (see Debusk, 2000; Johnson & Houghton, 2006; Selman et al., 2007; Sotile, 1992; Thorson, 2003 for more on managing the impact of heart disease). They had always enjoyed an active sexual relationship. They stopped having intercourse about a year ago. Lily is often very short of breath and does not like to be hugged or kissed. Herman has replaced these signs of affection with putting lotion on her feet, ankles, and calves, which are often very dry and swollen. Recently, Lily allowed Herman to bathe her because she could no longer do this herself. Herman wanted more physical intimacy with his wife. Lily felt that she "owed" this to him because she had been unable to have children. Individual sessions with Lily focused on her feeling obligated to be physically intimate. It was important to determine whether she felt coerced in any way. She explained that she did feel this was her wifely duty but admitted with some embarrassment that she did enjoy and miss the sexual contact. Her sense of entitlement to remain a sexual person was validated and affirmed. Couples sessions established that Lily liked having her feet gently touched and she was unconcerned if it was Herman' fingers or his palms that were touching her (see De Villers, 2002 for more on massage). The palliative social worker identified that massaging her feet could become more erotic for both of them.

At an individual session Herman shared the idea of rubbing his penis on the bottoms of Lily's feet (see Kaufman, Silverberg, & Odette 2007; Jones & Barlow, 1990 for further adaptive interventions). He was embarrassed to share that he had thought about doing this for a while but thought it was selfish and "dirty" of him to think about it at all. The palliative social worker encouraged Herman to share his thoughts with Lily to find out how she felt about his idea. Lily was discharged home with Herman. They had tried it twice since her discharge and he reported they both found their new sexual practices enjoyable. In a telephone contact with Lily, she shared with the palliative social worker that she and Herman have found a way to feel more close to each other. She felt it added something for her to look forward to in her life. The palliative social worker helped Herman and Lily consider building on the physical closeness they already had through the bathing (see Gallo-Silver, 2006 for more on the use of bathing). Herman was given permission and his desires were normalized and redefined as loving rather than as "selfish." Lily felt "like a real wife" because Herman was able to reach orgasm by rubbing his penis in between her toes. Soon after, they added a vibrator to enable Lily to experience small, manageable, and pleasurable orgasms (see Kaufman, Silverberg, & Odette 2007 for more on the use of sex toys).

The sex-positive stance of the palliative social worker integrated into counseling made it easier for Herman and Lily to express their feelings and their needs. The concept of "dirtiness" was reality tested against the palliative social worker's presentation that there was nothing "wrong" in them sharing more intimate contact with each other (see Horden & Street, 2007 for more on health care communication). The humanity of their sharing enjoyment of each other's bodies became more apparent to them as they

---

Box 24.2 (Contd.)

experimented with expanding Lily's comfort on the touch continuum (see Maltz, 2003 for more information on the touch continuum).

Serious illness can diminish the patient's sensitivity to touch, especially at affected parts of the body. As we are covered with skin made sensitive by blood and nerve endings, there is almost always an area of the body that will remain open to feeling the stimulation of touch. For Lily it was the bottom of her feet; for others, it could be any part of the "unaffected" body. As her sensual feelings increased, she wanted to go further and added a vibrator (also called a sex toy) to make her contact with Herman more erotic (Horden & Street, 2007).

Physical intimacy must be consensual. Sadly, vulnerable people are abused sexually and those receiving palliative care are not exceptions (see Bonomi et al., 2009; Zoloter, Denham, & Weil 2009; for more on family violence). It is crucial for the palliative social worker to determine that there is a sense of mutuality, respect, and caring before making specific interventions for physical contact.

Sex toys are sometimes able to compensate for sexual activities that the patient can no longer manage (Horden & Street, 2007).

Box 24.3
Patient/Family Narrative: James

James (32 years old) was diagnosed with cancer of the tongue and was treated with surgery and radiation (see Monga, Tan, Ostermann, & Monga, 1997 for more information on head and neck cancer patients). The side effects of these treatments resulted in James being fed through a feeding tube. He and his partner of 5 years, Gary age 29, demonstrated their caring for each other through oral sex (fellatio). Given James' medical condition, this was no longer plausible. They were reluctant to add a sex toy to their relationship, but the palliative social worker pointed out that perhaps the addition of a sex toy might be preferable to not having a sexual relationship with each other (see Nieman, 2002 for more on empowerment). Together James and Gary selected a sex toy that approximated the sensations of oral sex for Gary. James would manipulate the toy while Gary was able to fellate James in the traditional way (Kaufman, Silverberg, & Odette 2007).

Box 24.4
Patient/Family Narrative: Jerry

Jerry is a 71-year-old man of Irish descent married for 50 years to Theresa, age 68, who was from an Italian family. They are devout Roman Catholics. They were both each other's first and only sexual partner. They have been married for 50 years. Jerry was diagnosed with COPD/Obstructive Pulmonary Disease/emphysema (see Haas & Haas, 2000; Hardin, Meyers, & Louie, 2008; Lynn et al., 2000; Walbroehl, 1992 for more on pulmonary issues). They began their relationship with the palliative social worker around Jerry's career issues. He was the chief financial officer for a large nonprofit organization connected to the Church. Jerry did not want to retire or go out on disability. Yet he was unable to travel to work on some days and people were noticing changes in him such as weight loss,

a change in his gait, and obvious shortness of breath. Theresa was angry with him and feared he would get hurt because of his "pride." At the point when they needed each other the most they were at odds with each other. When it became clear he would need continuous portable oxygen to even attempt the commute to work, he knew he had to tell the Executive Director and Board of Directors about his condition. The palliative social workers helped Jerry find the words he felt most comfortable using to disclose that he was ill and needed to take Family Medical Leave (FMLA).

Assessment

The marital relationship continued to be strained and stressed often by Jerry's mood swings. He indicated to the palliative social worker that he wanted to return to being sexual active. This had consisted of mutual masturbation in the recent past (see Hulbert & Whittaker, 1991; Jones & Barlow, 1990; for more on masturbation). The palliative social worker assessed that they were not as emotionally intimate as they needed to be for this to be a reasonable goal. Currently the couple rarely kissed and slept in separate rooms. They were engaged in a process of reminiscing by reviewing why they chose each other, the circumstances of their wedding, the birth of their child, and other couple's milestones. Their emotional intimacy improved as the couple's discussion changed from Jerry's body/drugs/doctors to the things they have and still do share in common. This then set the stage for mutual feelings of desire and arousal specifically connected to their increased emotional intimacy (see Basson, 2001 for more on emotional intimacy).

Research

The palliative social worker acquired a general knowledge base in understanding COPD through discussions with the health care team and patient rounds. The social worker obtained more specific information germane to Jerry's condition from his physical and respiratory therapists. Further research through a literature search and lung-specific organizations provided additional information that focused on the impact of COPD on sexual functioning. Specific areas that needed medical clarification before the palliative social worker could proceed were as follows: the reason for his mood swings and how they could be managed; Jerry's exercise tolerance as sexual activity impacts on the heart and lungs as a physical exercise; oxygen needs and how they might be increased by sexual activity; body positioning that would not further hamper Jerry's breathing; and environmental issues such as room temperature and the timing of meals (see Gallo-Silver, 2006 for more on obstacles to physical intimacy). Jerry's mood swings were attributed to a reaction to the dosages of steroid medication he was prescribed. This was managed by his physician. For specific help with erectile dysfunction, an urologist with this specialty was identified.

Education

The palliative social worker was now better prepared to educate the couple about the research results. As partners, the couple and social worker reviewed the information together. Interpreting the information that was useful and understandable to the couple enabled them to contribute to suggestions and strategies. The enhanced emotional intimacy created by Jerry and Theresa enabled this level of participation in the process. Information from the health care team indicated that Jerry no longer had the exercise tolerance for the mutual masturbation he had shared with Theresa. Medications and fatigue rendered Jerry much less reactive to being touched and touching. Physical tiredness and

Box 24.4 (Contd.)

distress had dampened down Theresa's reactivity as well (see Eckberg, Griffith, & Foxfall, 1986, for more on caregiver burden). A referral was made to the urologist that specialized in erectile dysfunction and Jerry was prescribed an injectable medication.

Strategies

Jerry and Theresa needed to find some common level of touching and being touched that built on the level of physical communication with which they were comfortable. As in many partner/caregiver relationships, Theresa was already participating in helping Jerry bathe. As Jerry was using his upper chest muscles to breathe, he often experienced soreness in his shoulders. A shoulder rub for Jerry was added to bathing. Theresa suggested that she might enjoy having Jerry point the shower massage to various parts of her body and also wanted him to watch her masturbate (see Frohlick & Meston 2005; Hulbert & Whittaker 1991; Jones & Barlow 1990; for more on fantasy and arousal). As Jerry was able to sit in his shower chair outside the tub, he was able to manipulate the shower massage for brief periods of time. At times Jerry would become partially erect and Theresa would guide his hand in masturbatory strokes. If desired, Jerry was able to achieve a full erection using a medication injected into the shaft of his penis. Education on the use of this medication was provided by the urologist specialist. Injected erectile dysfunction medications act locally and do not have the side effects of oral medications.

Sustainment

Jerry's condition continued to deteriorate and his care became increasingly more complex. Rather than abandon their reclaimed physical and emotional intimacy, the palliative social worker supported them in trying to adapt to their changing situation. This support used counseling, further research, and additional education for the couple. Theresa could continue to masturbate in front of Jerry and his shoulder massage became moisturizing his skin with lotion (De Villers, 2002). It is important to test lotions and oils on a small patch of skin before ever using them on any large areas or near any mucus membranes. Patients can develop all sorts of sensitivities that they may or may not have presented when medically well (Kaufman, Silverberg, & Odette 2007).

Box 24.5
Patient/Family Narrative: Esther

Esther, a 46-year-old African American woman with recurrent ovarian cancer had struggled with obstructions, infections, fatigue, and pain. When her symptoms were managed by the palliative care team, her overall comfort and energy level increased (see Wilmoth, 2007; Woodhouse & Baldwin, 2008; for more on quality of life). She talked wistfully about how affectionate her husband, Kelvin, age 47, of 20 years had been. Now she was either patted on the shoulder or kissed on the forehead by him. She missed the long kisses he used to give her, the way he nuzzled her neck, and the way his lips used to brush her closed eyes. The palliative social worker asked her how she communicated her wish for this type of affection and physical intimacy (see Gallo-Silver, 2000, 2006; Katz, 2005, 2007; Melby, 2009; for more on enhancing communication). To indicate her interest, she would gently touch his behind, which was their special signal. Within counseling she

contemplated what would happen if she gave her husband the signal. Would he be revolted, horrified, or frightened by it? She wanted to either avoid or at least protect herself from the rejection she feared would be his response. The palliative social worker normalized her fears as well as reality tested them against Esther's 20-year knowledge base about her husband. Esther believed she needed to act on her feelings if only because her condition remained serious and would likely destabilize again. The next time Kelvin kissed her forehead, she reached around and gave him the signal. Kelvin's response was to sob on her shoulder. He never thought that anything could ever return to normal. After comforting him, Esther shared her work with the palliative social worker. Kelvin needed additional help to reconnect to his own sexual and sensual feelings. The palliative social worker developed a series of reconnecting exercises that could be accomplished while bathing (Gallo-Silver, 2000, 2006). Using different sponges and types of lotion soaps, Kelvin was encouraged to try self-exploration of what felt pleasurable. They also began to read erotica to each other that stimulated both of them (see Gallo-Silver, 2000, 2006; Kaplan, 1974; Kaufman, Silverberg, & Odette, 2007; for more information on using erotica). As a result, a more passionate level of affection reentered their relationship.

a caregiver. This, coupled with the break in the couples' typical sexual routines, can desexualize as much as serious illness has desexualized the patient (Gallo-Silver, 2000, 2006). Addressing the partner's needs as in Esther's and Kelvin's relationship (see Box 24.5) was the key to restoring an important aspect of their relationship and enhancing quality of life for both.

The management of serious illness is traumatizing to the body. Many patients can feel disconnected from their bodies as well as angry and betrayed by it. The rejection of the body is then projected outward, with the patient believing that the partner or potential partner will reject or be disgusted by him or her. In addition to the struggle with body image issues, there is a shutdown of the body's overall responsiveness to touch in any pleasurable way. Attempts at physical closeness are closely self-observed and negatively evaluated by the patient in a particularly damaging version of "spectatoring." *Spectatoring* is a term introduced by Helen Singer Kaplan, who used the word to describe a person's separation from the body and sensation (Kaplan, 1974, 1983). Spectatoring is a self-conscious monitoring of one's body and behavior during sexual activity that drains pleasure and spontaneity from the moment (see Box 24.6). This prevents the person from being able to perceive and receive the emotional closeness of sex.

Conclusion

Quality of life is self-defined by each palliative care patient. For some patients this includes remaining a sexual person in a way that is consistent with their medical condition. Palliative

---

Box 24.6
Patient/Family Narrative: Henry

Henry, a 26-year-old successful certified public accountant of East Indian descent from Trinidad, was engaged to be married when he was diagnosed with hepatitis. During his treatment his fiancée's family withdrew their support for the marriage and his girlfriend ended their relationship. He experienced liver failure and began work with a palliative care team. He informed the palliative social worker that he was very lonely, knew that he would always be alone, and shared his experience with his former girlfriend. He explained that because of his illness, he was no longer marriageable within his segment of his East Indian Caribbean community. Counseling with the palliative social worker addressed the loss of his girlfriend, self-esteem issues, and body image concerns. He was able to experience a longer interval of renewed strength through experimental treatments. He became more comfortable with himself; had his hair frosted in the style of the day; and dental veneers applied to his teeth. These were ways to help him feel more confident about his appearance. He met an East Indian woman from Guyana, named Sharda, at a public Diwali Festival, a Hindu holiday of lights that is celebrated by the East Indian Community. Months later, he and Sharda became engaged and soon after married. He told her about his illness after their third date. Henry did not overwhelm Sharda with information on their first date but waited a bit for them to get to know each other a little better. Sharda wanted a life with Henry no matter how long or short his life might be. Their first attempts at intercourse, using safe sex to protect Sharda's health, were hampered by Henry's concerns about how he looked, his ability to perform sexually, and whether Sharda would think he was a good lover. These concerns and spectatoring prevented him from being emotionally present. In addition to counseling with the palliative social worker, he was referred to a psychiatrist who specialized in sexual issues. An injected erectile dysfunction medication gave Henry renewed confidence without further affecting his liver functions. When Henry died, his wife was at his side. Henry had a short yet full life.

---

social workers need to be open to these patients and integrate a sex-positive approach that does not deny the possibilities for sexual expression for the chronically and seriously medically ill. Palliative care optimizes physical comfort and functional abilities to enjoy life's activities. This addresses the realms of eating, sleeping, parenting, work, recreation, and creativity among many others. Palliative care is committed to helping patients retain the healing, loving, comforting, caring, emotionally intimate, sensual, and sexual aspects of being touched and touching.

LEARNING EXERCISES

- Close your eyes and ask a friend or colleague to trace a three- or four-letter word on the palm of your hand. Try to guess the word. This is a skin sensitivity exercise devised by Wendy Maltz (2001).

- Write down the details of your most recent sexual experience, including masturbation. Reflect on what kind of difficulties you would have sharing this with a health care professional. Determine under what circumstances you would be comfortable sharing your information.

- Place a piece of your favorite food in your mouth. Write down all of the sensations you are experiencing from the candy. Include taste, texture, aroma, images, and memories. This will enable you to understand the concept of sensuality.

- Write down one physical aspect of your body you like and why. Name two people: one who agrees and one who disagrees with your opinion. Write down one physical aspect of your body you do not like and why. Name two people: one who agrees and one who disagrees with your opinion. This will make you more aware of body image and the potential for distortion.

ADDITIONAL SUGGESTED READINGS

Altman, C. (1997). *You can be your own sex therapist*. San Francisco, CA: Casper Publishing.

Britton, P. (2005). *The art of sex coaching*. New York, NY: W. W. Norton & Company.

De Villers, L. (2002). *Love skills*. Marina Del Rey, CA: Aphrodite Media.

Haas, F. & Haas, S. S. (2000). *The chronic bronchitis and emphysema handbook*. New York, NY: John Wiley & Sons, Inc.

Kaplan, H. S. (1987). *The illustrated manual of sex therapy*. New York, NY: Brunner/Mazel.

Kaufman, M., Silverberg, C., & Odette, F. (2007). *The ultimate guide to sex and disability*. San Francisco, CA: Cleis Press, Inc.

Schover, L. R. (1997). *Sexuality and fertility after cancer*. New York, NY: John Wiley & Sons.

Sotile, W. M. (1992). *Heart illness and Intimacy: How caring relationships aid recovery*. Baltimore, MD: Johns Hopkins University Press.

ADDITIONAL RESOURCES

American Cancer Society. (2004). *Sexuality and cancer: For the woman who has cancer and her partner*. Atlanta, GA: American Cancer Society Publications.

American Cancer Society. (2004). *Sexuality and cancer. For the man who has cancer and his partner*. Atlanta, GA: American Cancer Society Publications.

WEB SITES

American Association of Sex Educators, Counselors, and Therapists: http://www.aasect.org
Hosts, sponsors, and provides continuing education credits for a number of training programs throughout the United States for professionals at various levels of skill development.

Web sites for sex education: Illness/condition specific with sex
education materials. Please note that many conditions have
their own specific Web sites, and this list addresses the
conditions described in this chapter.
American Cancer Society: http://www.cancer.org
American Heart Association: http://www.americanheart.org
American Lung Association: http://www.lungusa.org
American Spinal Cord Association: http://www.spinal_cord.org
Hepatitis Foundation International: http://www.hepfi.org
Online shopping for sex toys: These are a sample of the commercial
sites for these products. It is advisable to shop in person for
these products if possible.
Discreet-Romance Products: http://www.discreet-romance.com
Eve's Garden: http://www.evesgarden.com
My Pleasure Products: http://www.mypleasure.com
Toys in Babeland: http://www.babeland.com

REFERENCES

Andrews, W. C. (2000). Approaches to taking a sexual history. *Journal of Women's Health and Gender-Based Medicine,* 9(Suppl.), S21–S24.

Annon, J. (1976). The PLISSIT model: A proposed conceptual scheme for the behavioral treatment of sexual problems. *Journal of Sex Education and Therapy, 2,* 1–15.

Basson, R. (2001). Human sex response cycles. *Journal of Sex and Marital Therapy, 27,* 333–343.

Bonomi, A. E., Anderson, M. I., Reid, R. J., Rivara, F. P., Carrell, D., & Thompson, R. S. (2009). Medical and psychosocial diagnosis in women with a history of intimate partner abuse. *Archives of International Medicine, 169*(18), 1692–1697.

Bowden, G., & Bliss, J. (2009). Does a hospital bed impact on the sexuality expression in palliative care? *British Journal of Community Nursing, 14*(3), 122–126.

Cagle, J. G., & Bolte, S. (2009) Sexuality and life-threatening illness: Implications for social work and palliative care. *Health and Social Work, 34*(3), 223–232.

Cort, E., Munroe, B., & Olviere, D. (2004). Couples in palliative care. *Sexual and Relationship Therapy, 19*(3), 337–354. doi:10.1080/14681990410001715454

De Villers, L. (2002). *Love skills.* Marina Del Rey, CA: Aphrodite Media.

Debusk, R. F. (2000). Evaluating the cardiovascular tolerance for sex. *American Journal of Cardiology, 86*(Suppl. 2A), F51–F56.

Eckberg, J., Griffith, N., & Foxfall, M. (1986). Spouse burn-out syndrome. *Journal of Advanced Nursing, 11*(2), 1146–1154.

Esmail, S., Yashima, E., & Munro, B. (2002). Sexuality and disability: The role of health care professionals in providing options and alternatives for couples. *Sexuality and Disability, 9*(4), 267–282.

Fairbairn, W. R. D. (1952). *Psychological studies of the personality.* London, England: Routledge & Kegan Paul.

Freud, S. (1922). *Beyond the pleasure principle.* London, England: International Psycho-Analytic Press.

Frohlick, P. F., & Meston, C. M. (2005). Tactile sensitivity in women with sexual arousal disorder. *Archives of Sexual Behavior, 34*(2), 207–217.

Gallo-Silver, L. (2000, January/February). The sexual rehabilitation of persons with cancer. *Cancer Practice: A Multidisciplinary Journal of Cancer Care, 8*(1), 10–15.

Gallo-Silver, L. (2006). Human sexuality and physical intimacy. In S. Gehlert & T. A. Browne (Eds.), *Handbook of health social work* (pp. 335–366). Hoboken, NJ: John Wiley & Sons.

Haas, F. & Haas, S. S. (2000). *The chronic bronchitis and emphysema handbook.* New York, NY: John Wiley & Sons.

Hardin, K. A., Meyers, F., & Louie, S. (2008, August). Integrating palliative care in severe chronic obstructive lung disease. *Journal of Chronic Obstructive Pulmonary Disease, 5,* 207–220. doi:10.1080/15412550802237366

Hazan, C., & Shaver, P. (1987). Romantic love conceptualized as an attachment process. *Journal of Personality and Social Psychology, 52,* 511–524.

Holland, J. C., & Lewis, S. (1999). *The human side of cancer.* New York, NY: Quill, HarperCollins Publishers.

Horden, A. J., & Street, A. F. (2007). Let's talk about sex: Risky business for cancer and palliative care clinicians. *Contemporary Nurse, 27*(1), 49–60.

Howlett, C., Swain, M., Fitzmaurice, N., Mountford, K., & Love, P. (1997). Sexuality: The neglected component in palliative care. *International Journal of Palliative Nursing, 3*(4), 218–221.

Hulbert, D. F., & Whittaker, K. E. (1991). The role of masturbation in marital satisfaction: A comparative study of female masturbators and non-masturbators. *Journal of Sex Education and Therapy, 17,* 272–282.

Jones, J. C., & Barlow, D. H. (1990). Self-reported frequency of sexual urges, fantasies and masturbatory fantasies in heterosexual males and females. *Archives of Sexual Behavior, 19,* 269–279.

Johnson, M. J., & Houghton, T. (2006). Palliative care for patients with heart failure. *Palliative Medicine, 20,* 211–214.

Kaplan, H. S. (1974). *The new sex therapy: Active treatment of sexual dysfunction.* New York, NY: Brunner/Mazel.

Kaplan, H. S. (1983). *The evaluation of sexual disorders: Psychological and medical aspects.* New York, NY: Brunner/Mazel.

Katz, A. (2005). The sounds of silence: Sexuality information for cancer patients. *Journal of Clinical Oncology, 23*(1), 238–241.

Katz, A. (2007). *Breaking the silence on cancer and sexuality: A handbook for healthcare providers.* Pittsburgh, PA: Oncology Nursing Society Publishing Division.

Katzin, L. (1990). Chronic illnesses and sexuality. *American Journal of Nursing, 90*(1), 181–189.

Kaufman, M., Silverberg, C., & Odette, F. (2007). *The ultimate guide to sex and disability.* San Francisco, CA: Cleis Press.

Kroll, K., & Klein, E. L. (2001). *Enabling romance: A guide to love, sex, and relationships for people with disabilities.* Horsham, PA: No Limits Communications.

Latona, J., & Stricklin, G. J. (1999). *Love is a journey: Couples facing cancer.* Fort Collins, CO: Greyrock Publishers.

Lemieux, L., Kaiser, S., Periera, J., & Meadows, L. M. (2004). Sexuality in palliative care: Patient perspectives. *Palliative Medicine, 18,* 630–637.

Lynn, J., Eli, E. W., Zhong, Z., Landrum, K., Dawson, N., Connors, A., Jr., Desbiens, N., Claessens, M., & McCarthy, E. (2000). Living and dying with chronic obstructive pulmonary disease. *Journal of the American Geriatric Society, 48,* 91–S100.

Maltz, W. (2001). *The sexual healing journey: A guide for survivors of sexual abuse.* New York, NY: HarperCollins.

Maltz, W. (2003). Treating sexual intimacy concerns of sexual abuse survivors. *Contemporary Sexuality, 37*(7), i–viii.

Masters, W. H., & Johnson, V. E. (1966). *Human sexual response.* Boston, MA: Little, Brown.

McCabe, M. P. (1994). The interrelationship between intimacy, sexual functioning and sexuality among men and women in committed relationships. *Canadian Journal of Human Sexuality, 8*, 31–38.

McCabe, M. P., & Taleporos, G. (2003). Sexual esteem, sexual functioning and sexual behavior among people with disability. *Sexuality and Disability, 17*(2), 157–170.

McInnes, R. A. (2003). Chronic illness and sexuality. *Medical Journal of Australia, 179*(5), 263–266.

Melby, T. (2009, April). Reviving sex after cancer strikes. *Contemporary Sexuality, 43*(4), 4–6.

Monga, U., Tan, G., Ostermann, H. J., & Monga, T. N. (1997). Sexuality in head and neck cancer patients. *Archives of Physical and Medical Rehabilitation, 78*(3), 298–304.

Nieman, S. (2002). *Sexuality, cancer and palliative care: Researching perceptions and practice of social work staff in a central London hospital.* Social Work Monographs, Monograph 192, Norwich, Great Britain: UEA Press.

Post, M. W., Bloemen, J., & DeWitte, L. P. (2005). Burden of support for partners of persons with spinal cord injuries. *Spinal Cord, 43*(5), 311–319.

Selman, L., Harding, R., Beynon, T., Hodson, F., Coady, E., Hazeldine, C., Gibbs, L., & Higginson, I. J. (2007). Modelling services to meet the palliative care needs of chronic heart failure patients and their families: Current practice in the UK. *Palliative Medicine, 21*, 385–390.

Schover, L. R. (2000). Sexual problems in chronic illness. In S. R. L. Lieblum & R. C. Rosen (Eds.), *Principles and practice of sex therapy* (pp. 57–81). New York, NY: Guilford Press.

Shell, J. A. (2008). Sexual issues in the palliative care population. *Seminars in Oncology Nursing, 24*(2), 131–134.

Small, D. M., Zatorre, R. J., Dagher, A., Evans, A. C., & Jones-Gotman, M. (2001). Changes in brain activity related to eating chocolate: From pleasure to aversion. *Brain, 124*, 1720–1733.

Sotile, W. M. (1992). *Heart illness and intimacy: How caring relationships aid recovery.* Baltimore, MD: Johns Hopkins University Press.

Taylor, B., & Davies, S. (2006). Using the Extended PLISSIT model to address sexual healthcare needs. *Nursing Standards, 21*(11), 35–40.

Thorson, A. I. (2003). Sexual activity and the cardiac patient. *American Journal of Geriatric Cardiology, 12*, 38–40.

Walbroehl, G. S. (1992). Sexual concerns of the patient with pulmonary disease. *Postgraduate Medicine, 91*, 455–460.

Wilmoth, M. C. (2007). Sexuality: A critical component of quality of life in a palliative care context. *Nursing Clinics of North America, 42*, 507–514.

Woodhouse, J., & Baldwin, M. A. (2008). Dealing sensitively with sexuality in a palliative care context. *British Journal of Community Nursing, 13*(3), 20–25.

Zoldbrod, A. (2003). Assessing intrapsychic blocks to pleasure using the Milestones of Sexual Development Model. *Contemporary Sexuality, 37*, 7–14.

Zoloter, A. J., Denham, A. C., & Weil, A. (2009). Intimate partner violence. *Obstetrical and Gynecological Clinics of North America, 36*(4), 847–860, XI.

25

John G. Cagle and Terry Altilio

The Social Work Role in Pain and Symptom Management

I felt like I had been broken into a million pieces; it was like a blur.
I could not understand what had happened to me.
—Jennifer, 57-year-old woman, reflecting on her experience of severe cancer pain

Key Concepts

- *Palliative social workers have an instrumental role to play in the assessment and management of physical symptoms.*
- *Pain and symptoms occur within and are influenced by a complex interplay of physical, cognitive, behavioral, emotional, social, cultural, and spiritual dimensions.*
- *Social workers who are vigilant about physical symptoms inquire about them during every patient contact.*
- *Although additional research is needed, a number of promising evidence-informed interventions are available for social workers to employ with patients experiencing symptom distress.*

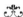

Introduction

Providing relief from pain and symptoms is a central component of high-quality palliative care and a priority for patients, families, and providers (National Consensus Project [NCP], 2004; National Quality Forum [NQF], 2008; Steinhauser et al., 2000). Unfortunately, life-threatening illness is too often accompanied by debilitating physical symptoms such as pain, shortness of breath (dyspnea), fatigue, nausea, and agitation. The presence of these and other symptoms can diminish an individual's quality of life, disrupt relationships, and contribute to mental health risks and social withdrawal (Brummel-Smith et al., 2002; Mulder, 2006). As core members of the palliative care team, social workers have a shared responsibility to contribute to pain and symptom management by using evidence-informed psychosocial strategies to effect relief. In this chapter, we do the following: *(1)* further refine the emerging role of the palliative social worker in pain and symptom management; *(2)* review some of the pertinent ethical, cultural, and medical complexities social workers are likely to encounter; *(3)* provide examples of validated measures that can be used to monitor the presence, type, and severity of various symptoms; and *(4)* identify specific, evidence-supported psychosocial strategies that social workers can use to evaluate symptoms and contribute to symptom relief. We concentrate our efforts on three prevalent symptoms that are commonly encountered in hospice and palliative care settings: pain, dyspnea, and fatigue. For other less common symptoms, the examples we provide here may serve as a template to guide social workers as they identify the relevant associated social, spiritual, and psychological dimensions and intervene accordingly. The focus in this chapter is on physical symptoms, but it is important to acknowledge that physical distress occurs within larger psychosocial-spiritual and environmental frameworks—a familiar social work maxim and one that we emphasize throughout the chapter.

Background

Despite the rapid proliferation of hospice and palliative care, many patients continue to experience substantial pain and symptom-related discomfort in their final days of life (Costello, Wiseman, Douglas, Batten, & Bennett, 2001; Fromme, Tilden, Drach, & Tolle, 2004; Jack, Hillier, Williams, & Oldham, 2003; McMillan, 1996; SUPPORT, 1995; Teno et al., 2004). To help minimize the prevalence of distress and discomfort over the course of a life-threatening illness, clinicians, advocates, and researchers have called for more attention to be paid to the social, psychological, cultural, and spiritual dimensions of pain and symptoms to complement the current, primarily medical and pharmacologic approach to enhancing comfort (Lloyd-Williams, 2003; Rustoen, Fossa, Skarstein, & Moum, 2003). As core members of hospice and palliative care teams, and with their extensive education in social and psychological dynamics, social workers are in a unique position to address these dimensions (National Association of Social Workers [NASW], 2003a; Parker-Oliver, Wittenberg-Lyles, Washington, & Sehrawat, 2009; Project on Death in America, 2004).

Although historically social work has had limited involvement in the treatment of pain and symptoms, numerous leaders and scholars have identified the need for a more pronounced participation by practitioners in the assessment and management of pain and other symptoms (Altilio & Otis-Green, 2005; Bern-Klug, Gessert, & Forbes, 2001; Csikai & Raymer, 2005; Glajchen, Blum, & Calder, 1995; Mendenhall, 2003; NASW, 2003b; Raybould & Adler, 2006). However, social work's role as advocates and clinicians in the identification, assessment, and treatment of pain in palliative care settings often remains unclear and ill defined (Parker-Oliver et al., 2009). The purpose of this chapter is to further the process of articulating this role within the context of palliative care.

An Interdisciplinary Framework

Patients and families receiving palliative care have many physical, psychological, social, and spiritual needs. To meet these varied needs, palliative care involves a team-based approach, which incorporates the knowledge and expertise of professionals from a wide-range of disciplines, including medicine, nursing, chaplaincy, pharmacy, social work, occupational therapy, physical therapy, and nutrition, to name only a few. Each of these disciplines brings a unique and valued perspective to address the holistic (e.g., biopsychosocial-spiritual) needs of the patient and his or her family. Ideally, team members work together as a synergistic whole to address the complex issues that arise during serious illness. This involves collaborative decision making and power sharing, while acknowledging that the patient and/or family are key contributors to care planning, as well as the ultimate authority when determining the goals of care. Palliative care teams, however, face a number of challenges when providing care, particularly when dealing with intractable pain or symptoms. Health care team members often have competing values, communications difficulties, role overlap or ambiguity, and differing ideas about the best way to approach care (Lickiss, Turner, & Pollack, 2004; Speck, 2006). These differences can add an additional layer of complexity. Social workers can help overcome these challenges by facilitating communication between providers and the family, taking an active role in team meetings, and working with fellow team members to understand how cultural issues can influence care and care preferences. One interdisciplinary model for symptom management in palliative care utilized social workers to conduct thorough psychosocial assessments, inventories of care-related resources, and interviews to broach the subject of advance directives (Strasser et al., 2004), although other palliative care practice models are beginning to emerge.

An Ethical Context

Social workers have an ethical obligation to maintain an active role in pain and symptom management. In fact, an NASW news brief stated that "social workers in all practice settings should be aware of pain and symptoms. Across all practice settings, a social worker's ability to empathize with those experiencing pain is critical, so that they can intervene to improve their client's quality of life" (NASW, 2003b, p. 3). For palliative social workers, this attention to physical symptoms is especially relevant. According to the *NASW Standards for Social Work Practice in Palliative and End-of-Life Care* (NASW, 2003a), "the physical, psychological, and spiritual manifestations of pain" (Standard #2) is a topic of core knowledge for palliative social workers.

Johnson (2001) wrote in the *Journal of Law, Medicine and Ethics* that:

> *Human dignity requires and demands that unnecessary, treatable pain be relieved. Severe or chronic pain blocks or seriously impedes the realization of almost all other human values. Relief from unrelenting pain is required to allow the human being to reflect, to enjoy human relationships, and even to think and function on a most basic level. (p. 11, emphasis added)*

This quote reflects the uniqueness of pain in the human experience. It is a sensation that is universal. It is subjective and culturally and spiritually infused in a way that separates it from all other symptoms. Complicating this uniqueness is the attention paid to pain by regulators, law enforcement, legislators, advocates, and the media—an attention that is driven by the fact that pain is undertreated and often managed with medications that are controlled, and potentially abuseable, substances. This sociopolitical context adds another layer of complexity to an already difficult to understand phenomena, and for these many reasons, it invites social work involvement (Altilio, 2006). At the same time the ethical mandate described by Johnson is the rationale by which all undesirable symptoms demand our professional attention.

Johnson's words reflect core values of the social work profession. We hear the appeal for dignity and worth, and a validation of the importance of human relationships, language that is directly reflected in our code of ethics. In addition, the mandate to manage pain is driven by the ethical principles of beneficence (i.e., actions that benefit others), nonmaleficence (i.e., doing no harm), and social justice (i.e., working to ensure equitable treatment of all individuals) (Lo, 2000). There is a vast literature that documents the undertreatment of pain in specific populations, including groups such as our elders, children, the cognitively impaired, persons of color, and the poor—a reality that pleads for advocacy in order that we remain congruent with our profession's commitment to social justice. The subject of pain and symptom management in palliative care is infused with ethical and moral principles. Although physicians and nurses are often asked to justify themselves when their behaviors and judgments are not in harmony with their commitment to relieve pain and suffering, social work has yet to be held to that same level of accountability. At the same time, we are called to action by the National Association of Social Workers (NASW, 1999) *Code of Ethics*, which describes *social justice, dignity and worth of the person* and the *importance of human relationships* as fundamental values.

These values are central to the shared responsibility in palliative and end-of-life care for impeccable assessment and treatment of pain and symptoms. Additionally, our commitment to service is defined as helping people in need and addressing social problems. Patients with uncontrolled pain or who are struggling with breathlessness are in need as are their families. In these cases, the capacity for self-determination and to engage in meaningful relationships and decision making becomes seriously compromised because symptoms can limit one's physical capability and impede cognitive and emotional functioning. Pain, with its complex and dynamic social, cultural, economic, and political correlates, is a social problem. Social work integrity demands that we act responsibly, and within the context of palliative care this includes accepting the covenant that working to relieve pain and suffering is a shared responsibility. Our commitment to the core value of competence requires that we pursue the skills and expertise needed to provide excellent care to patients and families who are dealing with pain and other symptoms (NASW, 1999).

Disparities in Pain and Symptom Management

An Institute of Medicine (Smedley, Stith, & Nelson, 2003) report entitled *Unequal Treatment Confronting Racial and Ethnic Disparities in Health Care* identified disturbing differences in health, health care, and access to health care among minority populations. Moreover, a report by the Hastings Center (Jennings, Ryndes, D'Onofrio, & Baily, 2003) and two systematic reviews of the literature (Anderson, Green, & Payne, 2009; Cintron & Morrison, 2006) confirm what was found in the IOM report, namely that minority populations continue to have disproportionately undertreated pain across the continuum of care. This is a multifaceted problem wherein factors such as socioeconomic inequalities, clinician biases and fears, lack of universal health coverage, education, gender, cultural beliefs, and patient preferences and fears may converge to limit access to effective, equitable treatment for pain and symptoms. Those at increased risk include individuals who are Hispanic, African American, female, very young (especially neonates), elderly, less educated, less affluent, or have a history of adverse effects to medications (Bonham, 2001, Cintron & Morrison, 2006; Palos, Mendoza, Cantor, Aday, & Cleeland, 2004; Portenoy, Ugarte, Fuller, & Haas, 2004). However, some disparities in the identification and treatment of pain may be more attributable to socioeconomic status than factors such as race or ethnicity (Portenoy et al., 2004).

Social workers can help minimize these apparent inequalities with increased vigilance, knowledge, and advocacy about pain and disparities in treatment. Social workers have been charged with advocating on behalf of vulnerable populations, including those living with untreated, or undertreated, pain (NASW, 2003a; NASW, 2003b). This requires our best assessments of the multiple factors that are at the nexus of this troubling reality.

The Synergy of Symptom Management, Palliative Care, and Social Work

Social work is a profession that has been historically committed to caring for the whole person, seeking to understand his or her view of the world and relationship to the environment, family, intimate network, and community. Symptoms are experienced through, and influenced by, a complex and dynamic interplay of biologic, social, behavioral, cultural, emotional, psychological, and spiritual dimensions. However, our understanding of how these dimensions interact with one another to create the symptom experience of the individual is poorly understood. Coexisting conditions such as depression or anxiety are, for example, known to exacerbate pain and complicate its treatment. Uncontrolled pain can also have devastating ripple effects that can erode one's sense of identity and self-worth (Mulder, 2006). Additionally, our fears and expectations about pain may create a dynamic of apprehension that influences its intensity and prevalence and results in a preoccupation with pain, even when pain is absent. Because of the connection between emotional states, perceptions, and other multidimensional factors on pain and symptoms, these are probably best addressed with proactive social work involvement *and* a holistic, family-centered, interdisciplinary team-based approach that targets these influential dimensions—an approach congruous with social work's commitment to the person in his or her environment. We begin where the patient is and, from there, seek to understand, with the patient, his or her experiences, hopes, and beliefs. Palliative care honors similar values, and symptom management, at its best, involves the same kind of comprehensive, multifocal assessment and understanding.

Definition and Scope

Pain is typically a normal and adaptive response that alerts us when we are being exposed to a potentially harmful physical stimulus. The International Association for the Study of Pain (IASP, 2010) defines pain as "an unpleasant sensory and emotional experience associated with actual or potential tissue damage" or "described in terms of such damage." We see in this definition the physiologic perspective and an acknowledgement of the emotional aspects of a pain experience. Another construct of pain and one that has been firmly established within the hospice and palliative care lexicon is Saunders' (2001) concept of *Total Pain*, which includes the physical, emotional, cognitive, and spiritual realms, thus capturing a more comprehensive sense of "suffering" (Fig. 25.1). In this same broader context, Cassell (1992) described "suffering" as distress brought about by an actual or perceived impending threat to the integrity or continued existence of the whole person. Based on this definition, suffering may or may not involve pain or other symptoms because it is rooted in a larger concept of personhood. More recently, Turk, Monarch, and Williams (2002) argued that the extensive literature on the assessment and treatment of chronic pain is

applicable to palliative care settings and those living with life-threatening illness. The literature on chronic pain includes a major focus on the subjective experience, incorporating sensory input, genetic composition, prior learning, cognitive appraisal, mood states, expectations, and sociocultural environment. All of these perspectives of pain, suffering, and symptomology converge to both challenge and channel our understanding of what it means to experience pain. Although there is no consensus-based definition of pain, these selected conceptualizations are a starting place for a comprehensive assessment that values the whole person, his or her physical, emotional, cultural, cognitive, behavioral, and spiritual selves and the reciprocal relationships with family, caregivers, and their environment (Turk, Monarch, & Williams, 2002).

Patients, of course, are often most knowledgeable about how a particular symptom is being experienced, its impact on their lives, personal preferences about treatments, and historically what treatments may or may not have worked. In the context of life-threatening illness or end of life, the ability to recover or express this knowledge may be compromised and needs to be enriched by collateral contacts, perhaps with family, caregivers, and health care clinicians who have a prior history with the patient.

Clinicians need to listen carefully to patients, family members, and fellow team members because the meanings ascribed to a presenting illness and its symptoms can be as important as the illness itself. When symptoms are difficult to manage, there may be a tendency to downplay or dismiss the patient's expressions of pain, or even blame him or her for the predicament. For example, when pain management is challenging (e.g., difficult to control, concerns about addiction, or concurrent psychological symptoms), patients may be labeled as "whiners," "drug seekers," having adopted a "sick-role," "dependent," or trying to gain special attention or

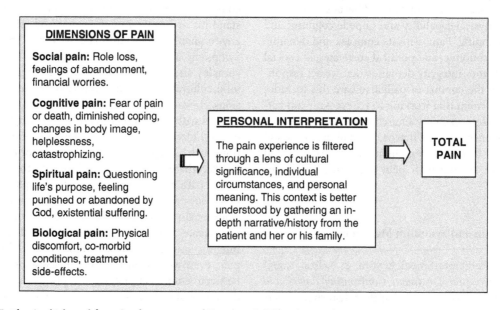

Figure 25.1. Total pain. (Adapted from Sanders, 2001, and Twycross & Wilcock, 2001.)

benefits (MacDonald, 2000; Mendenhall, 2003). Similarly, when the cause of a symptom is elusive, patients and families may attribute catastrophic meaning to the symptom, which may or may not be reflective of the medical reality. Clinicians also ascribe meaning to patients' behavior. For example, a patient who has successfully learned to distract himself from pain by engaging with friends or family may have his pain minimized or delegitimized by staff or family who see this behavior as a sign that the patient is either feigning discomfort or no longer has pain. In these situations, while affirming that patients are the experts on their own symptom experience, it is equally important to consider these attributions as important clinical data that need to be deconstructed and fully considered when crafting the appropriate intervention(s) to assist not only the patients but also their family and the staff. For example, it may be necessary to explore, affirm, or possibly correct the catastrophic attribution of family just as it would be important to explore accusations of drug seeking to either defuse the concern or validate the need for further assessment by the appropriate specialist.

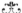

Assessment

Assessment of pain, dyspnea, or fatigue begins with attention to the current level of discomfort to determine whether an acute situation exists that must be emergently addressed by the medical team. In a symptom crisis, advocating for timely medical management is of primary importance, perhaps demanding an abbreviated assessment, which would then be followed up by a more comprehensive assessment once the patient is more comfortable. Using pain as a model for other symptoms, a comprehensive assessment considers the presenting illness, the etiology of the symptom, the goals of care, and prognosis. In addition to the uniqueness of the medical interventions, pain and other symptoms have symbolic significance. Chest pain, which is a common precursor to a heart attack, has a different meaning than neuropathic pain resulting from chemotherapeutic toxicity. Pain occurring in an imminently dying person is experienced and interpreted differently than postsurgical pain from an intervention that removed a tumor from the spinal cord. Palliative sedation, which involves sedation to treat an intractable symptom, may be a consideration in an imminently dying person but may be ethically and medically inappropriate in someone who has months of life remaining. As in many aspects of palliative care, understanding of context is essential to developing a plan of care that is respectful of the unique circumstance of the patient.

In addition to a clinical interview to uncover the relevant meanings, and biopsychosocial-spiritual aspects and impact of pain, there are numerous, well-validated assessment tools available for use (Table 25.1). Some of these instruments simply measure the intensity level of a single symptom, while others are more multidimensional and explore the symptom's impact

on factors such as mood and function. Commonly used pain scales include numeric rating scales, which quantify pain intensity on a scale from zero for "no pain" to 10 for "the worst pain imaginable," and verbal descriptor scales, which range from no pain through mild, moderate, and severe. Visual analog scales require a patient to place a mark to indicate pain intensity on a 10-point scale. One end of the continuum is labeled "no pain" and the other end is "worst pain." The Wong-Baker Faces of Pain scale (National Palliative Care Research Center, 2010; Wong & Baker, 1988) presents pictures of faces expressing a range of emotion from joy to tearfulness. This scale is particularly useful and well validated in children; and it is ostensibly applicable to persons with cognitive impairment. Multidimensional pain scales assist clinicians to assess the broader pain and symptom experience, including mood and function. A tool such as the Memorial Symptom Assessment Scale (MSAS; Portenoy et al.,1994) and its shorter version the MSAS-SF (Chang, Hwang, Feuerman, Kasimis, & Thaler, 2000) invite patients to rate symptoms such as pain, fatigue, and affective states such as worry and sadness and concurrently rate the level of distress associated with each symptom, thus guiding clinicians to prioritize interventions. The Brief Pain Inventory (BPI; Cleeland, 1989; Mendoza, Mayne, Rublee, & Cleeland, 2006) uses a patient-reported pain rating. It inquires about the location(s) of pain through a drawing and asks about the degree to which pain interferes in multiple life domains. The Psychosocial Pain Assessment Form (Otis-Green, 2005, 2006) is an eight-page assessment and guided interview form that measures the impact of pain on five domains: economics, social support, activities of daily living, emotional problems, and coping behaviors as perceived by the interviewer, patient, and significant other and is currently available in both English and Spanish (available online at City of Hope Professional Resource Center Web site: http://prc.coh.org).

Table 25.1. **Internet Resources for the Assessment of Pain and Symptoms**
Information on how to select a measure:
http://www.chcr.brown.edu/pcoc/TOOLKIT.htm
Four trusted Web sites with useful, publicly accessible tools and measures for evaluating pain and other symptoms in palliative care settings:
City of Hope Professional Resource Center: http://prc.coh.org/res_inst.asp
International Association for Hospice & Palliative Care: http://www.hospicecare.com/resources/pain-research.htm
National Palliative Care Research Center: http://www.npcrc.org/resources/
Promoting Excellence in End-of-Life Care: http://www.promotingexcellence.org/tools/

Whether due to medication effects or disease progression, many palliative care patients will experience some level of cognitive impairment that may impact their ability to report or describe their own symptoms. When this occurs, it is incumbent on social workers and other caregivers to look for nonverbal signs of pain, symptoms, or other distress. Observable pain behaviors such as grimacing, guarding, or rubbing are useful when attempting to understand pain in infants, children, or those who are cognitively impaired. Assessing pain in older adults who are unable to verbally report requires knowledge and collaboration with colleagues and family who know the patient or observe them over time. While self-report of pain is considered the gold standard for assessment, when faced with cognitive challenges, other approaches, such as observational and surrogate report, are necessary. A review of the literature by Herr, Bursch, and Black (2008) identified and evaluated existing tools for recognizing and assessing pain to provide clinicians and researchers with the information they need to enhance best practice for this vulnerable population. Included in the review were the Abbey Pain Scale (Abbey), the Assessment of Discomfort in Dementia (ADD) Protocol, and the Pain Assessment in Advanced Dementia (PAINAD) Scale.

A comprehensive assessment may be hindered by a reluctance to discuss pain with family and practitioners (Glajchen et al., 1995). For example, patients may fear that reporting pain will create added stress for their families, or they may worry that increasing levels of pain is a sign of advancing illness—which they may not want validated by their physician. There are times when a patient's report of pain may appear incongruous with the patient's behaviors. For example, patients who are raised in cultures where stoicism is valued or assertiveness is considered impolite may deny pain while at the same time their expressions and behaviors seem to contradict their words. If they accept medications, they may feel disloyal to their heritage or ashamed because they were not strong enough to tolerate the pain. At other times staff or family members may differ in their assessment of a patient's pain, sometimes minimizing the report of pain or, in other cases, believing that the patient has more pain than he or she will acknowledge. These discrepancies are important clinical data and part of the complexity that surrounds assessment of subjective phenomena like pain. Exploring these discrepancies is essential to ensure that treatment is focused on the right symptom and in accordance with the patient's preferences. For example, a staff member who minimizes a report of pain may inadvertently challenge a patient's credibility, thereby diminishing self-esteem, jeopardizing rapport, while contributing to an environment of mistrust—which would then become a focus for intervention.

Family members who report a higher level of pain than the patient may understand that the patient feels diminished by the fact that he or she is unable to bear the pain. At other times a higher pain report signifies that the family member may be assessing pain through his or her own emotions and suffering, requiring interventions that are uniquely separate from medications directed toward physical pain. These many challenges invite social workers to use their clinical skills to listen and facilitate effective communication between the patient, family, and providers, which is essential for a comprehensive pain assessment and exemplary palliative care (Bern-Klug et al., 2001).

Anxiety and depression may preexist pain and other symptoms or be a consequence of living with symptoms and life-threatening illness. Comprehensive assessment includes exploring anxiety and depression, preexisting psychiatric illness, anticipatory anxiety related to treatments such as painful dressing changes, and depressive symptoms such as hopelessness, guilt, and loss of interest or pleasure. Anxiety often accompanies pain, dyspnea, or cardiac symptoms and at times is related to medications such as corticosteroids or psychostimulants designed to manage distressing symptoms. Depression may decrease tolerance for pain or increase the consequent suffering. Living with life-threatening illness and the associated existential and psychosocial concerns can create depressive and anxious feelings that can exacerbate both symptoms and suffering. Furthermore, unrelenting pain is also a risk factor for suicide (Abrahm, 2005; Fisher, Haythornthwaite, Heinberg, Clark, & Reed, 2001); thus, when a patient's pain control is inadequate or discomfort is intractable, an ongoing assessment for suicidal ideation is warranted.

Although we recommend that social workers learn and use evidence-informed assessment strategies and interventions, it is equally important to avoid formulaic or "cookie cutter" practice approaches. While validated assessment tools and empirically tested treatment strategies are beneficial and can help guide social work practice, they are not one size fits all. Rather, palliative care treatment plans emphasize the uniqueness and diversity of individuals by taking into account patient/family goals, cultural considerations, spiritual orientation, and family dynamics. We believe that the core social work values of self-determination and patient centeredness take precedence over uniform assessment and treatment.

In addition to an instrument-based assessment, observational strategies, open-ended interview questions, or the use of journal and diaries can be used to inform assessment, provide better depth and understanding, while simultaneously serving as a potential treatment modality. These interventions are flexible and can be used by patients, family members, and caregivers. They can be adapted to accommodate a person's communication needs and writing style using voice recordings, handwritten paragraphs, outlines, or texting to document the symptom experience over a period of time, which may encompass days, weeks, or months depending on the clinical goal. These modalities provide a link to the clinical team, which, for some, has therapeutic value. In addition to documenting and sharing aspects of the pain and symptoms, diaries create a history of recorded data as well as the in-the-moment thoughts, attributions, feelings, fears, and beliefs of the writer (see Box 25.1). There are many models of diaries and the format and focus used depends on the clinical assessment and goal.

Box 25.1
Patient/Family Narrative: Mitchell

Mitchell is a 57-year-old man being treated for melanoma. He was referred to the pain clinic in a major cancer center for management of symptoms including leg pain, weakness, dry eyes and mouth, and anxiety. He is single and identifies himself as a practicing member of the Orthodox Jewish religion. His father and brother are his major support system. During conversations with the palliative social worker, Mitchell has shared that he expects to die from the melanoma and is especially frightened that his intensifying symptoms are indicative of disease progression. This belief, and his fear of death, has preoccupied Mitchell's thoughts, creating heightened anxiety and distress. Although, objectively, the spread of the melanoma appears to be contained for the time being, an expectation that something catastrophic will happen and the resulting anxiety and fear about this has taken over his life—more so than the physical limitations of the disease itself. As part of the psychosocial pain treatment plan, Mitchell is asked to keep a diary focusing specifically on his symptoms, their frequency and intensity and his daily activities. He is asked to write a brief comment about his interpretation of the symptoms, including his emotional response. He initially refused, but after further negotiation and a little encouragement from the palliative care team, he agreed to try the diary for 2 weeks. The following is a summary of the information gleaned from his diary, which informed the team's understanding of Mitchell' personhood and guided subsequent interventions and outcomes.

According to the diary, Mitchell was spending most of his days either sleeping or lying down watching television. It was also apparent that his social network had become limited to personnel working within the medical system. In response to this information, the palliative social worker explored prior sources of socialization and suggested he resume his social and political activities. The social worker helped Mitchell reconsider the attributed meaning of his leg pain, from a pervasive dread of disease progression to consider alternate meanings such as a lack of physical conditioning. The team also recommended that he return to the physical fitness center which he previously attended to increase exercise and add to opportunities for socialization.

The diary also revealed that Mitchell's car had been towed away during the week that he had begun the diary. His response to the incident was one of activity and initiative rather than the passivity and helplessness that pervaded many of his days and much of his interaction. Upon learning this, the social worker encouraged his curiosity and thoughtfulness as to the meaning of his response to the towing of his car. She validated his ability to act when he felt exploited or motivated by areas of his life that had meaning. She also explored aspects of his pre-diagnosis life that brought meaning and value to his days. He identified dancing (an opportunity for socializing and exercise), study of the Talmud (an opportunity to explore meaning and religious beliefs and understanding that might diminish his fear as well as inform his current existential experience), and political action (an opportunity to socialize and contribute to the world outside of self). The team advised Mitchell to prioritize his activities, teaching him the concept of pacing and suggesting that he carefully consider introducing these sources of meaning back into his life. Potential barriers to these activities were also explored to maximize the possibility of creating a positive outcome.

Interventions

The evidence base for social work interventions that are designed to relieve pain is currently limited. Nevertheless, several promising treatment strategies have demonstrated modest efficacy for reducing pain severity and may also help to address some of the social and psychological dimensions of suffering. Cognitive distractions, education, cognitive-behavioral interventions, relaxation techniques, guided imagery, hypnosis, and diaries are several strategies that are evidence informed and may be useful tools for palliative social workers (International Association for the Study of Pain [IASP], 2008-2009; National Cancer Institute [NCI], 2010). However, these social and psychological interventions are not substitutes for medication or other palliative interventions. They are best used as adjuncts, complementary and integrative strategies that may help minimize the experience of pain and/or the associated distress or improve coping.

- *Distraction.* Redirecting a patient's attention away from the pain experience can help to alleviate its severity. Using conversation, music, challenging tasks (e.g., crosswords or Sudoku), video games, or television allows patients to focus on activities other than the discomfort.
- *Education.* There are numerous studies, many focused on cancer pain, that have demonstrated the usefulness of education as a tool to improve outcomes. On a day-to-day basis the education is within the clinical relationships that support patients and their families through written materials. Education about the multiple aspects of pain and symptom management may be intended to decrease anxiety, promote acceptance of a treatment plan, or engage families who are ambivalent about medications and potential side effects such as confusion or sedation.
- *Cognitive-behavioral therapy (CBT).* Cognitive and behavioral treatment approaches seek to identify thought patterns and behaviors that contribute to the pain experience (NCI, 2010). When working with patients and families in palliative care settings, social workers can use self-talk coaching to foster coping (e.g., "I can use a focused breathing exercise to help manage this pain flare") and self-efficacy (e.g., "I am able to distract myself by imagining a comfortable, safe place"). They can also work with patients and families to identify any negative beliefs, thoughts, or unrealistic expectations that increase distress and may interfere with coping with pain or other symptoms.
- *Relaxation.* Relaxation strategies such as focused or deep breathing exercises may be especially helpful during brief, episodic pain. Progressive muscle relaxation, for example, involves the tensing and relaxing of muscle groups, while passive muscle

relaxation involves only the release of tension. Both types of exercise teach patients to control and relax various muscle groups to help diminish pain and anxiety (IASP, 2004).

- *Guided imagery.* Self-guided imagery may begin as a shared experience with a clinician later to become a skill independent of another. This technique involves focusing on a pleasant, calming, or distracting scene and redirecting one's attention to the sights, sounds, smells, and tastes of the imagined experience. As patients practice this skill, they may use it to divert attention from pain or other procedures such as dressing changes that may cause anxiety or distress. These exercises can be recorded, thus giving the patient the opportunity to access the clinician's voice and guidance whenever they would like. Interventions such as diaries and recorded exercises often become symbolic of the clinical relationship, perhaps similar to the dynamic reflected in Winnicott's concept of the transitional object (Winnicott, 1971). This has the potential to extend the therapeutic relationship beyond the actual time we are able to share with patients and their families.

- *Hypnosis-based CBT.* A trained therapist provides specific suggestions designed to bring the patient into a deep state of relaxation. Once this state is achieved, depending on the goal the therapist might use systematic desensitization techniques to help the patient control pain. As patients achieve success in using therapist-guided suggestions for pain control, they are typically taught self-hypnosis so that they can use this skill in a variety of daily pain-related situations (IASP, 2008–2009).

- *Diaries and journals.* As previously mentioned, keeping a pain diary may be beneficial for some patients. It can help patients explore the meaning of their pain and process the social and psychological impact of its manifestation. In addition, by keeping track of one's pain, the diary helps to identify what activities exacerbate the pain or help to relieve it.

The National Cancer Institute (2010) and the International Association for the Study of Pain (2008–2009) Web sites provide detailed pain-related information, including the status of the evidence supporting these interventions as well as many sample exercises. Social workers can learn these treatment approaches and apply them to their unique practice settings and the individual needs of their patients and families. In addition to intervening directly, advocating for excellence in pain and symptom management requires knowledge about the efficacy of integrative techniques and a respect for the healing modalities used in different cultures and faith-based communities. These may include prayer, acupuncture, mediation, massage, music, chanting, heat, and cold, which may be integrated into a care plan.

Barriers to Pain Management

Previous studies suggest the leading barriers to effective pain management in palliative settings are the knowledge, beliefs, and attitudes of patients, informal caregivers, and health care providers (Agency for Healthcare Research and Quality [AHRQ] 2008; Berry & Ward, 1995; Johnson, Kassner, Houser, & Kutner, 2005; Letizia, Creech, Norton, Shanahan, & Hedges, 2004; Randall-David, Wright, Porterfield, & Lesser, 2003; Ward, Berry, & Misiewicz, 1996). Macro barriers include those that are systemic (e.g., access to care), economic (e.g., the affordability of medications), and political (e.g., regulations that hinder effective pain management). Because many of the barriers to good pain management are psychosocial, spiritual, or cultural in nature, they are ideal targets for micro-level social work assessment and intervention (Altilio, 2004; Parker-Oliver et al., 2008; Parker-Oliver et al., 2009). Based on our extensive review of the literature, we highlight eight specific barriers which social workers can help to identify and address: addiction, side effects, stoicism, stigma, burden, tolerance, fears of overdose, and fatalism (AHRQ, 2008; Berry & Ward, 1995; Johnson et al., 2005; Letizia et al., 2004; Randall-David et al., 2003; Ward et al., 1996).

- *Addiction* is a primary, chronic, neurobiologic disease, with genetic, psychosocial, and environmental factors influencing its development and manifestations. It is characterized by behaviors that include one or more of the following: impaired control over drug use, compulsive use, continued use despite harm, and craving (Savage et al., 2002). The person with the disease of addiction seeks to achieve drug effects other than pain or symptom relief (McCaffery & Pasero, 1999). Others may use or abuse substances to treat such symptoms as anxiety, depression, or despair. These common concerns expressed by patients, caregivers, and providers require a comprehensive response that includes assessment, education, and appropriate interventions. While patients frequently require an increase in their pain medication over time, this does not equate with addiction but may instead be a sign of progression of disease or the development of physical tolerance to the medication. Note: *physical dependence,* which is often confused with addiction by both health care professionals and the public, is a state of adaptation that manifests as a withdrawal syndrome and can be brought on by a variety of factors, including, but not limited to, stopping one's medication abruptly. Thus, it is important to ensure that patients do not discontinue their medications without first consulting the palliative care team. This type of dependence is not specific to opioids because this adaptation is also observed with other medications such as steroids and beta-blockers (American Pain Society, 2006).

- *Tolerance* is a decline in drug effectiveness at a given dosage over a period of time. True tolerance is rare, but patients frequently require minor adjustments in the dose, scheduling, or type(s) of drug over the course of illness. Patients and caregivers may worry that using a medication early in the disease process will interfere in the management of pain as disease progresses and they can be helped by interdisciplinary education to dispel this fear.
- *Stoicism* is a willingness to endure pain or other usually undesirable symptoms. Stoicism may be especially valued among men, elders, and cultural groups who may not want to burden others or be perceived as weak. This can contribute to a patient's reluctance to report pain. Stoic patients may minimize the prevalence or intensity of their pain, thereby complicating the process of assessment and diagnosis and possibly impacting the disease outcome. Social workers can help patients by reframing the report of pain and other symptoms as a way of assisting the palliative care team in providing comprehensive care rather than as a sign of weakness. Reporting pain is not always followed by an acceptance of treatment, however. Personal, cultural, and spiritual values may influence the types of treatments that are acceptable. Respecting the cultural values and beliefs while presenting new information to expand and enrich those beliefs and negotiating a collaborative treatment plan often requires the involvement of the physician and the family, as well as social work skills.
- *Fatalism* is the belief that pain is a necessary and expected part of life, aging, and coping with serious illness. This may represent common spiritual or cultural beliefs, or in some cases it may be symptomatic of a potentially problematic mood disorder. While research tells us that pain is not always inevitable and that it can be effectively treated, the understanding and meaning of fatalism in the life of the patient or the patient's family requires careful assessment to inform potential intervention.
- *Side effects* are the unintended secondary effects of a treatment. Common fears associated with pain medications include being too drowsy, confused, feeling "knocked out," or having constipation. Some worry that pain medications will hasten death. Side effects, just as symptoms, have meaning to patients and their families. For example, drowsiness in a person who is imminently coming to the end of his or her life may rob the person of precious time to be interactive with family. For others, drowsiness is a relief because it protects them from experiencing the suffering around them. A patient's concern about side effects can be so great that he or she may choose to tolerate pain in order to avoid certain side effects such as drowsiness. With good patient, family, and provider communication and clinical skill, often unwanted side effects can be successfully avoided or managed. Constipation, a side effect of opioid pain medications that impacts a patient's sense of control and self-efficacy, for example, can be treated with laxatives and stool softeners.
- *Stigma* is the perceived disapproval of others that is often associated with taking pain medication. Many patients and caregivers report that they do not want to be viewed as "junkies" or "drug seeking" and, as result, may be hesitant to report pain or request additional medication to adequately control the pain. Social workers can intervene with patients and their families to acknowledge and explore fears, seeking to understand their etiology while clarifying misconceptions and educating, over time and repeatedly, about the difference between addiction, physical dependence, and tolerance. It is sometimes helpful to observe the difference in outcomes because using opioids to manage pain generally makes life better as opposed to the addictive use of drugs, which devastates the life of the person and often their families. When appropriate to the patient and family, education can focus on the role of opioids and other classes of medication in managing pain in life-threatening illness. This can provide reassurance of the clinical staff's ongoing commitment to assist in assessment, to value their observations, and to work to create a treatment plan that incorporates opioids, adjuvant medication, and other modalities such as physical therapy, music, massage, and relaxation.
- *Burden* refers to the belief that by reporting pain or asking for help, patients or caregivers are imposing on others, such as staff, family, or caregivers. To address concerns about being a burden, palliative social workers can assess the etiology of this perception in order to formulate an appropriate intervention and treatment plan. For example, in families where the cost of care is depleting financial resources the intervention is different than in a family where caregiver exhaustion has forced the patient to stop asking for help. Ensuring that patients and families understand that pain management is an integral aspect of palliative care may obviate the fear that they are burdening us as well.
- *Fear of overdose* is a concern that the patient will take, or be given, too much medication and experience severe side effects or cause or hasten death as a result of the dose. Overdosing on pain medication, however, is an unlikely occurrence when medications are prescribed properly and then taken as prescribed. Depending on the setting, health care providers or family are observing patient responses, and in instances where patients are taking their own medications if somnolence develops it can act to prevent the patient from taking additional doses. Patients and families require education to understand that medications can be adjusted if needed and that relief of pain is not a signal to stop medications. Persistent pain requires scheduled medications to keep it under control. If pain

Table 25.2.
Selected Social Work Assessment and Treatment Approaches for Common Symptoms

Symptom	Description	Selected Assessment Instruments	Treatment Approaches
Agitation	A state of heightened physical tension and increased irritability; often associated with mental illness, dementia, drug or alcohol withdrawal, or advanced terminal illness[1]	• Agitated Behavior Scale (ABS)[2] • Cohen-Mansfield Agitation Inventory (CMAI; Cohen-Mansfield, 1991)[3] • Positive and Negative Syndrome Scale Excited-Component (PANSS-EC)[4]	• Calm, soothing voice • Warn before touching • Apologize for causing distress • Keep person warm, covered • Companion if response is positive • Calm the environment • Experiment with light music • Touch gently, observe response • Provide continuity of staff[5]
Dyspnea	Shortness of breath or "air hunger;" a common and often debilitating symptom often experienced by persons with end-stage COPD*, cancer, and heart disease[6]	• Visual Numeric Scale[7] • Numeric Rating Scale (NRS)[7] • Modified Borg Scale[8] • Japanese Cancer Dyspnea Scale (CDS)[9] • Baseline Dyspnea Index (BDI)[10]	• Cognitive-behavioral therapy • Relaxation therapy • Art therapy • Massage therapy • Guided imagery[6, 11-12]
Fatigue	Persistent tiredness; commonly experienced by patients with COPD*, heart failure, and advanced cancer[6]	• One-item scale[7] • Brief Fatigue Inventory (BFI)[13] • Fatigue Symptom Inventory (FSI)[14] • Functional Assessment of Chronic Illness Therapy–Fatigue Scale (FACIT-F)[15]	• Cognitive-behavioral therapy • Expressive group therapy • Supportive therapy • Educational interventions • Group psychotherapy • exercise[6, 16, 17]
Nausea	An unpleasant feeling that precedes vomiting; experienced by nearly 80% of persons undergoing chemotherapy[6, 16]	• Visual Analog Scales (VAS)[18] • Analog Continuous Chromatic Scales (ACCS)[19] • Numerical Rating Scales (NRS)[7] • Verbal Categorical Scales (VCS)[20]	• Symptom monitoring • Progressive muscle relaxation • Systematic desensitization • Hypnosis • Cognitive distraction[6, 16]
Pain	Physical discomfort; a displeasing sensory and affective experience associated with real or potential somatic damage[21]	• Brief Pain Inventory (BPI)[22] • Memorial Symptom Assessment Scale (MSAS)[23] • Edmonton Symptom Assessment Scale (ESAS)[7] • Wong-Baker Faces of Pain Scale[24]	• Cognitive-behavioral therapy • Relaxation • Guided imagery, visualization • Hypnosis • Coping skills training • Problem solving • Systematic reminders[6, 21, 25]

1. Twycross & Wilcock, 2001; 2. Corrigan, 1989; 3. Cohen, Mansfield, 1991; 4. Chaichan, 2008; 5. Kong, Evans, & Guevara, 2009; 6. Brunnhuber, Nash, Meier, Weissman, & Woodcock, 2008; 7. Nekolaichuk, Watanabe, & Beaumont, 2008; 8. Mador, Rodis, & Magalang, 1995; 9. Bausewein, Farquhar, Booth, Gysels, & Higginson, 2007; 10. Dorman, Byrne, & Edwards, 2007; 11. Buckholz & von Gunten, 2009; 12. Zhao & Yates, 2008; 13. Mendoza et al., 1999; 14. Hann et al., 1998; 15. Cella, Lai, Chang, Peterman, & Slavin, 2002; 16. American Psychosocial Oncology Society, 2006; 17. NCCN, 2005; 18. Grunberg, Boutin, Ireland, Miner, Silvera, & Ashikaga, 2005; 19. Hesketh, 2005; 20. Saxby, Ackroyd, Callin, Mayland, & Kite, 2007; 21. IASP, 2010; 22. Cleeland, 1989; 23. Portenoy et al., 1994; 24. Wong & Baker, 1988; 25. NCI, 2010.

*COPD, chronic obstructive pulmonary disease.

medication is discontinued prematurely, the patient who is physically dependent may experience withdrawal symptoms in addition to the likely return of pain, an experience which is physically and emotionally distressing.

As an illness progresses and debilitation increases, patients become more reliant on family caregivers to identify discomfort and administer pain treatments. Recent research in hospice settings suggests that family caregivers frequently have concerns about pain and pain management particularly with administering analgesic medications (Letizia et al., 2004; Parker-Oliver et al., 2008) and that these concerns may be overlooked by palliative care providers (Parker-Oliver et al., 2008). Social workers have a clear role to evaluate for potential barriers to pain and symptom management and, when identified, to provide interventions to dispel myths, correct misconceptions, and explore caregiver expectations to see whether they are congruent with the scope and limitations of provider services. Social workers are also charged with being active participants in team conferences, advocating on behalf of patients and families, and ensuring that fellow team members are aware of caregiver concerns and potential barriers to pain and symptom management (NASW, 2003a; Parker-Oliver et al., 2009).

Additional Symptoms

The following sections provide a general overview of how social workers can help to identify and address two prevalent symptoms in palliative care: dyspnea and fatigue. These sections are noticeably shorter than the previous section on pain because (1) there is less literature on these topics and (2) many of the principles and practice approaches proposed for pain may be applicable to these symptoms. For example, readers will likely notice a striking number of commonalities between the assessment and treatment of pain and the suggested strategies with which to approach dyspnea and fatigue. These include their multidimensional nature, the importance of understanding the symptom within a cultural context, the availability of standardized instruments, and a dearth of evidence regarding the effectiveness of integrative interventions. Table 25.2 provides information on five of the most distressing symptoms experienced by palliative care patients—agitation, dyspnea, fatigue, nausea, and pain—with possible strategies for social work screening and intervention.

Dyspnea

Dyspnea, or shortness of breath, is a prominent symptom among palliative care patients, particularly those who are nearing death. Despite its prevalence, some evidence suggests that dyspnea may be underdiagnosed and undertreated due, in part, to a patient's diminished ability to communicate in the latter stages of a serious illness and a lack of well-validated instruments with which to measure observable signs of breathlessness (Campbell, Templin, & Walch, 2009). Like pain, dyspnea is a complex, multidimensional symptom that is largely subjective and uniquely experienced. More so than pain, breathing difficulties may be more directly linked to anxiety and existential suffering (Thomas & von Gunten, 2003). It is well known, for example, that a panic attack can trigger a dyspneic episode, leaving a patient frightened and gasping for breath.

A number of assessment instruments are available for the evaluation of dyspnea, but few seem to capture the symptom's multidimensional nature. Two systematic reviews of clinical instruments identified Visual Numeric Scale (VNS) (sometimes referred to as the Visual Analog Scale [VAS]) as the

most clinically relevant screen for palliative care (Bausewein, Farquhar, Booth, Gysels, & Higginson, 2007; Dorman, Byrne, & Edwards, 2007). Other potentially useful tools were identified as the modified Borg Scale (Mador, Rodis, & Magalang, 1995), Japanese Cancer Dyspnea Scale (CDS), and Baseline Dyspnea Index (BDI). During assessment, social workers are encouraged to be especially sensitive to the likelihood that lengthy conversations may exacerbate symptoms in patients experiencing breathlessness. Using close-ended questions that require only brief responses (e.g., yes/no questions), providing nonverbal means of communication such as a notepad and pen, or relying on proxy informants can reduce the potential burden of prolonged patient discussions.

Numerous psychosocial and environmental interventions have been proposed to provide relief to those suffering from dyspnea, but the effectiveness of these interventions is less clear (Buckholz & von Gunten, 2009). In a review of nonpharmacological treatments for the management of breathlessness in patients with lung cancer, Zhao and Yates (2008) identified two promising evidence-supported intervention strategies: one that enhanced patient–provider communication (Moore et al., 2002) and another that used a tailored approach consisting of an (1) individualized assessment; (2) education and family support; (3) an exploration of the meaning of the symptoms and disease as interpreted by the patient/family; (4) a combination of progressive relaxation, cognitive distraction, and breathing-control training; (5) goal setting to support coping strategies; and (6) identification of problems requiring medical or pharmacological interventions (Bredin et al., 1999). The latter of these intervention strategies showed improvements in breathing, functional performance, and depression. For practitioners interested in learning more about how to guide their patients through breathing exercises, Gallo-Silver and Pollack (2000) provide readers with clear, easy-to-implement instructions for teaching diaphragmatic breathing, a behavioral technique that has demonstrated efficacy in a number of studies (including Bredin et al., 1999) and can be taught easily and quickly. The choice of intervention, as with pain and other symptoms, is context driven and based on an individualized assessment and goals of care.

Other psychosocial strategies have been proposed and may also be useful to social workers attempting to relieve feelings of breathlessness. These include creative therapies such art and music, cognitive techniques, relaxation techniques (if patient is capable), massage therapy, and pacing. In many cases, patients may find solace using their own spiritual practices such as meditation, mindfulness activities, or prayer. Simple environmental changes may also help patients breathe easier; for example, a bedside fan directed at the patient's face (Rousseau, 1996) or elevating the head of the bed to a preferred height have been known to provide relief from feeling short of breath (Bruera, 2009). The effectiveness of these approaches in noncancer populations and those palliative care patients with diagnoses such as congestive heart failure or progressive neurologic disease remains unknown.

However, according to Buckholz and von Gunten (2009), "even though the evidence base is weak for many of these therapies, the low risk profile and the potential to avoid additional medications makes them attractive options" (p. 101).

Social workers can rely on their clinical judgment and patient/family preferences to tailor their intervention approaches. For example, a patient who is acutely short of breath may need immediate medical attention. Depending on patient and family preferences, breathlessness may require medication, oxygen, or even intubation. In other less emergent contexts, intervention may begin with an assessment focused on understanding the factors contributing to the environment of distress, only one of which may be the patient's symptom. In the case of dyspnea, portraying a calm demeanor and asking focused questions that can be answered by one word or with the nod of the head demonstrates awareness that the shortness of breath interferes with speaking while at the same time acknowledging the importance of patient input. Assisting a patient with a focused breathing or guided imagery exercise and proposing environmental interventions such as opening a window or asking family to allow physical space around the patient have the potential to lessen feelings of helplessness and anxiety—both of which may exacerbate the symptom experience for patients and the families. This is an example of starting where the patient and family are and then, over time, expanding clinical understanding by exploring fears, thoughts, and emotions that lead to a comprehensive and individualized plan of care. If the symptom is part of a dying process, intervention includes immediate attention to the emotional, spiritual, and informational needs of the family. Where dyspnea is related to fluid overload, medical staff may need to reduce fluid intake while simultaneously treating the symptom pharmacologically.

Fatigue

Fatigue is a persistent lack of energy or feeling of tiredness that is not easily remedied by the typical means of rejuvenation such as rest or nourishment (National Comprehensive Cancer Network [NCCN], 2005). Sometimes described as a "flu-like" feeling, it is a common symptom among patients with cancer, chronic obstructive pulmonary disease (COPD), and congestive heart failure (CHF). It is particularly prevalent in the advanced stages of illness and often lingers well beyond the conclusion of curative treatment (Mota & Pimenta, 2006). Similar to pain and dypnea, fatigue is influenced by, and has an impact upon, multiple dimensions of a person's life. It is thought to be caused by anemia, pain, emotional disturbances, insomnia, nutrition, or poor thyroid gland functioning (NCCN, 2005). The presence of fatigue can have a devastating impact on a patient's social, psychological, and physical functioning. In fact, among cancer patients, fatigue has been reported as the most frequent and distressing of all symptoms (Cella, Davis, Breitbart, Curt, & Fatigue Coalition, 2001).

While there is no gold standard for the assessment of fatigue, when patients are capable, self-report measures are preferred over observational measures (Mota & Pimenta, 2006). The one-item, 0–10 screening question for fatigue is recommended by the NCCN (2005). However, several other validated instruments are available including the Brief Fatigue Inventory (BFI; Mendoza et al., 1999), the Fatigue Symptom Inventory (FSI; Hann et al., 1998), and the Functional Assessment of Chronic Illness Therapy-Fatigue Scale (FACIT-F; Cella, Lai, Chang, Peterman, & Slavin, 2002). When assessing for fatigue, clinicians should be aware that it has been linked to depression and, therefore, may be a co-contributing factor (see Jacobsen, Donovan, & Weitzner, 2003 for information on distinguishing between fatigue and depression). A comprehensive fatigue assessment also includes an evaluation of the onset, known triggers, a functional assessment, responsiveness to past treatments, its impact on relationships, meaning and cultural significance, and a discussion of sleep patterns. Fatigue may also be an indication of disease progression, perhaps signaling the need for a family to re-evaluate the goals of care and day-to-day priorities. As with pain and dyspnea, the symptom of fatigue has meaning in the context of the illness, and interventions should follow from an understanding of the medical and diagnostic realities.

Systematic reviews of psychosocial interventions for fatigue suggest that education, supportive therapy, exercise, and energy conversation can minimize fatigue and its effect on important life activities (Jacobsen, Donovan, Vadaparampil, & Small, 2007; Mitchell & Berger, 2006). Patient and family education includes normalizing fatigue as common medically related occurrence; exploring fears, concerns, and ascribed meaning; informing them of possible causes (e.g., anemia, lack of rest, pain, or nutrition); and developing a patient-centered plan to treat and monitor the fatigue. In the early stages of a cancer diagnosis and for those undergoing curative treatment, aerobic exercise has demonstrated some efficacy in reducing fatigue (Radbruch et al., 2008). However, the evidence is weaker for those with advanced cancer or functional disability. An alternative approach may be to conserve one's energy (i.e., pacing) to ensure that energy is spent on aspects of life that are most meaningful. In a sample of cancer patients beginning treatment, behavioral management strategies such as prioritizing activities (e.g., pacing) and limiting exertion have proven successful for reducing fatigue (Mitchell & Berger, 2006). In some cases, patients may be experiencing *attentional fatigue*, which is a reduced ability to focus or concentrate (NCCN, 2005). To help address this, social workers can guide their patients to pursue attention-restoring activities, such as reading a book or magazine, gardening, swinging on a porch swing, or painting a picture (NCCN, 2005).

Conclusion

Palliative social workers who work in direct contact with seriously ill individuals are likely to encounter a myriad of physical symptoms with varying etiologies, severities, and treatment regimens. Although not addressed in this chapter, social workers can also have a prominent role in helping patients and families cope with other symptoms associated with serious illness such as sleep disturbances, loss of appetite (anorexia), dramatic weight loss (cachexia), constipation, and delirium. While further research is needed to develop and evaluate psychosocial strategies to identify and address the gamut of physical symptoms, a variety of promising and potentially effective interventions do exist for palliative social workers to use with their patients and families. The challenge for social workers is to establish competency and expertise in implementing these techniques.

Within our companion disciplines of nursing and medicine there have been widespread system-level efforts to treat patient pain as the "fifth vital sign." As social workers, we must adopt a similar professional vigilance by (1) making the alleviation of patient suffering an unwavering priority and (2) having the assessment and treatment of physical symptoms become routine practice. As Mendenhall (2003) argued, "Social workers are called, by their professional values: to be proactive in work to increase the priority status of pain management, promote the consideration of patients' holistic needs, and build collaboration into relationship models" (p. 44). In addition, social workers, in their roles as advocates and clinicians, are poised to join with interdisciplinary colleagues to overcome the social, psychological, cultural, political, and economic barriers to pain control (Mendenhall, 2003; Parker-Oliver et al., 2008). This includes macro-level advocacy to ensure that regulations do not hinder, but rather facilitate patient access to palliative care services and necessary pain treatments, including medication.

LEARNING EXERCISES

- *Symbolic significance of pain and conflicting goals.* During an initial evaluation, a hospice patient reports experiencing a high level of pain (a "7" on a 0–10 rating scale). However, he adamantly refuses any pharmacological interventions. The social worker and nurse explore his thoughts and feelings about pain, and he reports, "The pain reminds me that I'm alive." His wife does not like seeing her husband in pain and cries openly, expressing that she hopes hospice can do something to help alleviate his suffering. He is 49 years old, Caucasian, married with no children, and an atheist. He has been diagnosed with end-stage pancreatic cancer and given a prognosis of 3 months by his physician.

Narrative Questions: In this narrative, what are the relevant questions you would ask? What biopsychosocial-spiritual issues need to be considered? How would you differentiate the suffering of the patient from that of his wife? What are the pertinent ethical considerations? How might you intervene?

- *Sammy and Helen: Symptoms and suffering as redemptive constructs.* During a palliative care consultation you encounter a married couple dealing with the wife's new diagnosis of advanced lung cancer. During your interview, you discover that she is experiencing heightened levels of pain and dyspnea. The husband informs you that, according to their spiritual belief system, this illness is punishment for his wife's past transgressions. They are open to palliative interventions, but they ask that their spiritual beliefs be respected.

Narrative Questions: In this narrative, what are the relevant questions you would ask? What might this exchange signify about this couple's relationship? What biopsychosocial-spiritual issues need to be considered? What are the pertinent ethical considerations? How might you intervene? What variables would you consider as you evaluate the potential risk and benefit of intervening with the marital relationship and the spiritual constructs being expressed?

ADDITIONAL RESOURCES

Keefe, F. J., Ahles, T. A., Sutton, L., Dalton, J., Baucom, D., Pope, M.S., ... Scipio, C. (2005). Partner-guided cancer pain management at the end of life: A preliminary study. *Journal of Pain and Symptom Management, 29*(3), 263–272.

Keefe, F. J., Ahles, T. A., Porter, L. S., Sutton, L. M., McBride, C. M., Pope, M. S., ... Baucom, D. H. (2003). The self-efficacy of family caregivers for helping cancer patients manage pain at end of life. *Pain, 103,* 157–162.

Keefe, F. J., Lipkus, I., Lefebvre, J. C., Hurwitz, H., Clipp, E., Smith, J., & Porter, L. (2003). The social context of gastrointestinal cancer pain: A preliminary study examining the relation of patient pain catastrophizing to patient perceptions of social support and caregiver stress and negative responses. *Pain, 103,* 151–156.

PAIN WEB SITES

Alliance of State Pain Initiatives: http://www.aspi.wisc.edu
American Pain Foundation: http://www.painfoundation.org
City of Hope Pain and Palliative Care Resource Center: http://www.cityofhope.org/PRC
EPERC (End of Life/Palliative Education Resource Center) Fast Facts: http://www.eperc.mcw.edu/ff_index.htm
NCCN Clinical Practice Guidelines in Oncology Supportive Care Guidelines (Adult & Pediatric Cancer Pain): http://www.nccn.org/professionals/physician_gls/f_guidelines.asp?button=I+Agree
National Palliative Care Research Center: http://www.npcrc.org/

Pain and the Law: http://www.painandthelaw.org/

Partners Against Pain: http://www.partnersagainstpain.com

Social Work Palliative and End-of-Life Listserv SW-PALL-EOL@ PEACH.EASE.LSOFT.COM

Stop Pain: Department of Pain Medicine and Palliative Care, Beth Israel Medical Center, New York, NY: http://www.stoppain.org/

REFERENCES

Abrahm, J. L. (2005). *A physician's guide to pain and symptom management in cancer patients* (2nd ed.). Baltimore, MD: Johns Hopkins University Press.

Agency for Healthcare Research and Quality (AHRQ). (2008). *Improving the quality of care through pain assessment and management*. Rockville, MD: AHRQ Publication No. 08-0043. Agency for Healthcare Research and Quality (AHRQ) with support from the Robert Wood Johnson Foundation.

Altilio, T. (2004). Pain and symptom management: An essential role for social work. In J. Berzoff & P. R. Silverman (Eds.), *Living with dying: A handbook for end-of-life healthcare professionals* (pp 380–408). New York, NY: Columbia University Press.

Altilio, T. (2006). Pain and symptom management: Clinical, policy and political perspectives. *Journal of Psychosocial Oncology*, 24(1), 65–79.

Altilio, T., & Otis-Green, S. (2005). "Res Ipsa Loquitur" … it speaks for itself … social work-values, pain, and palliative care. *Journal of Social Work in End of Life and Palliative Care*, 1(4), 3–6.

American Pain Society. (2006). *Definitions related to the use of opioids for the treatment of pain*. Retrieved from: http://www.ampainsoc.org/advocacy/opioids2.htm

American Psychosocial Oncology Society. (2006). *Quick reference for oncology clinicians: The psychiatric and psychological dimensions of cancer symptom management*. Charlottesville, VA: IPOS Press.

Anderson, K. O., Green, C. R., & Payne, R. (2009). Racial and ethnic disparities in pain: Causes and consequences of unequal care. *Journal of Pain*, 10(12), 1187–1204.

Bausewein, C., Farquhar, M., Booth, S., Gysels, M., & Higginson, I. J. (2007). Measurement of breathlessness in advanced disease: A systematic review. *Respiratory Medicine*, 101(3), 399–410.

Bern-Klug, M., Gessert, C., & Forbes, S. (2001). The need to revise assumptions about the end of life: Implications for social work practice. *Health and Social Work*, 24(1), 38–48.

Berry, P. E., & Ward, S. E. (1995). Barriers to pain management in hospice: A study of family caregivers. *Hospice Journal*, 10(4),9–33.

Brunnhuber, K., Nash, S. E., Meier, D. E., Weissman, D., & Woodcock, J. (2008). Putting evidence into practice: Palliative care. *BMJ Clinical Evidence*, 1–88.

Bonham, V. L. (2001). Race, ethnicity and pain treatment: Striving to understand the causes and solutions to the disparities in pain treatment. *Journal of Law, Medicine and Ethics*, 29, 52–68.

Bredin, M., Corner, J., Krishnasamy, M., Plant, H., Bailey, C., & A'Hern, R. (1999). Multicentre randomised controlled trial of nursing intervention for breathlessness in patients with lung cancer. *British Medical Journal*, 318, 901–904.

Brummel-Smith, K., London, M. R., Drew, N., Krulewitch, H., Singer, C., & Hanson, L. (2002). Outcomes of pain with frail older adults with dementia. *Journal of the American Geriatrics Society*, 50(11), 1847–1851.

Buckholz, G. T., & von Gunten, C. F. (2009). Nonpharmacological management of dyspnea. *Current Opinions in Supportive Palliative Care*, 3, 98–102.

Campbell, M. L., Templin, T., & Walch, J. (2009). Patients who are near death are frequently unable to self-report dyspnea. *Journal of Palliative Medicine*, 12(10), 881–884.

Cassell, E. J. (1992). The nature of suffering and the goals of medicine. *New England Journal of Medicine*, 306, 639–645.

Cella, D., Davis., K., Breitbart, W., Curt, G., & The Fatigue Coalition. (2001). Cancer-related fatigue: Prevalence of proposed diagnostic criteria in a United States sample of cancer survivors. *Journal of Clinical Oncology*, 19(14), 3385–3391.

Cella, D., Lai, J., Chang, C., Peterman, A., & Slavin, M. (2002). Fatigue in cancer patients compared with fatigue in the general United States population. *Cancer*, 94, 528–538.

Chaichan, W. (2008). Evaluation of the use of the positive and negative syndrome scale-excited component as a criterion for administration of p.r.n. medication. *Journal of Psychiatric Practice*,14(2), 105–113.

Chang, V. T., Hwang, S. S., Feuerman, M., Kasimis, B. S., & Thaler, H. T. (2000). The memorial symptom assessment scale short form (MSAS-SF). *Cancer*, 89(5), 1162–1171.

Cintron, A., & Morrison, R. S. (2006). Pain and ethnicity in the United States: A systematic review. *Journal of Palliative Medicine*, 9(6), 1454–1473.

Cleeland, C. S. (1989). Measurement of pain by subjective report. In C. R. Chapman & J. D. Loeser (Eds.), *Advances in pain research and therapy: Issues in pain measurement* (Vol. 12, pp. 391–403). New York, NY: Raven Press.

Cohen-Mansfield, J. (1991). Instruction Manual for the Cohen-Mansfield Agitation Inventory (CMAI). Rockville, MD: The Research Institute of the Hebrew Home of Greater Washington.

Corrigan, J. D. (1989). Development of a scale for assessment of agitation following traumatic brain injury. *Journal of Clinical and Experimental Neuropsychology*, 11(2), 261–277.

Costello, P., Wiseman, J., Douglas, I., Batten, B., & Bennett, M. (2001). Assessing hospice inpatients with pain using numerical rating scales. *Palliative Medicine*,Csikai, E. L., & Raymer, M. (2005). Social workers' educational needs in end-of-life care. *Social Work in Health Care*, 41(1), 53–72.

Dorman, S., Byrne, A., & Edwards, A. (2007). Which measurement scales should we use to measure breathlessness in palliative care? A systematic review. *Palliative Medicine*, 21(3), 177–191.

Fisher, B. J., Haythornwaite, J. A., Heinberg, L. J., Clark, M., & Reed, J. (2001). Suicidal intent in patients with chronic pain. *Pain*, 89, 199–206.

Fromme, E. K., Tilden, V. P., Drach, L. L., & Tolle, S. W. (2004). Increased family reports of pain or distress in dying Oregonians: 1996 to 2002. *Journal of Palliative Medicine*, 7(3), 431–442.

Gallo-Silver, L., & Pollack, B. (2000). Behavioral interventions for lung cancer-related breathlessness. *Cancer Practice*, 8, 268–273.

Glajchen, M., Blum, D., & Calder, K. (1995). Cancer pain management and the role of social work: Barriers and interventions. *Health and Social Work*, 20, 200–206.

Grunberg, S. M., Boutin, N., Ireland, A., Miner, S., Silvera, J., & Ashikaga, T. (2005). Impact of nausea/vomiting on quality of life as a visual analogue scale-derived utility score. *Supportive Cancer Care, 4*(6), 435–439.

Hann, D. M., Jacobsen, P. B., Azzarello, L. M., Martin, S. C., Curran, S. L., Fields, K. K., … Lyman, G.(1998). Measurement of fatigue in cancer patients: Development and validation of the Fatigue Symptom Inventory. *Quality of Life Research, 7*, 301–310.

Herr, K., Bursch, H., & Black, B. (2008). *State of the art review of tools for assessment of pain in nonverbal older adults: Project overview update.* Retrieved from the Pain Resource Center Web site: http://prc.coh.org/PainNOA/OV.pdf

Hesketh, P. J. (2005). *Management of nausea and vomiting in cancer and cancer treatment.* Boston, MA: Jones & Bartlett Publishers.

International Association for the Study of Pain (IASP). (2007). *IASP pain terminology.* Retrieved from: http://www.iasp-pain.org/AM/Template.cfm?Section=Pain_Definitions&Template=/CM/HTMLDisplay.cfm&ContentID=1728#Pain

International Association for the Study of Pain. (2008-2009). *Psychosocial interventions for cancer pain.* Retrieved from: http://www.iasp-pain.org/AM/Template.cfm?Section=Home&Template=/CM/ContentDisplay.cfm&ContentID=7193

International Association for the Study of Pain (IASP). (2010). *IASP pain terminology.* Retrieved from http://www.iasp-pain.org/AM/Template.cfm?Section=Pain_Definitions&Template=/CM/HTMLDisplay.cfm&ContentID=1728#Pain

Jack, B., Hillier, V., Williams, A., & Oldham, J. (2003). Hospital based palliative care teams improve the symptoms of cancer patients. *Palliative Medicine, 17*(6), 498–502.

Jacobsen, P. B., Donovan, K. A., Vadaparampil, S. T., & Small, B. J. (2007). Systematic review and meta-analysis of psychological and activity-based interventions for cancer-related fatigue. *Health Psychology, 26*(6), 660–667.

Jacobsen, P. B., Donovan, K. A., & Weitzner, M. A. (2003). Distinguishing fatigue and depression in patients with cancer. *Seminars in Clinical Neuropsychiatry, 8*, 229–240.

Jennings, B., Ryndes, T., D'Onofrio, C., & Baily, M. A. (2003). Access to hospice care: Expanding boundaries, overcoming barriers (Special Supplement). *Hastings Center Report, 33*(2), S3–S59.

Johnson, D. C., Kassner, C. T., Houser, J., & Kutner, J. S. (2005). Barriers to effective symptom management in hospice. *Journal of Pain and Symptom Management, 29*(1), 69–79.

Johnson, S.H. (2001). Relieving unnecessary, treatable pain for the sake of human dignity. *Journalof Law, Medicine & Ethics, 29*, 11–12.

Kong, E. H., Evans, L. K., & Guevara, J. P. (2009). Nonpharmacological intervention for agitation in dementia: A systematic review and meta-analysis. *Aging and Mental Health, 13*(4), 512–520.

Letizia, M., Creech, S., Norton, E., Shanahan, M., & Hedges, L. (2004). Barriers to caregiver administration of pain medication in hospice care. *Journal of Pain and Symptom Management, 27*(2), 114–124.

Lickiss, J. N., Turner, K. S., & Pollack, M. L. (2004). The interdisciplinary team. In D. Doyle, G. Hanks, N. Cherny, & K. Calman (Eds.), *Oxford textbook of palliative medicine* (pp. 42–46). Oxford, England: Oxford University Press.

Lloyd-Williams, M. (Ed.). (2003). *Psychosocial issues in palliative care.* Oxford, England: Oxford University Press.

Lo, B., (2000). *Resolving ethical dilemma: A guide for clinician.* Philadelphia, PA: Lippincott Williams & Wilkins.

MacDonald, J. (2000). A deconstructive turn in chronic pain treatment: A redefined role for social work. *Health and Social Work, 25*(1), 51–58.

Mador, J. M., Rodis, A., & Magalang, U. J. (1995). Reproducibility of Borg scale measurements of dyspnea during exercise in patients with COPD. *Chest, 107*, 1590–1597.

McCaffery, M., & Pasero, C. (1999). *Pain: A clinical manual.* New York, NY: Mosby.

McMillan, S. (1996). Pain and pain relief experienced by hospice patient with cancer. *Cancer Nursing, 19*(4), 298–307.

Mendenhall, M. (2003). Psychosocial aspects of pain management: A conceptual framework for social workers on pain management teams. *Social Work and Health Care, 36*(4), 35–51.

Mendoza, T. R., Mayne, T., Rublee, D., & Cleeland, C. S. (2006). Reliability and validity of a modified Brief Pain Inventory short form in patients with osteoarthritis. *European Journal of Pain, 10*(4), 353–361.

Mendoza, T. R., Wang, X. S., Cleeland, C. S., Morissey, M., Johnson, B. A., Wendt, J. K., & Huber, S. L. (1999). The rapid assessment of fatigue in cancer patients: Use of the Brief Fatigue Inventory. *Cancer, 85*, 1186–1196.

Mitchell, S. A., & Berger, A. M. (2006). Cancer-related fatigue: The evidence base for assessment and management. *The Cancer Journal, 5*, 374–387.

Moore, S., Corner, J., Haviland, J., Wells, M., Salmon, E., Normand, C., … Smith, I.(2002). Nurse led follow up and conventional medical follow up in management of patients with lung cancer: Randomised trial. *British Medical Journal, 325*, 1–7.

Mota, D. D., & Pimenta, C. A. (2006). Self-report instruments for fatigue assessment: A systematic review. *Research and Theory for Nursing Practice, 20*(1), 49–78.

Mulder, J. (2006). Comprehensive pain assessment. In K. Doka (Ed.), *Pain management at the end of life bridging the gap between knowledge and practice* (pp. 79–87). Washington, DC: Hospice Foundation of America.

National Association of Social Workers (NASW). (1999). *Code of ethics.* Retrieved from http://www.socialworkers.org/pubs/code/default.asp

National Association of Social Workers (NASW). (2003a). *NASW standards for social work practice in palliative and end of life care.* Retrieved from http://www.socialworkers.org/practice/bereavement/standards/default.asp

National Association of Social Workers (NASW). (2003b). *End of life care practice update: Social workers in hospice and palliative care settings.* Retrieved from http://www.socialworkers.org/practice/bereavement/updates/EndOfLifeCare-PU0204.pdf

National Cancer Institute. (2010). *Pain: Physical and psychosocial interventions.* Retrieved from http://www.cancer.gov/cancertopics/pdq/supportivecare/pain/HealthProfessional/page5

National Comprehensive Cancer Network (NCCN). (2005). *Cancer-related fatigue and anemia: Treatment guidelines for patients. Version III.* Atlanta, GA: American Cancer Society.

National Consensus Project (NCP). (2004). *National consensus project for quality in palliative care.* Retrieved from http://www.nationalconsensusproject.org

National Palliative Care Research Center (NPCRC). (2010). *Measurement and evaluation tools*. Retrieved from http://www.npcrc.org/resources/resources_list.htm?cat_id=1246

National Quality Forum (NQF). (2008). *NQF framework*. Retrieved from http://www.nationalconsensusproject.org/NQF_Framework.asp

Nekolaichuk, C., Watanabe, S., & Beaumont, C. (2008). The Edmonton Symptom Assessment System: A 15-year retrospective review of validation studies (1991–2006). *Palliative Medicine, 22*(2), 111–122.

Otis-Green, S. (2005). Psychosocial pain assessment form. In K. K., Kuebler, M. P. Davis, & C. D. Moore (Eds.), *Palliative practices: An interdisciplinary approach* (pp. 462–467). St. Louis, MO: Elsevier Mosby.

Otis-Green, S. (2006). Psychosocial pain assessment form. In K. H. Dow (Ed.), *Nursing care of women with cancer* (pp. 556–561). St. Louis, MO: Elsevier Mosby.

Palos, G. R., Mendoza, T. R., Cantor, S. B., Aday, L. A., & Cleeland, C. S. (2004). Perceptions of the analgesic use and side effects: What the public values in pain management. *Journal of Pain and Symptom Management, 28*(5), 460–473.

Parker-Oliver, D., Wittenberg-Lyles, E., Demiris, G., Washington, K., Porock, D., & Day, M. (2008). Barriers to pain management: Caregiver perceptions and pain talk by hospice interdisciplinary teams. *Journal of Pain and Symptom Management, 36*(4), 374–382.

Parker-Oliver, D., Wittenberg-Lyles, E., Washington, K., & Sehrawat, S. (2009). Social work role in hospice pain management: A national survey. *Journal of Social Work in End of Life and Palliative Care, 5*(1-2), 51–74.

Portenoy, R. K., Thaler, H. T., Kornblith, A.B., Lepore, J. M., Friedlander-Klar, H., Kiyasu, E., … & Scher, H. (1994). The Memorial Symptom Assessment Scale: An instrument for the evaluation of symptom prevalence, characteristics and distress. *European Journal of Cancer, 30*(9), 1326–1336.

Portenoy, R. K., Ugarte, C., Fuller, I., & Haas, G. (2004). Population-based survey of pain in the United States: Differences among white, African-American, and Hispanic subjects. *Journal of Pain, 5*(6), 317–328.

Project on Death in America. (2004). *Transforming the culture of dying: The Project on Death in America 1994-2003*. Retrieved from http://www.soros.org/resources/articles_publications/publications/transforming_20040922

Radbruch, L., Strasser, F., Elsner, F., Gonçalves, J. F., Løge, J., Kaasa, S., … Stone, P. (2008). Fatigue in palliative care patients: An EAPC approach. *Palliative Medicine, 22*(1), 13–32.

Raybould, C., & Adler, G. (2006). Applying NASW standards to end-of-life care for a culturally diverse, aging population. *Journal of Social Work Values and Ethics, 3*(2). Retrieved from http://www.socialworker.com/jswve/content/view/38/46/

Randall-David, E., Wright, J., Porterfield, D. S., & Lesser, G. (2003). Barriers to cancer pain management: Home-health and hospice nurses and patients. *Supportive Care Cancer, 11*(10), 660–665.

Rousseau, P. C. (1996). Nonpain symptom management in terminal care. *Clinical Geriatrics Medicine, 12*, 313–327.

Rustoen, T., Fossa, S. D., Skarstein, J., & Moum, T. (2003). The impact of demographic and disease-specific variables on pain in cancer patients. *Journal of Pain Symptom Management, 26*, 696–704.

Saunders, C. (2001). Social work and palliative care: The early history. *British Journal of Social Work, 31*, 791–799.

Savage, S. R., Covington, E. C., Heit, H. A., Hunt, J., Joranson, D., & Schnoll, S. H. (2002). *Consensus document: Definitions related to the use of opioids for the treatment of pain. The American Academy of Pain Medicine, The American Pain Society, and the American Society of Addiction Medicine, 2002*. Retrieved from http://www.ampainsoc.org/advocacy/opioids2.htm

Saxby, C., Ackroyd, R., Callin, S., Mayland, C., & Kite, S. (2007). How should we measure emesis in palliative care? *Palliative Medicine, 21*(5), 369–383.

Smedley, B. D., Stith, A. Y., & Nelson, A. R. (Eds.). (2003). *Unequal treatment confronting racial and ethnic disparities in health care*. Washington, DC: National Academies Press.

Speck, P. W. (2006). *Teamwork in palliative care: Fulfilling or frustrating?* Oxford, England: Oxford University Press.

Steinhauser, K. E., Christakis, N. A., Clipp, E. C., McNeilly, M., McIntyre, L., & Tulsky, J.A. (2000). Factors considered important at end of life by patients, family physicians, and other care providers. *Journal of the American Medical Association, 284*, 2476–2482.

Strasser, F., Sweeney, C., Willey, J., Benisch-Tolley, S., Palmer, J., & Bruera E. (2004). Impact of a half-day multidisciplinary symptom control and palliative care outpatient clinic in a comprehensive cancer center on recommendations, symptom intensity, and patient satisfaction: A retrospective descriptive study, *Journal of Pain and Symptom Management, 27*(6), 481–491.

SUPPORT Principal Investigators. (1995). A controlled trial to improve outcomes for seriously ill hospitalized patients: Study to Understand Prognoses and Preferences for Outcomes and Risks of Treatments (SUPPORT). *Journal of the American Medical Association, 275*(16), 1632.

Teno, J. M., Clarridge, B. R., Casey, V., Welch, M. A., Wetle, T., Shield, R., & Mor, V. (2004). Family perspectives on end-of-life care at the last place of care. *Journal of the American Medical Association, 291*(1), 88–93.

Thomas, J. R., & von Gunten, C. F. (2003). Management of dyspnea. *Journal of Supportive Oncology, 1*, 23–34.

Turk, D. C., Monarch, E. S. & Williams, A. D. (2002). Cancer patients in pain: Considerations for assessing the whole person. *Hematology Oncology Clinics of North America, 16*, 511–525.

Twycross, R. G., & Wilcock, A. (2001). *Symptom management in advanced cancer* (3rd ed.). Abingdon, UK: Radcliffe Publishing.

Ward, S. E., Berry, P. E., & Misiewicz, H. (1996). Concerns about analgesics among patients and family caregivers in a hospice setting. *Research in Nursing and Health, 19*(3), 205–211.

Winnicott, D. W. (1971). *Objects and transitional phenomena in playing and reality*. Harmondsworth, UK: Penguin.

Wong, D., & Baker, C. (1988). Pain in children: Comparison of assessment scales. *Pediatric Nursing, 14*(1), 9–17.

Zhao, I., & Yates, P. (2008). Non-pharmacological interventions for breathlessness management in patients with lung cancer: A systematic review. *Palliative Medicine, 22*, 693–701.

26 *Nancy Sherman*

The Whys and Wherefores of Support Groups: Helping People Cope

Please keep the groups going. They are helpful and give people strength to carry on with the daily duties of life.

—45-year-old woman participating in group for young widows

Key Concepts

◆ *Support group participation can increase one's sense of self-worth, purpose, and control.*
◆ *For many, social support and interconnectedness are helpful in managing life-threatening illness, caregiving responsibilities, and/or loss.*
◆ *Participation in groups allows not only for the participant to receive and benefit from support and education but also to gain something from providing this to others.*
◆ *Group leaders determine group composition and facilitate group process to maximize benefits to participants.*

Introduction

Intense and difficult situations such as illness and loss can bring out profound emotions, which for many lead to a strong desire to talk with others. Doing so provides a way for people to develop a better understanding of their situation, to counter what is often isolation or even shame over their illness and/or their reactions, to explore their thoughts and feelings, and to perhaps learn new ways of approaching problems. A social phenomenon designed to encourage these goals is the concept of support groups. This chapter will address the value of this method of coping and understanding, as well as provide suggestions for structuring, leading, promoting, and facilitating.

Support Groups: A Rationale

"A support group is comprised of a group of people who gather voluntarily on a regular basis to meet certain needs they share in common" (Miller, 1998, p. 8). While it can most definitely be therapeutic, it is distinct from therapy groups in that it does not focus on the psychological growth of the individual members, as most therapy groups would. Most support groups could be characterized as psychoeducational, defined as having the following: *(1)* a strong and formal educational component; *(2)* a trained group leader; *(3)* a unifying theme and purpose; and *(4)* structure and direction. Their main purpose is to provide information and guidance about the disease, condition, or situation; to encourage and empower those attending to gain some control over and improve the quality of their lives; to provide an emotional support system that decreases alienation and isolation, moderates despair, and increases hopefulness and personal responsibility; helps members derive a greater sense of joy and satisfaction from life as it is with all its barriers, constraints, setbacks, and disappointments; and provides opportunities to practice and learn new ways of behaving and relating (Brown, 2003).

Because we live in a society that often frowns upon those who express "too much" emotion and because many people live far from family, groups can offer people a supportive environment in which to work through some of their feelings and concerns. For many there are few places in their lives where they can get reliable support and be themselves. By introducing people to others who are going through a similar situation, support groups offer a way in which to normalize their illness experience. Groups offer participants opportunities to learn new roles, problem-solving techniques, and/or coping skills in a safe setting with the help of a facilitator and by the sharing of experiences with other members. Groups may have a specific focus, such as loss or caregiving, while others are disease/diagnosis specific such as Multiple Sclerosis or Amyotrophic Lateral Sclerosis (MS or ALS) or the American Cancer Society's "I Can Cope" psychoeducational group (http://www.Cancer.org). Experience has shown that people who are struggling emotionally benefit from the opportunity to reach out and help others (Coward, 1990; Krause, Herzog, & Baker, 1992; Schwartz & Sendor, 1999), and participation in a group not only offers members the chance to be helped but also the chance to help others. Since the 1980s, support groups have been shown to be a potent and cost-effective form of psychosocial intervention for patients with cancer, showing positive effects on psychosocial adjustment (Spiegel, Bloom, & Yalom, 1981). Psychological assessments of participants in a cancer support group showed significant improvement in cancer patients' self-concept, hospital adjustment, and knowledge of disease in comparison to matched control subjects (Cain, Kohorn, Quinlan, Latimer, & Schwartz, 1986). Other studies showed that, while not prolonging survival rates, women with metastatic breast cancer who participated in supportive-expressive groups had improved mood and decreased perception of pain (Goodwin et al., 2001), while a subsequent study with the same population assisted group members to confront and cope with their disease-related stress and helped reduce distress (Classen et al., 2001). A study of breast cancer patients who participated in a 26-session supportive intervention demonstrated that they showed a reduced risk of breast cancer recurrence and death. The authors suggest that "if efficacious psychologic interventions to reduce stress are delivered early, they will improve mental health, health and treatment-relevant behaviors, and potentially, biologic outcomes" (Anderson et al., 2008, p. 3458). One study of cancer patients found that two-thirds of those participating expressed a need to talk with others, as well as to a close friend or family (Kuczynski, 2008). Davison, Pennebaker, and Dickerson (2000) conclude, through their investigation of groups and social phenomenon, that "support groups are particularly valued by individuals whose lives and social identities have been put at risk" (p. 216). While the benefit of groups continues to be investigated, one study (comparing social support groups to experiential-existential groups) suggests that, while unable to find a reduction in psychosocial distress in women with a primary breast cancer who attended either group, they still

---

Box 26.1
Patient/Family Narrative: Lisa

Lisa is a 43-year-old woman whose husband died of cancer just months after his diagnosis, leaving her with five children between the ages of 7 and 23. She called a grief center for help because she felt "hopeless, in despair, no life left in me." She expressed the feeling that she could not mother her children, that she did not want to go on, and that her heart was broken. She described her experience with the group as though someone took her by the hand and taught her to breathe again. She met "the most amazing women" in her grief group, who cried with her, laughed with her, and were not afraid to tell her what she needed to hear. "The love and support in that room was unbelievable and I looked forward to each and every week." At the end of this group experience she expressed the feeling that the members and experience had been a lifesaver.

---

recommend offering this type of support because it was clear that the women who were studied thought the intervention was helpful (Vos, Visser, Garssen, Duivenvoorden, & de Haes, 2007, p. 57).

Support groups are a cost-effective way of providing services to numbers of people and expanding the reach of clinical care when resources are limited. They may also be the preferred therapeutic method depending on the clinical goal and needs of patients and families. They have the potential to provide a safe place in which to express emotion and oftentimes to "try out" new ideas or new ways of behaving. Groups can create an environment in which new friendships develop and where people have a chance to laugh, learning that all struggle and challenge need not be sad and painful (see Box 26.1).

Assessing Need and Structuring Programs

Conducting a needs assessment allows you to determine services that are available within your agency and community, to assess the effectiveness of these services, and to identify unmet needs. This assessment will help guide the design of programs that are relevant and meaningful and thus more likely to be successful. There are a variety of ways in which groups are organized to meet the assessed needs of patients and families. Each has pros and cons and much depends on your resources, the mission of your organization and the resources of your community.

An *open group* generally serves greater numbers and a more diverse population with whom members can relate and from whom they may learn. The major feature of an open or unstructured group is that it has no predetermined end. While it meets at a set place and time, there is no regular attendance commitment. Participants may decide to attend steadily over a period of time, attend sporadically, or participate in one meeting and never return (Hughes, 1995). This structure suggests that people will be at various stages in their coping and adaptation and perhaps be able to use their experience in a targeted way to help others who are at a different stage of the process. For participants, an open group provides the freedom to choose when they attend. For some people who are struggling with an illness or significant responsibilities, a regular commitment from one week to the other can be difficult. Open groups provide less opportunity for bonding and continuity and may present more challenges for the facilitator because each group meeting may include new participants coming with different needs and at different places in their process of adaptation.

Closed or structured groups are closed ended and designed to cover certain topics or achieve certain goals for a designated population over an established period of time (Hughes, 1995). This modality allows for more bonding among members, which means they may trust and share more, and there is a greater likelihood of developing friendships that last outside the group. A closed group presumes clinical decision making about structure and membership. In addition, facilitators often have to make decisions about when and whether new members join, evaluating both the needs of the group as a whole and the needs of individual members.

Some programs offer monthly sessions, a type of one-time group meeting where people receive support within a targeted experience, which may focus on a range of experiences including sharing their stories or learning new skills such as relaxation techniques. This kind of program provides an interim supportive experience perhaps until the next series of group sessions begins. Additionally, this structure may be a helpful introduction to the experience of group for people who are uncertain about participation and may benefit those who chose a brief, one-time session to ask a few questions or clarify a few issues. Groups may be organized around certain diagnoses, age groups, gender, loss experiences, or roles such as caregivers. For some members, joining a group with a beginning and predetermined end provides a structure and a predictable termination process that is more comforting and/or fits the structure of their lives and responsibilities. However, others find that even the planned and expected ending of the group feels "too soon" and they are left with a lingering need for more connection. Closed groups tend to have more structure to each session, but whether open or closed, most groups have some planned structure that guides how a group starts, progresses, and ends and is guided by the leadership style and clinical skills of the facilitator.

Building Successful Programs

It is suggested that location is very important to a groups' success. The location should be barrier free, easy to find, with adequate parking, good lighting, and good signage to guide members to the meeting room. Seating that is movable allows

people to rearrange the room in response to members' needs, program focus, and clinical goals. Although it may seem obvious, seating should also be comfortable, not so low or soft that some people may have a struggle getting into or out, or so hard to be uncomfortable. It is crucial to ensure that the room is without distractions, private, and of a comfortable temperature that can be adjusted according to the needs of members. The space that is created to welcome group members is symbolic and demonstrates how the organizers value and respect the program they are offering and the group members who will attend. Details are noticed by people who are coming to be "taken care of," so a clean room with needed supplies and visual appeal becomes very important.

Group size varies, but it is commonly felt that a group is best with a minimum of 4 people and a maximum of 12 (Hermann, 2005; Wolfelt, 2004). When considering initial size, it is often beneficial to begin with a larger number of members because often participants will drop out during the beginning stages of a closed group. Some facilitators might run groups with as few as 3–4 people but only after preparing members and reinforcing their commitment to attendance, because one absent member can have a major impact on group process when there are so few members.

Timing may impact the success of a group. One aspect of needs assessment is to ask potential participants about the best time to organize programs. The key in planning is to have flexible response to the needs of those who are being served. In addition to timing, another program decision is whether to charge fees. Depending on the nature of the group, some clinicians will bill insurances for therapeutic group services. Many not-for-profit programs, while not charging a fee, will encourage member donations, which might include financial support or help with marketing by writing letters to the editor or speaking to community organizations about the value of the services to their lives. Some programs charge a fee for all groups, while some consider fees only for "special" programs and others pursue community sponsors and grant support to cover costs. Many agencies and hospitals provide free support programs that are open to the community as part of community service responsibilities.

Ussher, Kirsten, Butow, and Sandoval (2008) suggest, based on their research, that there is a need to educate people about the purpose and functioning of groups to reduce the stigma, because for some, groups are thought to be negative or fearful experiences. These authors also reinforce the importance of addressing some of the barriers to attending groups posed by participants, such as transportation, provision of respite care, varying times of day to suit people who work, and so forth.

Marketing Group Programs

There are many opportunities to let patients, families, the public, and professional communities know about the group programs that are offered through your organization, your institution, or your professional practices. The words that are chosen to publicize groups are important because they establish the first contact with potential members; the language and message of any marketing tools must be chosen with care.

The following activities and resources offer options for marketing group programs:

- Media, such as newspapers, radio, television, and the Internet can offer opportunities for extensive and free marketing. Although posting public service announcements (PSAs) or calendar listings is a good idea, more attention is created when efforts are made to garner a "story" of newsworthy items such as announcement of new staff, programs, grants received, and staff honored. Additionally, stories related to particular illness or clinical situation, such as caregiving, integrative therapies for pain, and symptom management, or a moving narrative about patients or families sometimes hold special interest for the media. Personalizing these stories with interviews with patients and families can be very helpful. This requires clinical staff to carefully screen and prepare those who are willing to speak with the media so the experience does not inadvertently cause distress and patients and families are not exposed in a manner that diminishes or surprises them.

- Newsletters published by organizations, community groups, and church groups often accept announcements of programs or articles. These can be more meaningful to readers if they include narratives and testimonials from persons who have benefited from your group interventions.

- Brochures and flyers created to promote specific events and programs can be mailed or posted in churches/synagogues, senior centers, hospitals, nursing homes, libraries, work places, and physician offices.

- When targeting a specific population such as gay and lesbian bereaved persons, various cultural groups, or when promoting a specific workshop, placing paid, donated, or sponsored ads in population specific newspapers can be helpful.

- Offering a speakers' bureau provides education and information and can also be used as a forum for promoting other services.

- Organizational and institutional Web sites and e-mail communication groups provide extension opportunities for marketing programs at no expense.

- When reaching out to persons who may be ambivalent about attending groups, confidentiality must be respected. Consequently, the referring source would need to contact the prospective member for written permission before sharing any clinical or identifying information.

Group Facilitation

While there are differing opinions on whether the facilitator should be a trained "professional," peer counselor, or volunteer, there are certain qualities needed by any facilitator (Helgeson, Cohen, Schulz & Yasko, 1999; Solomon, 2004). A peer support group, usually comprised of people with a similar diagnosis, loss, or situation such as caregivers, is defined by Mead, Hilton, and Curtis (2001) as "a system of giving and receiving help founded on key principles of respect, shared responsibility, and mutual agreement of what is helpful" (p. 135). They are thought to benefit those who lack support of a naturally occurring network, but research has been inconclusive in demonstrating positive effects for peer support (Helgeson, Cohen, Schulz, & Yasko, 2000). Toseland (1990) found that, after 1 year, peer-led and professionally led groups were more effective than no intervention for helping caregivers of frail elders reduce stress and increase competence, but they found no differences between the two types of groups. It has been argued that peer-led groups may be especially helpful and appropriate when attempting to respond to cultural variations and needs. Monahan, Green, and Coleman (1992), for example, found that groups conducted in Spanish were attended more regularly than groups for Latinos which were conducted in English. This suggests that, if a group is designed to serve a particular cultural population, peers representing that culture may be perceived as more understanding or helpful. A program created at the City of Hope National Medical Center in California, the Transitions Program, was designed to address a number of elements of end-of-life care within their large medical complex of services. The recognition that roughly a third of those served are Latino led easily to the suggestion that providing services solely in English would be neither respectful nor helpful to a significant number of their patient population. They obtained grant funding to develop a Spanish-speaking bereavement support group in collaboration with a local hospice (Otis-Green, 2006). This demonstrates the opportunity to be creative in networking, partnering, and/or developing resources in order to be responsive to the needs of a particular community or population.

Box 26.2
Patient/Family Narrative: Mary

Mary, a 45-year-old hearing impaired women, lost her mother after a long illness. She wished to join a bereavement support group for adults who have lost a parent, but she is unable to read lips well enough to understand what is being said in a group, nor is she able to speak clearly enough for participants to understand her. To be welcoming and beneficial to Mary, the organization providing the group worked with her to locate an American Sign Language interpreter and assist in paying for the services.

The decision about whether you use professional staff or volunteers, or some combination of this, is up to each individual agency and based in clinical judgment about the intended purpose and expected outcome of the group. Regardless of this decision, the following are important characteristics of a group facilitator:

- Knowledge of the topic (specific disease or symptom, caregiving, grief and loss)
- Understanding of group dynamics and how to respond to and manage group process
- An attitude that is accepting and nonjudgmental
- Skill at listening as well as communicating and teaching
- Ability to demonstrate compassion, empathy, respect, and authenticity
- Comfort with silence as well as conflict
- Ability to set boundaries for the members of the group but also for self
- Ability to be flexible and to adjust plans and process as needed
- Awareness of community resources
- Openness to learning and supervision and an awareness of when to seek help (Hughes, 1995).

Some Thoughts on Group Process

Most sessions begin with a welcome and any necessary "housekeeping comments." Some have an opening ritual followed by an invitation for members to introduce themselves and share their expectation for group participation. In follow-up meetings, participants may be asked to share events, thoughts, or feelings of related significance since the last session, soliciting questions they might have from the previous meeting. Facilitators of an open group often require a different structure because there is no stable membership and each meeting can be thought of as an entity in itself rather than as part of a series of ongoing sessions. Depending on the purpose of the group, each session will require introductions and always time for the facilitator to summarize and close each meeting.

It is generally helpful and necessary during initial sessions to review some basic "rules" or guidelines related to group process. Members often feel safer when they understand the structure, what is expected, and how they can count on the facilitator. Written guidelines can be reviewed and taken home as a reminder of their participation.

The following are some ideas that may be included in guidelines:

Confidentiality: Whatever is shared within the group remains confidential. Share with others outside the group only what you have learned about yourself.

Respect: It is important to respect your own feelings and process as well as that of the other members. Every situation is different; therefore, people will respond differently. This is ok, and it is also why coping with illness and loss can sometimes feel like a lonely process. There is no one or simple path to follow. Everyone moves through this process in his or her own way. While we can compare feelings, thoughts, and experiences, we work not to judge.

Beepers and cell phones: Respect the time you and others are giving to the work within the group by turning off beepers and cell phones or, if necessary, setting them on vibrate.

Advice: Sharing personal feelings and current concerns is not the same as fixing problems. You are welcome to ask questions and share what has been helpful to you, but we cannot know what is right for anyone but ourselves, so offering suggestions or support instead of "should do" or "must do" is most helpful.

Freedom to speak: You may choose to share or remain silent. No one will be put on the spot or forced to talk. Everyone who feels comfortable sharing will be given that chance. Make every effort not to interrupt when someone is speaking. At times, the facilitator may intervene to insure that everyone has the opportunity to share and be heard.

Feelings: Feelings are neither right nor wrong: They just are.

When you miss a session: We will be concerned if you miss a session and do not let us know. Please call if you will be missing a session or decide not to continue. The number to call is......

Group facilitators sometimes choose to begin a group with an exercise that helps to focus discussion and contain anxiety. For example, asking participants to work together to build a list on a flip chart of the most and least helpful things people have said or done for them can generate a range of comments, some of which are shared and validated. Other comments, brought forth within the group, may take on new or different meaning when the intention of these communications is explored. Strategizing together to consider a reframed meaning and possible responses can produce practical ideas, bring about much laughter, and empower those who may have felt helpless. When clinically indicated, these responses can sometimes be practiced within the groups, allowing members to experiment with new modes and manner of behavior and communication.

Following are some questions that can generate good dialogue:

- How are friends and family responding to your situation?
- Where are you finding the support you need?
- Can you share some of your fears?
- What do you wish you had done or could do differently?
- Are there times when it doesn't seem real? What is that like and how do you deal with it?

- What coping tip works best for you?
- What have you learned that has helped your family or friends understand how you are feeling?
- What is the biggest challenge your illness has presented for you? And how have you managed thus far?
- What brings meaning to your life now and in the past?

While many groups just seem to have a "perfect" flow, with people respectfully and meaningfully bonding and connecting, there are times when, as a facilitator, we are faced with some challenges. Typically these occur when people with fixed agendas and complex personalities participate in a group. These people may need more help than a group can offer, may have needs which are not appropriate or possible for a group, or just may not have the ability or social skills to participate in a way that is helpful to group process. Because there are unique complexities to the challenges these situations can create, facilitators use clinical judgment about how to intervene both to protect the group process as well as the dignity and integrity of the group member whose participation may be troublesome.

Group Activities

For a group to be most successful, planning is essential, bearing in mind that there must be room for flexibility to accommodate the evolving needs of the members during the meeting. The therapeutic purpose of the group and interests of participants will guide the nature of the activities that are used to enhance the process. Some groups provide refreshments and some do not. Others provide refreshments at the last meeting as a shared ritual. Some create, over time and with consent, a "buddy" system, where members call during the week between meetings to support each other and encourage relationship building.

It is very important to have necessary supplies to support the activities of the group because this preparation is a symbol of the facilitator's commitment to the members. Supplies might include pen and paper, name tags, tissues, and needed equipment for videos or music.

Many groups begin each session with a ritual chosen based on the clinical goal. For example, caregivers might be helped by a ritual such as a poem or a "centering" experience such as a focused breathing exercise to "shut out" or leave behind the stresses and responsibilities of their daily lives for a bit and focus on the time they will spend together. Some may find this kind of ritual uncomfortable and the clinical task is to select a ritual that is appropriate to everyone's comfort level.

Group activities are selected to meet clinical goals and also in relation to factors such as gender, age, culture and setting. A group focused on female caregivers will function quite differently than a group of widowers grieving the loss of their spouse. The following are a sampling of activities that may contribute to and enhance clinical outcomes:

- Stress management and self-care assessments to assist members to determine their stress level or how well they take care of themselves. This assessment is followed by a sharing of suggestions for self-care with the goal of having members practice selected behaviors and identify obstacles and potential intended and unintended consequences. For example, a 5-minute stress management exercise for a mother with young children may frustrate unless the potential obstacles are predicted and planned for. These behaviors may be practiced during the week with follow-up discussion during the next meeting.
- Teaching stress management techniques such as gentle stretching, deep breathing, meditation, and gentle yoga where there are no medical contraindications
- Expressive arts activities such as creating collages which might represent the present, the past and an envisioned future. This activity can be done as "homework" or done together as a group activity. For some, having a group activity on which to focus creates an environment that makes talking and sharing feelings a bit easier. For others, having a significant "homework" task can be intimidating, so group input into the best process of creating the collage will help build cohesion and a meaningful outcome. A comfortable compromise may be for people to prepare their materials, such as photos, poems, pictures, or pieces of jewelry, at home and assemble the collage together.
- Self-nurturing activities based on Alan Wolfelt's "Five Realms of Nurturing Yourself" include the *physical, emotional, cognitive, social, and spiritual* (2004). This activity helps members to focus on themselves as "whole persons" and asks participants either as a group or in subgroups to consider each category, how their situation impacts each, and what they might do to enhance self-care.
- Cognitive inquiry to identify thoughts and beliefs that impact coping and adaptation during meetings and/or between meetings through the use of diaries
- Use of journals and life review as clinical tools to explore meaning and to enhance insight and adaptation
- Facilitator-led discussions of agreed-upon topics, articles, or videos shared within the group
- Guest speakers to address member interests insuring both time for presentation and group discussion.

Group Endings

As each group nears the end of a session, the facilitator allows time for summing up, pointing out any significant points made or things learned. Many groups end, just as they begin, with a ritual.

For the last session of a closed group, preparation starts a number of weeks before and may include establishing a group consensus about the activities that will occur during the last meeting to acknowledge its significance. In addition to decisions about refreshments and shared ritual, it is important to create a process that summarizes what has taken place during the weeks of the group. Point out some of the key topics discussed, as well as significant ideas or insights people have shared. If appropriate, recognize progress and reinforce the optimism and hope most people have gained if this is congruous with their experience. Validate that there will likely be difficult days, but these do not have to be viewed as a setback but rather as an invitation to use some of the coping skills acquired over the life of the group. Some ending rituals, such as the lighting of a candle, if setting allows, provide a transitional object that remains with members and is invested with the memory of the group experience.

In addition to group input, clinical judgment influences the focus and therapeutic mileau created at the last session. For example, setting an expectation for exchange of addresses and phone numbers may create much discomfort for some but not for others. Suggesting that members bring refreshments to share may create a hardship and embarrassment for someone of minimal resources. Framing a last session as a "graduation" or celebration may be congruous with the feeling state of some and incongruous with others. As with the initial planning, clinical judgment and sensitivity to the group as a whole and to individual members is essential to meaningful endings.

Group Evaluation

While some programs use pre- and posttesting to evaluate group outcomes, many find that asking participants to evaluate their experience in a group or workshop is a useful way to learn what is working and what needs modification. Consider the following questions:

- What was the most helpful part of the group?
  - Least helpful?
- Would you recommend any changes and if so what?
- How would you rate the facilitator overall?
  - On a scale from 1 to 5 with 1 being least helpful and 5 being most helpful
  - Or excellent, good, fair
- Were written materials or readings helpful?
- Would you have preferred a different day or time of day?
- Were the location and room comfortable and accessible?

Questions that inquire about the participants' perceived changes in their feelings and well-being as a consequence of group participation can be helpful. This approach to evaluating outcome is reflected in the questions: How did you feel when you started the group? How do you feel now? Some typical responses have been as follows:

Before: Helpless, hopeless, alone, and isolated. Sometimes panicky about being alone.
After: Sitting in a quiet room with other people with the same feelings made me feel not so alone.
Before: Confused, guilty, and angry.
After: I feel so grateful to have had the opportunity to come to this group. I feel so much better now.
Before: Lost, alone, in denial, very tearful, afraid, life not worthwhile—I isolated myself.
After: Not less sad yet, but less alone due to the wonderful women in my group. I realize there are many people out there who feel and suffer as I do.

It can also be useful to send an evaluation or conduct a phone survey with people who start but do not finish a group. One study (Fowler et al., 2002) found that there was a greater response rate to phone versus mail surveys—66% versus 46%, respectively—suggesting that, if possible, phone surveys may provide more useful information and feedback. Inviting their feedback as to what might have been done differently will help determine the factors that influenced the outcome and isolate any changes that might have been made to enhance their participation.

Creative Programming

Groups and Technology

Alternatives to the more traditional support groups have proliferated as technology allows creation of online chats and telephone support groups. Telephone support groups require participants to call a central number to join with others, and a facilitator guides the process. The facilitator listens to words and intonation, but he or she is without the benefit of being able to observe nonverbal behaviors. The telephone experience can be complemented by mailing and e-mailing of readings, assessment, and evaluation tools. People can participate without leaving home, allowing access to a group modality when transportation, caregiver demands, or physical limitations make in-person participation a challenge. While the cost of arranging the phone service may be a disadvantage for agencies and the absence of personal interaction uncomfortable for some, others may feel freer to participate because of this same lack of personal contact. In addition, there is some evidence that these groups help meet needs of those where distance issues as in rural areas, cultural factors, or caregiver concerns preclude in-person participation (Bank,

Arguelles, Rubert, Eisdorfer, & Czaja, 2006; Brown et al., 1999; Colon, 1996).

Expanding Group Services

One very successful option for many organizations is educational workshops, which can be one-time offerings or a short series. While workshops may have a supportive and therapeutic element, their primary focus is educational. Most workshops run for 2–3 hours.

Topics may include the following:

- Coping with the holidays
- Talking to children about serious illness
- Spirituality and serious illness
- Managing fatigue
- Managing pain and other symptoms

A workshop series may encourage participants to attend all of the programs in a series, while others may be organized to allow attendees to attend based on their interest and availability. Some series ideas, in addition to topics listed earlier, include the following:

Expressing emotions creatively, which can create legacy or memory as well as healing by means of creative expression:

- Healing through creative writing
- Art as healer
- Quilting
- Therapeutic and healing experience of music

Mastering new roles:

- Financial management
- Shopping and cooking to support well-being.

Respecting Culture and Gender

Creative programming responds to gender, cultural, and generational preferences. For example, African American women coping with breast cancer received a great deal of comfort from family and friends, maintaining a positive attitude and relying on prayer (Henderson, Gore, Davis, & Condon, 2003). This might suggest a group incorporating family and friends, utilizing a spiritual and/or prayer element, or focusing on ways to stay positive would all be especially useful if serving this population. Another program for Mexican Americans with diabetes used Spanish language videotapes, resulting in statistically significant improvements in knowledge of their disease (Brown & Hanis, 1995). A study of Alzheimer's caregivers (Wood & Parham, 1990) found that white caregivers attended support groups more frequently than did blacks, while blacks had available, and used extensively, a more informal support network, again suggesting that incorporating family and perhaps church networks would prove more

beneficial and make programs more accessible and attractive. Morano and Bravo (2002), after studying and creating a program for Hispanic Alzheimer's caregivers, suggest that a psychoeducational model works best also incorporating practical assistance with needs such as transportation and respite. They suggest that bilingual facilitators are essential, and they comment on the need to recognize the relevance and importance of food and perception of time with this population. In planning programs that are culturally responsive, it is important to be aware of values and beliefs of the particular culture programs are designed to serve. A study by Stacciarini, O'Keefe, and Mathews (2007), looking at group therapy for depressed Latina women, concluded that cultural factors are important considerations for this population, including incorporating Latino values, using bilingual and bicultural group facilitators, decreasing barriers to participation, and recognizing family and religious themes, among others. Some cultures have spiritual or cultural beliefs that preclude discussions of death. Some may believe it is respectful and appropriate to avoid eye contact or to meet other's needs before their own. Many have beliefs and practices related to nontraditional or folk remedies (Altilio & Colon, 2007).

Traditional support groups do not meet the needs of many men who are less likely to join groups than are women (Krizek, Roberts, Ragan, Ferrara, & Lord, 1999). This is thought to be due to social norms of traditional masculinity, which makes help seeking more difficult because of both an inhibition related to emotional expressiveness and a socialization to be independent and conceal vulnerability (Davies et al., 2000; Moller-Leimkuhler, 2002). This may therefore require different modalities, such as programs focusing on education rather than support. One study (Zhang, Galenek, Strauss, & Siminoff, 2008) found that men are in fact willing to join groups and to adhere to them once they have committed, in particular to groups that focus on solving problems (2008). Youngmee, Loscalzo, Wellish, and Spillers (2006) studied husband caregivers of women with cancer and found that they had greater stress when their wives had poorer psychosocial functioning. It was concluded that these men will benefit from programs designed to educate them to effectively assist with their wife's adjustment to cancer.

A men's breakfast or dinner club creates an opportunity for men to meet over a meal, often in a restaurant, while talking about what is going on in their lives. Some organizations facilitate social gatherings such as the Meal and More programs, which meet monthly. After a meal and an hour of socializing, a program is planned that may include professional or community speakers or continued socialization around a game or activity.

Creative Programming

Book clubs require participants to read assigned books relevant to many aspects of the experience of illness and loss. Members convene with a facilitator to discuss the book and individual responses to the reading. The goals of these types of programs are to provide an avenue for socializing with others who share a similar situation and assist in understanding and coping with illness, caregiving, or loss. This modality may be very useful for people who tend to process experience in a more intellectual fashion. The following is a list of books that may be helpful depending on the population and intended therapeutic goal:

Tuesdays with Morrie, by Mitch Albom
The Lovely Bones, by Alice Sebold
When Bad Things Happen to Good People, by Harold Kushner
The Tao of Pooh, by Benjamin Hoff
For One More Day, by Mitch Albom
The Memory Keeper's Daughter, by Kim Edwards

This same modality, bibliotherapy, can be used to help parents and children together or separately to facilitate clinical work related to illness, loss, and adaptation (Altilio, 2002).

Since exercise is known to be helpful for stress reduction, offering a class that may include yoga, tai chi, meditation, or relaxation exercise can be helpful to patients, families, and staff. One study found that yoga may have a role in managing psychological distress and modulating circadian patterns of stress hormones in early breast cancer patients (Raghavendra et al., 2009). Yet another studied cancer outpatients who participated in a weekly meditation group lasting 1.5 hours for 7 weeks and found that it was effective in decreasing mood disturbance and stress symptoms in both male and female patients with a wide variety of cancer diagnoses, states of illness, and ages (Speca, Carlson, Goodey, & Angen, 2000). For those who are able, a walking club can be helpful and provide an activity around which participants can interact and share thoughts and feelings.

Conclusion

While there are a variety of ways in which people coping with illness, caregiving, and/or loss can gain support,

information, and assistance, the value of support groups for many is unmistakable. They offer an important and cost-effective alternative for reaching and supporting people living with a variety of life challenges. Groups offer people an opportunity to work through feelings associated with their situation, to reduce isolation that often results from being ill or from the responsibilities of being a caregiver and/or from grieving a loss, and to obtain information, resources, and tools for managing their situation. A group may be most effective and beneficial when it evolves and takes on some of its own characteristics and identity, thereby reflecting the needs and personalities of its members. The core concepts offered in this chapter can serve to guide the formation, implementation, and evaluation of any group. Facilitating a support group can be both a humbling and inherently rewarding experience, enabling growth not only for the participants but also for the facilitators.

LEARNING EXERCISES

- Think about a type of group you would like to offer and then create a list of sources for promoting your group, ways in which you can let people know about your group, and an outline of sessions and activities you would integrate to implement this group.
- Conduct a role play of a group session. Start by incorporating a visioning exercise whereby participants, with eyes closed, envision themselves in the doctor's office being given a diagnosis (for themselves or as a caregiver) of a serious illness. Ask them to envision their reaction, their first thoughts, ideas about what they will do, feelings they experience, and so forth. Then have them open their eyes and role play the first session of a support group they have joined for this new diagnosis or situation, where participants review group guidelines and then introduce themselves and tell their story.

ADDITIONAL RESOURCES AND WEB SITES

Caring Connections: http://www.caringinfo.org
A site of the National Hospice and Palliative Care Organization offering information, resources for planning, living with illness, being a caregiver, and coping with loss.
Daily Strength: http://www.dailystrength.org
Online support groups based on numerous disorders, diseases, and conditions.
Family Caregiver Magazine: http://www.familycaregiver.org
Connecting caregivers through resources, message boards, and online support, with a goal of empowering caregivers.
Disease/disorder-specific Web sites, most of which offer resources and information, and many of which offer support group information.
National Me/FM; Benefits of Support Groups; www.mefmaction.net
WillowGreen: http://www.willowgreen.com

Box 26.3
A Community Narrative: A Community Advisory Committee

A local hospice agency, recognizing the numbers of Latino and Russian people living in their area, formed advisory committees comprised of members of each of these communities, encouraging their input and ideas regarding knowledge of best ways to reach the members of their community with regard to end-of-life concerns and services. Additionally, they provided education about hospice, palliative care, and loss, and then utilized committee members as spokespersons in their communities, offered educational programs, and conducted workshops and groups.

Provider of support and materials (CDs, videos, books) to inspire and inform on life transitions, such as coping with illness, grief, and loss.

SUGGESTED READINGS

Berzoff, J., & Silverman, P. (Eds.). (2004). *Living with dying: A handbook for end-of-life healthcare practitioners*. New York, NY: Columbia University Press.

Johnson, D. W., & Johnson, F. P. (2008). *Joining together: Group theory and group skills*. Upper Saddle River, NJ:Pearson.

Kurtz, L. F. (1997). *Self-help and support groups: A handbook for practitioners*. Thousand Oaks, CA: Sage.

Lauria, M., Clark, E., Hermann, J., & Stearns, N. (2001). *Social work in oncology: Supporting survivors, families, and caregivers*. Atlanta, GA: American Cancer Society.

Nichols, K., & Jenkinson, J. (2006). *Leading a support group*. Berkshire, England: Chapman and Hall

National Hospice and Palliative Care Organization (NHPCO). (2007). *Social work guidelines*. Alexandria, VA: Author.

Raymer, M., & Gardia, G. (2007). *What social workers do: A guide to social work in hospice and palliative care*. Alexandria, VA: National Hospice and Palliative Care Organization.

Schiff, H. (1996). *The support group manual: A session by session guide*. New York, NY: Penguin Books Inc.

Schopler, J., & Galinsky, M. (1996). *Support groups: Current perspective on theory and practice*. New York, NY: Routledge.

Shaw, M. E. (1981). *Group dynamics: The psychology of small group behavior*. New York, NY: McGraw Hill.

Wuthnow, R. (1994). *Sharing the journey: Support groups and America's new quest for community*. New York, NY: Free Press.

REFERENCES

Altilio, T. (2002). Helping children, helping ourselves: An overview of children's literature. In J. Loewy & A. F. Hara (Eds.). *Caring for the caregiver: The use of music and music therapy in grief and trauma* (pp. 138–146). Silver Spring, MD: American Music Therapy Association Inc.

Altilio, T., & Colon, Y. (2007). Cultural perspectives in pain management: Implications for social workers and other psychosocial professionals. *The Pain Practitioner, 17*(2), 25–29.

Anderson, B., Yang, H., Farrar, W., Golden-Kreutz, D., Emery, C., Thornton, L., & Carson, W., 3rd, (2008). Psychologic intervention improves survival for breast cancer patients: A randomized clinical trial. *Cancer, 113*, 3450–3458.

Bank, A., Arguelles, S., Rubert, M., Eisdorfer, C. L., & Czaja, S. (2006). The value of telephone support groups among ethnically diverse caregivers of person with dementia. *The Gerontologist, 46*(1), 134–138.

Brown, N. (2003). *Psychoeducational groups: Process and practice*. New York, NY: Brunner-Routledge.

Brown, R., Pain, K., Berwald, C., Hirschi, P., Delehanty, R., & Miller, H. (1999). Distance education and caregiver support groups: Comparison of traditional and telephone groups. *Journal of Head Trauma Rehabilitation, 14*(3), 257–268.

Brown, S. A., & Hanis, C. L. (May-*June* 1995). A community-based, culturally sensitive education and group-support intervention for Mexican Americans with NIDDM: A pilot study of efficacy. *Diabetes Education, 3*, 203–210

Cain, E., Kohorn, E., Quinlan, D., Latimer, K., & Schwartz, P. (1986). Psychosocial benefits of a cancer support group. *Cancer, 57*, 183–189.

Classen, C., Butler, L, Koopman, C., Miller, E, DiMicelli, S., Giese-Davis, J, ... Spiegel, D. (2001). Supportive-expressive group therapy and distress in patients with metastatic breast cancer. *Archives of General Psychiatry, 58*, 494–501.

Colon, Y. (1996). Telephone support groups: A nontraditional approach to reaching underserved cancer patients. *Cancer Practice, 4*(3), 156–159.

Coward, D.(1990). The lived experience of self-transcendence in women with advanced breast cancer. *Nursing Science Quarterly, 3*(4), 162–169.

Davies, J., McCare, B., Frank, J., Dochnahl, A., Pickering, T., Harrison, B., ... Wilson, K. (2000). Identifying male college students' perceived health needs, barriers to seeking help, and recommendations to help men adopt healthier lifestyles. *Journal of American College Health, 48*, 259–267.

Davison, K., Pennebaker, J., & Dickerson, S. (2000). Who talks? The social psychology of illness support groups. *American Psychologist, 55*(2), 205–217.

Fowler, F., Gallagher, P., Stringfellow, V., Zaslavsky, A., Thompson, J., & Cleary, P. (2002). Using telephone interviews to reduce non-response bias to mail surveys of health plan members. *Medical Care,40*(3), 190–200.

Goodwin, P., Leszcz, M., Ennis, M., Koopmans, J., Vincent, L., Guther, H., ... Hunter, J. (2001). The effect of group psychosocial support on survival in metastatic breast cancer. *New England Journal of Medicine, 345*(24), 1719–1726.

Helgeson, V., Cohen, S., Schulz, R., & Yasko, J. (1999). Education and peer discussion group interventions and adjustment to breast cancer. *Archives of General Psychiatry, 56*(4), 340–347.

Helgeson, V., Cohen, S., Schulz, R., & Yasko, J. (2000). Group support interventions for women with breast cancer: Who benefits from what? *Health Psychology, 19*(2), 107–114.

Henderson, P., Gore, S., Davis, B. L., & Condon, E. (2003) African American women coping with breast cancer: A qualitative analysis. *Oncology Nursing Forum, 30*(4), 641–647.

Hermann, J. (2005). *Cancer support groups: A guide for facilitators*. Atlanta, GA: American Cancer Society.

Hughes, M. (1995). *Bereavement and support: Healing in a group environment*. Philadelphia, PA: Taylor and Francis.

Krause, N., Herzog, A. R., & Baker, E. (1992). Providing support to others and well-being in later life. *Journal of Gerontology, 47*(5), 300–311.

Krizek, C., Roberts, C., Ragan, R., Ferrara, J. J., & Lord, B. (1999). Gender and cancer support group participation. *Cancer Practice, 7*, 86–92.

Kuczynski, K. (2008). Life-threatening illness and the nature of social support: Brief research report. *Journal of Psychosocial Oncology, 26*(3), 113–123.

Miller, J. (1998). *Effective support groups*. Fort Wayne, IN: Willowgreen Publishing.

Mead, S., Hilton, D., & Curtis, L. (2001). Peer support: A theoretical perspective. *Psychiatric Rehabilitation Journal, 25*,134–141.

Moller-Leimkuhler, A. (2002). Barriers to help-seeking by men: A review of socio-cultural and clinical literature with particular reference to depression. *Journal of Affective Disorders, 71*(1), 1–9.

Monahan, D. J., Greene, V. L., & Coleman, P. D. (1992). Caregiver support groups: Factors affecting use of services. *Social Work, 37*, 254–260.

Morano, C., & Bravo, M. (2002). A psychoeducational model for Hispanic Alzheimer's disease caregivers. *The Gerontologist, 42*(1), 122–127.

Otis-Green, S. (2006). The transitions program: Existential care in action. *Journal of Cancer Education, 21*(1), 23–25.

Raghavendra, R., Vadiraja, H. S., Nagarathna, R., Nagendra, H. R., Rekha, M., Vanitah, N., ... Kumar, V. (2009). Effects of a Yoga program on cortisol rhythm and mood states in early breast cancer patients undergoing adjuvant radiotherapy: A randomized controlled trial. *Integrative Cancer Therapies, 8*(1), 37–46.

Schwartz, C., & Sendor, M. (1999). Helping others helps oneself: Response shift effects in peer support. *Social Science and Medicine, 48*(11), 1563–1575.

Solomon, P. (2004). Peer support/peer provided services underlying processes, benefits, and critical ingredients. *Psychiatric Rehabilitation Journal, 27*(4), 392–401.

Speca, M., Carlson, L., Goodey, E., & Angen, M. (2000). A randomized, wait-list controlled clinical trial: The effect of mindfulness meditation-based stress reduction program on mood and symptoms of stress in cancer outpatients. *Psychosomatic Medicine, 62*, 613–622.

Spiegel, D., Bloom, J., & Yalom, I. (1981). Group support for metastatic cancer patients: A randomized prospective outcome study. *Archives of General Psychiatry, 38*, 527–534.

Stacciarini, J. P., O'Keefe, M., & Mathews, M. (2007). Group therapy as a treatment for depressed Latino women: A review of the literature. *Issues in Mental Health Nursing, 28*, 473–488.

Toseland, R. (1990). Long-term effectiveness of peer-led and professionally led support groups for caregivers. *Social Service Review, June*, 308–327.

Ussher, J., Kirsten, L., Butow, P., & Sandoval, M. (2008). A qualitative analysis of reasons for leaving, or not attending a cancer support group. *Social Work in Health Care, 47*(1), 14–29.

Vos, P., Visser, A., Garssen, B., Duivenvoorden, H., & deHaes, H. (2007). Effectiveness of group psychotherapy compared to social support groups in patients with primary, non-metastatic breast cancer. *Journal of Psychosocial Oncology, 25*(4), 37–60.

Wolfelt, A. (2004). *The understanding your grief support group guide*. Fort Collins, CO: Companion Press.

Wood, V., & Parham, I. (1990). Coping with perceived burden: Ethnic and cultural issues in Alzheimer's family caregiving. *Journal of Applied Gerontology, 9*(3), 325–339.

Youngmee, K., Loscalzo, M., Wellisch, D., & Spillers, R. (2006). Gender differences in caregiving stress among caregivers of cancer survivors. *Psycho-Oncology, 15*(12), 1086–1092.

Zhang, A., Galanek, J., Strauss, G., & Siminoff, L. (2008). What it would take for men to attend and benefit from support groups after prostatectomy for prostate cancer: A problem-solving approach. *Journal of Psychosocial Oncology, 26*(3), 97–112.

27 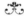 *Katharine M. Campbell*

Social Work and Technology: The Software and Hard Drive of Patient and Family Care

I feel less alone now that I am part of an online family of people going through the same thing I am. I can e-mail my social worker with questions when I am not strong enough for the drive, and I even used the Internet to find an acupuncturist in my area who specializes in pain management for my disease.

—*A cancer patient*

Key Concepts

- *Technology impacts the way patients and families obtain information and make decisions.*
- *Technology impacts how providers deliver care and perform services.*
- *Ethical and legal concerns arise due to technological advances.*
- *Professional boundaries can be challenged by electronic communication.*
- *Appropriate direction and guidelines are essential to assist patients, families, and providers to access reputable online resources.*

Introduction

High-tech palliative care may seem like a bit of a contradiction. When one thinks about palliative care, one may envision a hospice patient, discussion of a life-limiting diagnosis, enhancing quality of life, or termination of life-sustaining treatments. All of these are components of palliative care, but they are often integrated in a new way with today's technological advances. Internet searching, text messaging, instant messaging, e-mailing, Web sites, social media, and more play an integral role in how a palliative care plan is developed, provided, and received. Patients, who are working with palliative care clinicians or considering how palliative care might contribute to their lives, are often learning what the concept means and what services are available to them through use of technology. Health care systems and providers are attempting to meet patients' demands for technological advancements and conveniences by converting to electronic medical records, digital scans, blogs, and Web sites as mainstream avenues for storing and providing information.

Working with clients who face a life-threatening illness is both challenging and rewarding. Your practice setting, clientele, available resources, and your own knowledge base will guide your experiences as a palliative social worker. Your experience, now more than ever, is also influenced by the growing number of patients and families who are utilizing technology for accessing information, tapping into resources, adapting to new situations, broadening their social support system, and building their strategies for coping. Understanding technological advances is critical to effectively informing, empowering, and supporting patients and families within today's societal norms. Nevertheless, the appropriate incorporation of technology into palliative social work practice requires an understanding of all relevant implications for both the patient and the social worker.

Rather than focus on the technical aspects and definitions, this chapter will concentrate on the clinical aspects of how technology influences patients and social workers within the world of palliative care. The framework and principles of this chapter are built upon the definition of *technology* in the *Standards for Technology and Social Work Practice* (2005): "any electronically mediated activity used in the conduct of competent and ethical delivery of social work services" (p. 3). Technology has affected the realm of palliative care in two prominent domains that will be figuratively referred to as the "software" and "hard drive" of care (G. Brown, personal communication, July 10, 2009). These are defined as the ways in which patients and their families access information (the software of patient/family care) and the ways in which social workers provide services (the hard drive of patient/family care).

The Software of Patient/Family Care: Seeking Information and Support

The software of patient care describes how patients and their families access information, and how social workers can incorporate technological resources into their practice in a competent manner. Our world has embraced technology such that many people have cell phones and Internet access in modern society. It is estimated that 24% of the worldwide population uses the Internet. Within North America and Europe, 73% and 50% of their populations, respectively, access the Internet (Internet World Stats, 2009). According to Sillence and Briggs (2007), "Eighty per cent of adult Internet users have gone online in search of health information" (p. 347). The concept of patients seeking information through the virtual community and knowing how to seek out Internet resources is so common that the term "e-patient" is being used on blogs, Internet sites, and online dictionaries to describe these patients/family members. The psychosocial needs of e-patients (and all patients we work with) are dynamic and often shift over time as illness and its impact evolves. Technology can only be harnessed as a tool to inform and bridge these processes and serve as beneficial when accompanied by a thorough assessment of the patient's beginning point, his or her goals, the tools accessible to the patient, and the patient's knowledge base on how to appropriately utilize those tools. The search for understanding and meaning when dealing with a life-threatening illness can have a broad reach, reflecting the complexity of a person's life experiences, coping, and process of adaptation.

Seeking Information

When an illness affects one's life, for many the need for information and to make meaning of experiences is vital. More and more today, the Internet has become an avenue

for patients and families to seek out information about diagnoses and expectations of the physical changes one may undergo. According to the Pew Internet and American Life Project (2009), "Eight in ten internet users have looked online for health information. Many e-patients say the internet has had a significant impact in the way they care for themselves or others" (http://www.pewinternet.org/topics/Health.aspx). And today's resources are encouraging patients and families to educate themselves, seek online information, and take an active role in their health care (Foley et al., 2005). It can be a vehicle to share experiences, seek answers to specific concerns, and locate additional resources. The Internet has proven to be extremely helpful in allowing patients and their families to gain a better understanding of all their experiences, and for social workers to identify and locate resources to help their patients. At the same time, a vast amount of information available may be misleading or inaccurate.

Palliative social workers need to be effective as brokers of information within their specialty. Professionals need to be cognizant of what information is available, know how to guide their patients and families to appropriate sites, and know how to assess sites to determine whether they are inappropriate. Social workers are best positioned to assist patients in refining what they are looking for, as well as guiding them through and distilling the potentially overwhelming amount of information they receive. An excessive amount of information—especially from contradictory sources—can result in patients and their families feeling more hopeless and unable to make decisions effectively. In an analysis of information overload, Kim, Lustria, Burke, and Kwon (2007) found that results of the National Cancer Institute's Health Information National Trends Survey revealed "that in 2003, seven in ten Americans, or an estimated 149 million people, felt that there were so many recommendations about cancer information that they were confused" (http://informationr.net/ir/12-4/paper326.html). Anderson and Klemm (2008) detail how the Internet can be beneficial and empowering, but it can also lead to a patient feeling annoyed, dismayed, and anxious (see Box 27.1).

Seeking Support

Foley et al. (2005) noted a client statement that "there is an online computer site ... I go in there and talk to a lot of women ... that helps me a lot" (p. 95). The need for social support when facing a life-limiting illness is vital. Support for the patient as well as the family can allow for difficult dialogue to take place, and it can alleviate the patient's sense of isolation. Many patients seek support through technological avenues such as telephone and Internet support groups, social media Web sites, and videoconferencing services. In addition, the use of these resources also allows support to be found from the comfort of one's home.

Box 27.1
Patient/Family Narrative: Ms. Mosely

Martin, a junior social worker at an outpatient oncology clinic, has been working with Mrs. Mosely for about 6 months. Mrs. Mosely presented with stage IV breast cancer with metastasis. Her physician explained, in the initial consultation, that palliative care would be the objective because Mrs. Mosely was experiencing a great deal of pain that was diminishing her quality of life. Previous treatment regimens directed at the cancer had not been beneficial. The focus of social work assessment and intervention was Mrs. Mosely's anxiety—its contribution to her pain experience and impact on her quality of life. After a routine visit with the doctor, Mrs. Mosely brought the social worker a number of articles she found on the Internet about an herbal remedy that she was planning to try. This served as an invitation for the social worker to explore Mrs. Mosely's goals and hopes, as well as guiding her on how to assess the validity and reputation of the Web sites Mrs. Mosley was using to obtain information. The social worker requested a team meeting with the patient and the physician to ensure adequate communication, review prior treatments and decisions and to weigh the benefits of seeking all treatment options, including integrative options.

Box 27.2
Patient/Family Narrative: Mr. Jaminson

Mr. Jaminson is a stage IV colon cancer patient who has been referred to a local hospice program and informed that there are no additional disease-modifying treatment options available to him. As he talks with Mike, his palliative social worker, about his feelings of isolation and loss of hope, he shares that he has found a great deal of support in an online support group; however, he has not been fully honest with the group about his prognosis. Mike takes this opportunity to talk to Mr. Jaminson about his online identity versus his in-person identity. Mike probes further into his lack of full disclosure, exploring both the emotions and thoughts contributing to his decision and its impact on his group experience.

Technology has enabled patients and their families to communicate with multiple people at one time by use of social media sites. In addition to social networking sites such as Facebook, MySpace, and Twitter, there are a number of health care–specific sites designed for patients to share medical updates. Some find it easier, faster, and less emotionally draining to communicate electronically (see Box 27.2). A list of such sites has been included in the Additional Resources section at the end of this chapter.

The Hard Drive of Patient and Family Care: Providing Social Work Services

Technological advances are increasingly shaping the role of palliative social workers and influencing the methods that they use. Health care systems are turning to electronic medical records and data management programs, and patients and their families are accessing various technological options for their psychosocial care as well. Use of services such as online therapy, blogs, social networking sites, and listservs are on the rise. In addition, palliative social workers have more resources available to them as practitioners to increase their own knowledge base and improve their professional skills, including listservs, discussion boards, online educational services, and professional networking sites. Social workers can increase their provision of effective case management online by pulling together resources from government, pharmaceutical, and insurance Web sites, for example. However, this dynamic new realm of service provision within the electronic world does not come without challenges.

Ethical and legal issues are rising in proportion to concerns regarding online privacy, authenticity, and boundaries.

Legal and Ethical Issues

With the vast array of ethical and legal concerns that can arise with technological advances, the National Association of Social Workers (NASW) and Association of Social Work Boards (ASWB) have devised standards for technology and social work practice that serve as guidelines for practitioners (NASW/ASWB Standards, 2005). Palliative social workers who elect to take advantage of technology for providing services have an obligation to ensure they continue to provide competent care. This includes taking extra measures for ensuring information security, as well as safeguarding patient privacy and confidentiality. Performing competent assessments is additionally challenging when performed electronically versus in person. The NASW Code of Ethics (NASW, 2009) still applies under all circumstances, and special consideration must be given regarding ethical standard 1.07: Privacy and confidentiality, and ethical standard 3.04: Client records. Therapeutic engagement within the world of technology requires social workers to be well informed about electronic data interchange (EDI), which can be described as "the automatic, seamless and instantaneous exchanging of information between separate organizations based on predetermined data definitions, standards and protocols" (Finn, McNutt, Patterson, Regan, & Schoech, 2008). Standards for authentication, privacy, and confidentiality through EDI continue to improve. However, information shared is still subject to the same legal regulations and ethical guidelines as person-to-person contact. The practitioner is responsible for properly self-identifying as well as verifying the patient's identity prior to therapeutic engagement. Gathering contact information and consent, explaining ones' duty to warn, crisis intervention strategies, and verification of the patient's physical location in case of emergency are also important considerations that are recommended in providing online services (Mallen, Vogel, & Rochlen, 2005).

Professional Boundary Issues

Another challenge that has arisen due to the advances in technology is that of appropriate online boundaries. More and more organizations are engaging in social media, blogs, and listservs as a way to reach clients. And more organizations are encouraging social workers to participate in these online activities (see Box 27.3). Ethical considerations regarding the level of self-disclosure and appropriate boundaries for each contact with the social worker are heightened when interacting electronically. When considering self disclosure, palliative social workers consider questions such as:

- Does this information benefit the patient/family? How?
- Why is this information being shared?
- Is this information professional or personal?
- Would this information be shared if this were a face-to-face interaction?
- Is this information enabling rather than empowering the patient/family?

Mallen, Vogel, and Rochen (2005) note how "a therapist may be very skilled in verbalizing empathy during FtF (Face to Face) sessions; however, text-based online counseling renders those verbalizations irrelevant … and outcome of the session could be negatively impacted" (p. 787). They go on to recommend that practitioners ensure they obtain appropriate education, skills, and supervision for computer-based communication. In electronic communication, linguistics becomes more prominent as nonverbal cues are lost. Many social media sources use the term "friending" to allow someone access into your personal domain. During a practitioner–client interaction, are you becoming one's friend? Moreover, how do you establish and define the appropriate boundaries to the patient/family member with whom you are conversing electronically?

As providers are asked to engage more and more with online communities, issues of confidentiality, privacy, legal responsibilities/regulations, and professional boundaries come into play. Understanding one's legal and ethical responsibilities regarding electronic communication (whether providing counseling or basic information) is vital to safeguarding the worker and the workplace. Palliative social workers should familiarize themselves with their company's policies, the Standards of Technology set forth by the NASW and ASWB, and their own skill level of electronic communication.

EXERCISE

Based on the narrative in Box 27.3, answer the following questions:

- Because postings from patients or family members are public to all of those who have viewing rights, what level of privacy is possible?

Box 27.3
Patient/Family Narrative: Amy

Amy is a palliative social worker whose organization has created a Facebook page (social media Web site), and her administrator is asking each social worker to have a presence on the page. Amy's patients and their families have now been sending her a number of messages wanting to "friend" her and asking her therapeutic advice, including how to communicate with their children about their prognosis, and where they can seek integrative treatments. Patients have also sent messages complaining about their medical providers. Amy now has to determine ways to best address these circumstances.

- Whose privacy does Amy consider: the patient's posting, the viewers', or the company's?
- What ethical obligations does she have in regard to confidentiality?
- What are her responsibilities in regard to professional boundaries?
- What are her responsibilities to the medical providers being discussed?

Appropriate Direction and Guidelines

Although technological advances are prevalent, there is a need to recognize that not all populations and geographic areas have advanced at the same rate. Understanding the population one is serving and the resources available is vital to providing appropriate and effective care. For many rural, minority, immigrant, and/or low-income communities, technology is largely underused or entirely inaccessible. Creativity and resourcefulness still serve as strong assets to palliative social workers in any setting—knowing where and how to direct patients and families to access technological tools or services can be beneficial for all. Many county and city governments offer free Internet access at libraries and other public facilities. However, even then it is important to understand that a large percentage of the information on the Internet is in English, or written in language too complex to be truly accessible to those of any education level and background. The individual may also not be technologically experienced or savvy enough to distinguish what is a reputable source.

For those who are capable and wish to access information electronically, palliative social workers can best guide patients and their families by providing a list of reputable Web sites and relevant search terms for information. Recommending appropriate Web sites and Internet resources should be a standard of practice just as recommending appropriate books or videos that address patient needs. However, it is also important for the palliative social worker to know and be able to teach patients and their families basic techniques for evaluating Internet information so they can be empowered to explore independently. Understanding some of the fundamentals for evaluating Web sites can be critical to screening and filtering the immense amount of material that is available. Foley et al. (2005) provided a list of considerations for evaluating a Web site that include the following:

- Who runs and pays for the site?
- What is the purpose of the site?
- Where does the information come from?
- What type of information is being provided, and how relevant is it?
- Does the site collect personal information? If so, why?
- How does the site interact with its users?

Social workers can provide patients with these questions to use as screening tools, and social workers themselves can apply these questions whenever they are seeking online information.

Summary

The "software" and "hard drive" of patient and family care is an extremely important and fast-evolving topic within palliative social work. Technology has influenced nearly every aspect of society, and advanced tools for information gathering, communication, and service delivery can significantly influence how one lives and copes with a life-limiting illness. Technology is also transforming the field of palliative social work by offering new challenges and opportunities to assist patients and their families in seeking information and support. Palliative social workers must have a heightened awareness to issues that arise from the use of technology. It is vital to understand what tools patients and their families are using, and what corresponding challenges come with using those tools.

Clinical, ethical, and legal obligations must be considered prior to the application of any technology. Use of the Internet, including any electronic communication, brings about a degree of anonymity and yet eliminates confidentiality at the same time. Identity is gained and lost simultaneously. Patients and families can find solace across the Internet because isolation is quickly alleviated. Yet ironically there is the potential for the patient to feel further isolated by using the Internet as a substitute for "low-tech," in-person support or to feel overburdened with a superfluous and unfiltered amount of troubling or confusing information. As patients and their families increasingly access information online, there is the potential for them to become empowered by it or disabled by oversaturation, a dynamic that is especially challenging for patients and families who become increasingly vulnerable as they are informed of fewer or no disease-modifying treatments and seek hope in the form of alternative treatment modalities. Looking to the Internet for ways to elevate pain and suffering, physical and emotional, can result in a flood of information and support. As a palliative social worker, the task at hand is to assist in defining what one is searching for

and seeking the most beneficial ways to meet these needs. Sometimes the Internet offers that option and sometimes the Internet can contribute to anxiety, confusion, and an increased sense of powerlessness.

Palliative social workers have the opportunity and duty to work closely with patients and families in assessing what information they are seeking and finding, leading them to appropriate online resources, offering techniques for evaluating Web sites, and processing emotionally and cognitively the information that has been discovered. The provider may be able to enhance service delivery by offering and employing online tools in practice but must strictly adhere to standards of ethics, safeguard privacy and confidentiality, ensure information security and authenticity, and maintain appropriate competencies and professional boundaries with patients. With proper guidance from their social worker, patients and their families can ultimately use technology as effective, central tools to research treatment options, investigate additional services and resources available to them, communicate with service providers, and gain invaluable support from those with shared experiences.

ADDITIONAL RESOURCES FOR
SOCIAL WORKERS

The American Cancer Society: http://www.cancer.org
A community-based health organization devoted to eradicating and preventing cancer through research, education, advocacy, and service.
The Center to Advance Palliative Care (CAPC): http://www.capc.org
The CAPC's purpose is to increase quality palliative care services to those who are ill by providing tools and training for health care professionals.
Compassion and Choices: http://www.compassionandchoices.org
A nonprofit organization that supports and counsels individuals and their loved ones experiencing end of life, and educates the public and health care professionals on how to appropriately deal with patients coping with end of life.
The Department of Pain Medicine and Palliative Care Beth Israel Medical Center: http://www.stoppain.org
Offers therapies and treatments for individuals who experience any sort of chronic pain. The Department includes highly skilled medical professionals with experiences in neurology, rehabilitation, medicine, anesthesiology, and psychology.
The International Association for Hospice and Palliative Care (IAHPC): http://www.hospicecare.com
The IAHPC's purpose is to enhance the quality of life of patients with serious health conditions and their families, and to improve hospice and palliative care programs, education, research, and policies.
The National Association of Social Workers (NASW): http://www.socialworkers.org
The largest membership organization of professional social workers in the world, with 150,000 members. NASW works to enhance its members' professional growth and development, maintain professional standards, and advance social policies.
The National Cancer Institute (NCI): http://www.cancer.gov

Conducts and supports research, training, health information dissemination, and other programs with respect to the cause, diagnosis, prevention, and treatment of cancer, rehabilitation from cancer, and the continuing care of cancer patients and their families.

The National Hospice and Palliative Care Organization (NHPCO): http://www.nhcpo.org

The largest nonprofit membership organization representing hospice and palliative care programs and professionals in the United States. NHPCO is dedicated to improving end-of-life care, increasing access to hospice care, and enhancing quality of life for people dying and their loved ones.

The World Health Organization: Palliative Care: http://www.who.int/cancer/palliative/en

Provides leadership and technical support regarding cancer to countries. *Cancer Pain Release* is the publication of the World Health Organization global communications program to improve cancer and HIV pain control and palliative care.

ADDITIONAL RESOURCES FOR PATIENTS AND FAMILIES

The American Cancer Society: http://www.cancer.org/docroot/CLP/CLP_1.asp

"My calendar" helps you keep track of events, appointments, and American Cancer Society–related activities. Reminders can be sent to you and your friends and family.

Cancer Compass: http://www.cancercompass.com

A Web site for sharing common experiences, discussing cancer news, and voicing your thoughts and opinions. Access is granted to those who join to an active group of community message boards.

Carepages: http://www.carepages.org

An online community of millions of people coming together to share the challenges, hopes, and triumphs of anyone facing a life-changing health event. CarePages is the place to be for patients who want to journal their experience or connect with others facing similar circumstances.

Caring Connections: http://www.caringinfo.org

A Web site sponsored by the National Hospice and Palliative Care Organization (NHPCO) providing resources, information, state-specific advance directives, and publications about care at the end of life and expressing one's wishes.

Caring Bridge: http://www.caringbridge.com

Provides free Web sites that connect family and friends during a serious health event, care, and recovery. Caring Bridge's Web site is personal, private, and available 24/7.

Lotsa Helping Hands: http://www.lotsahelpinghands.com

Created to support family caregivers and volunteers by empowering their community who are eager to help those in need. They provide communication resources to caregivers.

Planet Cancer: http://www.planetcancer.org

An online community of young adults with cancer in their 20s and 30s. Planet Cancer is a place to share insights, explore fears, and laugh.

REFERENCES

Anderson, A. S., & Klemm, P. (2008). The internet: Friend or foe when providing patient education? *Clinical Journal of Oncology Nursing, 12*(1), 55–63.

Finn, J., McNutt, J. G., Patterson, D. A., Regan, J. R., & Schoech, D. (2008). *Encyclopedia of social work.* Washington, DC: National Association of Social Workers and Oxford University Press, Inc.

Foley, K., Back, A., Bruera, E., Coyle, N., Loscalzo, M., Shuster, J., … VonRoenn, J. (Eds.). (2005). *When the focus is on care: Palliative care and cancer.* Atlanta, GA: American Cancer Society Health Promotions.

Internet World Stats. (n. d.) *World internet users and population stats.* Retrieved from http://www.Internetworldstats.com/stats.htm

Kim, K., Lustria, M., Burke, D., & Kwon, N. (2007). Predictors of cancer information overload: Findings from a national survey. *Information Research, 12*(4), paper 326. Retrieved from http://InformationR.net/ir/12-4/paper326.html

Mallen, M., Vogel, D., & Rochlen, A. (2005). The practical aspects of online counseling: Ethics, training, technology and competency. *The Counseling Psychologist, 33*, 776–818.

McKenna, K., & Seidman, G. (2005). You, me and we: Interpersonal processes in electronic groups. In Y. Amichai-Hamburger (Ed.), *The social net: Human behavior in cyberspace* (pp. 191–217). New York, NY: Oxford University Press.

National Association of Social Workers. (approved 1996, revised 1999). *Code of Ethics of the National Association of Social Workers.* Retrieved from http://www.naswdc.org/pubs/code/code.asp.

National Association of Social Workers/Association of Social Work Boards (NASW/ASWB). (2005). *NASW & ASWB standards for technology and social work practice.* Retrieved from http://www.aswb.org/pdfs/TechnologySWPractice.pdf

Pew Internet & American Life Project. (n. d.). *Health.* Retrieved from http://www.pewinternet.org/topics/Health.aspx

Sillence, E., & Briggs, P. (2007). Examining the role of the Internet in health behaviour. In A. Joinson, K. McKenna, T. Postmes, & U-D. Reips (Eds.), *The Oxford handbook of internet psychology* (pp. 347–359). New York, NY: Oxford University Press.

28

Nancy F. Cincotta

Bereavement in the Beginning Phase of Life: Grief in Children and Their Families

All I wanted to do was see the body, so I hung around near the coffin hoping someone would open it—but no one did.

—8-year-old child whose father died

Key Concepts

♦ *There are unique developmental considerations that need to be recognized in order to assist children facing the loss of any significant member of their world: sibling, parent, grandparent, other relative, teacher, caregiver, or friend.*

♦ *The loss of a sibling or parent and the parental loss of a child present particular clinical issues that must be identified.*

♦ *The concept of "family memory" and the creation of family memories are valuable constructs when working with children facing illness and death in their families.*

♦ *Therapeutic rituals and interventions assist children who have a loved one facing death and those who have had a death of someone significant in their lives.*

Introduction

This chapter focuses on the experiences of children who have had a sibling or a parent die, and touches on the experiences of parents who have lost a child. However, the concepts articulated in losses for children and parents extend to the lives of children who have lost treasured or significant relationships with grandparents, aunts, uncles, caretakers, trusted teachers, and others. It is intended to inform the work of clinicians working directly with children as their primary focus and those who have access to families in any health care setting, including such diverse settings as the intensive care unit, the outpatient clinic, extended care facilities, or mental health clinics. The work of assisting families to help children with illness, death, and dying is implicit in the clinical skill set of palliative and hospice social work.

Children experience grief within the context of their physical age and level of development and require age-appropriate interventions. Death can have a profound impact on children and can serve as an impediment to development. Understanding and making connections in the worlds of grieving children can positively influence the bereavement course and help them move forward towards positive resolution of their grief. Grieving parents are in the position of simultaneously recognizing and addressing both their own needs and the needs of their children.

> *I find that myself and many other kids my age share the same view about this whole thing. That we are different and we can't do anything to change that. At first, it is a very hard thing to overcome, that you just can't change what just happened. It is a very painful thing to overcome, but once you do, you become a better person because of it. One thing that is also very hard is that when you are at school, it is very hard to avoid questions. What happened? Was it cool to watch him die? Why do you not want to talk about this? Questions like this can be very sensitive topics, and most of the time, the stuff they say is very insensitive.*

There is no way of avoiding these questions, and most of the time, you just want to curl up in a ball and cry.

—13 year-old boy, age 8 when his brother died

Bereaved children are first and foremost children, and they must be recognized for their strengths and capabilities. At each age they understand and experience grief and the circumstances that lead to loss differently, and they can benefit from interventions that are sensitive to their age and level of development (Christ & Christ, 2006). Their normal days are filled with physical activity, learning, joyful experiences, and whimsy, which may at first seem inconsistent with grief. Yet these components of childhood are overriding forces in the resolution of their losses; their daily activities sustain them and provide them balance and continuity. Interventions designed to meet children within this context will prove to be the most effective tools in aiding them on their bereavement journey (see Table 28.1). Understanding and managing loss and grief in childhood cannot be considered out of the context of the family, the school, and the community in which a child lives. The reactions of those who play influential roles in the world of the child affect how the child copes and continues to grow.

Whether the child is present at the time of death of a loved one or learns about the death after the fact, the actual moment of death and the moments before and after will be remembered throughout the child's life. There are no correct answers as to whether the child should be present at the time of death. Some children will express a sense of loss at not being part of that family moment, whereas others will have regrets at having been present. Consideration of the developmental level and emotional makeup of the child, as well as his or her family's religious and cultural beliefs, will help inform decisions about the child's participation. How a family has shared experiences and information in the past will influence what they do during this crisis period.

Two brothers described sitting in the back seat of the car with their brother knowing that he had died en route to the hospital; there were no words to describe the enormity of what they felt. In a bereavement group they discussed in great detail the events of that evening, provoking the others in the group (ages 13–19) to share the experience of the moments when their siblings died. These scenes remain fixed in their minds, along with a sense that they cannot share them with others who cannot understand. It can be years before they discuss these memories.

There is an emotional intensity and vulnerability that exists during the days surrounding death. It is a surreal, transitional time, as family members begin to envision the reality of the death of their loved one.

As his brother lay dying, a boy fell asleep in the hospital room with his parents. Even though he was more than aware of the circumstances, he was devastated when he

---

Table 28.1.
What Bereaved Children Need

Understanding that the experience of the death changes as the child's age, cognition, and emotional maturity develop, bereaved children need the following:

- Honest and open explanations of what happened to the person who died and what will happen now

- Creation of an avenue of communication in which the child feels heard, loved, understood, and taken care of

- Someone to understand and assess their fears and concerns and to answer their questions

- Validation of their feelings about the loss

- The ability to participate in choices that impact on their lives

- Opportunities for the expression of emotions and the meaning of the loss

- Acceptance that they face and deal with things differently than their parents

- Inclusion in family rituals and ceremonies

- Their family unit to be kept intact and other activities constant

- Time to heal with their family

- Role models in dealing with grief

- Acknowledgment of their value in the family

- To have a role and responsibility in the rebuilding of the family

- Opportunities for the deceased to be present in their lives

- Acceptance of how their world actually changed, and how they perceive it changed

- Permission to move on from their grief

---

awakened and learned of his brother's death while he was asleep. He felt that although he had been in the room, he was not present. For the first 2 years after his brother died, he could not speak about it. After that he would cry when he tried to speak and could not express himself, but he was able to participate in therapeutic activities, including a balloon launch and the painting of a rock for his brother. Five years later he is able to speak about that evening with remorse and is able to remember happier times with his brother.

The moment of death is a private one, but there are aspects of the ensuing rituals that are public. Maintaining a family's privacy and offering guidance regarding children's roles at the funeral are exceptionally helpful to bereaved families (Horsley & Patterson, 2006). If it is planned that children are to see the body, they need preparation, a supervised visit, and resources available to them afterwards.

The first time anyone, especially a child, sees a dead body, there is a degree of associated discomfort (Fristad, Cerel, Goldman, Weller, & Weller, 2001). Talking about it, creating a ritual for the child such as a special candle-lighting ceremony, offering physical comfort, and allowing for tears or overwhelming outbursts of grief, or simply addressing the feelings that can be provoked in this circumstance can all be of assistance. For some children there will be a natural curiosity about death, regardless of who the person is who died.

Special considerations surround the death of a child. A child's funeral is the last act of public parenting and the first act of parenting in a newly constituted family. Attending the funeral of a sibling can be very powerful for children because of their emotional reactions to the loss. In addition, they witness the magnitude of their parents' grief. They may fear that it is so great that their parents will no longer be able to take care of them, and they may feel that their parents could never love them as much as they loved their sibling.

For many bereaved children, the loss may be the first that they are experiencing. Not only are they dealing with their grief in the current situation, but they are also learning to deal with loss and grief in general. Feeling abandoned, both by the person who has died and the people around them can leave children emotionally vulnerable. Rebuilding trust and managing grief is a slow process; it is not a process of replacing a lost object, but rather learning to live without that person, and about growing to create and accept the new rhythm of life (Christ & Christ, 2006).

Sibling Death

The hardest part of the bereavement experience for me is witnessing the pain of my other children.

—Bereaved father of three

Sibling relationships are, in many situations, the longest relationships that people will have in life. Adult sibling relationships endure longer than those with parents, and withstand more than most friendships. In *Drums, Girls, and Dangerous Pie*, a book for middle school-aged children, Jason Sonnenblick (2005) portrays the plight of a sibling of a child with cancer and captures issues of anxiety, jealousy, and how family life changes. There is sadness, loneliness, and at times confusion and anger.

In a support group for siblings of children with cancer, a number of children felt that their parents truly cared about their siblings more than them. Regardless of any redirection on my part, the children were convinced that there was no way that their parents cared about them as much. When asked the question, "What if you got cancer, how do you think your parents would react?" One retorted, "Then I would be the second child in the family with cancer and it wouldn't be as important that I had cancer!"

Sibling bereavement may lead to crises of identity formation. Children grow alongside their siblings and need to learn to develop in their absence, while grieving for them. According to Packman and colleagues (2006), the impact of sibling death can be summarized by four general responses: "I hurt inside"; "I don't understand"; "I don't belong"; and "I'm not enough [to make my parents happy]." The time that led up to the sibling's death, the experience of the death, and the intense mourning period after the death are all profound factors in sibling adjustment. In addition, the effect on the surviving child involves not only the death of the sibling but also the loss of those experiences throughout life that change without the presence of that sibling.

Sibling loss has been dubbed a "double loss," not only due to the death of a sibling but also the loss of parental support, because parents may be less emotionally available due to the depth of their own grief. Children are perceptive and worry about their parents. If the grief of those around them is overpowering, children may retreat from the expression of their own emotions. They may suppress their own feelings and not want to do or say things that might further upset their parents (Balk, 1983; Horsley & Patterson, 2006).

A bereaved sibling remarked, "My mother went away for almost a year with my sister while she was having a bone marrow transplant. Then she came back and wanted everything to go back to how it was before she left. There was no way that was going to happen. She left me. I'm not going to depend on her now."
—19-year-old girl whose sister died

When living in a household in which a family member has died, children come to understand that bad things happen, and they are no longer naïve. They may become wiser and at times interested in different things than their peers, which can become an isolating factor. Surviving children may also become autonomous earlier, because they may have been separated emotionally and physically from other family members during the period preceding the death. Parents often regret this lost time, wishing that they could turn the clock back on their surviving children's development. Parents, children, grandparents, and others close to the family may need assistance with "reentry" into family life following the death.

I was sent to detention 17 times, and my parents never knew. I wanted to hurt people because I wanted them to understand how much my sister hurt.
—13-year-old boy whose sister died

For fear of upsetting them, and for fear of not getting attention from them, children do not always ask their parents for help after a family member dies.

> I did not feel prepared to take on the role of the older sibling to my sister. So, I go out itching for something, to a place where I know that there will be some action.
> —17-year-old boy whose sister died

> He always protected the younger kids. Now I feel that responsibility falls to me.
> —15-year-old boy whose cousin died

When a sibling dies, components of reality change, even birth order: You can become the oldest, the youngest, or the only. There may also be certain responsibilities, roles, rules, or privileges that change. Some children, latency age and older, needing an outlet for their emotions, may find themselves lashing out and trying to hurt others as a way of managing their own anger and hurt feelings. Such children need support, guidance, and redirection of their pain. They need to be reminded that parents and other relatives care about them and can be trusted to help them.

> My father is trying to shield me from bad things, but I already know that the worst can happen.
> —15-year-old girl whose sister died

As protective of children as parents are, children also learn to be protective of their parents, regardless of the dynamics after the death. The ongoing relationship parents have with the deceased child is complicated. Deceased children often become immortalized; their imperfections vanish. Surviving children have to live through the illness and death of their siblings, and they subsequently may have to live up to their legacies. Children may feel that they are competing with their deceased siblings for the attention of their parents.

Siblings consistently point out that if they could give one message to their parents, it would be that they are still alive. Although suffering the loss themselves, bereaved siblings need to know that their parents love them, that they are as important as the sibling who died, and that life is still worth living because of them. A feeling that "we are in this together" is desirable to help mitigate the loneliness and confusion engendered by the loss.

> One of my friends ... from camp once told me that her friend tried to compare her situation with herself, saying that her sister had just gone off to college. Things like this, I find, make you feel worse than you already feel. But even if your friends do stuff like this, you have to forgive them very quickly, because although things like this may make you angry, mad, sad, or all of the above, you have to believe that they are trying to help, not hurt you.
> —13-year-old boy, age 8 when his brother died

Adults may encourage a surviving child to go back to school immediately following the death of a family member, yet everything has changed. There is little to no expectation that adults will get on with their lives directly after a loss. Alternatively, when children do want to resume normal activities with friends, parents may resist, feeling that their children are not experiencing or expressing "enough grief."

Unique Considerations

> In response to the question in a children's bereavement group, "What do you wish for?" a girl replied, "I would want my little brother back and I would also want to keep our adopted sister." She was very specific in her wish, because she knew that her family would not have adopted the baby had her brother not died.

There are siblings who will be *born mourning*, born after the death of a sibling or parent. They will never know their siblings, yet they will come to learn of the legacy of the child through the stories and the grief of family members. In other situations, there are children who come to learn that they were adopted or conceived after the death of a sibling, and that they would not have been born otherwise. This realization can provoke an existential crisis for the "surviving" child.

The uniqueness of twin loss is readily apparent. Of particular note is the loss of a co-twin during adolescence, because maturing children are already seeking to develop their own identity and now must proceed in the absence of a critical component present since birth (Withrow & Schwiebert, 2005). For grieving parents, the loss of a twin means living with one child who is a constant reminder of the other. Each birthday celebration, each new accomplishment is also a marker of the loss.

Developmental Considerations

> Two days after the Germans marched into Budapest, my mother called the pediatrician. "Would you come to see Gabi," she requested, "he has been crying almost without stop since yesterday morning." "I'll come, of course," the doctor replied, "but I should tell you: all my Jewish babies are crying." Now, what did Jewish infants know of Nazis, World War II, racism, genocide? What they knew—or rather, absorbed—was their parents' anxiety.... They inhaled fear, ingested sorrow. Yet were they not loved? No less than children anywhere. (Maté, 2010)
>
> A mother in a support group reported that her 4-year-old daughter, from the time when she started speaking, kept saying to her, "Not mommy," which gradually changed to, "You are not my mother." Finally,

the mother found the courage to ask her daughter why she kept saying this. The child replied, "When I was a baby, my mommy went away for a long time and sent that other woman [i.e., you] back." (When the child was 11 months old, her brother was diagnosed with leukemia. Her mother abruptly stopped breastfeeding and left to be with the brother in the hospital for an extended period of time.)

Issues of loss and grief in childhood cannot be managed in a linear way or on an exclusively verbal plane. Children express themselves both verbally and nonverbally. Infants may not be able to express grief in a way that is easily understood, but they will certainly feel the affective climate in the household in which they live.

Language is a very important component of communication. Even when not being spoken to, children hear the language around them. One 4-year-old boy whose father died in Iraq thought he died on a rock. Another 5-year-old child thought that when the doctor came to "take blood" it was all the blood in someone's body. A 4-year-old boy was sad, because he did not understand how he could be his sibling's bone marrow donor, because he was afraid that he could only be helpful if he had "a bow and arrow."

Upon learning that she would be going to heaven to be with her grandmother, Vicky, age 5, innocently asked, "Do I need to bring another dress? Do I have to brush my teeth in Heaven?" She told me that she knew that people did not live forever, and that she knew people in Heaven. Then she asked, "Where do you go after Heaven? When you die there, where do you go?" She saw Heaven as one step in a continuum with successive deaths. (Cincotta, 2004)

When talking with bereaved children, it must be clear that they understand what is being said, both from semantic and cognitive perspectives. Young children are concrete and literal in their interpretations (Speece & Brent, 1992). At times of stress, children may be unable to make sense of what is happening and will require simple, unambiguously worded explanations.

Children force adults to think about issues that they may not be ready to address. However, if children are able to ask, adults need to respond. When speaking with children, it is most effective to answer the questions they are asking rather than impose adult thoughts and concerns.

After his mother died unexpectedly following routine surgery, an 8-year-old boy was having trouble sleeping and began bed-wetting. In bereavement counseling, in a medical play session, he set up a play hospital bed with characters. Once he set up the scene, he would throw the little boy and his toys out of the bed, as if to discard them. I would place them back in the bed and he would throw them out. He was very creative in the very many ways he threw the boy out of the room. He told me, "After things die, they get thrown away." In real life, he

had given his mother his blanket for security when she went to the hospital. Because of concerns about infection, the blanket was thrown out after his mother died. I explained that sometimes things get thrown away, but not people. People are loved forever. This is a conversation that could never have been had in the first person. After multiple sessions of reenactment, his bed-wetting and sleep issues subsided. There were many themes of "protection" in this work. The child could not protect his mother, even having given her his blanket; she could not protect the blanket; and her death could not protect him. (Cincotta, 2004)

The use of metaphor can be an effective way to give children information and to help them construct a reality that they can understand and accept (Mills & Crowley, 1986). Children's books can also serve as tools to help children understand and relate to the death of a sibling, a parent, a grandparent, a friend, or other significant people and pets (Altilio, 2002). Children's literature is very comforting, because it is often a staple of everyday life and something with which children can explore ideas and feelings related to a death experience (e.g., *Badger's Parting Gifts, The Tenth Good Thing about Barney, The Fall of Freddie the Leaf,* and *My Grandpa Died Today,* each of which uses animals and plant life to explore death-related issues).

An 11-year-old girl would not engage in conversation about her mother's death and was not moved to tears in the initial months. She would, however, sing in the loudest voice, assuring that everyone could hear, a song from church that contained the line, "Sometimes I feel like a motherless child." It was both a personal, public, and cultural refrain.

Grief is uncomfortable, and children must find ways to make it tolerable. Adults need to respect the creativity and innocence with which children approach the bereavement process.

I wanted to go ice-skating after the funeral, but nobody thought that I should go. It seemed unfair that my mother had died and that I could not go ice-skating.
—12 year-old girl

After the death of a significant family member, children need to know that their basic needs will be met and understand who will meet them (Christ & Christ, 2006). Their inherent narcissism helps them survive emotionally. Bereavement groups for children are an effective intervention, allowing children to be children and providing a controlled venue for reacting to loss. When children do not have to explain themselves to each other, they feel safe: A burden is lifted.

A child, in responding to her parent's decision not to celebrate the Christmas holidays shortly after the death of her brother asserted, "But I didn't die." She did not feel comfortable raising this issue with her parents, but she was comfortable discussing it in a bereavement group.

Bereaved children carry the burden of their grief through everyday life. Since the world most children live in is generally antithetical to loss and suffering, it can be a very difficult place for bereaved children to discuss their true feelings. They may find it easier to keep their thoughts private. When children are on active cancer treatment, it is not uncommon for them to wear a hat or a wig to compensate for the fact that they are bald. Similarly, bereaved children, actively grieving, want to hide their grief from others, so that they do not have to admit to being different or vulnerable.

I thought that my mother was crazy for decorating and having parties at the grave. It made me think about her differently, and it gave me great peace to know that other mothers were doing the same thing.
—18-year-old teen whose brother died

Children strive to be like their peers and by the time they reach adolescence, they want to avoid anything that might make them seem different. Adolescents who experience the loss of a sibling, in particular, may experience a crisis which can result in a search for new meaning in life and increased spirituality at a time when they are already burdened by new developmental tasks (Batten & Oltjenbruns, 1999). Teenagers are also profoundly affected when confronted with the loss of a peer (Ringler & Hayden, 2000).

Understanding the timeline of a child's grief can be complicated. It does not necessarily follow a progressive path; it follows a developmental continuum. What may seem resolved in the context of one age can unravel at the next. At each age, more is understood about life, illness, and death, and children need to work through the feelings of that particular developmental stage (Slaughter, 2005). As opposed to losses in adult life, which can be expected to lessen with time, losses in childhood are revisited throughout life into adulthood.

Continuing Bonds

A teenager began working on the concept of continuing a bond with her father after her death. She told her father that she would send him a postcard from Heaven after she died. Although the postcard has not arrived yet, the concept has been a great help to her father.

During the early part of the twentieth century, the idea took hold that for the bereaved to achieve closure and successfully grieve, they needed to disengage emotionally and detach themselves from the deceased. More recent models have focused on adaptation to the world without the loved one, while maintaining a continuing bond with the deceased (Field, Gao, & Paderna, 2005; Klass, Silverman, & Nickman, 1996). Some children use the deceased person referentially at times of decision making or during life's stresses and successes (Hogan & DeSantis, 1992).

The nature of the child's relationship with the surviving parent is the single most important factor influencing a child's response to death (Haine, Ayers, Sandler, & Wolchik, 2008). Family caregivers can model adaptive behaviors to encourage the development of healthy continuing bonds between their children and the deceased by being present, listening empathically, and offering consolation. Surviving children need encouragement so they do not feel guilty about continuing their own lives. There should be no preconceived notion that continuing bonds emerge immediately at the time of death; they may take time to develop (Packman et al., 2006).

A young man, who had lived with his illness for 22 years, was an accomplished saxophone player. His recordings became even more important after his death. In each of them you could hear his breathing between certain notes. For his mother this was the way she held on to the reality of his life while mourning his loss. Captured in his music, his breath, a true symbol of his essence, was very much alive.

Preserving handprints, voices, or handwritten items helps children hold onto "signature" pieces of loved ones as reminders of their presence on earth. Continuing bonds are not limited to family members. The enduring nature of loss between friends may sometimes be overlooked.

A 24-year-old recounted how she both named her child after a classmate who had died 10 years previously and got married on the anniversary of his death. Because the wedding was on that day, she felt at peace and that her childhood friend was telling her that all would be well and work out.

Models of Intervention

Individual counseling, children's bereavement groups, family treatment, parent guidance, parents' support groups, and family retreats are all interventions that can help bereaved children or those anticipating the death of a significant person (Horsley & Patterson, 2006). The goals for such interventions are to help the child and family cope during the later stages of the illness, to work on activities and experiences that will help the child feel engaged and connected to the person who is ill, and to ultimately work toward continued growth and positive resolution of the loss. Family bereavement retreats (see Table 28.2) represent a model of intervention that meets many of the underlying needs of bereaved children.

My last thing is coming up with ways to tell kids about going to camp [bereavement sessions]. This is hard, but something that I have found that works is being straightforward with them. If they are your friends, then they will respect you for who you are, and they will be the ones that you can talk to, confide in, and do

Table 28.2.
Key Attributes of a Bereavement Retreat

A bereavement retreat that is helpful to children and their families will do the following:

- Allow families to meet others in similar situations
- Normalize an abnormal situation
- Allow for sharing ideas on how to cope
- Allow for connections to be made with a diverse group of people
- Minimize the feelings of isolation and of being "ostracized" by peers
- Allow for age-appropriate activities that include fun as part of the process
- Give permission for laughter and tears
- Provide hope, as the bereaved meet others ahead of them on the journey
- Provide solace, as other families "seem normal," indicating that the bereaved might be as well
- Provide a safe environment to talk about painful situations
- Provide an environment to talk about things that might otherwise seem odd (e.g., the desire to dream about the deceased, no longer being afraid to die)
- Offer ceremonies and rituals for a family to share and then replicate at home if they choose
- Create a place where death is comfortable
- Have access to and promote the use of support groups
- Have access to programming for groups of children who are the same age
- Present opportunities for growth
- Support strengths and communication
- Encourage families to have fun together, even though they have experienced a loss
- Provide role modeling for grieving
- Build family memories
- Honor the deceased
- Connect children with other children; facilitate friendships
- Allow professionals to see not just individual concerns, but population-based concerns, and allow for program development

whatever else you need to. If they hear that "I am going to camp over the weekend," and you tell them about it and then they laugh, then they are not your real friends. I have lost a lot of "friends" this way, but it has taken a turn for the better. If this life-changing situation hadn't happened, then I wouldn't know who my real friends are.
—Bereaved brother, age 13

Many of the children who return to bereavement retreats feel as though they are places of true friendship and understanding. However, they are sometimes met with sarcasm from their friends, teachers, and coaches who do not understand why they would need or want to go to such a program. As a culture, we would like to believe that grief is more time limited.

What I like about camp is that I do not have to explain myself because everyone understands.
—Bereaved sister, age 12

I love Camp Sunshine, because it gave my son back his childhood.
—Mother of three bereaved children

Bereaved Parents

As a counselor, in a cabin of girls with cancer, I found myself captive as they braided my hair. During this time, they began a discussion about who would take care of their parents after they died. They talked about their wishes for the epitaphs on their tombstones and how they thought their parents would do, and what they would need for help. When they were ready to move on, my hair was done. Each of these children went on to die (after which I did share their discussions with their parents). (Cincotta, 2004)
"Perhaps the reason I came to know other kids who have died is so that I will know people when I get there." This teen turned her grief for friends who died of cancer into preparation for her own death. Dealing with your own mortality is within the purview of more advanced development. This teenager was able to grieve for the loss of her own life, while helping her sibling and parents on their journey toward her death.

One of the primary concerns for children who are aware of their own impending deaths is how their parents will function afterwards. Children embody the hopes of the future; therefore, the dreams of parents are lost when their child is lost. When the natural order of life is disrupted and a child becomes gravely ill, the homeostasis of the family changes, and the lives of all family members are altered forever.

Parents report that the visceral response to grief changes, but that the sense of loss and of longing never fades; it is a loss with which they may never come to terms. Lannen and colleagues (2008) investigated the consequences of unresolved grief in 449 parents who had lost a child to cancer 4 to 9 years previously. Those who felt that they had worked through their grief reported fewer physical and psychological problems than those with unresolved grief. Li and coworkers (2003) examined Danish national registries of population statistics and identified 21,082 parents whose children had died and 293,746 controls in which family structures matched the identified families whose children had died. There was an excess mortality rate from natural causes in mothers 10 to 18 years after the child's death and from non-illness-related causes (including suicide) in both mothers and fathers. The same group found that there was a relative risk of 1.67 for psychiatric hospitalization for bereaved parents compared to controls and that mothers were at greater risk than fathers (Li, Laursen, Precht, Olsen, & Mortensen, 2005). In addition, a child's death may create a difficult emotional climate between parents (Schwab, 1992). They experience both the loss of the child and the loss of each other for support, as each is caught up in his or her own grief (Barrera et al., 2007; Rando, 1983). Although parents have been found to cope differently, the assumption that there is a higher divorce rate in this community has been called into question (Schwab, 1998).

Utilizing qualitative analysis of structured interviews, Barrera and colleagues (2007) investigated patterns of bereavement in 20 parents who had experienced the loss of a child to cancer, congenital heart disease, meningitis, or drowning. They found that 13 parents expressed uncomplicated *integrated grief*, 5 mothers were *consumed by grief*, and 1 mother and 1 father displayed *minimal grief*. Those who had integrated grief well identified their remaining children as objects of hope and purpose in life, were well supported by friends and family, and kept busy with work, as well as physical routines and exercise. Mothers who were consumed by grief were so overwhelmed by the loss that it interfered with daily life. They sought out reminders of their deceased children to feel connected with them and found it difficult to reframe their losses. Those with remaining children found difficulties in parenting them, while the two who had lost their only child found it difficult to be around other children and their families. In general, they felt socially isolated. The two parents who experienced minimal (i.e., inhibited) grief demonstrated restricted affects, but they scored lowest on an inventory of depression. They tended to busy themselves with family and other responsibilities. Of note, each had lost a child to unexpected illness, i.e., drowning and meningitis (Barrera et al., 2007).

It is reported by some that mothers are more vulnerable and have more adverse reactions after the death of a child than do fathers (Florian & Krulik, 1991; Schwab, 1996; Sidmore, 1999). Role definitions and functions for mothers create a bond which when broken by illness or death can create inner turmoil regarding their purpose and function in life. In a recent study of 219 Dutch couples who had lost a child, Wijngaards-de Meij and coworkers (2005) also found that mothers reported more grief and depression than did fathers. Fathers may experience social isolation, while at the same time deliberately isolating themselves. They are not unamenable to support services, however (Aho, Tarkka, Astedt-Kurki, & Kaunonen, 2009). By their inclusive nature, retreat programs that involve the entire family are well positioned to serve fathers.

The death of a child imposes a "crisis of meaning" for many parents (Miles & Demi, 1983–84). Over the past few decades attempts have been made to understand the parameters that impact the course of adult bereavement following a child's death. In a 2004 paper, Goodenough and colleagues studied Australian parents who had lost a child to cancer and learned that bereaved fathers exhibited greater psychological distress if their children had died in the hospital rather than at home (Goodenough, Drew, Higgins, & Trethewie, 2004). In a comparative study of 203 bereaved parents, Wheeler (1993–94) found lower "purpose in life" scores for adults who were more newly bereaved, suffered the loss of a child to suicide, lost an only child, or lost more than one child. In situations in which an only child dies, parents must face not only the loss of the child but also issues of personal identity with regard to parenthood. However, Wheeler's study is hopeful for the future of bereaved parents, in that 57% said they had some reinvestment in life and 74% reported that their life was worth living (Wheeler, 1993–94).

Keesee and colleagues (2008) studied 157 bereaved parents in an effort to identify risk factors for grief severity. They examined the degree to which bereaved parents were able to make sense of an incomprehensible loss, often in spiritual or philosophical terms, as well as assessing their ability to find some benefit from the process (e.g., different sense of life's meaning, greater sense of compassion). Sense making was the strongest predictor of grief severity, not unexpected given that some of the children had met accidental or violent deaths, whereas benefit finding was not a factor.

Recognizing that there is variability in how people respond to and live with chronically stressful situations, it becomes important to understand factors that may serve to be protective during the process. Over decades, investigators have consistently found that bereaved individuals with higher religious affiliations seem to have less severe grief reactions and less fear of death (Bohannon, 1991; Sormanti & August, 1997). However, in a study of 621 respondents who had lost a child some time in their lives, Higgins (2002) found only weak associations between levels of depression and religiosity but documented lower levels of depression among married women and men with higher levels of education.

As they tolerate the intolerable, bereaved families find value in helping others through sharing their death experiences (Hynson, Aroni, Bauld, & Sawyer, 2006). The more parents expect the loss, the easier the journey of grief is; the more parents share the loss, the less isolating the reality of the death becomes (Wijngaards-De Meij et al., 2008).

Table 28.3.
Themes in Parents' Bereavement Groups

Longing for the child and the awareness of the length of time that one will have to live without a deceased child	*I cannot imagine that I might have to live another 50 years.*
Role confusion	*I have been taking care of her for 10 years; I don't know what else I can do.*
Circumstances around the child's death and coming to terms with the end of the child's life	*I wish we had done an autopsy so that we could understand why she died.*
Impact of the death on relationships with family members, friends, and associates at work	*Many people stopped talking to us.*
Not being understood	*Aren't you over this yet?*
Reframing one's own role in the world (the number of children you now have)	*If I say I have one child, I feel like I am denying the life of my daughter who died. If I say I have two children, but one died, I am in for a conversation I do not want to have.*
The need to talk and the inability of others to engage in the ongoing conversation	*Most people think that I should be done with it. I will never be done with it.*
The decisions that parents make about the "worldly" goods of their child	*I still have her room exactly as it was.*
The passage of time	*Is she aging in Heaven? Do I think of her at the age when she died, or the age that she would be now?*
The meaning of life now and in the future, the existential journey	*What would he have gone on to do with his life? What would he want me to do with my life?*
Connections to the natural world in relationship to your child. The concern does not stop because you have buried your child; you are still a parent.	*I worry that she will be cold and wet when it snows. (As a nonbereaved parent you do not always think about things in this context and it is uncomfortable to hear and relate to.)*
The needs of their surviving children	*Am I half the parent I used to be?*
The ongoing relationship with sleep, a common problem in the group	*A father's feeling was that he had to protect his family. He often had sleepless nights and checked in on all the remaining family members as they slept.*
The ongoing relationship with the deceased child, how they think about that relationship, and how that impacts the relationships with their other children	*On a number of occasions, a mother got up and sang a song to honor her deceased daughter. The needs of her living daughter were so apparent to other parents in the group that the group challenged her to see them. On the last night of the program, the mother got on stage and dedicated a song to the daughter who was present with her. The group had done its work.*
The meaning of symbols and messages in the lives of parents	*A father asked a dying relative to meet with his son in Heaven and to ask him drop a penny near his dad whenever he was around. Now each time this father sees a penny, he feels the presence of his son.*

Family Memory

Family memory is a component of the emotional armor that defines each family (Cincotta, 1989). Interwoven within the fabric of our minds are those memories that we share with family members that are derived during early childhood and times of family transitions. As time goes on, these shared memories serve as intellectual and emotional pillars, enabling strong family bonds. They define a component of the culture of a family. Adults and children carry this wealth of knowledge about the past and are able to bring it into conscious memory at critical moments in the present. It serves as a vehicle for understanding one's role in the family and the connections among family members (Cincotta, 2008). Clinicians working with families at all stages of illness are in a unique position to help them create special moments and activities, knowing that these memories will stay with a family for years to come. A regular time might be established when the child and adult read a particular book, eat ice cream together, or play a game. Time is a precious gift, at any stage of life, for a child.

One of the things that happens when a family member is diagnosed with a life-threatening illness is that family life changes. Sections of that memory bank become consumed by memories of illness. Often spending inordinate amounts of time apart from one another causes family members' experiences to become separate. The volumes of memories begin to have different chapters. Illness and death take away the ability of families to share the past in the future.

Among the times that families share are those days, hours, and moments when death is imminent. The focus is often on the tasks at hand and not necessarily the lasting memories, yet memory making is important. "Emotional gift giving"— simple moments, words, gestures, and kind acts—will help children to come to terms with the loss of the person who is dying. The death experience will influence the way children remember the deceased and will inform their coping with death later in life.

Organized retreat programs are but one avenue in which clinicians can create nurturing, hopeful, safe, honest, inclusive environments, affording opportunities consonant with normal child development and the building of future family memories. The actual environment serving the family when a family member is ill (hospital room, clinic, home hospice) can be made to feel safe, friendly, and even fun, so that children can feel comfortable. At times when children cannot be present with family members who are ill, such as during a flu epidemic, the use of computer-based communication tools, such as Skype, means that the hospital experience does not have to remain invisible to a child. In many schools, children who are not able to attend can still be present in their classrooms via Webcams, and there are hospital programs such as Starbright that connect hospitalized children with each other.

To serve as a buffer against the intense memories in the days before someone dies, it is useful to help families to have memorable moments that will last forever.

A child and her family created a new costume for her to wear when her doctor made nightly rounds. This kept both the family and the staff in an active, creative place facing her impending death, and created a legacy (Cincotta, 2004).

Rituals and Therapeutic Activities

Enabling hope is an important goal in working with children facing life-limiting illness and end-of-life issues in their families. There are many rituals that families create while their children are growing up. Once a family member is diagnosed with a life-limiting illness, these rituals and activities become even more important. Taking the time to create an opportunity with a child, to sit and read a book, to draw a picture, or to write a note, can all seem "burdensome" during an illness period. Helping families to recognize the value in these activities as well as others, such as taking photos, creating albums, journals, and innovative ways to "record time," can be fulfilling during the illness period and afterwards.

In one family, every time they came home from the hospital, mother and son would bake something. Years later, it is the baking that the child remembers.

Responses to death are often learned in childhood, because children see how the adults around them grieve and endeavor to comfort themselves and their loved ones. For children especially, boundless grief is too difficult to understand and endure. Rituals and activities can begin to restore order and provide a framework in which children can experience grief in a time-limited, focused way. They can serve as symbols of hope and healing. They honor and keep the memory and spirit of the deceased alive, offer support to those engaged in the process, and give a greater message to all involved that should they die, they will be remembered.

Children worry that they will forget the person who died. Activities focused on remembering, creating tangible items, or ways to document the relationship can facilitate children's coping and mitigate against the "surreal" feeling bereaved children can experience. Religious and cultural rituals also offer comfort and structure to children and their adult family members and should be identified as a resource to enhance coping.

Expressing, reenacting, releasing, and visiting complex feelings can enable children as they accompany those who are important to them on their journey through illness. For all bereaved children, regardless of who died in their lives, it is in the combination of things—activating old memories, creating new memories, experiencing present emotions about the deceased, and having positive experiences with others who have shared similar experiences—that serve as catalysts to help enable children and their families to come to peace with their losses. In the quest for meaning and a greater understanding of life and death, children can be leaders in identifying activities that meet their needs.

Conclusion

Children are basically resilient and have many natural support structures in their families, their schools, their communities, their religious organizations, and throughout their lives that can help them deal with their losses and work through their grief. Social workers are in a unique position, whether as providers of services or as referral sources to appropriate programs and agencies, to recognize and address the needs of children dealing with illness and loss in their lives. Such service can make a difference in the lives of children who have experienced losses, while they are children, and for decades to come.

LEARNING EXERCISES

In working with children, social workers can find themselves in a position to engage in therapeutic activities or to enable parents to work with their children in such activities. These may not only facilitate adaptation to illness and death but also provide the social worker with useful information about the child and the child's adjustment to the situation. Within the safety of these exercises, students, clinicians, and parents can learn to deal with and grow from the complicated issues they face in dealing with a child's reaction to illness and death.

- Find an open space for a biodegradable helium balloon release. Whether balloons are released alone or in a group (as a wish for someone who is living with an illness or to honor someone who has died), they can provide an emotional venue for expression, release, and catharsis. Having participants write on the balloons—a message to the loved one, an emotion, or something they would like to dispense with—adds another dimension to this activity. The action of writing on the balloons, the fluidity of magic markers, and the "impermanence" of the balloons allow for a more visceral expression of emotion on the part of the writer. The period before the balloon launch can be one of personal reflection, while the time after can be one of reminiscing, regrouping, and even relief. The physical separation with the balloon can help children with a visual portrayal of being connected, moving on, and letting go. Watching the balloon go off, and ultimately walking away from the spot where the balloon is released, can move children toward feelings of reconciliation with the loss.
- Drawing can be helpful, but one particular activity that has proved valuable is "drawing your family in three dimensions: in the past, in the present, and in the future" (Cincotta, 2003). The use of three time periods accesses emotional content that exposes a multi-dimensional sense of self (and is easy to achieve by folding the paper in thirds). It allows children to reflect on a younger age and project to an older age, affording them another avenue to conceptualize and understand themselves.
- A very common activity is to write a letter to the person who died, either saying something that might not have been said, or reinforcing something that was said. It is not unusual for a child to want such letter to go in the casket. Another venue for letter writing is the use of edible paper (available at candy stores, not stationery stores). Children can write something that may (or may not) feel threatening and, having expressed it, they can consume it. Something that might be too difficult or private to record for posterity might be better "served" on edible paper. Rather than being consumed by the emotion, the child can consume the words. These activities also give children permission to let others know that they have private thoughts and feelings about the deceased.
- Bibliotherapy, the art of using books in a therapeutic way, is an effective avenue for helping children understand and manage their feeling about illness and death (Altilio, 2002). Invariably, any library or bookstore that has a children's section will have a number of books that parents can read through with their children.
- The idea for the "Healing Circles" program was derived from a recurring clinical concern raised by parents about what to with their deceased children's clothing. Bereavement quilting becomes something that parents do for their deceased children. However, the process requires an ability to be present in a situation of great intensity. It engages families in decision making about their child once again. Touching, being near the clothing, and simply having the clothing out in public, can be complicated, painful, and wonderful. Each step is fraught with caution, discovery, and ultimately satisfaction, accomplishment, and closure. The items created can have many emotional lives, can serve as "transitional objects" of sorts with the person who died, and can serve as a bridge to the future, giving new meaning and purpose to the cherished items.
- Planting a tree or flowers, or creating a memorial garden can serve emotional and existential purposes, symbolically connecting someone who is dying or has died to something that is alive, that can still grow and be nurtured. The planting itself can be something from which other rituals and emotional outlets grow. When working outdoors, the weather should be seen as an asset: Whatever it adds serves as a reminder that the weather, like life itself, is something that cannot be controlled. The nurturing of indoor plants can be an easy, meaningful activity in which social workers can engage in an office or that family members can continue at home. Taking care of something at a time when someone they love is ill can afford even young children a feeling of control and mastery over a situation involving living things.
- When working with children, clinicians can turn virtually anything into creative activities, given the time and enthusiasm. For instance, elephants are associated with themes that resonate with bereavement work: elephants never forget (as people are never forgotten) and the theme of "the elephant in the room"

(the loneliness and pain associated with grief is difficult to share).

In a bereavement group for parents, the concept was to speak of the most personal issues that symbolized the elephant in the room, nurtured by gifts of small elephants for participants. In children's groups, the idea of elephants never forgetting prevailed. Younger children made papier-mâché elephants and elephants from rocks. In a communal syringe art painting (another component of medical play), a hidden elephant emerged under layers of paint. The image that emerged, and ensuing conversations, facilitated a creative expression for grief.

ADDITIONAL RESOURCES

READINGS

Doka, K. J. (1995). *Children mourning, mourning children.* New York, NY: Routledge.

Grollman, E. A. (1991). *Talking about death: A dialogue between parent and child.* Boston, MA: Beacon Press.

Grollman, E. A. (1993). *Straight talk about death for teenagers: How to cope with losing someone you love.* Boston, MA: Beacon Press.

Mehren, E. (1997). *After the darkest hour the sun will shine again: A parent's guide to coping with the loss of a child.* New York, NY: Fireside.

Miller, S., & Ober, D. (2002). *Finding hope when a child dies: What other cultures can teach us.* New York, NY: Fireside.

Rosof, B. D. (1995). *The worst loss: How families heal from the death of a child.* New York, NY: Henry Holt and Company.

Schaefer, C. E. (1989). *The therapeutic use of child's play.* Lanham, MD: Jason Aronson.

Schaefer, C. E. (1992). *Therapeutic powers of play.* Lanham, MD: Jason Aronson.

Silverman, P. R., & Kelly, M. (2009). *A parent's guide to raising grieving children: Rebuilding your family after the death of a loved one.* New York, NY: Oxford.

Strongin, L. (2010). *Saving Henry.* New York, NY: Hyperion Books.

Webb, N. B. (2010). *Helping bereaved children, third edition: A handbook for practitioners.* New York, NY: Guilford Press.

Wolfelt, A. D. (2001). *Healing a child's grieving heart: 100 practical ideas for families, friends and caregivers.* Fort Collins, CO: Companion Press.

WEB SITES

Art with Heart: http://www.artwithheart.org
An organization that focuses on healing kids through creativity.

Camp Sunshine: http://www.campsunshine.org
Retreat center for children with life-threatening illnesses and their families, as well as bereaved families.

Care Notes: http://www.carenotes.com
Helping You Help Others: messages of hope and compassion to those in need.

The Center for Grieving Children: http://www.cgcmaine.org/
Provides support, education, and information to grieving children and their families.

The Center for Loss & Life Transition: http://www.centerforloss.com/
The Center for Loss is dedicated to "companioning" grieving; an educational resource and professional forum.

Compassion Books: http://www.compassionbooks.com
Books, videos, and audios to help children and adults through serious illness, death and dying, grief, bereavement, and losses of all kinds.

The Compassionate Friends: http://compassionatefriends.org
Support and information for a family after a child dies.

The Dougy Center for Grieving Children and Families: http://www.dougy.org
Provides support groups, education, and training for children, teens, young adults, and their families.

The Grieving Center:
A Web-based television channel devoted to assisting those who have lost loved ones, created through Continuum Hospice Care at its Bereavement Center. The Center reaches out with a series of mailings that discuss such issues; it also offers informative workshops and makes individual counseling and support groups available.

National Air Disaster Alliance Foundation: http://planesafe.org/planesafe_archive/books/bereavementlibrary.shtml
Resources for sudden loss or tragic death.

Open to Hope: http://www.opentohope.com
Finding hope after loss through information and resources for those who have experienced a loss, and educational grants and networking support for those whose studies are focused on improving the care of people who grieve.

Solace House: http://www.solacehouse.org
A center for grieving children and their families.

SuperSibs!: http://www.supersibs.org/the-sib-spot/bereaved-main.html
Resources for siblings of children with cancer (bereaved and nonbereaved).

REFERENCES

Aho, A. L., Tarkka, M. T., Astedt-Kurki, P., & Kaunonen, M. (2009). Fathers' experience of social support after the death of a child. *American Journal of Men's Health, 3*(2), 93–103.

Altilio, T. (2002). Helping children, helping ourselves: An overview of children's literature. In J. V. Loewy & A. F. Hara (Eds.), *Caring for the caregiver: The use of music and music therapy in grief and trauma* (pp. 138–147). Silver Springs MD: American Music Therapy Association.

Balk, D. (1983). Adolescents' grief reactions and self-concept perceptions following sibling death - a study of 33 teenagers. *Journal of Youth and Adolescence, 12*(2), 137–161.

Barrera, M., D'Agostino, N. M., Schneiderman, G., Tallett, S., Spencer, L., & Jovcevska, V. (2007). Patterns of parental bereavement following the loss of a child and related factors. *Omega-Journal of Death and Dying, 55*(2), 145–167.

Batten, M., & Oltjenbruns, K. A. (1999). Adolescent sibling bereavement as a catalyst for spiritual development: A model for understanding. *Death Studies, 23*(6), 529–546.

Bohannon, J. R. (1991). Religiosity related to grief levels of bereaved mothers and fathers. *Omega*, 23(2), 153–159.

Christ, G. H., & Christ, A. E. (2006). Current approaches to helping children cope with a parent's terminal illness. *Ca-A Cancer Journal for Clinicians*, 56(4), 197–212.

Cincotta, N. (1989). Quality of life: A family decision. In J. van Eys (Ed.), *Cancer in the very young*. Springfield, IL: Charles Thomas.

Cincotta, N. (2003). Drawing in three dimensions: Transcending time. In H. G. Kaduson & C. Schaefer (Eds.), *101 favorite play therapy techniques* (Vol. 3, pp. 36–37). Northvale, NJ: Jason Aronson.

Cincotta, N. (2004). The end of life at the beginning of life: Working with dying children and their families. In J. Berzoff & P. R. Silverman (Eds.), *Living with dying: A handbook for end-of-life healthcare practitioners* (pp. 318–347). New York, NY: Columbia University Press.

Cincotta, N. (2008). Childhood cancer survivorship: The family's journey forward. *Archived Leukemia Teleconferences, The Leukemia and Lymphoma Society*. Retrieved from http://www.leukemia.org/all_page?item_id=556138

Field, N. P., Gao, B., & Paderna, L. (2005). Continuing bonds in bereavement: An attachment theory based perspective. *Death Studies*, 29(4), 277–299.

Florian, V., & Krulik, T. (1991). Loneliness and social support of mothers of chronically ill children. *Social Science Medicine*, 32(11), 1291–1296.

Fristad, M. A., Cerel, J., Goldman, M., Weller, E. B., & Weller, R. A. (2001). The role of ritual in children's bereavement. *Omega-Journal of Death and Dying*, 42(4), 321–339.

Goodenough, B., Drew, D., Higgins, S., & Trethewie, S. (2004). Bereavement outcomes for parents who lose a child to cancer: Are place of death and sex of parent associated with differences in psychological functioning? *Psycho-Oncology*, 13(11), 779–791.

Haine, R. A., Ayers, T. S., Sandler, I. N., & Wolchik, S. A. (2008). Evidence-based practices for parentally bereaved children and their families. *Professional Psychology-Research and Practice*, 39(2), 113–121.

Higgins, M. P. (2002). Parental bereavement and religious factors. *Omega-Journal of Death and Dying*, 45(2), 187–207.

Hogan, N., & DeSantis, L. (1992). Adolescent sibling bereavement: An ongoing attachment. *Qualitative Health Research*, 2(2), 159–177.

Horsley, H., & Patterson, T. (2006). The effects of a parent guidance intervention on communication among adolescents who have experienced the sudden death of a sibling. *American Journal of Family Therapy*, 34(2), 119–137.

Hynson, J. L., Aroni, R., Bauld, C., & Sawyer, S. M. (2006). Research with bereaved parents: A question of how not why. *Palliative Medicine*, 20(8), 805–811.

Keesee, N. J., Currier, J. M., & Neimeyer, R. A. (2008). Predictors of grief following the death of one's child: The contribution of finding meaning. *Journal of Clinical Psychology*, 64(10), 1145–1163.

Klass, D., Silverman, P. R., & Nickman, S. L. (1996). *Continuing bonds: New understandings of grief*. Philadelphia, PA: Taylor & Francis.

Lannen, P. K., Wolfe, J., Prigerson, H. G., Onelov, E., & Kreicbergs, U. C. (2008). Unresolved grief in a national sample of bereaved parents: Impaired mental and physical health 4 to 9 years later. *Journal of Clinical Oncology*, 26(36), 5870–5876.

Li, J., Laursen, T. M., Precht, D. H., Olsen, J., & Mortensen, P. B. (2005). Hospitalization for mental illness among parents after the death of a child. *New England Journal of Medicine*, 352(12), 1190–1196.

Li, J., Precht, D. H., Mortensen, P. B., & Olsen, J. (2003). Mortality in parents after death of a child in Denmark: A nationwide follow-up study. *Lancet*, 361(9355), 363–367.

Maté, G. (2010). *In the realm of hungry ghosts: Close encounters with addiction*. Berkeley, CA: North Atlantic Books.

Miles, M. S., & Demi, A. S. (1983–84). Toward the development of a theory of bereavement guilt: Sources of guilt in bereaved parents. *Omega*, 14(4), 299–314.

Mills, J. C., & Crowley, R. J. (1986). *Therapeutic metaphors for children and the child within*. New York, NY: Brunner/Mazel.

Packman, W., Horsley, H., Davies, B., & Kramer, R. (2006). Sibling bereavement and continuing bonds. *Death Studies*, 30(9), 817–841.

Rando, T. A. (1983). An investigation of grief and adaptation in parents whose children have died from cancer. *Journal of Pediatric Psychology*, 8(1), 3–20.

Ringler, L. L., & Hayden, D. C. (2000). Adolescent bereavement and social support: Peer loss compared to other losses. *Journal of Adolescent Research*, 15(2), 209–230.

Schwab, R. (1992). Effects of a child's death on the marital relationship: A preliminary study. *Death Studies*, 16(2), 141–154.

Schwab, R. (1996). Gender differences in parental grief. *Death Studies*, 20(2), 103–113.

Schwab, R. (1998). A child's death and divorce: Dispelling the myth. *Death Studies*, 22(5), 445–468.

Sidmore, K. V. (1999). Parental bereavement: Levels of grief as affected by gender issues. *Omega-Journal of Death and Dying*, 40(2), 351–374.

Slaughter, V. (2005). Young children's understanding of death. *Australian Psychologist*, 40(3), 179–186.

Sonnenblick, J. (2005). *Drums, girls, and dangerous pie*. New York, NY: Scholastic Press.

Sormanti, M. E., & August, J. (1997). Parental bereavement: An exploration of parents' spiritual connections with their deceased children. *American Journal of Orthopsychiatry*, 67(3), 460–469.

Speece, M., & Brent, S. (1992). The acquisition of a mature understanding of three components of the concept of death. *Death Studies*, 16, 211–229.

Wheeler, I. (1993-94). The role of meaning and purpose in life in bereaved parents associated with a self-help group: Compassionate friends. *Omega*, 28(4), 261–271.

Wijngaards-De Meij, L., Stroebe, M., Schut, H., Stroebe, W., van den Bout, J., van der Heijden, P., & Djikstra, I. (2005). Couples at risk following the death of their child: Predictors of grief versus depression. *Journal of Consulting and Clinical Psychology*, 73(4), 617–623.

Wijngaards-De Meij, L., Stroebe, M., Stroebe, W., Schut, H., Van den Bout, J., Van der Heijden, P. G. M., & Djikstra, I. (2008). The impact of circumstances surrounding the death of a child on parents' grief. *Death Studies*, 32(3), 237–252.

Withrow, R., & Schwiebert, V. L. (2005). Twin loss: Implications for counselors working with surviving twins. *Journal of Counseling and Development*, 83, 21.

29

Susan Gerbino and Mary Raymer

Holding On and Letting Go: The Red Thread of Adult Bereavement

I have never felt so shattered, so broken, and so alone in my life. Everyone tells me things like I should let go and move on, I should get some medication, I'm young and will love again. Everyone tells me what I should be doing ... all I want to do is to cry. There must be something wrong with me.

—35-year-old woman 1 year after the death of her husband

Key Concepts
♦ *Bereavement is a universal process, but each journey is unique.*
♦ *Grief is a normative process.*
♦ *Many long-held assumptions regarding grief and bereavement are not supported by empirical research.*
♦ *Grief and bereavement are influenced by numerous variables, including culture, gender, and spirituality.*
♦ *The efficacy of bereavement interventions is unclear.*

Introduction

Palliative social workers across all practice settings will confront the phenomenon of grief and bereavement. Patients and their significant others are intimately acquainted with numerous emotional and physical losses due to serious illness long before death occurs. A grief and bereavement assessment needs to begin at the first social work visit.

Bereavement is commonly defined as the state of loss resulting from death (Parkes, 1997). Grief is the emotional response associated with loss (Stroebe, Stroebe, & Hansson, 1993). Grief as opposed to bereavement can be in response to any loss, not just death. It can affect whole groups or systems like families, schools, communities, and countries. Physical vulnerability, loss of control, divorce, and inability to fulfill important goals are just a few examples of life events that can stimulate a grief response. Grief is a multidimensional process with numerous symptoms that affect people physically, emotionally, cognitively, socially, and spiritually. It can be one of the most distressing times in people's lives. Mourning can be defined as the public display of grief (Stroebe, Hanssson, Schut, & Stoebe, 2008). However, in this chapter, mourning is defined as the intrapsychic processes and the attempts at coping that accompany a loss from a death (Rando, 1993).

Social workers need the most current information available in order to assess accurately and provide the appropriate interventions to help people cope. Determining the difference between normal grief and depression or other clinical disorders is crucial. When it comes to grief and loss, the words of Marie Von Ebner-Eschenbach ring true, "Nobody knows enough, but many know too much."

Challenging Assumptions

Normal grief is not pathology. It is often a challenging process that requires people to work to find a healthy "new normal." There are no tidy and predictable stages, but there may be intense feelings, disturbing thoughts, and life challenges that need to be addressed in a proactive manner. One important social work role is to educate people regarding the nature of normative grief and its variability.

There are many long-held assumptions about grief and bereavement that are not supported by empirical research. These stubbornly persist and can create more pain for grieving individuals when they apply them to their own process. Because of this, effective social workers need to explore what people have heard and believe in order to clear up any false information. Many people have reported feeling abnormal or inadequate when in fact they were grieving normally. This can cause harm during an already painful and difficult time.

One of the most common sayings about grief is that time heals. While this can be true for some, for others the passing of time can actually exacerbate their pain. Many people say they feel worse before they feel better. When they hear that time heals, they become frightened since the passage of time has only intensified their grief, not reduced it. Others believe that if they just "grit their teeth" and "hang on" that grief is supposed to automatically get better. When appropriate, we can help people employ proactive coping skills and behaviors such as social support, problem solving, and spiritual practices, and we can validate that what they are feeling is normal.

The belief that it takes 1 year after a death to resolve grief is a related assumption. Many people report the second year may actually be harder in some ways than the first because the finality of the loss is unavoidable and often social support wanes. Because of the "1 year rule," their anxiety is intensified when at the end of that first year they are still struggling. One of the most difficult aspects of grief for many people is that there is not a set timeline for feeling better. Skilled social workers assist individuals by helping them look at how they have historically dealt with losses and review what actions helped and did not help them cope previously.

Individuals are often told not to make any major decisions during the first year after a loss. This has become a mantra that many people believe they must follow to the letter. While it is wise to delay some decisions, it is not always practical or realistic to delay all major decisions. If, for example, a person holds onto a house he or she cannot afford, he or she could face bankruptcy. Effective social workers help people practice good critical thinking and weigh the pros and cons of decisions to determine whether making change is rational and necessary.

At one time it was also believed that all losses were the same. However, every loss is unique with different experiences and impact even if the relationship and manner of death are the same. When diverse types of loss such as suicide, the expected death of a parent, homicide, and so forth are compared, the trajectory and experience of grief can be very different.

People often hear that the goal of getting through grief is to forget and "let go." While this may be the goal for some types of grievers, others ask how it is possible to forget a significant relationship and let it go. Certainly we learn to carry the relationship differently, but that is not letting go. This assumption increases anxiety significantly because people often perceive it as the need to forget the person who has died. Even in difficult or ambivalent relationships there are insights and lessons learned that people can carry forward for healthier future function.

The most common assumption of all is that grief occurs in predictable stages. Grief is not a linear process, and there are many differences influenced by factors such as gender, culture, spirituality, and so forth. Grief is more like a roller coaster. People frequently fear they are not grieving correctly if they have not experienced specific stages with the final endpoint of acceptance. Many people also believe that expressing or venting emotions is the main aspect of healing, but talking about a loss is not helpful to everyone. Effective social work intervention focuses on helping our clients with their unique journey through loss; respecting and honoring difference; and helping people decide what will help them heal.

With the increase of grief therapists and counselors has grown the belief that grieving people require psychotherapy. People do not require therapy to get through normal grief nor do they require medication unless they have a prolonged grief disorder that is not responding to support and interventions, a preexisting condition, or their sleep deprivation is severe. Many grieving people in the United States are placed on antidepressants after loss when, in fact, they are not depressed. Others who are depressed are told they are just grieving. Since the symptoms may be similar, impeccable assessment is essential. Depression is not an inevitable aspect of grief. Depression is a clinical condition that may result due to a prolonged grief disorder. Depression requires therapy from a skilled social worker or other practitioner, and in some cases medication may be indicated. Grief, on the other hand, requires validation, education, connection, and support for healthy changes. Grief fluctuates: Physical symptoms come and go, emotions are charged and all over the board, pleasure is fleeting at first but comes in glimpses, and the individual is focused on how the loss has impacted him or her. In depression the focus is usually on the self and feelings of worthlessness. Emotions are fixed, self-destructive behaviors are relatively persistent, and there is prolonged and marked functional impairment and psychomotor retardation. Depression must be treated before an individual can assess and find his or her way of coping with grief.

Bereavement Research and Theory

There have been seismic shifts in bereavement research and theory in the last 10–15 years. Many long-held beliefs have been challenged, often leaving social workers uncertain about the efficacy of our work with bereaved individuals and families. Despite this confusion, the picture that is emerging is a more nuanced one, allowing social workers to tailor their interventions to the unique needs of each individual and family, rather than trying to fit people into a theoretical trajectory or presumed stages in the grief process.

Despite the dominance of stage theories which began emerging in the late 1960's and a range of taken-for-granted assumptions in the professional literature, many of us who were working with bereaved persons in recent decades were hearing stories from our clients that did not fit the model. Our personal experiences of mourning also shook us, because often they did not bear much resemblance to the theory we were reading about and learning. Now, theory is beginning to catch up to the lived experiences of the bereaved, primarily because some researchers began to let go of preconceived notions of mourning and to simply ask people to tell their own stories of grief.

> "The loss of my mother runs like a red thread through my life"
>
> —Ernst Freud, Freud's grandson

This quote (cited in Kaplan, 1995 p. 66) is from an interview with the adult Ernst Freud; his mother died when he was 5 years old. The red thread is a helpful metaphor when we consider the myriad ways people react to and cope with loss. Significant deaths bring the pain of separation, but "thread" tends to signify connection. There is an ancient Chinese proverb about a silk red thread of destiny that connects one person with another; this magical cord may stretch or become tangled, but it can never break. The proverb suggests we are all connected to those we love by an unbreakable red thread. Some of the bereaved with whom we work need to hold it tightly, some allow it to stretch, some become tangled in it, and some sew it carefully into their hearts, where it resides forever, invisible to the eye.

If we were looking at the narratives in Box 29.1 through the lens of bereavement theory 10 or 15 years ago, all the people, with the possible exception of Joan, would have been diagnosed as suffering from "pathological grief," requiring professional help. Looking at these stories now, only Miss Havisham's extreme reaction stands out, yet even she has much to teach us. Who among us has not wanted to stop the clocks when confronted with a life-altering loss? Auden's "Funeral Blues," begins:

> Stop all the clocks, cut off the telephone,
> Prevent the dog from barking with a juicy bone,
> Silence the pianos and with muffled drum
> Bring out the coffin, let the mourners come.
> (Auden & Isherwood, 1936)

Box 29.1
Patient/Family Narratives

Hannah's partner, Marie, died 3 years ago. She grieved intensely the first year but is doing quite well now. She occasionally worries about their three young adult daughters but knows they did a great job as parents and this gives her peace. Hannah has a secret. She writes to Marie—long letters telling her what is happening and how their girls are doing. She continues to do this even as she moves into her new life with passion and creativity and a sense of resilience.

Jerry's daughter, Pat, age 20, died suddenly 4 years ago. He still feels very sad, but he does not cry every day like he used to. He feels close to his daughter when looking at her pictures and sitting in her bedroom. He feels his wife, Joan, has moved on too quickly, wanting to do new things, explore new horizons, and "get on with living." His crying upsets her. He worries about their marriage; perhaps Joan did not love Pat as much as he did. He feels guilty at the thought and more alone than ever. Joan also feels lonely; she thinks she has failed her husband and fears she will lose him as well.

Sarah's husband, Lenny, died 18 months ago. She keeps busy and feels her life is moving forward. She misses Lenny and has done her share of crying, but she does not want to talk about her feelings; in fact, she feels she does best when she avoids reminders of him. She comes to counseling because she attended a widow/widower's bereavement group and felt so different from everyone else. Is she really as okay as she thinks? Everyone tells her she will eventually "crash."

Laura's son, John, a rookie police office, was killed on September 11th in the World Trade Center. No part of his body was ever recovered. It is 8 years since his death and she wonders why her friends and family are worried about her. She goes to work each day, sees family and friends when up to it, and volunteers at the local school. Her daughter thinks her preoccupation with making sense of what happened that day is morbid, but Laura still needs to ask why. She feels exhausted and demoralized by dreams that continue to be filled with death and destruction, "the nightmare that never ends." She wonders whether her friends and family are right. "I haven't reached the stage of acceptance," she says. "I'm not getting any better … I must be crazy … I will never accept what happened … nothing makes sense anymore."

Finally, a fictional character: Miss Havisham from Great Expectations (Dickens, 1861/2002). Jilted by her fiancé at exactly twenty to nine on their wedding day, she has stopped all the clocks at that exact hour and remains forever in her home, dressed in her wedding gown.

Joan Didion, in her 2005 memoir *The Year of Magical Thinking*, wonders about time as she grieves the death of her husband, John. She and John had lived a great deal of their time alternating between homes in California and New York. John dies in New York and she writes:

> I found myself wondering, with no sense of illogic, if it had also happened in Los Angeles. I was trying to work out what time it had been when he died and whether it was that time yet in Los Angeles. Was there time to go back? Could we have a different ending in Pacific Time? (p. 31)

Time can stop and start and stop again when we are grieving—following no fixed timetable and no linear course.

For many years the prevailing paradigm in the professional bereavement literature endorsed the idea that letting go and moving on is at the core of "successful" mourning. This concept has its earliest roots in Freud's famous essay "Mourning and Melancholia" (1917/1957). However, for many grievers, mourning is an intricate dance between holding on and letting go. Freud himself affirmed the endurance of his bonds to his own daughter and grandson, in a letter to a friend who had just lost his son:

Although we know that after such a loss, the acute state of mourning will subside, we also know that we shall remain inconsolable and will never find a substitute. No matter what will fill the gap, even if it be filled completely, it nevertheless remains something else. And, actually this is how it should be. It is the only way of perpetuating that love which we do not want to relinquish. (1929/1975, p. 386)

Hannah writes letters to her partner. Years ago, she would likely have been diagnosed as having "chronic grief." She is not moving on; rather, she is clinging to a relationship with Marie that no longer exists. Continuing bonds theory (Klass, Silverman, & Nickman, 1996) gives us a new window into Hannah's mourning. Many mourners, but not all, find ways of staying connected to the person who has died—constructing an ongoing, internal relationship with their loved one while accommodating to a world without that person. Writing letters is one way of continuing the bond; talking to, praying to, or naming someone after a loved one are others. Once Hannah was reassured that writing letters was fine, she felt no need for grief counseling. Hannah finds comfort holding tightly to the red thread, while at the same time moving forward in her life.

Sarah's story cautions us that we should also be wary of how continuing bonds should "work" for the bereaved. Sarah stays busy, does not want to talk about feelings, and avoids reminders of her husband. This is not to say she has not constructed a continuing internal relationship with him—she may have in her own way. In the past, she might have been seen as having "avoidant grief" and encouraged to "talk about her feelings." However, so-called avoidant mourners can do as well as, and sometimes better than, those who mourn like Hannah (Bonanno &Kaltman, 2001; Bonanno, Keltner, Holen, & Horowitz, 1995). Sarah is doing well, feels well, and is taking good care of herself. Concepts like "grief work" and "working through feelings" are not helpful to mourners like Sarah. Sarah needed to be given "permission" to grieve in her own way. She left the bereavement group and grief counseling and is doing fine. She has sewn the red thread into her heart, where it can hopefully live undisturbed by notions about the "right way" to grieve.

Jerry and Joan, a loving couple, are mourning in disparate ways. Stroebe, Schut, and Stroebe (2005) describe the "dual process" model of mourning. This model suggests that mourning includes loss-oriented activities and restoration-oriented activities; grieving is understood as involving an oscillation between the two. Loss-oriented activities can include crying, looking at pictures, talking about the person who died, and yearning or pining for the person. Restoration-oriented activities can include doing new things, taking on new roles and responsibilities that previously belonged to the deceased, and sometimes creating new rituals. Loss-oriented activities and restoration-oriented activities lie on a continuum. However, Jerry fell more on the loss-oriented end of the continuum and Joan fell more on the restoration-oriented end. Helping each spouse to understand this and join the other on his or her side of the continuum was important. Jerry agreed to try some new things with Joan, and Joan agreed to spend more time talking to Jerry about Pat. Both were relieved to hear that their ways of mourning had nothing to do with the amount of love they felt for their daughter. They are learning how the red thread can be stretched between them, in ways that honor their separation as well as their connectedness.

One way that grieving can be understood is that of an evolving process involving an ongoing tension between holding on and letting go. In his 2002 essay, David Browning, a social worker whose mother died when he was 13, spent many years trying to figure out why he did not seem to be "succeeding" in grief therapy. In his essay, "Saying good-bye, saying hello–A grief sojourn," he writes:

In retrospect, I believe concepts like "saying good-bye," "finding closure," and "moving on" became stumbling blocks. All the knowledge I garnered from therapy, from the culture, and from my own professional training, made me feel that "successful" grieving required me to say good-bye to Mom. I knew I needed to say good-bye in one sense, but in a more important sense, what I needed most was help in saying hello. When I could say good-bye to my grief without saying good-bye to Mom, I was free to love more fully in the present. I say good-bye to the dominion of grief in my life. I say hello to my friends, my loved ones and the infinite possibilities. And I say hello, in a new and tender way, to Mom. (p. 465)

The process of holding on and letting go is often quite complicated and painful. Judy Ryan lost her only son, Sean, at the age of 23:

I have had to find ways to sustain an emotional link to Sean, which does not lead to intolerable longing for him … To hold onto him when he is forever missing creates unbearable yearning; not to be able to hold him internally is equally unbearable. … My preoccupation with him can feel invasive, and can undermine the joy that life still holds. But I have feared losing him, since if I let him go—as I can my daughters—I can no longer find him in the real world. (Glennon, 2005, pp. 532–533)

Finally, there is Laura, who is mourning a loss that is relatively new to us in this country: death due to terrorism.

Laura, like Judy Ryan, speaks about the intolerable yearning for her son, coupled with a search for meaning. Laura might have been diagnosed with "unresolved grief" and her search for meaning seen as perseveration. However, there are mourners who, after a senseless death, search for meaning for a long, long time. Neimeyer (2001) has described the process of meaning making as the ability to make sense of the death, often in some larger spiritual, psychological, or existential framework. Attig (1996) has described it as "relearning the world." Making sense of a loss often includes the reconstruction of identity; indeed, Laura wonders just who she is now, given the violent death that has torn her world asunder.

In many ways Laura may have the hardest journey of all the mourners described in this chapter, particularly if she cannot make sense of the loss. Some beginning research has shown that mourners who search for meaning and do not find it, may not fare well and are at risk for complicated mourning (Davis, Nolen-Hoeksema, & Larson, 1998; Davis, Wortman, Lehman, & Silver, 2000; Keesee, Currier, & Neimeyer, 2008).

The death of Laura's son was violent and traumatic; this will complicate Laura's journey as well. One can see the trauma aspects in her dreams of destruction and violence. Laura also reminds us that stage theories do not do justice to certain kinds of loss, and that acceptance may not always be a feasible or realistic goal. Maciejewski, Zhang, Block, and Prigerson (2007) found that while some mourners go through stages of grief, there is not a linear progression from disbelief to acceptance. They also found that yearning is often the predominant emotion, not depression. This is important to keep in mind when working with people like Laura. Despite all of this, Laura is persevering: She is clinging to the red thread, no matter how tangled.

The current terms used to describe Laura's mourning include *complicated mourning, prolonged grief disorder,* and *traumatic grief.* The distinctions between these terms are not always clear. Laura is an example of someone whose journey through her grief is complicated by the violence of her son's death and her search for meaning. Laura's grief is also traumatic, because of its horrific nature and its suddenness—her son literally vanished into thin air. Mourning can be complicated because of the nature of the death, the type of loss, and other factors that are specific to the mourner. Except for Ms. Havisham, the narratives in this chapter all describe loving relationships. However, complicated mourning can also be seen following the death of someone with whom the relationship was more ambivalent, such as the death of a former partner. These losses can also be disenfranchised, a concept that will be discussed further later in this chapter.

Complicated mourning interferes with functioning over an extended period of time and leaves the mourner with little pleasure in life, particularly pleasure in the things the mourner enjoyed before the death. It is most often described as lasting more than 6 months, and its signature symptoms include intense yearning and intrusive thoughts and feelings of emptiness and loneliness. It can lead to substance use and abuse and suicidal thoughts.

Prolonged grief disorder is the newest term for this type of mourning, and it is being considered for inclusion as a diagnosis in the 2012 *Diagnostic and Statistical Manual, 5th edition* (Prigerson et al., 2009). The proposed criteria for the diagnosis require a reaction to a significant loss that involves the experience of yearning and at least five of the following nine symptoms experienced at least daily or to a disabling degree: feeling emotionally numb, stunned, or that life is meaningless; experiencing mistrust; bitterness over the loss; difficulty accepting the loss; identity confusion; avoidance of the reality of the loss; or difficulty moving on with life. Symptoms must be present at least 6 months after the death and be associated with functional impairment.

Social workers hear many stories from clients about resilience and growth following bereavement, including after traumatic losses. Bonanno (2009) writes about these positive emotions—emotions other than sadness—that can include a new sense of meaning in life and the stronger connection to others.

Hope and resilience are illustrated in this story told by Rabbi Kenneth Cohen in *Embracing Life and Facing Death: A Jewish Guide to Palliative Care* (Brenner, Blanchard, Hirschfield, & Fins, 2005):

> When my mother died, I inherited her needlepoint tapestries. When I was a little boy, I used to sit at her feet as she worked on them. Have you seen needlepoint from underneath? All I could see was chaos, strands of thread all over, with no seeming purpose. As I grew, I was able to see her work from above. I came to appreciate the patterns, and the need for dark threads as well as bright and gaily colored ones. Life is like that. From our human perspective, we cannot see the whole picture. But we should not feel despair or feel there is no purpose. There is meaning and purpose, even for the dark threads, but we cannot see that right away. (p. 34)

Variables Influencing the Grief Process

There are many variables that affect the grief process, including the mourner's relationship to the deceased, attachment and loss history, prior history of depression and anxiety, and concurrent stressors. All of these, plus the mourner's support system, are part of the assessment process.

Spirituality

Spirituality is a key variable that is often linked to the construction of meaning. It can include both religious faith and a sense of connectedness and meaning. Some people will define themselves as spiritual but not religious, so our assessment should always include questions about both. Spirituality can be defined as "the aspect of humanity that refers to the way individuals seek and express meaning and purpose and the way they experience their connectedness to the moment, to self, to others, to nature, and to the significant or sacred" (Puchalski et al., 2009, p. 887). Religion can include spirituality but also a set of institutionalized beliefs, worship practices, and rituals.

A spiritual assessment includes asking the bereaved to share his or her religious and spiritual beliefs and his or her own definition of spirituality. For some, their spirituality is a source of strength; for others the loss has led to spiritual distress and a sense of meaninglessness and hopelessness. Thomas Lynch (1997) speaks of "deaths that took," referring to deaths that shake us and shatter our assumptions about the world. These deaths can also affect our faith in God and our sense of meaning. For Laura, the death of her son at the World Trade Center was a "death that took." Somewhat religious but always very spiritual, she is struggling to find her way back to spiritual well-being. Identifying this as an important aspect of her grieving and spending time in counseling looking at ways to "restore my faith" have been essential.

Culture

Grief is a universal process, but there are many pathways through grief, and culture plays an important role. Concepts such as "continuing bonds," "avoidant grief," and "holding on and letting go" may have little relevance in some cultures. Very often what passes for "cultural competence" is a list of traits that characterize the person we are working with as "the other." We all bring our culture to every clinical encounter and exploring culture should be a two-way conversation.

Tervalon and Murray-Garcia (1998) make a distinction between cultural competence and cultural humility, which requires health care professionals to "continually engage in self-reflection and self-critique as lifelong learners and reflective practitioners" (p. 118). Cultural humility does not negate increasing our knowledge about bereavement practices and rituals. Rather, it asserts that this is the beginning, not the endpoint. It means that we do not become comfortable in this knowledge but are humble enough "to say that we do not know when we truly do not know" (Tervalon & Murray-Garcia, 1998, p. 119). With true humility, the clinical encounter can reduce power imbalances and privilege the voice of the bereaved as the expert.

Gender

Interpreting the differences in how men and women grieve has led to debate (see McGoldrick, 2004 for a review of the research). While women report more symptoms of psychological distress than men, bereaved men have a greater mortality rate than bereaved women (McGoldrick, 2004). Harris (2009) suggests that both men and women can be oppressed by social expectations and that we must be vigilant not to gender stereotype the responses of our clients. Both Pat and Sarah reported feeling judged by their friends and families because of their "more masculine" way of grieving. Jerry was told he was "crying too much."

Martin and Doka (2000) have suggested a more gender-neutral paradigm, which they call instrumental and intuitive:

Instrumental grievers tend to have tempered affect to a loss. While intuitive grievers are more likely to experience their grief as waves of affect; instrumental grievers are more likely to describe it in physical or cognitive terms. While intuitive grievers often need to express their feelings and seek the support of others, instrumental grievers are more likely to cognitively process or immerse themselves in activity. (Martin & Doka, 2000, p. 5)

It is important to consider the intersection of gender and culture. Many cultures have prescribed ways of grieving for men and for women, which can require a pronounced emotional response such as weeping or a more "stoic" response. Some of these expectations may bring comfort to the mourner or may feel oppressive. Exploring these expectations in a respectful manner is an essential part of our work with the bereaved.

Disenfranchised Grief

Doka describes disenfranchised grief as that which cannot be openly acknowledged or is not socially sanctioned. Often these grievers are not accorded the right to grieve. Pat, Jerry and Sarah who are described in the narratives in Box 29.1, experienced disenfranchised grief because of the way that they grieved.

As noted above, grief can also be disenfranchised because the relationship of the mourner to the deceased is not socially sanctioned (e.g., death of a former spouse, death of a same-sex partner). Hannah, who is "out" in most spheres or her life, but not in her work life, had to take vacation days after Marie's death, because her employer's bereavement policy did not give time off for the death of a "friend." She also experienced far less social support at work, when she compared the reactions of her coworkers to her loss to their reactions to the loss of a coworker's wife. This is consistent with the literature on caregiving and grief among lesbians and gay men (Bent & Magilvy, 2006; Smolinksi & Colon, 2006). (For more information see Chapter 35)

Stigmatized deaths such as suicides or violent deaths can also lead to disenfranchisement. Laura has heard people say they are tired of hearing about September 11, that the mourners have received too much media attention, as well as a lot of money. This angers her but also makes her reluctant to seek social support for her loss.

Recognizing, validating, and naming the experiences of these disenfranchised mourners are essential parts of the helping process.

Bereavement Interventions

There is a growing controversy in the field of grief and bereavement about the efficacy of bereavement interventions, particularly with uncomplicated mourning (Currier, Neimeyer, & Berman, 2008; Jordan & Neimeyer, 2003; Larson & Hoyt, 2007; Schut & Stroebe, 2005). There is also debate about whether people "recover" from bereavement and whether the term itself has relevance (see "Special Issue on Bereavement, Outcomes and Recovery," *Death Studies*, Volume 32, 2008). Although it is beyond the scope of this chapter to address this issue, there is beginning evidence for some interventions targeted at people with complicated mourning (Kissane et al., 2006; Shear, Frank, Houck, & Reynolds, 2005).

Both authors have worked with hundreds of bereaved people, many who would fall into the category of "uncomplicated." It is our experience that psychoeducation, particularly dispelling any assumptions about the "right way to grieve," and offering support on a short-term basis have been helpful. Social workers need to be knowledgeable about the myriad of ways people grieve, especially the assumption that talking about feelings is always helpful. Until the research is clearer, we should proceed with caution, always taking our cues from the mourners.

Moving Forward

The field of grief and bereavement is evolving. It will be crucial that social workers stay current with and participate in related research as it emerges and adjust their practice accordingly. In the meantime, recognizing and respecting the differences that people exhibit during bereavement will strengthen the quality of our interventions. Impeccable assessment is key. Eliciting information about past losses, coping mechanisms, cultural and spiritual beliefs and practices and differentiating normal grief from a prolonged grief disorder will help us provide meaningful tools for the people we serve. Working with grief and bereavement requires that we do not become complacent in our practice. This work will challenge us in many ways, both clinically and personally. It will trigger our own losses, some times more than others. Self-awareness and self-care will help to ensure that our own issues do not cloud our clinical judgment or compassion. Some people are bound to touch us more than others, and it is imperative that

we look at our reactions so they do not get in the way of effective interventions. Maybe the person we are working with is near our age or the person reminds us of someone in our life, thus triggering a more emotional response. Using supervision or professional therapeutic intervention will help us identify our reactions so we can take the necessary action to help ourselves. Self-care will help us build our resilience so that we can continue to do the work. Exercise, nutrition, and rest are the basics. Seeking to consistently and consciously live our values keeps us intact and resilient. Surrounding ourselves with healthy people with similar values also helps us manage stress. Cultivating humor provides perspective. No matter how much we "know," if we do not know ourselves or take care of life in a healthy manner, our practice with patients and colleagues will be impacted negatively. The field of bereavement forces us to live every day with the full knowledge of mortality, suffering, and loss. Successful palliative social workers will use that knowledge to care for ourselves today, to develop ourselves as we fully experience the joys and sorrows of life. It is then that we are at our most effective at helping others.

"Smooth seas do not make skillful sailors."
—*African proverb*

Grief Awareness Exercises for Social Work Practitioners

1. How might my own experiences or lack of experiences with the death of significant others impact my practice with grieving individuals and family members?
2. Are there specific traditions or beliefs that might challenge me more than others?
3. What has been the most significant death you have experienced in your life?
4. What were the many losses that were included with the death of this person?
5. What were your personal emotional, physical, social, and spiritual experiences?
6. What actions (by you or others) gave you the most comfort?
7. Were there things people said or you did that were not helpful?
8. What was the most surprising aspect of your grief?
9. Were there traditions or rituals that helped you adjust?

ADDITIONAL SUGGESTED READINGS

Berzoff, J. (2003). Psychodynamic theories in grief and bereavement. *Smith College Studies in Social Work*, 73(3), 273–298.

Berzoff, J., & Silverman, P. (Eds.). (2004). *Living with dying*. New York, NY: Columbia University Press.

Blank, J. W. (1998). The death of an adult child: A book for and about bereaved parents. Amityville, NY: Baywood Publishing Company Inc.

Boelen, P. A., & Prigerson, H. G. (2007). The influence of symptoms of prolonged grief disorder, depression, and anxiety on quality of life among bereaved adults: A perspective study. *Eus Auch Psychiatry Clinical Neuroscience, 257*(8), 444-452.

Bonanno, G. (2001). Grief and emotion: A social-functional perspective. In M. Stroebe, R. O. Hansson, W. Stroebe, & H. Schut (Eds.), *Handbook of bereavement research: Consequences, coping, and care.* (pp. 493-515). Washington, DC: American Psychological Association.

Bowman, T. (1999). Literary resources for bereavement. *Hospice Journal, 4*(1), 39-54.

Browning, D. (2003). Pathos, paradox and poetics: Grounded theory and the experience of bereavement. *Smith College Studies in Social Work, 73*(3), 325-336.

Callahan, B. N. (1999). *Grief counseling: A manual for social workers.* Denver, CO: Love Publishing.

Canine, S. L. (1996). Counseling techniques for helping the bereaved. *The psychosocial aspects of death and dying* (pp. 253-264). Stamford, CT: Appleton & Lange.

Corwin, M. D. (1995). Cultural issues in bereavement therapy: The social construction of mourning. In *Session: Psychotherapy Practice, 1*(4), 23-41.

Dane, B. (1989). Middle-aged adults mourning the death of a parent. *Journal of Gerontological Social Work, 14*(3/4), 75-89.

Davidson, K. W., & Foster, Z. (1995). Social work with dying and bereaved clients: Helping the workers. *Social Work in Health Care, 21*(4), 1-16.

Fitzpatrick, T. R., & Tran, T. V. (2002). Bereavement and health among different race and age groups. *Journal of Gerontological Social Work, 37*(2), 77-92.

Gilbert, K. R. (1996). "We've had the same loss, why don't we have the same grief?" Loss and differential grief in families. *Death Studies, 20*(3), 269-283.

Irish, D. P., Lundquist, K. F., & Nelson, V. J. (Eds.). (1993). *Ethnic variations in dying, death and grief: Diversity in universality.* Washington, DC: Taylor & Francis.

Kissane, D. W., & Bloch, S. (1994). Family grief. *British Journal of Psychiatry, 164*(6), 720-740.

Kissane, D. W., & Bloch, S. (2002). *Family focused grief therapy: A model of family-centered care during palliative care and bereavement.* Buckingham, England: Open University Press.

Liken, M., & Collins, C. (1993). Grieving: Facilitating the process for dementia caregivers. *Journal of Psychosocial Nursing, 31*(1), 21-26.

Lord, B., & Pockett, R. (1998). Perceptions of social work intervention with bereaved clients: Some implications for hospital social work practice. *Social Work in Health Care, 27*(1), 51-66.

Malkinson, R. (2001). Cognitive-behavioral therapy of grief: A review and application. *Research on Social Work Practice, 11*(6), 671-698.

McBride, J., & Simms, S. (2001). Death in the family: Adapting a family systems framework to the grief process. *American Journal of Family Therapy, 29*(1), 59-73.

McNeil, J. (1995). Bereavement and loss. In Beebe L. (Ed.) *Encyclopedia of social work* (19th ed., pp. 284-291). Silver Springs, MD: National Association of Social Workers.

Parkes, C. M., Laungani, P., & Young, B. (Eds.). (1997). *Death and bereavement across cultures.* London, England: Routledge.

Rando, T. A. (1984). *Grief, dying and death.* Champaign, IL: Research Press Co.

Raphael, B. (1983). *Anatomy of bereavment.* New York: Basic Books.

Raymer, M. (1999). When is it not normal? Differentiating between normal and complicated grief. In S. Olson (Ed.), *Your gift* (pp. 113-125). Traverse City, MI: Seasons Press.

Schneider, J. (1994). *Finding my way.* Colfax, MI: Seasons Press.

Segal, D. L., Chatman, C., Bogaards, J. A., & Becker, L. A. (2001). One-year follow-up of an emotional expression intervention for bereaved older adults. *Journal of Mental Health and Aging, 7*(4), 465-472.

Segal, D. L., Bogaards, J. A., Becker, L. A., & Chatman, C. (1999). Effects of emotional expression on adjustment to spousal loss among older adults. *Journal of Mental Health and Aging, 5*(4), 297-310.

Stroebe, M. S., Hansson, R. O., Stroebe, W., & Schut, H. (Eds.). (2001). *Handbook of bereavement research. Consequences, coping, and care.* Washington, D.C: American Psychological Association.

Walsh-Burke, K. (2000). Matching bereavement services to level of need. *The Hospice Journal. 15*(1), 77-86.

Weinberg, N. (1995). Does apologizing help? The role of self-blame and making amends in recovery from bereavement. *Health and Social Work, 20*(4), 294-299.

WEB RESOURCES

The Center for the Advancement of Health (CFAH): http://www.cfah.org

Conducts research, communicates findings, and advocates for policies that support everyone's ability to benefit from advances in health science.

The Center for Loss: http://www.centerforloss.com

Dedicated to "companioning" grieving people as they mourn transitions and losses in their lives. The Center also helps professional caregivers and lay people, by serving as an educational resources and professional forum.

The Hospice Foundation of America: www.hospicefoundation.org/griefAndLoss

The Hospice Foundation of America provides leadership in the development and application of hospice and its philosophy of care with the goal of enhancing the U.S. health care system and the role of hospice within it.

Journey of Hearts: http://www.journeyofhearts.org/jofh/grief/cope

Designed to be a Healing Place with resources and support to help those in the grief process following a loss, crisis, or a significant life change. This Web site contains a variety of different resources to help visitors to the site to help in the education process.

The National Hospice and Palliative Care Organization (NHPCO): http://www.nhpco.org

The largest nonprofit membership organization representing hospice and palliative care programs and professionals in the United States. The organization is committed to improving end-of-life care and expanding access to hospice care.

REFERENCES

Attig, T. (1996). *How we grieve: Relearning the world.* New York, NY: Oxford University Press.

Auden, W. H., & Isherwood, C. (1936). *The ascent of F6*. London, England: Faber and Faber.

Bent, K., & Magilvy, J. (2006). When a partner dies: Lesbian widows. *Issues in Mental Health Nursing*, *27*(5), 447–459.

Bonanno, G. A. (2009). *The other side of sadness: What the new science of bereavement tells us about life after loss*. New York, NY: Basic Books.

Bonanno, G. A., & Kaltman, S. (2001). The varieties of grief experience. *Clinical Psychology Review*, *21*(5), 705–734.

Bonanno, G. A., Keltner, D., Holen, A., & Horowitz, M. J. (1995). When avoiding unpleasant emotions might not be such a bad thing: Verbal-autonomic response dissociation and midlife conjugal bereavement. *Journal of Personality and Social Psychology*, *69*(5), 975–989.

Brenner, D., Blanchard, T., Hirschfield, B., & Fins, J. J. (2005). *Embracing life and facing death: A Jewish guide to palliative care*. New York, NY: CLAL.

Browning, D. M. (2002). Saying goodbye, saying hello: A grief sojourn. *Journal of Palliative Medicine*, *5*(3), 465–469.

Currier, J., Neimeyer, R., & Berman, J. (2008). The effectiveness of psychotherapeutic interventions for bereaved persons: A comprehensive quantitative review. *Psychological Bulletin*, *134*(5), 648–661.

Davis, C. G., Nolen-Hoeksema, S., & Larson, J. (1998). Making sense of loss and benefiting from the experience: Two construals of meaning. *Journal of Personality and Social Psychology*, *75*(2), 561–574.

Davis, C. G., Wortman, C. B., Lehman, D. R., & Silver, R. C. (2000). Searching for meaning in loss: Are clinical assumptions correct? *Death Studies*, *24*(6), 497–540.

Dickens, C.(2002). *Great expectations*. London, England: Penguin Classics. (Original work published in 1861).

Didion, J. (2005). *The year of magical thinking*. New York, NY: Alfred A. Knopf.

Doka, K. J. (2002). *Disenfranchised grief*. Champaign, IL: Research Press.

Freud, S. (1957). Mourning and melancholia. In J. Strackey (Ed. & Trans.), *The standard edition of the complete psychological work of Sigmund Freud*. (Vol. 14). New York, NY: Norton. (Original work published in 1917).

Glennon, S. S. (2005). Psychoanalysis and mourning—Two distinct views: Commentary on papers by Martin Stephen Frommer and Mary V. Sussillo. *Psychoanalytic Dialogues*, *15*(4), 529–538.

Harris, D. (2009). Gender stereotyping and oppression in grief. *The Forum*, *35*(2), Deerfield, IL: Association for Death Education and Counseling.

Jordan, J., & Neimeyer, R. (2003). Does grief counseling work? *Death Studies*, *27*, 763–786.

Kaplan, L. J. (1995). *No voice is ever wholly lost*. New York, NY: Touchstone.

Keesee, N. J., Currier, J. M., & Neimeyer, R. A. (2008) Predictors of grief following the death of one's child: The contribution of finding meaning. *Journal of Clinical Psychology*, *64*(10), 1145–1163.

Kissane, D., McKenzie, M., Bloch, S., Moskowitz, C., McKenzie, D., & O'Neill, I. (2006). Family focused grief therapy: A randomized controlled trial in palliative care and bereavement. *American Journal of Psychiatry*, *163*(7), 1208–1218.

Klass, D., Silverman, P., & Nickman, S. (Eds.). (1996). *Continuing bonds: New understandings of grief*. Washington, DC: Taylor and Francis.

Larson, D., & Hoyt, W. (2007). What has become of grief counseling? An evaluation of the empirical foundations of the new pessimism. *Professional Psychology: Research and Practice*, *38*(4), 347–355.

Lynch, T. (1997). *The undertaking: Life studies from the dismal trade*. New York, NY: W.W. Norton & Company.

Maciejewski, P. K., Zhang, B., Block, S. D., & Prigerson, H. G. (2007). An empirical examination of the stage theory of grief. *Journal of American Medical Association*, *297*(7), 716–723.

Martin, T. L., & Doka, K. (2000). *Men don't cry … women do: Transcending gender stereotypes of grief*. Philadelphia, PA: Brunner Mazel.

McGoldrick, M. (2004). Gender and mourning. In F. Walsh & M. McGoldrick (Eds.), *Living beyond loss*. New York, NY: W. W. Norton.

Neimeyer, R. (Ed.). (2001). *Meaning reconstruction and the experience of loss*. Washington, DC: American Psychological Association.

Parkes, C. M. (1997) *Bereavement: Studies of grief in adult life* (3rd ed.). Madison, WI: International Universities Press.

Prigerson, H. G., Horowitz, M. J., Jacobs, S. C., Parkes, C. M., Aslan, M., … Maciejewski, P. K. (2009) Prolonged grief disorder: Psychometric validation of criteria proposed for *DSM-V and ICD-11*. *PLoS Med 6*(8), journal.pmed. e1000121, 1–12.

Puchalski, C, Ferrell, B.,Virani, R. N. C., Otis-Greene, S., Baird, P., Bull, J., … Sulmasy, D. (2009). Improving the quality of spiritual care as a dimension of palliative care: The report of the consensus conference. *Journal of Palliative Medicine*, *12*(10), 885–904.

Rando, T. (1993).*Treament of complicated mourning*. Champaign, IL: Research Press.

Shear, K., Frank, E., Houck, P., & Reynolds, C. (2005). Treatment of complicated grief: A randomized controlled trial. *Journal of American Medical Association*, *293*, 2601–2608.

Schut, H., & Stroebe, M. (2005). Interventions to enhance adaptation to bereavement. *Journal of Palliative Medicine*, *8*(Suppl. 1), 140–147.

Smolinski, K., & Colon, Y. (2006). Silent voices and invisible walls: Exploring end-of-life care with lesbians and gay men. *Journal of Psychosocial Oncology*, *24*(1), 51–64.

Stroebe, M. S., Stroebe, W., & Hansson, R. O. (1993). *Handbook of bereavement: Theory, research and intervention*. Cambridge, England: Cambridge University Press.

Stroebe, M. S., Hansson, R. O., Schut, H., & Stroebe, W. (2008). *Handbook of bereavement, research and practice: Advances in theory and intervention*. Washington, DC: American Psychological Association.

Stroebe, M., Schut, H., & Stroebe, W. (2005). Attachment in coping with bereavement: A theoretical integration. *Review of General Psychology*, *9*(1), 48–66.

Tervalon, M., & Murray-Garcia, J. (1998).Cultural humility versus cultural competence: A critical distinction in defining physician training outcomes in multicultural education. *Journal of Health Care for the Poor and the Underserved*, *9*(2), 117–125.

IV
Population-Specific Practice

For Lena

*The recreation room has too many people
Its convivial confusion frightens you with too many old ones
too important with their plans and purpose.*

*You journey a careful distance to my floor.
Each day you wear the same shabby yellow dress and the
worn out shoes.*

*You show me your wrinkled photos:
You as a cigarette girl in your husband's night club:
You with the shy curls cascading down your bare shoulders
with your long legs, in your slinky black dress, siren of the
thirties with movie style glamour of another age.*

*You smooth the pictures like petting a stray cat or any living
thing.
You still have the newspaper clippings when you were mugged
The past is real and tangible, the present is dusty and dim*

*Yesterday becomes impossible to remember.
You forget the son who calls daily, the woman who visits
weekly.*

*I gave you a small task to call the blind man.
He lived in a cluttered collection of debris and despair
You never met him but you knew his sadness.
"I know what it's like to be lonely," you said.
You did your best to provide comfort, in your still sensual
voice: buoyant and young seductive as a call to an
upscale bordello.*

One day, I closed the door where I worked,
Gently, I borrowed your cane and held it in a horizontal way.
"Lena, all these years you have been holding the cane wrong."
I did the soft shoe, assisted with your cane. You smiled in
memory.
You remembered the Yiddish folk songs of your youth, over
sixty years ago.

We forgot the peeling ceiling, and the dingy wall.
We became joy; it was some other country, some other time.
The room filled with sound. We sang and sang.

Constance H. Gemson LMSW
New York, NY

30

A. Marlene Lockey, Diane Benefiel, and Margaret Meyer

The Collaboration of Palliative Care and Oncology Social Work

I didn't know what I was getting into.

—Patient receiving cancer treatment

Key Concepts

- *Oncology social work requires the ability to work with existential suffering.*
- *Psychosocial assessment is the beginning of social work intervention.*
- *Palliative interventions start with cancer diagnosis.*
- *Oncology social workers and palliative social workers share many skills.*

Introduction

For many cancers, scientific advances have increased the number of persons cured or have lengthened the time between diagnosis and death. The hospital oncology social worker has opportunities to meet and to reconnect with patients and their family members as they are admitted and readmitted to the hospital. Patients will include those receiving cancer therapies, undergoing surgery, receiving care for disabilities and/or chronic symptoms resulting from cancer and treatment, and those who are dying.

Increasingly hospitals offer the specialized services of a palliative interdisciplinary team to patient and families with complex medical and psychosocial needs. A palliative team is trained to assist across the continuum of care, and a palliative social worker is often one of the interdisciplinary team members. Interdisciplinary teams work collaboratively as a whole with frequent coordination of team interventions. In contrast, oncology social workers are often one of several disciplines comprising a multidisciplinary team in which each discipline provides care as requested by the physician. Progress notes may be the primary communication between multidisciplinary team members while palliative care clinicians often share information through team meetings. More about the differences between these two types of teams is discussed later in this chapter.

Depending on patient and family needs, a palliative interdisciplinary team may supplement or replace the services of a multidisciplinary team. Oncology social workers share many skills with palliative social workers, and this creates an opportunity for collaboration and sharing to avoid duplication of services and confusion for patients, families, and staff.

Comprehensive Oncology Social Work

A hound started a hare from her form, and pursued her for some distance; but as she gradually gained upon him, he gave up the chase. A rustic who had seen the race met the hound as he was returning, and taunted him with his defeat. "The little one was too much for you," said

he. "Ah, well," said the hound, "don't forget it's one thing to be running for your dinner, but quite another to be running for your life."
—Aesop's Fables: The Hare and The Hound

Rare is a newly diagnosed cancer patient who does not feel he is running for his life. A cancer diagnosis startles a patient out of familiar routines and emotional equilibrium. Fears of the worst-case scenario hound him until initial biopsy and test results are complete. Psychosocial relationships throughout the patient's and his family's life are impacted by the diagnosis because treatment and symptoms will disrupt family roles and schedules (Adler & Page, 2007; Baider, Cooper, & Kaplan De-Nour, 2000). Regardless of whether a patient knows what palliative care is, it will be an integral part of treatment from initial diagnosis. Its purpose will be to provide comfort from symptoms, not treatment for cancer. The psychosocial dynamics of illness and the psychosocial interventions are subjects of expertise for the oncology social worker. From her initial meeting with a patient and his family, the oncology social worker will be providing palliative care. Even if treatment achieves a remission, the patient can feel the "hound," that is, cancer recurrence, is waiting to renew pursuit (Miller, Merry, & Miller, 2008).

Palliative care embraces both the patient and his family, acknowledging the suffering of both. If a cancer patient's family is hurting, the patient is hurting for them. The suffering of family is felt in an excerpt from a wife's poem paying tribute to her husband, a cancer patient. The poem was pasted on a homemade heart and taped to his hospital door. An excerpt from the poem asks: "Do you know about losing one so dear? When you see me do you see the tears?" The role of the oncology social work is not just to see the tears; it is to provide care to the patient's family as well as the patient.

Changing perspectives about life's meaning, time, and mortality are characteristics of a cancer patient's experience that contribute to oncology social work as a rewarding career (Moadel et al., 1999; Rohan & Baush, 2009). When faced with a life-threatening illness, a cancer patient looks beyond extraneous concerns to focus on the basics that provide meaning to his life. A sense of personal meaning and a perception of personal resources available to meet the challenge of cancer provide the base for a patient's coping abilities and social support (Moss & Dobson, 2006). Of the myriad of psychosocial changes resulting from a cancer diagnosis, the most profound is a heightened awareness of mortality. To help patients define their meaning of illness and face the reality of their mortality is to work in a setting with existential depth (Moadel et al., 1999; Steinhauser et al., 2001). Cancer patients for whom all treatment options have failed have a different perspective of time. For a patient who has only months or weeks to live, today is a greater percentage of his life than it is for a person who has years to live. This perspective can bring an uncommon depth to interactions with care providers (Block, 2001).

In this setting of profound life experiences, the oncology social worker is in her workplace—one that encompasses functional agendas, including productivity data, documentation deadlines, discharge pressures, and large caseloads. Additionally, a hospital is a highly technical and challenging setting 24 hours a day, 7 days a week. Interactions that convey a sense of unhurried calm and attentiveness can easily be neglected and can become merely perfunctory. Interventions include psychosocial assessment to identify potential challenges to accessing care, locating resources to address identified needs, providing counseling focused on emotional distress, grief and changes associated with diagnosis, treatment and prognosis and assisting with discharge planning.

A component of palliative care is the acknowledgement that clinicians need to guard against becoming emotionally drained from their work. It is unrealistic to step day after day into the stream of emotional intensity that is part of working with cancer patients without strategies for personal renewal (Simon, Pyrce, Roff, & Klemmack, 2006). Suffice it to say, the oncology social worker needs activities and interests beyond work with patients and a way to release the grief that accumulates from her work. Personal strategies of renewal may include exercise, outdoor activities, handcrafts, hobbies, as well as vacations, personal retreats, and meditation. Interdisciplinary palliative care has also been called upon to incorporate strategies for the care of staff as well as patients (National Consensus Project, 2007). The oncology social worker in a multidisciplinary setting will need to incorporate her own self-care strategies into her life.

Assessment

A hound who had served his master well for years, and had run down many a quarry in his time, began to lose his strength and speed owing to age. One day, when out hunting, his master started a powerful wild boar and set the hound at him. The latter seized the beast by the ear, but his teeth were gone and he could not retain his hold; so the boar escaped. His master began to scold him severely, but the hound interrupted him with these words, "My will is as strong as ever, master, but my body is old and feeble. You ought to honor me for what I have been instead of abusing me for what I am."
—Aesop's Fables: The Old Hound

Regardless of the age at which a patient's health becomes fragile from treatment or disease, there remains an obligation to honor his place in his family and his community. When a person is diagnosed with cancer, he faces many losses. The greatest danger is the loss that may occur when a unique individual becomes a "patient" because a medical team knows little about the person's identity outside the medical setting. Other team members may provide brief psychosocial information but none equal the level of detail or depth of a social worker's assessment. Social work assessments reflect a patient's place in a broader environment of relationships, resources, and coping history available to him as he struggles to integrate his prognosis and meets the demands of treatment. A thorough assessment communicates that the social worker is interested in the patient as a person who has a valued life beyond cancer treatment.

Assessment is also the starting point of treatment and the process can establish rapport between patient, family, and social worker. It includes demographic information as well as noting the coping styles, emotional strengths, spirituality, and relationships that support the patient (Nicholas & Veach, 2000). Challenges in these dimensions can impede and/or complicate a patient's medical care. In addition, practical resources for accessing treatment need to be explored, such as transportation, housing, work status, financial resources, and availability of others to help with care. Failure to overcome a significant challenge can literally mean life or death. Among the competencies applied to assessment is knowledge of how cultural and ethnic customs, as well as gender, age, and place in a family life cycle, may influence the patient when faced with difficult medical realities. Social work's understanding of behavior in the social environment provides a valuable perspective to the medical team for finding strengths others miss. The narrative in Box 30.1 integrates this perspective in a manner that enriched collaboration with palliative care colleagues arranging discharge plans.

Assessments can reveal previous problems which have the potential to resurface when a patient experiences the stress that accompanies a life-threatening illness. Oncology social workers not only need skills in basic psychosocial assessment but also specific screening tools for substance abuse, suicide risk, spirituality, neglect and physical abuse, and complicated grief. Through the use of appropriate screening, the oncology social worker can alert the medical team to problems that might arise during treatment and enlist the necessary resources for help.

Once a patient understands the purpose of an assessment is to help him achieve his goals, he is typically open with sharing information about his intrapersonal life such as how he and his family are emotionally responding to his diagnosis, treatment plans, and prognosis. Inquiring as to whether a patient has completed advance directives can be an avenue for assessing the cultural and family context of illness as well as creating an opportunity for a patient to discuss end-of-life concerns. Past experiences with cancer provide insight into present and future reactions of the patient and his family to his cancer. Whether family members were cured, obtained lengthy remissions, or died, and whether cancer deaths were miserable or peaceful are personal experiences that set up expectations for what his experience might be like. Understanding what a patient knows about his disease and his cancer experience shapes the social worker's wording of further questions. For example, if the oncology social worker knows that a patient has been diagnosed with metastatic disease but remains hopeful for a cure, this hope is taken into

Box 30.1
Patient/Family Narrative: Doug

An anxious palliative care team newly assigned to a patient paged the oncology social worker to collaborate about a safe discharge plan for Doug, a 69-year-old man with advanced metastatic prostate cancer who lived alone on his boat in a marina. Doug told the palliative team that he did not have—and did not need—anyone to help him. He did not want hospice and said that he wanted to leave against medical advice to return to his boat. Although he had no living family, he had a strong network of friends composed of his sailing and drinking buddies who were unmarried. He received a small retirement check and had little savings. Sailing was his whole life; his adventures and boat were the envy of his friends.

Hospice was the best discharge plan; however, his friends would need to be his caregivers and Doug would have to allow them to care for him. The palliative care team expressed concern whether men who are not family members would be reliable caregivers. Familiar with Doug's visitors and his blustery refusals to disgruntled approvals when asked about accepting help from others, the social worker having the benefit of history, provided an assessment of the relational strengths and availability of those in his network of friends. A longtime friend stepped forward, offering to care for the patient and to coordinate the help of others. Grumbling that he could take care of himself, Doug agreed to hospice. The palliative care team eyed the discharge plan with skepticism and worried that the patient to be back in the emergency room within 24 hours. Despite progressive deterioration, Doug remained at home longer than expected. When he did return, he was admitted to the hospital's palliative care unit, where his nurses observed that he had been well cared for by his friends. To the end, his friends visited, reminisced, and laughed with him about sailing and manly adventures.

account while assessing the coping abilities and spiritual and personal support networks that may be available in the event his hope is not realized.

Each change in a patient's condition, including remission, cure, progression, recurrence, and nonresponse to treatment, calls for reassessment because each change can present new challenges to his ongoing care and coping abilities. These changes also offer opportunities for a patient to rethink his definition of quality of life and rediscover personal meaning and purpose.

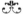

Interventions

A thirsty crow found a pitcher with some water in it, but so little was there that, try as she might, she could not reach it with her beak, and it seemed as though she would die of thirst within sight of the remedy. At last she hit upon a clever plan. She began dropping pebbles into the pitcher, and with each pebble the water rose a little higher until at last it reached the brim, and the knowing bird was enabled to quench her thirst.

—Aesop's Fables: The Crow and the Pitcher

The stakes are so high, the physical and emotional suffering often so intense, that cancer patients and their families can feel too overwhelmed and exhausted to bring forth interior strength or call on others to support them. By assessing the circumstances, the oncology social worker helps the family add "pebbles" to increase the level of support reachable by those who feel depleted. Pebbles can be as simple as encouraging a walk in a hospital garden, visiting the hospital chapel, taking time for meditation or guided imagery, or calling long-time friends or other family members to come be with them.

The consequences of a cancer diagnosis can be devastating on multiple psychosocial levels (Adler & Page, 2007). With treatment might come financial crisis, disabilities, changes in sexual functioning, or chronic symptoms. The earlier psychosocial interventions can be introduced and the longer they can be maintained, the greater their likelihood of benefiting the patient and his family (Rehse & Pukrop, 2003). Aided by assessment, interventions are formulated to help with adjustment to the requirements and consequences of each stage of cancer. There is no set of basic interventions that will help every patient and family. Different circumstances call for different interventions and techniques. An appropriate counseling approach might be cognitive behavioral, problem solving, brief therapy, crisis intervention, grief counseling, relaxation techniques, or guided imagery (Rehse & Pukrop, 2003). Different symptoms such as fatigue, pain, shortness of breath, or difficulty sleeping respond better to certain interventions more than to others (Newell, Sanson-Fisher, & Savolainen, 2002). Interventions may also involve linkage to community resources or advocating for assistance. With practice and experience, an oncology social worker selects interventions that bring comfort and clarity to the cancer patient and his family (Rehse & Pukrop, 2003; Smith, Walsh-Burke, & Crusan, 1998). To guide her choices, psychosocial researchers are striving to increase understanding of the effectiveness of specific interventions (Folkman & Greer, 2000; Helgeson, 2005; Newell et al., 2002). The social worker will benefit her patients by staying abreast of current research. Maintaining access to a university library's online journals, subscribing to and reading professional journals, and attending conferences and workshops are several ways to follow research on evidence-informed psychosocial interventions.

Some patients find that creative interventions help them to express feelings that underlie their emotional response to cancer and treatment (Serlin, Classen, Frances, & Angell, 2000). These include journaling, art therapy, expressive movement, scrapbooking, and writing poetry. Patients facing a poor prognosis might find it meaningful to make video or audiotapes for loved ones or to prepare cards to be given after their death at significant milestones in others' lives (Romanoff & Thompson, 2006; Unruh, 1983). A tangible creative expression can remind a patient that his life has been meaningful and that he will be remembered. The example in Box 30.2 shows how an artistic activity kept a family interacting as a mother was dying.

Box 30.2
Patient/Family Narrative: Shu

Newly transferred to a hospital palliative care unit, Shu, a young mother of Asian descent, was visibly deteriorating but still responsive. Her children, ages 9 and 11, visited but she would close her eyes and avoid talking with them. She did the same when offered counseling. Her husband explained that her family did not talk about dying because it was bad luck.

The occupational therapist learned that Shu could write Japanese calligraphy. The multidisciplinary team knew he had found a culturally sensitive intervention this family could use to open communication. He gathered the necessary supplies, and on the children's next visit, invited the patient to write calligraphy for her children. The children were fascinated and stood close by their mother's bedside as she wrote a special symbol for each child and explained what she had chosen. Communication was reestablished. With this activity, Shu left her children with an emotional and tangible memory of closeness and warmth. She never talked about her dying on later visits; instead, the children would eagerly ask her about the things she knew how to do and how she learned them.

A cancer diagnosis affects the whole family profoundly, and there are special needs for families with minor children along the continuum of illness and at the end of life. Children, like adults, will experience stress related to their parent's cancer, their own losses, and grief. Parents with cancer are concerned about how to talk with their children, how much to tell them, and/or guardianship issues. Children's needs and understanding are age specific, and interventions should be adjusted accordingly. In general, children understand more than they are credited with, and their fears and concerns can be worse than reality (Christ et al., 1993; Forrest, Plumb, Ziebland, & Stein, 2006). Many adults have been surprised by the maturity of children when discussing the impact of cancer on their family. Through the trajectory of cancer children may experience considerable suffering as shown in Box 30.3.

Spirituality is a significant part of the cancer experience. Spiritual suffering for many is addressed within a specific religious context that provides comfort and meaning. For some, their religious understanding of illness and suffering may be disquieting. Regardless of whether within a religious context, patients who question the meaning of their illness, their suffering, or their life are addressing dimensions of spirituality. If a patient shares these questions with his social worker, particular sensitivity is needed (Kelly, 2004; Miovic, 2004; Puchalski, Lunsford, Harris, & Miller, 2006; Weaver & Flannelly, 2004). An oncology social worker needs to be comfortable with the breadth of spiritual expression. When receptive, patients and family members need to be offered a referral to the hospital chaplain or a community pastor.

To give meaning and purpose to his life and cancer experience, a patient may reminisce or reflect on the past. This has the potential to reduce depression and anxiety and to diminish suffering (Chochinov et al., 2005; Hultman,

---

Box 30.3
Patient/Family Narrative: Children Describe What Is the Hardest When a Parent Has Cancer

An oncology hospital social work department held a family support group once a month. Patients, caregivers, younger children, and teens held separate groups. In one session of the younger children's group attended that evening by children ages 6 to 9, the social worker asked, "What is the hardest part about your parent having cancer?" One boy mentioned that his older brother went out of control emotionally and would hit his dad (the patient) and had been sent to a residential home. A girl responded, "You lose your house." Another boy said that his parent sat and cried when watching the television show "Touched by an Angel" (a television drama series in which angels brought messages from God to help people with their problems).

Reder, & Dahlin, 2008). This process has various names, including life review, reminiscence, and life reflection (Parker, 1999; Staudinger, 2001). It need not be a formal process but one that can be encouraged by the social worker because of its potential benefit. It can be as simple as having siblings tell stories of shared experiences with the patient. Or a social worker might say to a patient, "Tell me your story." Some patients when reflecting on life begin to analyze choices and relationships. This can be an entrée into a patient's desire to reconcile with persons and events in his life, which is another aspect of healing and one in which the oncology social worker and hospital chaplain might collaborate.

Ethical issues can arise when a patient and family's understanding of life and illness differ in a significant way from those of his health care providers. Ethical conflicts can also occur around issues of treatment and discharge. The oncology social worker may find herself a key team member in contributing her understanding of a patient/family in efforts to negotiate ethical conflict. Even when resolved, tensions can remain between medical team members and the family that challenge the social worker's capacity to maintain a nonmoralistic stance (Shannon, 1997; Spano & Koenig, 2003).

For many patients, information is a coping strategy. It reduces anxiety from uncertainty and can empower a patient to make choices that support his treatment preferences (Charles, Gafni, & Whelan, 1999; Quill & Brody, 1996; van der Molem, 2001). A family conference is an effective intervention both for providing a patient and family members with the information needed for decisions and a forum for the patient to voice his preferences. It can be particularly helpful to patients and families when disease-related information is disappointing. When participating in a family conference, the oncology social worker provides a supportive presence to the patient, sees that psychosocial needs are taken into account in a plan of care, and intervenes to enhance group process when needed. The significance of the family conference is considerable and has warranted a chapter of its own (for more information see Chapter 22).

One of the most difficult transitions for a cancer patient occurs when he is told that no more treatments are indicated for his cancer. He views his world and relationships through a new timeframe and his thoughts may shift to maintaining quality of life. This is a significant time for a family conference to be held. Often, not all family members have yet understood or accepted the patient's medical condition and only do so when supported by the patient and other family members. Watching their family member discuss terminal illness with the physician can open communication within the family regarding end-of-life issues that were previously avoided.

When a cancer patient's health takes a sudden turn for the worse and death is imminent, his family may have difficulty accepting the rapid change. The oncology social worker provides a supportive presence that allows the family to express a range of emotions, including shock and anxiety. Family members may or may not be present at the moment of death and either scenario requires skilled clinical intervention and anticipatory guidance to assist the family as they integrate the death. Saying goodbye to a loved one for the last time is among the hardest things people ever do.

Following a patient's death, the oncology social worker continues to provide a supportive presence that allows the family to work toward acceptance, notify others, and say final goodbyes. If possible, practical matters such as funeral arrangements should be completed earlier, but this is another area in which the social worker can provide sensitive assistance and support.

The career of an oncology social worker offers many opportunities to develop expertise. Each of the interventions noted earlier requires further training and supervision to enhance a social worker's effectiveness. The expertise developed by an oncology social worker may include clinical treatment, ethics consultation, pain and symptom management, survivorship needs, patient advocacy, end-of-life care, bereavement, or research. All of these relate to palliative care when they aim to relieve the distress and suffering of patients and their families.

Models of Hospital Palliative Oncology Social Work

The moon once begged her mother to make her a gown. "How can I?" replied she. "There's no fitting your figure. At one time you're a new moon, at another time a full moon; and between whiles you're neither one nor the other."

—Aesop's Fables: The Moon and Her Mother

No one description completely fits the hospital oncology social worker because provision of psychosocial services differs from hospital to hospital. In some hospitals, the oncology social worker and case manager role are the same; in others, the social worker fills the role of psychosocial counselor; or there is a blend of the two roles. The oncology social worker may cover the oncology unit in a general hospital, or she may work in a cancer hospital. She may work in an oncology clinic and follow patients admitted to the hospital, or she may work entirely with hospitalized patients and collaborate with a clinic social worker or private practice clinician.

Oncology acknowledges the significant role that psychosocial dynamics play in the treatment of cancer patients. Oncologists have many "tools" to manage the symptoms of their patients that may include team members such as social workers, psychiatric nurse specialists, nurse educators, chaplains, and others. Some symptoms and psychosocial needs, however, require more specialization to manage. Interdisciplinary palliative care programs are being established within hospitals as a resource to manage the care of complex cases. Interdisciplinary and multidisciplinary teams work together differently.

The hospital oncology social worker typically works as a member of a multidisciplinary team. Multidisciplinary team members individually assess and provide services to a patient, and the oncologist uses their information to develop a plan of care for his patient. The multidisciplinary medical team manages palliative needs along the continuum of illness and transitions to solely palliative interventions when no further disease modifying treatment is recommended. However, if a palliative care team is available, its services might be requested for management of intractable symptoms or complex end-of-life care. If the palliative team includes a social worker, a handoff or collaboration of social work services will occur between palliative and oncology social workers. The transition to the palliative team is with the intent of enhancing care. This transfer between medical teams and social workers requires sensitive communication to avoid inadvertently leaving a patient and his family feeling abandoned by the team that had been "fighting" along with him during treatment.

The palliative social worker is a member of a team. Each member of an interdisciplinary team assesses the patient and family referred to their care. Unlike a multidisciplinary team, an interdisciplinary team comes together with the physician to review their assessments and to discuss interventions and care options, and it will involve the patient and family in developing a plan of care. Team members have advanced training and certification in interventions for symptom management and for end-of-life issues. The interdisciplinary team will meet regularly to review interventions and plan ongoing care.

The emergence of new models for palliative care brings shifting roles for hospital social workers. With changes in the delivery of palliative care, the inpatient oncology social worker will need a collaborative relationship with the palliative social worker. Both will need a clear understanding of their separate but complementary roles, and they will need to educate families and staff to the role of each social worker.

Conclusion

As practice supported by research provides increased understanding of effective palliative interventions, changes and enhancement of the delivery of palliative care in hospitals will occur. The presence of both an oncology social worker and palliative social worker in a hospital setting can identify patients and families with complex palliative care needs and provide the level of intervention effective for reducing suffering in these families. Collaboration in transitions between oncology and palliative social workers can reassure a patient that his needs and those of his family are understood and a plan to help has been employed.

LEARNING EXERCISES

Exercise 1: A Web of Gratitude

This exercise can be used with a patient, his family, and friends to express gratitude for knowing the patient. It can also be used as a team-building exercise. The group facilitator has a large ball of yarn. The group forms a circle. The facilitator explains that the ball of yarn represents gratitude. Each person throws the ball to another person in the group while expressing what they are grateful for. Example: I'm grateful to know [patient] because _____. Or I'm grateful to work with this team because _____. By the end of the exercise, the yarn has formed a web that connects everyone in the group. The facilitator tells the people in the group that they are now connected by their gratitude for the patient or for working with this team.

Exercise 2: Psychosocial Stress and the Family Life Cycle

Identify the psychosocial stresses likely for each patient. What end-of-life issues does each face?

Patient A: Laura, a 39-year-old, is diagnosed with metastatic ovarian cancer. She is married and has three young children. Laura has carried the family health insurance so that her husband, Nathan, could start his own business. Laura's and Nathan's extended families live out of state.

Patient B: George is 70 years old and diagnosed with end-stage colon cancer. He has been married 52 years and has one daughter, Susan. Susan is 43 years old, single, lives at home, and receives disability income due to schizophrenia, which is controlled. George and his wife, Catherine, are active in a local church. Catherine is 67 years old and in good health except for occasional arthritis pain in her shoulders.

Exercise 3: Circumstances and Intervention Selection

Patient: Patricia is a 43-year-old female diagnosed with acute myeloid leukemia. She is hospitalized for chemotherapy and has achieved a remission. Her oncologist has just told her that because she is in remission, he would like to proceed with a donor stem cell transplant in 2 weeks. Patricia is verging on a panic attack over how to make arrangements so quickly. The oncology social worker, Martha, has been paged to counsel her. What intervention might be used if *(a)* this is Martha's first time to meet Patricia, and Patricia is scheduled to be taken for magnetic resonance imaging (MRI) in 45 minutes; *(b)* Patricia is known to Martha, who is aware of Patricia's anxious personality. Martha can visit as long as she needs with Patricia.

ADDITIONAL SUGGESTED READINGS

Groopman, J. (2005). *The anatomy of hope: How people prevail in the face of illness*. New York, NY: Random House.

Papero, D. (1990). *Bowen family systems theory*. Needham Heights, MA: Allyn & Bacon.

REFERENCES

Adler, N. E., & Page, A. E. (Eds.). (2007). *Cancer care for the whole patient: Meeting psychosocial health needs*. Washington, DC: Institute of Medicine, The National Academies Press.

Aesop. (2005). *Aesop's fables*. New York, NY: Barnes & Noble Classics.

Block, S. (2001). Psychological considerations, growth, and transcendence at the end of life: The art of the possible. *Journal of the American Medical Association, 285*(22), 2898–2905.

Baider L., Cooper C. L., & Kaplan De-Nour A. (Eds.). (2000). *Cancer and the family* (2nd ed.). New York, NY: John Wiley & Son Ltd.

Charles, C., Gafni, A., & Whelan, T. (1999). Decision-making in the physician-patient encounter: Revisiting the shared treatment decision-making model. *Social Science and Medicine, 49*, 651–661.

Christ, G. H., Siegel, K., Freund, B., Langosch, D., Hendersen, S., Sperber, D., & Weinstein, L. (1993). Impact of parental terminal cancer on latency-age children. *American Journal of Orthopsychiatry, 63*(3), 417–425.

Chochinov, H. M., Hack, T., Hassard, T., Kristjanson, L. J., McClement, S., & Harlos, M. (2005). Dignity therapy: A novel psychotherapeutic intervention for patients near the end of life. *Journal of Clinical Oncology, 23*(24), 5520–5525.

Folkman, S., & Greer, S. (2000). Promoting psychological well-being in the face of serious illness: When theory, research and practice inform each other. *Psycho-Oncology, 9*, 11–19.

Forrest, G., Plumb, C., Ziebland, S., & Stein, A. (2006). Breast cancer in the family—children's perceptions of their mother's cancer and its initial treatment: A qualitative study. *BMJ* Advance online publication. doi:10.1136/bmj.38793.567801.AE.

Helgeson, V. (2005). Recent advances in psychosocial oncology. *Journal of Consulting and Clinical Psychology, 73*(2), 268–271.

Hultman, T., Reder, E. A., & Dahlin, C. M. (2008). Improving psychological and psychiatric aspects of palliative care: The national consensus project and the national quality forum preferred practices for palliative and hospice care. *Omega, 57*(4), 323–339.

Kelly, J. (2004). Spirituality as a coping mechanism. *Dimensions of Critical Care Nursing, 23*(4), 162–168.

Miller, K., Merry, B., & Miller, J. (2008). Seasons of survivorship revisited. *The Cancer Journal, 14*(6), 369–374.

Miovic, M. (2004). An introduction to spiritual psychology: Overview of literature, east and west. *Harvard Review Psychiatry, 12*(2), 105–115.

Moadel, A., Morgan, C., Fatone, A., Grennan, J., Carter, J., Laruffa, G., … Dutcher, J. (1999). Seeking meaning and hope: Self-reported spiritual and existential needs among an ethnically diverse cancer patient population. *Psycho-Oncology, 8*, 378–385.

Moss, E. L. & Dobson, K. S. (2006). Psychology, spirituality, and end of life care: An ethical integration? *Canadian Psychology, 47*(2), 284–299.

National Consensus Project. (2007). *Clinical practice guidelines for palliative care*. Retrieved from http://www.scribd.com/doc/36275/Clinical-Practice-Guidelines-for-Quality-Palliative-Care-National-Consensus-Project.

Newell, S. A., Sanson-Fisher, R. W., & Savolainen, N. J. (2002). Systematic review of psychological therapies for cancer patients: Overview and recommendations for future research. *Journal of the National Cancer Institute, 94*(8), 558–584.

Nicholas, D. R., & Veach, T. A. (2000). The psychosocial assessment of the adult cancer patient. *Psychosocial Psychology: Research and Practice, 31*(2), 206–215.

Parker, R. G. (1999). Reminiscence as continuity: Comparison of young and older adults. *Journal of Clinical Geropsychology, 5*(2), 147–157.

Pulchalski, C. M., Lunsford, B., Harris, M. H., & Miller, T. (2006). Interdisciplinary spiritual care for seriously ill and dying patients: A collaborative model. *The Cancer Journal, 12*(5), 398–416.

Quill, T. E., & Brody, H. (1996). Physician recommendations and patient autonomy: Finding a balance between physician power and patient choice. *Annals of Internal Medicine, 125*(9), 763–769.

Rehse, B., & Pukrop, R. (2003). Effects of psychosocial interventions on quality of life in adult cancer patients: Meta analysis of 37 published controlled outcome studies. *Patient Education and Counseling, 50*, 179–186.

Rohan, E., & Baush, J. (2009). Climbing Everest: Oncology work as an expedition in caring. *Journal of Psychosocial Oncology, 27*, 84–118.

Romanoff, B. D., & Thompson, B. E. (2006). Meaning construction in palliative care: The use of narrative, ritual, and the expressive arts. *American Journal of Hospice and Palliative Care, 23*(4), 309–316.

Serlin, I. A., Classen, C., Frances, B., & Angell, K. (2000). Support groups for women with breast cancer: Traditional and alternative expressive approaches. *The Arts of Psychotherapy, 27*(2), 123–138.

Shannon, S. E. (1997). The roots of interdisciplinary conflict around ethical issues. *Critical Care Nursing Clinics of North America, 9*(1), 13–28.

Simon, C. E., Pyrce, J. G., Roff, L. L., & Klemmack, D. (2006). Secondary traumatic stress and oncology social work. *Journal of Psychosocial Oncology, 23*(4), 1–14.

Smith, E. D., Walsh-Burke, K., & Crusan, C. (1998). Principles of training social workers in oncology. In J. C. Holland (Ed.), *Psycho-oncology* (pp. 1061–1069). New York, NY: Oxford University Press.

Spano, R. N., & Koenig, T. L. (2003). Moral dialogue: An interactional approach to ethical decision making. *Social Thought, 22*(1), 91–103.

Staudinger, U. M. (2001). Life reflection: A social-cognitive analysis of life review. *Review of General Psychology, 5*(2), 148–160.

Steinhauser, K. E., Christakis, N. A., Clipp, E. C., McNeilly, M., Grambow, S., Parker, J., & Tulsky, J. A. (2001). Preparing for the end of life: Preferences of patients, families, physicians, and other care providers. *Journal of Pain and Symptom Management, 22*, 727–737.

Uhruh, D. R. (1983). Death and personal history: Strategies of identify preservation. *Social Problems, 30*(3), 340–351.

Van der Molem, B. (2001). Relating information needs to the cancer experience: 1. Information as a key coping strategy. *European Journal of Cancer Care, 8*(4), 238–244. doi:10.1046/j.1365-2354.1999.00176.x.

Weaver, A. J., & Flannelly, K. J. (2004). The role of religion/spirituality for cancer patients and their caregivers. *Southern Medical Journal, 97*(12), 1210–1214.

31 *Teri Browne*

Palliative Care in Chronic Kidney Disease

No one ever told me that I could stop dialysis. Everything about coming to dialysis makes me hurt, but I am afraid to tell my doctor or my family. What should I do?
                    —"Florence," 72-year-old hemodialysis patient

Key Concepts

♦ *Chronic kidney disease patients have many palliative care concerns, including but not limited to pain, advance care planning, high mortality, and end of life.*

♦ *Every dialysis and kidney transplant center has a master's-level social worker who can integrate the eight domains of palliative care into the practice.*

♦ *Chronic kidney disease patients have the right to start, refuse, or discontinue dialysis at any time.*

♦ *Kidney disease interdisciplinary teams need more education and familiarity with palliative care.*

♦ *There are unique issues related to hospice provision for chronic kidney disease patients.*

Spectrum of Chronic Kidney Disease and Related Palliative Care Overview

Chronic kidney disease (CKD) leads to kidney failure (end-stage renal disease [ESRD]) and requires lifelong medical treatment with dialysis or kidney transplantation. There are two types of dialysis: peritoneal dialysis and hemodialysis. Peritoneal dialysis is performed by patients themselves every day and involves the use of a catheter that is placed above the navel to "exchange" fluids in the peritoneum cavity to remove toxins and fluids. Hemodialysis can be performed by patients at home, or it can be conducted in outpatient dialysis centers. Hemodialysis involves cleaning a patient's blood in a machine to remove toxins and fluids. This is achieved through a catheter or an "access" (fistula or graft) in a patient's arm that allows needles to be inserted and is hooked up to tubes and the hemodialysis machine. Most ESRD patients receive dialysis in outpatient centers, and they usually receive treatment three times per week with each treatment taking about 4 hours total. Kidney transplant patients can receive a kidney from a deceased donor, or a living donor, and remain on immunosuppressant medication for the life of the organ.

An ESRD patient's kidneys stop processing fluids and toxins, resulting in the need for a restricted diet and fluid consumption. Most of CKD is a result of hypertension or diabetes; however, kidneys may also fail because of lupus, cancer, chemotherapy, or hereditary kidney diseases. With sufficient work credits, all dialysis and kidney transplant patients have automatic eligibility for Medicare. Chronic kidney disease is a public health crisis in the United States. According to the U.S. Renal Data System Annual Data Report (2009), Medicare expenditures for this population were $57.5 billion (not accounting for Medicaid or private insurance spending), and 368,544 individuals had ESRD (U.S. Renal Data System, 2009). It is projected that by 2030 the number of ESRD patients will increase to 2.24 million (U.S. Renal Data System, 2002).

Issues related to palliative care are critically important in the CKD population and are considered a clinical priority (Davison, 2001). Kidney disease patients may have the same symptom burden, quality of life, and psychological distress as patients with terminal cancer (Saini et al., 2006). According to Jablonski (2008, p. 206) and other experts, "there is an urgent need to incorporate palliative care into the treatment of patients with end-stage renal disease (ESRD)." Patients with CKD are faced with many different palliative care issues, including enhancing quality of life, advance care planning, pain issues, decision making, end-of-life concerns, a high mortality rate, and hospice needs. At any point in their treatment, it is a kidney disease patient's right to refuse to start or to discontinue dialysis.

Many kidney disease patients can live long and successful lives. However, those with ESRD and particularly dialysis patients have far lower life expectancy than the general population (see Fig. 31.1). At least 21% of deaths in dialysis patients are preceded by a patient decision to withdraw dialysis (U.S. Renal Data System, 2002); attention to the palliative care needs in this population is critical. Also important is the demographic composition of the ESRD population. The rates of elderly patients, age 75 and older, have doubled since 1997 (U.S. Renal Data System, 2009), and older patients are more likely to have other comorbid illnesses and conditions that also diminish their life expectancy and quality of life.

Despite the high death rate, quality-of-life concerns, pain issues, and advance care planning needs of this population, kidney disease patients underutilize palliative care services, and many kidney disease teams are ill equipped to address patients' palliative needs. Because of this, the kidney disease community has made strides in addressing these critical patient needs, starting with the publication of the *Clinical Practice Guideline on Shared Decision-Making in the Appropriate Initiation of and Withdrawal from Dialysis* (Renal Physicians Association, 1999). In 2002, the Kidney End-of-Life Coalition was also created, with the mission of promoting "effective interchange between patients, families, caregivers, payers, and providers in support of integrated patient-centered end-of-life care of chronic kidney disease (CKD) patients" (Kidney End-of-Life Coalition, 2010).

In addition, the most recent Medicare Conditions for Coverage, which dictate the scope of care and required services provided to every dialysis patient in the United States, now require that every dialysis patient receive information about the fact that refusing any treatment is a patient right, and that every patient must be informed about advance directives (Federal Register, 2008). An important part of these conditions mandates that every dialysis and kidney transplant program must have an interdisciplinary team that includes a master's-level social worker, nephrologists (kidney doctors), surgeons, nurses, dietitians, and patient care technicians. Therefore, social workers in CKD facilities need to be knowledgeable about the domains of palliative care relevant to their patients and families, and social workers in palliative care programs, hospices, and other health settings need to be knowledgable about the unique palliative care needs of patients with CKD.

The components of an ideal renal palliative care program include attention to pain and symptom management, advance care planning, psychosocial and spiritual support to patients

| | General U.S. population, 2004 All races | | | | ESRD patients, 2007 | | | | | |
	All	M	F	All	Dialysis All	M	F	Transplant All	M	F
0–14	71.4	68.8	73.9	71.8	19.8	20.5	19.1	55.0	54.7	55.6
15–19	61.6	59.1	64.1	62.0	17.6	18.5	16.6	42.4	42.0	43.0
20–24	56.9	54.4	59.2	57.2	14.9	15.8	13.9	38.4	38.0	39.1
25–29	52.1	49.7	54.4	52.5	13.2	13.9	12.3	35.1	34.7	35.9
30–34	47.4	45.1	49.5	47.7	11.4	11.8	10.8	31.3	30.8	32.2
35–39	42.7	40.4	44.7	42.9	9.9	10.3	9.5	27.8	27.2	28.8
40–44	38.0	35.8	40.0	38.3	8.6	8.8	8.4	24.3	23.7	25.4
45–49	33.5	31.4	35.4	33.7	7.4	7.5	7.3	21.1	20.5	22.3
50–54	29.2	27.2	30.9	29.3	6.5	6.6	6.4	18.1	17.4	19.3
55–59	25.0	23.1	26.5	25.1	5.6	5.7	5.6	15.5	14.8	16.7
60–64	21.0	19.3	22.4	21.0	4.8	4.8	4.9	13.1	12.4	14.2
65–69	17.2	15.7	18.5	17.3	4.1	4.0	4.1	10.8	10.2	11.8
70–74	13.8	12.5	14.8	13.8	3.4	3.4	3.5	8.9	8.4	9.8
75–79	10.8	9.7	11.5	10.7	2.9	2.8	2.9	7.5	7.0	8.3
80–84	8.2	7.3	8.7	8.1	2.4	2.3	2.5			
85+	4.4	3.9	4.6	4.3	1.9	1.9	2.0			
Overall	25.2	23.4	26.6	25.3	5.9	6.0	5.9	16.4	15.8	17.4

Figure 31.1. Expected remaining lifetimes (years) of the U.S. population and of dialysis and transplant patients, by age, gender, and race (U.S. Renal Data System, 2009)

and families, and ethical issues in dialysis decision making (Moss et al., 2004). Because the goal of any palliative care program is to enhance patient quality of life, this is congruent with the ESRD care provision that all patients must have their quality of life measured every year (Federal Register, 2008), and it relates directly to the finding that patient quality of life can independently predict morbidity and mortality (DeOreo, 1997; Knight, Ofsthun, Teng, Lazarus, & Curhan, 2003).

Psychosocial Issues in Chronic Kidney Disease Related to Pain Management

Episodic, acute, and chronic pain are very common among patients with CKD and can negatively impact patient quality of life and increase depression (Devins et al. 1990; Weisbord et al., 2005). Iacono (2003, 2004) found that 60% of dialysis patients have chronic pain, and that 66% of these patients were using prescription medication for pain. Germain, Cohen, & Davison (2007) found that 50% of patients with CKD had chronic pain. Many patients with ESRD also have significant pain prior to their death (Cohen et al. 2005). Despite these facts, only 48% of more than 1000 dialysis professionals reported having discussions with patients about pain (Weiner, 2008). Patients may have pain related to kidney disease and treatment-related issues, in addition to pain caused by comorbid conditions. Lori Hartwell (2002, p. 8), a patient with ESRD and an advocate, describes her experiences with procedure related pain as follows:

> *During my many medical procedures, I've had to endure hundreds of needle pricks. When I was younger, I would never complain about the number of sticks the nurses made. Consequently, they repeatedly told me what a good patient I was. In reality, those needles hurt! I wanted to cry and scream at the person who kept poking me. Most often I was silent and tried to be as accommodating as possible.*

This quote captures the complex relationships and reality of the patients who depend on their care providers, who may cause pain to patients to achieve a positive outcome.

Nephropathy, calciphylaxis, dry skin, itching, calcific uremic arteriolopathy, dialysis-related amyloidosis, and renal osteodystrophy are all conditions that cause pain related to kidney disease. Patients with polycystic kidney disease may have pain related to the cysts on their kidneys. Restless legs syndrome, in which patients have persistent tremors in their extremities, is also common in patients with ESRD. Pain can also result from cramping and headaches during dialysis, and from the needle sticks required for hemodialysis. Hemodialysis access surgery may leave patients with "steel hand syndrome" or other nerve damage and pain. The pain of a hemodialysis patient may be caused or exacerbated by sitting in the hemodialysis chair for hours

at a time. Peritoneal dialysis patients may have severe pain from a common infection, peritonitis. Transplant patients may have pain from kidney disease complications, as well as from the transplant surgery. Pain related to comorbid conditions includes complications from diabetic neuropathy, peripheral vascular disease, amputation, arthritis, lupus, and gout.

Treating pain in kidney disease patients is a challenge. Because of their kidney failure, patients cannot metabolize medications like other individuals, and prescribers must be cautious not to prescribe pain medications that are toxic to patients or dialyze out of their system during treatments. This is particularly the case for dialysis patients; transplant patients have better kidney function to process the medications. The Mid-Atlantic Renal Coalition (2009) published the booklet *Clinical Algorithm and Preferred Medications to Treat Pain in Dialysis Patients* to assist medical teams in assessing pain and treating it appropriately. For dialysis patients, this guideline recommends that the following pain medications not ever be used in dialysis patients because of the potential for toxicity: morphine, codeine, meperidine, and propoxyphene. Because of the complexities of pain management in kidney disease patients, it is recommended that dialysis teams consult with palliative care experts in this area to determine the proper strategy for pain management for individual patients.

Oral medication self-management is also challenging in kidney disease patients, because recent research concluded that these patients have the highest pill burden of any chronically ill patients (Chiu et al., 2009). Chiu and colleagues discovered that more than one-quarter of hemodialysis patients take at least 25 pills per day (median = 19), and 62% of patients did not take their oral medications as prescribed. Therefore, teams need to explore the unique reasons for this outcome in individual patients and prescribe in an effort to decrease burden and enhance successful treatment. Acupuncture and physical therapy may also be helpful for patients in managing their pain. Kidney disease patient Lori Hartwell recommends that patients manage pain by seeking support from social networks and spiritual counselors, and by integrating relaxation techniques, massage, stretching, and exercise into their treatment plan (Hartwell, 2002).

Disturbingly, patients with kidney disease may not mention pain symptoms to their team (Brown, 2007), and renal teams underestimate or may not be aware of their patients' pain. (Weisbord et al., 2007). Teams can use pain assessment tools to assess pain and related distress and intervene accordingly. Because hemodialysis patients may have treatment or transportation delays, clinicians can encourage patients to have their pain medication with them at all times to maximize their comfort. Teams must build in routine pain assessment of home dialysis and kidney transplant patients, because they do not have regular contact as they do with in-center hemodialysis patients. Social workers can assist in assessing patients' pain on a routine basis, and they can intervene with education, cognitive-behavioral techniques, and supportive counseling for patients and families when pain is a concern. Social workers and team members can also collaborate with palliative care specialists to address unresolved symptoms. (For more information, see Chapter 5.)

Psychosocial Issues in Chronic Kidney Disease: To Start or Stop Dialysis

When a patient is first diagnosed with kidney failure, he or she has the choice to not receive any renal replacement therapy. After patients start dialysis, they have the right to stop dialysis at any time. If patients do not receive dialysis and they have ESRD, they will die. Without dialysis, the median number of days that patients will survive is 8 days; however, patients routinely live even longer (Germain et al., 2007). A research study of 115,239 deceased dialysis patients found that 96% of patients who stopped dialysis died within a month (Murray, Arko, Chen, Gilbertson, & Moss, 2006). Death from ESRD is not usually painful (National Kidney Foundation, 2007). It is the shared work of nephrology social workers and their interdisciplinary teams to engage patients in informed consent discussions about starting or stopping dialysis (Brown, 2007).

The Decision Not To Start Dialysis

In the United States, less than 5% of patients do not start dialysis (Germain et al., 2007). Kidney disease teams are encouraged to discuss realistic expectations of prognosis and quality-of-life issues related to starting this life-extending treatment. Russ, Shim, and Kaufman (2007) recommend that nephrologists have frank discussions with their patients about their prognosis, how long they can expect to live on dialysis, and how dialysis will impact their quality of life and that of their families.

Taking into account that the fastest growing and greatest population of patients who start dialysis is older adults, it is important to consider the consequences of starting dialysis in elderly patients. A study of all nursing home patients in the United States suggests that starting dialysis in these patients may be associated with a significant decline in functional status, and that 58% of these patients died within 1 year of starting dialysis (Tamura et al., 2009). A study of other older adults determined that patients over 75 years with comorbid illnesses (particularly ischemic heart disease) had little survival advantage compared to patients who did not start dialysis (Murtagh et al., 2007). These results are similar to the work of Smith et al. (2003), who found no survival benefit of dialysis with patients who are elderly with significant comorbid complications. Recent research has suggested that kidney failure in the elderly is also related to faster cognitive decline (Buchman et al., 2009). These findings

need to be taken into account by the nephrologist and the renal team when deciding the most clinically and culturally appropriate way of sharing, in a direct and compassionate manner, prognostic information as well as the benefit and burden of dialysis.

Moss et al. (2004) suggest that when talking to patients about not starting dialysis, teams should take the following factors into account and attend to them in their discussions: realistic patient prognosis, patient survival with and without dialysis, the details of what dialysis treatment would require (surgery for an access, diet and fluid restrictions, time required every week), explanation of palliative and hospice resources available in the community, assurance that the nephrologist will not "abandon" the patient if the patient decides not to start dialysis, and inclusion of the patient's support network in such discussions.

The *Clinical Practice Guideline on Shared Decision-Making in the Appropriate Initiation of and Withdrawal from Dialysis* recommends that providers take the following steps when working with patients about a dialysis decision (Galla, 2000):

- Establish and nurture a patient–provider relationship that encourages shared decision making that includes the patient's support system
- Maximize the patient's informed consent by providing full disclosure of the patient diagnosis and prognosis, including life expectancy and quality-of-life expectations
- Talk about the possibility of a "trial run" of dialysis to see how the patient responds to dialysis if the patient is interested
- Talk about end-of-life resources such as hospice
- Facilitate conflict resolution if necessary between the patient and family about this decision
- Help and encourage patients to complete advance directives
- Ensure that patient receives palliative care regardless of his or her decision

Taking these steps may alleviate the fears and misconceptions that patients have about starting or stopping dialysis and provides a basis upon which ongoing discussions can occur.

The Decision to Stop Dialysis

If a patient indicates that he or she wants to stop dialysis, the social worker and dialysis team first insure that the patient has the capacity to make the decision and involve the patient's health care power of attorney if the patient does not (King, 2007). The patient's motivation and understanding of the benefits and burdens of the decision needs to be explored to determine whether it is due to depression, treatable problems with the dialysis experience, feelings of being a burden to family, mental illness, or other factors that are remediable. The social worker can secure the psychiatric, psychological, or spiritual counseling necessary to assist the patient's decision-making process. Likewise, if a patient is talking about stopping treatment because a hemodialysis regime is too intrusive or painful, the patient might want to try home dialysis or consider a kidney transplant. It is important to also take into consideration a patient's ethnicity culture and spiritual, personal, and family beliefs about stopping or not starting dialysis. In one study, black dialysis patients were found to be about three times less likely to choose to withdraw from dialysis treatment (Leggat, Swartz, & Port, 1997), and in another, black and Hispanic patients were found to be half as likely to discontinue dialysis (Germain et al., 2007). Although there is no formal evidence that any organized religion or spiritual system suggests that stopping dialysis is morally problematic because it may hasten death, patients may think this is the case. Social workers can explore these belief systems, work with the patient and/or family, the patient's spiritual leader, along with a chaplain, to explore this concern.

There are medical events that might serve as an invitation to rediscuss the overall treatment plan and benefit and burden of continued dialysis. They include frequent infections, numerous hospitalizations, significant weight loss, poor nutrition, significant hemodialysis and peritoneal dialysis access problems, chest pain, shortness of breath, malignancy, or other comorbid causes of decline (Brown, Chambers, & Eggeling, 2008). It is critical that dialysis teams help patients link to hospice services whenever patients refuse to start or stop dialysis.

The Pulitzer Prize–winning author Art Buchwald's experience with discontinuing dialysis is enlightening for kidney disease patients and teams. He says of his decision to stop dialysis:

> I agreed to continue dialysis, as I was not getting much support from my loved ones for the dying option, which I personally thought was best. I tried dialysis twelve times and decided I didn't like it. "That's it," I said. "I don't see a future in this and I don't want to do it anymore!" I had discovered the idea of the hospice by then, and knew I had an alternative. Dr. Newman said, "It's your choice. You're the only one who can decide." I knew the entire family was against the idea of stopping dialysis. Everybody warned me that I was signing my own death certificate. (Buchwald, 2006, pp. 15–16).

Mr. Buchwald actually ended up living almost a year after he stopped dialysis, and he had a very good experience with hospice services. However, Pruchno, Lemay, Field, and Levinsky's 2006 study of 291 hemodialysis patients discovered that patients were reluctant to discontinue dialysis because they feared end-of-life suffering. This and other research suggests the kidney disease community has more work to do to help patients know they will not be left to suffer.

Psychosocial Issues in Chronic Kidney Disease Related to Advance Care Planning

An important role for nephrology social workers is to faciltate advance care planning, whether oral or written, and discussions with patients about their treatment wishes in case of an emergency such as respiratory arrest. Social workers can educate their team members about optimal advance care planning. If introduced early, these discussions, held over time, invite a collaborative relationship and can increase patient and family comfort with the concepts and process (Moss et al, 2004). Davison (2006) recommends that frank discussions about the patient's prognosis and expectations for dialysis treatment be part of an ideal advance care planning process in the CKD setting and be revisited as part of a routine global assessment about ongoing care and evolving needs. Social workers trained in family, cultural, and spiritual asessment can insure that these conversations respond to the unique needs of the patient and family.

One aspect of advance care planning is the completion of oral or written advance directives. Research has indicated that a majority of patients with CKD do not have advance directives (Cohen, McCue, Germain, & Woods, 1997), nor have they had advance care planning discussions with their kidney disease teams. A 2003 National Kidney Foundation survey of hemodialysis patients reported that the issue least discussed by their team was end-of-life care (Weiner, 2008). Research conducted by Davison, Jhangri, Holley, and Moss (2006) concluded that only 39% of 360 patients with CKD perceived themselves as very well prepared to make end-of-life decisions. In a 2007 survey of 182 hemodialysis patients across the country, more than half (54%) of the respondents said that they never had a conversation with their dialysis team about palliative care and advance care planning, despite the fact that 76% reported they wanted to have these conversations with their teams (Weiner, 2008).

Nephrology social workers are the experts in the area of advance care planning in their dialysis units. In research conducted by Rabetoy and Blair (2007), only 25% of nurses discussed advance care planning with patients, compared to 82% of social workers. In 2008, Medicare mandated that all dialysis patients need to have discussions with their teams about advance directives (Federal Register, 2008). These regulations likewise mandate that if dialysis facilities are legally unable to honor a patient's advance directives (for example, a do not resuscitate [DNR] request), they must have a protocol in place to transfer the patient to a unit that will honor the patient's wishes. With regard to DNR orders, dialysis teams need to be sure that they are in compliance with state laws because some require a dialysis-only DNR order while others can be guided by the order on file at a hospital or nursing home. Educating dialysis staff includes increasing awareness of who has a DNR order and what will occur in case of a patient adverse event such as cardiac arrest. Dialysis teams who work collaboratively to create a plan to intervene with patients who die with a DNR order need to consider how they will respond to the needs of other patients in the unit and how they will create a bereavement ritual for themselves and other patients. Additionally, staff should have contact information for the patient's funeral home, be knowledgeable of local laws and regulations related to patients who die at the center with a DNR order, have up-to-date emergency contact information for all patients, and have a practiced routine of what will happen to the patient's body after death (see Box 31.1).

The National Kidney Foundation of Michigan has been successful in using a patient peer mentoring program to educate patients about advance care planning (Perry, 2007). Dialysis patients in 22 dialysis units across Michigan were trained to be peer mentors and discussed their own experiences related to advance care planning with fellow patients. This intervention significantly increased dialysis patients' desire, completion, and comfort with advance directives. Interestingly, black patients were significantly more likely than white patients to complete advance directives. This study, in which patients were placed in control or experimental groups, and controlled for effects of literacy and education, suggests that black dialysis patients may respond better to oral information provided by peers rather than written materials.

Any advance care planning education should integrate the findings of national research studies that suggest that kidney disease patients' families *may not be* aware of patients' end-of-life wishes. In a study of 291 hemodialysis patients and their spouses, patient preferences related to continuing dialysis were only moderately correlated ($r = .33$) with their spouses' judgment of what the patient desired (Pruchno et al., 2006). Likewise, Song et al.'s 2009 study indicated that the patient's end-of-life treatment preferences differed from that of the person appointed to make decisions for the patient should they become incapacitated. These studies suggest that dialysis social workers include such findings in education and involve the patient's family and appointed health care agents in discussions about the patient's treatment wishes; the psychological, spiritual, and cultural variables that inform the decisions; and the potential impact on the family.

Nephrology Social Work Collaboration with Hospice Teams

Research suggests that a majority of dialysis patients who discontinue treatment and die at home receiving hospice care have better deaths (Cohen et. al., 2000). Patients who withdraw from dialysis usually have a very short life expectancy and may choose to be cared for at home with hospice or, if indicated, in an inpatient setting. Dialysis patients who have a prognosis of 6 months or less, depending on the diagnoses, might be better served if referred to hospice services as early as possible (Holley, 2005). However, the majority of kidney disease patients who die after stopping dialysis do not benefit from hospice services and often die in a hospital or receive very short-term hospice services. One study concluded that only 13.5% of all dialysis patients who die used hospice services (Murray et al., 2006), and another study found that less than 50% of patients who withdrew from dialysis received hospice services prior to their death (Murray et al., 2006). A study of all of the 2002 hospice claims in the United States determined that patients who had previously received dialysis represented 55% of all hospice patients, and the researchers concluded that patients did not receive hospice services until very shortly before their death (Connor, Elwert, Spence, & Christakis, 2007). In settings where patients are admitted to a hospital at any time along the continuum of illness and at the end of life, referral to palliative consult teams can enrich the care of patients and their families. Patients who are cared for at home will of necessity have a short experience with hospice providers given the limited life expectancy following withdrawal from dialysis. In both settings, collaboration between social work clinicians is essential to insure that potential feelings of abandonment are diminished.

Box 31.1
Patient/Family Narrative: Mr. Jones

Mr. Jones is a 26-year-old married black chronic kidney disease patient who attended an educational seminar for patients newly diagnosed with kidney disease. At this workshop, the social worker, dietitian, nurse, and physician all present information to patients in a group setting. The social worker's presentation includes a talk about advance care planning, and in the context of this discussion, Mr. Jones informs the social worker that he wants to have a do not resuscitate (DNR) order when he comes to dialysis. A few months later when Mr. Jones starts dialysis, he requests a DNR order. The social worker reviews family history, values, and beliefs that inform this decision and works with him to consider the impact of his decision on his wife and family. She explains exactly what a DNR order means, exploring the medical context in which he would want it activated and encourages him to discuss this with his wife, offering a joint meeting, if needed, to assist Mrs. Jones. The social worker consults with the nephrologist to obtain a signed DNR order and, with the charge nurse, reviews the document with Mr. Jones. At the monthly staff meeting in which all DNR patients are reviewed with all staff, several nurses and patient care technicians disagree with this patient choosing DNR because of his young age. The social worker takes the opportunity to share the thoughts, values, and beliefs that informed his decision and provides team education about the patient's right to participate in these care decisions. In addition to exploring feelings and thoughts about this choice, the social worker processes their feelings about not intervening to resuscitate a patient who has a cardiac arrest in the dialysis unit. The social worker revisits this issue every month and works with the nurse manager and physician to regularly review all patients' advance care plans and their current wishes related to this topic.

One barrier to referring dialysis patients to hospice is related to reimbursement and payment for services (Germain & Cohen, 2007; Germain et al., 2007). Because dialysis is considered a life-sustaining medical treatment, there are misconceptions about dialysis patient eligibility to receive hospice services, particularly if the patient chooses to continue dialysis. If a patient is eligible for hospice due to a non–kidney disease diagnosis (for example, malignant cancer), the patient can usually choose to continue dialysis and still receive hospice services consequent to the hospice diagnosis of cancer. Other diagnoses, such as "failure to thrive" or diabetes, are an obstacle for hospice organizations who may not get paid for their services if the patient continues dialysis. This has resulted in confusion and misinformation in the kidney disease and hospice communities about dialysis patients' eligibility for receiving hospice services. In response to this confusion, the National Hospice and Palliative Care Organization (2009) created a flowchart that summarizes hospice eligibility for patients with chronic kidney disease (see Fig. 31.2).

Nephrology social workers can collaborate with their hospice peers to advocate for patients and educate payers about patient eligibility. In addition to such skills as family assessment and interventions, psychological assessment, and resource finding, on kidney disease interdisciplinary teams, social workers have been found to be the most knowledgeable about patient eligibility for Medicare hospice benefits

(Thompson, Bhargava, Bachelder, Bova-Collis, & Moss, 2008).

Nephrology Social Work Collaboration with the Kidney Disease Team

As an essential member of kidney disease teams, master's-level social workers play an important role on the interdisciplinary team in helping patients and their families with palliative care issues. Social workers can provide patient education, intervene with pain and symptom management, provide supportive and grief counseling, assist with advance care planning and adaptation to illness, and provide referrals to palliative and hospice teams. This role extends from the CKD setting before patients start treatment, to the outpatient dialysis clinics and transplant centers where individual and group modalities can be employed to assist patients and their families.

Social workers with appropriate skill sets are often the experts in palliative care in dialysis units, and they can educate their team members about patient and family needs with the goal of responding to their multidimensional experience. Research suggests that nephrologists and nurses are not as informed as social workers about the role of palliative care in patients with kidney disease. Holley et al.'s research (2003)

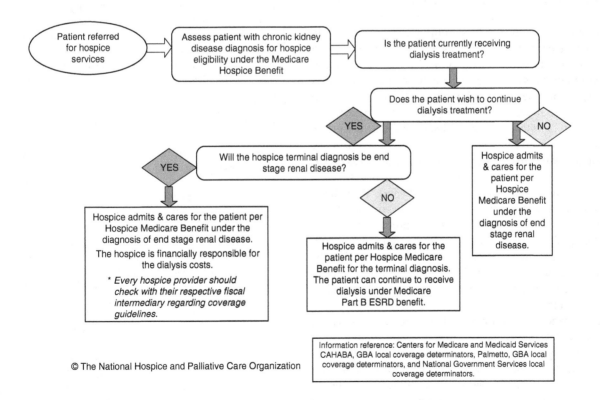

Figure 31.2. Determining hospice eligibility for chronic kidney disease—Medicare Hospice Benefit. (Reproduced with permission from The National Hospice and Palliative Care Organization.)

discovered that only 22% of nephrology fellows received training in managing patient end-of-life needs. Nephrologists may not have the time or the inclination to discuss palliative care issues with patients (Burns & Carson, 2007).

Research indicates that patients are in significant need of assistance from their teams when considering the choice to discontinue dialysis. Bhargava, Germain, Kitsen, Cohen, and Meyer (2009) found that 51% of patients who withdrew from dialysis did not actively participate in discussions with their care teams about this withdrawal. Burns and Carson (2007) suggest that patients with CKD contemplating choices related to dialysis treatment may be swayed by the concern that their physicians will discontinue all care if they do not want dialysis. Social workers can help physicians with these challenging discussions and also be available to explore these concerns individually with patients and their families. They can also help teams, patients, and their social support network with conflict resolution and care planning as options are explored and goals of care are reformulated (see Box 31.2). (For more information, see Chapter 38.)

There are specific suggestions in the literature for ways that kidney disease teams can approach the domain of palliative care that relates to end of life. First, the dialysis team should be very aware of their reactions to death and dying (King, 2007). Kidney disease teams are also encouraged to regularly revisit patient and family discussions about pain, advance care planning, and dialysis as a treatment choice, because patient decisions may change over time. The 2008 Conditions for Coverage of Dialysis (Federal Register, 2008) require that patient status and care plan is reassessed frequently, and dialysis teams can easily add these components to their regular assessment process. As nephrology social workers need to measure quality of life at least annually, they can create an opportunity to assess palliative domains of care such as social and spiritual aspects of quality of life. These conditions of coverage also mandate that dialysis teams help patients and their families with psychosocial issues and create a private area where sensitive discussions can be held. Teams can take advantage of this mandate and use these private areas to have patient family discussions about palliative case issues.

As a team, discussions that routinely review the patient's condition can identify changes in medical condition, family concerns, or increasing disability that provide impetus to explore goals of care. Robust research has found that asking a nephrologist the question, "Would I be surprised if this patient died in the next year?" (Moss et al., 2008) or "Would I be surprised if this patient died in the next six months?" (Cohen, Ruthazer, Moss, & Germain, 2010) can significantly identify patients who are at high risk for early mortality. Kidney disease teams may use these assessment questions to screen their patient population and first focus efforts on palliative care for the patients who may die within 6 months and then those who may die within a year. If the kidney disease team's selected focus is on care planning and dialysis decision making, dialysis social workers and teams can begin discussions with patients by exploring whether there might be any

---

Box 31.2
Patient/Family Narrative: Mrs. Blake

Mrs. Blake is a 74- year-old white, widowed, dialysis patient. She has been on hemodialysis for 2 years consequent to diabetes, which has resulted in two above-the-knee amputations. She is on insulin, is legally blind, and has resided in a skilled nursing facility (SNF) for 5 years because she is unable to live independently. She has three grown children and seven grandchildren. Her children and all but one grandchild live out of the state and visit the patient about once a year. Her out-of-town families call her on the telephone about once a week for a brief chat. She has one 30-year-old grandson who visits at least monthly. Her essential, continuous support system includes the care teams at her residence and at the dialysis center. Her Kidney Disease Quality of Life score is very low, as is her laboratory value for albumin (which indicates she is poorly nourished and will have low energy and a higher likelihood of being hospitalized or dying). During her hemodialysis treatments she has become increasingly restless and uncomfortable. She cannot transfer independently from wheelchair to the dialysis chair, and a Hoyer lift must be used. She is obese, so the transfer is sometimes difficult and uncomfortable for the patient and stressful for the staff. At the SNF, she refuses many meals and does not participate in any activities other than watching television. She often refuses her medications. Her physicians have diagnosed her with depression; however, antidepressants and counseling have proved ineffective. There are no residences that can address her needs and provide dialysis in residence. She receives hemodialysis through an access in her arm that has been very problematic. It is difficult to stick with the hemodialysis needle and the nurses often have to try several times to place the needles in her arms for dialysis. Several times her access has been infiltrated, leaving her with significant bruises and pain. These medical and access problems have resulted in caring clinicians having to hurt Mrs. Blake in an effort to continue the care she has chosen. Her dialysis treatments often result in cramping and hypotension, because her fluid consumption is in excess of the recommendations and the treatment needs to extract sometimes as much as 6 kilograms from her body in 3 hours. She has great difficulty with the strict fluid restrictions imposed on dialysis patients, and she often drinks more fluid than the amount she is allowed, resulting in high fluid weight gains between treatments. Furthermore, the Medicaid van that transports Mrs. Blake to and from dialysis is often an hour late. During her hemodialysis treatments, Mrs. Blake reports continuous pain and discomfort, both from the treatment itself as well as sitting in a dialysis chair for 3 hours. Mrs. Blake has been telling her doctor, nurses, and social worker, that she does not want to come to dialysis anymore and that she "has had enough." As her disability has increased the interventions that had been beneficial have become increasingly burdensome.

The dialysis team has explored all of these issues with Mrs. Blake, her grandson, and the SNF staff. The team has ruled out depression and suicidal ideation, has tried various methods of pain relief, and other ways to make dialysis more comfortable. Mrs. Blake's two daughters and son have come into town to have a patient care conference with the dialysis team to talk about Mrs. Blake's request to stop dialysis. They meet with the dialysis social worker, the nephrologist, the dialysis nurse, the grandson, and the patient to talk about the treatment options. Initially, Mrs. Blake's son refused to talk about stopping dialysis, and told Mrs. Blake

Box 31.2 *(Contd.)*

that she "would just be giving up on everyone and would be a quitter." These words reflected his anger and disappointment that his mother would make a choice that would result in her death and in her leaving her children. Mrs. Blake's oldest daughter expressed the belief that Mrs. Blake "would go to hell for committing suicide," which invited exploration of the religious values that often infuse these discussions. The nephrology social worker actively listened to all of the children's concerns and helped Mrs. Blake explain what was involved in dialysis and how much pain she was in. None of the children had ever visited Mrs. Blake while she received dialysis, so the nurse and social worker explained all of the issues and problems that Mrs. Blake was having related to dialysis and her other medical problems. The social worker validated the grandson's feelings, encouraging him to share his unique experience and perspective about his grandmother's suffering and poor quality of life. The distress of other family members was also acknowledged. The family was helped to understand that Mrs. Blake was cared for by dialysis and nursing home staff who observed her changed quality of life and the coherence of her request to discontinue dialysis. The nephrologist explained what was likely to occur as dialysis was discontinued, the prognosis with or without dialysis, and the likely process of her death. A chaplain was asked to join the discussion to explore the religious conflict expressed by the son, and time was spent differentiating suicide from decisions that allowed death to occur. The social worker provided the family with information about how the local hospice organization could help the patient with a chaplain, pain and symptom management, and support for the patient and family if the patient decided to stop dialysis. This had been reviewed previously with the patient who wanted to see how her children would respond to these discussions. The social worker also offered to help the family and patient talk to their family priest and reviewed the process by which the patient had reached the decision to stop dialysis.

The social worker acknowledged feelings of grief and loss, and provided empathetic listening, reframing the patient's decision as a wish for relief of suffering rather than a sign of weakness or a wish to leave her children. Mrs. Blake's children did agree to a meeting with hospice to discuss the services they could provide the patient in the comfort of the nursing facility with familiar staff providing care. The nephrology social worker attended this meeting at the SNF to support a seamless transition and integration of the hospice clinicians into Mrs. Blake's care. After this consultation, the patient did choose hospice care and discontinued dialysis. Mrs. Blake died 6 days later, in her room with her children and grandchildren at her side. The nephrology social worker sent a sympathy card to the family on behalf of the dialysis unit after the patient's death, and a year after the death in memory of the patient.

circumstances in which they would not want to continue with dialysis (Hackett & Hackett, 2007). If the chosen focus of the kidney disease team is on advance care planning, patients can be asked who they might want to make medical decisions for them if something occurred that prevented direct communication with the patient. Another way to start

these discussions is by asking patients: "Would it be OK with you if we talk about what you might want to happen to you in case of emergency?" Finally, dialysis teams may want to ask patients whether they have "more bad days than good days" to assess ongoing quality of life and reaffirm treatment choices.

Kidney transplant teams also have many opportunities to address patient quality of life and goals of care. Although transplant patients have better mortality and morbidity rates than dialysis patients, these discussions are appropriate along the continuum of illness, not just in emergencies or at end of life. Also, patients who receive an organ from a deceased donor may experience coping issues related to the death that was necessary for them to receive the transplanted organ. Transplant social workers can help patients acknowledge and process this grief. In some transplant centers, letters are written by transplanted patients to the family of the deceased donor thanking them for the "gift of life." The National Kidney Foundation has many different programs and services for families of organ donors that can also help transplanted patients cope with the fact that someone had to die in order for them to receive a transplant.

After a patient's death, the dialysis social worker can lead the team to create processes to mourn patients and help staff, other patients, and family members cope with the death. As hemodialysis patients often see the dialysis team, and other patients, more than even their own family members and friends because of all the time involved in the treatment, it is essential that dialysis teams address the loss of a patient in a dialysis unit. This is also true for home dialysis patients or transplant patients. Taking into account HIPPA privacy laws, this can be done by staff debriefing after a death, an annual memorial service for patients, a card sent to the family after the death, or in many other ways (Cohen, 2004; Holley, 2005; King, 2007). Staff grieving can be facilitated by the social worker in a staff meeting or be the shared work of the team to honor both their work and the life of the patient who has died. Dialysis teams can routinely assess the quality of pain management and the death experiences of patients in their monthly Quality Assessment and Performance Improvement (QAPI) meetings that Medicare mandates in all facilities (Federal Register, 2008), thus providing a regular setting to acknowledge the loss of specific patients.

Conclusion

Attention to palliative care for patients with kidney disease from the moment they are diagnosed with kidney failure will benefit patients and can enhance their quality of life and quality of dying. Every dialysis and kidney transplant center must have a master's-level social worker on its interdisciplinary team, and these social workers are uniquely situated to help their teams, patients, and families in areas related to pain management, advance care planning, psychosocial-spiritual interventions, treatment decision making, and hospice care. While additional research is needed in the areas of palliative care for children and younger patients with kidney disease, ethnic minorities, and the unique palliative care needs of home dialysis and kidney transplant patients, there is a breadth of knowledge to inform and enrich the daily practice of nephrology social workers and palliative social workers who provide services to patients with kidney disease and their families.

LEARNING EXERCISES

- Using the National Association of Social Workers (NASW) Code of Ethics, identify four areas in the Code of Ethics that relate to the "Mrs. Blake" family narrative and discuss how the social worker did or did not adhere to the Code of Ethics.
- Imagine you are a dialysis social worker, assigned to a new patient. This patient is 21 years old, just started dialysis after a kidney transplant was rejected, and informs you in your first meeting with him that he does not want to come to dialysis anymore and would "rather die." What should your next steps be as the social worker providing services to this patient?
- Contact a local hospice provider in your area and ask them about their hospice services available to patients with kidney disease. What are the possibilities for care if the patient has less than a 6-month prognosis because of the diagnosis "failure to thrive" and the patient wants to continue dialysis? What services is the patient eligible for? Consider contacting different hospice organizations and then compare the answers. As a group of classmates or colleagues, discuss these answers and what you can do as advocates to help patients on a local and national level to access hospice services.

ADDITIONAL SUGGESTED READINGS AND RESOURCES

Cohen, L., Poppel, D., Cohn, G., & Reiter, G. (2001). A very good death: Measuring quality of dying in end-stage renal disease. *Journal of Palliative Medicine*, 4(2), 167–172.

Dialysis Quality of Dying APGAR. This is a tool developed to determine a dialysis patient's quality of dying, and it can be found in the appendix of the Cohen article listed above.

Kidney End-of-Life Coalition: http://www.kidneyeol.org

Resources for patients, families, and professionals on all aspects of palliative care for kidney disease patients.

Mid-Atlantic Renal Coalition: http://www.kidneyeol.org/painbrochure9.09.pdf

Clinical algorithm and preferred medications to treat pain in dialysis patients. Can be ordered from by calling 1-804-794-3757.

Mid-Atlantic Renal Coalition: http://www.kidneyeol.org/ACPOrderForm10-09.pdf

Advance care planning for the dialysis patient and their family. Can be ordered from by calling 1-804-794-3757.

National Kidney Foundation: http://www.kidney.org/atoz/content/AdvanceDirectives.cfm

Advance directives a guide for patients and their families. Can be ordered from the National Kidney Foundation 1-800-622-9010.

National Kidney Foundation: http://www.kidney.org/ATOZ/pdf/IfYouChoose.pdf

If you choose not to start dialysis treatment. Can be ordered from the National Kidney Foundation 1-800-622-9010.

National Kidney Foundation: http://www.kidney.org/atoz/pdf/StopDialysis.pdf.

When stopping dialysis treatment is your choice. Can be ordered from the National Kidney Foundation 1-800-622-9010.

Promoting Excellence in End-of-Life Care (2002). *End-stage renal disease workgroup recommendations to the field*. Missoula, MT: The Robert Wood Johnson Foundation.

The Renal Physicians Association (RPA). Wrote the position paper, *Quality Care at End of Life*, which led to the RPA and the American Society of Nephrology (ASN) publishing an evidence-based clinical practice guideline, *Shared Decision Making*, which addresses withholding and withdrawal of dialysis.

REFERENCES

Bhargava, J., Germain, M., Kitsen, J., Cohen, L., & Meyer, K. (2009). Ethics: Knowledge and participation of front-line dialysis facility staff in end-of-life discussions. *Nephrology News and Issues*, 8, 10–13.

Brown, E. A. (2007). Epidemiology of renal palliative care. *Journal of Palliative Medicine*, 10(6), 1248–1252.

Brown, E. A., Chambers, E. J., & Eggeling, C. (2008). Palliative care in nephrology. *Nephrology Dialysis and Transplant*, 23(3), 789–791.

Buchman, A. S., Tanne, D., Boyle, P. A., Shah, R. C., Leurgans, S. E., & Bennett, D. A. (2009). Kidney function is associated with the rate of cognitive decline in the elderly. *Neurology*, 73(12), 920–927.

Buchwald, A. (2006). *Too soon to say goodbye*. New York, NY: Random House.

Burns, A., & Carson, R. (2007). Maximum conservative management: A worthwhile treatment for elderly patients with renal failure who choose not to undergo dialysis. *Journal of Palliative Medicine*, 10(6), 1245–1247.

Chiu, Y-W., Teitelbaum, I., Misra, M., de Leon, E. M., Adzize, T., & Mehrotra, R. (2009). Pill burden, adherence, hyperphosphatemia, and quality of life in maintenance dialysis patients. *Clinical Journal of the American Society of Nephrology*, 4(6), 1089–1096.

Cohen, L. (2004). Planning a renal palliative care programme and its components. In E. J. Chambers, M. Germain, & E. Brown (Eds.), *Supportive care for the renal patient* (pp. 27–34). New York, NY: Oxford.

Cohen, L. M., Germain, M. J., Poppel, D. M., Woods, A. L., Pekow, P. S., & Kjellstrand, C. M. (2000). Dying well after discontinuing the life-support treatment of dialysis. *Archives of Internal Medicine*, 160, 2513–2518.

Cohen, L., McCue, J., Germain, M., & Woods, A. (1997). Denying the dying. Advance directives and dialysis discontinuation. *Psychosomatics, 38*(1), 27–34.

Cohen, L. M., Ruthazer, R., Moss, A .H., & Germain, M. J. (2010). Predicting six-month mortality for patients who are on maintenance hemodialysis. *Clinical Journal of the American Society of Nephrology, 5,* 72–79.

Connor, S. R., Elwert, F., Spence, C., & Christakis, N. (2007). Geographic variation in hospice use in the United States in 2002. *Journal of Pain and Symptom Management, 34*(3), 277–285.

Davison, S. N. (2001). Quality end-of-life care in dialysis units. *Seminars in Dialysis, 15*(1), 41–44.

Davison, S. N., Jhangri, G. S., Holley, J. L., & Moss, A. H. (2006). Nephrologists' reported preparedness for end-of-life decision-making. *Clinical Journal of the American Society of Nephrology, 1*(6), 1256–1262.

DeOreo, P. B. (1997). Hemodialysis patient-assessed functional health status predicts continued survival, hospitalization, and dialysis-attendance compliance. *American Journal of Kidney Diseases, 30*(2), 204–212.

Devins, G. M., Mandin, H., Hons, R. B., Burgess, E. D., Klassen, J., Taub, K., Schorr, S., Letourneau, P. K., & Buckle, S. (1990). Illness intrusiveness and quality of life in end-stage renal disease: Comparison and stability across treatment modalities. *Health Psychology, 9*(2), 117–142.

Federal Register (2008). Conditions for Coverage for End Stage Renal Disease Facilities, 42 CFR Part 405, Subpart U, April 2008. Washington, DC: U.S. Government Printing Office.

Galla, J. (2000). Clinical practice guideline on shared decision-making in the appropriate initiation of and withdrawal from dialysis. *Journal of the American Society of Nephrology, 11,* 1340–1342.

Germain, M., & Cohen, L. M. (2007). Renal supportive care: View from across the pond: The United States perspective. *Journal of Palliative Medicine, 10*(6), 1241–1244.

Germain, M. J., Cohen, L. M., & Davison, S. N. (2007). Withholding and withdrawal from dialysis: What we know about how our patients die. *Seminars in Dialysis, 20,* 195–199.

Hackett, A. S., & Kackett, S. G. (2007). Withdrawal from dialysis in end-stage renal disease: Medical, social, and psychological issues. *Seminars in Dialysis, 20*(1), 86–90.

Hartwell, L. (2002). *Chronically happy.* San Francisco, CA: Poetic Media Press.

Holley, J. L. (2005). Palliative care in end-stage renal disease: Focus on advance care planning, hospice referral, and bereavement. *Seminars in Dialysis, 18*(2), 154–156.

Holley, J. L., Carmody, S. S., Moss, A. H., Sullivan, A. M., Cohen, L. M., Block, S. D., & Arnold, R. M. (2003). The need for end-of-life care training in nephrology: National survey results of nephrology fellows. *American Journal of Kidney Diseases, 42*(4), 813–820.

Iacono, S. A. (2003). Coping with pain: The dialysis patient's perspective. *Journal of Nephrology Social Work, 22,* 42–44.

Iacono, S. A. (2004). Chronic pain in the hemodialysis patient population. *Dialysis and Transplantation, 33*(2), 92–101.

Jablonski, A. (2008). Palliative care: Misconceptions that limit access for patients with chronic renal disease. *Seminars in Dialysis, 21*(3), 206–209.

Kidney End-of-Life Coalition. (2010). Kidney end-of-life coalition home page. Retrieved from http://http://www.kidneyeol.org/.

King, K. (2007). Withdrawal from dialysis: The literature, DOPPS, and implications for practice. *Journal of Nephrology Social Work, 26,* 45–53.

Knight, E. L., Ofsthun, N., Teng, M., Lazarus, J. M., & Curhan, G. C. (2003). The association between mental health, physical function, and hemodialysis mortality. *Kidney International, 63*(5), 1843–1851.

Leggat, J. E., Swartz, R. D., & Port, F. K. (1997). Withdrawal from dialysis: A review with an emphasis on the black experience. *Advances in Renal Replacement Therapy, 4*(1), 22–29.

Mid-Atlantic Renal Coalition. (2009). *Clinical algorithm and preferred medications to treat pain in dialysis patients.* Midlothian, VA: Author.

Moss, A., Holley, J., Davison, S., Dart, R., Germain, M., Cohen, L., & Swartz, R. D. (2004). Core curriculum in nephrology palliative care. *American Journal of Kidney Diseases, 43*(1), 172–185.

Moss, A. H., Ganjoo, J., Sharma, S., Gansor, J., Senft, S., Weaner, B., … Schmidt, R. (2008). Utility of the "surprise" question to identify dialysis patients with high mortality. *Clinical Journal of the American Society of Nephrology, 3*(5), 1379–1384.

Murray, A., Arko, C., Chen, S., Gilbertson, D., & Moss, A. (2006). Use of hospice in the United States dialysis population. *Clinical Journal of the American Society of Nephrology, 1,* 1248–1255.

Murtagh, F. E. M., Marsh, J. E., Donohoe, P., Ekbal, N. J., Sheerin, N. S., & Harris, F. E. (2007). Dialysis or not? A comparative survival study of patients over 75 years with chronic kidney disease stage 5. *Nephrology, Diaysis, and Transplantation, 22*(7), 1955–1962.

National Kidney Foundation. (2007). *If you choose not to start dialysis treatment.* New York, NY: Author.

National Hospice and Palliative Care Organization (2009). *Determining Hospice Eligibility for Chronic Kidney Disease – Medicare Hospice Benefit.* Retrieved from http://www.nhpco.org/files/public/InfoCenter/Access/ESRD_Eligibility_decision_tree.pdf

Perry, E. (2007). *Peer mentoring in nephrology.* Retrieved from http://www.bkwfriends.org/Peer_Mentoring.pdf

Promoting Excellence in End-of-Life Care. (2002). *End-stage renal disease workgroup recommendations to the field.* Missoula, MT: The Robert Wood Johnson Foundation.

Pruchno, R. A., Lemay, E. P., Field, L., & Levinsky, N. G. (2006). Predictors of patient treatment preferences and spouse substituted judgments: The case of dialysis continuation. *Medical Decision Making, 26*(2), 112–121.

Rabetoy, C. P., & Bair, B. C. (2007). Nephrology nurses' perspectives on difficult ethical issues and practice guideline for shared decision making. *Nephrology Nursing Journal, 34*(6), 599–606.

Renal Physicians Association. (1999). Clinical practice guideline on shared decision-making in the appropriate initiation of and withdrawal from dialysis. *Journal of the American Society of Nephrology, 11,* 1340–1342.

Russ, A. J., Shim, J. K., & Kaufman, S. R. (2007). The value of "life at any cost": Talk about stopping kidney dialysis. *Social Science and Medicine, 64*(11), 2236–2247.

Saini, T., Murtagh, F. E. M., Dupont, P. J., McKinnon, P. M., Hatfield, P., & Saunders, Y. (2006). Comparative pilot study of symptoms and quality of life in cancer patients and patients with end stage renal disease. *Palliative Medicine, 20*(6), 631–636.

Smith, C., Silva-Gane, M. D., Chanda, S., Warwicker, P., Greenwood, R., & Farrington, K. (2003). Choosing not to dialyse: Evaluation of planned non-dialytic management in a cohort of patients with end-stage renal failure. *Nephron Clinical Practice, 95*(2), 40–46.

Song, M. K., Ward, S. E., Happy, M. B., Piraino, B., Donovan, H. S., Shields, A. M., & Connolly, M. C. (2009). Randomized controlled trial of SPIRIS: An effective approach to preparing African-American dialysis patients and families for end of life. *Research in Nursing and Health, 32*(3), 260–273.

Tamura, M., Covinsky, K. E., Chertow, G. M., Yaffe, K., Landefeld, C. S., & McCulloch, C. E. (2009). Functional status of elderly adults before and after initiation of dialysis. *New England Journal of Medicine, 361*(16), 1539–1547.

Thompson, K. F., Bhargava, J., Bachelder, R., Bova-Collis, R., & Moss, A. H. (2008). Hospice and ESRD: Knowledge deficits and underutilization of program benefits. *Nephrology Nursing Journal, 35*(5), 461–502.

United States Renal Data System. (2002). *USRDS 2002 annual data report: Atlas of end-stage renal disease in the United States.* Bethesda, MD: National Institutes of Health.

United States Renal Data System. (2009). *USRDS 2009 annual data report: Atlas of end-stage renal disease in the United States.* Bethesda, MD: National Institutes of Health.

Weiner, S. (2008). End-of-life care discussions: A survey of dialysis patients and professionals. *The Journal of Nephrology Social Work, 28*, 52–60.

Weisbord, S. D., Fried, L. F., Arnold, R. M., Fine, M. J., Levenson, D. J., Peterson, R. A., & Switzer, G. E. (2005). Prevalence, severity, and importance of physical and emotional symptoms in chronic hemodialysis patients. *Journal of the American Society of Nephrology, 16*(8), 2487–2494.

Weisbord, S. D., Fried, L. F., Mor, M. K., Resnick, A. L., Unruh, M. L., Palevsky, P. M., … Arnold, R. M. (2007). Renal provider recognition of symptoms in patients on maintenance hemodialysis. *Clinical Journal of the American Society of Nephrology, 2*(5), 960–967.

32 *Robin Rudy Lawson and Kelly M. McHenry*

Emerging Opportunities for Palliative Social Workers

Health is a state of complete physical, mental, and social well-being, not merely the absence of disease or infirmity.

—World Health Organization, 1946

Key Concepts

- ◆ *Palliative care usually begins for patients with organ failure or neurological illness at the end of life.*
- ◆ *Unique challenges exist for patients and caregivers due to the progressive nature of these illnesses and the impact on physical, emotional, and cognitive functioning.*
- ◆ *Palliative social workers can play a key role beginning at time of diagnosis and through the end of life for patients and families dealing with these chronic, progressive disorders.*
- ◆ *Specific interventions can enhance outcomes for patients, families, and caregivers living with the uncertainty of progressive, incurable illness.*

General Introduction

The purpose of this chapter is to identify the unique challenges that patients and families face when diagnosed with either a neurodegenerative disease, heart failure, or pulmonary disease and to illustrate disease-specific palliative social work interventions. These disease categories cover a broad range of illnesses, from progressive illnesses such as congestive heart failure (CHF) or dementia, to acute illness events such as heart attack or stroke. This chapter will focus on five specific illnesses in order to provide a concise clinical picture of the diversity of progressive illness. Palliative care is typically utilized at the end of life for illness such as CHF, chronic obstructive pulmonary disease (COPD), and neurodegenerative illnesses like amyotrophic lateral sclerosis (ALS) and dementia. The evolution of palliative care will create opportunities for social workers to intervene at time of diagnosis with patients and families who face these illnesses and to enhance the quality of care throughout the continuum of illness.

Introduction to Heart and Lung Disease

Due to their chronic nature and ambiguous prognosis, CHF and COPD are complex illnesses for patients and families to manage. Patients and families may experience multiple episodes of acute exacerbations followed by periods of lingering stability with the possibility of death occurring at any time, thus making it difficult to plan for the future (Lynn, Chaudhry, Simon, Wilkinson, & Schuster, 2007). Recovery is typically slower with each episode and is marked by a lower level of functioning (National Heart, Lung, and Blood Institute, 2009).

Congestive Heart Failure

Heart disease (HD) is the leading cause of death in the United States, and CHF, also known as heart failure (HF), is the culprit causing many of these deaths (Centers for Disease Control and Prevention [CDC], 2009a). Congestive heart failure can either be a functional or structural disorder that encumbers the heart ventricle from filling up with or ejecting blood (ejection fraction), resulting in what is referred to as fluid congestion or ascites and/or a compromised cardiac output (Teuteberg, 2008). Other common symptoms of CHF are dyspnea, fatigue, pain, nausea, anxiety, and depression (Teuteberg, 2008). There is no cure for CHF, and once diagnosed a majority of patients will take medications to help manage the disease for the remainder of their lives. Prior to developing CHF, many patients will have risk factors such as chronic hypertension, coronary artery disease, and diabetes (CDC, 2006). In addition, age significantly impacts the risk of developing HF with an estimated "doubling in incidence with each decade of ageing" (Davis, Hobbs, & Lip, 2000).

Each year in the United States, 550,000 new cases of HF are diagnosed, and this number is climbing (CDC, 2006). A common misconception of HD is that men are most affected; however, in 2005 women accounted for 51% of HD-related deaths (CDC, 2009a). Heart failure is the leading cause of death among American Indians, Alaska natives, Blacks, and Latinos who also present with high rates of the previously identified risk factors (CDC, 2009).

Chronic Obstructive Pulmonary Disorder

The incidence of COPD has significantly increased over the last 30 years (Jemal, Ward, Hao, & Thun, 2005). Chronic obstructive pulmonary disorder is a result of prolonged exposure to social and environmental risk factors such as first- and second-hand tobacco smoke and pollution (American Lung Association, 2009). Also referred to as chronic bronchitis or emphysema, COPD is damage of lung tissue from inhaled toxins (Rocker, Curtis, & Simpson, 2008). It is considered to be preventable, as well as treatable; however, there is no cure with the rare exception of lung transplant. Jones et al. (2004) state that progressive COPD is marked by dyspnea, chronic cough, sputum production, and recurrent hospitalizations, eventually leading to intractable dyspnea (respiratory failure).

An estimated 10.2 million people were diagnosed with COPD in 2007 (American Lung Association, 2009) with most being middle age or elderly (National Heart Lung and Blood Institute, 2009). A significant increase in mortality rates is correlated with increasing age (American Thoracic Society, 2009) and prolonged exposure to environmental or industrial toxins. One study reports that 19% of COPD cases can be attributed to occupational hazards (American Thoracic Society, 2009). Eighty percent to 90% of COPD deaths were related to smoking, with men being 12 and women 13 times more likely to die from COPD than nonsmokers (American Lung Association, 2009).

Introduction to Neurological Illnesses

Every year, roughly 6.8 million people die worldwide as a result of neurological disorders (World Health Organization [WHO], 2007). Patients living with neurological disease face a long-term, degenerative illness with an accumulation of both physical and cognitive disabilities. The age distribution for neurological diseases varies greatly, with people experiencing their first symptoms of multiple sclerosis (MS) between the ages of 20 and 40 (National Institute for Neurological Disorders and Stroke, 2009) and people over the age of 65 experiencing nearly three-quarters of all strokes (CDC, 2009). Cognitive impairment, a common symptom in progressive neurological illnesses, makes assessment and management of disease symptoms troublesome (Gofton, Jog, & Schulz, 2009); undertreatment of pain in both dementia (Sachs, Shega, & Cox-Hayley, 2004) and stroke patients (Addington-Hall, Lay, Altmann, & McCarthy, 1995) is common.

Gofton et al. (2009) assert the need to improve advance care planning and prognostication, and to augment symptom management and support for patients and families by introducing palliative care principles into neurological care earlier in the illness continuum. Despite varying disease trajectories, emerging research indicates that there are similar psychosocial and physical needs of patients and families who suffer from progressive, neurological illness (Gofton et al., 2009).

Dementia

Most dementias, particularly in the elderly, are the result of neurodegenerative changes that occur over an extended period of time and culminate in a complete loss of independence (Volicer, 2004). Dementia impacts memory, thinking, orientation, comprehension, calculation, learning capacity, language, and judgment (Cahill, Macijauskiene, Nygard, Faulkner, & Ingen, 2007). Behavioral and psychological symptoms in dementia include disinhibition, mood disorders, hallucinations and delusions, and inappropriate behavior (Cahill et al., 2007). Alzheimer's disease accounts for more than 65% of all cases and is by far the most common type of dementia followed by vascular dementia (Cahill et al., 2007).

Stroke

A stroke occurs either when the blood supply to part of the brain is blocked or when a blood vessel in or around the brain bursts, causing damage to a part of the brain (CDC, 2009). Physical and emotional symptoms include muscle weakness (paresis), loss of consciousness, confusion, bowel and bladder problems, difficulty communicating, nutritional compromise, pain, depression, and anxiety (Hamann, Rogers, & Addington-Hall, 2004). The Centers for Disease Control and Prevention (2009) report that stroke is the third leading cause of death in the United States. Stroke death rates are higher for African Americans than for Caucasians, even at younger ages (CDC, 2009).

Multiple Sclerosis

Multiple sclerosis is the most common inflammatory demyelinating disorder of the central nervous system (Borasio, Lorenzl, Rogers, & Voltz, 2010). The median age of onset for MS is 31 years, and the disease is three times as common in women as men (Mcdonald & Ron, 1999). Specific problems caused by multiple sclerosis include muscle weakness and spasticity, tremor, fatigue, urinary disorders, bowel dysfunction, visual problems, pain, and risks involving skin breakdown (Macleod & Formaglio, 2004). Typically underrecognized, 50%–80% of patients with MS have pain, depression, and fatigue (Kumpfel et al., 2007), and approximately 50% will have some cognitive impairment (Edmonds, Vivat, Burman, Silber, & Higginson, 2007).

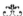

The Picture of Progressive Illness

In Box 32.1 and Box 32.2 are two patient/family narratives that briefly describe common clinical presentations for organ failure and neurology patients. They are followed by an in-depth examination of the specific psychosocial issues that palliative social workers will face when working with patients and families dealing with progressive illnesses.

Assessment

While the NYHA classifications (Heart Failure Society of America, 2006) provide a general model for outlining the progressive nature of CHF, they do not concurrently address the global impacts that emanate from a diagnosis of CHF. As represented in Box 32.1, the multidimensional effects of CHF on an individual's and family's life create vast opportunities for palliative social work involvement. Mr. Payton's frustration with medication efficacy and his recurring CHF symptoms altered his role in the family causing disequilibrium and role adjustments. His symptoms limited participation in activities and may have contributed to an undiagnosed depression. Symptoms such as dyspnea and pain and medications such as beta-blockers for his heart can cause fatigue (Teuteberg, 2008). Patients who struggle with the delicate balance of medication and diet management may not only suffer with a debilitating disease but are also at risk of being stigmatized by both health care providers and family alike,

---

Box 32.1
Patient/Family Narrative: Mr. Payton and Congestive Heart Failure

Mr. Payton is a 68-year-old white male who was diagnosed with congestive heart failure (CHF) 3 years ago. He and his wife of 41 years are Catholic and have three children and four grandchildren, none of whom live in the immediate area but visit when possible. At diagnosis his symptoms were mild fatigue and fluid congestion in his feet and ankles. For 2 years Mr. Payton met the criteria for New York Heart Association (NYHA) Class I heart failure: He was able to control his symptoms with medication management and regular appointments with his cardiologist, and he had no limitations on his activities. The NYHA provides a functional and therapeutic classification for recommended physical activity for cardiac patients.

Mr. Payton's first hospital admission was 8 months ago when he presented to the emergency department (ED) with chest pain, mild abdominal fluid congestion, and increased shortness of breath that developed while doing chores around his home (NYHA Class II heart failure). When describing his chest pain, he said he was unable to catch his breath and stated, "It feels like someone is standing on my chest." Mr. Payton was admitted to the hospital for 4 days to treat ascites and his diuretic was titrated until his symptoms improved. In additional to several medication changes at discharge, he was prescribed a new medication for anxiety and provided with literature on diet changes to reduce fluid congestion. Since Mr. Payton's first admission he was admitted to the hospital seven times for symptom exacerbation. Each time he returned home from the hospital he reported feeling less able to perform normal daily activities and was disinterested in seeing friends or family.

After his last hospitalization he began using a shower chair for baths, and at times he required some assistance with transfers. Mrs. Payton reports to the medical team that her husband requires more assistance and that she feels overwhelmed and finds the transfers physically straining on her back and legs. His application for home care services was declined due to his "high level of functioning," even though Mr. Payton states that on most days he does not feel like getting out of bed and that he is frustrated that the eight medications he takes do not seem to help control his symptoms. Since his last appointment he lost 12 pounds. He is unable to walk to the exam room without assistance, and he has begun to use oxygen but still feels short of breath at rest (NYHA Class IV heart failure).

Mr. Payton died in the hospital 2 days after being rehospitalized with symptoms of dyspnea, fluid congestion, and pain.

---

labeled as nonadherent or blamed for not managing their disease appropriately. All of these aspects of care invite social work attention and intervention.

Interventions

Palliative social work interventions over the course of Mr. Payton's admissions would focus on the challenges of adapting to life with a debilitating illness and progressive functional decline and exploring the patient's and family's understanding of prognosis. Mr. Payton might have been helped to see that his physical decline did not preclude his participation in decision making, and he might have been taught how to use his energy for aspects of his life that have the most meaning. Interventions to assess and normalize Mr. Payton's experience with symptoms and side effects might have impacted related anxiety and any feelings of self-blame that either the patient or spouse may have experienced related to the challenges of managing diet and medications. Mr. and Mrs. Payton could have been helped by learning how environmental interventions such as position changes, the use of a fan, or the opening of a window can reduce the perception of breathlessness, thus providing Mr. Payton with a way he can contribute to controlling his own symptoms. Both diaphragmatic and pursed-lip breathing are specific self-management techniques patients can use to manage their dyspnea (McCoy, 2009). In collaboration with the palliative care team, Mr.'s Payton's fears and internal dialogue related to uncontrolled breathlessness could have been explored to understand his priorities and to reassure him that his symptoms could be managed. In addition, a focus that includes a gradual awareness of prognosis could help Mr. and Mrs. Payton integrate and prepare their extended family, children, and grandchildren as illness progressed.

Frequently hospitalized patients may be cared for on different floors and moved from floor to floor based on their medical needs, with the result that highly stressed patients and families are asked to form new relationships with clinical staff and answer the same questions repeatedly. The palliative social worker's rapport with patients and families and clinicians and the provision of "continuity of relationship" can help Mr. and Mrs. Payton through these transitions by bridging communication gaps and providing patient and family history to new clinicians while orienting patients and families to new settings.

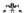

Caregiver Distress

Caregivers of patients facing either progressive organ failure or neurological illness constantly adapt to continuous losses, robbing them of any respite and jeopardizing their own physical and emotional health. Caregiver distress in this population differs from oncology due to the accumulation of functional impairments, multiple hospitalizations for CHF or COPD patients, and the added distress of cognitive impairment for dementia or stroke patients. Similar to advanced dementia patients, those in the late stages of COPD are often housebound yet receive little or no support from community health services (Rocker et al., 2008).

Social workers can assist caregivers to protect and maximize their own physical and emotional health both for themselves and to lessen the patient's sense that his or her needs are causing harm to family and caregivers. Providing

supportive counseling and accessing resources such as psychological services, support groups, home health services, and Web and telephone supports are essential contributions to the well-being of caregivers and patients. Encouraging the caregiver to communicate with the physician or nurse regarding the disease process, including distressing symptoms and the uncertainty of the disease trajectory, can help facilitate goals of care conversations between the patient, family, and the primary and palliative care teams.

Impact of Equipment on the Environment

The functional impairment caused by CHF, COPD, and neurology disorders requires patients and families to rely on equipment such as oxygen to help with dyspnea, a walker to assist with mobility, and letter boards to enhance communication for patients whose disease interferes with their ability to speak. The presence of equipment such as wheelchairs, commodes, canes, walkers, and oxygen encroaches on a person's personal space and is a constant reminder of his or her illness. The symbolic significance of these pieces of equipment to patients and their families are a focus of therapeutic inquiry and intervention. Environmental interventions that may include sleeping upright in a chair to improve dyspnea in COPD or CHF patients mean that they no longer sleep with their partners. The addition of equipment symbolizes a loss of function, and this may be accompanied by feelings of anger, sadness, and anxiety. Palliative social workers can provide supportive counseling through these transitions and adaptations, as well as practical suggestions such as storing or camouflaging equipment not in use to maintain some normalcy in the physical environment.

Mental Health

Loss of independence due to functional impairment and distressing symptoms such as dyspnea or cognitive impairment can lead to depression and anxiety in patients. Depression can have a major impact on decision making and treatment preferences, suggesting that frequent and ongoing assessment is required (Stapelton, Nielsen, Engelberg, Patrick, & Curtis, 2005,). The prevalence of depression and anxiety in patients with CHF and COPD is high, affecting 40%–50% of all patients; both can aggravate symptoms such as pain and dyspnea (Mikkelsen, Middelboe, Pisinger, & Stage, 2004). Multiple sclerosis is unique in that depression is also related to the "cerebral pathology of the disease and steroid treatment" (Borasio et al., 2010, p. 932). The risk of suicide is increased in patients with MS (Borasio et al., 2010) and CHF (Senior Journal, 2009). Risk factors for suicide or requests for euthanasia among MS patients were not physical symptoms but rather social isolation, unemployment and a lack of psychosocial support (Borasio et al., 2010).

Palliative social workers with strong clinical assessment skills can identify depressive and anxious symptoms in patients, advocate for pharmacologic management, and intervene with treatments such as relaxation/imagery techniques and supportive counseling and psychotherapy. Linking patients and families to community organizations like the Alzheimer's Association and the American Heart Association decreases social isolation and increases their support network. A psychosocial intervention program for spouse-caregivers of Alzheimer's patients who were depressed showed that treated caregivers who received counseling and participated in support groups were less depressed by the eighth month of the program compared to those in the control group (Mittelman et al., 1995).

Assessment

In an initial meeting, Mr. Nesbit is observed sitting on his wife's bed, holding her hand. It is apparent from their body language and facial expressions that they are both devastated

---

Box 32.2
Patient/Family Narrative: Mrs. Nesbit and Stroke

Mrs. Nesbit is a 70-year-old African-American female with a history of hypertension and diabetes who is taken to the emergency department (ED) by her spouse of 45 years after experiencing weakness on her left side, sudden vision problems, and dizziness. A computed tomography (CT) confirmed that Mrs. Nesbit had suffered an ischemic stroke caused by a blocked artery. While still in the ED, Mr. Nesbit notices that his wife seemed confused, and he is having difficulty understanding her words. Mrs. Nesbit is admitted to an acute stroke unit within the hospital.

During the course of her hospitalization, she lost her ability to speak, and left-sided weakness left her unable to get out of bed. A bladder catheter was inserted to manage urinary incontinence. In addition to feeling embarrassed, the catheter represented the loss of normal body function. Normally a very active woman, she became depressed about her loss of function and dependence on staff. Her inability to swallow led to nutrition problems, and her increasing confusion worried her husband and the multidisciplinary stroke team.

The nurse on the unit recommended that a palliative care consultation be called to assist Mr. and Mrs. Nesbit with adjustment to this sudden, devastating illness, pain management issues related to shoulder/hand syndrome, concerns about artificial nutrition and hydration, and the lack of written advance directives. The unit social worker, responsible for 20–25 patients, was occupied with transfers of patients to extended care facilities and discharges home. She had begun an initial assessment and in a meeting with the palliative social worker provided the following information: Mrs and Mr. Nesbit had been married for 45 years, were both born and raised in the South, had no children, and had no other family living in the area. Mr. Nesbit, age 75, had Parkinson's disease, which was responding well to medications.

---

by the impact and uncertain trajectory of the stroke. Mr. Nesbit feels that the unit staff avoids talking to him about prognosis, stating that the course is uncertain. He observes that the staff ignores Mrs. Nesbit when they come into the room and only talk to him.

Both express concerns about the increasing shoulder and arm pain and the discomfort she feels when repositioned in bed. Mrs. Nesbit's inability to swallow is causing secretions to build in her throat. Her husband believes the secretions leave her with a choking sensation, increasing her anxiety about her condition and his fears that she is dying.

Mrs. Nesbit appears sad and confused, and she avoids eye contact. Mr. Nesbit believes his wife is depressed as demonstrated by frequent crying and the fact that she has stopped squeezing his hands to signal "yes" and "no" answers. Mr. Nesbit asks to speak to the palliative social worker outside his wife's room. Through tears he explains that he is terrified about the possibility of his wife dying because they are both only children and he is scared of being alone. He also describes an enmeshed relationship as evidenced by his dependence on her for all decision making. Mrs. Nesbit was a ballet dancer, and Mr. Nesbit believes the debilitating effects of the stroke are particularly depressing to her because her physical ability has been an important aspect of her identity and she is a very neat, orderly, and private person.

He reports that his wife informed him at a friend's funeral 3 years ago that she would want everything done at the end of life to keep her alive and that it was the Lord's decision when her time was up. He believes she would want artificial nutrition if she is unable to eat and that she would want to be resuscitated under all circumstances.

Interventions

During the palliative care consultation team meeting, a plan of care is developed that reflects the combined assessments of the social worker, physician, and nurse. In response to the symptom distress, a pain regimen and an antidepressant is initiated and the unit staff will be alerted to the discomfort experienced upon movement with the plan to offer Mrs. Nesbit a short-acting pain medication prior to movement. Medication will be provided to reduce secretions, and the social worker will explore the relationship between symptoms and anxiety with both patient and husband who may be responding in a manner that exacerbates Mrs. Nesbit's anxiety. Education will be provided related to symptoms, anxiety, and thoughts that contribute to distress; and focused breathing and imagery exercises will be offered. To address the uncertainty surrounding prognosis and the perceived lack of communication with the stroke team, the palliative social worker coordinates a meeting with the stroke team, the palliative care team, and Mr. and Mrs. Nesbit to discuss prognosis, treatment issues such as hydration and nutrition, and care options upon discharge from the hospital. In an effort to maximize Mrs. Nesbit's participation, a capacity assessment is done and a communication board is provided to assist Mrs. Nesbit, who expresses a desire to participate in the meeting. Mrs. Nesbit's "neat and orderly" approach can be integrated into planning for her care by organizing meetings and decision-making processes with the goal of enhancing her participation both to relieve Mr. Nesbit of profoundly difficult decisions and to ensure that care decisions reflect her values as they relate to her current medical condition. In addition to exploring Mrs. Nesbits' previously articulated wishes, the meeting will create an opportunity to encourage either oral or written advance care directives to guide future decisions. The palliative social worker also requests that the team chaplain see Mrs. Nesbit because she is a religious person who may benefit from her presence and participation. Because studies have shown that music therapy can help with social functioning and participation in rehabilitation (Nayak, Wheeler, Shiflett, & Agostinelli, 2000), music therapy staff see both Mr. and Mrs. Nesbit. Daily meetings are held with Mr. Nesbit to explore his concerns and fears, with a focus on his social isolation and high bereavement risk. Mr. Nesbit's inability to see a future without his spouse prompts the palliative social worker to utilize cognitive restructuring for his negative self-statements and to conduct a suicide risk assessment. She also provides Mr. Nesbit with resources on stroke and rehabilitation, identifies support groups for people with Parkinson's disease that are close to his home, and explores his relationship with his spiritual network.

Functional Impairment

Many of the physical symptoms that occur in patients with either organ failure or neurological illnesses impact their ability to perform activities of daily living (ADLs). Functional impairment also impacts a patient's mood and ability and willingness to participate in rehabilitation or therapy programs (Volpe, 2001). The spasticity caused by diseases such as ALS and MS increases fatigue and reduces mobility (Macleod & Formaglio, 2004), further isolating patients from social supports. Fatigue in CHF is a marker for progressive disease and can be related to the disease itself or medications (Teuteberg, 2008). Mobility problems in patients with stroke can cause skin breakdown and pressure sores (Volpe, 2001), which then can raise the risk of infection and pain.

A comprehensive clinical assessment by a palliative social worker can identify whether function or mobility problems are impacting a patient's mood, or their adherence to medication or therapy programs. Communication and collaboration between the patient's primary care team (cardiology, for example) and the palliative care team can help foster an overall, global perspective on the patient's condition and enhance continuity of care for patients and their caregivers. This same kind of collaboration and inclusion of rehabilitation services (see Chapter 45) validate their essential

contribution to patients with cardiac disease, stroke, or progressive neurological illnesses like MS (Tookman, Hopkins, & Scharpen-von-Heussen, 2004) and help patients adapt to new levels of function.

Cognitive Impairment and Communication

Cognitive impairment contributes significantly to the burden of illness and impacts a person's ability to work, drive, care for children, and manage finances, and it leaves one unable to advocate for oneself. Cognitive impairment ranges from disorientation and confusion in the COPD patient with hypoxemia (Incalzi et al., 2003) to the pervasive impairment of the advanced dementia patient. The loss of decision-making ability in patients with neurological illness presents significant challenges to caregivers and clinicians because decisions about nutrition (artificial hydration), breathing (tracheostomy in ALS patients), and the use of certain medications (antibiotics in patients with end-stage dementia) are made by family members who may be unaware of their loved one's wishes. For COPD patients with severe dyspnea, communication problems can arise when they are suddenly intubated, sedated, and put on ventilators and become unable to participate in making decisions about their care.

The loss of self that occurs in patients with dementia and stroke impacts relationships and social role, and it is devastating to loved ones who lose essential aspects of their partner or parent. Feelings of loneliness and isolation are common in caregivers of patients with cognitive impairments. In the early to middle stages of dementia, patients may feel unwanted, isolated, and unable to participate in conversations with family and friends due to an inability to follow the conversation. Rogers and Addington-Hall's work (as cited in Hamann et al., 2004) regarding care on an acute stroke unit in the United Kingdom discovered that patients with stroke who are unconscious are in danger of a "social death" because they are ignored by clinical staff and treated as nonpersons. Palliative social workers can help mitigate this tendency by encouraging families to share pictures, accomplishments, interests, and stories about the person and by assisting staff to connect with the whole person they are caring for.

Cognitive impairments introduce a unique set of symptoms that support the case for the palliative social worker to become involved early in order to advocate for technology that enhances communication while at the same time assisting patients and families to integrate a changed reality. Encouraging alternate ways of communicating invites patients and families to honor and maximize the time available, enhancing opportunities to share through writing, music, or other expressive arts (see Chapter 48). Encouraging advance care planning discussions and helping caregivers of cognitively impaired patients to partialize the complex decision making regarding life-prolonging treatments can enhance their sense of control. Social work interventions can also be focused on providing support and education to caregivers about cognitive deficits and ways to help the patient manage his or her environment to minimize distress for all.

Conclusion

Palliative care is essential to enhance care for patients and families with chronic, progressive illnesses such as COPD and MS due to the accumulation of physical impairments, distressing symptoms, and the impact on caregiver physical and mental health. Palliative social workers can play an integral role in early intervention with these patients and families utilizing their expertise in clinical assessment of the multidimensional impact of life-limiting illnesses. By bridging gaps in communication, we facilitate collaboration among the many providers of patient care. Working with patients and families at time of diagnosis through the end of life, the palliative social worker can assist with transitions through targeted clinical interventions and ensure comprehensive and person-centered care.

LEARNING EXERCISES

- Using the narrative on stroke in this chapter (see Box 32.2), role play an advance care planning meeting between Mr. and Mrs. Nesbit and the palliative care team. The role play could be broken into three different parts: care planning right after a stroke, during the recovery phase, and at the end of life. How might you adapt the process and communication to maximize Mrs. Nesbit's ability to participate?
- Thinking about the challenges that patients with progressive illness and their caregivers face from time of diagnosis through end of life, how would you, as a palliative social worker working in an outpatient primary care practice, advocate for earlier involvement with these patients and families?
- Write and rehearse a relaxation exercise for a COPD patient who has anxiety related to anticipation of his or her next episode of severe shortness of breath. Practice this exercise with a colleague imagining that you are an inpatient palliative social worker. Please refer to the Keefe and Altilio publication listed in the Additional Suggested Readings section for examples.

ADDITIONAL SUGGESTED READINGS

Keefe, F. and Altilio, T. (2006) American Pain Foundation. *Treatment options: A guide for people living with pain.* Retrieved from http://www.painfoundation.org/learn/publications/.

Berkman, B. (2006). *Handbook of social work in health and aging.* New York, NY: Oxford University Press.

Cox, C. B. (2007). *Dementia and social work practice: Research and interventions.* New York, NY: Springer Publishing Company, LLC.

Silver, M. (2002). *Success with heart failure: Help and hope for those with congestive heart failure.* Cambridge, MA: Perseus Books Group.

REFERENCES

Addington-Hall, J. M., Lay, M., Altmann, D., & McCarthy, M. (1995). Symptom control, and communication with health professionals, and hospital care of stroke patients in the last year of life as reported by surviving family, friends, and officials. *Stroke, 26*(12), 2242–2248.

American Lung Association. (2009). *Chronic obstructive pulmonary disease (COPD)* (Fact Sheet). Retrieved from http://www.lungusa.org/site/aps.nlnet

American Thoracic Society. (2009). *COPD guidelines: Epidemiology.* Retrieved from http://www.thoracic.org/clinical/copd-guidelines/index.php

Borasio, G. D., Lorenzl, S., Rogers, A., & Voltz, R. (2010). Palliative medicine in non-malignant neurological disorders. In G. Hanks, N. I. Cherny, N. A. Christakis, M. Fallon, S. Kaasa, & R. K. Portenoy (Eds.), *Oxford textbook of palliative medicine* (pp. 1267–1279). Oxford, England: Oxford University Press.

Cahill, S., Macijauskiene, J., Nygard, A-M., Faulkner, J. P., & Hagen, I. (2007). Technology in dementia care. *Technology and Disability, 19*(2-3), 55–60.

Centers for Disease Control and Prevention (CDC). (2006). *Fact sheets at-a-glance reports: Heart failure fact sheet.* Retrieved from http://www.cdc.gov/DHDSP

Centers for Disease Control and Prevention (CDC). (2009a). *Heart disease facts and statistics.* Retrieved from http://www.cdc.gov/heartdisease/statistics.htm

Centers for Disease Control and Prevention (CDC). (2009b). *Stroke facts and statistics.* Retrieved from http://www.cdc.gov/stroke/stroke_facts.htm

Davis, R. C., Hobbs, F. D. R., & Lip, G. Y. H. (2000). ABC of heart failure history and epidemiology. *British Medical Journal, 320,* 39–42.

Edmonds, P., Vivat, B., Burman, R., Silber, E., & Higginson, I. J. (2007). Loss and change: Experiences of people severely affected by multiple sclerosis. *Palliative Medicine, 21*(2), 101–107.

Gofton, T. E., Jog, M. S., & Schulz, V. (2009). A palliative approach to neurological care: A literature review. *Canadian Journal of Neurological Science, 36*(3), 296–302.

Hamann, G. F., Rogers, A., & Addington-Hall, J. (2004). Palliative care in stroke. In S. Gilman (Series Ed.) & R. Voltz, J. L. Bernat, G. D. Borasio, I. Maddocks, D. Oliver, & R. K. Portenoy (Vol. Eds.), *Palliative care in neurology* (pp. 13–26). Oxford, England: Oxford University Press.

Heart Failure Society of America. (2006). *The stages of heart failure–NYHA Classification.* Retrieved from http://www.abouthf.org/questions_stages.htm

Incalzi, R. A., Marra, C., Giordano, A., Calcagni, M. L., Cappa, A., Basso, S., … Fuso, L. (2003). Cognitive impairments in chronic obstructive pulmonary disease. *Journal of Neurology, 250*(3), 325–332.

Jemal, A., Ward, E., Hao, Y., & Thun, M. (2005). Trends in the leading causes of death in the United States, 1970-2002. *Journal of the American Medical Association, 294*(10), 1255–1259.

Jones, I., Kirby, A., Ormiston, P., Loomba, Y., Chan, K. K., Rout, J., ... Hamilton, S. (2004). The needs of patients dying of chronic obstructive pulmonary disease in the community. *Family Practice, 21*, 310–313.

Lynn, J., Chaudhry, E., Simon, L. N., Wilkinson, A. M., & Schuster, J. L. (2007). *The common sense guide to improving palliative care.* New York, NY: Oxford University Press.

Kumpfel, T., Hoffmann, L. A., Pollmann, W., Rieckmann, P., Zettl, U. K., Kuhnbach, R., ... Voltz, R. (2007). Palliative care in patients with severe multiple sclerosis: Two case reports and a survey among German MS neurologists. *Palliative Medicine, 21*(2), 109–114.

Macleod, A. D., & Formaglio, F. (2004). Demyelinating disease. In S. Gilman (Series Ed.) & R. Voltz, J. L. Bernat, G. D. Borasio, I. Maddocks, D. Oliver, & R. K. Portenoy (Vol. Eds.), *Palliative care in neurology* (pp. 27–36). Oxford, England: Oxford University Press.

McCoy, K. (2009). Breathing techniques for COPD patients. Retrieved from http://www.everydayhealth.com/copd/breathing-techniques-for-copd.aspx

McDonald, W. I., & Ron, M. A. (1999). Multiple sclerosis: The disease and its manifestations. *Philosophical Transactions of the Royal Society of London B, 354*, 1615–1622.

Mikkelson, R. L, Middelboe, T., Pisinger, C., & Stage, K. B. (2004). Anxiety and depression in patients with chronic obstructive pulmonary disease (COPD). A review. *Nordic Journal of Psychiatry, 58*(1), 65–70.

Mittelman, M. S., Ferris, S. H., Shulman, E., Steinberg, G., Ambinder, A., Mackell, J. A., & Cohen, J. (1995). A comprehensive support program: Effect on depression in spouse-caregivers of AD patients. *The Gerontological Society of America, 35*(6), 792–802.

National Heart Lung and Blood Institute. (2009). *What Is COPD?* Retrieved from http://www.nhlbi.nih.gov/health/dci/Diseases/Copd/Copd_WhatIs.html

National Institute for Neurological Disorders and Stroke. (2009). *NINDS Multiple Sclerosis Information Page.* Retrieved from http://www.ninds.nih/gov/disordersmultiple_sclerosis.htm

Nayak, S., Wheeler, B. L., Shiflett, S. C., & Agostinelli, S., (2000). Effect of music therapy on mood and social interaction among individuals with acute traumatic brain injury and stroke. *Rehabilitation Psychology, 45*(3), 274–283.

Rocker, G., Curtis, R. J., & Simpson, C. (2008). Chronic obstructive pulmonary disease. In C. P. Storey, Jr. (Series Ed.) & S. Levine & J. W. Shega (Vol. Eds.), *The hospice and palliative medicine approach to selected chronic illnesses: Dementia, COPD, and CHF–U9* (3rd ed., pp. 37–53). Glenview, IL: AAHPM.

Sachs, G.A., Shega, J. W., & Cox-Hayley, D. (2004). Barriers to excellent end-of-life care for patients with dementia. *Journal of General Internal Medicine, 19*(10), 1057–1063.

Senior Journal. (2009). *Some common illnesses may increase suicide risk for elderly people.* Retrieved from http://www.seniorjournal.com/NEWS/Eldercare/4-06-15illness.htm

Stapelton, R. D., Nielsen, E. L., Engelberg, R. A., Patrick, D. L., & Curtis, J. R. (2005). Association of depression and life sustaining treatment preferences in patients with COPD. *Chest, 127*(1), 328–334.

Teuteberg, W. G. (2008). Congestive heart failure. In C. P. Storey, Jr., (Series Ed.) & S. Levine & J. W. Shega (Vol. Eds.), *The hospice and palliative medicine approach to selected chronic illnesses: Dementia, COPD, and CHF–U9* (3rd ed., pp. 53–72). Glenview, IL: AAHPM.

Tookman, A. J., Hopkins, K., & Scharpen-von-Heussen, K. (2004). Rehabilitation in palliative medicine. In D. D. Doyle, G. Hanks, N. I. Cherny, & K. Calman (Eds.), *Oxford textbook in palliative medicine* (pp. 1021–1032). Oxford, England: Oxford University Press.

Volicer, L. (2004). Dementias. In S. Gilman (Series Ed.) & R. Voltz, J.L. Bernat, G.D. Borasio, I. Maddocks, D. Oliver, & R. K. Portenoy (Vol. Eds.), *Palliative care in neurology* (pp. 59–67). Oxford, England: Oxford University Press.

Volpe, B. T. (2001). Palliative treatment for stroke. *Neurologic Clinics, 19*(4), 903–920.

World Health Organization (WHO). (2007). *Neurological disorders affect millions globally: WHO report.* Retrieved from http://www.who.int/mediacentre/news/releases/2007/pro4/en/index.html

33 *William Goeren*

Social Work, HIV Disease, and Palliative Care

At first, I dealt with my AIDS every few months, just going to the doctors, then it was every month. Now I am sick and it became every week, then every few days. The sicker I get, I have to deal with something going wrong every day. Now it is hour to hour and soon it will be minute to minute because of all the things going wrong with my body.

—Curt, who died in 1989

Key Concepts

- *Human immunodeficiency virus (HIV) was first identified in the early 1980s, with a few cases of rare and specific diseases.*
- *Initially affecting gay men in the major urban cities of New York, San Francisco, and Los Angeles, it is now a chronic pandemic, affecting millions worldwide.*
- *Social workers have been at the forefront of caring for people with HIV since the beginning of the epidemic, providing care, organizing support, initiating education and awareness, and changing policy at all levels.*
- *This chapter reviews the interface of social work, HIV disease, and palliation, providing interventions for the future of that interface.*

Introduction

In 1981, the world was first introduced to a new disease conundrum, a viral syndrome that seemed to initially infect only homosexual men (later classified as MSM or men who have sex with men to include men who do not identify as gay), intravenous (IV) drug users, then Haitians and hemophiliacs. At first called GRID (gay-related immune deficiency syndrome) because of the association with and proportion of gay men initially diagnosed, "by September of 1982, the Centers for Disease Control and Prevention (CDC) had published a case definition, using the current designation of acquired immune deficiency syndrome (AIDS) in print, and it was rapidly adopted by researchers" (University of California San Francisco [UCSF], 2008, p. 2). The cause was a virus, passed via body fluids, which led to a progressive destruction of the immune system, leaving the patient vulnerable to a spectrum of medical conditions and diseases. What started as a few, uncommonly related cases in unrelated, marginal populations heralded a wave of unprecedented public concern, fear, and amazement. Patients had no concept of why they were ill, and their caregivers and medical and psychosocial staffs were at a loss as to how to help the growing number of the sick and, ultimately, dying. Loved ones became the advocates for those whose voices were being silenced, joining the efforts of medicine and psychosocial disciplines to provide comfort, ease pain, relieve suffering, and hopefully to address the physical, emotional, and spiritual needs of the afflicted. It was the beginning of HIV palliative care. Selwyn states that "at the beginning, HIV care was palliative care" (Selwyn, 2005, p. 2).

AIDS Epidemiology

Science now knows, however, that the emergence of human immunodeficiency virus (HIV) into society predates its presence as a medical phenomenon by at least two decades. "Researchers examining the earlier medical literature identified cases appearing to fit the AIDS surveillance definition as early as the 1950s and 1960s" (Huminer, Rosenfeld, & Pitlik, 1987, p. 1102).

From 1981 until the mid-1990s, the infection and death rates from HIV expanded at alarming rates, increasingly impacting all societal segments and reaching beyond all cultural and national boundaries. In the United States, "AIDS cases increased rapidly in the 1980s and peaked in 1992 (an estimated 78,000 cases diagnosed) before stabilizing in 1998 (as a result of the impact of early HAART treatment and prevention); since then, approximately 40,000 AIDS cases have been diagnosed annually" (CDC, 2006, p. 590). In the mid 1990s, a new class of medication was introduced called HAART (highly active antiretroviral therapy), ARV, or ART (antiretroviral treatment), and prevention policies and education had been put in place.

Globally, epidemiological data indicate the spread of HIV appears to have peaked in 1996, when 3.5 million (3.2–3.8 million) new HIV infections occurred. The number of people living with HIV worldwide continued to grow in 2008, reaching an estimated 33.4 million (31.1–35.8 million). The total number of people living with the virus in 2008 was more than 20% higher than the number in 2000, and the prevalence was roughly threefold higher than in 1990. (United Nations AIDS [UNAIDS] & World Health Organization [WHO], 2009, p. 7)

"Worldwide, over 60 million people have contracted HIV and 22 million have died of AIDS since the epidemic began in the late 1970s" (Hall, 2007, p. 57). In 2008 alone, "the estimated number of adults and children newly infected with HIV was approximately 2.7 million people (2.4–3.0 million) while the estimated deaths of adults and children due to AIDS in 2008 was approximately 2.0 million" (1.7–2.4 million) (UNAIDS & WHO, 2009, p. 8).

In developing countries, heterosexual activity remains the primary mode of transmission of the virus, particularly in Africa ... the center of the AIDS epidemic for more than 20 years ... although UNAIDS (2003) estimates that there are at least one million HIV infected people in China and that this number could grow to 20 million by 2010. (Hall, 2007, p. 57)

In the United States, HIV/AIDS continues to present at racially and culturally disproportionate rates, similarly to when it first emerged publicly in the late 1970s. "While African Americans represent 12.3% of the U.S. population, they account for 50% of HIV/AIDS diagnoses and are more than 15 times more likely in their lifetime to be diagnosed with HIV compared to whites" (Hall, An, Hutchinson, & Samson, 2008, p. 295). This chronic disproportion of HIV/AIDS in relation to the percentage of populations affected has multifaceted causes, including, but not limited to, health

care access and disparity, HIV/AIDS awareness, education and stigma, HIV testing availability, cultural mistrust and suspicion of healthcare, as well as internecine beliefs and influences about HIV. "Hispanics, who represent 12.5% of the population, account for 20%" (CDC, 2006, p. 590).

Among HIV/AIDS cases reported during 2001–2004, the most common route of HIV infection is attributed to male-to-male contact (MSMs) at 44%, followed by heterosexual contact at 34%, injection drug use (IDU) at 17%, MSM/IDU at 4% and perinatal (children being infected in utero, during birth or by being breast fed) at 0.6%. (CDC, 2006, p. 590)

"Among women of child-bearing age, HIV/AIDS is the leading cause of mortality world-wide" (Barclay, 2009, p. 1).

HIV/AIDS is a global development emergency and continues to spread unabated in many parts of the world where it is wiping out the developmental gains achieved over the past decades, threatening the peace and stability of nations and regions. Whether in developed countries or third world countries, HIV affects and adds to, the plight of the marginalized, stigmatized and disempowered. (Hall, 2007, p. 56)

"The death rate from AIDS continues to be significant: approximately 15,000–16,000 per year in the United States" (AIDS National Resource Center [AETC], 2009, p. 1).

Historically, HIV presented the global medical community, in those first years of the epidemic, with a spectrum of diagnosis and treatment challenges and obstacles as well as host of unknowns. With no known available or reliable treatments, the medical profession was at a loss to resolve the medical conundrum or to address the patient's "total pain" (Carroll-Johnson, Gorman, & Bush, 1998, p. 16), the myriad and layered medical, social, emotional, psychiatric, and spiritual complexities that AIDS patients presented. These issues included, but were not limited to the following: stigma; fear of contagion; abandonment of partner, spouses, friends, family, and employers; loss of income; psychological complications, including anxiety spectrum disorders, depressive disorders, suicidality, AIDS-related dementia; chronic, progressive disability and illness; and debilitating and unrelenting pain. Cassell noted that suffering is "personal and subjective ... and includes a threat to personal integrity" (Cassell, 1982, p. 641). This concept of integrity cycles back to the model of "total pain," a term first coined by the Cecily Saunders, founder of the modern hospice movement, to describe the holistic (physical pain, affect or emotional discomfort, interpersonal conflicts, nonacceptance of one's own dying) impact of terminal illness on the total person (Leleszi & Lewandowski, 2005, p. 56). HIV presented as the epitome of that total threat and an amalgam of losses. In addition to the dilemma of the HIV patients and adding to the medical complexities were the dynamic issues of those friends, partners, spouses, and families who remained in the lives of the patients as they traveled their AIDS journey. Many of the issues of these "others" paralleled the issues of the patient: stigma; fears of contagion; loss of community; family upheaval and destabilization; psychological responses; illness and death of a loved one; and bereavement and grief; to name but a few.

Considering, in these early days of AIDS, the quantity of HIV patients and the quality of the losses patients endured, medicine incorporated other disciplines into primary treatment teams: nurses, social workers, pastoral counselors, psychiatrist/psychologists, case managers, and nutritionists. The palliative care team, first described in 1975, had now moved into the forefront of HIV patient care.

This comprehensive framework of care addresses and emphasizes a balance of patient needs with the unpredictability of HIV disease. The continuum of care for HIV patients was now altered to incorporate a team of providers to address the burden and impact of HIV disease on the patient and the patient's personal support system. Within this continuum of care model, comfort and supportive treatment eventually and ultimately replace curative treatment as the patient progresses to end of life. The patient may, finally, be referred for hospice care, if there is physician designation of 6 months or less to live. This designation allows the hospice benefit system to be accessed, whether through most private insurance, HMOs, Medicaid, or Medicare.

> *My husband told me if I ever came home with HIV he would kill me. He will. He has beat me before. I am 32, I have three young children. My family is in the DR (Dominican Republic). Where am I to go?*
> — *Rosa, in 2002, upon learning that she is HIV positive*

Social Workers in HIV Palliative Care

In 1999, Dr Peter Selwyn, chair of family medicine at Montefiore Medical Center in the Bronx, New York, in cooperation with the School of Public Health, Columbia University, established an HIV Palliative Care Program. This 3-year demonstration program was sponsored by HRSA as a federally funded Special Project of National Significance (SPNS) pilot to determine the efficacy of palliative care for people with HIV in a large, urban, teaching, medical center, whose patient demographic was primarily disenfranchised, working class, poor, and minority. Dr. Selwyn and the Columbia team designed the program as interdisciplinary. Included in the primary team was a physician, nurse practitioner, social worker, outreach worker, pastoral counselor, and a data entry technician. A palliative care psychiatrist was hired on a part-time basis. The program was designed to offer palliative care services to the broad, HIV patient population of Montefiore

Medical Center, with referrals coming from inpatient services, the outpatient infectious disease clinic, nine community-based primary care clinics, and four outpatient substance abuse treatment programs. The goal was to provide the broadest spectrum of palliative services to ensure the broadest spectrum of patient referrals and patient consents for care. Patients, who consented to receive palliative care, were followed throughout the trajectory of their illness and would be seen at home, at the clinics or substance abuse treatment programs, or as inpatients. Patients were followed from time of enrollment to death or, in some cases, until the end of the study. Much work was done to facilitate cooperation and coordination with existing service providers in order to create a sense of team work, inclusion, and collaboration rather than alienation, competition, and territoriality. The palliative social worker strove to be incorporated into existing social work services, including hospital discharge planners and outpatient clinic staff.

The palliative social worker, the nurse practitioner, and outreach worker conducted initial, baseline psychosocial assessments as well as a monthly follow-up, which included psychosocial assessments, the Memorial Symptom Assessment Scale (MSAS), Mini-Mental Status Examination (MMSE), Karnofsky score, and Rapid Disability Rating Scale (RDRS) (Selwyn et al., 2002). The function of the social worker was multifaceted and dyadic, that is, to provide a normative range of psychosocial support and services while simultaneously fulfilling the requisite components of the study.

Social Work: Pre-HAART and HAART Eras

The current history of HIV is divided into two distinct eras: pre-HAART-era HIV and HAART-era HIV. There are, however, few differences in the scope and complexity of HIV palliative social work services. While few, these distinctions are monumental.

> *In the pre-HAART era, AIDS was a uniformly fatal, relentlessly progressive illness, characterized by multiple opportunistic infections, swift decline, and death within months of diagnosis. [In the HAART era, treatment] has meant the possibility of full return of function and health, while for others ... the survival time from diagnosis to death has lengthened [and survival] has shifted to a trajectory more typical of chronic, progressive illnesses ... with much more variability in outcomes. (Selwyn et al., 2002, p. 5)*

Consequent to the changes just described, the functions of the HIV palliative social worker in the HAART era have broadened to include levels of psychosocial complexity not confronted before. While numbers of deaths have dropped significantly, there arrives with that progress, a series of other complicating factors associated with HIV work.

Pre- and HAART-Era HIV Palliative Social Work Assessment for Potential Interventions

1. Education of patient and/or family and intimate network focused on the following:
   - Wellness, self-care, caregiving, stress management
   - Basics and myths about HIV, HIV routes of transmission, sexual history, and safer sex education
   - Basic functions of the immune system, CD4 and viral counts, HIV antibody testing, HIV positive versus AIDS, infection versus disease
   - Knowledge of HIV and possible course of illness, with and without HAART—a realistic appraisal of the potential for illness as well as chronic versus acute illness
   - Knowledge of other treatments and comorbid diseases
   - Importance of supporting adherence in light of the changing face of HIV treatments, health disparities and challenges to continuity of care
   - Knowledge of and referrals to palliative and hospice care, education of the similarities and differences, including scope of multidisciplinary services
   - AIDS phobia—fears based on cultural, religious, societal, familial, intrapsychic beliefs, and attitudes. Includes HIV stigma, discrimination, as well as homophobia
   - Resources and supports pre- and post-HIV disclosure issues that may enhance coping with HIV disease. Includes the realities and ethics of confidential versus anonymous approaches as well as education and support for sero-discordant relationships.

2. Comprehensive and ongoing assessments of the following:
   - Client's and caregiver's "total pain," including biopsychosocial issues and benefits structure
   - Counseling and appropriate legal, mental health, and substance abuse referrals.

3. Dying and death/grief and bereavement include the following:
   - Education and counseling related to needs, beliefs, and attitudes of patient, family, and intimate network
   - Assessments of issues related to multiple AIDS-related illnesses and deaths of others.

4. Palliative social workers provide the following:
   - Ongoing self-assessment and awareness of AIDS burnout and the impact of complex patient care and cumulative AIDS-related deaths.

I used to be the gay man who stood on the soap box yelling about safe sex, staying negative, not getting infected. And then one night … I can't believe this. I have HIV and I got it at 40 and I know better. I am on meds and my health is great, but I feel like a failure. I am depressed and I can't tell anyone because I am ashamed and a failure. Who will want me?
—Jeff in 2009

HAART-Era Additions to Palliative Social Work Assessment for Potential Interventions

1) Recovery into wellness:
   - Many patients expected and even prepared themselves and/or others for death. Now healthier due to HAART, there are conflicted and multiple reactions to a return to health, including but not limited to a redefinition of identity, relationships, profession, benefits structure, and goals.
   - Patients may or may not continue to receive palliative care services.

2) Recovery into chronic illness:
   - Many patients who remain in a state of chronic, unrelenting illness continue to receive palliative care services and live in fear that their stable chronic condition is temporary.

3) Adherence to lifelong treatment:
   - With the advent of HAART, many patients must stay on their medication regimens, daily, for life. This may compromise the patient's quality of life (QoL).
   - Palliative clinicians can assist patients by assessing the myriad of factors, in the short term and the long term, that influence adherence, including organization, side effect management, literacy, and capacity to work with numbers. Ongoing adherence counseling and assessments by the palliative care team are essential.

4) Fear of failure of HAART:
   - Described as one of the major sources of psychological and emotional upset. Ongoing assessment and intervention are essential to assisting patients with poor adherence or the medical failure of HAART.

5) Failure of HAART with no options:
   - A prominent and profound moment for the patient, loved ones, and the palliative care team
   - Interventions involve ongoing reviews of a patient wishes, goals and advance directives, including do not resuscitate (DNR) and do not intubate (DNI)
   - End-of-life preferences and legacy building

6) Lazarus syndrome:
- A situation when a patient is close to death, expecting and preparing to die.
- With HAART, there is a remarkable and profound recovery.

7) Emerging long-term survivor medical conditions:
- Science is now learning that long-term survivors are beginning to present with a spectrum of illnesses and conditions previously not seen, including non-HIV-related cancers, neurological symptoms such as peripheral neuropathies, and cognitive changes such as short-term memory loss.

8) Sero-conversion after three decades of HIV prevention, awareness, and education:
- Recent sero-conversion, that is, being newly infected with HIV, during the HAART era, can bring an array of reactions, including intense guilt, shame, remorse, anger, and depression, primarily because transmission prevention information is readily available and known.
- Conversely, the positive efficacy of HAART has created a false sense that HIV infection is relatively inconsequential, resulting in increases in new sero-conversions as well as other sexually transmitted diseases (STDs).

Patient Family Narratives

The patient/family narratives in Boxes 33.1–33.3 were documented by the Montefiore Medical Center HIV Palliative Care Team.

Palliative care as a modality of care in HIV disease has been instrumental in establishing innovative approaches

---

Box 33.1
Patient/Family Narrative: Miss J.

Miss J., a 34-year-old, Latina, married, mother of three, was referred to the Palliative Care Program after her husband of 18 years had left her upon her learning that she was HIV positive. He refused to get tested, to speak about the issue, and verbally attacked his wife for the infection. Miss J., 8 years sober but no longer attending Alcoholics Anonymous, reports that since marriage to him, he was her only sexual encounter and wonders whether he was with other women or on the down low with men, but she is afraid to ask. Her two daughters, ages 15 and 13, were beginning to display psychological and behavioral symptoms related to their mother's HIV issues, the stressors of the marital conflict, the abandonment by their father, and their mother's resulting depression and concerns for alcohol relapse. Miss J.'s CD4 had recently dropped to dangerous levels and she needed to begin HAART. Being informed of her fragile health and the need to

---

begin HAART exacerbated her depression and fears that she was going to die and abandon her daughters.

The palliative care team intervened to assist both the mother and children. The physician worked closely with the psychiatrist to improve her CD4 and reduce her viral load while simultaneously addressing her depression. The palliative social worker and adherence counselor provided support to Miss J. and her daughters, working to understand how her adherence issues related to self-blame, guilt, hopelessness, depression, and family conflict. Custody planning, should Miss J. die, was a predominant focus both to reinforce a sense of security for the children, demonstrate to the father the potential consequence of abandonment, and to reinforce Miss J.'s continuing role as mother and primary parent. Seen on a weekly basis, the social worker created a supportive environment for Miss J. to explore the multifaceted medical and psychosocial issues related to her HIV infection, the potential course of her disease with HAART versus without HAART, obstacles to adherence, and the stressors of her AIDS diagnosis on her marriage and her children. The palliative social worker became the bridge for Miss J.'s other palliative care services as well as an advocate to collateral resources and external support systems. Today, Miss J. remains sober, her health is improved, and her family structure is stable, with ongoing negotiations to bring her husband home.

Box 33.2
Patient/Family Narrative: Louis

Louis, a 25-year-old, gay, biracial (white and Latino) male returned to live at his mother's home when his HIV symptoms became unmanageable. He was then hospitalized with severe, unrelenting headaches of unknown origin. While an inpatient, he became paraplegic and had to be transferred to another hospital, to diagnose the cause of his paralysis. His primary physician, an attending in the outpatient HIV clinic, referred him to the palliative care team who were able to make home visits; from that time on, he received all of his medical care at home. His CD4 was in the single digits and viral load in the six figures. The etiology of his paraplegia remained a mystery to his primary physician and the palliative team. Louis could also not tolerate HAART. The palliative nurse practitioner provided his medical care at home. He was seen weekly by the palliative social worker, who also provided counseling sessions to his mother and adult siblings as requested. The social work goals were to assist with the ongoing assessment of Louis's total pain—his multiple losses, including independence, ability to self-care, intimate relationships, and future hopes and dreams—as well as monitor his progressive decline, increased physical pain, cognitive changes and, finally, prepare both Louis and his family for his eventual death. The palliative care psychiatrist and minister came on an "as-needed" basis. For 1 year, the team worked with the client and assisted the family to cope with his declining health. As Louis entered into an active dying phase, the family discussed this process with the team. The morning Louis died, the family called to ask that someone from the palliative care team be there with the family to witness his death. After the client's death, bereavement counseling services were provided to the family for a year after his death.

Box 33.3
Patient/Family Narrative: Nancy

Nancy, a 59-year-old, single, gay, former intravenous drug-using female, was referred to the palliative care program by her primary physician after numerous trials of HAART had failed, leaving Nancy with no treatment options. Her CD4 was 2 and she had just been diagnosed with stage 4 lung cancer. Nancy lived alone in a single-room apartment. Her mother, with whom she was extremely close, had recently died and her surviving sister lived in Puerto Rico. Nancy was initially reluctant to invest in and trust the palliative care team, believing that this was "death squad" who came in to her home to "hurry up her death." She began to see the palliative social worker, psychiatrist, and minister in her home but chose to continue to see her primary physician at her clinic, since this physician had also cared for her mother. Her relationship with her primary physician was valued and supported because it was exceedingly important to her; trust in the medical profession was an issue that was of great significance. Over time, she began to look forward to the home visits by the team and eventually entrusted them with her losses, secrets, and wishes. As she neared death, she discussed her burial with the palliative care team, even directing what clothes she wanted to be buried in. It gave her great comfort to have these conversations, knowing that her extended family would not and could not have them. The palliative care team was at the bedside of the patient as she died, along with extended family. Bereavement services were offered to the family, but they declined.

---

throughout the life of the patient. With the advent of HAART, HIV disease has been redefined as a potentially chronic condition, providing patients newly infected the opportunity to remain symptom free and, in some situations, allowing those with long-term infection, compromised immune systems, and/or a history of opportunistic infections to reclaim health and, hopefully, quality of life. These accomplishments, however, do not mean that palliative care as the modality of service should be abandoned. There is evidence that, because of the positive responses of HAART, some of the commitment to palliative care is waning. The HAART-era HIV assessment interventions listed earlier point to the ongoing need for the integration of active treatment and palliative care.

The Department of Health Resources and Services Administration (HRSA) reports that their "goal is to achieve 100% access to health services and 0% disparity in healthcare" (HRSA, 2009, and O'Neil & Marconi, 2001, p. 452). In reference to HIV, a component of that goal is the recommendation that "individuals with HIV whose living situations are stabilized ... may see their health improve. Pain relief and other palliative services may then need to be integrated for several years with curative treatments" (Sebuyira, Gwyther, Merriman, & Schietinger 2006, p. 15). HAART has, hopefully, changed the terminal face of HIV in the United States, creating hope that a once fatal syndrome can now be managed as a chronic, if incurable, condition. "Combined [more than two HAART medications used simultaneously] antiretroviral therapy appears to have cut the average mortality rate

by half in HIV patients ... [and this] mortality reduction was translated into a 5% increase in 5-year survival for (combined therapy) initiation" (Douglas, 2010, p. 123). The report provides the caveat that "the impact on overall mortality, however, remains unclear" (Douglas, 2010, p. 123).

The Future: Social Work, HIV/AIDS, and Palliative Care

With appropriate adherence, HAART provides the person with HIV the potential to transform the disease trajectory into *conditional chronicity* with palliative care remaining the standard of interdisciplinary care. While not curative in the purest definition, meaning infection free, HAART does provide the opportunity to remain disease free, at this time.

Conclusion

"The number of people needing palliative care is projected to grow dramatically over the next few years while the number of people who will provide care is expected to decrease" (Von Gunten, 2005, p. 694). O'Neil and Marconi have outlined elements, not prerequisites or determinants, to advance palliative care for vulnerable populations, which includes people with HIV/AIDS:

- The knowledge, attitudes, training, and experience of health professionals and staff to interact appropriately ... with populations with advanced disease
- The importance of collaboration between medical and supportive services in achieving high-quality palliative care
- The appropriateness of the organizational characteristics of ... palliative care services. Characteristics ... include participation of clients ... in shaping clinical services, appropriate eligibility requirements of care, availability of on-site or easily accessible ancillary services, and adoption and support of clinical care guideline.
- The responsiveness of palliative care service delivery systems ... including the types of services offered ... the extent to which health and support service organizations maintain regular contact ... and the adoption of standards of care
- The flexibility of the health policy environment to support palliative care services for all populations. In the United States, both federal and state reimbursement policies are critical factors. Current issues that limit access include interstate variations in Medicaid and Medicare and immigration and welfare reforms (O'Neil & Marconi, 2001, p. 454).

Social work has been an integrated and integral component of HIV palliative care since the beginning of the epidemic, and social workers certainly have been and will continue to be participants in advocating for the essential elements outlined by O'Neil and Marconi. The profession is the major psychosocial contributor to the comprehensive palliative care provided to persons living with HIV/AIDS. It is the responsibility of the individual social worker and the discipline of social work to place their work and field on par with that of the medical disciplines. "Social workers in palliative care need to make themselves heard ... social workers need to make themselves visible ... need to speak the language of social work, the medical model and advocacy for the patient—all at once" (Meier & Beresford, 2008, pp. 11–12). Without a social work presence, HIV palliative care is reduced to a primary medical model, with narrowed and reduced holistic goals. Social workers who gain and retain leadership roles in their HIV palliative care programs contribute to a balanced and cohesive approach to patient quality of life and goals of care. Social work commitment to advocate means that they advocate just as passionately for the profession in HIV palliative care, as they do for their HIV palliative care patients. The primary goal of palliative care is the improvement of the patient's quality of life, mutually supported by collaborative, interdisciplinary care providers with the patient and the family. HIV palliative social workers have been, and continue to be, leaders in achieving those goals.

LEARNING EXERCISES

Based on the following narratives, provide a psychosocial palliative care points assessment, plan interventions, and consider possible goals of care.

- *A 45-year-old, white, gay male client, who has been infected with HIV for 25 years, is considered to have experienced the Lazarus syndrome. HAART is no longer effective and there are no other HIV treatment options. He is in a sero-discordant relationship with a 35-year-old African American man. The relationship is 2 years old. Both are Jewish and have been renounced by their families because of their sexual orientation and relationship. The client's family does not know of his HIV-positive status. He has refused to accept the finality of the situation.*

- *An 82-year-old African American woman refuses to acknowledge or discuss with her medical team that she has HIV/AIDS. Despite numerous attempts by various members of the multidisciplinary team, she remains adamant that she is unaffected. Her medical reports indicate that she needs to begin HAART and is in fragile health. She is exceedingly religious, goes to Church every Sunday, and believes that God performed a miracle by saving her from a terminal illness (cirrhosis of the liver) 20 years ago. Both her children died as adults, one*

of cancer. The death of the other child is something that the client refuses to speak about. She takes care of her 100-year-old mother.

- *A 32-year-old African American young woman arrives at your office with her home attendant. She has a very low CD4 count and her viral load is exceedingly high. She is unable to tolerate the side affects of her HAART medication. She needs this to boost her immune system so that she can tolerate the chemotherapy for her vaginal cancer, which was diagnosed 3 years ago. She has been diagnosed with epilepsy. She has a history of substance abuse and prostitution. She states she has seven children in foster care, with whom she has no contact. Her mother, with whom she recently reconnected, has just died of cancer. She also reports that she is being sexually abused by her boyfriend.*

ADDITIONAL RESOURCES

READINGS

Allen, D., & Marshall, E. (2008). Children with HIV/AIDS: A vulnerable population with unique needs for palliative care. *Journal of Hospice and Palliative Nursing, 10*(6), 359–367.

Aranda-Naranjo, B. (2004). Quality of life in the HIV-positive patient: Implications and consequences. *Journal of the Association of Nurses in AIDS Care, 15*(5), 20–27.

Becchetti, R. (2003). Difficult conversations–The reality of end-of-life palliative care. *Oncology Issues, 18*(1), 36–39.

Bogart, L., Catz, S., Kelly, J., Gray-Berhardt, M., Hartmann, B., Otto-Salaj, L., Hackl, K., & Bloom, F. (2010). Psychosocial issues in the era of new AIDS treatments from the perspective of persons living with HIV. *Journal of Health Psychology, 5*(4), 500–516.

Breitbart, W. (2003). Pain. *A clinical guide to supportive care for HIV/AIDS 2003 edition.* Retrieved from http://hab.hrsa.gov/tools/palliative/chap4.html

Byock, I. (2002). The meaning and value of death. *Journal of Palliative Medicine, 5*(2), 279–288.

The Center for Palliative Care Education (CPCE). (2006). *Overview of HIV/AIDS palliative care. Northeast AIDS Education and Training Center.*

Curtis, J.R. (2003). Patient-clinician communication. *A clinical guide to supportive care for HIV/AIDS 2003 edition.* Retrieved from http://hab.hrsa.gov/tools/palliative/chap21.html

Education Development Center. (2002). *Innovations in end-of-life care.* Retrieved from http://www.edc.org/lastacts

Harding, R., Karus, D., Easterbrook, P., Raveis, V., Higginson, I., & Marconi, K. (2005). Does palliative care improve outcomes for patients with HIV/AIDS? A systematic review of the evidence. *Sexually Transmitted Infections, 81,* 5–14.

Matheny, S. (2001). Clinical dilemmas in palliative care for HIV infection. *Journal of the Royal Society of Medicine, 94,* 449–451.

Mazanec, P., Daly, B., Pitorak, E., Kane, D., Wile, S., & Wolen, J. (2009). A new model of palliative care for oncology patients in advanced disease. *Journal of Hospice and Palliative Nursing, 11*(6), 324–331.

Mount, B. (2003). Existential suffering and the determinants of healing. *European Journal of Palliative Care*, *10*(2), 40–42.

National Association of Social Workers (NASW). (2004). *NASW standards for palliative and end of life care*. Washington, DC: Author.

National Association of Social Workers (NASW). (2009). *NASW standards for social work practice in palliative and end of life care*. Washington, DC. Retrieved from http:www.socialworkers.org/practice/bereavement/standards/default.asp

Nord, D. (1997). *Multiple AIDS-related loss: A handbook for understanding and surviving a perpetual fall*. Washington, DC: Taylor & Francis

O'Hare, T., Williams, C., & Ezoviski, A. (1996). Fear of AIDS and homophobia: Implications for direct policy and advocacy. *Social Work: Journal of the National Association of Social Workers, 41*(1), 51–58.

Oliviere, D., Hargreaves, R., & Monroe, B. (1998). *Good practices in palliative care*. Burlington, VT: Ashgate.

O'Neill, J., & Barini-Garcia, M. (2003). HIV and palliative care. *A clinical guide to supportive care for HIV/AIDS 2003 edition*. Retrieved from http://hab.hrsa.gov/tools/palliative/chap1.html

O'Neill, J., Marconi, K., Surapruik, A., & Blum N. (2000). Improving HIV/AIDS services through palliative care: An HRSA perspective. *Journal of Urban Health, 77*(2), 244–254.

Robinson, L., Dugger, K., Fong, G., Heintzman, T., Hnizdo, S., Libby, J., McDaniels, J., Miles, J., Rempel, H., Taylor, A., & Warshaw, M. (2006). Palliative home nursing interventions for people with HIV/AIDS: A pilot study. *Journal of the Association of Nurses in AIDS Care, 17*(3), 37–46.

Schaffner, B. (May 22, 1993). *The crucial and difficult role of the psychotherapist in the treatment of the HIV-positive patient*. Paper presented to the American Academy of Psychoanalysis, San Francisco, CA.

Selwyn, P., & Rivard, M. (2003). Palliative care for AIDS: Challenges and opportunities in the era of highly active anti-retroviral therapy. *Journal of Palliative Medicine, 6*(3), 475–483.

Shippy, R. A., & Karpiak, S. E. (2005). The aging HIV/AIDS population: Fragile social networks. *AIDS Community Research Intiative (ACRIA), 9*(3), 246–254.

Treisman, G., & Angelino, A. (2004). *The psychiatry of AIDS*. Baltimore, MD: The Johns Hopkins University Press.

Twycross, R. G. (2004). Care of the terminally ill patient. *Triangle, 31*(1), 1–7.

United Nations AIDS (UNAIDS) & World Health Organization (WHO). (2009). *09 AIDS epidemic update*. Retrieved from http://www.unaids.org

UNAIDS Technical Update. (2000). *AIDS palliative care*. Retrieved from http://www.unaids.org

United Nations General Assembly Special Session (UNGASS). (2001). *Review of the problem of HIV/AIDS in all its aspects*. Special Session of the General Assembly on HIV/AIDS: Report of the Secretary General, 16

United States Department of Veterans Affairs. (2009) *Palliative care of patients with HIV*. Retrieved from http://www.hib.va.gov/vahiv?page=cm602_palliative

Winiarski, M. (Ed.). (1997). *HIV mental health for the 21st Century*. New York, NY. New York University Press.

World Health Organization (WHO). (2010). *HIV/AIDS–palliative care*. Retrieved from http://www.who.int/hiv/topics/palliative//PalliativeCare/en/

RESOURCES AND WEB SITES

The Body: http://www.thebody.com
Uses the Web to lower barriers between patients and clinicians, improve patients' quality of life, demystify HIV/AIDS and its treatment, and foster community through human connection.

The AIDS Action Europe clearinghouse: http://www.hivaidsclearinghouse.org
A central point where nongovernmental organizations, policy makers, networks, and other stakeholders in Europe and Central Asia can share key documents and good practice materials.

AIDS Education Global Information Systems (AEGIS): http://www.aegis.com
A database for information on AIDS that presents published materials.

Americans for Better Care of the Dying (ABCS): http://www.abcd-caring.org
By sharing expertise and building collaborative networks and public commitment, ABCD seeks to achieve substantive health care reform through improved policy, professional practice, and care reimbursement.

The American Medical Association (AMA): http://www.ama-assn.org
Promotes the art and science of medicine and the betterment of public health. Members, medical societies and other physicians, medical students, and staff play an integral role in the AMA and contribute to its success.

The Center to Advance Palliative Care (CAPC): http://www.capc.org
Provides health care professionals with the tools, training, and technical assistance necessary to start and sustain successful palliative care programs in hospitals and other health care settings.

The Centers for Disease Control and Prevention (CDC): http://www.cdc.gov
One of the major operating components of the U.S. Department of Health and Human Services.

Dying Well: http://www.dyingwell.org
Provides resources for people facing life-limiting illness, their families, and their professional caregivers.

The Elizabeth Glaser Pediatric AIDS Foundation: http://www.pedaids.org
Seeks to prevent pediatric HIV infection and to eradicate pediatric AIDS through research, advocacy, and prevention and treatment programs.

The Gay Men's Health Crisis: http://www.gmhc.org
Provides HIV/AIDS prevention, care, and advocacy.

Hospice Education Institute: http://www.hospiceworld.org
An independent, not-for-profit organization, serving members of the public and health care professionals with information and education about the many facets of caring for the dying and bereaved.

The Hospice Foundation of America: http://www.hospicefoundation.org
Provides leadership in the development and application of hospice and its philosophy of care with the goal of enhancing the U.S. health care system and the role of hospice within it.

Last Acts: http://www.lastacts.org
A highly acclaimed Robert Wood Johnson Foundation national program that came to a close in 2005. However, *Last Acts* created a wealth of useful Web content—for health care

consumers, health care practitioners, policy makers, and employers.

National AIDS Hotline: http://www.AIDS.gov

Provides access to federal HIV/AIDS information through a variety of new media channels and supports the use of new media tools by federal and community partners to improve domestic HIV programs.

The National Association of Social Workers (NASW): http://www.naswdc.org/

The largest membership organization of professional social workers in the world, with 150,000 members. NASW works to enhance members' professional growth, to maintain professional standards, and to advance social policies.

The National Center for Death Education at Mount Ida College: http://www.mountida.edu Promotes knowledge and understanding in the field of thanatology. The Center assists caregiving professionals and students in acquiring current knowledge and skills for providing care associated with end of life, bereavement, and loss.

The National Center for HIV, STD, and TB Prevention: http://www.cdc.gov/nchhstp/

Maximizes public health and safety nationally and internationally through the elimination, prevention, and control of disease, disability, and death caused by HIV/AIDS, viral hepatitis, STDs, and TB.

The National Family Caregivers Association: http://www.thefamilycaregiver.org/

Educates, supports, empowers, and speaks up for the more than 50 million Americans who care for loved ones with a chronic illness or disability or the frailties of old age.

The National Hospice Foundation: http://www.national hospicefoundation.org

In partnership with the National Hospice and Palliative Care Organization, raises funds for programs that affect the lives of the patients and families served by NHPCO's membership of more than 3400 hospice and palliative care providers.

The National Hospice and Palliative Care Organization (NHPCO): http://www.nhpco.org

A nonprofit membership organization representing hospice and palliative care programs and professionals in the United States. The organization is committed to improving end-of-life care and access to hospice care.

Promoting Excellence in End-of-Life Care: http://www.promotingexcellence.org

A national program of the Robert Wood Johnson Foundation dedicated to improve health care for dying people and their families; it no longer operates. Results of the program are archived by Growth House, Inc.

The Social Work in Hospice and Palliative Care Network: http://www.swhpn.org

A network of social work organizations and leaders who seek to further the field of end-of-life and hospice/palliative care.

The WHO HIV Testing and Counseling: http://www.who.int/HIV/topic/vct/en

Provides information and guidance for provider-initiated HIV testing and counseling (PITC) in health facilities to increase uptake and improve access to HIV health services.

The World Health Organization Palliative Care: http://www.who.int/cancer/palliative/

Provides leadership and technical support regarding cancer to countries. *Cancer Pain Release* is the publication of the World Health Organization global communications program to improve cancer and HIV pain control and palliative care.

REFERENCES

AIDS National Resource Center (AETC). (2009). *Palliative care and HIV*. Retrieved from http://www.aids-etc.org/aidsetc?page=cm-602_palliative

Barclay, L. (2009). *WHO issues new HIV recommendations*. Medscape Medical News. Retreived from http://www.medscape.com/viewarticle/713121

Carroll-Johnson, R. M., Gorman, L., & Bush, N. (1998). *Psychosocial nursing care along the cancer continuum*. Pittsburgh, PA: Oncology Nursing Press.

Cassell, E. J. (1982). The nature of suffering and the goals of medicine. *New England Journal of Medicine, 306,* 639–645.

Centers for Disease Control and Prevention (CDC). (2006). Epidemiology of HIV/AIDS–United States, 1981-2005. *Morbidity and Mortality Weekly Report*. Retrieved from http://www.cdc.gov/mmwr/preview/mmwrhtml/mm5521a2.htm

Douglas, D. (2010). Combination antiretroval therapy has halved mortality in HIV patients since 1996. *AIDS 2010, 23,* 123–137.

Hall, H. I., An, Q., Hutchinson, A., & Samson, S. (2008). Estimating the lifetime risk of a diagnosis of the HIV infection in 33 states, 2004-2005. *Epidemiology and Social Sciences, 49*(3), 294–297.

Hall, N. (2007). *We care don't we? Social workers, the profession and HIV/AIDS*. Binghampton, NY: The Haworth Press.

Health Resources and Services Administration (HRSA). (2009). *A guide to primary care for people with HIV/AIDS*. Retrieved from http://www.hab.hrsa.gov/tools/primarycareguide/index.htm

Huminer, D., Rosenfeld, J. B., & Pilik, S. S. (1987). AIDS in the pre-AIDS era. *Infectious Disease Review, 9*(6), 1102–1108.

Kearney, M. (1996). *Mortally wounded*. New York, NY: Touchstone.

Krouse, R. (2008). Palliative care for the cancer patient: An interdisciplinary approach. *Cancer and Chemotherapy Reviews, 3*(4), 152–160.

Leleszi, J., & Lewandowski, J. (2005). Pain management in end-of-life care. *Journal of American Osteopathic Association, 105*(3), 56.

Meier, D., & Beresford, L. (2008). Social workers advocate for a seat at the palliative care table. *Journal of Palliative Medicine, 11*(1), 10–14.

O'Neil, J., & Marconi, K. (2001). Access to palliative care in the US: Why emphasize vulnerable populations. *Journal of the Royal Study of Medicine, 94,* 452–454.

The President's Emergency Plan for AIDS Relief, Office of the US Global AIDS Coordinator (2006). *HIV/AIDS palliative care guidance #1 for the United States government in-country staff and implementing partners*. Retrieved from http://www.cdc.gov/nchstp/od/gap/strategies

Reith, M., & Payne, M. (2009). *Social work in end-of-life and palliative care*. Chicago, IL: Lyceum Books.

Sebuyira, L., Gwyther, L., Merriman, A., & Schietinger, H. (Eds.). (2006). *A clinical guide to supportive and palliative care for HIV/AIDS in sub-Saharan Africa*. The African Palliative Care Association. Retrieved from http://www.theworkcontinues.org/docs/news/apca

Selwyn, P. (2005). Why should we care about palliative care for AIDS in the era of antiretroviral therapy? *Sexually Transmitted Infections, 81,* 2–3.

Selwyn, P., Rivard, M., Kappell, D., Goeren, B., LaFosse, H., Schwartz, C., & Farber-Post, L. (2002). Palliative care and HIV/AIDS at a large urban teaching hospital: Clinical challenges and program description. *Journal of Palliative Medicine, 5*(2), 4–33.

University of California, San Francisco (UCSF). (2008). *Palliative care of patients with HIV.* Retrieved from http://www.hivinsite.ucsf.edu/InSite?page=kb-03-03-05

Von Gunten, C. F. (2005). Innovations in palliative care. *Journal of Palliative Medicine, 8*(4), 694–695.

World Health Organization (WHO). (1990). *Cancer pain relief and palliative care. Report of a WHO expert committee.* Publication # 1100804. Retrieved from http://www.who.int/cancer/Palliative/definition/en

World Health Organization (WHO). (2005). *The HIV/AIDS programme at WHO.* Retrieved from http://www.who.int/hiv

34 *Sarah Gehlert and Teresa Moro*

Palliative Care with Vulnerable Populations

*It's scary when you're sick and you really don't even have a place to call your own. Hope helps
you hang on, but sometimes it is hard to find anything to hold onto.*

—Anonymous

Key Concepts

◆ *Consumers who have life-threatening illness are vulnerable by
virtue of their illnesses, yet factors such as mental illness, social
isolation, homelessness, immigration, and intellectual and
developmental disability increase their vulnerability.*

◆ *Individuals from vulnerable populations have unique and
complex care needs and present additional challenges for social
workers.*

◆ *Social workers who care for individuals from vulnerable
populations will need to work in concert with a myriad of care
providers from different disciplines and settings, such as hospitals,
shelters, community groups, and other mental health
practitioners.*

Introduction

Although life-threatening illness itself confers vulnerability,
a number of conditions increase that vulnerability and present challenges to social work practice in palliative care. These
conditions include mental illness, social isolation, homelessness, immigration, and intellectual and developmental disability. Individuals with these conditions may or may not be
underserved in terms of health care insurance coverage and
the ability to pay for services. Even in the presence of
resources, however, these conditions challenge one's ability
to maximally use services to maintain functioning in the face
of life-threatening illness.

Two ongoing, intersecting trajectories create a cadre of
persons in the United States who are particularly vulnerable
in the face of life-threatening illness. The first trajectory is an
increase in life expectancy, or survival, in the face of serious
illness. Advances in medicine and biotechnology have
enabled many people to live longer with life-threatening illnesses that previously would have been fatal. The relative
5-year survival rate for all cancers, for example, increased
from 50% between 1974 and 1976 to 64% between 1995 and
2000, which is a statistically significant difference (Jemall
et al., 2005).

The second trajectory is an increase in the gap between
population groups within the United States, arguably making
some people more vulnerable than others to developing and
coping with life-threatening illness. Health disparities by
race and ethnicity have continued to increase through time.
As an example, data collected by the National Cancer Institute on cancer mortality demonstrate a significant and
enduring black/white disparity in deaths from all cancers in
both men and women from 1975 to 2004 (Ries et al., 2007).
Black women currently are 37% more likely to die from
breast cancer than their white counterparts, and the gap continues to increase. Not coincidentally, the number of persons
living in poverty also has increased. According to the United
States Census Bureau (DeNavas-Walt, Proctor, & Smith,
2008), the official poverty rate rose from 11.3% in 2000 to
12.5% in 2007. In addition, 45.7 million Americans were
uninsured in 2007 (Robert Wood Johnson Foundation,

2009). Lastly, more Americans are socially isolated than in the past. McPherson, Smith-Lovan, and Brashears (2006) found that the number of persons saying they had no one with whom to discuss important matters nearly tripled between 1985 and 2004.

In this chapter, we outline the special challenges to individuals and their significant others experiencing life-threatening illness that is conferred by mental illness, social isolation, homelessness, immigration, and intellectual and developmental disability. We then review best practices for working with individuals and families facing life-threatening illness who have increased vulnerability by virtue of having one or more of these conditions. For each, we offer recommendations for practice.

Mental Illness and Palliative Care

The Challenge

Persons with existing mental illness are no more immune to life-threatening illness than are any other members of the population. In addition, palliative care patients without pre-existing mental illnesses may develop those conditions in response to their illness. This chapter outlines challenges to providing palliative care to persons with preexisting mental illnesses and to those that develop mental illness in response to the diagnosis of a life-threatening illness such as cancer.

Persons with serious mental illnesses, such as schizophrenia or bipolar disorder, experience life-threatening illnesses at around the same rates as the general population—that is to say that they are no more nor less likely to develop life-threatening illnesses than people who do not have serious mental illnesses. Although the prevalence of schizophrenia and other serious mental illnesses is low (the lifetime prevalence of schizophrenia, for example, is estimated to be between 0.5% and 1% [American Psychiatric Association, 2000]), these illnesses present enormous challenges to palliative care providers (see Box 34.1). Life-threatening illnesses can be particularly distressing to persons with serious mental illnes, who may be *(1)* unable to understand why they are experiencing pain and *(2)* distrustful of providers and their suggestions for treatment.

By all accounts, palliative care patients have moderate to high levels of mental illness. In a meta-analysis of psychiatric disorders among persons with advanced cancer, Miovic and Block (2007) found that about 50% of patients met the diagnosis of a mental disorder, and 7.5% to 35% of patients had more than one mental disorder. The most common disorders reported in studies reviewed by the authors were adjustment disorders (11% to 35%), major depression (5% to 26%), and anxiety disorders (6% to 8.2%). The Institute of Medicine (2001) reports that 10% to 15% of cancer patients develop major depression at some point during the course of their illness. Durkin, Kearney, and O'Siorain (2003), found that

> **Box 34.1**
> **Patient/Family Narrative: James**
>
> *James is a 35-year-old man who received a diagnosis of bipolar I disorder when he was 20 years old. For 13 years he was successfully treated with lithium. Two years ago, however, James' sister died. She was the only family member with whom he had contact and he was devastated by this loss. Shortly after her death, he took his medication less regularly and visited his doctor only sporadically. For the last 6 months, James has not taken lithium at all. During this time, as his mood swings have returned, he began to miss work and has quit paying his bills. Three months ago, James lost his job and was evicted from his apartment. He has been living off and on in a homeless shelter. A few months ago James began experiencing extreme fatigue, foot swelling, and trouble sleeping. A social worker at the homeless shelter convinced James to seek treatment and he was diagnosed with chronic kidney disease.*

almost two-thirds (62%) of the patients in a palliative care unit in Ireland met diagnostic criteria for mental illness. Ninety-one percent of those patients were symptomatic at the time of admission to the unit. It is alarming to note that 35% were receiving treatment deemed by the authors to be incorrect or inadequate.

Recommendations for Practice

Persons with serious mental illnesses, such as schizophrenia and bipolar disorder, who are in stable treatment relationships with mental health care providers have a markedly better chance of doing well than those who lack such relationships. This is because the trust in providers and the more favorable notion of treatment that is implied by working closely with mental health care providers can form the basis for similar positive outcomes, namely trust in palliative care providers and the expectation that participating in treatment will lead to foreseeable positive outcomes. In addition, providers who are familiar with patients and their families will be able, with permission, to share this knowledge with palliative care providers, thus setting the stage for a more functional relationship.

Communication between mental health care and palliative care providers is essential for achieving successful outcomes of the palliative care among persons with serious mental illness. Establishing this communication is a prime role for social workers, who are well suited by virtue of their training to serve as the conduits between the two systems of care. Setting up in-person meetings or teleconferences between the groups of providers ultimately conserves time and other resources and heightens the chance of coordinated care, such as the avoidance of deleterious drug–drug interactions.

The high percentage of persons with life-threatening illnesses who develop mental disorders makes it imperative that these disorders are diagnosed as early as possible and treated adequately. Barraclough (1997) laments that mental disorders like depression and anxiety often are considered natural reactions to life-threatening illness, and therefore not afforded the consideration and treatment that they require. Cancer Care Ontario's Program on Evidence-Based Care (Rodin et al., 2007) recommends using a structured clinical interview for diagnosing depression in palliative care patients. The program also recommends using a predefined cut-off point on a validated depression assessment scale. *The Hospital Anxiety and Depression Scale* (Zigmond & Snaith, 1983) is one such validated assessment scale that has been widely used to diagnose mental disorders among palliative care patients (Le Fevre, Devereux, Smith, Lawrie, & Cornbleet, 1999; Miovic & Block, 2007; Moorey et al., 2009).

Both pharmacologic and psychotherapeutic techniques have been used to treat mental illness among palliative care patients, at times in conjunction. Rodin and colleagues (2007) developed treatment guidelines for Cancer Care Ontario's Program on Evidence-Based Care, for instance, that includes a combined modality approach of psychosocial and pharmacologic interventions. The Institute of Medicine (2001) report on palliative care in cancer cautions that some pharmacologic agents can cause serious side effects in the face of concurrent life-threatening illness (McCoy, 1996), increasing the importance of effective, evidence-based psychotherapeutic treatments. A number of psychotherapeutic techniques have been shown to improve symptoms of mental illness among patients with life-threatening illnesses.

As was stated earlier, adjustment disorders, depression, and anxiety are the three most prevalent mental disorders among palliative patients. The central feature of an adjustment disorder is "the development of clinically significant emotional or behavioral symptoms in response to an identifiable stressor or stressors that results in the development of clinically significant emotional or behavioral symptoms" (American Psychiatric Association [APA], 2000, p. 629). According to Miovic and Block (2007), the symptoms of adjustment disorders may result in increased reliance on caregivers among patients in palliative care.

Adjustment disorders, as is the case with major depression and anxiety, respond to individual and group therapy that is problem focused and provides support and opportunity for emotional expression. Barbara Anderson and colleagues (2008) found that a group treatment that includes progressive muscle relaxation for stress reduction, problem solving for common difficulties, identifying supportive family members or friends capable of providing assistance, using assertive communication to get psychological and medical needs met, and practical strategies for dealing with side effects is significantly effective in reducing symptoms of anxiety and depression among women with breast cancer. The group treatment package also increased survival time for women who participated compared to women in the assessment-only arm of the study.

Cognitive-behavioral therapies have received the most attention among psychotherapeutic treatment modalities and have undergone more rigorous empirical testing than have other modalities (Miovic & Block, 2007; Moorey et al., 2009). Two clinical studies found cognitive-behavioral therapy to be both acceptable to patients and feasible for palliative care clinicians, such as nurses, to provide (Anderson, Watson, & Davidson, 2008; Moorey et al., 2009).

Other treatment modalities have proved effective for reducing mental symptoms among patients. Miller and Hopkinson (2008) found relaxation through guided visualization to be effective in reducing anxiety. Horne-Thompson and Grocke (2008) conducted a randomized clinical trial of a single music therapy session in reducing anxiety among palliative care patients. Symptoms such as pain, tiredness, and drowsiness were significantly lower among patients in the experimental compared to the control condition. (For additional information see Chapter 14)

Social Isolation and Palliative Care

The Challenge

Americans are becoming more socially isolated through time. The number of persons reporting that they had no confidants nearly tripled between 1985 and 2004, while social network size decreased by almost a third (McPherson, Smith-Lovan, & Brashears, 2006). Although the decrease was true for both relative and nonrelative social ties, it was more pronounced for the latter. The number of persons listing a neighbor as confidant, for example, decreased by more than half from 1985 to 2004.

Social isolation has been linked to a number of adverse health outcomes across a number of population groups. A seminal review by House, Landis, and Umberson (1988) noted an association between social integration and life expectancy across populations as diverse as Evans County, Georgia, blacks and residents of Eastern Finland, with relative risks ranging from 1.08 to 4.00. In recent years, social isolation has been linked to a number of health outcomes, including first occurrence of myocardial infarction, recurrence of stroke, and death among stroke patients (Boden-Albala, Litwak, Elkind, Rundek, & Sacco, 2005), mortality among patients with coronary artery disease (Brummett et al., 2001), and a number of adverse disease outcomes in the elderly (Tomaka, 2006), raising the specter of comorbidities among palliative care patients.

Social isolation may add to the burden of persons with life-threatening illnesses in two major ways. First, those who are isolated from supports may have difficulty in caring for themselves within their homes, as well as difficulties in getting to medical appointments. Payne and colleagues (2001) found traveling a distance for care contributed to feelings of social isolation and loneliness. Secondly, social isolation, and its psychological component, felt loneliness, have been significantly linked to depression and anxiety in empirical studies (Cacioppo & Patrick, 2008).

Recommendations for Practice

An important practice concern for social workers and other providers working with isolated and lonely persons is that these individuals may be particularly susceptible to the power and influence of providers. This may cause patients to agree to suggestions for care with which they normally would not have agreed, without questioning or completely understanding their potential impact. This may lead to further distress and discomfort. It is imperative then that social workers are cognizant of this possibility when working with socially isolated patients with life-threatening illnesses. Social work interventions are very helpful when focused on creating an environment that encourages questions, enhances the patient's comfort with decisions, and allows sufficient time for treatment choices to be discussed and questions to be re-asked and addressed.

The palliative plan of care for isolated and lonely patients may include a focus on opportunities that offer the possibility of interaction with others. This might include group psychotherapy, support groups, and adult day care. Isolated, lonely patients may benefit from networks or groups that meet electronically or by telephone. These resources may be more accessible and comfortable for patients with limited mobility or those who may be uncomfortable with in-person group experiences. When individuals who desire social networks find themselves without them as they face serious illness, it may be necessary for social workers and other providers to try to reconstruct prior social networks, when feasible, or create new ones that are virtual (i.e., by computer) or arranged through health care or social service agencies who serve patients with life-threatening illnesses.

Homelessness and Palliative Care

The Challenge

The homeless, estimated to be 2.3 to 3.5 million persons a year (Kushel & Miaskowski, 2006), develop life-threatening illnesses with at least the same frequency as the nonhomeless. In fact, they are overrepresented among persons with cancer, HIV/AIDS, and diabetes (Podymow, Turnbull, & Coyle, 2006). Providing palliative care to homeless persons with life-threatening illnesses is a challenge, for a number of reasons. These include lack of stable housing and social supports and inadequate insurance coverage. More than half of homeless persons lack health insurance, with others covered mainly by Medicaid, Medicare, and Veterans Administration benefits (Kushel, Vittinghoff, & Haas, 2001). In addition, many homeless persons have problems with substance use/abuse and mental illness.

Little has been written about the palliative care needs of the homeless. Podymow and colleagues (2006) followed 28 consecutive homeless persons who were admitted to a shelter-based palliative care unit in Ottawa. Forty-three percent had liver disease, 25%, HIV/AIDS, and 25% cancer with metastasis. An alarming 82% were addicted to alcohol or drugs or had mental illness. Eighty-two percent eventually died in the unit and 18% died in hospitals, with an average time of admission to the palliative care unit to death of 4 months. An expert panel was convened to consider alternative care locations and concluded that shelter-based palliative care produced enormous cost savings while meeting the palliative care and emotional needs of patients. The authors concluded that "many confirmed that they would not have wanted tertiary or palliative hospitalization, preferring to die in the shelter system to which they had become familiar" (p. 85).

Kushel and Miaskowski (2006) note two additional challenges to homeless persons with life-threatening illnesses, namely safely storing medications and finding transportation to health care appointments. Challenges to providers include pain management among persons concurrently using illicit drugs, adherence to medications, and the legal issues that accompany the latter challenge.

Recommendations for Practice

Although shelter-based palliative care units exist in a number of other countries, they are infrequent in the United States. In the United States, services often are provided by hospitals and hospices that serve uninsured or underinsured patients. In the absence of family members or close friends, as is the case with homeless persons (Norris, Nielson, Engelberg, & Curtis, 2005), making medical decisions for homeless terminally ill patients may become the responsibility of the health care team, which implies a profound ethical and moral responsibility. To further complicate the situation, a survey by the American Bar Association found that only eight states have enacted statutory authorization for physicians to assume default surrogacy without judicial involvement (Karp & Wood, 2003).

The hospital or hospice social worker often is in the position of helping physicians and other members of health care teams to understand and coordinate care for homeless persons at the end of life. Understanding the impact of medical decision making and providing care on various providers and seeking information to enhance these processes for team members can pave the way for improved quality of life of dying homeless patients. The National Health Care for the Homeless Council (http://www.nhchc.org) is a valuable resource for social workers who provide services to homeless persons with life-threatening illnesses.

Palliative Care with Immigrants

The Challenge

According to the Center for Immigration Studies (Camarota, 2007), the immigrant population of the United States was

37.9 million in 2007, representing one in eight U.S. residents. Thirty-one percent of adult immigrants were without a high school diploma and 31% lacked health insurance. In 2007, one out of every three immigrants was undocumented. Undocumented immigrants are even less likely than documented immigrants to have graduated from high school or to be insured, and more likely to have limited or no English skills (Marcus, 2003).

Although no definitive data are available on the health status of immigrants, there is evidence that the two groups use health care services differently. Immigrants access health services less frequently. Undocumented immigrants receive the vast majority of their care through emergency departments and the remainder through community health centers and public clinics (Goldman, Smith, & Sood, 2006). Lack of health insurance, lower levels of formal education and health literacy, and decreased access to primary health care have major implications for palliative care. Cultural beliefs about illness and its treatment may affect when and how immigrants access health care. In the book *The Spirit Catches You and You Fall Down*, Fadiman (1997) describes a conflict between physicians and the family of a young immigrant child about the cause and appropriate treatment of her epilepsy that resulted in the two sides watching impotently as the child's condition deteriorated to the point of serious disability.

In the end, immigrants are diagnosed with life-threatening illnesses later in the disease course, (Lasser, Himmelstein, & Woolhandler, 2006; Lauderdale, Wen, Jacobs, & Kandula, 2006) are less likely to understand or accept explanations of their illnesses, and are less likely to be able to afford palliative care services. There often is no recourse for undocumented immigrants who lack health insurance, because state governments lack a consistent policy on the provision of health care services to the undocumented.

Recommendations for Practice

Social workers can help to address the needs of immigrants with life-threatening illnesses in a number of ways. When they become aware that immigrants' and families' understanding is incongruent with their providers, social workers can help to interpret one group to the other group until an accord is reached. Kleinman (1980) provides a list of questions for use in determining patients' health care beliefs that can serve as a tool for social workers. These are as follows: *(1)* What do you think caused the problem? *(2)* How severe do you think the problem is? *(3)* Do you think its course will be short or long? *(4)* What difficulties is the problem causing for you? *(5)* With what are you most concerned? *(6)* What treatment do you think is most warranted for your problem? and *(7)* What benefits do you expect to receive from treatment?

Another way in which social workers can help is to facilitate the services of a professional medical interpreter (Gehlert, 2005). Professional medical interpreters take a spoken message and render it into another spoken language. This differs from interpreters, who deal with written rather than spoken language. The services of professional medical interpreters are mandated for all health care facilities that receive Department of Health and Human Services funding, which is enforced by the federal Office of Human Rights. A number of features are known to enhance the accuracy of medical interpretation. The American Association of Medical Colleges (http://www.aamc.org/students/medstudents/interpreterguide.htm) provides a valuable set of guidelines for how to engage in conversations with patients through an interpreter.

Perhaps the greatest challenge for social workers in palliative care working with immigrants, especially those who are undocumented, is helping them to find providers who will treat them with only partial reimbursement or in the absence of reimbursement. Large public hospitals that traditionally provided palliative services to undocumented immigrants have discontinued those services. Grady Memorial Hospital in Atlanta, for example, will no longer provide renal dialysis for undocumented immigrants. Although there is no easy solution to this dilemma, keeping in touch with other social workers who work with immigrant populations allows the exchange of information on immigrant palliative care services. The American Immigration Lawyers Association is a resource for obtaining information on the rights of immigrants (http://www.aila.org).

Intellectual and Developmental Disability and Palliative Care

The Challenge

Over 22 million people in the United States have some form of cognitive disability (Braddock, Hemp, & Rizzolo, 2008). This number includes people with intellectual and developmental disability (I/DD); severe, persistent mental illness; traumatic brain injury; and stroke. The over 4 million individuals with I/DD (Braddock et al., 2008) continue to be one of the most disenfranchised groups in terms of health care and inclusion in research (Marks, Sisirak, & Hsieh, 2008; Tuffrey-Wijne, Hogg, & Curfs, 2007).

Intellectual disability, previously referred to as mental retardation, occurs before the age 18 years and "is characterized by significant limitations both in intellectual functioning and in adaptive behavior as expressed in conceptual, social, and practical adaptive skills" (Schalock et al., 2007, p. 118). Developmental disabilities represent a diverse collection of severe and chronic conditions that occur before the age of 21 years of age and may result from a wide array of mental and/or physical impairments (Centers for Disease Control and Prevention, 2004). In recent decades, the life expectancy of individuals with I/DD has increased, such that persons with mild I/DD now have a life expectancy equal to that of the population as a whole (Patja, Molsa, & Livanainen, 2001). Although persons with I/DD qualify for public assistance in the form of Social Security Disability Insurance or Medicare and Medicaid (Braddock et al., 2008), this nonetheless may limit their access to and choice of providers (Marks et al., 2008).

Individuals with I/DD are more likely than the general population to be misdiagnosed or to experience delays in treatment (Marks et al., 2008), often due to problems with communication. Arguably, the inability to comprehend and communicate information is the primary barrier to optimal health care for individuals with I/DD. Individuals with I/DD may, for example, have difficulty communicating their symptoms and other crucial information to health care providers (Regnard et al., 2007; Tuffrey-Wijne et al., 2007). For example, many individuals exhibit atypical responses to pain, such as engaging in self-injurious behaviors, and thus pain and other physical symptoms may be attributed to their I/DD and therefore not appropriately assessed and addressed by caregivers or health care professionals (Tuffrey-Wijne et al., 2007).

Providers tend to overattribute disease symptoms to I/DD, thus delaying treatment for medical conditions (Tuffrey-Wijne et al., 2007). And, even after appropriately diagnosing conditions, clinical staff may fail to adequately explain diagnoses, offer a full range of treatment options, or include persons with I/DD in health care decision making (O'Regan & Drummond, 2008; Tuffrey-Wijne et al., 2007).

Recommendations for Practice

Social workers can contribute to the quality of health care for persons with I/DD who have life-threatening illnesses in a number of ways. One of the most significant is by facilitating the bidirectional communication of medical information. Communication to persons with I/DD may be facilitated through the use of nonverbal strategies, such as visual representations (Marks et al., 2008). In addition, it may help to reduce stress if persons with I/DD are introduced to health care providers prior to medical examinations or procedures (Prater & Zylstra, 2006). Likewise, some tools are available to inform and enhance the communication of important information to providers. Regnard and colleagues (2007) created the Disability Distress Assessment Tool (DisDAT) to help document signs and behaviors associated with distress in individuals with I/DD. The authors found that the majority of people with I/DD have idiosyncratic patterns of distress, and that identifying these patterns and conveying them to providers expedites the exchange of vital information.

Perhaps the most important element for improving care is to facilitate open and truthful communication, at an appropriate level, between health care providers, individuals with I/DD, and their families, friends, or community caregivers (O'Regan & Drummond, 2008; Tuffrey-Wijne et al., 2007). Communication is essential in all areas of care, but it is particularly important when delivering a diagnosis and providing care options, in particular because caregivers play such an essential role in working with individuals with I/DD as they traverse their illnesses. Caregivers often provide essential support such as administering medications, helping the individual adhere to treatment regimens, and transporting them to medical appointments. Nonrelative caregivers, such as staff in group homes, in addition to providing formal care, may become essential members of the social networks of people with I/DD. Thus, it is important that social workers recognize them as such and provide support to them when patients are diagnosed with a life-threatening illness.

Unfortunately, health care providers in hospitals, clinics, hospices, and nursing homes often have limited or no experience in working with individuals with I/DD and their significant others (Sowney & Barr, 2006; Tuffrey-Wijne et al., 2007). Although a number of manuals and programs are available to train health care providers and residential and community caregivers, few of these programs have undergone rigorous testing to determine their effectiveness (Tuffrey-Wijne et al., 2007). Thus, more research is needed.

Conclusion

Life-threatening illnesses in and of themselves confer vulnerability. Yet for millions of Americans, physical and biological characteristics and life circumstances add additional vulnerability and present particular challenges to coping with, and finding treatment for, life-threatening illnesses. Palliative social workers, by virtue of their skills and training, are in a particularly good position to advocate creatively and assertively for marginalized individuals and groups, at multiple levels of influence. Our commitment to social justice mandates that every effort be made to secure care for the most vulnerable. In addition to advocacy and resource finding, palliative social workers can provide training and support for health care providers who serve these individuals and groups. This chapter provides a beginning guidance and direction for palliative social workers to work within their systems and teams to meet the needs of these patients and their families.

LEARNING EXERCISES

- Read the narrative in Box 34.2. Since chronic kidney disease is linked to increased risk of heart disease and stroke and, if untreated, can lead to permanent kidney failure, it is essential that James begin to make lifestyle changes. He will need to monitor his blood glucose and seek regular visits with his physician. However, he will not be able to resume lithium because it has been linked to kidney disease. As the social worker working with James in the homeless shelter, what services would you connect him to? How would you do this? How

Box 34.2
Patient/Family Narrative: Olivia

Olivia is a 22-year-old mother of three children, all of whom are under 5 years of age. She and the children's father live in a rural community approximately 100 miles from a large urban center. Nine months ago, Olivia was diagnosed with stage III cervical cancer. She immediately underwent surgery to remove both ovaries, fallopian tubes, and her uterus. She also underwent radiation and chemotherapy treatments. She had to drive 2 hours to the nearest major hospital in order to receive her radiation treatments. Since her partner could not take off work, it was necessary for Olivia to drive herself to the hospital. As a result of the side effects of her treatment, including nausea and fatigue, Olivia's partner, who already had two jobs, became responsible for the care of the two children and the household. Olivia's mother lives in the same town but has severe rheumatoid arthritis and has difficulty caring for the children.

Olivia's health insurance covers her surgery and some of her treatment costs; however, she exceeded her insurance policy limit prior to the completion of her treatment. In addition, Olivia missed so many days of work that she lost her job. Her partner is not eligible to receive health insurance, because neither of his jobs is full time. Yesterday, Olivia found out that her cancer had progressed to stage IVB and had metastasized to her liver, pancreas, and lymph nodes.

would palliative care service be beneficial for James? How might you work with his grief surrounding the death of his sister? What would your role be in working with James? What would be the elements of your treatment plan?

- Stage IVB cervical cancer means that it has metastasized, in this case to Olivia's liver, pancreas, and lymph nodes. Neither surgery, chemotherapy, nor radiation was successful in slowing the progression of her cancer, and no further disease-modifying treatments are available. Although palliative care services would focus on her comprehensive needs, Olivia is uninsured and unable to access these services. As the hospital social worker, you met Olivia when she was in for her surgery. Olivia has asked you as her social worker for guidance in how to manage her pain and assist her family. What would you suggest? What would your role be in working with Olivia? What would be the elements of your treatment plan?

- Think about the vulnerable populations with whom you work. How does their vulnerability impact their palliative care needs? What is your role in working with individuals with both life-threatening conditions and additional social vulnerabilities? Now challenge yourself: Create a service provider guide for yourself and your colleagues comprised of Internet and community resources that will benefit a variety of individuals that you work with. As you do this, think about how to distinguish helpful Web sites from those that may not be ideal and put a reference list together

for clients. Also consider ways that you can connect with community and medical resources now in order to have access to them when you have clients in need.

ADDITIONAL RESOURCES

American Association on Intellectual and Developmental Disabilities (AAIDD): http://www.aamr.org

American Immigration Lawyers Association: http://aila.org/

The National Health Care for the Homeless Council: http://www.nhchc.org

National Resource Center on Diversity in End of Life Care: http://www.nrcd.com/NRCDPublications.htm

The Surgeon General's Call to Action to Improve the Health and Wellness of Persons with Disabilities: http://www.surgeongeneral.gov/library/disabilities/

University of Washington Medical Center: http://depts.washington.edu/pfes/CultureClues.htm

REFERENCES

American Psychiatric Association (APA). (2000). *Diagnostic and statistical manual of mental disorders* (4th ed., text rev.). Washington, DC: Author.

Anderson, B. L., Yang, H-C., Farrar, W. B., Golden-Kreutz, D. M., Emery, C.F., Thornton, L. M., … Carson III, W. E. (2008). Psychologic intervention improves survival for beast cancer patients: A randomized clinical trail. *Cancer, 113*(12), 3450–3458.

Anderson, T., Watson, M., & Davidson, R. (2008). The use of cognitive behavioural therapy techniques for anxiety and depression in hospice patients: A feasibility study. *Palliative Medicine, 22*(7), 814–821.

Barraclough, J. (1997). ABC of palliative care: Depression, anxiety, and confusion. *British Medical Journal, 315*, 1365–1368.

Boden-Albala, B., Litwak, E., Elkind, M. S. V., Rundek, T., & Sacco, R. L. (2005). Social isolation and outcomes post stroke. *Neurology, 64*, 1888–1892.

Braddock, D., Hemp, R. E., & Rizzolo, M. C. (2008). *The state of the states in developmental disability* (7th ed.). Washington, DC: American Association on Intellectual and Developmental Disabilities.

Brummett, B. H., Barefoot, J. C., Siegler, I. C., Clapp-Channing, N. E., Lytle, B. L., Bosworth, H. B., & Mark, D. B. (2001). Characteristics of socially isolated patients with coronary artery disease who are at elevated risk for mortality. *Psychosomatic Medicine, 63*, 267.

Cacioppo, J. T., & Patrick, W. (2008). *Loneliness: Human nature and the need for social connection.* New York, NY: W. W. Norton & Company.

Camarota, S. A. (2007). *Immigrants in the United States, 2007: A profile of America's foreign born.* Retrieved from http://www.cis.org/articles/2007/bac2007.pdf

Centers for Disease Control and Prevention (CDC). (2004). *Developmental disabilities.* Retrieved from http://www.cdc.gov/ncbddd/dd/dd1.htm

DeNavas-Walt, C., Proctor, B. D., & Smith, J. C. (2008). *Income, poverty, and health insurance coverage in the United States*

(P60-235). Washington, DC: Government Printing Office. Retrieved from http://www.census.gov/prod/2008pubs/p60-235.pdf

Durkin, I., Kearney, M., & O'Siorain, L. (2003). Psychiatric care in a palliative care unit. *Palliative Medicine, 17,* 212–218.

Fadiman, A. (1997). *The spirit catches you and you fall down: A Hmong child, her American doctors, and the collision of two cultures.* New York, NY: Noonday Press.

Gehlert, S. (2005). Communication in health care. In S. Gehlert & T. Arthur Browne (Eds.), *Handbook of health social work* (pp. 252–281). Hoboken, NJ: John Wiley & Sons.

Goldman, D. P., Smith, J. P., & Sood, N. (2006). Immigrants and the cost of medical care. *Health Affairs, 25*(6), 1700–1711.

Horne-Thompson, A., & Grocke, D. (2008). The effect of music therapy on anxiety in patients who are terminally ill. *Journal of Palliative Medicine, 11,* 582–590.

House, J. S., Landis, K. R., & Umberson, D. (1988). Social relationships and health. *Science, 241,* 540–545.

Institute of Medicine. (2001). *Improving palliative care for cancer.* Washington, DC: National Academy Press.

Jemall, A., Murray, T., Ward, E., Samuels, A., Tiwari, R. C., Ghafoor, A., & Thun, M. J. (2005). Cancer statistics, 2005. *CA: A Cancer Journal for Clinicians, 55,* 10–30.

Karp, N., & Wood, E. (2003). *Incapacitated and alone: Health care decision making for the unbefriended elderly.* Washington, DC: American Bar Association Commission on Law and Aging.

Kleinman, A. (1980). *Patients and healers in the context of culture: An exploration of the borderland between anthropology, medicine, and psychiatry.* Berkeley, CA: University of California Press.

Kushel, M. B., & Miaskowski, C. (2006). End-of-life care for homeless patients: "She says she is there to help me in any situation." *Journal of the American Medical Association, 296,* 2959–2966.

Kushel, M. B., Vittinghoff, E., & Haas, J. S. (2001). Factors associated with the health care utilization of homeless persons. *Journal of the American Medical Association, 285,* 200–206.

Lasser, K., Himmelstein, D., & Woolhandler, S. (2006). Access to care, health status, and health disparities in the United States and Canada: Results of a cross-national population-based survey. *American Journal of Public Health, 96*(7), 1300–1307.

Lauderdale, D., Wen, M., Jacobs, E., & Kandula, N. (2006). Immigrant perceptions of discrimination in health care: The California health interview survey 2003. *Medical Care, 44*(10), 914–920.

Le Fevre, P., Devereux, J., Smith, S., Lawrie, S. M., & Cornbleet, M. (1999). Screening for psychiatric illness in the palliative care inpatient setting: A comparison between the Hospital Anxiety and Depression Scale and the General Health Questionniare-12. *Palliative Medicine, 13,* 399–407.

Marcus, E. N. (2003, April 8).When a patient is lost in translation. *New York Times,* p. D7.

Marks, B., Sisirak, J., & Hsieh, K. (2008). Health services, health promotion, and health literacy: Report from the state of the science in aging and developmental disabilities conference. *Disability and Health Journal, 1,* 136–142.

McCoy, D. M. (1996). Treatment considerations for depression in patients with significant medical comorbidity. *Journal of Family Practice, 43,* S35–S44.

McPherson, M., Smith-Lovan, L., & Brashears, M. E. (2006). Social isolation in America: Changes in core discussion networks over two decades. *American Sociological Review, 71,* 353–375.

Miller, J., & Hopkinson, C. (2008). A retrospective audit exploring the use of relaxation as an intervention in oncology and palliative care. *European Journal of Cancer Care, 17,* 488–491.

Miovic, M., & Block, S. (2007). Psychiatric disorders in advanced cancer. *Cancer, 110,* 1665–1676.

Moorey, S., Cort, E., Kapari, M., Monroe, B., Hansford, P., Mannix, K., & Hotopf, M. (2009). A cluster randomized controlled trial of cognitive behavioral therapy for common mental disorders in patients with advanced cancer. *Psychological Medicine, 39,* 713–723.

Norris, W. M., Nielson, E. L., Engelberg, R. A., & Curtis, J. R. (2005). Treatment preferences for resuscitation and critical care among homeless persons. *Chest, 127,* 2180–2187.

O'Regan, P., & Drummond, E. (2008). Cancer information needs of people with intellectual disability: A review of the literature. *European Journal of Oncology Nursing, 12,* 142–147.

Patja, K., Molsa, P., & Livanainen, M. (2001). Cause-specific mortality of people with intellectual disability in population-based, 35-year follow-up study. *Journal of Intellectual Disability Research, 45*(1), 30–40.

Payne, S., Jarrett, N., Jeffs, D., & Brown, L. (2001). Implications of social isolation during cancer treatment. *The implications of residence away from home during cancer treatment on patients' experiences: A comparative study. Health and Place, 7*(4), 273–282.

Podymow, T., Turnbull, J., & Coyle, D. (2006). Shelter-based palliative care for the homeless terminally ill. *Palliative Medicine, 20,* 81–86.

Prater, C. D., & Zylstra, R. G. (2006). Medical care of adults with mental retardation. *American Family Physician, 73*(12), 2175–2183.

Regnard, C., Reynolds, J., Watson, B., Matthews, D., Gibson, L., & Clarke, C. (2007). Understanding distress in people with severe communication difficulties: Developing and assessing the Disability Distress Assessment Tool (DisDAT). *Journal of Intellectual Disability Research, 51*(4), 277–292.

Ries, L. A. G., Melbert, D., Krapcho, M., Mariotto, A., Miller, B. A., Feuer. E. J., & Edwards, B.K. (2007). *SEER cancer statistics review, 1975–2004.* Washington, DC: National Cancer Institute. Retrieved from http://seer.cancer.gov/csr/1975_2004/results_merged/topic_annualrates.pdf

Robert Wood Johnson Foundation (2009). *At the brink: Trends in America's uninsured: A state by state analysis.* Princeton, NJ: Author. Retrieved from http://covertheuninsured.org/files/u15/State_by_State_Analysis_2009.pdf

Rodin, G., Katz, M., Lloyd, N., Green, E., Mackay, J. A., & Wong, R. K. S. (2007). Treatment of depression in cancer patients. *Current Oncology, 14,* 180–188.

Schalock, R. L, Luckasson, R. A., Shogren, K.A., Borthwick-Duffy, S., Bradley, V., Buntinx, W. H., & Yeager, M. H. (2007). The renaming of mental retardation: Understanding the change to the term intellectual disability. *Intellectual and Developmental Disabilities, 45*(2), 116–124.

Sowney, M., & Barr, O. G. (2006). Caring for adults with intellectual disabilities: Perceived challenges for nurses in accident and emergency units. *Journal of Advanced Nursing, 55*(1), 36–45.

Tomaka, J. (2006). The relation of social isolation, loneliness, and support to disease outcomes among the elderly. *Journal of Aging and Health, 18,* 359–384.

Tuffrey-Wijne, I., Hogg, J., & Curfs, L. (2007). End of life and palliative care for people with intellectual disabilities who have cancer or other life-limiting illness. *Journal of Applied Research in Intellectual Disabilities, 20,* 331–344.

Zigmond, A. S., & Snaith, R. P. (1983). The hospital anxiety and depression scale. *Acta Psychiatrica Scandinavica, 67*(6), 361–370.

35 *Kathryn M. Smolinski and Yvette Colón*

Palliative Care with Lesbian, Gay, Bisexual, and Transgender Persons

Whenever I see new health care providers, I have to deal with invisibility. My life is invisible to them. I constantly have to decide if it's safe to come out to new providers. I wish that my life was reflected at the doctor's office or the clinics where I receive health care, in their questions and forms. I wish I didn't have to decide to disclose my sexual orientation and the context in which I live my life. I wish I didn't have to explain about my family of choice. Straight people don't have to do that. Why do I?

—37-year-old lesbian patient

Key Concepts

- *Social workers working with lesbian, gay, bisexual, and transgender (LGBT) patients need to understand both the patient's family of origin and family of choice and their respective relationships and patterns of communication with each other.*
- *The psychosocial needs of LGBT patients and their caregivers in a palliative care setting may include issues of disclosure, privacy, and disenfranchised grief.*
- *There are unique legal and financial considerations of LGBT patients that commonly arise in a palliative care setting.*
- *LGBT individuals have higher risks of certain diseases, stress-related mental health problems, and substance abuse.*
- *Health care and personal assistance services are more complex for persons who are transgender, and finding culturally sensitive health care providers is particularly difficult.*

Introduction

Social workers have the aptitude, skills, and compassion to address the unique challenges presented by lesbian, gay, bisexual, and transgender (LGBT) patients in a palliative care setting. There exists a high probability of working with LGBT individuals in a palliative care setting. An attitude survey of lesbian and gay adults related to end of life reported that a majority (86%) preferred palliative care and advance care planning as special interests (Stein & Bonuck, 2001). While the entire interdisciplinary team must be sensitive to the needs of this patient population, the social worker is especially skilled in identifying and intervening with issues of disclosure, communication, family composition, finances, and legal concerns that are endemic to LGBT patients and their caregivers.

LGBT individuals have the same basic health needs as the general population, but they experience health disparities because of continuing discrimination and lack of knowledge related to sexual orientation or gender identity (Gay and Lesbian Medical Association, 2006). No consideration of LGBT health can overlook the experiences of stigma and prejudice that impact health and the ability of health care professionals to provide comprehensive palliative care services.

LGBT Health Concerns

Like the general population in the United States, LGBT individuals and families are quite diverse in terms of age, education, income, cultural background, and ethnic or racial identity. However, there are important issues particular to LGBT populations that can negatively affect access to appropriate palliative care services. There are gaps in health care services and systemic biases in employment, health care, health insurance, and public entitlements for LGBT persons. There is a lack of knowledge about LGBT health among health care providers. Transgender care is not taught in U.S. medical schools (Gay and Lesbian Medical Association, 2006). Although much has been written about HIV/AIDS and its impact on the LGBT communities in particular, little research has addressed other LGBT health concerns (Boehmer, 2002). LGBT individuals often face financial, personal, and cultural barriers when attempting to access health care. Despite numerous disparities, many medical providers are not aware of specific health issues impacting LGBT individuals or are not skilled in making their practices welcoming and inclusive of LGBT patients (Gay and Lesbian Medical Association, 2006).

In addition to the prevalence of diseases that affect all Americans (Heron et al., 2009), LGBT people as a whole have a higher risk for certain diseases. Evidence suggests that the rates of tobacco use among LGBT men and women may exceed those of the general population, ultimately leading to increased rates of lung disorders and smoking-related diseases (Engels et al., 2008). In addition, LGBT individuals are at increased risk for certain forms of cancers, including cervical and breast cancer, Hodgkin lymphoma, non-Hodgkin lymphoma, Kaposi sarcoma, and anal, lung, and liver cancers due to a higher prevalence of smoking, being overweight, inadequate risk assessment, health care screenings, and early detection (Engels et al., 2008). Individuals with chronic diseases such as these are the very patients who can benefit from palliative care interventions.

LGBT individuals have increased risk of stress-related mental health problems and substance abuse (Harcourt, 2006). LGBT adults and youth are more likely to avoid routine health care due to discomfort of coming out to health care providers (Mayer et al., 2008; Meckler, Elliott, Kanouse, Beals, & Schuster, 2006). They may withhold personal information about sexual orientation, gender identity or expression, sexual practices, and behavioral risks from health care providers due to fear of discrimination. Given these multiple factors, it is apparent that social workers can play a pivotal and critical role in education about and access to palliative care services and interventions. Furthermore, coping with stress has led to higher rates of alcohol and drug dependence among lesbians and gay men, and reports suggest that LGBT individuals are more likely to attempt suicide than their non-LGBT peers (Harcourt, 2006; Paul et al., 2002). These ineffective coping behaviors, coupled with a chronic illness, illustrate the importance of early social work intervention in the palliative care setting.

Transgender Individuals

Transgender is an umbrella term for people whose gender identity and/or gender expression differs from the sex they were assigned at birth (Gay and Lesbian Alliance Against Defamation [GLAAD], 2007). Transgender people may or may not decide to alter their bodies hormonally and/or surgically. Transgender persons face many unique challenges in life, including stigma, discrimination, harassment, and violence. Finding culturally sensitive health care providers is particularly difficult. Health care and personal assistance services are more complex for persons who are transgender (Gay and Lesbian Medical Association, 2006). Apparent mismatch between genital anatomy and gender of presentation can result in difficulty in obtaining medical services, practical nursing care, or even appropriate funeral arrangements. Persons who undertake gender transition during mid to late life are more likely than their younger peers to experience difficulties related to physical health status, and transgender elders as a group are particularly "invisible" (Witten, 2002). Social workers and case managers can best assist transgender clients by providing information about the importance of routine health care and preventive services, arranging referrals to providers who are empathic and supportive to members of the transgender community, and educating medical, nursing, and other colleagues involved in clients' (palliative) care (Witten, 2002).

Myths and misconceptions abound: that transgender people are confused or really gay, that being transgender is a choice or something that can be "cured," or that all transgender people have surgery (Human Rights Campaign, 2005). Avoiding offensive and problematic terms like "lifestyle," "sex change operation," "transvestite," and "transgenders/transgendered" (GLAAD, 2007) can provide positive communication and create a welcoming environment. Transgender individuals should be identified with the pronoun that corresponds with the gender with which they identify. It is appropriate to respectfully ask their name and what pronoun they prefer that you use.

Family of Origin and Family of Choice

Jennifer is sitting beside Lucy's hospital bed on the oncology unit. Both women are in their mid-thirties and are visibly exhausted with this now third hospitalization in just the past month. While Lucy is finally resting, Jennifer is hoping to be able to get an update from the health care team on the status of Lucy's cancer and the next steps in the care plan. An unfamiliar admitting nurse walks in and asks Jennifer, "Are you her family?"

Such a routine question can be emotionally charged for Jennifer and Lucy as a lesbian couple. Jennifer indeed sees herself as Lucy's "family," but in a state that does not recognize same-sex unions, Jennifer is Lucy's "family of choice," distinguished from the law's view of what constitutes a "family of origin" (Hash, 2006). A health care provider may inadvertently inform the partner that she is indeed not the "official next-of-kin," setting up a barrier to the partner's support, invalidating the authenticity of the relationship, and negating the very real existence of the "dual family concept," which recognizes both the "family of choice" and the "family of origin" (Hash, 2006). In palliative care, where support networks provide essential resources to patients and their caregivers, it is imperative that the interdisciplinary team understand the composition of a patient's network. Thus, being aware of both types of families for LGBT individuals can be extremely beneficial in working together to create the optimal palliative care plan. It is important that the team not assume a lack of support from the family of origin (Hash, 2006), but rather, be aware of the existence of and then follow up with an assessment of the level of acceptance, communication, and support that is (or is not) available between the families. As importantly, however, a social worker must extend his or her assessment beyond the families to the health care teams. This is essential because health care professionals may or may not be supportive of the relationship between patient and partner, as evidenced in research with LGBT patients in a medical setting that indicates "conflict is much more likely between the family and the medical team than among family members" (Werth, 2007, p. 853). In fact, it has been reported while only up to 24% of LGBT patients have internal family conflicts, almost half (40%–48%) endure conflicts with the health care team (Werth, 2007).

However, it is imperative that the LGBT patient and his or her partner disclose the nature of their relationship (commonly referred to as "coming out") only if they desire to do so. This can present a challenging situation for a social worker, as well as the rest of the team, in trying to complete a comprehensive assessment and subsequently develop a care plan. Nevertheless, as one study highlights, "disclosing one's sexual orientation is a phenomenon that is unique to LGB[T] people. Heterosexual populations need not worry about disclosure, for heterosexuality is almost inevitably assumed" (Neville & Henrickson, 2006, p. 409). Such a presumption of a patient's sexual orientation among health care professionals and society in general is referred to as "heteronormativity" and "describes the powerful heterosexual structure and normative principle [referring] to the assumption that heterosexuality is a universal norm, i.e., that heterosexuality is the only sexuality of individuals and society" (Rondahl, Innala, & Carlsson, 2006, p. 374). Such heteronormativity is "communicated in waiting rooms, in patient documents and when registering for admission" (Rondahl, Innala, & Carlsson, 2006, p. 373).

Surrounded by such information, not counterbalanced by LGBT-friendly materials, many LGBT patients may not feel "culturally safe" (Neville & Henrickson, 2006) in disclosing their primary relationship and thus may not speak candidly about it. One intervention to assist in providing a more culturally safe environment is the use of the Gay Affirmative Practice Scale (Crisp, 2006) as a measure of assessing cultural sensitivity with gay and lesbian clients. The scale is designed to assess practitioners' beliefs and behaviors in practice with gay and lesbian individuals and help health and human services staff evaluate the policies and procedures of their organization (Hash & Netting, 2007).

Palliative care practitioners can further promote an atmosphere of acceptance by using more neutral terms that allow for the patient and caregiver to disclose the nature of their relationship in a way that is most comfortable to them. Participants in Neville's (2006) study suggested specific questions to ask that can allow the team to retrieve the appropriate information and give permission for the LGBT patient to disclose if he or she desires. Examples of such questions are, "Who lives in your household? Are you in a relationship with someone you do not live with? Who is most likely to visit with you while you are in [the] hospital?"

Additionally, Rondahl, Innala, and Carlsson (2006) point out, if a patient or his or her caregiver is open about their relationship, further questions to provide more specific information should be asked such as, "How open are you? Do you have the support of friends and family? Does your partner communicate with your parents and siblings?" And, most important, the team should ask what the patient wants the staff to call his or her partner and how to document it within the medical record (Rondahl et al., 2006; Smolinski & Colón, 2006). Such demonstrations of sensitivity and inclusion will allow the couple the freedom to be more involved in the care plan. Supportive professionals were described as those who "bent the rules and treated partners as immediate family as far as policies and decision-making were concerned" (Hash, 2006, p. 133). Finally, professionals should be cognizant of LGBT resources in the community, make them visible in waiting areas and other resource locations, and direct patients to them.

Clinical Interventions, Issues of Intimacy, and Disenfranchised Grief

While it may be challenging for LGBT patients to disclose their sexual orientation to the palliative care team, the clinical benefits to them and their partners can be very rewarding. Trusting the team with such information allows interventions to be tailored appropriately. For example, in suggesting palliative interventions such as massage to alleviate pain or to enhance sexual intimacy to reduce isolation, the social worker can be much more effective teaching skills to the partners together if he or she is aware of their relationship. Furthermore, as "sexuality is about who we are and how we express that aspect of ourselves to the outside world" (Redelman, 2008, p. 367), creating an environment that encourages a patient to fully express himself or herself informs a comprehensive and authentic palliative plan of care that includes supportive listening, clinical interventions, and directed community resources. Although health care professionals agree that sexuality is an important issue for patients in their overall care plan, they recognize that it is inadequately addressed in the palliative care setting (Redelman, 2008). Not only does the health care system seem insensitive to the privacy required for intimacy, but even the individual practitioner can be uncomfortable and inadequate in addressing this need (Cagle & Bolte, 2009; Redelman, 2008). The failure to address sexuality in the palliative care setting, coupled with the denial of who shares intimate relationships, can impact the LGBT couple's trust within the system and prevent disclosure of relevant details that would help the team to provide comprehensive palliative care that enhances the quality of life along the continuum of illness for both patient and partner. (For more information, see Chapter 24)

Disenfranchised grief may be experienced by LGBT individuals during the course of the illness and at the end of life. Defined as isolated grieving, as it fails to be acknowledged or recognized because the relationship is not validated, disenfranchised grief can complicate the mourning process (Doka, 1989). The hallmark of palliative care is proactive alleviation of symptoms and suffering as opposed to reactive interventions. As Redelman (2008) observes, "If touching and hugging cannot be open, if true sadness and grief cannot be displayed, then extra pain is suffered" (p. 369). Disenfranchised grief may take many forms of isolation for the LGBT patient and his or her partner. From the time of diagnosis of a critical illness when patients (and their partners) feel the immediate "loss" of life the way it was before the illness, neither patient nor partner can be supported as a couple if the relationship is not known. Not being able to express one's authentic self to the team is an unnecessary loss that can engender an even more profound sense of isolation. Furthermore, during the course of treatment, clinical interventions are focused differently if the nature of the relationship is known and the partner more fully participates. Otherwise a persistent sense of sadness and isolation can permeate the relationship for the couple.

> When Lucy is experiencing pain and could benefit from some relaxation, distraction, or massage, the social worker who is aware that Jennifer is her partner may discuss using these techniques within the context of an intimate relationship rather than a friendship. Upon Lucy's death, if the relationship has not been acknowledged, Jennifer may be excluded from being mentioned in obituaries, participating in planning the funeral or memorial service, or being supported by the larger community as having experienced the death of a life partner.

Using excellent assessment and supportive counseling skills, the social worker can identify those at risk for complicated mourning and work with the couple, the extended family, and support network in the palliative care setting to anticipate and mitigate such distressing outcomes (Smolinski & Colón, 2006).

Financial and Legal Considerations

When serious illness occurs and a palliative care team is added to the care of the patient, the assessment may include inquiries about financial and legal affairs. One of the key roles of the palliative social worker is to guide patients and their caregivers to relevant information, resources, and community supports, including those focused on financial and legal issues. Common examples include assistance with family and medical leave requests, disability paperwork, insurance issues, wills, and advance directives. Many times, the threat of serious illness becomes the catalyst which motivates individuals to begin to address such matters for the first time in their lives. This situation is especially true when working with LGBT patients and their caregivers:

> Research has shown that the people who are most likely to need legal protection—men and women in same-sex partnerships who have not disclosed their relationship to their family—are less likely to have engaged in advance care planning, which is obviously problematic from both psychological and legal perspectives. (Werth, 2007, p. 854)

While most social workers in palliative care are cognizant of these common financial concerns, many are not aware of how they can uniquely affect LGBT individuals. For example, financial protections that are afforded to legal spouses are not granted to same-sex partners. These include eligibility for Social Security benefits and legal rights to shared properties. Older LGBT people in same-sex relationships are at high risk of economic devastation due to an absence of Medicaid spend-down protections afforded to legal partners. Medicaid is a state-administered medical assistance program for low-income people. Individuals can qualify for Medicaid if they "spend-down" their income by paying their medical bills and subsequently meet the income requirement set by their state Medicaid eligibility criteria. This process of subtracting those medical bills from an individual's income is called a Medicaid "spend-down" (Center for Medicaid and Medicare Services, 2009). Compared to heterosexual couples, LGBT couples are at a disadvantage in computing the spend-down amount and what assets get protected for the "community spouse," that is, the spouse that is still living in the community if the patient enters a nursing home. Many same-sex couples (all those living in the majority of states that do not recognize same-sex marriage) cannot qualify as the "community spouse" and retain some of the household assets, family home, and family car as a heterosexual spouse could while continuing to live in the community. Furthermore, many LGBT individuals are not eligible for other types of medical insurance because many insurance companies and employers do not provide for domestic partnership benefits (Human Rights Campaign (2009). In fact, in 1997 and again in 2004, the U.S. General Accounting Office issued a report identifying over 1000 benefits, rights, and privileges that are contingent on marital status and therefore not available to unmarried same-sex couples. Additionally, despite the legality of same-sex marriage in a handful of states, the Defense of Marriage Act still denies federal benefits to LBGT couples whose unions have been legally sanctioned at the state level (U.S. General Accounting Office, 2004).

LGBT patients and caregivers themselves may not be aware of the benefits to which they may or may not be entitled and simply assume that certain benefits are unavailable to them. This can be especially true if they have never had a discussion with a knowledgeable lawyer, financial planner, or tax consultant about how illness and death may impact their partner's financial situation. For example, in Jennifer and Lucy's case, Jennifer may not be considering the very real fact that her employer may not automatically grant her up to 12 weeks under the Family Medical Leave Act (FMLA) to care for Lucy.

A gay couple will pay significantly more over their lifetimes for extra costs related to health care, legal affairs, and other issues; in a worst-case scenario, it could be as much as $467,000 (Bernard & Lieber, 2009). In calculating this dollar amount, the authors created a same-sex couple whose real-life counterpart was a heterosexual couple. The authors chose three states with the largest LGBT populations (California, New York, and Florida) and analyzed annual gross incomes and various cost of living expenses to determine a hypothetical picture. The biggest expenses that same-sex couples faced were health care costs, payment of estate taxes, and inability to transfer any Social Security benefits to the healthy partner.

The palliative social worker may need to be very proactive in probing about financial status and concerns with LGBT couples to determine, for example, whether an employer is progressive and does extend FMLA benefits to all employees regardless of legal relationship status. It is imperative that social workers do not err in giving misinformation about common financial benefits that may not be available to the LGBT family. A thorough assessment is the social worker's best intervention to begin addressing financial concerns and limitations that may complicate the palliative care plan for an LGBT couple.

When provided early, palliative care allows the time and advance care planning to utilize the health care system, community resources, and personal relationships to maximize an individual's quality of life and health status for the remainder of his or her illness. Therefore, it is a prime opportunity, especially at the beginning of the assessment process, to identify and address the legal aspects of care. Lack of legal relationship recognition is harmful for women in same-sex relationships and affects both direct and indirect health care issues (American College of Obstetricians and Gynecologists, 2009). Although lesbian partners may have legal documents in place, discrimination still occurs. For example, Jennifer may be prevented from seeing Lucy in the hospital or may not be able to give consent for medical care. Social work staff needs to assess the environment of the health care setting because even well-executed documents may not

compensate for homophobia or insensitivity among the health care providers. The social worker can be active in ensuring continuous quality care in a supportive and inclusive environment for all patients, including those in LGBT relationships, by helping staff create awareness and eliminate discriminatory behaviors.

Palliative social workers are all too familiar with the shortcomings of inadequate advance directives or living wills. This can become increasingly stressful in the case of LGBT patients because default legal protections such as "next of kin" or "family visitation" do not automatically apply. However, extensive advance care planning can be a useful tool in securing the wishes and treatment preferences of patients prior to subsequent crisis points in their plan of care. This is especially true in LGBT families because legal documents such as a power of attorney for health care may be the only way a partner is able to make decisions on behalf of the patient. For example, Jennifer may only be allowed to make treatment decisions for Lucy if a durable power of attorney was duly executed while Lucy had capacity to make such a choice. Unlike married couples where the law commonly allows for the automatic right of the spouse to become a patient's decision maker, LGBT couples are not afforded this privilege. Therefore, a social worker in a palliative care setting needs to be sure to discuss such legal ramifications with the patient and family to avoid unnecessary heartache and disruption if the family of origin is not supportive of the relationship. However, if the opportunity was not available, and social workers find themselves in a situation where an LGBT patient has not executed an advance directive, there is still hope that the legal system will support the couple's relationship.

Such was the case with Sharon Kowalski, a lesbian who ultimately was reunited with her partner as her caregiver after 18 years of a prolonged legal battle. Sharon Kowalski and her partner Karen Thompson had lived together in Minnesota for 4 years and had had a commitment ceremony. In 1983, a drunk driver hit the car Kowalski was driving. Her nephew was injured, her niece was killed, and Kowalski was left comatose and then severely disabled by a head injury. When Thompson informed Kowalski's family that she and Kowalski had been lovers, they reacted harshly. In 1985, Kowalski's father acquired legal guardianship without a court hearing, moved Kowalski to a skilled nursing facility 200 miles from her home, and left orders forbidding Thompson from seeing her partner. While there may be legal barriers that could impede these actions today, the prejudices that motivated them still exist.

Although Kowalski continually typed messages (the only way she could communicate after many years of rehab) saying she wished to live with Thompson, her parents and the court considered her incompetent to decide her own future. Thompson waged a long, expensive battle to bring Kowalski home. In September 1988, Kowalski was tested for competency and the court found that she was capable of understanding and communicating her wishes. Thompson was allowed to visit her partner for two weekends each month. The courts, however, continued attempts to award guardianship to a "neutral third party." In 1991, the courts determined that Kowalski had stated a clear preference for Thompson to be her guardian; Kowalski and Thompson won their case and the court allowed Thompson to bring Kowalski home (Charles, 2003). The case established Kowalski's lesbian partner as her legal guardian and highlighted the importance of durable power of attorney for same-sex couples wishing to name each other guardian. This case set a legal precedent and was seen as a victory for the gay rights movement.

Given the lack of routine legal protections for LGBT couples and families, advance directive documents (e.g., will, living wills, health care proxy, and financial power of attorney) are particularly important. However, same-sex couples cannot be sure that their health care decisions will be respected or that naming a partner as a health care proxy will ensure that their wishes will be followed. Unfortunately, while state laws give spouses in heterosexual relationships decision-making authority many states do not afford gay couples the same authority. LGBT individuals, therefore, must put their legal affairs in order as best they can to cover aspects of care already assumed and protected for heterosexual couples under state law. Such matters should at least consist of legally designating the following:

- A partner or some other person who is not a legal relative is authorized to make medical and financial decisions for an LGBT individual who is not able to speak for himself or herself.
- A same-sex partner is authorized to make hospital visits and be given medical information regarding an LGBT individual.
- A same-sex partner can be legally entrusted to raise minor children.
- A same-sex partner can be authorized to make medical, educational, and financial decisions for minor children.

More and more emphasis has been placed on ensuring that these legal protections are in place, yet LGBT families may still be reluctant to complete these documents. Although the majority of the 1000 lesbian, gay, bisexual, and transgender respondents aged 50–61 who were surveyed in 2006 had begun the process of advance planning, there were still those who had not completed or executed any formal documents (MetLife Mature Market Institute, Lesbian and Gay Aging Issues Network of the American Society on Aging, & Zogby International, 2006) While only about 15%–25% of all American adults have executed an advance directive, married heterosexual individuals have many more legal protections in place as secondary support that are not universally available to LGBT partners (Salmond & David, 2005). As noted by Hash and Netting (2007), "Because they are not afforded many of the protections that come with legal marriage, gay and lesbian couples cannot be confident that their plans and wishes will be respected" (p. 73).

Conclusion

Hospitals and other palliative care settings do not always recognize same-sex partners as family because of homophobia, inadequate staff training, or other policy barriers. LGBT patients and families often encounter less than optimal health care and confront financial and legal factors that can affect access and treatment to palliative care. They may experience a number of challenges, including stigma and discrimination, that exacerbate suffering and impact their ability to navigate a complicated health system successfully. A domestic partnership registration, civil union, or same-sex marriage in states that recognize them still does not guarantee that same-sex couples will be treated as family. These practical and psychosocial challenges provide palliative social workers ongoing opportunities to tailor interventions specific to the LGBT population and promote care that is inclusive and sensitive. Changing local hospital policies, educating the palliative care team and other health care providers, and advocating for LGBT families who are discriminated against are all part of the compassion and skills that a palliative social worker can provide. Palliative social workers are in key positions to affect LGBT patients' and families' experiences in health care and are well positioned to impact LGBT-supportive practices across the health care system.

LEARNING EXERCISES

- Distribute the Gay Affirmative Practice (GAP) Scale in your setting to provide a means for practitioner self-assessment. The palliative care team can use it as a guide for practice evaluation, their commitment to cultural sensitivity and humility, and a tool to develop sound policies and procedures that will contribute to the provision of excellent and appropriate services that are inclusive of LGBT clients.
- Review and revise intake forms, health history forms, and other documents to reflect more inclusive choices regarding LGBT patients and their families, such as using the terms "partner" instead of "husband or wife" and "relationship status" instead of "marital status." Create a more welcoming environment by displaying LGBT-related media (magazines, newsletters) and LGBT symbols in waiting areas, patient libraries, and patient care units. Display brochures or flyers about LGBT health topics or concerns.
- Update the palliative care resource binder or database in your office or clinic by including local LGBT resources. If no resources are local, evaluate national online and telephone resources. Reach out to LGBT-friendly services (e.g., attorneys, financial planners, accountants, clinical social workers/psychotherapists/counselors, health care providers, community organizations, businesses) so that you will be ready to

provide appropriate information and referrals to your LGBT clients.

- Plan and conduct an LGBT sensitivity training for your palliative care team. Include content on sexual orientation and gender identity, consider LGBT health issues, and define commonly used LGBT terms and inclusive language. Describe barriers faced by LGBT individuals and families when accessing the health care system. Review how to document appropriately and how to maintain privacy and confidentiality. List ways to help your staff and services become more culturally sensitive.

ADDITIONAL RESOURCES

The Gay Affirmative Practice (GAP): http://sites.google.com/site/ccrisp002/gayaffirmativepracticescale
A two-dimensional, 30-item scale developed to assess practitioners' beliefs and behaviors when working with gay and lesbian clients. If you are interested in additional information about the GAP Scale and/or would like to use it in a study you are conducting, please contact the author for additional information. The full article is available publically at http://www.safeguards.org/wordpress/wp-content/uploads/GAP%20Article.pdf
Gay and Lesbian Alliance Against Defamation Media Reference Guide, 7th Edition: http://www.glaad.org/Document.Doc?id=25
The Gay and Lesbian Alliance Against Defamation (GLAAD) promotes fair, accurate, and inclusive news media coverage and expanding public awareness and understanding of LGBT lives. It provides a media guide to help meet the informational and educational needs of reporters, writers, editors, and others.
Gay and Lesbian Medical Association: http://www.glma.org
Works to maximize the quality of health services for lesbian, gay, bisexual, and transgender people and to foster a professional climate in which their diverse members can reach their full potential.
Healthy People 2010 Companion Document for Lesbian, Gay, Bisexual, and Transgender (LGBT) Health: http://www.lgbthealth.net/downloads/hp2010doc.pdf
A massive collaborative effort coordinated by the Gay and Lesbian Medical Association, with involvement of dozens of LGBT health experts and the recently formed National Coalition for LGBT Health, has yielded the first-ever comprehensive document on the state of LGBT health.
Human Rights Campaign: http://www.hrc.org
A bipartisan organization that works to advance equality based on sexual orientation and gender expression and identity, to ensure that gay, lesbian, bisexual, and transgender Americans can be open, honest, safe, and healthy at home, at work, and in the community.
The Journal of Gay and Lesbian Social Services: http://www.informaworld.com/smpp/title~content=t792304012~db=all
Dedicated to the development of knowledge that meets the practical needs of lesbian, gay, bisexual, and transgender people in their social context and provides empirical knowledge and conceptual information related to sexual minorities and their social environment.

LGBT Healthy Families Initiative: http://www.lgbthealthinitiative.com
Created to help promote an awareness of family health history for LGBT families and help them understand how health, family history, health beliefs, healthy living, and genetic background are an important part of future health.
Mautner Project: the National Lesbian Health Organization: http://www.mautnerproject.org/
Committed to improving the health of women who partner with women, including lesbian, bisexual, and transgender individuals, through direct and support service, education, and advocacy.
The National Coalition for Lesbian, Gay, Bisexual and Transgender Health: http://www.lgbthealth.net/
Committed to improving the health and well-being of lesbian, gay, bisexual, and transgender individuals and communities through public education, coalition building, and advocacy that focus on research, policy, education, and training.
Tools for Protecting Your Health Care Wishes—Lambda Legal: http://data.lambdalegal.org/publications/downloads/ttp_your-health-care-wishes.pdf
Provides a guide to help create the right documents that will help make sure wishes are respected.
World Professional Association for Transgender Health: http://www.wpath.org
An international multidisciplinary professional association that works to promote evidence-based care, education, research, advocacy, public policy, and respect in transgender health.

READINGS

Appleby, G. A., & Anastas, J. W. (Eds.). (1998). *Not just a passing phase: Social work with gay, lesbian, and bisexual People.* New York, NY: Columbia University Press.
Clifford, D., Hertz, F., & Doskow, E. (2007). *A legal guide for lesbian and gay couples.* Berkeley, CA: Nolo Press.
Laird, J., & Green, R. J. (Eds.) (1996). *Lesbians and gays in couples and families: A handbook for therapists.* San Francisco, CA: Jossey-Bass Publishers.

FILMS

Anderson, J., Coolidge, M., & Heche, A. (2000). *If These Walls Could Talk 2 [Motion picture].* United States: HBO Home Video
A portrait of three women from three generations (all who occupied the same house at various times) tells the stories of women who love women. The first story, taking place in 1961, shows a woman "widowed" when her partner of 50 years dies suddenly. The 1972 story shows a young woman who finds dealing with the sexual politics of the gay community increasingly more complex when she falls in love with a boyish woman. The most modern piece, taking place in 2000, portrays a contemporary lesbian couple determined to have a baby.
Anderson, J. (2003). *Normal [Motion picture].* United States: HBO Home Entertainment.
The relationship of a devoted couple in rural Illinois is deeply challenged when the husband confesses to his wife that he's a woman trapped in a man's body and he must face their

children, friends, and coworkers with the new way of life he has planned.

Davis, K. (2001). *Southern Comfort.* [Motion picture]. United States: New Video Group.

Southern Comfort is a documentary that chronicles the last year of the life of Robert Eads, a female-to-male transgender person who succumbs to ovarian cancer. The film shows Robert and his adopted transgender family living in rural Georgia. The film's title comes from an annual gathering that Robert describes as "the cotillion of the trans community, the coming-out party—an event part convention, part high school prom."

REFERENCES

American College of Obstetricians and Gynecologists. (2009). *Legal status: Health impact for lesbian couples. Obstetrics and Gynecology, 113*(2), 469–472.

Bernard, T. S., & Lieber, R. (2009, October 2). The high price of being a gay couple. *New York Times.* Retrieved from http://www.nytimes.com/2009/10/03/your-money/03money.html

Boehmer, U. (2002). Twenty years of public health research: Inclusion of lesbian, gay, bisexual, and transgender populations. *American Journal of Public Health, 92*(7), 1125–1130.

Cagle, J. G., & Bolte, S. (2009). Sexuality and life-threatening illness: Implications for social work and palliative care. *Health and Social Work, 34*(3), 223–233.

Center for Medicaid and Medicare Services. (2009). *Medicaid.* Retrieved from http://www.cms.hhs.gov/home/medicaid.asp

Charles, C. (2003). *The Sharon Kowalski case: Lesbian and gay rights on trial.* Lawrence, KS: University Press of Kansas.

Crisp, C. (2006). The gay affirmative practice Scale (GAP): A new measure for assessing cultural competence with gay and lesbian clients. *Social Work, 51*(2), 115–126.

Doka, K. (1989). *Disenfranchised grief: Recognizing hidden sorrow.* Lexington, MA: Lexington Books.

Engels, E. A., Biggar, R. J., Hall, H. I., Cross, H., Crutchfield, A., Finch, J. L.,… Goedert, J. J. (2008). Cancer risk in people infected with human immunodeficiency virus in the United States. *International Journal of Cancer, 123*(1), 187–194.

Gay and Lesbian Alliance Against Defamation (GLAAD). (2007). *Media reference guide* (7th ed.). Retrieved from http://www.glaad.org/Document.Doc?id=25

Gay and Lesbian Medical Association. (2006). *Guidelines for care of lesbian, gay, bisexual, and transgender patients.* San Francisco, CA: Author.

Harcourt, J. (Ed.) (2006). *Current issues in lesbian, gay, bisexual and transgender (LGBT) health.* New York: Harrington Park Press.

Hash, K. (2006). Caregiving and post-caregiving experiences of midlife and older gay men and lesbians. *Journal of Gerontological Social Work, 47*(3/4), 121–138.

Hash, K., & Netting, F. (2007). Long-term planning and decision-making among midlife and older gay men and lesbians. *Journal of Social Work in End-of-Life & Palliative Care, 3*(2), 59–77.

Heron, M., Hoyert, D. L., Murphy, S. L., Jiaquan, X., Kochanek, K. D., & Tejada-Vera, B. (2009). Deaths: Final data for 2006. *National Vital Statistics Reports, 57*(14), 1–135.

Human Rights Campaign. (2005). *Gender visibility: A guide to being you.* Retrieved from http://www.hrc.org/documents/transgender_visibility_guide.pdf

Human Rights Campaign. (2009). *Answers to questions about marriage equality.* Retrieved from http://www.hrc.org/documents/HRC_Foundation_Answers_to_Questions_About_Marriage_Equality_2009.pdf

Mayer, K. H., Bradford, J. B., Makadon, H. J., Stall, R., Goldhammer, H., & Landers, S. (2008). Sexual and gender minority health: What we know and what needs to be done. *American Journal of Public Health, 98*(6), 989–995.

Meckler, G. D., Elliott, M. N., Kanouse, D. E., Beals, K. P., & Schuster, M. A. (2006). Nondisclosure of sexual orientation to a physician among a sample of gay, lesbian, and bisexual youth. *Archives of Pediatric Adolescent Medicine, 160*(12), 1248–1254.

MetLife Mature Market Institute, Lesbian and Gay Aging Issues Network of the American Society on Aging, & Zogby International (2006). *Out and aging: The MetLife study of lesbian and gay baby boomers.* Westport, CT: MetLife Market Institute. Retrieved from http://www.asaging.org/networks/LGAIN/OutandAging.pdf

Neville, S., & Henrickson, M. (2006). Perceptions of lesbian, gay and bisexual people of primary healthcare services. *Journal of Advanced Nursing, 55*(4), 407–415.

Paul, J. P., Catania, J., Pollack, L., Moskowitz, J., Canchola, J., Mills, T., … Stall, R. (2002). Suicide attempts among gay and bisexual men: Lifetime prevalence and antecedents. *American Journal of Public Health, 92*(8), 1338–1345.

Redelman, M. (2008). Is there a place for sexuality in the holistic care of patients in the palliative care phase of life? *American Journal of Hospice and Palliative Medicine, 25*(5), 366–371.

Rondahl, G., Innala, S., & Carlsson, M. (2006). Heterosexual assumptions in verbal and non-verbal communication in nursing. *Journal of Advanced Nursing, 56*(4), 373–381.

Salmond, S. W., & David, E. (2005). Attitudes toward advance directives and advance directive completion rates. *Orthopaedic Nursing, 24*(2), 117–129.

Smolinski, K. M., & Colón, Y. (2006). Silent voices and invisible walls: Exploring end of life care with lesbians and gay men. *Journal of Psychosocial Oncology, 24*(1), 51–64.

Stein, G. L., & Bonuck, K. A. (2001). Attitudes on end-of-life care and advance care planning in the lesbian and gay community. *Journal of Palliative Medicine, 4*(2), 173–190.

United States General Accounting Office. (2004). *Defense of Marriage Act: Update to prior report.* Retrieved from http://www.gao.gov/new.items/d04353r.pdf

Werth, J. (2007). Some personal aspects of end-of-life decision making. *University of Miami Law Review, 61*, 847–860.

Witten, T. M. (2002). Geriatric care and management issues for the transgender and intersex populations. *Geriatric Care and Management Journal, 12*(3), 20–24.

36

Barbara L. Jones, Stacy S. Remke, and Farya Phillips

Social Work in Pediatric Palliative Care

When you come and just sit with me, I know how much you care.
—Adolescent male to his pediatric social worker

Key Concepts

◆ *The developmental, legal, and ethical issues in pediatrics ensure that pediatric palliative care is unique from adult palliative care.*

◆ *Children and families have a right to have consistent, compassionate care.*

◆ *Social workers play an integral role in the interdisciplinary team supporting children and families in pediatric palliative care.*

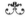

Introduction

Pediatric palliative care (PPC) involves the provision of medical, psychosocial, and spiritual care for a child with a life-limiting or life-threatening condition and the child's family by an interdisciplinary team. Social workers play an integral role in the interdisciplinary PPC team and in supporting children with life-limiting conditions and their families. This chapter will provide the overview of PPC and discuss the role of social work in providing that care.

Pediatric palliative care is both a philosophy and an organized method for delivering competent, compassionate, and consistent care to children with chronic or life-threatening conditions and their families. Such care involves an interdisciplinary care team—generally consisting of doctors, a variety of physicians, nurses, a social worker, therapists, a child life specialist, and chaplain. Ideally, PPC is a relationship that starts at the time of diagnosis and continues through death and bereavement. Pediatric palliative care focuses on enhancing quality of life, minimizing suffering, optimizing function, and providing opportunities for personal and spiritual growth. Planned and delivered through the collaborative efforts of an interdisciplinary team with the child, family, and caregivers at its center, PPC can be provided along with curative treatment or as the main focus of care. The rise of PPC has occurred simultaneously and symbiotically with the focus on family-centered care (FCC), also called patient- and family-centered care. Family-centered care, which emphasizes the importance of the family voice in decision making and care, is synergistic with PPC and has been universally recognized as a standard of care that results in better health care, safety, patient/family satisfaction, staff satisfaction, and quality outcomes for patients (American Academy of Pediatrics [AAP], 2003; Lewandowski & Tesler, 2003).

The American Academy of Pediatrics (2000) calls for an integrated model of palliative care in which the components of palliative care are offered at diagnosis and continued throughout the course of the illness. They recommend an integrated interdisciplinary approach in which the child and family's physical, emotional, psychosocial, and spiritual domains of distress are addressed. Palliative care for children represents a unique, although closely related field to adult palliative care. The World Health Organization's (WHO) definition of palliative care appropriate for children and their families is as follows (1998):

- Palliative care for children is the active total care of the child's body, mind, and spirit, and it also involves giving support to the family.
- It begins when illness is diagnosed and continues regardless of whether a child receives treatment directed at the disease.
- Health providers must evaluate and alleviate a child's physical, psychological, and social distress.
- Effective palliative care requires a broad multidisciplinary approach that includes the family and makes use of available community resources; it can be successfully implemented even if resources are limited.
- It can be provided in tertiary care facilities, in community health centers, and even in children's homes.

It is estimated that there are over 88,000 children living with life-limiting or life-threatening conditions in the United States (Friedrichsdorf, Remke, Symalla, Gibbon, & Chrastek, 2007). These conditions can include congenital anomalies (e.g., Trisomy 13 or 18, anencephaly), hematologic or oncologic conditions, progressive degenerative conditions (e.g., spinal muscular atrophy, Duchene's muscular dystrophy), fragility that results from traumatic injuries, static conditions that render children medically fragile (e.g., cerebral palsy, birth asphyxia), or chronic diseases from which children will potentially die before reaching adulthood (e.g., certain cancer conditions, cystic fibrosis) (The Association for Children with Life Threatening or Terminal Conditions, 2003). When a child is diagnosed with one of these conditions, the entire family experiences a shock and must respond to the demands, fears, and hopes of treatment and beyond.

In childhood, serious illness is often actively treated. The dual concepts of "hoping for the best, preparing for the worst" are everyday realities for these families and the professionals who care for them. While death may not be unexpected, it is fought aggressively. Prognostic uncertainty and continued hope for survival make the shift from active treatment to pure palliative care difficult for children, families, and providers (De Graves & Aranda, 2005). The burdens of decision making for all parties are compounded by emotional intensity, rapid advances in the frontiers of medicine, and the pediatric culture that emphasizes doing all that can be done for children. In many cases, shifting the focus of care from efforts for a cure to a focus upon palliation occurs over time and gradually as awareness and acceptance grow (De Graves & Aranda, 2005; Hutton, Jones, & Hilden, 2006). The emotional, psychological, spiritual, relational, and practical aspects of coping are complex and multifaceted. Families and children are emotionally and psychologically able to delve into evolving issues at different stages of the disease

trajectory. A therapeutic relationship available over time, offering continuity and access to the needed expertise, is well positioned to be helpful to seriously ill children and their families, as well as to the health care team. The palliative social worker can function as a clinical specialist, focusing efforts on these evolving needs over time, and offering continuity of relationship at the same time.

Pediatric versus Adult Palliative Care

Pediatric palliative care differs from palliative care delivered to adults in several important ways. Children with palliative care needs range in age from prenatal to those adults whose conditions are followed by pediatric subspecialists and so whose developmental and/or physical challenges are better served by pediatricians. Thus, PPC teams must be able to care for patients with wide-ranging diagnoses whose understanding of illness and decision making changes significantly throughout the developmental spectrum (Friebert, 2009). Because the causes of illness and death for children are so different from those of adults, PPC goals and treatments are also different.

The most commonly perceived barrier to PPC is uncertain prognosis, a concept cited more frequently in pediatric literature than in adult literature (Davies et al., 2008). Children with life-limiting illnesses suffer from a diverse range of conditions for which it is difficult to predict accurately overall prognosis or disease trajectory. This uncertainty impedes providers' ability to predict accurately treatment responses or overall chances for the child's survival. Uncertainty may confuse the goals of care and affect decision making, reinforcing the dichotomy of cure versus palliative care thinking, rather than encouraging the collaboration and concurrent application of these two types of therapies. Uncertainty in prognosis encourages parents' pursuit of curative treatments until the medical staff are "sure" of the child's imminent death, which may confine palliative care efforts to late in the course of disease (Davies et al., 2008). Uncertainty, if not handled appropriately, may delay initiation of the psychosocial support and respite from suffering that a palliative approach could offer. Therefore, an uncertain prognosis should serve as a signal to initiate PPC services rather than to avoid it, even if end-of-life care is not yet appropriate. Reserving PPC for children who have exhausted all other curative treatment would mean those children and their families would miss out on the benefits palliative care has to offer.

Pediatric palliative care must also focus on the family structure more than is common in adult palliative care. Children may not legally consent to treatments, so parents and caregivers become their surrogate decision makers. This poses both an ethical and legal claim on the health care professionals to engage with the parents as part of the care team. Parents may need emotional support as they struggle with changing medical status, physical and psychological responses of the child, and the potential of disability and/or death. Other young children in the home are dramatically impacted by the illness of a sibling and often experience isolation, confusion, anger, and hurt (Labay & Walco, 2004; Murray, 1999; Nolbris, Enskär, & Hellström, 2007; Williams et al., 2009). The PPC team is continually required to assess the family unit and attend to the unique, evolving needs of the various members.

Pediatric clinical models of care delivery, funding mechanisms, research paradigms, educational initiatives, communication strategies, ethical concerns, and staffing ratios and management are all significantly different from those that are effective for adult patients (Friebert, 2009). These need to account for the variety of issues and challenges facing the family as they deal with their child's life-threatening condition, as they work with multiple subspecialists, navigate the complex system of care, and also attend to family demands like work and sibling care, and interface with schools and the larger community. The context of care is challenging not only for families but also for professionals providing care (Periyakoil, 2008). These situations are often complex, emotionally compelling, and by their nature fraught with uncertainty. Team care is considered critically important, and yet effective strategies to prevent burnout and enhance long-term resilience are not clear. Social workers as members of the interdisciplinary team can be in a unique position to identify, name, and attend to individual and system dynamics that can result from this stressful work. Social work knowledge regarding group and system dynamics, as well as long-established professional practices, including clinical supervision and consultation, can offer helpful strategies for other disciplines as well. Normalization of the pressures on practitioners, and the importance of attending to self-care and team functioning, can help promote healthy practice patterns as well as retention of valued and seasoned experts in the field. This may prove to be an important area for social work leadership as the field evolves.

Demographics

According to the Annual Summary of Vital Statistics (Martin et al., 2008), in 2005 (the most recent year for which complete data are available) there were 2.5 million deaths in the United States. While still relatively small, the number of patients receiving hospice care has been increasing. In fact, 1.2 million U.S. patients received hospice care in 2005 and 1.3 million in 2006. Thus, 36% of all patients who died in the United States in 2006 were under the care of a hospice program. There were 53,552 total deaths of children aged 0–19 years, which accounted for 2.2% of all deaths in 2005. Slightly more than half of childhood deaths occur in infancy. Beyond infancy, there were 25,018 deaths in children ages 1–19 years. Causes of death in 2005 for children beyond infancy in descending order were as follows: accidents, assault, malignancy, suicide, congenital malformations/deformations, chromosomal anomalies, and heart disease. Approximately 27% of these deaths were preventable or sudden (accidents, assault, etc.). Cancer (malignancies) remains the leading cause of disease-related death in childhood. The causes of death in descending order for children with chronic conditions are as follows: malignancy, 43%; neuromuscular (neurologic, neurodegenerative), 23%; and cardiovascular, 17% (Friebert, 2009).

Overall the prevalence of children living with life-limiting conditions is increasing due to advances in pediatric medical and surgical care, as well as emergency responsiveness. However, the overall number of deaths in children with these chronic conditions declined between 1989 and 2003 (Feudtner, Feinstein, Satchell, Zhao, & Kang, 2007). It is obvious that children with chronic illness and complex health care needs are living longer and will continue to require innovative care to meet their unique needs, and the PPC team is best equipped to provide the holistic services these families will require.

There is evidence that children with life-limiting conditions and their families have faced significant suffering and distress at the end of life (Galloway & Yaster, 2000; Wolfe et al., 2000). In 2000, Wolfe and colleagues found that a significant number of children with cancer were dying in the intensive care unit (ICU) with poorly controlled pain and symptoms. Parents reported that these children were suffering from pain, dyspnea, fatigue, and anxiety. Bereaved parents who reported that their child's primary physician was not actively involved in end-of-life care were more likely to report that their child suffered a great deal from pain. Other studies show similar concerns regarding suffering among newborns (Abe, Catlin, & Mihara, 2001; Galloway & Yaster, 2000).

But there are also positive signs of change. In 2003, the Institute of Medicine (IOM) released *When Children Die* (Field & Behrman, 2003), a 712-page report that examines existing deficits and guides improvements in PPC (http://www.nap.edu/books/0309084377/html/index.html). Several public and private organizations have begun to address aspects of PPC, including clinical and behavioral research, public policy, and organizational and educational initiatives. For example, in 2000 the American Academy of Pediatrics (http://www.aap.org) issued a policy statement endorsing palliative care as a critical dimension of pediatrics. In 1997, Last Acts (http://www.lastacts.org), a coalition of professional and consumer organizations, adapted its Precepts of Palliative Care specifically for children from birth through adolescence. And Children's Hospice International (http://www.chionline.org) seeks to raise the standards for PPC worldwide.

Standards and policy statements cannot in themselves foster change. A deliberate effort must be made to transform the attitudes and beliefs of clinicians who care for children with life-threatening conditions. Such transformation is a prerequisite to the creation of interventions aimed at improving the quality of care for all children living with life-threatening conditions. Equally important are efforts to address the knowledge deficits of pediatric professionals, such as the Initiative for Pediatric Palliative Care (http://www.ippcweb.org), the National Hospice and Palliative Care Organization (http://www.nhpco.org), and the Pediatric End-of-Life Nursing Education Consortium (http://www.aacn.nche.edu/elnec).

Social Work's Role

As the field of PPC grows, the role of social work has become an important area for program planning and innovation. While consensus exists that social work is an essential component of the interdisciplinary team, the job description, domains of practice, and emergence of practice patterns are very much a work in progress. Social workers have long been integral to efforts to improve care for children and their families along the continuum of illness and have strived to address the unique needs of the dying child. These efforts are in line with the IOM report that defines quality care at the end of life as care that is consistent with the wishes of the dying patients and their families and meets established medical, cultural, and ethical standards (Field & Cassel, 1997). Quality palliative care is often hindered by a medical culture, health care system, and social policies that time and again dichotomize curative and life-sustaining intervention and quality of life and supportive care. For many palliative care clinicians a pervasive focus is to bridge this dichotomy. This view and its application to children were detailed in the later IOM report *When Children Die* (2003), which highlighted the need for PPC and for professional training and service options (Field & Behrman, 2003).

In 2002, a national Social Work Summit on Palliative and End-of-Life Care was convened. Social work leaders described state-of-the-art practice and core competencies for social work in palliative and end-of-life care for adult and pediatric populations. This comprehensive statement describes "individual, family, group, team, community and organizational interventions that extend across settings, cultures and populations, and encompasses advocacy, education, training, clinical practice, community organization, administration, supervision, policy and research" (Gwyther et al., 2005, p. 88). They further went on to describe competencies in knowledge and skills, as well as practice values and attitudes. They specified end-of-life care for children as a particular area in need of more research and development (Gwyther et al., 2005) (For additional information, see chapter 3).

In pediatrics, additional competencies have since been defined (see Table 36.1). These include developmental expertise and family systems knowledge focusing on younger families, in addition to knowledge regarding complex conditions and diseases of childhood, assessment and treatment of abuse and neglect, legal considerations for pediatric patients, and related issues. Also, boundary issues become

very complex and important to consider when providing PPC. In pediatrics, the engaging nature of children, legal and ethical issues, complex family and system dynamics, caregiver investments in their patients, and the emotional intensity that is inherent in these situations contribute to potential role conflicts and enmeshment. Social work has sensitivity to these aspects of relationships, as well as knowledge and expertise to guide interdisciplinary practice in this important area (Remke, 2006).

Table 36.1.
Pediatric Palliative Care Social Worker: Sample Job Description and Preferred Competencies

The social worker on the pediatric palliative care team provides skilled assessment and intervention for children with life-threatening conditions and their families, and he or she provides clinical consultation to the interdisciplinary care team. Additionally, the social worker attends to the system dynamics of the health care delivery network and advocates for interventions that can alleviate the burdens of disease and coping for the children and families that pediatric palliative care seeks to serve.

Qualifications

- Master's degree in social work (MSW)
- Demonstrated experience working with children and families in a clinical capacity
- Demonstrated experience working with life-threatening conditions, chronic disease, hospice and/or end-of-life care, and related situations
- Demonstrated experience working with family systems
- Licensure appropriate to the state and organizational guidelines for the location of practice

Activities

The social worker provides clinical services to children, families, and the team. These include the following:

- Psychosocial assessment, including family history, presenting concerns, and assessment of strengths, needs, and vulnerabilities from a family-centered care perspective
- Referrals to appropriate community services and resources
- Anticipatory guidance for coping with emotional, psychological, physical, and spiritual dimensions of the disease process from a family-centered perspective
- Assessment of child and family coping, and family system integrity
- Collaboration with family and team to identify options, goals, and priorities for care: advanced care planning
- Family counseling
- Mental health assessment and treatment as relates to coping with the child's health condition
- Facilitation of communication between family and team

Table 36.1. (*Contd.*)

• Conflict management • Cognitive-behavioral skills training to facilitate effective coping • Bereavement care planning and support • Training and education • Clinical supervision • Graduate student mentorship and field supervision
Knowledge base
The pediatric palliative care social worker provides services that require knowledge encompassing a range of issues: • Social worker role on an interdisciplinary team • Biopsychosocial, emotional, spiritual, and practical needs of client systems • Impact of illness, disease, and stress on individual and family, across disease trajectories • Signs, symptoms, diagnosis, and treatment of psychiatric disorders • Psychosocial dimensions of pain and symptom management • Religious, spiritual, and cultural values and expectations • Ethical and legal principles and guidelines for decision making • End-of-life preparation, loss, and bereavement • Justice and equity • State and community resources for care delivery and support • Standards of care • Multidimensional assessment • Treatment planning and intervention • Communication and counseling, psychotherapy, cognitive-behavioral therapy • Interdisciplinary teamwork • Mediation and conflict resolution • Supervision, leadership, and training • Child development • Attachment theory, effective parenting • Family systems: child as patient, impact of child loss • Communication with children • How death and illnesses are understood at different stages • Child maltreatment risk assessment, intervention, and prevention
Social work practice is governed by the Social Work Code of Ethics, the standards of practice established through state licensing boards, and the National Association of Social Workers. *Source:* Printed with permission from Children's Institute for Pain and Palliative Care, Children's Hospitals and Clinics of Minnesota, 2009.

In the 5 years since the Summit report emerged, there has been tremendous growth in the field of PPC in general, and social work presence and contributions to the field in particular, as more social workers specialize in this practice area. The role of social work continues to develop as a key

member of the PPC subspecialty team. Some tensions do exist in interprofessional practice. In some cases, budgetary constraints create pressure to utilize unit-based social work staff as ad hoc members of nascent PPC teams. While this can have benefits for enhancing continuity for families and job satisfaction for these social workers, there can also be problems with managing workloads and availability for the tasks required for PPC. In social work, where relationships are used with intention to effect change, and where both families and providers appreciate the value of continuity, these are important considerations. As is the case in adult models, pros and cons exist with both models (Meier & Beresford, 2008). Decisions may rest upon pragmatic considerations during program startup. However, it is advisable to plan ahead for growth, and they demand more sophisticated expertise as the following physician experience illustrates:

> A PPC physician who started his hospital-based program 2 years ago reported how he weighed whether to advocate for the money and staff time for a dedicated social worker at the start of the program, and he opted to use unit-based staff on an ad hoc basis instead. Now, 2 years later, he expressed regret that he had not insisted on a dedicated interdisciplinary team at the outset. While he appreciated the talents and dedication of the unit staff, the PPC team was always losing out to competing demands for the unit social worker's time, and they had not been able to develop as a team given the ad hoc model and the diversity of social work clinicians, which impacted the stability and cohesiveness of the core palliative care team. They had not seen the social work role in PPC develop to the same extent the physician and advanced practice nurse roles had over that same period of time, and it was a source of frustration for them.

It is important to consider how the subspecialty of PPC is emerging, and how that will impact the practice and integration of palliative care concepts in a variety of settings. For example, as knowledge grows, the field hopes to "raise the bar" around the palliative care needs for children and their families, and so endeavor to practice with greater sensitivity, continuity, and effectiveness across multiple care settings. Educational programs to enhance knowledge about palliative care are becoming more available. Social workers in settings such as oncology and are interested in developing more awareness and skills in order to better serve their pediatric patient populations. Patients who, over time, receive care from a particular service such as oncology, often appreciate the services and relationships that have been established with their unit social worker (Meier & Beresford, 2008). At the same time, specialist PPC is emerging and the challenge will be to avoid duplication, enhance collaboration, and insure that the patients and families receive the best care. This can sometimes create role confusion between palliative care clinicians and those who practice as a member of an established interdisciplinary care team all working with a common patient and family. While there is no doubt similarity between these focus areas, there are also distinctions that are becoming more defined as the field evolves. These two separate but related "tracks" are important to distinguish. Doing so will assist social workers working in these settings to define their scope of practice, communicate their focus, and assist in carving out collaborative practice strategies. As in many other areas of clinical social work practice, effective and respectful professional relationships with colleagues can enhance collaboration and create better systems of care for patients and families as the narrative in Box 36.1 illustrates.

Box 36.1
Patient/Family Narrative: Alex

The pediatric intensive care unit (PICU) social worker met Alex, a child with a complex cardiac condition diagnosed at birth, shortly after stage one repair of his heart at 6 months of age. She worked with his family to anticipate and describe what they could expect over the next few days, and how to manage their stay in the PICU most effectively. She also introduced the PICU chaplain, who prayed with the family. The family met a number of nurses and specialists over the next few days. They were very worried about how Alex was going to do with the surgery, and they also felt anxious knowing this was only the first step in a year-long process of attempts to repair his heart. The PICU social worker met with the parents almost daily, providing emotional support, anticipatory guidance, and assistance, accessing what they needed for their hospital stay, including meals and transportation, and planning for being away from home for long stretches of time. She also helped the parents to plan for care at home when the time came once again, helping them anticipate the future—this time planning for a seamless transition. After 4 days, Alex was improved and well enough to move up to the med-surg floor. A different social worker and chaplain covered that unit, as did a different and larger group of nurses and doctors.

The pediatric palliative care team (PPCT) social worker met Alex's family 1 month after this hospital stay when they were referred to the outpatient clinic for pediatric palliative care in light of his serious heart defect and the long road of treatment he and his family would face. His family was hopeful for his eventual recovery and long-term survival, but they also recognized he could die from complications of his condition. They had been to the emergency room twice since the surgery. Alex had an infection, but he was now doing well again after treatment. The team worked with the family to identify their priorities for care and for their family life, and they also elicited their insights into the hopes they had and challenges they were anticipating. The team also made suggestions for promoting Alex's comfort and developmental progress. The PPCT social worker talked with the parents at length about how they were coping and their thoughts and feelings about Alex's condition and the impact it was having on their relationships and family. Since this was a period when Alex was doing better, they had energy to reflect and process the stressful sequence of events they had been through.

On subsequent hospitalizations, the PPCT social worker visited them as they moved through the various units in the hospital, maintaining continuity of relationship and providing the psychosocial-spiritual perspective that often gets fractured and disrupted as patients and families move through different settings. In addition to assisting the family in communicating their preferences and needs to the inpatient social worker and team, and observing the family's experiences as they navigated the complex care situation they were involved in, the PPCT social worker alerted the unit staff and palliative care physician about family concerns for Alex's comfort, modeling to the family how these issues could be addressed proactively. The inpatient social worker appreciated the background information that the PPCT social worker could provide and the continuity that the PPCT social worker could offer the family. The PCT social worker respected the fact that the inpatient social worker could help the family understand their immediate situation effectively, could advocate for the family's needs on the unit day to day, and could alert the PPCT social worker to issues that needed attention so they could work together with the family to identify solutions. The family developed positive relationships with several of the hospital social workers over time, and they continued to meet with the PPCT social worker in the clinic, as well as during hospital stays. Because the social workers took care to communicate effectively and thoroughly, no conflicts emerged.

The Case for a Clinical Specialist Social Worker

As in many aspects of PPC, the role of the social worker is developed from known practice specialty areas and defining best practice as the field evolves. For example, PPC social work practice has been informed by pediatric oncology, social work practice in neonatal intensive care units (NICUs), and adult hospice care. Social workers in PPC practice in medical settings in which their discipline is in the minority. These are settings where social workers contribute as part of an interdisciplinary team and routinely work with many of the core issues that PPC social workers face, including helping patients and families with adjustment and coping, managing the effects of their disease, the impact on families, parenting an ill or fragile child, anticipatory guidance, and negotiating the complex health care system dynamics that can complicate the burden of care on the individual and family. Given the cultural environment of the health care setting, it may be advantageous to adopt language that has meaning to those within that system, like that of "clinical specialist."

Just as is true with other areas of specialization, in PPC, the more one practices, the more experienced and expert one becomes (Jones, 2005). Advance care planning, discussions about changing prognosis or impending death, ethical considerations, untreated symptoms, and similar issues can be effectively addressed by social workers comfortable with these topics, in conjunction with their interdisciplinary team colleagues. Clinical social workers also bring their knowledge and skill in assessment, treatment planning, and intervention to the table, adapting sophisticated understanding of the situation to the constraints posed by the health care setting, and confounded by the unpredictable course of the child's life-threatening illness. This is a skill in itself: adapting the specialist clinical social work knowledge base in a host setting not only to ameliorate the impact of an overwhelming set of circumstances for the child and family but also to enhance the environment to be as responsive as possible to suffering children and their families.

Because subspecialty PPC teams are increasing, they are often in a position to provide care across settings and over time. In this way, they have a window on the experiences of children with complex, chronic conditions and their families that reflects a history and continuity that is not possible for those whose work is confined to a particular practice area. This vantage point informs assessments, anticipatory guidance, and interventions and, as in the patient/family narrative, can inform the work of new clinicians entering the lives of these children and their families. Conceptualizations of family dynamics and needs are informed by this history and palliative care that is provided over the continuum of illness. This structure may even offer opportunities for a social worker to observe strengths and needs that are not evident to those focused on a more narrow set of needs at a specific point in time. Some research indicates that unit-based teams develop their own culture and norms that can impact family experiences (McDonald, Liben, Carnevale, Rennick, & Cohen, 2007). Additionally, unit staff may have feelings of discomfort or a lack of confidence when dealing with complex palliative care needs, such as advanced care planning or complex decision making, including those for children at end of life (Jones et al., 2007). Feelings may be especially complex when clinicians have cared for children and families over time where the goal of care had been cure. Given these factors, it is important to consider that the emerging role of the palliative care social worker specialist may be very strategically useful. In essence, these practitioners may operate outside the culture and politics of a given specialty setting, and so are more autonomous in their work. Social workers in this role can facilitate difficult conversations and enhance family participation in critical care (De Graves & Aranda, 2005; Wolfe et al., 2000).

The NICU social worker explained a difficult encounter on her unit:

She was meeting with a family well known to her at their daughter's bedside. They expressed their awareness of their daughter's deteriorating condition, how hard it was to see her like this, and were wondering "when it was time to stop." The social worker talked with the family about their feelings and concerns and talked with the parents about how they wanted to address the issue. The social worker then went to get the physician so that they could discuss these important concerns with him. When she approached the doctor and described her encounter, the physician became angry

and stated that he was waiting for results from one more lab test, and then planned to bring it up himself. While they were able to talk it through, and then go respond to the family's questions, the social worker observed how disappointing and stressful the encounter had been and described reluctance to get into that situation again. As they debriefed this situation, the unit-based social worker described concerns about her future interactions with this physician colleague that the palliative care team social worker was not likely to encounter, being separate from the unit's politics and cultural environment. They discussed how they could help each other in future situations.

Social workers are often in a position to assist families in identifying and addressing their greatest concerns at a time of overwhelming stress, identifying the psychosocial, cultural, and family systems issues that influence and inform their responses and needs. The social work skill sets that include person-in-context assessment, therapeutic counseling, interpersonal skills, group facilitation, and systems knowledge are of great value in PPC situations. Tasks associated with defining goals of care and advance care planning are emerging as important "procedures" in PPC. This activity can be greatly enhanced by social work interventions such as family meetings, interprofessional coordinated care, and psychosocial assessment. This process involves both formal and informal steps, including elicitation of hopes, cultural and spiritual beliefs, priorities, values, and fears, as well as defining treatment options and facilitating assimilation of complex information over time in an emotionally charged situation. This process may become formalized through a document (Hays et al., 2006) or remain more fluid, characterized by a series of discussions between family and providers. In either case, the importance of good communication and clarity of goals cannot be understated. Social workers can be in a position to facilitate, to ensure that essential clinicians and family members are present, and to ensure that family-centered goals for care are addressed and respected.

The Social Work Role in Pain and Symptom Management

As the field advances, and interdisciplinary and transdisciplinary models for care delivery develop, the role of social work in pain and symptom management comes to be more prominent as well. Social workers can assist families in identifying and reporting signs of discomfort to those on the team who can address it, simultaneously teaching patients and their families how to understand pain management approaches and options. In pediatrics, the complex nature of the relationships between children and their parents can sometimes confound the assessment of escalating needs. Parents may underidentify escalating symptoms as a function of denial or wishful thinking. Children may underreport new symptoms out of concern for how their family or parents may react. In still other situations, families may fear that medications may create an addiction or rob their child of consciousness when communication and emotional connectedness are of profound importance (http://www. IPPCweb.org). In other situations parents may wish to have their child sedated to diminish psychological and existential suffering. At times, children and families present with mental health issues that complicate coping and communication efforts. This is a critically important juncture in which the social work skills for assessment, education, and counseling intersect and can be of immense benefit to the ill child, the family, and the treatment team itself to ensure that efforts are made to differentiate and respond to the holistic needs of the child and family as well as the pain.

Social workers may also develop skill sets that can assist in the direct treatment of pain and symptom management. Therapeutic counseling around the emotional, psychological, and spiritual issues related to the experience of pain can be one important aspect. Integrative methods, including clinical hypnosis, relaxation, meditation, and guided imagery training, can also be facilitated by effectively trained social workers (Jones, 2005; Loscalzo, 1996; Otis-Green, Lucas, Spolum, Ferrell, & Grant, 2008; Redd, Montgomery, & DuHamel, 2001; Syrajala, Donaldson, Davis, Kippes, & Carr, 1995).

Knowledge of family relationship dynamics and especially the vital role of attachment in personality development is another important social work perspective that can contribute to effective pain and symptom management. The social worker can focus on coaching parents on how to address their child's need for comfort. Also, parents can be empowered to remain engaged in spite of their child's distress, and to understand the role that parent–child dynamics can play in confounding cooperation with treatment or behavior management of the ill child. These are all important areas for attention and intervention. One of the core tasks in PPC involves assisting parents in the context of their child's life-threatening illness. Social work approaches can help to normalize these challenges, offer anticipatory guidance and specific suggestions, and so empower the family system to cope more effectively (Jones, 2005).

International Concerns

In recent years there has been growing concern about the impact of global health crises like HIV, the impact on children, and how the international community can be of assistance. (http://www.ICPCN.org.uk). While the social work role or presence in these areas has not yet been specifically addressed or defined, it is clear that the traditional concerns of social work are relevant here. In areas beset by high incidence of life-threatening disease, many children both affected by the disease and also orphaned or homeless as a

result of its sweep, PPC in general, and social work practice in particular, has much to offer. Social justice concerns emerge given the challenge of meeting high needs with limited resources. Practical considerations related to community organizing and service delivery planning abound. Advocacy for social justice may look very different in environments where pain and suffering emanate from unremitting hunger rather than from progression of a disease. Culturally appropriate anticipatory guidance, education, and therapeutic counseling are essential if we are to meet the needs of persons whose spiritual and cultural beliefs and values preclude open discussion of such issues as prognosis and death and where decision making is a family process. In PPC, where efforts are directed at simultaneously promoting growth and development to the extent the child is capable given his or her disease burden, the need to balance resources for treatment with opportunity to ameliorate the effects of disease becomes paramount and profoundly complex. The importance of access to PPC is underscored by moral arguments: "Since health care promotes health (normal functioning) and health contributes to protecting opportunity, then health care protects opportunity" (Blinderman, p. 107, 2009). The need to develop culturally sensitive and effective training resources for international work is likely to escalate in coming years, and social work will have much to offer in these important and developing areas.

Training and Professional Development Issues

At present, few formal training or education programs focused specifically for PPC social work exist (see Chapter 76 regarding education and training opportunities). The literature and knowledge base for PPC is expanding as the field grows and more programs develop. The professional contributions of social work to the interdisciplinary literature and into our specialty practice literature are essential to enrich, inform, and define the work of social work clinicians. At the present time, the well-established avenues for social work education and professional development apply here: mentorship, continuing education, active networking with peers, Internet education, graduate and postgraduate specialty programs, and clinical supervision are all helpful sources for training and professional development.

Conclusion

The field of PPC has made great advances in the past decade. A recent report by Wolfe and colleagues (2008) showed that children with cancer are receiving care that is more reflective of the recent recommendations from the Institute of Medicine. Parents reported more preparedness for the evolution of their child's illness and death and less suffering of their child (Wolfe et al., 2008). These advances are significant and have resulted from interventions from teams such as the Pediatric Advanced Care Team (PACT) in Boston, which includes a physician, nurse, and social worker. Emerging data suggest that parents and children receiving PPC are engaged in more conversations with providers; receive increased attention and intervention to facilitate goals of care and advance care planning; improved symptom management; and greater overall support (Wolfe et al., 2008). In coming years, as the field of PPC evolves, social work practice will be defined by the experiences and reflections of those providing care and those receiving care, and it will be informed by a growing body of knowledge. It is important that pediatric palliative social work practitioners reflect upon their experiences and lessons learned in the field, inform this body of knowledge, participate in research initiatives, and contribute stories and feedback from children and families to the growing literature. Going forward, the prism of social work perspectives, knowledge, and skills has much to contribute to our understanding of how best to care for children with life-threatening conditions and their families.

REFERENCES

Abe, N., Catlin, A., & Mihara, D. (2001). End of life in the NICU. A study of ventilator withdrawal. *American Journal of Maternal Child Nursing, 26*(3), 141–146.

American Academy of Pediatrics (AAP). (2003). *Family-centered care and the pediatrician's role.* Committee on Hospital Care and Institute for Family Centered Care. www.aap.org

American Association of Pediatrics. (2000). Palliative care for children. *Pediatrics, 106,* 351–357. doi:10.1542/peds.106.2.351

The Association for Children with Life Threatening or Terminal Conditions (ACT). (2003). *Royal College of Paediatrics and Child Health: A guide to the development of children's palliative care services* (2nd ed.). Bristol, England: ACT.

Blinderman, C. (2009). Palliative care, public health and justice: Setting priorities in resource poor countries. *Developing World Bioethics, 9*(3), 105–110. doi:10.1111/j.1471-8847.2009.00264.

Davies, B., Sehring, S. A., Partridge, J. C., Cooper, B. A., Hughes, A., Philp, J. C., … Kramer, R. F. (2008). Barriers to palliative care for children: Perceptions of pediatric health care providers. *Pediatrics, 121*(2), 282–288. doi:10.1542/peds.2006-3153.

De Graves, S., & Aranda, S. (2005). When a child cannot be cured: Reflections of health professionals. *European Journal of Cancer Care, 14*(2), 132–140.

Feudtner, C., Feinstein, J. A., Satchell, M., Zhao, H., & Kang, T. I. (2007). Shifting place of death among children with complex chronic conditions in the United States, 1983-2003. *Journal of the American Medical Association, 297*(24), 2725–2732.

Field, M., & Behrman, R. E. (2003). When children die: Improving palliative and end-of-life care for children and their families. In M. J. Field & R. E. Behrman (Eds.), Washington DC: Institute of Medicine.

Field, M., & Cassel, C. (1997). *Approaching death: Improving care at the end of life.* Washington DC: National Academy Press.

Friebert, S. (2009). *NHPCO facts and figures: Pediatric palliative and hospice care in America.* Alexandria, VA: National Hospice and Palliative Care Organization.

Friedrichsdorf, S., Remke, S., Symalla, B., Gibbon, C., & Chrastek, J. (2007). Developing a pain and palliative care program at a US children's hospital. *International Journal of Palliative Nursing, 13*(11), 534–542.

Galloway, K., & Yaster, M. (2000). Pain and symptom control in terminally ill children. *Pediatric Clinics of North America, 47*(3), 711–746.

Gwyther, P. L., Atilio, T., Blacker, S., Christ, G., Csikai, L. E., Hooyman, N., Kramer, B., … Howe, J. (2005). Social work competencies in palliative and end-of-life care. *Journal of Social Work in End-of Life and Palliative Care, 1*(1), 87–120.

Hays, R. M., Valentine, J., Haynes, G., Geyer, J. R., Villareale, N., McKinstry, B., … Churchill, S. S. (2006). The Seattle pediatric palliative care project: Effects on family satisfaction and health-related quality of life. *Journal of Palliative Medicine, 9*(3), 716–728.

Hutton, N., Jones, B., & Hilden, J. M. (2006). From cure to palliation: Managing the transition. *Child and Adolescent Psychiatric Clinics of North America, 15*(3), 575.

Jones, B. L. (2005). Pediatric palliative and end-of-life care: The role of social work in pediatric oncology. *Journal of Social Work in End-of-Life and Palliative Care, 1*(4), 35–61.

Jones, B. L., Sampson, M., Greathouse, J., Legett, S., Higgerson, R. A., & Christie, L. (2007). Comfort and confidence levels of health care professionals providing pediatric palliative care in the intensive care unit. *Journal of Social Work in End-of-Life and Palliative Care, 3*(3), 39–58.

Labay, L. E., & Walco, G. A. (2004). Brief report: Empathy and psychological adjustment in siblings of children with cancer. *Journal of Pediatric Psychology, 29*(4), 309–314. doi:10.1093/jpepsy/jsho32

Lewandowski, L. and Tesler, M. (2003) Family-Centered Care: Putting It Into Action, American Nurses Association.

Loscalzo, M. (1996). Psychological approaches to the management of pain in patients with advanced cancer. *Hematology/Oncology Clinics of North America, 10*(1), 139–155.

Martin, J. A., Kung, H-C., Mathews, T. J., Hoyert, D. L., Strobino, D. M., Guyer, B.,… Sutton, S. R. (2008). Annual summary of vital statistics: 2006. *Pediatrics, 121*(4), 788–801. doi:10.1542/peds.2007-3753.

McDonald, M. E., Liben, S., Carnevale, F. A., Rennick, J. E., & Cohen, S. R. (2007, June 24-28). *Office or Bedroom? A Disconnect Between the Family Culture and Professional Culture in the PICU.* Paper presented at the 5th World Congress on Pediatric Critical Care, Geneva, Switzerland.

Meier, D. E., & Beresford, L. (2008). Palliative care's challenge: Facilitating transitions of care. *Journal of Palliative Medicine, 11*(3), 416–421.

Murray, J. S. (1999). Siblings of children with cancer: A review of the literature. *Journal of Pediatric Oncology Nursing, 16*(1), 25–34. doi:10.1177/104345429901600104

Nolbris, M., Enskär, K., & Hellström, A-L. (2007). Experience of siblings of children treated for cancer. *European Journal of Oncology Nursing, 11*(2), 106–112. doi:10.1016/j.ejon.2006.10.002.

Otis-Green, S., Lucas, S., Spolum, M., Ferrell, B., & Grant, M. (2008). Promoting excellence in pain management and palliative care for social workers. *Journal of Social Work in End-of-Life and Palliative Care, 4*(2), 120–134.

Periyakoil, V. S. (2008). Growing pains: Health care enters "team"-age. *Journal of Palliative Medicine, 11*(2), 171–175.

Remke, S. (October, 2006). *Boundary issues in pediatric palliative care.* Paper presented at the International Congress on Palliative and End of Life Care, Montreal, Canada.

Redd, W. H., Montgomery, G. H., & DuHamel, K. N. (2001). Behavioral intervention for cancer treatment side effects. *Journal of the National Cancer Institute, 93*(11), 810–823.

Syrajala, K. L., Donaldson, G.W., Davis, M. W., Kippes, M. E., & Carr, J. E. (1995). Relaxation and imagery and cognitive behavioral training to reduce pain during cancer treatment: A controlled clinical trial. *Pain, 63,* 189–198.

World Health Organization (WHO). (1998). The World Health Report 1998. Life in the 21st century: A vision for health for all. Geneva, Switzerland: Author.

Williams, P. D., Ridder, E. L., Setter, R. K., Liebergen, A., Curry, H., Piamjariyakul, U., … Williams, A. R. (2009). Pediatric chronic illness (cancer, cystic fibrosis) effects on well siblings: Parents' voices. *Issues in Comprehensive Pediatric Nursing, 32*(2), 94–113.

Wolfe, J., Grier, H. E., Klar, N., Levin, S. B., Ellenbogen, J. M., Salem-Schatz, S., … Weeks, J. C. (2000). Symptoms and suffering at the end of life in children with cancer. *The New England Journal of Medicine, 342*(5), 326–333.

Wolfe, J., Hammel, J. F., Edwards, K. E., Duncan, J., Comeau, M., Breyer, J., …. Weeks, J. C. (2008). Easing of suffering in children with cancer at the end of life: Is care changing? *Journal of Clinical Oncology, 26*(10), 1717–1723.

37 *Daniel S. Gardner*

Palliative Social Work with Older Adults and Their Families

How beautifully leaves grow old. How full of light and color are their last days.

— *John Burroughs*

Key Concepts

◆ *Increased longevity and higher prevalence of chronic illnesses, functional limitations, and psychosocial challenges in later life suggest the importance of integrating palliative care and geriatrics.*

◆ *Older adults are at increased risk for multiple chronic physical and mental health conditions that can increase the need for medical management and hospitalization, limit independent functioning, and threaten quality of life.*

◆ *Ageist assumptions that illness, pain and discomfort, depression, anxiety, and functional decline are a natural result of aging can minimize the subjective experiences and marginalize older adults; these assumptions are also associated with misdiagnosis and undertreatment of chronic illnesses and conditions.*

◆ *All palliative social workers must possess competencies in working to assess and alleviate the biopsychosocial-spiritual challenges facing older adults and their families living with chronic and advanced illness.*

Introduction

Advances in public health, medicine, and biotechnology over the last 150 years have dramatically reduced the burden of acute disease and nearly doubled life expectancy in the United States. Americans are living longer and the population is aging rapidly. These trends are expected to continue well into the twenty-first century. By the year 2030 an estimated 72 million Americans—nearly 20% of the total population—will be aged 65 or older, with individuals aged 85 and older comprising the fastest growing demographic (He, Sengupta, Velkoff, & DeBarros, 2005). Although older adults are living longer, healthier lives, aging is highly associated with increased risk of developing chronic diseases and functional disabilities. An estimated 80% of elders have at least one chronic illness, and 50% have two or more conditions that require ongoing monitoring, medical treatment, and multiple hospitalizations (Centers for Disease Control & Prevention [CDC], 2003). Chronic and advanced illnesses are responsible for 70% of all deaths in the United States (CDC, 2009), and the majority (73%) of those deaths occur in individuals aged 65 or older (Kung, Hoyert, Xu, & Murphy, 2008). As a result, older adults and their families are the primary recipients of palliative and end-of-life care (Bolmsjo, 2008).

The pervasiveness of advanced chronic disease, functional limitations, and frailty in later life pose distinct health and psychosocial challenges to older patients, their families, and health care providers. While individuals with acute infections or injuries often experience rapid deterioration at the end of life, older adults are more likely to experience disease trajectories that are less predictable and involve extended progressions of illness, disability, and frailty (Amella, 2003; Covinsky, Eng, Lui, Sands, & Yoffe, 2003). Chronic illnesses commonly present differently in older adults and often manifest as functional decline (Beers & Berkow, 2000). Older adults with advanced chronic conditions also experience psychological, social, and cultural challenges that significantly affect their health and well-being. Despite their distinctive concerns, there has been relatively little empirical attention paid to the needs and experiences of older adults and their family caregivers in the field of palliative and end-of-life care (Bolmsjo, 2008; Goldstein & Morrison, 2005).

Palliative social work brings a family-centered, person-in-environment perspective to assessing and meeting the biopsychosocial and spiritual needs of older adults and their families living with chronic and life-threatening illnesses. To better understand and enhance the quality of care, this chapter describes the emerging subspecialty of geriatric palliative medicine; addresses the primary medical, psychosocial, and systemic challenges facing older adults and their families living with chronic illness and disability; and provides implications for future geriatric palliative social work practice, policy, and research.

Geriatric Palliative Care

As Sylvia's story (see Box 37.1) illustrates, older adults face multiple medical and psychosocial conditions that can limit mobility and diminish quality of life (Kapo, Morrison, & Solomon, 2007). Many of these challenges fall under the overlapping purviews of geriatrics and palliative medicine (Seymour, Clark, & Philip, 2001). Geriatric medicine focuses on health promotion, disease prevention, and treatment of disease and disability in later life (American Geriatrics Society [AGS], 2009). Palliative care aims "to prevent and relieve suffering and to support the best possible quality of life for patients and their families, regardless of the stage of the disease or the need for other therapies" (National Consensus Project for Quality Palliative Care [NCP], 2009, p. 6). There is a natural synergy between these two specialties, both of which aim to monitor and control chronic illness and geriatric syndromes, ameliorate suffering from pain and other symptoms, prevent frailty and enhance functional capacity, support family members and minimize burden among caregivers, and

---

Box 37.1
Patient/Family Narrative: Sylvia

Sylvia is an 84-year-old woman with chronic obstructive pulmonary disease (COPD) who lives alone in a one-room fourth floor walk-up apartment, in the urban neighborhood in which she has lived all of her life. Sylvia, who was widowed 12 years ago, has an adult son who lives with his family in a nearby suburb and a brother who lives over 350 miles away. She was recently discharged after 7 weeks of hospitalization and rehabilitation following a fall that fractured her leg in three places. During her hospitalization, Sylvia was diagnosed with chronic heart failure, a complication of her frequent lung infections. Although she can still walk, feed, dress, and bathe herself, Sylvia's shortness of breath, the pain in her back and legs, and swelling in her feet have made doing chores increasingly difficult, and she has ventured out of the apartment less and less.

---

promote informed decision making, quality of life, and independence of elders within the context of an interdisciplinary team approach (Hickman, Newton, Halcomb, Chang, & Davidson, 2007; Seymour, Clark & Philip, 2001). Given the multiple needs of chronically and progressively ill patients, geriatric palliative care fills a critical gap in the evaluation and treatment of a growing population of older adults and their families (Amella, 2003; Morrison & Meier, 2003).

Geriatric palliative physicians, nurses, and social workers do not view palliative care as synonymous with end-of-life care but as "a major focus of care throughout the aging process, regardless of whether death is immediately proximate" (Jerant, Rahman, Nesbitt, & Meyers, 2004, p. 54). The care plan for Sylvia, for example, includes evaluating and managing her pain, arranging and securing funding for home care supports, providing medical case management and education, helping her perform instrumental activities of daily living (IADLs), exploring alternative housing and long-term care options, and supporting her son and brother in order to help them remain involved in her care.

Chronic Illnesses and Conditions

As noted earlier, older adults like Sylvia are significantly more likely than those under the age of 65 to live concurrently with multiple chronic health conditions such as diabetes, cardiovascular disease (e.g., hypertension and coronary disorders), cancer, lower respiratory disease (e.g., chronic obstructive pulmonary disease and pneumonia), kidney disease, and Alzheimer's disease or other diseases that cause cognitive dementia. Chronic diseases and conditions are associated with diminished quality of life and increased pain, depression, and mortality (Kane & Kane, 2001; Lawton, 2001). Over 60% of all deaths of individuals aged 65 or older are related to heart disease, cancer, or stroke alone (CDC & Merck, 2007).

Co-occurring chronic and degenerative diseases often cause or exacerbate functional limitations that threaten an elder's ability to care for herself or live independently. Frailty—a condition defined by muscle weakness, limited mobility, and fatigue—becomes increasingly common with age and is associated with increased risks of falls, disability, hospitalization, and premature death (Feldt, 2004; Woods et al., 2005). Geriatric syndromes such as vision and hearing loss, balance and walking difficulties, falls, eating and nutritional problems, delirium, and incontinence can significantly limit an older adult's ability to carry out daily activities and reduce quality of life (Inouye, Studenski, Tinetti, & Kuchel, 2007).

Mental Health and Aging

Older adults are vulnerable to a broad range of mental illnesses that affect thinking, mood, emotions, and behavioral and social functioning. Although only 7% of elders report frequent mental distress (i.e., have experienced 14 or more days of poor mental health in the past month), over a quarter of people aged 65 or older are diagnosed with a mental disorder that is not a normal part of aging (Bartels & Smyer, 2002; CDC & National Association of Chronic Disease Directors [NACDD], 2008). The most common conditions include depression, anxiety, disorders of cognitive functioning, and substance abuse problems. Mental health problems may be longstanding conditions or may have developed in later life, including responses to illness, pain or other symptoms, medications, approaching death, or some combination of these factors. Mentally ill adults are at higher risk for a variety of physical problems, including obesity, diabetes, and hip fracture, which increase their risk of functional decline and mortality (Goy & Ganzini, 2003).

Depression and Anxiety

Late-life depression is a growing public health issue that impairs quality of life and increases the risks of physical, psychological, social, and functional impairment. Between 5% and 15% of older adults (1.7–5.0 million) have been diagnosed with major depression (Compton, Conway, Stinson, & Grant, 2006). Depressive symptoms and subsyndromal depression have been identified in up to 40% of chronically and terminally ill elders (Hybels & Blazer, 2003; Lander, Williams, & Chochinov, 2000). Depression affects overall health and functioning, and it can cause or complicate the course of other chronic health problems (Bruce, Seeman, Merrill, & Blazer, 1994; Chapman & Perry, 2008). For example, depressed elders have increased hospital admissions (Sullivan, Simon, Spertus, & Russo, 2002), take longer to recover from hip fracture or stroke, and have significantly higher mortality rates than nondepressed elders (Covinsky et al., 1999; Schulz et al., 2000).

Clinically depressed older adults are often underdiagnosed, misdiagnosed, and undertreated for a variety of reasons (Goy & Ganzini, 2003). Elders, caregivers, and health care professionals often assume that depression is a natural response to aging as opposed to a treatable disorder (Bartels & Smyer, 2002; Chapman & Perry, 2008). Older adults are also less likely than other adults to complain of sadness or unhappiness (Swartz & Margolis, 2004), and their depressive symptoms are often "masked" or expressed as cognitive impairment, psychomotor retardation or agitation (Chapman & Perry, 2008), somatic ailments, general malaise, or social withdrawal (Blazer, 2003). Furthermore, it can be difficult to distinguish depressive symptoms (i.e., depressed mood, lack of energy and decreased pleasure in daily activities, sleeping and eating changes) from the effects of comorbid chronic illnesses and dementia, medication effects, or a combination of these factors (Beers & Berkow, 2000).

Older Americans account for an estimated 16%–25% of deaths due to suicide, and they represent the age group at highest risk in the United States and internationally (Chapman & Perry, 2008; Conwell, 2001; Kennedy & Tannenbaum, 2000). American men over the age of 75 commit suicide almost 8.5 times as often as women in this age group, presumably due to higher rates of social isolation, status changes, and men's use of more violent methods (Kennedy & Tannenbaum, 2000). Researchers fear these numbers will rise as the baby boom generation, a cohort with unusually high suicide rates at all ages, moves into old age (Conwell, 2001). Late-life risk factors include past history of suicidal behavior, physical illness and functional impairment, chronic hopelessness, social isolation, and a current or past diagnosis of mood disorder. A history of mental illness, primarily depression, is present in an estimated 77% of older adults who die by suicide (Harwood, Hawton, Hope, & Jacoby, 2001).

Anxiety, characterized by psychological concerns (e.g., apprehension, worries, or rumination about health, finances, or safety) or physical manifestations (e.g., jitters, muscle tension, heart palpitations, or abdominal distress) is as common as depression among older adults, but it is not as well researched or understood (Kogen, Edelstein, & McKee, 2000). Prevalence rates vary widely from estimates of 0.7% to 19% (Sable & Jeste, 2001), depending on assessment and demographic differences among samples. Anxiety is highly associated with depression in older adults, and it can be triggered by delirium or endocrine disorders. Other risk factors include current or prior history of anxiety, substance abuse, chronic pain, dyspnea, and the use of a variety of medications commonly used by the elderly (Goy & Ganzini, 2003). As with depression, anxiety can be difficult to recognize in older adults, because elders often present with low-level symptoms that caregivers and professionals miss or minimize. Older adults are more likely to complain of "worries" or somatic symptoms such as palpitations or sleeplessness.

Despite the prevalence of mental illness in later life, older adults are far less likely than younger adults to receive mental health treatment in either community or institutional settings (Bartels & Smyer, 2002; Persky, 1998). Barriers to treatment include a shortage of trained geriatric mental health providers; inadequate knowledge about geriatric mental health among primary care providers and mental health professionals; a lack of culturally competent, multilingual services; stigma associated with mental illness; and elders' fears of losing their autonomy and independence. Late-life depression and anxiety have been found to be highly responsive to pharmacological and psychotherapeutic treatments (Bartels & Smyer, 2002; Gatz & Smyer, 2001).

Dementia and Neurodegenerative Disorders

Dementia is a syndrome of progressive decline in cognitive and intellectual functioning (including profound loss of memory, language, mobility, emotional and executive functioning, and personality and behavioral changes) that can last from 2 to 10 years (Shuster, 2000). Alzheimer's disease

(AD), the most common cause of dementia, and other disease-related dementias affect an estimated 4–5 million or 10% of individuals aged 65 or older, and 25% of those aged 85 or older (Beers & Berkow, 2000). By mid-century, the number is expected to grow to 14 million elders living with AD alone (Olson, 2003). Elders with dementia are particularly vulnerable to depression and anxiety, confusion, and geriatric syndromes such as urinary incontinence, eating problems, and risk of falls (Beers & Berkow, 2000). Progressive neurological disorders such as AD, vascular dementia, Parkinson's disease, multiple sclerosis, and amyotrophic lateral sclerosis (ALS) ultimately lead to total dependence and death.

Dementia can pose multiple challenges for older adults and their caregivers. Cognitively impaired elders may be unable to communicate their concerns, needs, and preferences as the disease progresses. Older adults with dementia also commonly experience periods of confusion, delirium, hallucinations, and agitation, all of which can significantly complicate their care (Shuster, 2000). As the elder loses cognitive functioning, family members must assume greater responsibility for daily care and adapt to a relationship with a loved one whose personality may have markedly changed, who may no longer recognize family members, and may exhibit restless, irritable, or agitated behavior. Although invariably fatal, dementia disorders are varied and unpredictable in course and progression (Olson, 2003). The resulting uncertainty complicates prognostication, prevents anticipatory planning, and fosters what Boss (1999, 2002) calls "ambiguous loss," where family members are unable to experience closure or begin to grieve the loss of a previously present and functioning parent, partner, or other relative.

Psychosocial Challenges

Older adults share many physical, psychological, social, and spiritual concerns that shape their aging and illness experiences, quality of life, and palliative care needs.

Life Transitions and Developmental Losses

Older adulthood is often a time of significant life transitions, often including the death of a partner and other loved ones, retirement, changing family roles, and declining health, functioning, autonomy, and independence. Research on emotions in later life suggests that over the life course, many elders develop greater cognitive and affective complexity, greater mastery in self-regulating emotions, and enhanced coping and adaptation to life stressors (Magai, 2001; Schulz & Heckhausen, 1997). While there is wide variability in how older patients experience chronic and progressive illness, some view a life-threatening diagnosis as an "expected" and developmentally consistent phenomenon.

Older adults think and talk about death more frequently and are less likely to report fear of death than younger adults (Cicirelli, 1999; Wilkinson & Lynn, 2001). This may reflect a cohort effect, because contemporary older adults were raised at a time when death and dying were viewed as natural aspects of life and were less medicalized and marginalized than they are today (Aries, 1974; Zimmerman & Rodin, 2004). Many older adults report that they fear the process of dying more than death itself; frequent concerns are the possibility of experiencing uncontrollable pain, growing incapacity, loss of autonomy and control, and becoming a burden on family members (Cicirelli, 1999; Gardner & Kramer, 2010).

While there is some evidence that acceptance of death increases with age, the findings have been inconsistent (Wilkinson & Lynn, 2001). Older adults who have or expect to experience more physical pain, who fear abandonment, or who lack social and spiritual support report having more difficulty coping with progressive illness and dying (Fortner & Neimeyer, 1999). One's acceptance of death and dying reflects differences in one's prior experience with illness and loss, cultural and spiritual values and beliefs, quality of care, and the depth and quality of social supports (Cicirelli, 1999).

Spirituality and the Search for Meaning

Older adults generally cope with advanced illness and the threat of dying by turning inward, engaging in life review, and seeking meaning in their lives by exploring spiritual or existential questions (Atchley, 2009; Werth, Gordon, & Johnson, 2002). Many engage in inquiry about life's meaning, one's legacy, and the afterlife, which can foster spiritual growth in later life (Bolmsjo, 2000; Nelson-Becker, 2005). Spiritual and religious engagement are generally associated with improved coping with illness and higher quality of life (Idler, 2002). Some older adults experience renewed faith or become committed to a larger purpose that can strengthen their connections to family and community, and help them adapt to loss, chronic illness, functional decline, dying, and death (Atchley, 2009).

Awareness of one's mortality often precipitates the developmental crisis that Erikson (1963) characterized as the final stage of psychosocial development, ego integrity versus despair. Life review is the process of reviewing one's "life career," revisiting accomplishments, failures, and disappointments, evaluating one's contributions and legacy, and pursuing self-acceptance and closure with oneself and others (Bohlmeijer, Smit, & Cuijpers, 2003; Butler, 1963). Erikson believed developing a coherent life narrative that acknowledges accomplishments and acceptance of past failures is a necessary step toward successful ego integrity in later life. Failure to resolve internal conflicts and find meaning in life can lead to despair and anxiety about impending death (Bohlmeijer, Smit, & Cuijpers, 2003; Haight, Michel, & Hendrix, 2000).

Tornstam's (1996, 2005) theory of gerotranscendence in later life expands beyond ego integrity. Gerotranscendent elders grow less self-occupied and more self-accepting, develop a deeper affinity for and acceptance of others, and face death with a clearer sense of purpose and spiritual connection with the world at large. In Akira Kurosawa's film *Ikiru* (1952), for example, an aging widower diagnosed with terminal stomach cancer realizes his 30 years of slaving at a deadening government job have alienated him from his adult children and left his life bereft of meaning. In his grief, he decides to use his expertise and professional network to build a playground for children in a neglected urban neighborhood. After overcoming many bureaucratic obstacles, he sits peacefully on a set of swings in the newly completed playground. His family and friends later mourn him as a venerated and generative man. In this simple and moving story, Kurosawa demonstrates how one man's impending death provides an opportunity to find purpose, self-worth, and transcendence.

Social Support

Feeling that one has reliable, reciprocal social supports and a community or social network (e.g., church congregations, friends, and extended family) is a significant predictor of health and well-being in later life (Berkman, 2000; Krause, 2006), and it may mediate the impact of serious illness and stressful life events (Cohen, 2004). Conversely, older adults who are socially isolated, live alone, and report few social resources are more vulnerable to illness, disability, and mortality (Lyyra & Heikkinen, 2006; Moren-Cross & Lin, 2006). Social interaction patterns and networks, however, tend to change with advanced age. Older adults living with chronic and progressive illness often lose connections with their social networks due to lack of mobility or transportation, pain or discomfort, depression, fatigue, or stigma. In addition, as individuals grow older they make fewer new social acquaintances, and their social networks often narrow to comprise small circles of close family and friends (Carstensen, Isaacowitz, & Charles, 1999).

Ageism and Marginalization

Contending with ageism can pose the most intractable challenges to quality of life in older adults. Butler (1969) defined ageism as a pervasive pattern of discriminatory beliefs, attitudes, and practices regarding aging and older people. American culture values youth, productivity, autonomy, and beauty, and equates aging with "decline," dependence, burden, and diminished social value. Older and chronically ill adults are largely marginalized and excluded in contemporary society (Cuddy, Norton, & Fiske, 2005; Otis-Green & Rutland, 2004) and experience disparities in health and long-term care due to ageism, paternalism, and subtle forms of health care

rationing (Kane & Kane, 2005; Keady, 1997). The negative social construction of aging can also damage older adults' self-esteem and self-worth if they internalize negative self-stereotypes (Cohen, 2001; Levy, Hummert, & Zebrowitz, 2003).

Ageist assumptions that illness, pain and discomfort, depression, anxiety, and functional decline are a normal result of aging can minimize the subjective experience and dignity of older adults, and they can lead to the underdiagnosis and undertreatment of chronic illnesses and conditions. For example, a growing literature identifies ageism as a factor in the undertreatment of older patients with a range of cancer diagnoses (Dale, 2003; Peake, Thompson, Lowe, & Pearson, 2003). There is, however, variation in the extent to which individuals and cultures internalize negative views of aging. Asian, Latino, and African American families, for example, traditionally demonstrate greater respect for and deference to their elders (Sung, 2001) and value familism, where the needs of the individual are subordinated to those of the family as a whole (Crist et al., 2009; Rozario & DeRienzis, 2008).

Family Roles and Dynamics

Family-centered care is a core precept of palliative medicine (Levine, 2003; NCP, 2009). Palliative care teams view families like Olivia and Walter's (see Box 37.2) as the focus of care and as partners in providing care. Families facing advanced, chronic or terminal illnesses experience intense emotional reactions and must adjust to changes in family roles, structure and process, new caregiving responsibilities, and living with increased uncertainty and ambiguity (Gardner, 2008; Waldrop, Kramer, Skretny, Milch, & Finn, 2005). Palliative social workers empower family members to be involved in directing the elder's care, stay informed about changes in health status and treatment developments, make informed decisions about chronic and end-of-life care, and prepare themselves emotionally and concretely for the dying process when death is imminent (NCP, 2009).

Box 37.2
Patient/Family Narrative: Walter and Olivia's Family

Walter and Olivia have been married for 47 years and live alone in a small suburban home. Olivia, who is 68 years old, has metastatic lung cancer and is being cared for at home by hospice. For several years, she has been the primary caregiver to her husband, Walter, 71, who has early-stage Alzheimer's disease (AD) with moderate cognitive impairment. Their children, Anna (age 45), Gio (age 43), and Edward (age 39) are concerned about how long they can manage their father at home. They want to keep their parents together in their own home as long as possible, but this is becoming increasingly difficult due to Olivia's escalating care needs and Walter's deteriorating function.

In Olivia and Walter's case, the social worker helped to ensure effective pain and symptom management for Olivia, plan for Walter's ongoing and future care needs, and support Anna, Gio, and Edward's efforts to care for their parents while managing other family and work responsibilities. The geriatric palliative social worker is well positioned to help the family make day-to-day and long-term decisions about treatment, take advantage of supportive services and informal caregivers, and weigh the potential benefits and risks of hospitalization and long-term care alternatives.

Family Caregiving

Due to the aging of the population and changes in health care over the past 20 years, the responsibility of care for chronically and terminally ill older adults has increasingly shifted onto families (Berkman, Gardner, Zodikoff, & Harootyan 2005). Approximately 29 million Americans are unpaid caregivers for their older family members (National Alliance for Caregiving [NAC]/AARP, 2004), at an estimated value of $306 billion of care each year (Arno, 2006). Family caregivers provide the bulk of care for chronically ill and dying elders (Rabow, Hauser, & Adams, 2004; Wolff, Dy, Frick, & Kasper, 2007) and play a significant role in providing hands-on day-to-day care, ensuring adherence with medications and care plans, and maintaining communication with health care team members, friends, and family about the patient's daily status, needs, and concerns (Glajchen, 2004; Hauser & Kramer, 2004; Waldrop et al., 2005). Over 60% of family caregivers are women, primarily adult daughters who have their own families and work at least part time (NAC/AARP, 2004).

Family caregivers share much of the emotional and physical strain of living with chronic and terminal illness, and often have unmet needs of their own (Hudson, Aranda, & Kristjanson, 2004; Waldrop, 2007). Despite the potential benefits of caring for one's aging relatives (Kramer, 1996), caregiving increases one's vulnerability to a range of mental and physical health problems (Braun, Mikulincer, Rydall, Walsh, & Rodin, 2007; Wagner, Bigatti, & Storniolo, 2006) and economic hardship (Emanuel, Fairclough, Slutsman, & Emanuel, 2000). In addition, caregivers themselves are aging; an estimated 13% of family caregivers are aged 65 or older and must contend with medical and functional concerns of their own (NAC/AARP, 2004). (For more information see Chapter 21)

Family Communication and Decision Making

Family decision making in palliative care is often viewed by providers and policy makers as synonymous with advance care planning (Radawany et al., 2009). However, families of chronically ill elders make countless decisions concerning all aspects of the elders' care for years prior to hospitalization, advanced illness, or death (Wackerbarth, 1999). Family

decision making about an older adults' living situation, ability to drive, medical treatment, choice of providers, utilization of support services, and settings of care (e.g., home, nursing home, hospice) can be challenging and emotionally charged for families. These decisions can become increasingly complex and difficult to negotiate as the elder's illness and functional decline progress, and require communication and problem-solving skills that many families do not have (Csikai, 2009). Palliative social workers can help by addressing goals and preferences for end-of-life care with families early in the disease course and facilitating better family communication, problem solving, and decision making.

Advance care planning (ACP) challenges families of older adults in several ways (Prendergast, 2001). Many families are uncomfortable discussing the older adults' death and their concerns about dying prior to the point when death is imminent (Gardner & Kramer, 2010). This discomfort may emanate from cultural, religious, or spiritual beliefs that preclude discussion of death. Discussions about ACP also involve communicating about subjects most families have not broached before, including anxieties about death and dying, values about the use or withdrawal of life-sustaining treatment, and the selection of a surrogate decision maker in the event that the elder becomes unable to communicate his or her preferences. End-of-life communication can be complicated by family dynamics, including role changes and role reversals among family members, boundary ambiguity, and conflicting perceptions about who holds decision-making authority, the nature of the illness and prognosis, the patient's needs, and appropriate or feasible treatment goals. Kramer and colleagues (2006) found that a history of prior family conflict, communication constraints, and having a family member assert undue control contributed strongly to family conflict at the end of life.

Older adults dying from advanced chronic disease often lack a critical incident or observable medical turning point when it becomes clear that medical treatment will no longer work. End-of-life decisions are therefore prompted less often by medical or physiological changes, but by subtle changes in the elder's quality of life (Teno, 2003).

Decision making in families of older adults with Alzheimer's disease and dementia can be particularly difficult and stressful, because decisions about daily care, medical procedures, and end-of-life preferences are often met with confusion on the part of the elder and with feelings of guilt and ambivalence in families (Feinberg & Whitlatch, 2002; Horton-Deutsch, Twigg, & Evans, 2007). The elder's impaired cognitive functioning can progressively limit decision-making capacity, and families must make decisions incrementally during an often long course of illness (Quill & McCann, 2003). Decisional capacity, the elder's ability to make decisions about his or her own care, changes over time and should be viewed as situation specific, as opposed to an all-or-nothing phenomenon (Baker, Lichtenberg, & Moye, 1998; Mezey, Kluger, Maislin, & Mittelman, 1996). Grisso and Appelbaum (1998) suggest decisional capacity can be assessed based on four capacities: *(1)* an understanding of one's medical situation and appreciation of the need to consider medical options; *(2)* the ability to comprehend relevant information, including the potential risks and benefits of available options; *(3)* the capacity to rationally consider and compare alternatives; and *(4)* the ability to communicate one's choice.

Systemic Factors in Palliative Care with Older Adults

Quality palliative care for chronically and progressively ill older adults and their families is shaped by evolving organizational, systemic, economic, political, and sociocultural contexts, some of which create barriers or facilitators to care (Morrison, 2005).

Health Care Financing and Delivery

The changing structures and delivery systems of health and long-term care have a significant impact on the provision of quality geriatric palliative care, and the health and well-being of older adults. Health care systems that are increasingly fragmented, privatized, and oriented toward profit impair the provision of quality care to older adults (Shi & Singh, 2009). Elders with multiple chronic health conditions are more likely to require care from many health care professionals and specialties in a greater array of health care settings (Berkman et al., 2005). Navigating among these often-disjointed services requires a working knowledge of health care systems and resources that can be daunting for older adults and their caregivers. Elders must cope with a growing number of care transitions, involving movement between health care providers and settings (i.e., inpatient acute and subacute care, ambulatory primary or specialty care, long-term care rehabilitation and nursing facilities, and home) during the course of an illness. These transitions often lack comprehensive planning and coordination, which creates barriers to continuity of care and communication about the patient's health status, needs, and care preferences (Coleman & Boult, 2003; Meier & Beresford, 2008).

The transformation from an acute, hospital-based care model to a primarily community-based outpatient care system has largely transpired in the absence of a medical reimbursement system that adequately covers the home, community, and long-term care needs of chronically ill elders (Anderson & Knickman, 2001; Morrison, 2005). Despite recent efforts to reform health care, Medicare costs for older adults with advanced chronic disease in their last years of life remain disproportionately high and are expected to continue growing as the population ages (Hogan, Lunney, Gabel, & Lynn, 2001; Shugarman, Lorenz, & Lynn, 2005). Despite soaring expenditures, Medicare and Medicaid, the primary funders of health care for older adults, do not adequately support home-based, chronic, or long-term care (Master &

Eng, 2001). Medicare reimbursement for palliative care services is negligible, notwithstanding a hospice benefit that only covers the care of terminally ill individuals during the last 6 months of life.

Health Care Disparities

Older Americans experience wide disparities in health and inequitable access to a wide range of health and mental health care services. African American, Latino, and Native American elders have higher rates of chronic illness, more frequent and longer hospitalizations, and shorter life expectancies than white elders (Smedley, Stith, & Nelson, 2003). Minority elders have the cumulative disadvantage of lifelong inequities based on race/ethnicity and socioeconomic status, lack of insurance, and language differences (Crystal & Shea, 1990; O'Rand, 1996). Hospice and palliative care continue to be underutilized and are often inaccessible to poor people, racial and ethnic minorities, people living in rural areas, and those with uncertain disease pathways (Cohen, 2008; Crawley et al., 2000). Very little empirical attention has been paid to the distinct needs of underrepresented populations, including gay, lesbian, bisexual, and transgender (GLBT) elders, with chronic illness and at the end of life (Stein & Bonuck, 2001).

Despite considerable advances in medical and supportive approaches to pain management, older adults with advanced illness continue to experience significant pain, discomfort, emotional, and spiritual distress across all care settings (Altilio, 2004; Bernabei et al., 1998; Teno et al., 2004). Documentation of pain and pain management for older adults has been found to be far below accepted medical standards (Chodosh et al., 2004; Feldt, 2004). Social workers, traditionally committed to promoting social justice and meeting the needs of underserved populations, must advocate for greater access to needed services to all geriatric palliative care patients.

Long-Term Care

Long-term and extended care provides a wide range of personal care, health care, and social services to chronically and terminally ill individuals, spanning from home care to adult day care, to assisted living, and skilled nursing facilities (For more information see Chapter 11). Although most older adults report they would prefer to die in their homes (Tang & McCorkle, 2003; Thomas, Morris & Clark, 2004), in 2005 less than a quarter (23%) died at home, while 42% died in acute care hospitals and 29% in nursing homes (CDC, 2008). This reflects a significant shift in place of death from hospitals to nursing homes over the past 20 years. Furthermore, an estimated 30% of elders who die in hospitals have recently been transferred from nursing homes (Johnson et al., 2005). This trend of transinstitutionalization is expected to continue, so that an estimated 40% of all deaths will occur in nursing homes within the next 10 years (Carter & Chichin, 2003).

Access to palliative care has, unfortunately, been limited and inconsistent in long-term care (Zerzan, Stearns, & Hanson, 2000). Nursing homes have been slow to integrate palliative care and overcome the cultural and systemic barriers to providing quality end-of-life care (Carter & Chichin, 2003; Travis et al., 2002). There is little consistency in the design, regulation, or financing of palliative care in long-term settings, and options such as assisted living and adult day care programs are even less consistent in their approach to managing advanced chronic disease (Hanson & Ersek, 2006). The need to develop innovative community-based, consumer-directed long-term and extended care services and to fund existing programs is critical (Holt, 1999; Wieland et al., 2000).

Lack of Skilled Geriatric Health Care Workforce

As the nation ages, the health and psychosocial care needs of the older adult population have begun to outstrip the capacity of the professional workforce to meet them. Studies by the Institute of Medicine (IOM, 2008) and the National Association of Social Workers (NASW, 2006) found a critical shortage of health care providers, including social workers who are skilled in assessing, treating, and improving the health of older adults, particularly those at the end of life. The IOM (2008) proposes three goals to meet this need: (1) recruit, train, and sustain the next generation of geriatric health specialists; (2) train all health care professionals in basic skills of working with older adults and their families; and (3) improve existing models and develop and implement new evidence-based interventions to improve the health and well-being of older adults.

Implications for Palliative Social Work with Older Adults

Although geriatric palliative care has a great deal in common with good palliative care in general, there are several areas of knowledge and expertise that are essential to effective social work practice with older adults and their families.

Knowledge about Aging, Health, and Palliative Care

It is essential that social workers in geriatrics and palliative care maintain a working knowledge of aging and human development, family systems, common geriatric health and functional problems, and principles of health promotion, illness prevention, and the impact of chronic and terminal illness on older individuals and their families (Berkman et al., 2005). Knowledge of mental health and illness, specifically regarding the ways in which psychopathology and symptoms present in later life (Ferry & Abramson, 2005) and

evidence-based behavioral and psychopharmacological interventions for mental health disorders such as depression, anxiety, and dementia are also essential.

Given the prevalence of chronic pain among older adults (Bernabei et al., 1998; Helm & Gibson, 2001), it is of paramount importance that social workers understand the complex nature of pain management in chronically ill elders. Multidimensional, biopsychosocial assessment of pain and other symptoms extends beyond physical distress to explore patient and family suffering and what palliative care providers call "total pain" (Saunders, 1967; Saunders & Baines, 1989). This construct situates the subjective individual experience of pain within the larger contexts of physical, psychological, social/cultural, and spiritual domains. Social workers are trained to identify and give voice to distinct and often ignored perspectives on pain, and they can help alleviate suffering in patients and family members from a wide range of cultural, racial, and socioeconomic backgrounds. Pain management skills play a particularly important role in practice with older adults living with dementia, who may not be able to verbalize the extent and quality of their pain (Feldt, 2004; Kapo et al., 2007). Palliative social workers must be well versed in assessment strategies, age-related pain and treatment considerations (e.g., pharmacologic and psychopharmacologic sensitivities, and medication interactions) in older patients, barriers to effective pain management, ethical considerations regarding treatment, and evidence-supported clinical interventions (e.g., cognitive-behavioral approaches, relaxation and guided imagery, advocacy, and supportive counseling) with elders, families, caregivers, and health care providers (Altilio, 2004; See also Chapter 25).

Geriatric palliative social workers must also possess a working knowledge of health care systems, financial structures, and care delivery processes (i.e., Medicare, Medicaid, prospective payment, and managed care systems), and the continuum of health and psychosocial supports and resources for chronically ill elders, including acute care, rehabilitation, and institutional and community-based long-term care. Social workers who are familiar with eligibility requirements for health care resources can effectively access appropriate services for older individuals and their caregivers (Gardner & Zodikoff, 2003).

Comprehensive Geriatric Assessment

Conducting a comprehensive assessment of an older adult's physical, psychological, social/environmental, and cultural functioning is critical to engagement, exploration, and the development of a care plan that responds to the unique needs and preferences of every patient and family. Multidimensional assessments can promote the early identification of elder and family needs; facilitate access to financial, health, and social services; demonstrate the need for and effectiveness of social work intervention; and ensure professional accountability (Berkman et al., 2005). Geriatric palliative social workers can draw on a wide variety of standardized measures to facilitate the process of evaluating different aspects of health and mental health in older adults (Geron, 2006; Osterwill, Brummel-Smith, & Beck, 2000).

Assessing older adults with multiple chronic illnesses is an active, ongoing process that requires establishing rapport, empathic listening, in-depth interviewing, and focused observation (Gallo, Fulmer, Paveza, Paveza, & Reichel, 2000; Richardson & Barusch, 2006). It is often difficult to disentangle the effects of comorbid conditions, functional changes related to aging, medication reactions, and cognitive or emotional functioning in geriatric assessment (Amella, 2003; Beers & Berkow, 2000). In addition, older adults tend to underreport or minimize symptoms such as pain and discomfort, identify vague symptoms, or have trouble remembering medical details due to confusion, cognitive impairment, or communication difficulties (Altilio, 2004). Palliative social workers conduct multidimensional biopsychosocial geriatric assessments that incorporate patient, family, and provider perspectives and integrate social, cultural, spiritual, and economic contexts in order to evaluate the elder's health and well-being.

Clinical Case Management and Care Transitions

Older adults with advanced chronic illness generally receive care from a variety of health and psychosocial service providers in a range of health care systems and settings. Geriatric case managers help to guide individuals and families through health care systems, gain access to and link patients with appropriate resources, and maintain continuity of care between systems and service providers (Ferry & Abramson, 2006). Clinical case managers in palliative care educate, counsel, and advocate for older adults and their caregivers in order to help them manage chronic health conditions and treatment, delay functional decline, and avoid unnecessary hospitalizations. In this way, palliative social workers help to maintain individuals in their communities, minimize the disruptions involved in transfers, and reduce health care costs (Berkman et al., 2005).

In an increasingly fragmented health care environment, geriatric case managers ensure integration and promote "seamless service" across the continuum of care (Gardner & Zodikoff, 2003). Older adults with multiple comorbidities often move more frequently between health care settings (e.g., home, hospital, outpatient clinic, rehabilitation, and skilled nursing facilities) and may be particularly vulnerable to "breakdowns" or gaps in service (Coleman & Boult, 2003; Naylor & Keating, 2008). Research on advance directives, for example, suggests that medical histories, care plans, and documentation of patient preferences often do not follow patients between settings such as home, hospital, and nursing home (Morrison, Olson, Mertz, & Meier, 2005). Lack of care coordination and follow-up around hospital discharge can put elders at risk and lead to avoidable rehospitalizations or premature

admissions to long-term care facilities (Halasyamani, 2006). Social workers' holistic person-in-environment approach, their integration across the continuum of health and mental health care settings, and their skills in working within and across institutional and community-based systems of care uniquely qualify them to provide continuity of care to older adults through multiple care transitions.

Family-Centered Practice

As the burden of caring for older adults with advanced chronic disease falls more on families, geriatric palliative social workers must be skilled in intervening with primary caregivers and other family members to reduce stress and alleviate burden, improve their efforts to care for elders, facilitate adaptation to changing roles and relationships, and enhance communication and information sharing between family members and the health care team (Gwyther et al., 2005). Family-centered practice incorporates family members in all aspects of care and views the family as partners in providing care as well as care recipients. Essential skills include ongoing family assessment, evaluation of the need for additional supports, developing family-centered care plans, providing individual, family, and group interventions, and linking caregivers with resources such as respite care, homecare assistance, geriatric care management, and caregiver support programs.

Family conferences that facilitate information sharing, care planning, and decision making are a vital component of family-centered palliative care (Hudson, Thomas, Quinn, & Aranda, 2009; for more information, see Chapter 22). Social workers use their clinical skills to help families partialize, prioritize, and clarify goals about treatment and palliative care, anticipate and make treatment decisions and develop strategies for effective communication and resolution of family conflict (Hudson et al., 2009; Kramer et al., 2006). In addition, geriatric palliative social workers advocate for family caregivers and help to identify, address, and communicate their unmet needs, care preferences, and cultural perceptions about the elder's health and well-being to the rest of the health care team (Altilio & Rigiglioso, 2004).

Cultural Diversity and Promoting Social Justice

Culturally sensitive assessment, care planning, and intervention are requisite skills in an increasingly diverse, aging society (Bonder, Martin, & Miracle, 2001). Maintaining ongoing awareness of one's own cultural beliefs, values, and practices—particularly in regard to aging, physical and mental illness, decision making, medicine, death and dying—and respect for diversity is essential to good social work practice. To engage with and understand minority elders and their families, palliative social workers must remain sensitive and open to cultural differences in coping with illness, loss, and grief, and know about health disparities and the pervasive effects of racism, xenophobia, language differences, sexism, ageism, economic oppression, and cumulative disadvantage. Multidimensional pain and symptom management, for example, is impossible without examining individual, familial, and cultural perceptions, values, and beliefs about pain, and developing interventions that respect the unique, individualized experiences of older patients and their families (Altilio, 2004; Davidhizar & Gige, 2004).

Social work's core value of respect for the dignity and self-worth of clients encourages attention to the dynamics of difference as they impact upon individuals, families, and organizations. Increasing awareness of the diverse cultural perspectives of older patients and family members, advocating for their needs and concerns, and educating members of the palliative care team about distinct beliefs and values regarding aging, illness, pain, and treatment can expand the reach and enhance the quality of palliative care (Del Rio, 2004). Social workers have a professional mandate to intervene on multiple levels (i.e., individual, familial, institutional, community, and societal) to ensure the provision of just and equitable care to older adults and their families (Harootyan & O'Neill, 2006) and advocate within health care systems to balance the desire for cost-efficiency and measurable outcomes with services that best meet the needs of older adults and their families.

Interdisciplinary and Ethical Practice

Interdisciplinary collaboration has been found to be an essential element in the provision of high-quality community-based care for older adults (Damron-Rodriguez & Corley, 2002; Geriatrics Interdisciplinary Advisory Group [GIAG], 2006; Hickman et al., 2007). The use of interdisciplinary teams is associated with improved health outcomes and psychosocial well-being, fewer hospitalizations, and increased social interaction among older adults (Mukamel et al., 2006; Sommers, Marton, Barbaccia, & Randolph, 2000). Social workers, who have long practiced in the context of community and institution-based healthcare teams, bring well-established skills of collaboration, advocacy, and leadership to their work with palliative physicians, nurses, and allied health professionals (Christ & Blacker, 2005; Meier & Beresford, 2008).

In palliative and end-of-life care, geriatric social workers serve as consultants, mediators, and advocates on teams around complex ethical dimensions of medical decision making, family conflict, and goals of care. Social workers are uniquely trained to address complex ethical dilemmas involving individual autonomy and quality of life, and to mediate among the individual needs, perspectives, values, and responsibilities of older adults, their family members, and health care providers (Csikai, 2009; Csikai & Chaitin, 2005).

Conclusion

In summary, palliative social workers have a great deal to contribute to the provision of high-quality, family-centered biopsychosocial care to chronically and terminally ill older adults and their caregivers in a wide variety of settings. Geriatric social workers have the educational training and professional expertise to provide a broad range of palliative care services that are critical in helping older adults and their families adjust to chronic and advanced illness, navigate complex health care and social service systems, participate actively in their care, and maintain choice, dignity, and quality of life. Social workers are uniquely skilled to assess older adults and families and to meet their psychological, emotional, and spiritual needs by providing crisis intervention and supportive and psychotherapeutic individual, group, and family counseling. They play an essential role in helping patients and families communicate about care preferences and goals, engage in advance care planning, make day-to-day decisions about care, and advocate for themselves within the health care system. A broad knowledge of social services and resources available from organizations, communities, and public programs, and a commitment to social justice help make palliative social workers a resource to patients, families, and health care teams. In order to continue meeting the needs of aging Americans in the twenty-first century, it is essential that we prepare a new generation of social workers to become skill geriatric palliative social work practitioners and future leaders in palliative care.

LEARNING EXERCISES

- View Akira Kurosawa's film *Ikiru* (1952; Japanese with English subtitles). Imagine that you are a palliative care social worker assigned to work with Mr. Watanabe. Based on the film, write a brief biopsychosocial assessment of Mr. Watanabe, making sure to answer the following questions:

  - What can you tell about Mr. Watanabe's psychosocial history, physical and mental health, living situation, familial and social relations, and financial status? What are his current concerns and needs? What strengths and challenges can you identify in his life? What questions might you ask him to complete your assessment?
  - How do you think Mr. Watanabe copes with the news that he has less than a year to live? What does his response tell you about his unique perceptions about life, work, and family? How might these perceptions be shaped by his age, culture, gender, socioeconomic status, and life in post-war Japan?
  - In what ways could palliative care help to enhance Mr. Watanabe's quality of life? What treatment goals

might you talk with him about, and what intervention strategies might help him to meet those objectives? What resources could you draw on to enhance his quality of life? What challenges do you think his children face, and how might you help them?

- Imagine yourself at 85 years old. What do you picture your life will be like? How do you imagine you will be functioning physically, cognitively, emotionally, and socially? What might a typical day involve? What do you think would be most challenging about your life? The most rewarding? How will others view and behave toward you? Write a brief biopsychosocial assessment of your future self.

REFERENCES

Altilio, T. (2004). Pain and symptom management: An essential role for social work. In J. Berzoff & P. Silverman (Eds.), *Living with dying: A handbook for end-of-life healthcare practitioners.* New York, NY: Columbia University Press.

Altilio, T., & Rigoglioso, R. (2004). The social worker's role as family caregiver advocate. In C. Levine (Ed.), *Always on call: When illness turns families into caregivers* (2nd ed., pp. 144–165). Nashville, TN: Vanderbilt University Press.

Amella, E. (2003). Geriatrics and palliative care: Collaboration for quality of life until death. *Journal of Hospice and Palliative Nursing, 5*(1), 40–49.

American Geriatrics Society (AGS), Foundation for Health in Aging. (2009). What is geriatrics? Retrieved from http://www.healthinaging.org/public_education/what_is_geriatrics.pdf

Anderson, G., & Knickman, J. (2001). Changing the chronic care system to meet people's needs. *Health Affairs, 20*(6), 246–260.

Ariès, P. (1974). *Western attitudes toward death: From the Middle Ages to the present.* Baltimore, MD: The John Hopkins University Press.

Arno, P. (2006, January 25-27). *Economic value of informal caregiving.* Presented at the Care Coordination and the Caregiving Forum, Dept. of Veterans Affairs, NIH, Bethesda, MD.

Atchley, R. (2009). *Spirituality and aging.* Baltimore, MD: Johns Hopkins University Press.

Baker, R., Lichtenberg, P., & Moye, J. (1998). A practice guideline for assessment of competency and capacity of the older adult. *Professional Psychology: Research and Practice, 29*(2), 149–154.

Bartels, S., & Smyer, M. (2002). Mental disorders of aging: An emerging public health crisis. *Generations, 26*(1), 14–20.

Beers, M. H., & Berkow, R. (2000). *The Merck manual of geriatrics* (3rd ed.). Whitehouse Station, NJ: Merck Research Laboratories.

Berkman, B., Gardner, D., Zodikoff, B., & Harootyan, L. (2005). Social work in health care with older adults: Future challenges. *Families in Society, 86*(3), 329–337.

Berkman, L. (2000). Social support, social networks, social cohesion, and health. *Social Work and Health Care, 31*, 3–14.

Bernabei R., Gambassi, G., Lapane, K., Landi, F., Gatsonis, C., Dunlop, R., Lipsitz, L., Steel, K., & Mor, V. (1998). Management of pain in elderly patients with cancer. *Journal of the American Medical Association, 279*(23), 1877–1882.

Blazer, D. (2003). Depression in late life: Review and commentary. *Journals of Gerontology, Series A: Biological and Medical Sciences, 58A*, M249–265.

Bohlmeijer, E., Smit, F., & Cuijpers, P. (2003). Effects of reminiscence and life review on late-life depression: A meta-analysis. *International Journal of Geriatric Psychiatry, 18*(12), 1088–1094.

Bolmsjo, I. (2008). End-of-life care for old people: A review of the literature. *American Journal of Hospice and Palliative Medicine, 25*(4), 328–338.

Bolmsjo, I. (2000). Existential issues in palliative care; Interviews with cancer patients. *Journal of Palliative Care, 16*, 20–24.

Bonder, B., Martin L., & Miracle, A. (2001). Achieving cultural competence: The challenge for clients and healthcare workers in a multicultural world. *Generations, 25*, 35–43.

Boss, P. (1999). *Ambiguous loss: Learning to live with unresolved grief.* Cambridge, MA: Harvard University Press.

Boss, P. (2002). Ambiguous loss from chronic physical illness: Clinical interventions with individuals, couples, and families. *Psychotherapy in Practice, 58*(11), 1351–1360.

Braun, M., Mikulincer, M., Rydall, A., Walsh, A., & Rodin, G. (2007). Hidden morbidity in cancer: Spouse caregivers. *Journal of Clinical Oncology, 25*(30), 4829–4834.

Bruce M., Seeman T., Merrill S., & Blazer D. (1994). The impact of depressive symptomatology on physical disability: MacArthur Studies of Successful Aging. *American Journal of Public Health, 84*, 1796–1799.

Burroughs, J. (1922). *The writings of John Burroughs.* Boston, MA: Houghton-Mifflin Co.

Butler, R. (1963). The life review: An interpretation of reminiscence in the aged. *Psychiatry, 26*, 65–70.

Butler, R. (1969). Ageism: Another form of bigotry. *Gerontologist, 9* (4 Pt. 1), 243–246.

Carstensen, L., Isaacowitz, D., & Charles, S. (1999). Taking time seriously: A theory of socioemotional selectivity. *American Psychologist, 54*, 165–181.

Carter, J., & Chichin, E. (2003). Palliative care in the nursing home. In S. Morrison & D. Meier (Eds.) *Geriatric palliative care* (pp. 357–375). New York, NY: Oxford University Press.

Centers for Disease Control and Prevention (CDC). (2003). Public health and aging: Trends in aging, United States and worldwide. *Morbidity and Mortality Weekly Report, 52*(06), 101–106.

Centers for Disease Control and Prevention (CDC). (2008). *Worktable 309: Deaths by place of death, age, race, and sex: United States, 2005.* National Health Statistics Program, National Vital Statistics Program. Retrieved from http://www.cdc.gov/nchs/data/dvs/Mortfinal2005_worktable_309.pdf

Centers for Disease Control and Prevention (CDC). (2009). *Healthy aging: Improving and extending quality of life among older Americans–At a glance: 2009.* Retrieved from http://www.cdc.gov/chronicdisease/resources/publications/AAG/pdf/healthy_aging.pdf

Centers for Disease Control, Prevention (CDC) & The Merck Company Foundation (Merck). (2007). *The state of aging in America: 2007.* Whitehouse Station, NJ: The Merck Company Foundation.

Centers for Disease Control, Prevention (CDC) & National Association of Chronic Disease Directors (NACDD). (2008).

Issue 1: What do the data tell us? The state of mental health and aging in America. Atlanta, GA: National Association of Chronic Disease Directors.

Chapman, D., & Perry, D. (2008). Depression as a major component of public health for older adults. *Preventing Chronic Disease, 5*(1), 1–9.

Chodosh, J., Solomon, D., Roth, C. P., Chang, J., MacLean, C., Ferrell, B., Shekelle, P., & Wenger, N. (2004). The quality of medical care provided to vulnerable older patients with chronic pain. *Journal of the American Geriatrics Society, 52*(5), 756–761.

Christ, G., & Blacker, S. (2005). Setting an agenda for social work in end-of-life and palliative care: An overview of leadership and organizational initiatives. *Journal of Social Work in End-of-Life & Palliative Care, 1*(1), 9–22.

Cicirelli, V. (1999). Personality and demographic factors in older adults' fear of death. *The Gerontologist, 39*(5), 569–579.

Cohen, E. (2001). The complex nature of ageism: What is it? Who does it? Who perceives it? *Gerontologist, 41,* 576–577.

Cohen, S. (2004). Social relationships and health. *American Psychologist, 59,* 676–684.

Cohen, L. (2008). Racial/ethnic disparities in hospice care: A systematic review. *Journal of Palliative Medicine, 11*(5), 763–768.

Coleman, E., & Boult, C. (2003). American Geriatrics Society Health Care Systems Committee: Improving the quality of transitional care for persons with complex care needs. *Journal of the American Geriatrics Society, 51*(4), 556–557.

Compton, W., Conway, K., Stinson, F., & Grant, B. (2006). Changes in the prevalence of major depression and comorbid substance use disorders in the United States between 1991–1992 and 2001–2002. *American Journal of Psychiatry, 163*(12), 2141–2147.

Conwell, Y. (2001). Suicide in later life: A review and recommendations for prevention. *Suicide and Life Threatening Behavior, 31*(Suppl.), 32–47.

Covinsky, K., Eng, C., Lui, L., Sands, L., & Yoffe, K. (2003). The last two years of life: Functional trajectories of frail older people. *Journal of the American Geriatrics Society, 51,* 492–298.

Covinsky, K., Kahana, E., Chin, M., Palmer, R., Fortinsky, R., & Landefeld, C. (1999). Depressive symptoms and 3-year mortality in older hospitalized medical patients. *Annals of Internal Medicine, 130*(7), 563–569.

Crawley, L., Payne, R., Bolden, J., Payne, T., Washington, P., & Williams, S. (2000). Palliative and end-of-life care in the African American community. *Journal of the American Medical Association, 284*(19), 2518–2521.

Crist, J., McEwen, M. Herrera, A., Kim, S., Pasvogel, A., & Hepworth, J. (2009). Caregiving burden, acculturation, familism, and Mexican American elders' use of home care services. *Research and Theory for Nursing Practice, 23*(3), 165–180.

Crystal, S., & Shea, D. (1990). Cumulative advantage, cumulative disadvantage, and inequality among elderly people. *The Gerontologist, 30*(4), 437–443.

Csikai, E. (2009). Communication related to end-of-life care and decisions. In J. Werth & D. Blevins (Eds.), *Decision making near the end of life* (pp. 169–188). New York, NY: Routledge.

Csikai., E., & Chaitin, E. (2005). *Ethics in end-of-life decisions in social work practice.* Chicago, IL: Lyceum Books.

Cuddy, A., Norton, M., & Fiske, S. (2005). This old stereotype: The pervasiveness and persistence of the elderly stereotype. *Journal of Social Issues, 61*(2), 267–285.

Dale, D. (2003). Poor prognosis in elderly patients with cancer: The role of bias and undertreatment. *The Journal of Supportive Oncology, 1*(Suppl. 2), 11–17.

Damron-Rodriguez, J., & Corley, C. (2002). Social work education for interdisciplinary practice with older adults and their families. *Journal of Gerontological Social Work, 39*(1/2), 37–55.

Davidhizar, R., & Gige, J. (2004). A review of the literature on care of clients in pain who are culturally diverse. *International Nursing Review, 51*(1), 47–55.

Del Rio, N. (2004). A framework for multicultural end-of-life care: Enhancing social work practice. In J. Berzoff & P. Silverman (Eds.), *Living with dying: A comprehensive resource for healthcare practitioners* (pp. 439–461). New York, NY: Columbia University Press.

Emanuel, E., Fairclough, D., Slutsman, J., & Emanuel, L. (2000). Understanding economic and other burdens of terminal illness: The experience of patients and their caregivers. *Annals of Internal Medicine, 132,* 451–459.

Erikson, E. H. (1963). *Childhood and society* (2nd ed.). New York, NY: Norton.

Feinberg, L., & Whitlatch, C. (2002). Decision-making for persons with cognitive impairment and their family caregivers. *American Journal of Alzheimer's Disease and Other Dementias, 17*(4), 237–244.

Feldt, K. (2004). The complexity of managing pain for frail elders. *Journal of the Amercan Geriatrics Society, 52,* 840–841.

Ferry, J., & Abramson, J. (2006). Toward understanding the clinical aspects of geriatric case management. *Social Work in Health Care, 42*(1), 35–56.

Fortner, B., & Neimeyer, R. (1999). Death anxiety in older adults: A quantitative review. *Death Studies, 23*(5), 387–411.

Gallo, J., Fulmer, T., Paveza, G., Paveza, G., & Reichel, W. (Eds.). (2000). *Handbook of geriatric assessment* (3rd ed.). London, England: Jones & Bartlett Publishers International.

Gardner, D. (2008). Cancer in a dyadic context: Older couples' negotiation of ambiguity and meaning in end-of-life. *Journal of Social Work in End-of-life and Palliative Care, 4*(2), 1–25.

Gardner, D., & Kramer, B. (2010). End-of-life challenges, fears and care preferences: Congruence in reports of low-income elders and their family members. *OMEGA: Journal of Death and Dying, 60*(3), 273–297.

Gardner, D., & Zodikoff, B. (2003). Meeting the challenges of social work practice in aging in the 21st Century. In B. Berkman & L. Harootyan (Eds.), *Social work and health care in an aging society* (pp. 377–392). New York, NY: Springer Publishing Co.

Gatz, M., & Smyer, M. (2001). Aging and mental health and aging at the outset of the 21st Century. In J. Birren & K. W. Schaie (Eds.), *Handbook of the psychology of aging* (5th ed., pp. 523–545). New York, NY: Academic Press.

Geriatrics Interdisciplinary Advisory Group. (2006). Interdisciplinary care for older adults with complex needs: American Geriatrics Society position statement. *Journal of the American Geriatrics Society, 54,* 849–852.

Geron, S. (2006). Comprehensive and multidimensional geriatric assessment. In B. Berkman (Ed.), *Handbook of social work in health and aging* (pp. 719–727). New York, NY: Oxford University Press.

Glajchen, M. (2004). The emerging role and needs of family caregivers in cancer care. *Journal of Supportive Oncology, 2*(2), 145–155.

Goldstein, N. E., & Morrison, S. (2005). The intersection between geriatrics and palliative care: A call for a new research agenda. *Journal of the American Geriatrics Society, 53*(9), 1593–1598.

Goy, E., & Ganzini, L. (2003). End-of-life in geriatric psychiatry. *Clinics in Geriatric Medicine, 19*, 841–856.

Grisso, T., & Appelbaum, P. (1998). *Assessing competence to consent to treatment.* New York, NY: Oxford University Press.

Gwyther, L., Altilio, T., Blacker, S, Christ, G., Csikai, E., Hooyman, N., Kramer. B. J., Linton, J., Raymer, M., & Howe J. (2005). Social work competencies in palliative and end-of-life care. *Journal of Social Work in End-of-Life and Palliative Care, 1*(1), 87–120.

Haight, B., Michel, Y., & Hendrix, S. (2000). The extended effects of the life review in nursing home residents. *International Journal of Aging and Human Development, 50*, 151–168.

Halasyamani, L., Kripalini, S., Coleman, E., van Walraven, C., Nagamine, J., Torcson, P., Bookwalter, T., Budnitz, T., & Manning, D. (2006). Transition of care for hospitalized elderly patients: Development of a discharge checklist for hospitalists. *Journal of Hospital Medicine, 1*(6), 354–360.

Hanson, L., & Ersek, M. (2006). Meeting palliative care needs in post-acute care settings: "To help them live until they die." *Journal of the American Medical Association, 295*(6), 681–686.

Harootyan, L., & O'Neill, G. (2006). National advocacy groups for older adults. In B. Berkman (Ed.), *Handbook of social work in health and aging* (pp. 817–822). New York, NY: Oxford University Press.

Harwood, D., Hawton, K., Hope, T., & Jacoby, R. (2001). Psychiatric disorder and personality factors associated with suicide in older people: A descriptive and case-control study. *International Journal of Geriatric Psychiatry, 16*, 155–165.

Hauser, J., & Kramer, B. (2004). Family caregivers in palliative care. *Clinics in Geriatric Medicine, 20*, 671–688.

He, W., Sengupta, M., Velkoff, V., & DeBarros, K. (2005). U.S. Census Bureau, current population reports, P23–209. 65+ in the United States: 2005. Washington, DC: U.S. Government Printing Office.

Helm, R., & Gibson, S. (2001). Epidemiology of pain in elderly people. *Clinics in Geriatric Medicine, 17*, 417–431.

Hickman, L., Newton, P., Halcomb, E., Chang, E., & Davidson, P. (2007). Best practice interventions to improve the management of older people in acute care settings: A literature review. *Journal of Advanced Nursing, 60*(2), 113–126.

Hogan, C., Lunney, J., Gabel, J., & Lynn, J. (2001). Medicare beneficiaries' costs of care in the last year of life. *Health Affairs, 20*(4), 188–192.

Holt, B. (1999). Community-based long-term care. In A. Kilpatrick & J. Johnson (Eds.), *Handbook of health administration and policy* (pp. 355–372). New York, NY: Marcel Dekker, Inc.

Horton-Deutsch, S., Twigg, P., & Evans, R. (2007). Health care decision-making of persons with dementia. *Dementia, 6*(1), 105–120.

Hudson, P., Aranda, S., & Kristjanson, L. (2004). Meeting the supportive needs of family caregivers in palliative care:

Challenges for health professionals. *Journal of Palliative Medicine, 7*(1), 19–25.

Hudson, P., Thomas, T., Quinn, K., & Aranda, S. (2009). Family meetings in palliative care: Are they effective? *Palliative Medicine, 23*, 150–157.

Hybels, C., & Blazer, D. (2003). Epidemiology of late-life mental disorders. *Clinics in Geriatric Medicine, 19*, 663–696.

Idler, E. (2002). The many causal pathways linking religion to health. *Public Policy and Aging Report, 12*, 7–12.

Inouye, S., Studenski, S., Tinetti, M., & Kuchel, G. (2007). Geriatric syndromes: Clinical, research and policy implications of a core geriatric concept. *Journal of the American Geriatrics Society, 55*(5), 780–791.

Institute on Medicine (IOM). (2008). *Retooling for an aging America: Building the health care workforce.* Washington, DC: The National Academies Press.

Jerant, A., Rahman, A., Nesbitt, T., & Meyers, F. (2004). The TLC model of palliative care in the elderly: Preliminary application in the assisted living setting. *Annals of Family Medicine, 2*(1), 54–60.

Johnson, K., Kuchibhatala, M., Sloane, R., Tanis, D., Anthony N. Galanos, A., & Tulsky, J. (2005). Ethnic differences in the place of death of elderly hospice enrollees. *Journal of the American Geriatrics Society, 53*(12), 2209–2215.

Kane, R., & Kane, R. (2001). Emerging issues in chronic care. In R. Binstock & L. George (Eds.), *Handbook of aging and the social sciences* (5th ed., pp. 406–425). New York, NY: Academic Press.

Kane, R., & Kane, R. (2005). Ageism in healthcare and long-term care. *Generations, 29*(3), 49–54.

Kapo, J., Morrison, L., & Solomon, L. (2007). Palliative care for the older adult. *Journal of Palliative Medicine, 10*(1), 185–209.

Keady, J. (1997). The tragedy of healthcare rationing by age. *British Journal of Nursing, 6*(7), 357.

Kennedy, G., & Tannenbaum, S. (2000). Suicide and aging: International perspectives. *Psychiatric Quarterly, 71*(4), 345–362.

Kogan, J., Edelstein, B., & McKee, D. (2000). Assessment of anxiety in older adults: Current status. *Journal of Anxiety Disorders, 14*(2), 109–132.

Kramer, B. J. (1996). Gain in the caregiving experience: Where are we? What next? *The Gerontologist, 37*(2), 218–232.

Kramer, B. J., Boelk, A., & Auer, C. (2006). Family conflict at the end of life: Lessons learned in a model program for vulnerable older adults. *Journal of Palliative Care, 9*(3), 791–801.

Krause, N. (2006). Social relationships in late-life. In R. Binstock & L. George (Eds.), *Handbook of aging and the social sciences* (6th ed., pp. 182–201). New York, NY: Academic Press.

Kung, H., Hoyert, D., Xu, J., & Murphy, S. (2008). Deaths: Final data for 2005. *National Vital Statistics Reports, 56*(10). Retrieved from http://www.cdc.gov/nchs/data/nvsr/nvsr56/nvsr56_10.pdf

Lander, M., Wilson, K., & Chochinov, H. (2000). Death and dying: Depression and the dying older patient. *Clinics in Geriatric Medicine, 16*, 335–356.

Lawton, M. P. (2001). Quality of life and the end of life. In J. Birren & K.W. Schaie (Eds.), *Handbook of the psychology of aging* (5th ed., pp. 593–616). New York, NY: Academic Press.

Levine, C. (2003). Family caregivers: Burdens and opportunities. In S. Morrison & D. Meier, (Eds.), *Geriatric Palliative Care.* (pp. 376–385). New York, NY: Oxford University Press.

Levy, B., Hummert, M., & Zebrowitz, L. (2003). Mind matters: Cognitive and physical effects of aging self-stereotypes. *The Journals of Gerontology, 58B*(4), P203–P211.

Lyyra, T., & Heikkinen, R. (2006). Perceived social support and mortality in older people. *Journals of Gerontology, 61B,* S147–S153.

Magai, C. (2001). Emotions over the life span. In J. Birren & K.W. Schaie (Eds.), *Handbook of the psychology of aging* (5th ed., pp. 399–426). San Diego, CA: Academic Press.

Master, R., & Eng, C. (2001). Integrating acute and long-term care for high-cost populations. *Health Affairs, 20*(6), 161–172.

Meier, D., & Beresford, L. (2008). Social workers advocate for a seat at palliative care table. *Journal of Palliative Medicine, 11*(1), 10–14.

Mezey, M., Kluger, M., Maislin, G., & Mittelman, M. (1996). Life-sustaining treatment decisions by spouses of patients with Alzheimer's disease. *Journal of the American Geriatrics Society, 44*(2), 144–150.

Moren-Cross, J., & Lin, N. (2006). Social networks and health. In R. Binstock & L. George (Eds.), *Handbook of aging and the social sciences* (6th ed., pp. 111–127). New York, NY: Academic Press.

Morrison, R. S. (2005). Health care system factors affecting end-of-life care. *Journal of Palliative Medicine, 8*(Suppl. 1), 79–87.

Morrison, S., & Meier, D. (Eds.). (2003). *Geriatric palliative care.* New York, NY: Oxford University Press.

Morrison, R. S., Olson, E., Mertz, K., & Meier, D. (2005). The inaccessibility of advance directives on transfer from ambulatory to acute care settings. *Journal of the American Medical Association, 274*(6), 478–482.

Mukamel, D., Temkin-Greener, H., Delavan, R., Peterson, D., Gross, D., Kunitz, S., & Williams, T. F. (2006). Team performance and risk-adjusted health outcomes in the Program of All-Inclusive Care for the Elderly (PACE). *The Gerontologist, 46,* 227–237.

National Alliance for Caregiving (NAC) & the American Association of Retired Persons (AARP). (2004). *Caregiving in the U.S.* Retrieved from http://www.caregiving.org/data/04finalreport.pdf

National Association for Social Workers (NASW), Center for Workforce Studies. (2006). *Assuring the sufficiency of a frontline workforce: A national study of licensed social workers.* Retrieved from http://workforce.socialworkers.org/studies/nasw_06_execsummary.pdf

National Consensus Project for Quality Palliative Care (NCP). (2009). *Clinical practice guidelines for quality palliative care, second edition.* Retrieved from http://www.nationalconsensusproject.org/Guidelines_Download.asp

Naylor, M., & Keating, S. (2008). Transitional care. *American Journal of Nursing, 108*(9), 58–63.

Nelson-Becker, H. (2005). Spiritual, religious, nonspiritual, and nonreligious narratives In marginalized older adults: A typology of coping styles. *Journal of Religion, Spirituality and Aging, 17*(1 & 2), 21–38.

Olson, E. (2003). Dementia and neurodegenerative disorders. In S. Morrisson & D. Meier (Eds.), *Geriatric palliative care* (pp. 160–172). New York, NY: Oxford University Press.

O'Rand, A. M. (1996). The precious and the precocious: Understanding cumulative disadvantage and cumulative advantage over the life course. *Gerontologist, 36,* 230–238.

Osterwil, D., Brummel-Smith, K., & Beck, J. (2000). *Comprehensive geriatric assessment.* New York, NY: McGraw-Hill.

Otis-Green, S., & Rutland, C. (2004). Marginalization at the end of life. In J. Berzoff & P. Silverman (Eds.), *Living with dying: A comprehensive resource for healthcare practitioners* (pp. 462–481). New York, NY: Columbia University Press.

Peake, M., Thompson, S., Lowe, D., & Pearson, M. (2003). Ageism in the management of lung cancer. *Age and Ageing, 32*(2), 171–177.

Persky, T. (1998). Overlooked and underserved: Elders in need of mental health care. *The Journal of the California Alliance for the Mentally Ill, 9,* 7–9.

Prendergast, T. (2001). Advance care planning: Pitfalls, progress, promise. *Critical Care Medicine, 29*(2), N34–N39.

Quill, T., & McCann, R. (2003). Decision making for the cognitively impaired. In S. Morrison & D. Meier (Eds.), *Geriatric palliative care* (pp. 332–341). New York, NY: Oxford University Press.

Rabow, M., Hauser, J., & Adams, J. (2004). Supporting family caregivers at the end of life. *Journal of the American Medical Association, 291*(4), 483–491.

Radawany, S., Albanese, T., Clough, L., Sims, L., Mason, H., & Jahangiri, S. (2009). End-of-life decision making and emotional burden: Placing family meetings in context. *American Journal of Hospice and Palliative Medicine, 26*(5), 376–383.

Richardson, V., & Barusch, A. (2006). *Gerontological practice for the twenty-first century: A social work perspective.* New York, NY: Columbia University Press.

Rozario, P., & DeRienzis, D. (2008). Familism beliefs and psychological distress among African American women caregivers. *The Gerontologist, 48,* 772–780.

Sable, J., & Jeste, D. (2001). Anxiety disorders in older adults. *Current Psychiatry Reports, 3,* 302–307.

Saunders, C. (1967). *The management of terminal illness.* London, England: Hospital Medicine Publications.

Saunders, C., & Baines, M. (1989). *Living with dying: The management of terminal disease* (2nd ed.). New York, NY: Oxford University Press.

Schulz, R., Beach, S., Ives, D., Martire L., Ariyo, A., & Kop, W. (2000). Association between depression and mortality in older adults: The Cardiovascular Health Study. *Archives of Internal Medicine, 160,* (12), 1761–1768.

Schulz, R., & Heckhausen, J. (1997). Emotions and control: A life-span perspective. In K. W. Schaie & M. P. Lawton (Eds.), *Annual Review of Gerontology and Geriatrics, 7*(7), 185–205.

Seymour, J., Clark, D., & Philip, I. (2001). Palliative care and geriatric medicine: Shared concerns, shared challenges. *Palliative Medicine 2001, 15,* 269–270.

Shi, L., & Singh, D. (2009). *Essentials of the U.S. health care system.* (2nd ed.). Sudbury, MA: Jones & Bartlett Publishers.

Shugarman, L., Lorenz, K., & Lynn, J. (2005). End-of-life care: An agenda for policy improvement. *Clinics in Geriatric Medicine, 21*(1), 255–272.

Shuster, J. (2000). Palliative care for advanced dementia. *Clinics in Geriatric Medicine, 16*(2), 373–386.

Sommers, L. S., Marton, K. I., Barbaccia, J. C., & Randolph, J. (2000). Physician, nurse, and social worker collaboration in primary care for chronically ill seniors. *Archives of Internal Medicine, 160,* 1825–1833.

Smedley, B., Stith, A., & Nelson, A. (Eds.). (2003). *Unequal treatment: Confronting racial and ethnic disparities in health care.* Institute of Medicine, Committee on Understanding and Eliminating Racial and Ethnic Disparities in Health Care. Washington, DC: National Academies Press.

Stein, G., & Bonuck, K. (2001). Attitudes on end-of-life care and advance care planning in the lesbian and gay community. *Journal of Palliative Medicine, 4*(2), 173–190.

Sullivan, M., Simon, G., Spertus, J., & Russo, J. (2002). Depression-related costs in heart failure care. *Archives of Internal Medicine, 162,* 1860–1866.

Sung, K. (2001). Elder respect: Exploration of ideals and forms in East Asia. *Journal of Aging Studies, 15*(1), 13–26.

Swartz, K., & Margolis, S. (2004). *The Johns Hopkins white papers: Depression and anxiety.* Baltimore, MD: Johns Hopkins Medical Institutions.

Tang, S., & McCorkle, R. (2003). Determinants of congruence between the preferred and actual place of death for terminally ill cancer patients. *Journal of Palliative Care, 19*(4), 230–237.

Teno, J. (2003). Advance care planning for frail older persons. In S. Morrison & D. Meier (Eds.), *Geriatric palliative care* (pp. 307–313). New York, NY: Oxford University Press.

Teno, J., Clarridge, B., Casey, V., Welch, L., Wetle, T., Shield, R., & Mor, V. (2004). Family perspectives on end-of-life care at the last place of care. *Journal of the American Medical Association, 291*(1), 88–93.

Thomas, C., Morris, S., & Clark, D. (2004). Place of death: Preferences among cancer patients and their careers. *Social Science and Medicine, 58,* 2431–2444.

Tornstam, L. (1996). Gerotranscendence: A theory about maturing into old age. *Journal of Aging and Identity, 1,* 37–50.

Tornstam, L. (2005). *Gerotranscendence: A developmental theory of positive aging.* New York, NY: Springer Publishing Company.

Travis, S., Bernard, M., Dixon, S., McAuley, W., Loving, G., & McClanahan, L. (2002). Obstacles to palliation and end-of-life care in a long-term care facility. *The Gerontologist, 42,* 342–349.

Wackerbarth, S. (1999). What decisions are made by family caregivers? *American Journal of Alzheimer's Disease, 14*(2), 111–119.

Wagner, C., Bigatti, S., & Storniolo, A. (2006). Quality of life of husbands of women with breast cancer. *Psycho-oncology, 15*(2), 109–120.

Waldrop, D. (2007). Caregiver grief in terminal illness and bereavement: A mixed-methods study. *Health and Social Work, 32*(3), 197–206.

Waldrop, D., Kramer, B.J., Skretny, J., Milch, R., & Finn, W. (2005). Final transitions: Family caregiving at the end of life. *Journal of Palliative Medicine, 8*(3), 623–638.

Werth, J., Gordon, J., & Johnson, R. (2002). Psychosocial issues near the end of life. *Aging and Mental Health, 6,* 402–412.

Wieland, D., Lamb, V., Sutton, S., Boland, R., Clark, M., Friedman, S., Brummel-Smith, K., & Eleazer, G. (2000). Hospitalization in the Program of All-Inclusive Care for the Elderly (PACE): Rates, concomitants, and predictors. *Journal of the American Geriatrics Society, 48*(11), 1373–1380.

Wilkinson, A., & Lynn, J. (2001). The end of life. In R. Binstock & L. George (Eds.), *Handbook of aging and the social sciences* (5th ed., pp. 444–461). San Diego, CA: Academic Press.

Wolff, J., Dy, S., Frick, K., & Kasper, J. (2007). End-of-life care: Findings from a national survey of informal caregivers. *Archives of Internal Medicine, 167*(1), 40–46.

Woods, N., LaCroix, A., Gray, S., Aragaki, A., Cochrane, G., Brunner, R., Masaki, K., Murray, A., & Newman, A. (2005). Frailty: Emergence and consequences in women aged 65 and older in the Women's Health Initiative Observational Study. *Journal of the American Geriatrics Society, 53*(8), 1321–1330.

Zerzan, L., Stearns, S., & Hanson, L. (2000). Access to palliative care and hospice in nursing homes. *Journal of the American Medical Association, 284*(2), 2489–2494.

Zimmermann, C., & Rodin, G. (2004). The denial of death thesis: Sociological critique and implications for palliative care. *Palliative Medicine, 18*(2), 121–128.

V
Collaborations in Palliative Care

A Philosophy

I believe...

That kindness goes a long way

That a commitment to collaborative communication is imperative

That transparent, transdisciplinary, transgenerational interactions offer infinitely more

That inclusivity is stronger than exclusivity

That passion is necessary

That words matter.

Shirley Otis-Green MSW, LCSW, ACSW, OSW-C
City of Hope National Medical Center
Duarte, CA

"This rich work ties us to the rest of humanity."

Julia A. Little LMSW
Project Coordinator
CancerCare for Kids

38 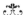 *Doretta Stark*

Teamwork in Palliative Care: An Integrative Approach

At the heart of the practice of hospice and palliative care is the notion of team.

—*Muir, 2008, p. 5*

Key Concepts

- *Palliative care consultation teams (PCCTs) have specific characteristics that infuse both organization and function.*
- *The social work role on palliative care teams is multifaceted and relates to relationships with team members as well as the collaborative relationships with referring clinicians and social work colleagues within the institution.*
- *Palliative care teams strive to function as an integrated whole and to consider the patient and family as the unit of care.*
- *Palliative care team members have shared skill sets as well as unique expertise that enriches the care of patients and families.*
- *There is emerging evidence that palliative care teams have the potential to impact cost and patient/staff satisfaction.*
- *Social work training and skill sets contribute to the ongoing function of the team and the comprehensive care of patients and families.*

Introduction

The palliative care consultation team (PCCT) strives to function as an integrated whole to ensure the best care for the patient and family whose needs are at the center of the team's purpose and function. There are different models of palliative care teams, and the model chosen often depends on resource availability within a particular institution. Medical facilities determine the team model usually based on the "… the hospital's size, culture, population served, financial commitment to palliative care, and access to existing professional resources in the facility" (Meier & Beresford, 2008b, p. 10). Some include a single physician, a nurse and physician, or a nurse or social worker alone. Models without an assigned social worker may focus primarily on physical symptom management and decision making in isolation. There are some teams that rely on the unit social worker to enhance the psychosocial perspective. Many would say that a single-practitioner model challenges the concept of team unless one broadens the perspective to include the referring sources and the clinicians who are primary caregivers to the patient and family. These approaches, while helpful, do not provide integrated holistic palliative care by a team whose specialized focus is guided by the Clinical Practice Guidelines for Quality Palliative Care (National Consensus Project, 2009). The focus of this chapter will be on the full palliative care consultation team model, as described in the Center to Advance Palliative Care's (CAPC) Program Model Options Chart (CAPC, 2009).

The fully staffed PCCT is minimally comprised of a physician, an advanced practice nurse, a master's prepared social worker, and a chaplain, all of whom are experienced in palliative care, bring an appreciation for collaborative work, and approach their colleagues with humility and respect for each discipline's expertise (Meier & Beresford, 2008b). This expertise includes excellent communication and interpersonal skills. This combination brings a biopsychosocial-spiritual approach to the care of patients and families. Some PCCTs also have volunteers, massage and expressive arts therapists, or others involved in their teams. At the center of the team's evolving plan of care are the patient, the patient's family, and their values, beliefs, and needs. The PCCT joins with patients and families to ensure their culture and values are respected and to provide guidance, support, and advocacy to promote the maximization of their treatment goals. Palliative care teams at their best are "characterized by self-awareness, cohesiveness and shared decision making, trust, respect, accountability, mutual support, self care, positive work environment, recognition of a job well done, and attention to retention and job satisfaction" (Meier & Beresford, 2008b, p. 677). In addition, teams that function well work toward "establishing consensus and clarity regarding goals, objectives, strategies; clear definition of tasks and responsibility/accountability and means for communication within teams; and competent leadership appropriate to the structure and function of the team … and procedures for evaluating the effectiveness and quality of team efforts" (Lickiss, Turner, & Pollock, 2004, p. 43).

The PCCT functions differently than the traditional multidisciplinary health care team. There are many types of teams found in medical care:

> Teams exist along a continuum from unidisciplinary (several members within a single discipline), multidisciplinary (typically a reactive model with ad hoc membership that uses a consultation format), to interdisciplinary (members are identified as working together proactively but often without shared leadership and decision-making authority), to transdisciplinary (in which members create a shared team mission, benefit from role overlap, and have integrated responsibilities, training, and leadership).
> (Otis-Green et al., 2009, p. 121)

In a tertiary acute care teaching hospital, teams are primarily interdisciplinary as are many palliative care teams. The PCCT often functions somewhere between interdisciplinary and transdisciplinary structures and possibly flows back and forth, depending on the task at hand, the membership, and the stage of development of the team. The primary interdisciplinary team relies on team communication and interaction to function for the good of the patient, and the individual disciplines may work independently, not always as a well-integrated whole (Leipzig, Hyer, Ek, & Wallenstein, 2002). This is reflective of the culture of the primary health care teams in many settings where there are multiple disciplines, shifts, of staff members and rotations of physicians who share the care of patients. In community facilities there is often a primary physician who makes rounds and then returns to the community or clinic, thus minimizing opportunities for regular communication with the hospital staff and with patients and families. This impedes integrated patient care and could be defined as the multidisciplinary team model. These systems issues impact not only the relationships and collaborations between health team members but most important the quality of care and cohesive communications with patients and families.

This chapter will examine PCCT functioning and hospital culture, role clarity within the team and between the palliative social worker and unit social workers, the role of the social worker on the team and with patients and families, and various integrative therapies, as potential components of palliative social work practice. Through patient and family narratives, team collaboration, cultural issues, and ethical issues will be explored. In addition, the impact of the PCCT on the holistic care of patients and families, on the health care setting, and on hospital finances will be considered. While the setting of this chapter is inpatient work, the concepts and challenges that infuse team collaboration and effectiveness are relevant across settings, whether one practices in an extended care facility, hospice, or outpatient palliative care clinic.

The Palliative Care Consultation Team and Hospital Culture

The culture of the tertiary acute care teaching hospital has unique characteristics that may or may not translate to other institutions. While settings may have different challenges, the essence of specialized palliative care is not setting specific and the commonalities will surface throughout the chapter.

There are many physicians, nurses, clinicians, and students of diverse disciplines involved in the care of patients. Medical teams rotate every few weeks, with the attending and staff physicians rotating even more frequently, depending on the disease-specific service. Each new team may come with different perspectives on the patient's plan of care or on the disease process. There are usually consult services involved, increasing the number of medical staff providing information to the patient and family, who can easily be confused about the plan of care and unclear as to which physician has the responsibility for the overall care of the patient and the most comprehensive information upon which they can make decisions. The pressure of rapid discharges can lead to decisions being made hurriedly without thorough consideration of diagnostic data and options for treatment and potential occurrences and outcomes. Anticipating possible occurrences such as increase in pain or disability which impact the person and family and possibly the illness itself is the role of informed clinicians. The primary team does not always have the time to give patients and families answers to their questions and then allow a respite to consider and make thoughtful decisions. In addition to the hurried nature of the environment, communication among primary team members and with consult services can be poor to contradictory. In contrast, the palliative care consult team is expected to use skillful communication to bring consistency, a holistic view, time, coordination, and a collaborative approach to developing a care plan in consultation with the primary team and other clinicians, To achieve this outcome and to create a healthy culture within the PCCT requires that the team members understand and are committed to the concept of a fully functioning integrated team (Meier & Beresford, 2008b). Most disciplines are not educated about team dynamics (Feinberg, Wenger, & Forrow, 2004). However, social work training includes communication and group skills that can serve to facilitate the process of evolving a team through role modeling, shared discussion, and joint learning about team work. This is easier to accomplish when all team members are starting at the same time. However, at any point in the developmental stage of the team, this process is critical. This dynamic, shared, and evolving experience will need frequent attention by all members to ensure that the team functioning remains optimal.

In many teams, membership changes consequent to the rotation of fellows who join to learn the specialty practice of palliative care. This creates a process of reorganization and change with stability and constancy revolving around the vision, structure, and permanent team members. The social worker, by training, may be most attuned to this process. However, all members of the team need to accept the shared responsibility for building team coherence through changes and disruption, enhancing trust and mutual respect (Junger, Pestinger, Elsner, Krumm, & Radbruch, 2007; Meier & Beresford, 2008b).

The goal is to have an interdependent team that works collaboratively, recognizes shared expertise as well as the specialty skills of each member, communicates well, and is comfortable relying on one another for the work and support (Meier & Beresford, 2008b).

The following questions capture some of the variables that infuse the building of a healthy team process over time. They can be used to stimulate discussion and foster thoughtfulness and shared decision making.

- How does the history and culture of a team and the larger institutional culture in which they function influence the members and the team process?
- What are the essential components of an effective palliative care team?
- What were members' previous experiences on health care teams? On any teams?
- In what ways might this type of team work differently?
- What expertise does each member bring, and in what ways can these talents be used to maximize collaborative assessment, intervention, and outcome for patients and families?
- How can the team ensure good communication? How can they recognize when there are problems?
- What methods of communication will be used to keep members informed? What should trigger communication? How frequently should the team communicate and in what format?
- What are the roles of each team member, and how will the team ensure role clarity and mutual respect?
- How will leadership be handled? Will leadership be shared, based on discipline, or determined by the specific needs of a patient and family?

- How can the team ensure a collaborative holistic patient/family care plan?
- What will be the process to decide who makes the initial contact with the referral source?
- What clinical guide will be used to determine who and how many team members will see the patient and/or family for an initial visit?
- How will the team handle confidentiality? What information is necessary to be shared?
- How will members support one another and recognize when the team and/or individual members are struggling?
- How will the team create an environment where groupthink is discouraged and critical thinking, disagreement, and struggle are valued?
- How will the team maintain healthy functioning and team cohesion; encourage differences of opinions and authenticity?
- For programs that include a palliative care clinic, how will continuity of care be encouraged across settings and through transitions?

Working together to consider these aspects of practice can be the beginning of building a team culture and establishing a precedent for ongoing team and individual development.

In contrast to most interdisciplinary and multidisciplinary medical team models, members of a transdisciplinary palliative care team represent their own discipline as well as the team itself. For instance, the social worker or chaplain may be the first to contact the referral source to explain what the PCCT can offer both to the referral source and to the patient and family. In their role as practitioner and team representative, they hear the issues from the primary team, gather basic medical information, see the patient and/or family to begin the assessment within the framework of their expertise, and then report back to the other team members. A well-functioning team can divide the workload when necessary to ensure that all of the patients/families are seen and referrals responded to in a timely manner

Role Clarity

Just as role clarity is vital within the palliative care team and between team members, it is equally important in collaborating with the primary team members. For the PCCT social worker and unit social worker, it is essential that they determine ways in which they can collaborate in the work with the patient/family. As Meier and Beresford (2008a) reflect in the article "Social Work Advocates for a Seat at the Palliative Care Table," the palliative social worker does not *take over*; but rather approaches the unit social worker with humility and respect for his or her role and relationships with unit staff and with the referred patient and family. In some situations, the unit social worker's caseload may be such that he or she would welcome the palliative social worker's involvement (McCormick, Engelberg, & Curtis, 2007) and in other situations, the unit social worker may wish to have the specialized expertise of the PCCT social worker in such areas as pain and symptom management, goal-of-care discussions, or ethical dilemmas (Christ & Sormanati, 2000; Zebrack & Walsh, 2008)In many cases, the unit social worker is providing excellent, comprehensive service to the patient and family and supporting that relationship is congruous with our commitment to continuity of relationship and nonabandonment. This does not necessarily exclude a role for the PCCT social worker, who may act in a consultative role or in some instances provide interventions such as clinical hypnosis, guided imagery, and/or relaxation techniques. These integrative therapies can be used in concert with clinical interventions to decrease anxiety, panic attacks, sleep disturbances, pain, nausea, and agitation (Liossi, 2006). The palliative social worker experienced in psychosocial pain assessments can provide relevant information to the primary team and unit social worker informing the symptom management care plan. "Persons from diverse cultures and ethnic backgrounds, … those with lower socio-economic status, women, pediatric and geriatric populations … are less likely to receive adequate treatment of pain" (Otis-Green et al., 2008). It is therefore important for the PCCT Social worker to assess these patients to ensure their pain is being addressed. In some settings the PCCT social worker is able to follow patients and their families as they move from unit to unit providing continuity which is usually not possible for social workers assigned to specific units. It is always the responsibility of the PCCT social worker, whether actively or peripherally involved with the referred patient and family, to seek information that keeps his or her team informed of the psychosocial care and discharge planning process.

Role clarity *within the team* needs to be explored at the beginning stages of team development and at other times when blurred boundaries and shared skill sets create the potential for duplication or competition. As all disciplines are expected to understand the psychosocial-spiritual aspects of palliative care, not all team members have the skill sets to intervene. Yet at times there are overlapping counseling skills, such as with the social worker, psychologist, or chaplain. This can provide an opportunity for collaborative work or a decision for one clinician to provide needed services in the setting of a trusting interdependence that ensures that the expertise of team members will be tapped when necessary. Whether clinicians work through joint counseling sessions or individually, it is essential that team members meet regularly to ensure their work is complementary. When there is role confusion or conflicts, the social worker might take the lead in bringing these tensions to the team's attention, understanding that unspoken conflict can erode the spirit and collaboration of the team, which will impact the care provided.

The Role of the Team Social Worker

Social work intervention in palliative care is driven by social work values of "starting where the patient is." Some situations require crises intervention such as an emergent medical situation where the immediate need might be for both medical intervention and decision making. In other instances the palliative social worker meets with referred patients and/or families to complete a psychosocial, behavioral assessment, which includes the usual domains of assessment as well as an additional focus on ethical concerns, goals of care, and pain or other symptoms that might lend themselves to integrative interventions. The assessment drives clinical interventions that are part of a care plan coordinated with the patient and family, the primary physician, and the PCCT. In addition to informed and regular communication with all clinicians, the social worker participates and sometimes leads patient/family conferences and provides education and consultation regarding the focus and function of the palliative care team. Because many patients referred to the PCCT experience anxiety, sleep disturbances, panic attacks, pain, nausea, and depression, integrative interventions can be very helpful in treating these symptoms (Liossi, 2006, p.47). It is also the role of the team social worker to participate in an assessment of the need for psychotropic medication, if appropriate. Therapeutic techniques based on rational emotive, cognitive-behavioral, person-in-environment, and family systems concepts in combination with medication are often most effective for managing major depression, anxiety and panic attacks, and agitation. These interventions can then be integrated into the palliative plan of care (Breitbart, Payne, & Passik, 2003).

The use of relaxation, guided imagery, progressive muscle relaxation, music, and/or other integrative techniques incorporated into the therapeutic process can be most efficacious (Levitan, 1997; Liossi, 2006). These therapies are simply additional tools which can be utilized to supplement existing clinical skills and are very specific complements to the work that is usually done by the unit social workers (see Box 38.1).

Referrals

Reasons for referrals can include assistance with symptom management, establishing goals and a plan of care, end-of-life decision making, discussion of code status, and giving "bad news." Delivery of "bad news" and code status discussions are frequent reasons for referral and require the team to decide whether this is best handled by a separate group of clinicians or in consultation with the referring sources both as an educational process and to diminish the potential for patients to feel abandoned by their primary providers. After discussion with the referral source and/or the primary team and the patient and family, it is essential to consider the need for a family conference incorporating the unique patient family system and cultural variables that need to be respected. Where deemed clinically and culturally appropriate, this will

---

Box 38.1
Patient/Family Narrative: Mrs. Green

Mrs. Green, 42-year-old Caucasian, Protestant, married mother of two teenage children, was diagnosed with a brain tumor. She was scheduled to remain in the hospital for radiation and chemotherapy treatments and was referred to the palliative care consultation team (PCCT) for treatment of claustrophobia and unmanageable anxiety, despite medication. She was experiencing progressive loss of vision and impaired mobility as a consequence of the brain tumor. In the course of the assessment, the PCCT social worker determined that the patient would be a candidate for clinical hypnosis, which was included in the team's care plan. The social worker provided education to assist the patient to overcome her initial uncertainty about using hypnosis, and she agreed to use this integrative approach to help her with claustrophobia, anxiety, and fears.

The patient loved the outdoors and enjoyed canoeing on the lake. This proved to be a wonderful destination for the trance work. Cognitive-behavioral interventions proved to be very helpful in reducing the patient's behavioral and psychological symptoms. An assessment of the environment revealed a table fan that was used as a trigger for entering trance, because the wind from the fan felt like a cool outdoor breeze. The social worker engaged the patient and her husband to help them in the adjustment to illness and to assist them in talking with their children, who were acting out as a result of their mother's illness, her absence from the home, and the challenge to family structure.

---

allow for an open discussion of the disease process and treatment options to set the stage for the patient and family to make decisions. The process of a joint family conference can demonstrate collaborative process, clarify information for the patient and family, and also be an opportunity for the PCCT to role model the ways in which this type of discussion can be facilitated. It is important that decisions about participants be based on clinical assessment and need as well as respect for the power imbalance that often exists between patients, families, and medical staff (Altilio, Otis-Green, & Dahlin, 2008) To provide balance and model the transdisciplinary process, it is helpful if one PCCT representative is from medicine or nursing and one is the social worker and/ or chaplain to reinforce the range of team involvement and scope of services for both the primary team and the patient and family. In addition, *A Family Conference Toolkit* developed by an interdisciplinary group at the University of Minnesota Medical Center 2003 can be downloaded from the Center to Advance Palliative Care's Web site (http://www.capc.org).

Integrating Cultural Sensitivity within and beyond the Palliative Care Team

Truth telling regarding the patient's diagnosis and disease process and respect for patient autonomy are two tenets of

ethical practice and considered "best practices" (Byock, 1994). However, "other cultures have different concepts of whether to share information with the patient, when it is shared, whom to tell, how much information is given, and what information is given to whom" (Kagawa-Singer, Martinson, & Munet-Vilaro, 1998, p. 1752). Kagawa and Blackwell (2001) in the article "Negotiating Cross Cultural Issues at End of Life" provide information from a number of studies that review the values of different cultures. It identifies elements such as worldview, value system, history of medical experiences, family system, and the family decision-making process as variables in the patient and family's experience that can impact aspects of care such as the medical decision-making process and perceptions related to pain and suffering. This leads to another important role for the PCCT in working with primary team members: to reinforce cultural respect and sensitivity. All health care providers need to recognize their own values to ensure they are not being imposed on others. However, as the majority medical values are based in Western values of autonomy and truth telling, it can be easy to assume that these values apply to everyone rather than taking the time to learn the unique perspective of each patient and family. With the PCCT's focus on holistic care, being sensitive and respectful in exploring the cultural aspects of the patient and family's world brings their cultural narrative into the illness experience and decision-making process. Meeting with the patient/family to hear what they need to ensure their values and beliefs are understood is critical. When the practices and values of the patient and family differ from the primary team's medical values, conflict can arise that can impact relationships and interfere in treatment decision making. Mediation is often helpful as is ensuring that language differences are not creating misunderstanding and discordance. These patient, family, and staff situations often involve those who speak a language other than English or whose primary language is one other than English. When patients/families and staff need to rely on interpreters, it is essential that the interpreter is trained in medical interpretation and that the team meet with them prior to patient family contact to be sure that they understand and can successfully translate the treatment and/or end-of-life terminology to be used in the discussion. It is critical that information is delivered unbiased and unfiltered. Use of family members to interpret, even when preferred by the patient, is very problematic because it is impossible for clinicians to know what is being said, what is being understood or misunderstood, or what is interpreted accurately or inaccurately. The patient narrative in Box 38.2 illustrates the need to address these issues.

The PCCT chose to view this experience as an invitation to advocate with the hospital interpreter department, requesting that they only provide staff from their department with the expectation that this would provide consistency. The interpreters and PCCT concluded that it would be mutually beneficial to create a tool that would translate complex medical and end-of-life terms for which there were no comparable

Mrs. Xiong, 54-year-old Vietnamese woman diagnosed with a progressing head and neck cancer, was referred to the palliative care consultation team (PCCT). The patient spoke Vietnamese and was a widow with no children. She was referred because she was refusing radiation treatment, a decision which confused and concerned her oncology team. The PCCT social worker and physician met with the patient and an outside agency interpreter because none of the hospital's Vietnamese interpreters were available. It appeared to the PCCT members that the interpreter was having extended conversations with the patient which seemed to exceed the amount of information the team was expecting to provide. Speaking with the interpreter following the meeting, the team discovered that the information given was being censored because the interpreter, assuming a role of cultural mediator, did not think it was in the patient's best interest, from a cultural perspective, to tell her all that was being said about her condition. In addition, there is no comparable term in Vietnamese for radiation therapy, so the interpreter used the term "burned." This focused the PCCT team on two immediate issues: to learn what information the patient was open to hearing in the context of her cultural beliefs and to find a better way to explain radiation therapy. It also became apparent that the immediate need to explain a therapy had dwarfed the importance of the basic assessment of the patient's cultural beliefs and her support system to determine who, if anyone, needed to be involved during this time.

terms in other languages. This tool was developed for languages that were most commonly spoken at the hospital (http://www.uofmmedicalcenter.org). Anecdotally, this joint process helped the interpreters to understand the important work they were doing and improved their ability to assist the hospital staff and their understanding of the patients and families. This is an example of extending the focus of palliative care beyond the formal team to invite participation of other departments and specialists to enhance both patient care and institutional culture.

Kagawa-Singer, Martinson, and Munet-Vilaro (1998) report that even when death is near, many Asian and Native American cultures value a positive and hopeful tone. So in addition to the appropriate language and tone, choice of words is an important and essential aspect of communication within and beyond the palliative care team. In many cultures, autonomy is not the primary value. Rather, the tribe, extended family, religious leaders, or elders are the decision

The Vietnamese interpreters found another way of describing radiation therapy. This important contribution, coupled with daily support, exploration, and active listening to what was important to the patient, created an environment of comfort and safety. She ultimately agreed to treatment.

makers. To promote patient/family-centered care, the PCCT must ensure that the patient/family are hearing information in a manner that allows them to receive support and make informed choices within their cultural framework.

Not only are values and beliefs important for understanding different approaches to illness, end of life, and death, but understanding the patient's and family's worldview is critical. This is particularly important when discussing advance directives, which are often a focus of palliative care. '... the medical and bioethics literature often suggests that cultural mistrust is a significant influence on the attitudes and the behaviors of African American patients toward advance directives and other end of life care issues"(Crawley, Payne, Bolden, Washington, & Williams, 2000, p.2518) A study by Wallace, Weiner, Pekmezaris, Almendral, and Cossiquien (2007) "correlates physicians own racial background, clinical experience and cultural sensitivity training, with their attitudes, perceptions, and knowledge of advance care planning issues for African-Americans patients" (p. 722). The article continues by illustrating that the low rates of completion of advance directives by African Americans reflected that many had distrust of the health care system, personal experiences with health disparities, and cultural and religious perspectives on death, dying, and suffering, which affected their decision making (see Box 38.3). There is also documentation

Mr. Jones, a 78-year-old, Baptist, African American widower diagnosed with end-stage congestive heart failure and chronic obstructive pulmonary disease, was referred to the palliative care consultation team (PCCT) for the discussion of advance directives, code status, and plan of care. The PCCT chose to use these facilitated discussions as an opportunity to educate the multitiered medical staff participating in Mr. Jones care, inviting then to participate in both the family and one-on-one meetings that were organized. The PCCT physician and social worker met with the patient, engaging him in discussions of his medical condition and his values and beliefs, creating a context in which Mr. Jones might share his thoughts on how to help him as his medical condition deteriorated. "I'm ready to cross over whenever the Lord wants me, but I'm not in any hurry!" He said that his life was in God's hands, not his. He felt that everything should be done and that God would decide when it was enough. The PCCT's work focused on improving Mr. Jones comfort by adjusting his medications and reassuring him that his wishes would be respected. This intervention was responsive to his need for symptom management and symbolically represented the staff's commitment to caring for him and joining with him until his God determined the outcome. The PCCT social worker was able to speak with the primary care team members to explain the value system from which the patient made the decision to be full code. Over time, through the collaborative work of the PCCT chaplain and social worker, the primary team understood that in addition to his religious beliefs, the patient's history with health care providers and the experiences of other

Box 38.3 *(Contd.)*

family members and friends led him to question the intention of health care providers. He wondered why they were offering him the option to forgo treatment. Were they trying to hasten his death by discussing code status and advance directives? These concerns of African American patients can influence their treatment and end-of-life decisions, especially for those who are older. They inform the need for PCCT and others to reinforce care that will be provided concurrently with discussions of options that may be deemed, under unique circumstances, to not be beneficial.

that the infamous Tuskegee Syphilis Study may continue to infuse African American patients' and families' health care decisions (Wallace et al., 2007).

Ethical Dilemmas

It is important to note that in addition to the ethical issues that relate to patients and families, each discipline represented on the team has its own unique code of ethics and its own values, religious and cultural, that impact perceptions and opinions. While the concept of teams implies collaborative decision making, mutual respect, and shared responsibility, there are different roles and unique responsibilities. For example, writing an order for palliative sedation or giving the sedating medication is not the same responsibility, ethically or legally, as participating in discussions, counseling, education, and support to staff and family throughout the decision-making process and during the time period when sedation is maintained. Administering pain medication has a different degree of responsibility than participating by providing education and relaxation techniques. Open discussion of these complex differences in responsibility is essential to authenticity in team function and relationships.

Ethical issues can often impede the patient/family and primary team from moving forward with a plan of care. "Despite advances in medicine, the nature of ethical dilemmas remains relatively unchanged. Issues of communication, family conflict, and futility continue to give rise to ethical quandaries" (Swetz, Crowley, Hook, & Mueller, 2007, p.686). The following ethical principles infuse the work of palliative care teams:

- *Beneficence*: Acting for the good of the patient
- *Autonomy*: Respecting the right of the patient to determine the course of his or her care, which naturally leads to considerations of the patient's capacity and competence to make decisions
- *Nonmaleficence*: "First do no harm"; balancing benefits versus burdens
- *Truth telling*: The duty to tell the truth
- *Distributive justice*: The equitable distribution of, and access to, resources

- *Confidentiality*: Maintaining the sanctity and privacy of information shared by the patient and family
- *Professional integrity*: The right of medical professions to determine standards of practice and to decline to violate those standards (Byock, 1994, p. 9; Aroskar, 1980 pp. 658–659)

Palliative care consultation teams often receive referrals to assist the primary teams with ethical dilemmas. This can include value conflicts between the primary team and the patient and family, thus affecting decisions regarding treatment and/or end-of-life care planning. These referrals may involve the weighing of benefit and burden, clarification of advance directives, exploring of family conflict, and clarifying understanding and communication between staff, patients, and family. Often palliative care clinicians bring objectivity or an alternative view that defuses conflict and allows decision making to proceed (see Box 38.4).

Box 38.4
Patient Family Narrative: Mr. Smith

Mr. Smith is a 43-year-old, Caucasian, devout Catholic with end-stage cancer, who is being cared for in the medical intensive care unit. He is in multisystem failure, unresponsive, and on a ventilator. He is married, with two teenage children and a large extended family. Mr. Smith was referred because of value discord with the family regarding the plan of care. The intensive care staff were frustrated because they believed that they were contributing to patient suffering and that continued intensive care interventions were nonbeneficial and doing harm. The family's religious beliefs were such that they believed a miracle might occur and that suffering was part of the patient's religious journey. The palliative care consultation team (PCCT) met and, after thorough review of the biopsychosocial-spiritual history and discussion with the referring team, developed a plan on how to formulate the clinical and ethical issues and how to assist the unit staff and the family. The team physician, social worker, and chaplain met with the family to understand the unique needs and perceptions of each as an individual and as a family, clarifying their goals and determining their understanding of the patient's condition. It became clear that the family's faith was the primary value guiding their decisions. After the team members were able to establish a trusting relationship, it was possible to guide the family reframing process, which gave them permission to acknowledge the patient's dire medical condition and the extent of his prior and current suffering. This invited them to weigh these observations in the setting of their religious values. The family members were then able to permit nonbeneficial treatments to be discontinued at the same time that active symptom management provided comfort during the dying process. The patient died peacefully with his family around him. These interventions helped the primary team to feel more comfortable in their care of the patient and preserved the belief system of the family, which would sustain them beyond the death. The PCCT supported and advocated for the patient and family while acknowledging the struggle and conflict of the clinical teams and helping them to understand the family's perspective.

In addition to the clinical interventions, it is important for the PCCT to know the facility's policies on such issues as futility, withdrawing or withholding of treatments, and the state laws regarding decision making at end of life. It is also helpful, when appropriate, to partner with the hospital ethics consultation service and ensure that the primary physicians are aware of their rights regarding providing treatment when it conflicts with their values.

Confidentiality: The Sanctity of Patient/Family Information

All health care professionals are bound by federal HIPPA requirements (Health Insurance Portability and Accountability Act, 1996, https://www.cms.gov/HIPAAGenInfo/Downloads/HIPAALaw.pdf), but this does not cover the use of information shared between health care clinicians providing care to the same patient and family. In Neil MacDonald's chapter on confidentiality in the *Oxford Textbook of Palliative Medicine* (2004, p. 58), he states that "central to a respect for personal autonomy is the concept that the privacy of individuals must be respected." The purpose of sharing private information must always be discussed with patients and families who need to be helped to understand that the PCCT works integratively to provide biopsychosocial-spiritual care, which implies that some information may need to be shared to maximize this care. This discussion includes a request for permission to share information. It is not necessary to share all information with all team members; rather a judgment is made as to what information is shared in order to assist others to do their work to the benefit of the patient and family. One must always discuss legally bound reporting responsibilities, including issues such as adult or child abuse and suicidal/homicidal threats. As in all interactions regarding the sharing of privileged information, it is necessary to use sound judgment, based on experience, and when necessary, consultation. It is equally important that written documentation include information that is based on fact and, once again, necessary to the provision of care to the patient. In the context of palliative care's commitment to including the family in the unit of care, it is important to consider that the medical chart is, in fact, the chart of the patient. To that end, family information becomes relevant when related to the patient plan of care. General assessments, plan of action, and recommendations are sufficient. Remember that the patient can request to read his or her chart.

Reduction of Hospital Costs and Improved Patient/Family and Staff Satisfaction

There are an increasing number of studies that have shown a reduction in hospital costs and improved outcomes, such as physical and psychological symptom management, health care team satisfaction, and family well-being, when consultation and care from a PCCT is provided.

In the "most comprehensive study to date," Morrison et al., found that

of the 2966 palliative care patients discharged alive ... [from eight hospitals] had an adjusted net savings of $1696 in direct costs per admission and $279 in direct costs per day including significant reductions in laboratory and intensive care unit costs compared with usual patients. The palliative care patients who died had an adjusted net savings of $4908 in direct costs per admission and $374 in direct cost per day including significant reductions in pharmacy, laboratory and intensive care unit costs compared with usual care patients. (Morrison et al., 2008, p. 1783)

Their conclusion was that

although others have postulated that palliative care programs could substantially reduce hospital costs this study is the first, to our knowledge, to empirically evaluate the actual effect of palliative care on U.S. hospital costs using a sample size to assure reliable results ... ." (Morrison et al., 2008, pp. 1786–1787)

There have been a number of single-site studies suggesting that clarifying goals and assisting patients and families to select treatments that meet these goals have reduced hospital and intensive care unit costs For example, in 2007, Ciemins, Blum, Nunley, Lasher, and Newman analyzed the care of palliative care patients in one large nonprofit academic facility. Their results showed daily costs "... reduced by 33% and length of stay reduced by 30%. The large reduction in daily mean costs and length of stay resulted in $2.2 million in the study hospital" (p. 1347). The study further found that patients receiving palliative care experienced significant improvements in their symptom status. In another study by Penrod et al. (2006) it was found that in two urban veteran's hospitals "palliative care was associated with significantly lower likelihood of intensive care unit costs compared with usual costs ... the total inpatient direct daily costs were $239 lower for palliative care patients than usual patients" (p. 855). In another single study by Bendaly, Groves, and Gramelspacher, (2008) found that their palliative care team efforts reduced the hospital's cost by $7,000 compared to the group which did not receive palliative care services.

The aforementioned studies add "... to the growing literature on the benefits of palliative care consultation by demonstrating that in addition to improved clinical care and patient/family and health care team satisfaction, these programs are associated with considerable reductions in hospital costs" (Morrison et al., 2008, p. 1789). This is added endorsement for earlier referrals to palliative care consultation teams and for hospitals to consider developing palliative care teams.

The Educational Role of the Palliative Care Consultation Team

In an acute care tertiary teaching hospital, education of all health care disciplines occurs alongside opportunities for patient/family care and research. The PCCT is no exception because this is a relatively new field that needs to continually clarify its focus and obviate the perception that palliative care is limited to end of life. Education is mutual and can occur informally as the PCCT members meet with health care team members to discuss referrals. These informal interactions provide the opportunity for role modeling as well as refining the understanding of the ways in which the PCCT can be helpful. This educational process is reciprocal as palliative clinicians reinforce their knowledge and learn from others within the same discipline and across disciplines. This is another example of PCCT members not only representing their discipline but also the team, because they assert not only their ability to teach but also a willingness to learn. Establishing more structured educational opportunities is also important. This can be journal clubs or monthly palliative care grand rounds where patient and family narratives or new research can be presented not only by the palliative care team but also by colleagues in other specialties with whom the PCCT shares responsibility for the care of patients and families.

Scheduled educational sessions with specific patient care units, disease-specific clinicians, or specific disciplines are other ways to structure palliative care education. Palliative care fellowships for physicians, nurses, and social workers provide intensive educational experiences for clinicians wanting to pursue this subspecialty. In addition, there are a number of continuing education, ongoing peer consultation, and support resources available to social workers already working in palliative care.

The palliative care consultation team functions very differently than a primary health care team. The expectations for the PCCT members are to work interdependently and to represent not only their individual disciplines but the PCCT as well. The team can bring a fresh perspective to patient and family care focusing on physical and psychological symptom management, cultural and value differences and conflicts, ethical dilemmas, and clarification of patient/family goals of care. The PCCT works to bring an integrated holistic approach to patient/family care. The social worker provides a comprehensive psychosocial-spiritual assessment, which includes pain and symptoms that might benefit from integrative/behavioral interventions, as well as appropriate clinical interventions to patients and families. Furthermore, the social worker educates and collaborates with primary team members, ensures good communication with the primary team and the patient and family, and coordinates roles with team members and the unit social workers. The social worker models good communication and collaborative skills, initiating discussions regarding role clarity, conflict and confusion and team functioning, and maintaining a pulse on the team's need to reclarify focus and take time out to debrief, grieve, and rejuvenate.

LEARNING EXERCISES

- You are sitting down with the new palliative care team as the social worker, how might you participate in the forming process?
- You are meeting with a unit social worker for the first time. How will you begin the conversation? How is this collaboration unique?
- A patient has been referred to the team who does not speak English, how might you ensure that the patient is receiving the information being shared?
- You have met with a patient and family, and you determine they would be open to integrative methods. How would you describe them, assess what might be helpful to them, and seek to provide assistance to them?
- What can you do on the team to facilitate attention to good team functioning and collaboration with team colleagues?

ADDITIONAL RESOURCES

The Language Services and Community Health Outreach, University of Minnesota

Medical Center, Fairview: http://www.uofmmedicalcenter.org click on interpreter services

Information on interpreter language tool for palliative and end-of-life terms.

The National Association of Social Workers Standards for Cultural Competence: http://www.naswdc.org/practice/standards/NASWCulturalStandards.pdf

Charges that social workers have the ethical responsibility to be culturally competent.

National Institutes of Health–Bioethics: http://Bioethics.od.nih.gov/

This Web site contains a broad collage of annotated Web links, and while this list is comprehensive, it is not totally inclusive. The listed resources provide background information and various positions on issues in bioethics.

ADDITIONAL SUGGESTED READINGS

Smith, T. J., Coyne, P., Cassel, B., Penberth, L., Hobson, A., & Hager, M. A. (2003). A high volume specialist palliative care unit and team may reduce in hospital end of life care costs. *Journal of Palliative Medicine*, 6(5), 699–705.

Otis-Green, S., Lucas, S., Spolum, M., Ferrell, B., & Grant, M. (2008). Promoting excellence in pain management and palliative care for social workers. *Journal of Social Work in End of Life and Palliative Care, 4*(2), 121–134.

Otis-Green, S., Lucas, S., Spolum, M., Ferrell, B., & Grant, M. (2008). Promoting excellence in pain management and palliative care for social workers. *Journal of Social Work in End of Life and Palliative Care, 4*(2), 121–134

Zebrack, B., Walsh, K., Burg, M. A., Maramaldi, P., & Lim, J. W. (2008). Oncology social worker competencies and implication for education and training. *Social Work in Health Care, 47*(4), 355–375.

Zhukovsky, D., … Bruera, E. (2004). Palliative care inpatient service in a comprehensive cancer center: Clinical and financial outcomes. *Journal of Clinical Oncology, 22*(10), 2008–2014.

ACKNOWLEDGMENTS

Special thanks to the UMMC- Fairview Palliative team: Mark Leenay, MD, Rudy Keimowitz, MD, Kerstin McSteen, RN, CNS, David Berg, MA, MDiv, and to my husband for his love and support.

REFERENCES

Altilio, T., Otis-Green, S., & Dahlin, C.(2008). Applying the national quality forum preferred practices for palliative and hospice care: A social work perspective. *Social Work and End of Life and Palliative Care, 4*(1) 3–16.

Aroskar, M. (1980). Anatomy of an ethical dilemma: Theory and practice. *American Journal of Nursing, 80,* 658–663.

Bendaly, J. S., Groves, J. B., & Gramelspacher, G. P. (2008). Financial impact of palliative care consultation in a public hospital. *Journal of Palliative Medicine, 11*(6), 1304–1308.

Byock, I. R. (1994). Ethics from a hospice perspective. *American Journal of Hospice and Palliative Care,* (July/August), 9–11.

Center to Advance Palliative Care (CAPC). (2009). Palliative care program model options chart. Retrieved from http://www.capc.org/building-a-hospital-based-palliative-care-program/designing/characteristics/program-model-chart

Christ, G., & Sormanati, M. (2000). Advancing social work practice in the end of life. *Social Work in Health Care, 30*(2), 81–99.

Ciemans, E. L., Blum, L., Nunley, M., Lasher, A., & Newman, J. M. (2007). The economic and clinical impact of an inpatient palliative care consultation service: A multifaceted approach. *Journal of Palliative Medicine, 10*(6), 1347–1355.

Crawley, L., Payne, R., Bolden, J., Washington, P., & Williams, S. (2000). Palliative end-of-life care in the African American community. *Journal of the American Medical Association, 284*(19), 2518–2521.

Feinberg, I. C., Wenger, N. S., & Forrow, L. (2004). Interdisciplinary education: Evaluation of a palliative care training intervention for pre-professionals. *Academic Medicine, 79*(8), 769–776.

Junger, S., Pestinger, M., Elsner, N., Krumm, N., & Radbruch, L. (2007). Criteria for successful multi professional cooperation in

palliative care teams. *Journal of Palliative Medicine, 21*(4), 347–354.

Kagawa-Singer, M., & Blackwell, L. (2001). Negotiating cross cultural issues at end of life. *Journal of the American Medical Association, 286*(23), 2993–3001.

Kagawa-Singer, M., Martinson, I. M., & Munet-Vilaro, F. (1998). A multi-cultural perspective on death and dying. *Oncology Forum, 25*(10), 1751–1756.

Leipzig, R. M., Hyer, K., Ek, K., & Wallenstein, S. (2002). Attitudes towards working in interdisciplinary health care teams: A comparison of disciplines. *Journal of the American Geriatric Society, 50,* 1141–1148.

Levitan, A. (1997). Oncology. In R. Temes (Ed.), *Medical hypnosis: An introduction and clinical guide* (pp. 107–114). :Churchill Livingston Publishers.

Lickiss, N. J., Turner, K. S., & Pollock, M. L. (2004). The interdisciplinary team. In D. Doyle, G. Hanks, N. Cherny, & K. Calman (Eds.), *Oxford textbook of palliative medicine* (pp. 42–46). Oxford, England: Oxford University Press.

Liossi, C. (2006). Hypnosis in cancer care. *Contemporary Hypnosis, 23*(1), 47–57.

MacDonald, N. (2004). Confidentiality. In D. Doyle, G. Hanks, N. Cherny, & K. Calman (Eds.), *Oxford textbook of palliative medicine* (3rd ed., pp. 58–61). Oxford, England: Oxford University Press.

McCormick, A., Engelberg, R., & Curtis, J. (2007). Social workers in palliative care: Assessing activities and barriers in the Intensive care unit. *Journal of Palliative Medicine, 19*(4), 929–937.

Meier, D., & Beresford, L. (2008a). Social work advocates for a seat at the palliative care table. *Journal of Palliative Medicine, 11*(1), 10–14.

Meier, D., & Beresford, L. (2008b). The palliative care team. *Journal of Palliative Medicine, 11*(5), 617–681.

Morrison, R., Penrod, J., Cassel, J., Caust-Ellenbogen, M, Litke, A., Spragens, L., & Meier, D. (2008). Cost savings associated with United States palliative care consultation programs. *Archives of Internal Medicine, 168*(16), 1783–1790.

Muir, J. C. (2008). Team, diversity, and building communities. *Journal of Palliative Medicine, 11*(1), 5–7.

National Consensus Project. (2009). *Clinical practice guidelines for quality palliative care, second edition.* Retrieved http://www.nationalconsensusproject.org/Guidelines_Download.asp

Otis-Green, S., Ferrell, B., Spolum, M., Uman, G., Mullan, P., Baird, P., & Grant, M. (2009). An overview of the ACE project-Advocating for Clinical Excellence: Transdisciplinary palliative care education. *Journal of Cancer Education, 24*(2), 120–126.

Penrod, J. D., Deb, P., Luhrs, C., Dellenbaugh, C., Zhu, C., Hochman, T., … Morrison, R. S. (2006). Cost and utilization outcomes of patients receiving hospital based palliative care consultation. *Journal of Palliative Medicine, 9*(5), 855–860.

Swetz, K. M., Crowley, M. E., Hook, C. C., & Mueller, P. S. (2007). Report of 2555 clinical ethics consultations and review of literature. *Mayo Clinic Proceedings, 82*(6), 686–691.

Wallace, M., Weiner, J., Pekmezaris, R., Almendral, A., & Cossiquien, R. (2007). Physician cultural sensitivity in African American advance care planning: A pilot study. *Journal of Palliative Medicine, 10*(3), 721–727.

39 *Becky A. Anderson, Louise E. Marasco, Julia Kasl-Godley, and Sheila G. Kennedy*

Social Work and Psychology

For weeks I have planned to stop by your unit to thank you for caring for my husband. He died a month ago. Somehow my car is able to bring me, but my feet refuse to go in the front door. Emotions I thought were under control resurfaced! I do thank you for managing to find a bed just before I left for those days of respite. Please know you have in us a family of grateful people. We especially appreciate the team, and their care of us. We were rather thrust upon you— something that embarrassed me but that I could not refuse. It was the team that most impressed us … it was clearly a team effort that put my husband's comfort first. That has meant so much to us during the roller coaster of emotions we've experienced.

—Widow of former palliative care patient "Mr. Z."
(detailed in patient narrative in Box 39.1)

Key Concepts

- ◆ *Effective collaboration between social workers and psychologists can improve psychosocial aspects of care.*
- ◆ *Organizational (contextual) and interpersonal and team (process) factors influence collaborative effectiveness.*
- ◆ *There are benefits as well as challenges for palliative social workers and psychologists working together.*

Introduction and Objectives

This chapter is intended for social work professionals and students working with psychologists in palliative care settings. Whether one is working within the context of a newly developed relationship or an established one, certain organizational and interpersonal factors can impinge on or facilitate ongoing collaboration. This chapter reviews some of these factors, in the hopes that awareness of these factors will increase the likelihood of successful collaboration and better delivery of palliative care by both social workers and psychologists at the micro, macro, and systems levels. We also provide a patient/family narrative that highlights the rich synergy and benefits of palliative social workers and psychologists working together as well as some of the potential challenges.

Palliative care providers within social work and psychology play a vital role in addressing the multidimensional nature of suffering and promoting coping and adaptation among patients and families dealing with advanced, life-limiting, or terminal illness. Professionals from both disciplines achieve these goals by drawing upon broad-based academic knowledge, specialized training in assessment and intervention, and models of human behavior, particularly the biopsychosocial-spiritual model.

The similarity in approach, combined with unique perspectives and skills, can be leveraged to provide more comprehensive psychosocial care to palliative care patients and their family members. It also has the potential of compromising care, if it consequently results in role confusion, unclear expectations, or turf battles (e.g., providers struggle with who "should" be doing various activities such as family therapy or bereavement support). However, to date, there is a paucity of literature examining either the relationship between psychologists and social workers providing palliative and end-of-life care or the outcomes of such collaboration. When looking to the literature on outcomes of collaboration between health care professionals in general, effective collaboration has been associated with improved use of medications, decreased length of hospital stay, decreased medical care costs (Zwarenstein, Goldman, & Reeves, 2009), increased job satisfaction, and improved care for patients (Baggs & Schmitt, 1997). Conversely, a failure of collaboration among health care professionals can result in poor patient care and an unhealthy work environment (Larson, 1999).

Extrapolating from this literature, we postulate that effective collaboration between social work and psychology should result in improved psychosocial care for palliative care patients and their families over that care provided by either discipline alone. However, collaboration requires institutional and personal commitment. Factors likely to influence collaboration and thus psychosocial care can be organized into (1) contextual factors, or characteristics of the context in which care is provided and (2) process factors, or factors that influence the "work" of working together.

Contextual Factors

Contextual factors include the venue of care and physical environment, organizational policies and procedures, funding, and attitudes and beliefs toward palliative care.

Aspects of the physical environment in which care is provided, be it within an inpatient hospital unit, an outpatient clinic, an intensive care unit, a skilled nursing facility, a prison, or a patient's home, can affect the degree to which social workers and psychologists can interact. These aspects include whether there is dedicated space available for meeting basic work needs (e.g. computers, phones) or fostering collaboration (e.g. joint visits, meetings).

In addition, when providers are seeing patients in multiple venues across a large coverage area, even if they have designated office space, their schedules rarely may overlap, which places increased importance on communication via text/page and e-mail. It may be helpful to elucidate the preferred mode of communication between the two providers as well as to set expectations about when and how often communication will occur (e.g., scheduling a regular time to touch base, making arrangements to check voice mail during the day, or verifying that text pages have been seen and acknowledged for follow-up). Providers may have to be creative in working around limitations for face-to-face meetings, such as requesting a meeting room at a local church or spiritual center or reserving a conference room at a local library when serving patients in home-based programs.

Policies governing the operation of the institution in which the palliative care program is housed or affiliated is another factor that can affect collaboration between social workers and psychologists. Policies can determine the scope of services offered as well as staffing, including the percent

FTE (e.g., full time, quarter time) designated for palliative care services. Thus, providers may have varying amounts of time to devote to direct clinical care, communication and coordination with other disciplines, or activities to build the collaborative relationship. The practical issue of availability and time may determine which provider sees the patient/family and when, as well as who can participate in care planning or family meetings. Directly addressing these practical issues can mitigate against unclear or unmet expectations. Policies also can dictate caseload requirements or expectations; furthermore, when the caseload is large and consists of high acuity of needs, providers may struggle to meet these needs adequately. When social workers and psychologists can divvy up responsibilities and coordinate care, they can potentially better serve patients. However, this sharing of responsibilities can be complicated by billing requirements and limitations on what can be billed.

The funding structure of palliative care services, which may include a combination of research grants, charity, direct hospital support, or fee for service, can affect collaboration. In many settings, psychologists are expected to generate billable hours and then are reimbursed for services (Lichtenberg et al., 1998). This arrangement may constrain the activities in which they can engage, such as attendance at team meetings or informal consultations if these activities are not billable. In contrast, palliative care social workers typically do not face the same billing constraints as palliative care psychologists given that their services most often are covered under the umbrella of patients' total care costs and are absorbed by the funding source. As a result, social workers may be under less pressure to define their roles and responsibilities, to prove the need for their interventions, or to see patients in shorter amounts of time. In comparison, psychologists may need to demonstrate more specifically how their time is used and/or the complexity of the patients they see.

However, if palliative care social workers were reimbursed for services, there may be a greater likelihood of increased competition between social work and psychology due to overlapping services. For example, some social work professionals working in outpatient palliative care settings already are able to bill as fee for service (Meier & Beresford, 2008) with reimbursement dependent upon state requirements (Cowen & Moorhead, 2006). It is important to note that whereas psychologists can bill under Medicare, "clinical social workers are currently reimbursed for psychotherapy services only under Medicare Part B. NASW is advocating for clinical social workers to receive reimbursement under Part A services, as well. Clinical social work services are bundled in hospitals and skilled-nursing facilities and, therefore, are not reimbursable at this time" (Coleman, 2010). More attention is needed to the topic of billing among social workers across palliative care settings, particularly because palliative care social workers collaborate with psychologists and may use similar diagnosis codes.

Other providers' attitudes and beliefs about palliative care and mental health care services provided within this context can affect collaboration by influencing referrals and potentially pigeon-holing social workers or psychologists. These attitudes can be reified by social workers and psychologists, thereby reinforcing divisions, but they also may present the opportunity for palliative care social workers and psychologists to educate other providers and model effective interdisciplinary care. The social worker and psychologist can work together to clarify misconceptions that may exist and to challenge stereotypes or the tendency to typecast the palliative care program and/or the respective disciplines.

Process Factors

Factors that affect the "work" of working together, such as team structure and dynamics and communication and conflict resolution skills, can influence collaboration between palliative care social workers and psychologists.

Palliative social workers and psychologists may find themselves joining an established team or a newly forming team, or functioning as a core member of, or consultant to, a team, with each scenario presenting different challenges for collaboration. Furthermore, the type of team in which the palliative care social workers and psychologists are working can affect collaboration. For example, in *multidisciplinary teams*, members of different disciplines work together but function independently, with minimal coordination or consultation with each other regarding care. Individual disciplines own their treatment plan, though they often integrate input from others. Multidisciplinary teams are hierarchically organized, and leadership and decision making are not shared (Lickiss, Turner, & Pollock, 2004; Zeiss & Gallagher-Thompson, 2003; Zeiss & Steffen, 1996, 1998). Decision making is vertical—so even if collaborative, one person has the final say, which can result in team members feeling ineffectual or undervalued.

Interdisciplinary teams are composed of providers from different disciplines who collaboratively and interdependently plan, implement, and evaluate outcomes of the care provided to patients and families. Division of tasks among team members is based more on patient problems and needs than on traditional role definitions (Zeiss & Gallagher-Thompson, 2003). Decision making and leadership are shared and flexible (Zeiss & Steffen, 1996, 1998). Team members have consensus and clarity regarding goals and strategies, recognize their shared responsibility for patients, and acknowledge the unique competencies, contributions, and roles of each discipline, as well as the areas of overlapping function (Lickiss, Turner, & Pollock, 2004; Zeiss & Steffen, 1998). While shared decision making is the ideal on interdisciplinary teams, it may be difficult to maintain equal contributions and responsibilities across all disciplines. Alternatively, when no clear answer to complex problems exists, responsibility may be diffuse across all team members.

Transdisciplinary teams are comprised of professionals from different disciplines who teach, learn, and work together across traditional disciplinary or professional boundaries. Members are familiar with the concepts and approaches of colleagues from different disciplines, as well as their own. Roles and responsibilities are shared, disciplinary lines are blurred, and there are few seams between the members' functions, often resulting in the phenomenon known as "role release" (Larson, 1993). These types of teams are less common, particularly when patients need the special skills of specific disciplines. Transdisciplinary teams may require more negotiation to decide which team member assumes responsibility for a task since the usual fall-back option of "this is the social worker role (or psychologist or nurse role)" is not invoked. In addition, teams may be transdisciplinary with respect to some tasks (e.g., case management, bereavement contacts, or QI projects) but interdisciplinary or even multidisciplinary with respect to other tasks (e.g., administrative responsibilities).

How members of the respective teams, in this case, social workers and psychologists, navigate conflict influences the degree of successful and sustainable collaboration. Conflict can result from a variety of factors such as personality clashes, large caseloads, deficiencies in communication, gatekeeping, clash of ideas, principles and values, poorly defined or disputed roles or role expectations (Lickiss, Turner, & Pollock, 2004; Oliver & Peck, 2006; Yeager, 2005), or unmet or inconsistent expectations (e.g., the social worker and psychologist do not know what to expect of each other) (Larson, 1993). To minimize conflict, social workers and psychologists may want to delineate clinical services that medically ill persons can receive from each discipline, deciding whether this delineation will be a generalized or specific to the patient/family situation. It may be helpful to identify what each professional is expected to provide, based on the professionals's respective training and specialized skills and knowledge, thereby defining unique skills and clarifying areas that can be a source of conflict because of overlap. This process can be facilitated when the social worker and psychologist take the time to ask about individual skill sets as well as training models and professional culture. Furthermore, collaboration can be fostered when differences of opinion are seen as complementary, rather than right or wrong, and as an opportunity to learn something about each provider. Some questions that help to elucidate these issues are as follows:

- What are the key differences distinguishing the roles of the social worker and the psychologist?
- How are these differences discipline specific?
- How are these differences distinctly individualized based upon a provider's particular educational background and specialized training?
- How will the palliative care social worker and psychologist negotiate the implementation of interventions, particularly when both are similarly prepared to provide certain treatments?

- How can the social worker and psychologist work together to educate others regarding their roles and relationship?
- What forums are available for an exchange of ideas and resources, and for continuing education relative to the overlap of roles and collaboration between disciplines?

Furthermore, collaboration requires a trusting and good working relationship. Several strategies can assist with relationship building: (1) identify shared interests with respect to patient and family outcomes and care coordination; (2) consider giving timely, frequent, concrete, nonjudgmental feedback about how the other's behavior affects you and why, while being open to the same feedback; (3) ask "What can I do differently that would make things better for the social worker/psychologist?" (4) build in meetings focused both on patient care and on working together; (5) conduct visits together when possible and clinically indicated and maintain regular, informal, brief communication; (6) provide empathy, praise, and celebration of personal events, professional accomplishments, and one other; and (7) be aware of your colleague's life beyond the work environment, including stressors in his or her personal life and provide appropriate support.

We recognize that some of these strategies require time that may not be compensated and is over and above direct clinical responsibilities, which can make it difficult to prioritize or schedule time devoted to collaboration and team development. However, as Ogland-Hand, and Zeiss (2000) note with respect to teams, attention to the collaborative process pays off. Team that develop a high level of effectiveness "become expert at using these processes to make decisions and get work done. At that point, the team members experience a sense of commitment and belonging and are well focused on their task." (p. 260)

Time and effort devoted in the short term may be time well spent in the long term, if future challenges are avoided or overcome more easily. We encourage you to consider what activities will build trust and support (i.e., meeting for lunch on a regular basis, facilitating social activities for the team, or planning a retreat) and to identify a preferred style of problem solving and ways of negotiating disagreements at the same time that you affirm what works well and where there are opportunities for improvement.

The narrative in Box 39.1 details several of the aforementioned contextual and process factors.

Patient/Family Narrative Comments

The patient/family narrative in Box 39.1 provides a glimpse at some of the contextual and process factors involved in effective collaboration throughout all stages of evaluation

---

Box 39.1
Patient/Family Narrative: Mr. Z.

Mr. Z. is an 88-year-old, Caucasian, married veteran, retired bank manager, atheist, and father of six adult children diagnosed with coronary artery disease, congestive heart failure, diabetes, and chronic pain. He was admitted to a 25-bed inpatient hospice and palliative care unit from home for extended respite while his wife recovers from back surgery. One of Mr. Z.'s sons has taken several months leave from his job out of state to help care for Mrs. Z.; in a telephone call with the social work fellow, he expressed caregiver fatigue related to his mother's situation and identified his own anxiety about his father returning home.

Upon initial interview with the social work fellow, Mr. Z. reports strain in his relationship with his children, identifying conflict, feelings of disappointment, and regret. He expresses doubt that his children would honor his wishes regarding his goals and plan of care, which includes his desire to return home with privately hired caregivers. Therefore, Mr. Z. has identified his wife as his primary durable power of attorney for health care and an alternate agent whom he describes as a "neutral business associate whom I trust to honor my wishes." However, Mr. Z. gave permission to contact his son who is caring for Mr. Z.'s wife. Mr. Z. also reports feeling frustrated about his declining physical function and increased dependence on others for activities of daily living and laments his diminished control over his situation.

Shortly after admission, Mr. Z. presents with intermittent periods of confusion and disorientation that was suspected to be delirium. A blood panel and urine analysis revealed a urinary tract infection, which resolved with antibiotics. However, Mr. Z. continued to evidence some mild cognitive impairment. The son expressed concern about these cognitive changes to the attending physician, implying that he thought the changes might preclude his father from returning home. The physician indicate to the son that she would ask the psychology fellow to evaluate Mr. Z.'s mental status.

In the interim, the social work fellow and psychology fellow met to discuss treatment planning and coordination of care, drawing on their respective assessments and observations from other team members. They identified the need for a formal cognitive and mood assessment and agreed to revisit possible intervention approaches once they had the results of their respective assessments. Given that the psychology fellow had extensive training in cognitive assessment, the social work and psychology fellow agreed that the psychology fellow would formally assess Mr. Z.'s cognitive function, share the results with the treatment team, and provide feedback to the patient and family. The social work fellow expressed interest in assessing Mr. Z.'s mood because she had clinical experience assessing mood in the context of physical illness and cognitive dysfunction and was in fact writing a manuscript on this topic. Both agreed that she would formally evaluate mood using a mood screen and diagnostic interview.

After presenting their plan at the palliative care team meeting, the physician indicated that she had told the family that the psychology fellow would be evaluating the patient and seemed to question the appropriateness of a social worker conducting a diagnostic interview. The psychology fellow thanked the physician for the referral while explaining the rationale for the decision and reaffirming the social work fellow's requisite competence, noting that mood assessment can be a skill of which both professionals.

Box 39.1 (*Contd.*)

Results of the neuropsychological screen indicated mild impairment in memory and abstraction that could be compensated for with the use of memory aids (e.g., written instructions/ reminders, memory notebook) and simple, concrete language. The mood assessment revealed elevated but subclinical depressive and anxiety symptoms, namely helplessness, worthlessness, dysphoria, anhedonia, and significant worry. The social work and psychology fellows met to discuss their respective findings and outline an integrated treatment plan based on differences in their individualized training and skill strengths as well as each clinician's time availability. As the psychology fellow had 50% dedicated time to the inpatient palliative care unit in comparison to the full-time social work fellow, they discussed how to best coordinate their schedules to follow up with Mr. Z. (e.g., to avoid "double booking" or too many visits on one day). The psychology fellow planned to provide feedback to the patient and family and discuss recommendations that capitalized on remaining strengths and compensated for impairments. The social work fellow planned to address depressive symptoms by using a combination of life review, behavioral activation/pleasant event scheduling, and cognitive restructuring; anxiety symptoms using a combination of supportive counseling (regarding fears, loss of control) and relaxation training; and family caregiver stress related to Mr. Z.'s desire to return home by facilitating communication around Mr. Z.'s goals of care and discharge planning.

They agreed to update one another regularly with phone calls after visits, to keep the larger treatment team abreast of their work, and to coordinate the education of the patient, family, and staff about the unique services they would offer in order to reduce the potential for confusion about roles. Each would speak with family members individually to provide updates while addressing related questions and concerns.

Despite these efforts, Mr. Z.'s son expressed to the social work fellow doubts about the findings from the neuropsychological assessment and subsequent conclusions. The social work fellow clarified his concerns, validated the difficulty of receiving the results, and offered to address these concerns in a joint meeting with the psychology fellow. The son agreed. In the meeting that followed, the psychology fellow nondefensively listened to the son's concerns, which after a lengthy discussion, seemed to reflect his lack of understanding of the psychology fellow's training in assessment as well as fears that the findings did not substantiate the son's perception that his father could not return home. The psychology fellow provided information to address his concerns and soon after, the son expressed doubts about the social work fellow's assessment of his father's mood. In examining these concerns and this repeated behavioral dynamic, it became clear that the son again was fearful of the implications of the assessment; that is, the findings did not agree with the son's assessment of his father's mood, and he worried that if Mr. Z. were to be discharged home, he would become clinically depressed with no easy access to treatment. The fellows inquired further to assess the reasons why the son thought his father was depressed and realized that he was misattributing some of his father's medical symptoms to depression. Interventions included psychoeducation, a review of the treatment plans, and brainstorming to identify ways that the son could build on the treatment plan at home. They also identified potential triggers and signs of worsening mood and a plan for responding,

including returning to the VA hospital for outpatient mental health care or pursuing community referrals. The fellows reflected the son's anxiety about his father returning home and reinforced his caregiving efforts, reassuring him that his father would not be discharged if the team determined he would be unsafe while at the same time underscoring the fact that the team had no such reservations at this time. The fellows also explored the possibility of obtaining additional support for both the son and his parents, acknowledging that their relationship had not always been easy, which can complicate caregiving.

and treatment planning. In this example, the social work and psychology fellows outlined the assessment and treatment needs of the patient and family, then divided the tasks based on the individual providers' skills and training, and time availability, while recognizing the overlap in who could provide what service. Although the social work and psychology fellows were comfortable with their care coordination and collaboration, the role overlap proved to be somewhat confusing to the family and care providers, as seen with the attending physician's assumption about who is qualified to conduct mood assessments. One strategy to avoid such confusion is to directly ask patients and family members, as well as team members, if they have questions regarding individual professionals' roles. This question can facilitate a conversation about overlapping skills and abilities and the benefits of collaboration.

Another challenge highlighted in this narrative, and in practice in general, is the possibility that patients or families will manipulate providers in order to feel in control of an overwhelming or frightening situation. We again emphasize the need for established rapport, trust, and communication in the relationship to best address the strain between professionals when such situations arise. Strategies for dealing with team splitting should be considered early as is demonstrated in the narrative by the social work and psychology fellows' decision to meet together with the son together.

Conclusion

Social workers and psychologists within the field of palliative care stand at an unprecedented juncture with the opportunity to join together in discovery of how their unique training, ethical codes, and histories as professions can infuse and inform collaboration for the future. We are not aware of any studies exploring the nature of this collaboration or measuring its effect on the care of patients and/or families.

In this chapter, we have argued that effective collaboration between palliative social workers and psychologists results in more comprehensive, improved psychosocial care. Collaboration is likely to be most effective when providers consider the influence of both (1) contextual factors, or characteristics of the context in which care is provided, and (2) process factors, or factors that influence the "work" of working together. In the words of Ira Byock, "By collaborating to care well for critically ill or injured patients and extend support for their families, the disciplines of ... palliative care can complete one another" (Byock, 2006, p. 420)

ADDITIONAL SUGGESTED READINGS

Abramson, J., & Rosenthal, B. (1995). Interdisciplinary and interorganizational collaboration. In A. Minahan (Ed.), *Encyclopedia of social work* (19th ed., Vol II, pp. 1479–1489). Silver Springs, MD: National Association of Social Workers.

Atwal, A. (2005). Do all health and social care professionals interact equally: A study of interactions in multidisciplinary teams in the United Kingdom. *Scandinavian Journal of Caring Sciences, 19,* 268–273.

Bronstein, L. R. (2003). A model for interdisciplinary collaboration. *Social Work, 46*(3), 297–306.

Corless, I., & Nicholas, P. (2004). The interdisciplinary team: An oxymoron? In J. Berzoff & P. Silverman (Eds.), *Living with dying: A handbook for health care practitioners* (pp. 161–170). New York, NY: Columbia University Press.

Crunkilton, D. D., & Rubins, V. D. (2009). Psychological distress in end-of-life care: A review of issues in assessment and treatment. *Journal of Social Work in End-of-Life and Palliative Care, 5,* 75–93.

D'Amour, D., Ferrada-Videla, M., Rodriguez, L. S. M., & Beaulieu, M. D. (2005). The conceptual basis for interprofessional collaboration: Core concepts and theoretical frameworks. *Journal of Interprofessional Care, 1,* 116–131.

Drinka, T. J., & Clark, P. G. (2000). *Health care teamwork: Interdisciplinary practice and teaching.* London, England: Auburn House.

Gardner, D. B. (2005). Ten lessons in collaboration. *OJIN: The Online Journal of Issues in Nursing, 10*(1), Retrieved from http://www.nursingworld.org/MainMenuCategories/ANAMarketplace/ANAPeriodicals/OJIN/TableofContents/Volume102005/No1Jan05/tpc26_116008.aspx

Hermsen, M. A., & Have, H. A. (2005). Palliative care teams: Effective through moral reflection. *Journal of Interprofessional Care, 19*(6), 561–568.

Hall, P. (2005). Interprofessional teamwork: Professional cultures as barriers. *Journal of Interprofessional Care, 1,* 188–196.

Higginson, I. J., Finlay, I. G., Goodwin, D. M., Hood, K., Edwards, A. G. K., Cook, A., ... Normand, C. E. (2003). Is there evidence that palliative care teams alter end-of-life experiences of patients and their caregivers? *Journal of Pain and Symptom Management, 25*(2), 150–168.

Jones, M. L. (1993). Role conflict: Cause of burnout or energizer. *Social Work, 38*(2), 136–141.

Junger, S., Pestinger, M., Elsner, F., Krumm, N., & Radbruch, L. (2007). Criteria for successful multiprofessional cooperation in palliative care teams. *Palliative Medicine, 21,* 347–354.

Karel, M. J., Smith, S., & Ogland-Hand, S. (2000). Training psychologists in long term care. In V. Molinari (Ed.), *Professional psychology in long term care* (pp. 349–371). New York, NY: Hatherleigh Press.

Lichtenberg, P. A. (1998). *Mental Health Practice in geriatric Health Care Settings.* New York, NY: Haworth Press.

Parker-Oliver, D., Bronstein, L. R., & Kurzejeski, L. (2005). Examining variables related to successful collaboration on the hospice team. *Health and Social Work, 30*(4), 279–286.

Reese, D. J., & Sontag, M (2001). Successful interprofessional collaboration on the hospice team. *Health and Social Work, 26,* 167–174.

Sheldon, F. M. (2000). Dimensions of the role of the social worker in palliative care. *Palliative Medicine, 14,* 491–498.

REFERENCES

Baggs, J. G., & Schmitt, M. H. (1997). Nurses' and resident physicians' perceptions of the process of collaboration in an MICU. *Research in Nursing and Health, 20,* 71–80.

Byock, I. (2006). Where do we go from here? A palliative care perspective. *Critical Care Medicine, 34*(11), 416–420.

Coleman, M. (2010). Enrolling in Medicare as a clinical social work provider. *NASW, (p 2),* Retrieved from: http://www.socialworkers.org/assets/secured/documents/practice/clinical/WKF-MISC-38710.ClinicalSW.pdf.

Martinez, J.A. (2006). Changing practice in hospice and palliative care: Recent changes and current issues. In P. Cowen & S. Moorhead (Eds.), *Current issues in nursing* (p. 196). Saint Louis, MO: Mosby, Inc.

Larson, D. G. (1993). *The helper's journey: Working with people facing grief, loss, and life-threatening illness.* Champaign, IL: Research Press.

Larson, E. (1999). The impact of physician-nurse interaction on patient care. *Holistic Nursing Practice, 13*(2), 38–46.

Lichtenberg, P. A., Smith, M., Frazer, D., Molinari, V., Rosowsky, E., Crose, R.,... Gallagher-Thompson, D. (1998). Standards for psychological services in long-term care facilities. *The Gerontologist, 38*(1), 122.

Lickiss, J. N., Turner, K. S., & Pollock, M. L. (2004). The interdisciplinary team. In D. Doyle, G. Hanks, N. I. Cherny, & K. Calman (Eds.), *Oxford textbook of palliative medicine* (3rd ed., pp. 42–46). New York, NY: Oxford University Press.

Meier, D. E., & Beresford, L. (2008). Social workers advocate for a seat at palliative care table. *Journal of Palliative Medicine, 11*(1), 10–14.

Ogland-Hand, S. M., & Zeiss, A. M. (2000). Interprofessional health care teams. In V. Molinari (Ed.), *Professional psychology in long term care* (pp. 257–277). New York, NY: Hatherleigh Press.

Oliver, D. P., & Peck, M. (2006). Inside the interdisciplinary: Team experiences of hospice social workers. *Journal of Social Work in End-of-Life and Palliative Care, 2*(3), 7–21.

Yeager, S. (2005). Interdisciplinary collaboration: The heart and soul of health care. *Critical Care Nursing Clinics of North America, 17,* 143–148.

Zeiss, A. M., & Gallagher-Thompson, D. (2003). Providing interdisciplinary geriatric team care: What does it really take. *Clinical Psychology: Science and Practice, 10,* 115–119.

Zeiss, A. M., & Steffen, A. M. (1996). Interdisciplinary health care teams: The basic unit of geriatric care. In L. L. Carstensen, B. A. Edelstein, & L. Dornbrand (Eds.), *The practical handbook of clinical gerontology* (pp. 423–450). Thousand Oaks, CA: Sage Publications.

Zeiss, A. M., & Steffen, A. M. (1998). Interdisciplinary health care teams in geriatrics: An international model. In A. S. Bellack & M. Hersen (Eds.) *Comprehensive clinical psychology: Clinical geropsychology* (Vol. 7, pp. 551–570). New York, NY: Elsevier Science.

Zwarenstein, M., Goldman, J., & Reeves, S. (2009). Interprofessional collaboration: Effects of practice-based interventions on professional practice and healthcare outcomes. *Cochrane Database of Systematic Review, 3.* Retrieved from http://www2.cochrane.org/reviews

40

 Laura Benson and Carolyn Messner

Social Work, Fund-Raising, and Philanthropy: It's Not Just about Money

I have always depended on the kindness of strangers.
—Blanche DuBois in the 1951 film adaptation of Tennessee Williams' play A Streetcar Named Desire

Key Concepts

- *This chapter will focus upon fund-raising and philanthropy in palliative social work.*
- *Emphasis will be placed upon cultivating key donors.*
- *The nuts and bolts of casting a wide net for donors and donations will be described.*
- *The importance of asking for funding as well as thanking funders will be highlighted.*
- *The authors will address philanthropic fund-raising.*
- *Ethical collaboration in fund-raising will be explicated.*

Introduction

Fund-raising has existed for thousands of years. In ancient Greece and Rome, people gathered money to provide food for the poor and homeless. During the eighteenth and nineteenth centuries, funds were continually raised for war efforts, as well as political and social endeavors. Universities, colleges, and religious and nonprofit institutions also rely heavily upon fund-raising tactics.

In palliative care, fund-raising provides support to enable the provision of a wide array of vitally important psychosocial care services for patients and their loved ones. It allows social workers to offer a host of practical, educational, and psychotherapeutic support services, as well as develop innovative programs to meet the changing needs of the palliative care population (Berzoff & Silverman, 2004; Boehm, 2006; Kash, Mago, & Kunkel, 2005). Philanthropic fund-raising insures the viability of organizations and departments and allows them to operate in ways that otherwise would not be fiscally possible (Bray, 2008; Edles, 2006; Preston, 2005).

Guiding Principles: "If You Don't Ask, You Won't Get"

Successful fund-raising is much like the work of providing palliative care. There are many different activities that you can undertake, but it only makes sense to provide the service that has the greatest impact on patient care. Fund-raising for your organization, much like patient care, is a continuous activity with ongoing assessments, evaluations, and adjustments along the way. This chapter offers some suggestions, hints, and tips that you can use in your efforts. It is written by an oncology nurse working in the pharmaceutical industry and an oncology social worker from a nonprofit institution as a model of interdisciplinary and institutional collaboration that is critically important in any fund-raising effort or appeal. The more members of the health care team as well as your institution's development, administrative, and fund-raising departments and donors that you can enlist to work with you on this endeavor, the greater its likelihood for success. Our hope is that you will tailor the recommendations provided in this chapter to your setting and circumstances.

The first major hurdle is to realize that *asking for help* in the form of donations and money might be outside your comfort zone. Many social workers find it difficult to ask for adequate funding for their projects. They are not taught the principles of fund-raising unless they major in administration. The majority of social workers are trained to provide direct service to patients and families. The fund-raising skill sets to sustain, grow, and develop programs, staff, and departments are not a major part of the generalist social work curriculum. But if you do not ask for help, donations, and services, you will never get anything (Burlingham, 1997; Desmet & Feinberg, 2003; Levy, 2008; Worley & Little, 2002, Yörük, 2009). The worst thing that someone can say is "no." In that spirit, forge ahead with the philosophy of "nothing ventured nothing gained." Learn how to describe the important work that you do and your ideas for new initiatives to others, so potential donors understand what you do that is so unique and invaluable to patients and their loved ones. Learn to sell what you do with compelling anecdotes that demonstrate the efficacy of your interventions. Individual as well as institutional donors often donate based on your ability to make what you do sound relevant to their interests (Bilodeau & Steinberg, 2006; Burnett, 2002; Fairfield & Wing, 2008). That being said, if you know that there is *no way* you will be able to perform the activities related to fund-raising, enlist the help of someone on your team who can. The viability of social work services in palliative care often depends upon collaboration, fiscal support, relationships with potential donors, and consistent acquisition of funds.

Make personal connections of all kinds and enlist others who are passionate about your cause (MacMillan, Money, & Downing, 2005)—for example, other health care professionals; families and friends of patients and former patients; national, state, and local businesses—especially those who provide goods and services to patients. Approach local pharmacies, durable equipment and homecare providers, taxi/car services, florists, restaurants, stationary stores, and grocers. Help potential donors to "connect the dots," and draw lines to how their involvement might impact their business (Cutlip, 1990; Mount, 1996). For example, pet care services might not be something that is associated with palliative care, but dog walking, kennel care, and pet respite might be things that a family dealing with serious illness might be interested in. Scouting groups can sometimes provide person power at tables and provide volunteer assistance at events. Social work training often does not provide the expertise and skill sets needed to ask for money from others to support their vital psychosocial delivery of services. Make a point of learning the art of fund-raising: take courses in fund-raising and public speaking, collaborate with the fund-raising department in your institution, consider getting an MBA, subscribe to fund-raising journals, and read about fund-raising strategies so that you acquire the skill sets needed.

Do not disregard someone you have approached because he or she has turned you down in the past (Grant et al., 2007). Keep and build a list of potential donors, create a database, and note each donor's specialties. Circumstances change over time. An appeal might be right the second, third, or fourth time you ask for help. Maintain a balance between being persistent and being a pest (Desmet & Feinberg, 2003; Greenfield, 2002).

Seek out a diverse pool of potential donors (Boland, 2009; Hager, Rooney, & Pollak, 2002). Cast a wide net when you seek to diversify your funding streams (Hruby & Marquardt, 2002; Pettey, 2001). Churches; schools; scouts; private, state, and federal charitable foundations; sisterhood and brotherhood organizations; unions; and any group known to become involved in local causes should not be overlooked.

Money is nice, but it is not the only form of donation (Rumsey & White, 2009; Sargeant, 2001). Potential donors may not be in a position to make a monetary contribution, but perhaps they can donate "gifts in kind"—goods and/or services. Donated items make great raffle items, are great for "goodie bags," or for use with patients in need. Consider pro bono work and other skilled services and donations of time. This is a great way to involve people who provide services such as legal work, advertising, financial planning, printing, and delivery and a path to enlisting volunteers into your palliative care service. A graphic designer or school might be able to develop a mailing, annual report, or advertisement that draws attention to your cause or event. It can save you time and money, and it can involve someone who might not otherwise have had a way to contribute (Hall, 2002).

Get to know your tax status. Understand if and when donations might be tax deductible, if you are a recognized charity, and what restrictions might apply (Lee, 2003; Rosen, 2005). Identify a person to turn to for the answers to these kinds of questions. This might be a great way to involve an attorney or tax consultant in pro bono work. Keep abreast of the latest regulations and rules regarding charitable donations (Beyel, 1997; Briscoe, 1994; Eikenberry, 2008). In recent years there has been an increase in government scrutiny in this area.

Understand what you can and cannot request from pharmaceutical companies, industry, and other corporate donors. Learn the art of negotiation, collaboration, and boundary setting. Educate industry partners about the standards of practice in palliative care, with a focus on enhanced delivery of care to patients, survivors, and caregivers. Social work practice adheres to a very thoughtful code of ethics, which serves social workers well in collaborating with funders. Become comfortable with the importance of seeking funding for your programs from diverse revenue streams. Collaborate with funders on the project's direction and focus to enhance patient care. Talk about constraints, your institution's fund-raising guidelines, ethics, and opportunities with your potential donors (Farr, 2002; Kidder, 2004). Most large companies have online request processes. Understand what they are looking for, how best to provide the information, and the nuances of each organization's request process. Know that for which you can, and just as important, cannot request funding. Ask questions for clarity.

Develop a relationship with your industry contacts and understand their priorities. Visualize how they fit into your organization's goals. Goals change over time. Invest the time and effort in building long-term relationships with potential donors (Cruz, 2008; Fairfield & Wing, 2008; Kay-Williams, 2000). Build your budget carefully. Most formal requests for funding to large organizations require the submission of a detailed proposal and budget (Chung & Shauver, 2008; Haas, 1998). It is important to factor in administrative costs and overhead to provide a clear and accurate picture of your fund-raising activities. Work collaboratively with your finance, administrative, and development departments.

Benchmark your organization. There are a number of Web sites that review the activities of charities (Kurzeja & Charheneau, 2000). They rank organizations based on their tax status, how much money is spent in administrative costs, and how much actually goes to patient services. Seek these sites out. Make sure their information is accurate. Every once in a while do an Internet search on your organization and see what pops up. Are you hard to find? Does the information portray your organization in a good or bad way? Can people figure out how to make a donation? Is that information readily available?

Get the message out. Build a mailing/contact/e-mail list and stay in touch with your donors and potential donors. Remind folks of the good work you do. Use the media to get your message out, including public service announcements (PSAs) for TV, local newspapers, and radio. Enlist the aid of your facility's public relations and communications departments (Burnett, 2002; Hall, 2002). Position your needs and events as public interest stories to increase coverage. Make them personal with local stories and anecdotes.

Do not rely on one medium alone. To cast a wide net, you need to consider all sorts of media to get your message out. Traditional paper-based mailings are good, but consider using e-mail and other ways of communicating. Use technology to your advantage. Social networking sites such as MySpace, Facebook, Twitter, and other viral media are important tools to use in staying connected and engaging new stakeholders (Comm & Burge, 2009; Gauba, 2009; Hart, 2002; Ingenhoff & Koelling, 2009; Sargeant, West, & Jay, 2007; Waters, Burnett, Lamm, & Lucas, 2009). Work with your Web teams to market the services that social work provides in the palliative care setting.

Don't forget to say "thank you" (Harmon, 2009). Find ways to memorialize/recognize people and donors (O'Neil, 2007). Examples include the following: a donation to a memory tree in your facility's lobby, a notice on your Web site, an article in a newsletter, names or logos on materials and tee shirts, or a personal thank-you letter for everyone who gives time, money, or gifts. Public recognition goes a very long way.

Make things fun! Although this might be work for you, volunteers are giving up their free time. Fund-raising is serious business and extremely important to you and your organization, but events should be inspiring, hopeful, and uplifting.

Lessons Learned

"Connectors, mavens, and salesman" (Gladwell, 2002) are key to all fund-raising efforts. They involve cultivation of relationships to key people who may not themselves give money but provide essential linkages to donors, foundations, and grants. Social workers in many ways are perfect fund-raisers, because they have excellent people skills and are adept at advocacy and working with others collegially to accomplish goals. Getting funding is another form of advocating—getting donors to support what you do. "Connectors" know lots of key people essential to getting support and are willing to introduce you to their connections. "Mavens" know a great deal more than most and are critically important in connecting with potential funding resources. "Salesmen" know how to market, sell, champion, and package your ideas to make them more fundable. A central theme that unites connectors, mavens, and salesmen is the passion they feel about the issues at hand. Their passion drives them to succeed and excel in their efforts. These three are a winning team to cultivate and grow the services you provide as well as innovate and conduct research. Fund-raising cannot be undertaken alone. To make it work, it is essential to enlist expert fund-raising colleagues, the interdisciplinary health care team, your colleagues, and a community of support from the large pool of potential donors. Given the changing needs of palliative care patients and their caregivers, it is the innovative social work staff, department, institution, and schools of social work that will be able to meet the future needs of this growing population (Messner, 2004).

ADDITIONAL RESOURCES
AND WEB SITES

Advancing Philanthropy: http://www.afpnet.org/
  Publications/?navItemNumber=506
The official journal of the Association of Fundraising Professionals,
  this bimonthly magazine contains how-to articles and reports
  on successful fundraising practice.
Crain Publications: http://www.crain.com/
An authoritative source of vital news and information to industry
  leaders and consumers. Weekly publications include Crain's
  Chicago Business, Cleveland Business, Detroit Business,
  Manchester Business, and New York Business.
The Foundation Center: http://foundationcenter.org/
A national nonprofit service organization recognized as the nation's
  leading authority on organized philanthropy, connecting
  nonprofits and the grant makers, supporting them with tools
  they can use and information they can trust.
Fundraising Success: http://www.fundraisingsuccessmag.com/

A magazine providing complete source for multichannel fund-
raising strategy and integration techniques.
The NonProfit Times: http://www.nptimes.com/
A leading business publication for nonprofit management.

REFERENCES

Berzoff, J., & Silverman, P. (2004). *Living with dying*. New York,
NY: Columbia University Press.
Beyel, J. (1997). Ethics and major gifts. *New Directions for
Philanthropic Fundraising, 16*, 49–59.
Bilodeau, M., & Steinberg, R. (2006). Donative nonprofit
organizations. *Handbook on the Economics of Giving,
Reciprocity and Altruism, 2*, 1271–1333.
Boehm, A. (2006). The involvement of social workers in
fundraising. *Journal of Social Science Research, 32*(3), 41–65.
Boland, J. (2009). Pulse. *Fundraising Success*. December, 2009.
p. 11–12.
Bray, I. (2008). *Effective fundraising for nonprofits: Real-world
strategies that work* .Berkeley, CA: Nolo.
Briscoe, M. (1994). Ethics and fundraising management. *New
Directions for Philanthropic Fundraising, 6*, 105–120.
Burlingame, D. F. (Ed.). (1997). *Critical issues in fund raising*.
New York, NY: John Wiley & Sons, Inc.
Burnett, K. (2002). *Relationship fundraising: A donor based
approach to the business of raising money*. San Francisco, CA:
Jossey-Bass.
Chung, K., & Shauver, M. (2008). Fundamental principles of
writing a successful grant proposal. *The Journal of Hand
Surgery, 33*(4), 566–572.
Comm, J., & Burge, K. (2009). *Twitter power*. Hoboken, NJ: John
Wiley & Sons, Inc.
Cruz, E. (2008, September 1). Framework; Fundraising for a cause.
BusinessWorld, p. S1/4.
Cutlip, S. (1990). Fund raising in the United States. *Society, 27*(3),
59–62.
Desmet, P., & Feinberg, F. (2003). Ask and ye shall receive: The
effect of the appeals scale on consumers' donation behavior.
Journal of Economic Psychology, 24(3), 349–376.
Edles, L. P. (2006). *Fundraising: Hands-on tactics for nonprofit
groups*. New York, NY: McGraw Hill.
Eikenberry, A. (2008). Fundraising in the new philanthropy
environment: The benefits and challenges of working with giving
circles. *Nonprofit Management and Leadership, 19*(2), 141–152.
Fairfield, K., & Wing, K. (2008). Collaboration in foundation
grantor-grantee relationships. *Nonprofit Management and
Leadership, 19*(1), 27–44.
Farr, L. (2002). Whose files are they anyway? Privacy issues for the
fundraising profession. *International Journal of Nonprofit and
Voluntary Sector Marketing, 7*(4), 361–367.
Gauba, R. (2009). The basics of online giving. *Fundraising Success*.
November, p. 18–19.
Gladwell, M. (2002). *The tipping point*. New York, NY: Little,
Brown and Company.
Grant, A., Campbell, E., Chen, G., Cottone, K., Lapedis, D., & Lee,
K. (2007). Impact and the art of motivation maintenance: The
effects of contact with beneficiaries on persistence behavior.
*Organizational Behavior and Human Decision Processes,
103*(1), 53–67.

Greenfield, J. (2002). *Fundraising fundamentals: A guide to annual
giving for professionals and volunteers*. New York, NY: Wiley.
Haas, M. (1998). How writers in nonprofit organizations develop
grant proposals. *New Directions for Philanthropic Fundraising,
22*, 49–58.
Hager, M., Rooney, P., & Pollak, T. (2002). How fundraising is
carried out in US nonprofit organizations. *International Journal
of Nonprofit and Voluntary Sector Marketing, 7*(4), 311–324.
Hall, M. (2002). Fundraising and public relations: A comparison of
programme concepts and characteristics. *International Journal
of Nonprofit and Voluntary Sector Marketing, 7*(4), 368–381.
Harmon, J. (2009). The fine (yet simple) art of "thank you."
Fundraising Success. November, p. 15
Hart, T. (2002). ePhilanthropy: Using the internet to build support.
*International Journal of Nonprofit and Voluntary Sector
Marketing, 7*(4), 353–360.
Hruby, L., & Marquardt, K. (2002). Cultivating diversity in
fundraising. *Chronicle of Philanthropy, 14*(7), 28.
Ingenhoff, D., & Koelling, M. (2009). The potential of Web sites as
a relationship building tool for charitable fundraising NPOs.
Public Relations Review, 35(1), 66–73.
Kash, K., Mago, R., & Kunkel, E. (2005). Psychosocial oncology:
Supportive care for the cancer patient. *Seminars in Oncology,
32*(2), 211–218.
Kay-Williams, S. (2000). The five stages of fundraising: A
framework for the development of fundraising. *International
Journal of Nonprofit and Voluntary Sector Marketing, 5*(3),
220–240.
Kidder, R. (2004). Foundation codes of ethics: Why do they matter,
what are they, and how are they relevant to philanthropy? *New
Directions for Philanthropic Fundraising, 45*, 75–83.
Kurzeja, K., & Charheneau, B. (2000, May). Need funding? Let the
net work for you! *Computers in Libraries*, 38–41.
Lee, S. (2003). The regulation of fundraising: In search of the
"public good" or an intractable problem of vested interest?
*International Journal of Nonprofit and Voluntary Sector
Marketing, 8*(4), 307–314.
Levy, R. (2008). *Yours for the asking*. Hoboken, NJ: John Wiley &
Sons, Inc.
MacMillan, K., Money, K., & Downing, S. (2005). Relationship
marketing in the not-for-profit sector: An extension and
application of the commitment-trust theory. *Journal of Business
Research, 58*(6), 806–818.
Messner, C. (2004). *Stories of innovation in oncology social work*.
Ann Arbor, MI: UMI: ProQuest.
Mount, J. (1996). Why donors give. *Nonprofit Management and
Leadership, 7*(1), 3–14.
O'Neil, J. (2007). The link between strong public relationships and
donor support. *Public Relations Review, 33*(1), 99–102.
Pettey, J. (2001). *Cultivating diversity in fundraising*. Hoboken, NJ:
John Wiley & Sons, Inc.
Preston, C. (2005). Effective fundraising for nonprofits: Real-world
strategies that work. *Chronicle of Philanthropy, 17*(14), 40.
Rosen, M. (2005). Doing well by doing right: A fundraiser's guide
to ethical decision-making. *International Journal of Nonprofit
and Voluntary Sector Marketing, 10*(3), 175–181.
Rumsey, G., & White, C. (2009). Strategic corporate philanthropic
relationships: Nonprofits' perceptions of benefits and corporate
motives. *Public Relations Review, 35*, 301–303.
Sargeant, A. (2001). Relationship fundraising: How to keep donors
loyal. *Nonprofit Management and Leadership, 12*(2), 177–192.

Sargeant, A., West, D., & Jay, E. (2007). The relational determinants of nonprofit Web site fundraising effectiveness: An exploratory study. *Nonprofit Management and Leadership, 18*(2), 141–156.

Waters, R., Burnett, E., Lamm, A., & Lucas, J. (2009). Engaging stakeholders through social networking: How nonprofit organizations are using Facebook. *Public Relations Review, 35*, 102–106.

Worley, D., &Little, J. (2002). The critical role of stewardship in fund raising: The Coaches vs. Cancer campaign. *Public Relations Review, 28*(1), 99–112.

Yörük, B. (2009). How responsive are charitable donors to requests to give? *Journal of Public Economics, 93*(9-10), 1111–1117.

41

Peter Beresford and Suzy Croft

Social Work, Self-Advocates, and Users of Palliative Care

I know that any changes that will be made as a result of what I say will probably come too late for me. I probably won't be here then. But for me, speaking up, giving my views, as someone who uses social work and palliative care, is a way I feel that I can pass something on. I can put something back. It is my bequest.

—*U. K. palliative care service user, 2004*

Key Concepts

- *Social work is being impacted internationally by a major new initiative related to self-advocacy, user or consumer involvement in the services people receive.*
- *Social work has been a pioneer of innovation in this field.*
- *This major development has begun to move forward into the context of palliative social work.*
- *Understanding the historical, policy, and the philosophical context will assist social workers to embrace collaboration with consumers of palliative care as a natural extension of the profession's commitment to advocacy.*
- *There are existing learning and positive experiences that provide a basis for moving forward to effectively engage consumers in the crafting of the palliative services to the benefit of recipients, practitioners, and policy makers.*

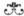

Introduction

Advocacy has always been a key aspect of the role of the social worker. This involves supporting people to achieve greater self-determination as well as to negotiate with other agencies. The global standards for professional social work education and training adopted by the International Federation of Social Workers (IFSW) and the International Association of Schools of Social Work (IASSW) highlight this. They include as core purposes of social work:

- Act with and/or for people to advocate for the formulation and targeted implementation of policies that are consistent with the ethical principles of the profession
- Act with and/or for people to advocate for changes in those policies and structural conditions that maintain people in marginalized, dispossessed, and vulnerable positions, and those that infringe upon the collective social harmony and stability of various ethnic groups, insofar as such stability does not violate human rights
- Encourage people to engage in advocacy with regard to pertinent local, national, regional, and/or international concerns
- An emphasis on the importance of advocacy and changes in sociostructural, political, and economic conditions that disempower, marginalize, and exclude people (IFSW & IASSW, 2004)

The idea and practice of advocacy have greatly enlarged internationally in recent years. Key to this has been the development of what has come to be known as "peer" or "self-advocacy." Self-advocacy means people speaking and acting on their own behalf, as well as gaining support from others through professional and legal advocacy. Self-advocacy takes both individual and collective forms, with people gaining skills and confidence to speak up for themselves as individuals as well as getting together to support their own empowerment and to work for broader social change. The emergence of self-advocacy is linked with a major development in modern societies, the growth of movements involving health and welfare service users. Such movements of disabled people, mental health service users, older people, and young people looked after in state care, those with learning difficulties and persons living with HIV/AIDS, and others have developed in different ways and at a different pace in countries around the world. They have, however, become international and indeed global developments, identified in both the Western and developing world.

This chapter reflects the professional and personal experience of one of the authors, Peter, who was a user of mental health services for 12 years and actively involved in the U.K. service user movement and its organizations at the local, national, and international levels. This has involved writing, researching, and campaigning for change from a "service user's" perspective. It is also a reminder that any of us may one day be users of social work services, including palliative care services.

The Growth of Service User Movements

The mobilization of health, welfare, and social care service user movements is a relatively recent development that can be traced to the last quarter of the twentieth century. It has led to major changes in ideas, culture, practice, and policy. Groups that had previously often been hidden have gained a greater individual as well as political and cultural presence in societies. In some countries, their viewpoints have begun to permeate mainstream discussion and developments (Aspis, 1997; Campbell & Oliver, 1996; Charlton, 1998; Coleridge, 1993; Morris, 1996; Oliver, 1993; Priestley, 1999). Each of these movements has its own particular history, character, culture, and traditions. However, they also seem to have some important things in common. All highlight the importance they attach to self-advocacy, people's human and civil rights, challenging discrimination, being part of mainstream life and communities, being able to take on responsibilities as well as securing entitlements, and having appropriate and adequate support with the proviso that they are able to exert greater choice and control (Beresford, 1999; Beresford & Harding, 1993; Campbell, 1996; Campbell & Oliver, 1996; Carter & Beresford, 2000). Some see them as "new social movements," and others see them as liberatory movements (Davis, 1993; Oliver, 1996; Oliver & Zarb, 1989; Shakespeare, 1993). Their members often identify with other new social movements, like the women's, black people's, and lesbian, gay, bisexual, and transgender movements, while user movement commentators and theoreticians focus on studying the relationships and links with these earlier movements (Campbell & Oliver, 1996; Morris, 1996).

Ideas of User Involvement

A new idea developed in public policy that is linked with the emergence of service user organizations and movements. This is the concept of user or consumer involvement. It has resonated with new public service ideas of the active citizen and public service consumer, which places an emphasis on individuals being able to play a more active role in services affecting them, rather than being passive recipients or claimants. There is no single meaning for service user/consumer involvement. It may have different meanings for different groups, at different times, in different countries. Terms like *partnership, engagement, self-advocacy,* and *participation* may be used rather than *user involvement.* Such user involvement, described in a variety of ways, can mean a wide range of things. It may mean the following:

- Consulting with and listening to what service users/consumers have to say
- Developing links with service user/consumer groups and organizations
- Involving service users/consumers in practice and policy organizations so these are better informed by them
- Encouraging service users/consumers individually and collectively to have more say over their lives and in services that they use
- Involving service users/consumers in "co-producing" policy and practice as a joint activity (Beresford & Croft, 1993)

User Involvement's Centrality in Social Work

These ideas have had particular resonance for social work, and in some countries the development of user involvement has been particularly advanced in this field. User involvement connects closely with and helps advance the goals and concerns of social work, as defined by the International Federation of Social Workers. These include promoting social justice, human rights, social change and people's empowerment, well-being, and social inclusion (IFSW, 2001).

Getting involved in service user/consumer organizations can help people solve the problems they face. It can enable them to gain new skills, greater self-confidence, and a better understanding of themselves. In this way it can offer a form of self-help that links with the positive goals of social work. Service users/consumers have placed an emphasis on the development of social approaches to understand and meet their rights and needs, like the "social model of disability." These reflect and reinforce the social and holistic approach of international social work. While such involvement is often particularly developed in more community-based and community-oriented social work approaches, it can also be very helpful in work with individuals and families.

Involvement and Advocacy in Palliative Care

Ideas of involvement and self-advocacy seem, however, to have been slow to come to palliative care. It is not difficult to see why. There have been concerns that people who may have little time left and many demands on it, and who may be experiencing discomfort and a range of symptoms would be unable and unwilling to play a more active role in their care. As the authors of one book summed it up in their title, they might well be "too ill to talk." They also raised ethical issues, fearing that patients and their families might be put under pressure to "get involved" at very difficult times (Small & Rhodes, 2000). There is also perhaps another issue at work, as *A Guide to Involving Patients, Carers, and the Public in Palliative Care and End of Life Care Services*, put it: "It was recognized that palliative and end-of-life care provision is very different from other parts of the care services. This is partly because there is a discomfort around discussing dying and death" (National Council for Palliative Care [NCPC] and National Health Service [NHS], 2008).

The report of the first national event in the United Kingdom, which brought together palliative care professionals and people with life-limiting illnesses and conditions who used such services, highlighted the value that service users placed on being more actively involved, even very near to the end of their lives, to improve the quality and suitability of services and support to meet their rights and needs (Beresford et al., 2000). What became clear was that if people were to be involved, then it would have to be done in ways which were as positive and comfortable as possible for participants. At this event, for example, sessions were short, there was a quiet room where people could rest and lie down if they wanted to, and nursing staff were on hand. Some participants were just a few weeks from the end of their lives, but they were able to make a valuable contribution from their unique perspective, based on "lived experience."

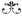

User Involvement and Collaboration with Palliative Social Work

Advocates and policy experts have identified three related constituencies in palliative care. These are people with life-limiting illnesses and conditions, those close to them and facing bereavement as family and friends, sometimes referred to as "carers" or caregivers, and the general public. In this chapter the focus is on collaboration of social workers with the first two groups, both of whom can be seen as palliative care service users, even though their needs may be different

and sometimes at odds with each other. Up to this point, involvement and engagement in palliative care have taken different forms. These include, for example, consultations and market research approaches to information gathering from patients and service users, helping to develop "stories" or "narratives" as well as enabling them to undertake creative activities to memorialize, share, and convey the meanings and accounts of their experiences (Gunaratnam & Oliviere, 2009; Jarrett, 2007). Social work has a long track record of seeking the views of service users and involving them (Meyer & Timms, 1970). As pioneers in the field of supporting individual and collective self-advocacy, social work has employed a wide range of approaches often interactive and participatory. Rather than simply seeking people's views, individuals have been actively engaged in activities and processes.

On an international level, within social work, there are four key areas in which service users, both individually and collectively, have begun to be involved:

- Social work education
- Social work practice
- Improving social work quality and standards
- Social work research and evaluation

Involvement in Education

In England, there is a requirement for service user and carer involvement in all aspects and all stages of qualifying and post-qualifying professional social work education. Thus, service users are involved in the recruitment of students and their assessment, in shaping the curriculum, and in teaching itself (Levin, 2004). A key criterion in the evaluation of a course is the nature and quality of such involvement (see Box 41.1).

Involvement in Practice

A picture emerged from a U.K. study of service users' experience of palliative social work practice that seemed to regard good practice as a participatory process—a kind of co-production between them and the people they worked with (Beresford, Adshead, & Croft, 2007). They sought to match their approach and interventions with the particular preferences and needs of individual service users. This could include individual case work, group work, or broader community-based approaches. It might also mean spending more time on a counseling approach or offering more practical support.

Involvement in Improving Quality

In recent years, there has been considerable policy emphasis internationally on improving quality and developing quality and performance indicators; targets; and standards in health,

---

Box 41.1

Service User Narrative: Getting Involved in Social Work Education: A Positive Experience

Mandy, a mother with a life-limiting illness, attends three sessions with social work students at one university and describes her experience.

We talked about the importance of user involvement and of listening to their views. I think it's important to help social workers see what things are like "from the other side." One of the students became my social worker for a while after she had qualified. She told me that the sessions were helpful because I would say things like how important it is for a service user that the social worker asks questions like, "How would you like this to be done?" or "How are things for you?" During the sessions I talked about what was really important to me—to have some "quality time," for example, help to go shopping for clothes for myself, and the students had never thought of things like that before. One student commented, "It helped me to see things differently." I enjoyed doing the sessions and because I am so obviously ill, but prepared to talk about those issues, it helped the students think about the importance of discussions about end of life. People want to talk about death and dying. I've got the chance of doing more training sessions in another university and would like to do it. I need to have goal posts to aim for and to keep busy. Keeping busy is what helps me (Mandy Paine, Member, Users and Carers Group, National Council for Palliative Care, 2009).

---

social work, and social care. Ideas have mainly come from policy makers, practitioners, and managers. They have tended to be managerially and bureaucratically based in inspiration and approach. We know that patients' and service users' concerns and priorities are not always the same as those of service providers. Quality and performance can mean very different things to the two groups. There is evolving pressure to include service users in both the development of quality standards and outcome measures and in evaluating and interpreting them. The work of Shaping Our Lives, the national independent user-controlled organization, on developing "user-defined" outcome measures has signified the beginnings of this process in the United Kingdom (*Shaping Our Lives*, 2003). It has made it possible to base social work on the standards that service users value (Harding & Beresford, 1996). The involvement of service users in palliative social work has provided an evidence base to take such a development forward, offering social workers insights into improving the quality of their practice, both how it is organized and how it is carried out.

Involvement in Research and Evaluation

There has been growing interest in user involvement in social work research from two key sources: first, service users themselves; and second, from social work researchers and research organizations (Kemshall & Littlechild, 2000). It is argued that such participation makes for better focused and better quality research, which is also likely to be more useful and effective (see Box 41.2). The Social Care Institute for Excellences, which has a responsibility in England to advance the knowledge base of social work and social care, places an emphasis on user knowledge and user involvement in research (Lowes & Hulatt, 2005). The 2008 research assessment exercise, which judged the quality of research in England, included user involvement as a key criterion of social work research quality. The U. K. government established an advisory body, *Involve*, which in 2009 published the findings of the first review of the impact of user involvement in research, which highlighted a wide range of positive effects (Staley, 2009).

Gains from Involvement and Supporting Self-Advocacy

Palliative social workers can engage with and involve service users as individuals, as groups, and as communities. Such involvement and engagement can be a way to reach out to groups who may historically have had less access to such social work support, for example, black and minority ethnic communities and people with learning difficulties (Gunaratnam, 2007). It can also be of great value to palliative social work itself. While social work's approach is strongly supportive of the holistic values underpinning the modern hospice movement, these continue to be vulnerable to powerful pressures toward the remedicalization of palliative and end-of-life care. Service users, however, make clear that they particularly value the social focus of palliative social work (see Box 41.3). They emphasize how helpful they find its concern with both the personal and the material; the individual, his or her social setting, and the relations between the two (Beresford et al., 2007).

Box 41.2

Getting Involved in Research: Research Narrative

A national research project in the United Kingdom studied service users' views of specialist palliative social work practice and how it could be improved. Two palliative care service users with life-limiting conditions were members of the advisory group that supported the project. Other groups of service users were formed locally to advise on progress and provide feedback as to how the research methods were working on a day-to-day basis. Some of these met more than once and had a rotating membership to respond to the deaths of those service users who had been involved and died during the course of the work. All these groups played an important part in shaping the final nature of the research project and ensuring that it was sensitive to the rights and needs of participating service users (Beresford et al., 2007).

Box 41.3
Group Narrative: A Group for Black African Women with HIV/AIDS

A hospice working with people with cancer, motor neuron disease, and HIV/AIDS attracted a growing number of black African women living with HIV/AIDS, some of them refugees and asylum seekers. They liked to participate in the hospice day center. They often felt that the men dominated things there and they did not have the space and opportunities they wanted. The social worker helped them to set up their own women's group, with their own time and place to meet. They felt that it gave them strength and confidence and made it "possible to be more involved in what happens to us and to have more control over our lives." They met at other times beyond the structured group and became involved in creative activities, collaborating with a playwright to perform a play that was broadcast on national radio. They felt the group gave support, practical help, the chance to learn from expert speakers, and helped them to empower themselves (Croft & the St John's Hospice Women's Group, 2007).

Box 41.4
Institutional Narrative: Involving Palliative Social Work Service Users in Planning for the Future

A voluntary hospice in a multiethnic city area was working out its development plans for the next 3 years. The social workers met with service users in advance to hear their views on what was needed for the future. Four service users participated and contributed to setting out their priorities for the future. Two were using the social work bereavement service. Another had both used the bereavement service and was a patient in her own right. One man living with HIV/AIDS used the day center as well as receiving social work support. They met with managers and other professionals offering detailed comments about the improvements they wanted to see and what they valued about hospice social work services. Their views were included in the report that fed into the development plan, and they were kept appraised of the evolving plans.

Developing New Skills

In the past, the length of time that social workers might be able to work with people with life-limiting illnesses and conditions could be short. As palliative care emerged to provides services along the continuum of life-threatening illness and medical innovations increased length of life, service users and their families might receive care over a correspondingly longer period with the expectation of improving quality of their life, and coping with and adapting to impending death and dying. This has important implications for user involvement. It strengthens the gains, as well as making user involvement more possible. It is now well established that user involvement can require new skills from both social work practitioners and service users. Working in a participatory way requires new ways of working (Beresford, Croft, Adshead, Walker, & Wilman, 2005).

Social work practitioners will need to learn both to overcome barriers and to discover successful ways of involving the wide range of service users they are likely to work with. Service users are also likely to need different skills and abilities if they are to make the most of opportunities to play a more active part in what happens to them and better shape their experience of services. In the United Kingdom, for example, there are now many courses and conferences where social workers can find out more about working in this way. At the same time, service users have come together locally and nationally in user groups, sometimes linked with palliative care services, sometimes with national bodies, building capacity, sharing new understandings, and identifying new skills.

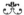

A Conclusion: The Importance of Evaluation

While user involvement has been welcomed as offering a positive route to enhancing palliative social work, we clearly need to know how to enhance effectiveness. This is highlighted in a guide to involvement in palliative care services:

Evaluation is a key phase in the palliative and end-of-life care public, patient involvement (PPI) wheel, but it is also the most challenging phase. Identifying the impact of involvement requires the use of a range of different outcome measures, including measures of patient and carer experience, which are not always simple to capture. Providing feedback to those who have been involved is the final phase of the wheel. The way in which organizations do this will influence how much trust and confidence patients, carers, and the public have and will also influence how prepared people are to continue to be involved in the future (NCPC & NHS, 2008, p. 5).

Evidence is now emerging about gains achieved through supporting the involvement of palliative care service users. Two research studies in cancer care in the United Kingdom have highlighted how this involvement can both be a positive for service users and providers (Cotterell, Morris, Harlow, Morris, & Beresford, 2009). User involvement can increase the insights of social workers, add to their knowledge base, extend the range of their practice and make it more effective, while improving the experience of service users and maximizing the support they receive (Beresford et al., 2007).

LEARNING EXERCISES

- *Involving service users.* The social workers in a palliative care service want to involve their service users more effectively. They contact a local disabled people's organization whose members assert the importance of making sure that involvement is a positive "zero-cost" activity, meaning that there is no financial, personal, and emotional or access burden or consequence to participants. What do you think could help make this so both for service users and the social workers involved?

As a first step, social workers discuss their goals and speak with individual palliative service users who consent to participate, including both people with life-limiting illnesses and those who are bereaved. These were some of the many options:

- Set up a "suggestions box"
- Put up a notice to bring attention to the idea of setting up a service user group
- Consult service users individually to check out what they find most helpful
- Design a questionnaire or checklist to do this
- Set up a meeting with interested service users, in a convenient, comfortable environment with pleasant refreshments
- Meet travel costs for people; offer child care
- Meet at times that are most convenient
- Provide advance information in an accessible and user-friendly way
- Let people know what can be done with their ideas and provide feedback
- Make clear how much it is valued
- Make sure there is absolutely no pressure on people to get involved

- *Enabling diverse involvement.* A community-based palliative social worker is concerned that her service is only reaching and engaging with the most "articulate" confident and assertive service users. She wants to be sure to be as inclusive as possible. What would help the social worker to ensure the involvement of such palliative care service users who would represent a wide range of views? The following groups have been identified as liable to be left out, "seldom-heard," or "hard to reach":

- People with learning difficulties
- Mental health service users
- People who do not communicate verbally
- Members of minority ethnic groups and communities
- People with experience of the criminal justice and prison system
- Homeless people
- People living in residential services

Improving access for seriously ill persons includes a commitment to enabling access and participation by providing the following:

- Physical and environmental accommodation so that people can be involved as easily as possible whether they have physical impairments or experience pain and discomfort
- Communication access, including use of interpreters, for those whose first language is other than the primary language of the clinicians or

institutions and those who use modalities such as sign language, picture language, and so forth
- Cultural respect and climate that is supportive of particular social and cultural needs and background

ADDITIONAL RESOURCES AND WEB SITES

SOCIAL WORK ORGANIZATIONS

The Association of Palliative Care Social Workers (United Kingdom): http://www.apcsw.org.uk/
Opened to qualified social workers, registered with the General Social Care Council, who work in a specialist palliative care setting.
The National Association of Social Workers (United States): http://www.socialworkers.org/research/naswResearch/EndofLifeCare/default.asp
The largest membership organization of professional social workers in the world, with 150,000 members. It works to enhance the professional growth of its members, to maintain professional standards, and to advance social policies.

PALLIATIVE CARE ORGANIZATIONS AND RESOURCES

The National Council for Palliative Care (United Kingdom): http://www.ncpc.org.uk/
The umbrella organization for all those who are involved in providing, commissioning, and using palliative care and hospice services in England, Wales, and Northern Ireland.
National Health Service (United Kingdom): End of Life Care Programme Web site: http://www.endoflifecare.nhs.uk/eolc
Aims to support the implementation of England's Department of Health's End of Life Care Strategy by sharing and providing health and social care staff information on a variety of aspects relating to end-of-life care.

WEB SITE ABOUT ARTWORK IN PALLIATIVE CARE

Rosetta Life: http://www.rosettalife.org
Artist-led residencies in hospices. This organization works in partnership with hospices and hospitals to deliver public artworks that create a voice for the palliative care community.
Shaping Our Lives National User Network (United Kingdom): http://www.shapingourlives.org.uk
An independent user-controlled organization, think tank, and network.

REFERENCES

Aspis, S. (1997). Self-advocacy for people with learning difficulties: Does it have a future? *Disability and Society, 12*(4), 647–654.

Beresford, P. (1999). Making participation possible: Movements of disabled people and psychiatric system survivors. In T. Jordan & A. Lent (Eds.), *Storming the millennium: The new politics of change* (pp. 34–50). London, England: Lawrence and Wishart.

Beresford, P., Broughton, F., Croft, S., Fouquet, S., Oliviere, D., & Rhodes, P. (2000). *Palliative care: Developing user involvement, improving quality*, Middlesex, England: Centre for Citizen Participation, Brunel University.

Beresford, P., Adshead, L., & Croft, S. (2007). *Palliative care, social work and service users: Making life possible*. London, England: Jessica Kingsley.

Beresford, P., Croft, S., Adshead, L., Walker, J., & Wilman, K. (2005). Involving service users in palliative care: From theory to practice. In P. Firth, G. Luff, & D. Oliviere (Eds.), *Loss, change and bereavement in palliative care* (pp. 119–132). Maidenhead, England: Open University Press.

Beresford, P., & Croft, S. (1993). *Citizen involvement: A practical guide for change*. Basingstoke, England: Macmillan.

Beresford, P., & Harding, T. (Eds.). (1993). *A Challenge to change: Practical experiences of building user led services*. London, England: National Institute for Social Work.

Campbell, J., & Oliver, M. (1996). *Disability politics: Understanding our past, changing our future*. Basingstoke, England; Macmillan.

Campbell, P. (1996). The history of the user movement in the United Kingdom. In T. Heller, J. Reynolds, R. Gomm, R. Muston, & S. Pattison (Eds.), *Mental health matters: A reader* (pp. 218–225). Basingstoke, England: Macmillan.

Carter, T., & Beresford, P. (2000). *Age and change: Models of involvement for older people*. York, England: York Publishing.

Charlton, J. I. (1998). *Nothing about us without us: Disability, oppression and empowerment*. CA: University of California Press.

Coleridge, P. (1993). *Disability, liberation and development*. Oxford, England: Oxfam in association with Action on Disability and Development.

Cotterell, P., Morris, S., Harlow, G., Morris, C., & Beresford, P. (2009). *Making user involvement effective: Lessons form cancer care*. London, England: Macmillan Cancer Support.

Croft, S., & The St John's Hospice Women's Support Group. (2007). The women's group. In L. Jarrett (Ed.), *Creative engagement in palliative care: New perspectives on user involvement* (pp. 89–93). Oxford, England: Radcliffe Publishing.

Davis, K. (1993). On the movement. In J. Swain, V. Finkelstein, S. French, & M. Oliver (Eds.), *Disabling barriers: Enabling environments* (pp. 285–293.). London, England: Sage in association with the Open University.

Gunaratnam, Y. (2007). Improving the quality of palliative care. Better health briefing 1. London, England: REU (Race Equality Unit).

Gunaratnam, Y., & Oliviere, D. (Eds.). (2009). *Narrative and stories in health care: Illness, dying and bereavement*. Oxford, England: Oxford University Press.

Harding, T., & Beresford, P. (Eds.), (1996). *The standards we expect: What service users and carers want from social services workers*. London, England: National Institute for Social Work.

International Federation of Social Workers (IFSW). (2001). *Definition of social work*. Retrieved from http://www.ifsw.org/en/p38000208.html

International Federation of Social Workers (IFSW) & International Association of Schools of Social Work (IASSW). (2004). *Core purposes of the social work profession*, Adopted at the General Assemblies of the IFSW and IASSW, Adelaide, Australia.

Jarrett, L. (Ed.). (2007). *Creative engagement in palliative care: New perspectives on user involvement*. Oxford, England, Radcliffe Publishing.

Kemshall, H., & Littlechild, R. (Eds.). (2000). *User involvement and participation in social care*. London, England: Jessica Kingsley.

Levin, E. (2004). *Common aims: A strategy to support user involvement in social work education*. London, England: Social Care Institute for Excellence.

Lowes, L., & Hulatt, I. (Eds.). (2005). *Involving service users in health and social care research*. London, England: Routledge.

Meyer, J. E., & Timms, N. (1970). *The client speaks: Working class impressions of casework*. London, England; Routledge.

Morris, J. (1996). *Encounters with strangers: Feminism and disability*. London, England: Women's Press.

National Council for Palliative Care/ National Health Service. (NCPC/NHS). (2008). *A guide to involving patients, carers and the public in palliative care and end of life care services*. London, England: National Council for Palliative Care and NHS National Centre for Involvement.

Oliver, M. (1993). *Social work with disabled people*. Basingstoke, England: Macmillan.

Oliver, M. (1996). *Understanding disability: From theory to practice*. Basingstoke, England: Macmillan.

Oliver, M., & Zarb, G. (1989). The politics of disability: A new approach. *Disability, Handicap and Society*, 4(3), 221–240.

Priestley, M. (1999). *Disability politics and community care*. London, England: Jessica Kingsley.

Shakespeare, T. (1993). Disabled people's self-organisation: A new social movement? *Disability, Handicap, and Society*, 8(3), 249–264.

Shaping Our Lives National User Network, Black User Group (West London), Ethnic Disabled Group Emerged (Manchester), Footprints and Waltham Forest Black Mental Health Service User Group (North London), & Service Users' Action Forum (Wakefield). (2003). *Shaping our lives–From outset to outcome: What people think of the social care services they use*. York, England: York Publishing.

Small, N., & Rhodes, P. (2000). *Too ill to talk. User involvement in palliative care*. London, England: Routledge.

Staley, K. (2009). *Exploring impact: Public involvement in NHS, public health and social care research*. Eastleigh, England: Involve.

42

 Maura Conry, Christopher M. Herndon, and Diane R. Jackson

Social Work and Pharmacy

My husband says I don't take my medications right. I don't know why I should have to take them because they cause too many side effects.

—Anonymous

Key Concepts

- ◆ *Social workers may be unaware of the role pharmacists play in palliative care, and the wide range of services they provide to enhance quality of life for clients.*
- ◆ *Consulting the readily available pharmacist is a direct, time-saving first step when medication related concerns are observed.*
- ◆ *This chapter describes a step-by-step process by which social workers may collaborate with pharmacists to streamline and coordinate care.*

Introduction

Palliative care is a dynamic process beginning at first diagnosis and proceeding through end-of-life care. The role of the social worker changes with every milestone as the client alternates between home, hospital, institution, and/or hospice. A social worker may initially engage a client at any stage in this process. Many clients refuse home care for long periods of time, seeking to manage independently. When services are requested, the social worker must coordinate a myriad of services focused on medical, emotional, family, community, and social service needs. Since pharmacy has not typically been included in the psychosocial evaluation as a medical resource, many social workers are unaware of the role of pharmacists in palliative care and the wide range of services pharmacists provide.

Nowhere are medication safety issues more urgent than in palliative care, where individuals at the end of life are possibly our most vulnerable client population. The need for medication accuracy and safety in palliative care can only be achieved with coordinated interdisciplinary efforts involving all members of the treatment team, including pharmacists (American Society of Health-Systems Pharmacists, 2002). Understanding medication-related problems, and how to solve them, becomes especially important for the social worker who may be the first professional encountered. Since the use of pharmaceuticals can be intense in palliative care, the imperative exists that social workers be able to interface with and utilize pharmacists as a readily available health care resource. This chapter provides social workers with an overview of the education and practice of pharmacy, models for collaboration, and recommendations for strengthening collaboration with pharmacists within interdisciplinary teams, as well as a step-by-step process by which social workers can help clients through increased collaboration (see Box 42.1).

Box 42.1
Patient/Family Narrative: Cecilia

Cecilia is a 68-year-old woman, presently hospitalized, who is nearing discharge. Cecilia and her husband have decided to refuse further disease-modifying treatment for metastatic lung cancer. Cecilia is determined to return to her home to be with her cat. The hospital social worker worked with the interdisciplinary team, including the pharmacist, and the family to facilitate discharge to home. The social worker reported to the pharmacist that she had learned from the patient's husband that Cecilia was not taking her medications regularly because she did not trust them, did not know what they were for, and thought they were giving her too many side effects. Prior to discharge, the team pharmacist provided medication counseling for the couple, dose adjustments to reduce side effects, and changed the medication schedule to make it easier for Cecilia and the family to remember. While Cecilia accepted her husband's assistance with medication management, she refused home health services but agreed to have a social worker visit her in a week for an assessment.

Barriers and Challenges to Collaboration between Social Workers and Pharmacists in Palliative Care

Professional barriers, for both social workers and pharmacists, include lack of knowledge of the training and expertise of the other profession, not understanding the professional jargon, and basic philosophical differences in their approaches to client care and treatment (Curran, Deacon, & Fleet, 2005). Professional stereotypes exist where social workers are thought of as "food stamp getters" and pharmacists as "pill counter merchants." These negative connotations can be reduced over time through formal education and interdisciplinary training. Social workers and pharmacists are often isolated from each other with limited opportunities for contact unless they proactively initiate them directly. Both professionals may feel intimidated or limited in their understanding of what the other does. Social workers may feel that it is out of their scope of care to even inquire about medications. Pharmacists may be reluctant to get too involved in the personal lives of clients or even fear opening a "Pandora's box" of emotions and personal issues.

For collaboration to occur, both professionals must agree that helping the client, reducing distress, and improving quality of life is the primary focus of their care. Professionals will need to understand and respect the benefits and treatment approaches of the other discipline. Professionals who embrace interdisciplinary client care will have one less obstacle to effective collaboration.

Social workers are trained to assess the client in his or her environment and intervene according to the assessed needs of the patient and family. They bring specific skills and knowledge in accessing community resources to resolve psychosocial–spiritual challenges to health care. They are

trained in communication, paying specific attention to nonverbal communication from the client, and cues from the environment (home, outpatient clinic, hospital) that may indicate barriers to effective palliative care. They often view non-adherence or medication misuse as behaviors that require assessment and inquiry as to the underlying beliefs, history, or fears that may influence patient and family attitudes and worries about medication. These skills are applicable to any palliative care setting, whether the home, long-term care facilities, institutions, or hospice.

Similarly, pharmacists have unique skill sets that lend themselves to the pharmacotherapy and other multidimensional issues frequently encountered by clients receiving palliative care (Thompson, 2008). Pharmacists, like social workers, have numerous different training environments, specialties, and practice settings. Most pharmacists have what is considered an entry-level professional degree. This may be a master of pharmacy (MPharm) degree in the European Union, doctor of pharmacy (PharmD) in the United States, or a diploma in pharmacy (DPharm) in India. It is important for social workers seeking to collaborate with pharmacists in their respective areas and practice settings to become familiar with the skills and knowledge base of the pharmacist available to them. While we might assume a basic skill set in these respective disciplines, a specialist-level skill set ought not to be assumed in either discipline. That said, basic skills all pharmacists should possess include medication record review for adherence assessment, anticipation of common adverse effects of medications, client education on the appropriate use of medications, and administration routes (see Box 42.2). Any pharmacist in any practice setting will likely have these basic minimum competencies. A growing number of pharmacists are becoming more specialized in clinical practice and may additionally possess the ability to diagnose and adjust pharmacotherapy in conjunction with a physician (American Society of Health-Systems Pharmacists, 2002). Pharmacists in these practice roles usually have additional training in the form of residencies, fellowships, apprenticeships, or advanced degrees. Credentialing or board certification in a specialized area may also provide the social worker with background on the pharmacist's abilities.

Practice Settings to Engage Pharmacists for Collaboration

Palliative care is provided to clients in a growing number of health care settings. Each of these settings may have a pharmacist responsible for the care of these clients. While not an exhaustive list, pharmacists are frequently available in hospitals, community pharmacies, specialized pharmacies serving hospice programs, and long-term care facilities. Given the setting the social worker's client is in may dictate the most appropriate pharmacist with whom to seek a collaborative

---

Box 42.2
Patient/Family Narrative: Cecilia at Home

A week later, the social worker makes a follow-up visit to the home. Cecilia left the hospital with a solid discharge plan in place with all medication problems resolved. During the in-home assessment, the social worker observes that prescription and non-prescription medications are everywhere. Cecilia has gone back to taking some of her old medications from different physicians and medications that were discontinued during Cecilia's hospitalization.

Polypharmacy, a common problem encountered in palliative care, may either refer to the sheer number of prescriptions taken simultaneously (oftentimes considered five to ten concurrent medications) or the use of prescriptions from more than one pharmacy or provider. Safe medication management requires a level of cognitive function and organizational skill that may deteriorate as the illness progresses. Until Cecilia is ready to allow home health or other in-home services, the social worker must discover available community pharmacy resources and guide the family to use them.

The first step is to understand the meaning of Cecilia's and her husband's behaviours related to medications. Are symptoms undertreated? Medications deemed ineffective? Are troubling side effects such as delirium being accurately or inaccurately attributed to medications? Is Cecilia struggling to regain independence in the marital relationship and using medications as a way to assert herself? This is a sampling of the social work assessment process that precedes decisions about interventions.

On a practical level to maximize safety and to enlist the pharmacist as a care partner, the family is encouraged to use a single pharmacy that ensures that all medications are in the same computer where drug interaction screens are done each time a prescription is filled. A pharmacist may easily transfer prescriptions from multiple pharmacies to one. No extra medical visits are required for this to occur. While using one pharmacy is easy to accomplish, selecting one pharmacist for care may be more difficult depending on the size and structure of the pharmacy. Smaller pharmacies may have just one or two pharmacists, making this process much easier. Additionally, ask what kind of additional educational or clinical services that pharmacy offers, such as specialty compounding, disease state group education, and one-on-one consultations with patients and caregivers.

In Cecilia's case, the social worker assisted the couple to choose a pharmacy that offered services that met the family's needs. Cecilia's husband brought a bag containing all of the prescription and non-prescription medications in the home to the pharmacy, where they were evaluated and organized for the family. The pharmacist transferred all prescriptions from other pharmacies to one place. This particular pharmacy had two pharmacists who rotated schedules, thus allowing a more consistent, ongoing support for Cecilia and her family throughout her care.

---

relationship. Unfortunately, most pharmacists do not cross practice settings for continuity of care, nor do they frequently communicate with pharmacists in the other areas. Examples of care settings, corresponding pharmacists available, and potential services are outlined in Table 42.1.

Opportunities for Social Work/Pharmacist Collaboration in Palliative Care

Networking with pharmacists is an invaluable resource for social workers who can benefit from their easy access, immediate problem solving, efficient physician interface, and medication counseling (Kilwein, 1991). Pharmacy is, by far, the most accessible of all the medical professions with most pharmacies open and staffed long hours (some 24 hours). Pharmacists interface with physicians throughout the day, and they are trained to evaluate and report medication problems to physicians for their patients as a standard part of daily practice. All clients who use prescription medications obtain them from pharmacists who are bound by law to assist with medication safety and counseling.

Pharmacists are particularly helpful when the social worker discovers a dangerous in-home situation called polypharmacy, which occurs when a client's prescription, non-prescription, over-the-counter drugs, home remedies, and health-store medicinal products are in confusion and disarray. Polypharmacy can, and all too often does, lead to accidental overdoses and medication emergencies which are on the rise. Pharmacists are trained to resolve chaotic polypharmacy situations to create clear, understandable, and safe medication regimens for their patients.

Social workers cannot ethically or legally make medication corrections on their own regardless of their level of perceived knowledge. When social workers call physicians directly with medication problems they can only report concerns from a social work perspective. Pharmacists, on the other hand, can consult physicians for new prescription orders; make changes in existing medications, dosages, and other medication-related issues while providing new medication at the same time. In most cases, calling the pharmacist is a rational, time-saving, first step. Consultation with pharmacists may save time, expense for the client, and potentially prevent further medical misadventures.

For these reasons, social workers will benefit from developing a network of pharmacist colleagues with whom collaboration is possible. Specific opportunities include transitions in care in which patient's medications may not be immediately available. Unfortunately there are numerous reports of pharmacies in specific areas failing to stock adequate supplies of opioids and other essential medications for the palliative care patient. Knowing which pharmacies frequently provide services to hospice organizations in the surrounding area may help avert a crisis due to lack of medication availability. Recommendations for requesting services from pharmacists are presented in Table 42.2 (Conry, 2001).

Table 42.1.
Settings for Collaborating with Pharmacists and Potential Services

Setting of Patient	Setting of Pharmacist	Triggers for Consultation	Services to Be Requested
Ambulatory or home health	• Community-based pharmacists	• Polypharmacy	• Review of all medications for potential drug interactions
	• Clinic-based pharmacists	• Multiple physicians	• Review of all medications for potential adverse effects
		• Multiple pharmacies	• Consolidation of all prescriptions to one pharmacy
		• Numerous non-prescription items and remedies	• Review and suggestion of lower cost alternatives when necessary
		• Suspected non- adherence issues • Medication expense	• Medication education for patient or caregiver
		• Concern regarding accessibility of medications from the pharmacy	• Provision of adherence tools and education (pill boxes, refill reminders, etc.)
Hospital	• Hospital pharmacists	• Home medication reconciliation	• Review home medication list for accuracy while inpatient • Review of medication list for drug interactions or adverse drug effects
	• Specialist pharmacists	• Discharge planning	• Discharge planning for continuation of appropriate medications, discontinuation of unnecessary medications, accessibility in community
		• Unresolved or unexpected symptoms or side effects	• Recommendations based on cost, efficacy, ease of adherence
Long Term Care Facilities (LTCF)	• Community-based pharmacists	• Unresolved or unexpected symptoms	• Review of patient chart for medication interactions or adverse effects
	• Consultant pharmacists	• Medication expense	• Recommendations for medication alteration for unresolved symptoms
		• Transitions: Are medication immediately available in receiving facility?	• Recommendations for discontinuation for unnecessary medications
Hospice	• Community-based pharmacists	• Unresolved or unexpected symptoms	• Recommendations for discontinuation of unnecessary medications
	• Consultant pharmacists	• Loss of usual administration route	• Review for potential medication interactions or adverse effects
	• Specialist pharmacists	• Suspected non-adherence issues	• Assistance with adherence / costs

Note: Community-based pharmacists are pharmacists who practice in a community, retail, or drugstore setting. Hospital pharmacists will usually practice as part of the general provision of medications to inpatients. Oftentimes specialist pharmacists will additionally work within the hospital environment in focused care areas such as pain management or palliative care. Consultant pharmacists are generally affiliated with a long-term care facility (LTCF), nursing home, or convalescent center. These pharmacists may be involved with the provision of medications, review of medication reconciliation records, and patient charts for identification of drug–drug or drug–disease interactions. In the United States, consultant pharmacists are required to review each LTCF patient's chart monthly.

Table 42.2.
Recommendations for Requesting Additional Services from Available Pharmacists

Medication counseling or education. Most pharmacists are willing and eager to educate patients and caregivers on prescription and nonprescription medications. Numerous studies link medication counseling with patient satisfaction and reduced symptom burden. It may take a patient advocate, such as the social worker, to request this service.

Educational materials. Pharmacists have easy-to-understand medication and disease information readily available, oftentimes in multilingual formats. This may be beneficial for the patient, the caregiver, and the social worker.

Adherence aids. Depending on the setting, pharmacists have adherence aids such as pill boxes to assist in the appropriate use of medications. Additionally, more advanced services are commonly available such as automated telephone call reminders for refills, Internet-based cellular phone text message reminders, and automatic refill and mailing. Pharmacies may offer a single-dose option called "blister packing," which is a form of a disposable pill box upon request.

Request pharmacist to simplify medication regimen. Complicated medication regimens make optimal patient outcomes difficult to achieve. If this is suspected, ask the pharmacist to recommend easier to administer options (i.e., once daily versus three or four times daily administration or once weekly for some medications).

Locate the specialist in your area of practice. Like social workers, oftentimes local pharmacists may gain advanced training in a particular area, such as pain management or palliative care. These individuals may serve as valuable resources when questions arise or more complex patient needs occur.

Conclusion

In summary, the social worker often through assessment, pain and symptom management interventions, and case management may identify problems before or as they arise in the palliative care population. Effective interdisciplinary collaboration is the centrepiece of every strong palliative care program, and pharmacist collaboration is a vital tool for achieving optimal client outcomes. By availing themselves of this resource, social workers may improve the quality of life and decrease the distress and symptom burden of their clients.

LEARNING EXERCISES

- Consider how many pharmacists you interact with regularly. How often do you utilize the recommendations from this chapter?
- Consider your last five to ten clients. Applying the recommendations from this chapter to those clients, list opportunities for each client in which a proactive collaboration with a pharmacist may have improved overall client care.
- A good learning exercise is to create medication safety in your own home first. Perhaps you have a chronically ill, or elderly, family member you could assist with medication safety?
- Consider the narrative of Cecilia and her husband. How might some of these problems have been overcome by engaging a pharmacist in this client's care? Using

Tables 42.1 and 42.2, develop a plan for collaborating with a pharmacist to address Cecilia's problems.

ADDITIONAL RESOURCES
AND WEB SITES

American Society of Consultant Pharmacists: http://www. seniorcarepharmacist.com
Offers patients and caregivers tips on safe medication use, information on polypharmacy, and a database to find consultant pharmacists in your area. Note that this searchable database is currently only available in Australia, Canada, Sweden, and the United States.
Case Management Society of America: http://www.cmsa.org
Provides guidelines and tools on assisting case managers on improving adherence to medication therapies.
Growth House: http://www.growthhouse.org
A wonderful resource for all professionals practicing in palliative care, several of the materials may assist the social worker in learning more about medications frequently used in palliative care.
International Association for Hospice and Palliative Care: http:// www.hospicecare.com
Provides a list of essential medicines used in palliative care.
National Council on Patient Information and Education: http://www.talkaboutrx.org
Provides both free and fee-based content on safe medication use.
National Network of Libraries of Medicine: http://www.nnlm.gov
Provides health, medical, and medication information for the consumer in over 10 different languages.
Needy Meds: http://www.needymeds.org
Provides consumers and social workers with access to additional prescription assistance programs and printable coupons for various prescription medications.

RX assist: http://www.rxassist.org
A Web site offered by a coalition of pharmaceutical companies to serve as a single source for patient assistance programs for those with difficulties obtaining medications due to financial challenges.

REFERENCES

American Society of Health-System Pharmacists. (2002). ASHP statement on the pharmacist's role in hospice and palliative care. *American Journal of Health-System Pharmacy, 59*(18), 1770–1773.

Conry, M. (2001). Your practice: Care teams provide model for community practice. *Geriatric Times, 2*(1), 21–25.

Curran, V. R., Deacon, D. R., & Fleet, L. (2005). Academic administrators' attitudes towards interprofessional education in Canadian schools of health professional education. *Journal of Interprofessional Care, 19*(Suppl. 1), 76–86.

Kilwein, J. H. (1991). Social workers in the community pharmacy: Why not? *American Pharmacist, NS31*(7), 60–61.

Thompson, C. A. (2008). Palliative care pharmacists consider patients' psychosocial issues. *American Journal of Health-System Pharmacy, 65*(6), 500–502.

43 *Ellen Goldring and Judith Solomon*

Social Work and Child Life: A Family's Journey with Childhood Cancer

Loss makes artists of us all as we weave new patterns in the fabric of our lives.
—*Greta W. Crosby*

Key Concepts

◆ *Family-centered care is at the core of effective psychosocial assessment and planning. The patient is assumed to be part of the family unit, and all members are assessed and worked with.*

◆ *Team collaboration emphasizes the unique role of each profession. The goal of the team is to ensure quality of life for the pediatric patient and his or her family coping with a life-threatening illness.*

◆ *Continuity of care allows the social worker and child life specialist to work with the patient/family in all units of the hospital, including inpatient and outpatient departments, from diagnosis to end of life, and bereavement, allowing professionals the opportunity to put into practice the components of palliative care.*

◆ *The social worker's role includes educating the medical/nursing staff about marginalized populations and its impact on patient and family's coping style to facilitate understanding, tolerance, and respect for the family and patient.*

◆ *The child life specialist focuses on the developmental needs of pediatric patients throughout all stages of treatment and therefore needs to be skilled in developmental interventions for the dying child or teen.*

◆ *Bereavement services offer the family the opportunity to share the impact of the loss and give the family the time they need to mourn with professionals who were connected to their child. Comfort is found in working with professionals who accompanied the family on their journey from diagnosis to death.*

The Interface of Social Work and Child Life in a Pediatric Oncology Setting

One of the most salient characteristics of pediatric oncology is the family-centered team approach. Beginning with the workup and diagnosis until the end of treatment and beyond, the interdisciplinary team provides expertise and helps children and their families receive the best medical care possible while learning to understand, accept, and cope with a life-threatening illness. Family-centered care has been described as follows: "Healthcare professionals who practice family-centered care tailor their approach to each patient and family. They respect differences, build on and seek to support each family's strengths, and help families secure the resources they need to compliment these strengths" (Bell, Johnson, Desai, & McLeod, 2009, p. 96). This definition serves as a guiding principle for the work of the social worker and child life specialist throughout the patient and family narrative, which is discussed on the following pages.

The social work profession has a long history of working with families. The work revolves around identifying the strengths of the family unit, focusing on their positive coping skills rather than focusing on their weaknesses. Social workers in a pediatric setting provide a safe, empathetic and supportive relationship within which parents are helped to identify their needs at stressful times and recognize the impact of their reactions on their children. Child life professionals are specifically trained to assess and meet the emotional needs of hospitalized children. Child life specialists focus on a child's strengths, optimize developmental levels, offer creative and play opportunities, prepare and accompany young patients to medical procedures, and help the child and family cope with their medical experiences. The child life specialist often models, for the parents, behaviors and skills that help to facilitate the child's adaptation to the hospital and to their illness and treatments (American Academy of Pediatrics, 2000).

It is thus appropriate for the professions of social work and child life to demonstrate the synergy of these disciplines through a patient and family narrative that exemplifies the principles of palliative care in a pediatric setting. The narrative in Box 43.1 describes the ongoing assessments that informed the work with a child and her family throughout the continuum of palliative care beginning at the day of her diagnosis at age 9 and spanning her treatment, posttreatment, school reentry, readjustment to "normal life," relapse, and end of life. Our work continues at the time of her death at age 14, as well as during the intense phase of bereavement. At this final stage, the social worker continued to provide a therapeutic relationship and support to the mother while the child life specialist/art therapist continued to provide therapy to the bereaved sibling. Weekly sessions revolved around the mother's extreme sadness and the void that Adrianna's death created in her life. Initially, the mother could only cry throughout the sessions, but eventually she began to verbalize her feelings, some of which related to childhood abandonment experiences that were reactivated by her child's death. Sessions with the sister focused on the intensity of the loss of her older sister and role model.

Box 43.1A
Patient/Family Narrative: Adriana and Family

I don't want her to become a grotesque monster on machines in a place where nobody knows us.

—Adriana's mother

At the time of initial diagnosis with T-cell acute lymphoblastic leukemia, Adriana was 9 years old. She transferred to our institution from another hospital in the city where the child and mother reside. The patient was the older of two children. Mother, Ms. Cruz, age 32, was a single parent, of Puerto Rican descent. She spoke English fluently and her daughters were raised in the United States. Ms. Cruz had recently begun to work, which allowed her to end her dependence on public assistance. She could not stay with the patient overnight because she had a younger child at home and had minimal extended family support. Ms. Cruz participated in meetings with the physician, nurse, and social worker. Early on she shared her concerns about signing consent for radiation and chemotherapy treatment. She had been informed that a secondary malignancy was a known potential side effect of one of the chemotherapy agents. She was also told about the dangers and side effects of cranial radiation. Her conflicts related to making difficult treatment decisions were exacerbated by the reality that Adriana's leukemia was aggressive in nature, and it needed to be treated accordingly. Although Ms. Cruz signed the consent, she would periodically share with the social worker the burden she felt for allowing the treatments that caused Adriana so much pain, discomfort, and isolation. Ms. Cruz alluded to a history of abuse by her mother as well as the father of her children. She had worked hard to remove herself and her daughters from these unhealthy relationships, and her job allowed her to care for herself and her family and be independent from those who abused her and from public assistance. Her abuse history made it difficult for her to form trusting relationships with adults, including the medical and psychosocial staff who reached out to Ms. Cruz consistently to discuss her daughter's care and foster mutual decision making. Eventually Ms. Cruz was able to trust the staff.

Adriana was often in the hospital for the next 2 years due to the aggressive nature of her illness and her treatment. Her mother would make short visits, because she was dependent on others for transportation and she lost income when she was unable to work. At times the staff would voice frustration that the mother could not be there for her daughter. The social worker advocated on Ms. Cruz's behalf, explaining the struggles that inner-city single parents face on a day-to-day basis (Livermore & Powers, 2006). Adriana would defend her mother, making up stories to tell the nurses about why she could not be present. Privately, in session, with child life specialist/creative arts therapist, she would voice ambivalence and anger toward her mother. This is a developmentally appropriate theme for adolescents who are working through their relationship with their parents. The added dependence that sometimes results from serious illness can compound this ambivalence and add to the complex feelings related both to illness and to the tasks of adolescence.

During treatment Adriana participated in music and art therapy sessions, which provided a forum for expression and gave her the opportunity to engage in developmentally appropriate activity not related to her illness (Councill, 2000). Adriana was unable to attend school; therefore, group creative arts sessions were one of her only sources of socialization.

Eventually, with much support from the physicians, nurses, social worker, and child life specialist, Adriana completed her medical treatment. After a lapse of 2 years, Adriana returned to school and faced a difficult transition. Due to learning challenges and missing so much school, Adriana was held back two grades. She struggled and found that she did not fit in with her classmates either academically or developmentally. The illness and treatment had taken a toll on the patient and family and had depleted them of much of their energy and resources. A school reentry visit was made to Adriana's school to help ease the transition. Members of the team met with faculty and students to increase their awareness and sensitivity to Adriana's needs. Eventually, life began to improve as the family adjusted to their old and new routines. Through supportive counseling, Ms. Cruz was able to continue her job and establish a supportive healthy relationship with a new partner. Adriana was still finding school work difficult, but she was adjusting to the school environment with the help of school reentry services provided by hospital staff. Her younger sibling appeared to be resuming age-appropriate activities, which had been curtailed because weekends revolved around Adrianna's illness. Also, living in an inner city, Ms. Cruz was comfortable with the two sisters going places together, but during Adrianna's treatment Ms. Cruz limited the younger daughter's outside activities. She did not want her on the streets of the city by herself. Now that Adrianna was home and feeling better they could go places together.

On a routine follow-up visit to the medical center, laboratory results determined that Adriana had leukemic blasts in her blood. She had developed a different type of leukemia, caused by a medication given during her initial treatment. Ms. Cruz's worst nightmare had come true. Her guilt about signing the original consent form resurfaced. However, this time, she had the support of a caring partner. She was frightened and needed the social worker's help in learning how to develop a healthy supportive relationship with a man. Previous relationships had been abusive, thus leaving Ms. Cruz fearful of being weakened and vulnerable to attack. Adriana also urged her mother to remain with her

Box 43.1A (*Contd.*)

boyfriend, demonstrating her desire to protect the future of the family unit.

Treatment options were explored, such as an unrelated donor bone marrow transplant in a distant hospital. However, chances of survival were small. This option was unacceptable to Ms. Cruz, who felt her child had suffered enough. "I don't want her to become a grotesque monster on machines in a place where nobody knows us." Ms. Cruz knew she was losing her daughter and knew they would need care from a team she had learned to trust. She decided to include Adriana, who was then 14 years old, in the decision-making process. While this is a principle recommended in the palliative care literature (Field & Behrman, 2003), Ms. Cruz intuitively understood the importance of engaging Adriana.

Palliative chemotherapy was offered and symptom management became the focus of her medical care. Simultaneously, great efforts were made to maximize quality of life and create meaningful and memorable experiences for the family. The social worker obtained financial assistance to send the family on a trip to Disney World and Adriana and her family traveled to Puerto Rico to visit with family members. This would be Adriana's last visit.

Psychosocial Team

The large majority of children with cancer are treated in pediatric oncology centers, which are located either in children's hospitals or in large university medical centers. Many of these pediatric oncology centers utilize the services of both social workers and child life specialists. Within our child life division, many staff members are also creative arts therapists. This additional training enables the child life team to integrate creative arts into their daily work with the children and teens, offering a variety of modalities for psychosocial care (Rode, 1995). These modalities include art, music, drama, and dance/movement therapies. In our setting, social workers focus primarily on the parents and the extended adult family members, while child life specialists focus on the patient and siblings. The unit of care is the family and each member is assigned a primary physician, nurse, social worker, and child life specialist. Psychologist and education liaisons are available as needed. This model allows us to develop treatment plans that are created by the entire psychosocial team. The treatment plan includes an integrated summary, which reviews medical information. Each member writes a summary of his or her assessment with sensitivity to cultural and spiritual issues; the goals, objectives, interventions, and outcomes are developed as a group. If a crisis or a medical change takes place, this team reviews the plan and makes necessary modifications. Should a child be coming to the end of life, the team reconvenes and develops an advanced illness treatment plan. In addition to these scheduled meetings, there are many less formal discussions. The social workers and child life specialists have developed a close collaboration that enables them to interact informally throughout the day, allowing for ongoing conversations that infuse the clinical work.

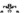

Child Life and Art Therapy

Both child life and art therapy were utilized with Adriana who was now an adolescent. "The essence of the child life intervention consists of establishing an intimate and therapeutic relationship with the adolescent" (Freyer et al., 2006, p. 705). For years, Adriana's life revolved around being a patient in the hospital; as a consequence, she was unable to meet the vital developmental need for socialization. Therefore, activities were scheduled to allow for fun, structure, and various kinds of nonmedical experiences. There were days when the child life specialist took Adriana to the hospital cafeteria for lunch or to the gift shop for an outing. She danced with the nurses in her hospital room and listened to favorite songs. If family were present, all participated in activities in an effort to create a familial atmosphere and replicate the family events that were not possible because of Adriana's long hospitalizations. These types of interventions are described in the child life literature. "For a child who is distressed because of the lack of appropriate developmental experiences, creatively arranging appropriate developmental activities may help. Child Life Specialists are expert at designing such interventions…" (McSherry, Kehoe, Carroll, Kang, & Rourke, 2007, p. 619).

Adriana requested and came to expect that the child life specialist would accompany her to most medical procedures. During the procedures, Adriana benefited from comforting behaviors such as having her hand held and being spoken to soothingly. Throughout Adriana's long hospital stays the child life specialist/creative arts therapist consistently provided art activities. Crafts were a favorite, providing a modality to enhance self-awareness and self-esteem while creating a product she could share with others. At other times she would allow herself to engage in more expressive art activities, using art supplies that would not necessarily ensure a finished product. Metaphor was a powerful tool for Adriana. She wrote and illustrated a book creating a fictional character with leukemia. The use of a cartoon character allowed Adriana to tell her own story from a distance, without being too overwhelmed by the painful emotions evoked. Choosing her diagnosis for her main character revealed her desire to process feelings. The creation of a mask allowed for an ongoing creative process, filled with imaginative inspirations. Initially she painted the mask with typical images, rainbow, clouds, and stars. But as the finished product emerged she painted tears on the mask, naming it the "Sad Voodoo Clown." This clown was crying for all the sick children in the world and was going to become a doctor to save them.

Art therapy can serve as a conduit for expressing overwhelming or repressed feelings and emotions that might be threatening to the individual (Jones & Weisenfluh, 2003). As her medical condition deteriorated, Adriana became more guarded about her sad feelings, but art provided a means of releasing intense emotions. Art was also used to strengthen the sibling bond by joint sessions with both sisters. In one session they made masks on each other's faces. Adriana's sister was able to tenderly show her affection by placing the petroleum jelly and wet plaster strips on her bed-ridden sister's face. Adriana was able to relax with this care and sisterly trust was shared. Continued art therapy sessions allowed Adriana to express herself through symbols without challenging her sense of hope, as in designing her perfect hospital room, which became a metaphor for positive change as well as a focus for the expression of complex feelings related to spending so much time in the hospital. Although given a choice of colors, Adriana chose to paint her fantasy hospital room deep colors of purple, red, and black, giving it a sense of enclosure and hinting at her impending death. The red emergency button she placed above the bed seemed to represent her desire to have access to staff in case she became overwhelmed with loneliness, fear, or pain (Rode, 1995).

End of Life and Bereavement

The following is an example of collaboration of social work and child life to meet the needs of a dying child and her family.

Box 43.1B
Patient/Family Narrative: Adriana and Family (continued)

How long will it take to get my wings?

—Adriana

As Adriana's disease progressed, she experienced more pain and required increasing doses of pain medications. The nursing staff was uncomfortable administering these doses of opioid medications, fearing that they may cause respiratory depression and hasten Adriana's death. The social worker and child life specialist brought this to the attention of the primary oncologist, who readily approached the nursing staff and care team to have an open discussion about the clinical, emotional, and ethical issues related to medications at the end of life, pain and suffering of the patient and family, and also the staff who were caring for a dying child they had cared for over an extended period of time. This discussion affirmed the impact of the impending death of a child who had been under their care for the past 5 years. "Professionals caring for children have special responsibilities for educating themselves and others about the identification, management, and discussion of the last phase of a child's fatal medical problem" (Institute of Medicine, 2003, p. 7).

As it became clear that the palliative treatment being offered was no longer producing any benefit, the focus of our interventions changed to preparation for end of life. According to Kane and Primomo (2001, p165), "the dying process calls for a shift in paradigm in the minds and hearts of the caregivers, a shift necessary to fulfill the needs of the terminally-ill child and his or her family." Before she became too weak, a shopping spree at the mall, funded by Make a Wish Foundation, took place. Adriana brought gifts for family and friends as a long-lasting confirmation

of their relationship. This served two important purposes for Adriana and her family, as the intervention was able "to restore her sense of personal integrity, dignity, autonomy, self-mastery and self-control" while also serving "to strengthen interpersonal relationships so that they may feel connected and part of each other"(Kane & Primomo, 2001, p. 166).

Adriana began making collages, using family photos. The entire family participated in designing these large collages, filled with images of special days, creating memories for the family to keep. Adriana took on the leadership role in making these collages, once again, recognizing her family's suffering and guiding them to participate in a ritual that acknowledges her impending death. She encouraged her mother to take on the important role of bringing in the photographs. She directed the child life specialist and art therapist to bring art supplies and frames, to ensure completion and permanence.

As Adriana became more ill and her pain increased, she and her mother spoke about her death and her becoming an angel. Although chronologically she was an adolescent, she was cognitively and affectively presenting as a latency age child. According to Jones and Weisenfluh, (2003) her responses reflected the coping style of a 6–11 year old, a developmental delay attributed to her illness and long hospitalizations. Cognitively Adriana comprehended her death in a very concrete manner, as reflected in her question to her mother, "How long will it take to get my wings?" This hopeful image may have also helped her cope with what might have been frightening and overwhelming feelings (Jones & Weisenfluh, 2003).

Books about death were introduced by the child life specialist and became a helpful therapeutic tool. One of her favorites described a caterpillar becoming a butterfly. Transitioning to a new life form seemed to be a reassuring image for Adriana, helping her to accept this final stage. As she came closer to the end of her life, pain control became more of a concern and radiation was offered as a palliative intervention. During these treatments the child life specialist would stay with Adriana before and after radiation. In line with Freyer et al. (2006), who emphasized the importance "of establishing and keeping an intimate and therapeutic relationship" with the child life specialist, the therapeutic alliance was maintained in differing ways throughout the progression of the disease. As Adriana's medical condition worsened, the intravenous pain medications compromised her ability to communicate, but she was able to squeeze the child life specialist's hand when she experienced pain and squeezing of the hand thus became a symbol of their recognition of one another.

Adriana lived longer than the medical staff had anticipated and her mother was able to be present with her during this last stage of life. Ms. Cruz's presence helped change the staff's perception of her as a mother. It was difficult for the nursing staff to understand why a mother would not be more present during her child's hospitalizations. Ms. Cruz believed that Adriana hung on purposely to help the staff understand her mother in a different way, and others believed that she hung on until she was convinced that her mother's relationship with her significant other was strong enough to survive her death. Yet others believed that she died when her heart could no longer sustain her life. Social work interventions included assuring the patient that she would continue to help and support her mother and family after her death. The social worker and mother's partner were present in the

Box 43.1B (*Contd.*)

room at the time this patient took her last breath. Ms. Cruz had briefly stepped out of the room and the social worker had just arrived. Perhaps this fulfilled Adriana's wishes to protect her mother, knowing that she would be taken care of by the social worker and boyfriend.

Ms. Cruz met with the social worker for weekly bereavement sessions and the child life specialist met with the sister, continuing to work together using art as the therapeutic modality. This bereavement plan was designed to maintain relationships to provide a continuum of family-centered care after the death. Both the mother and sister's mourning processes were complicated due to the history of abuse and loss, and they were eventually referred to bereavement mental health specialists. The social worker and child life specialist continued to remain available for support.

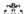

Conclusion

The communication among team members involved in the care of pediatric oncology patients and the day-to-day work of these teams is congruent with the definition of palliative care (Feudtner, 2007). At the time that this patient was treated, the literature on palliative care was sparse. We were, however, utilizing many of the basic tenets of this philosophy of care from the day of diagnosis and throughout treatment, including end of life and bereavement. Our model of care described in the patient family narrative is an example of how the social work and child life professions join with the medical team to support patient and family as they make decisions and enhance quality of life and relationships along the continuum of illness and through end of life. The trusting relationships developed during this period of time afforded us the opportunity to continue to help Adriana's mother and sister in their grief and bereavement processes. Ms. Cruz needed her own clinical support as she shared her life story and faced both her economic challenges and the serious illness of her daughter. These needs were addressed by her social worker. Adriana needed a professional who could travel with her during hospitalizations, understand her developmental needs, and support her through difficult times, especially since family could not always be present. The child life specialist met these needs. Because each member of the family had his or her own therapist, each was provided an opportunity to express feelings freely and be comforted by the knowledge that the others were being cared for. Our model, which was utilized throughout the continuum of care, allowed for ongoing assessments of family dynamics and the practice of "medicine with a heart" (Feudtner, 2007).

Many years have passed since we worked with Adriana and her family, yet this narrative continues to resonate. The conceptual framework of palliative care was in its early phase, but we drew from our professional training to implement what would become the basic tenets of palliative care. For us,

this patient/family narrative remains a model paradigm of interdisciplinary pediatric palliative care. Through the eyes of time we reflect that it was a willingness to share information and process our emotions that fostered growth as professionals and enhanced the interface of our disciplines.

We are grateful to the openness and resiliency of this patient and family who allowed us to journey with them. We thank the nurses, who remain role models of medical care with compassion. We are also appreciative of our medical director, who had the vision to employ both social workers and child life specialists and gave us the opportunity to provide in-depth ongoing palliative care services.

LEARNING EXERCISE

The following is a summary of the clinical issues and interventions used in the care of Adriana and her family. Consider a setting where you are the social worker and do not have the benefit of working collaboratively with a child life specialist. Imagine how this process would change; how would you complement and adapt your services in an effort to provide the most comprehensive care for Adriana and her family?

PRINCIPLES, CLINICAL ISSUES, AND INTERVENTIONS

- Family-centered care:

    Patient and family are part of the care team
    Psychosocial treatment plan for family

    Interventions: Inclusion of parents and patient in discussions about care

    Each family member is assigned to a child life specialist and social worker
    Rounding on inpatient unit

- Collaborative team approach

    Formal and informal collaborative meetings of psychosocial and medical staff
    Psychosocial treatment plan for family

    Interventions: Weekly patient care meeting of entire team

    Psychosocial team planning
    Rounding on inpatient unit

- Continuity of care

    Primary care team assigned upon diagnosis, through treatment, off treatment follow-up, end of life, bereavement
    Seamless care including outpatient, inpatient, and community

    Interventions: Follow patient on the continuum of care

Support through treatment transitions

- Compassionate care

    Preserving dignity of patient and family

    Interventions: Respect for patient and family as individuals

- Decision making

    Patient and family are part of the care team

    Interventions: Explore meaning of choices

    Support patient/family decisions

- Cultural competency

    Socioeconomic factors

    Single-parent families

    Interventions: Reducing biases

    Education of staff

- Developmental assessment of patient

    Cognitive

    Emotional

    Affective

    Social

    Interventions: Child Life Assessment Tools

- Provision of opportunities for expression for patient and family

    Interventions:

        Creative arts

        Individual sessions

        Family or group sessions

- Effective pain management

    Interventions:

        Assessment of pain needs

        Explore options

        Support of patient, family, and staff

        Child life and creative arts as distraction and relaxation

- End-of-life care

    Entering and living during the terminal phase
    Interventions:

        Wish fulfillment

        Art therapy

        Child life support

        Anticipatory grief counseling

        Sibling support

        Multidisciplinary psychoeducation about death process

- Bereavement

    Final separation and living with loss

        Interventions:
        Funeral arrangements
        Grief and loss counseling for family

    Art therapy

ADDITIONAL SUGGESTED READINGS

American Academy of Pediatrics. (2000). Palliative care for children. *Pediatrics, 106*(2), 351–357.

Corr, C. A., & Balk, D. E. (1996). *Handbook of adolescent death and bereavement.* New York, NY: Springer Publishing Company.

Jones, B. L. (2005). Pediatric palliative and end-of-life care: The role of social work in pediatric oncology. *Journal of Social Work in End-of-Life & Palliative Care, 1*(4), 35–62.

REFERENCES

American Academy of Pediatrics. (2000). Child life services. *Pediatrics, 106*(5), 1156–1159.

Bell, J., Johnson, B., Desai, P., & McLeod, S. (2009). Family-centered care and the implications for child life practice. In R. Thompson (Ed.). *The handbook of child life: A guide for pediatric psychosocial care* (pp. 95–115). Springfield, IL: Charles C. Thomas Publisher, Ltd.

Councill, T. (2000). Art therapy with pediatric cancer patients. In C. Malchiodi (Ed.), *Medical art therapy with children* (pp. 75–93). Philadelphia, PA: Jessica Kingsley Publishers Ltd.

De Graves, S., & Aranda, S. (2005). When a child cannot be cured–reflections of health professionals. *European Journal of Cancer Care, 14*(2), 132–140.

Feudtner, C. (2007). Collaborative communication in pediatric palliative care: A foundation for problem-solving and decision-making. *Pediatric Clinics of North America, 54*(5), 583–607.

Field, M. J., & Behrman, R. E. (2003). When children die: Improving palliative and end-of-life care for children and their families. Washington, DC: The National Academies Press.

Freyer, D. R., Kuperberg A., Sterken, D. J., Pastyrnak, S. L., Hudson, D., & Richards, T. (2006). Multidisciplinary care of the dying adolescent. *Child and Adolescent Psychiatric Clinics of North America, 15*(3), 693–715.

Jones, B., & Weisenfluh S. (2003). Pediatric palliative and end-of-life care: Developmental and spiritual issues of dying children. *Smith College Studies in Social Work, 73*(3), 423–443.

Kane, J. R., & Primomo, M. (2001). Alleviating the suffering of seriously ill children, American *Journal of Hospice and Palliative Care, 18*(3), 161–169.

Livermore, M., & Powers, R. (2006). Unfulfilled plans and financial stress: Unwed mothers and unemployment. *Journal of Human Behavior in the Social Environment, 13*(1), 1–17.

McSherry, M., Kehoe, K., Carroll, J. M., Kang, T. I., & Rourke, M. T. (2007). Psychosocial and spiritual needs of children living with a life-limiting illness. *Pediatric Clinics of North America, 54*(4), 609–629.

Petersen, M. F., Cohen J., & Parsons V. (2004). Family-centered care: Do we practice what we preach? *Journal of Obstetric, Gynecologic, and Neonatal Nursing, 33*(4), 421–427.

Rode, D. C. (1995). Building bridges within the culture of pediatric medicaine: The interface of art therapy and cild life programming. *Art Therapy: Journal of the American Art Therapy Association,12*(2), 104–110.

44

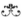 *Jimmie C. Holland and Anne Martin*

Social Work and Psychiatry

In trying to get my thoughts together about what makes treatment at your hospital special, the phrase that keeps coming to mind is the "team approach."
— *R. C., reflecting on her husband's psychosocial care after his treatment and death*

Key Concepts

- ◆ *Historical perspective of social work/psychiatry collaboration*
- ◆ *Creating a structure of collaboration within an institution*
- ◆ *Professional challenges in collaboration*
- ◆ *Benefits of collaboration on patient care*

Historical Perspective

The field of oncology provides an example of collaboration that has its roots in the very beginning of formal psychosocial care and research with the birth of psychosocial oncology. In the 1950s, the staff of a very few institutions in the United States were formally exploring the psychological impact of cancer on patients and their families. At the Massachusetts General Hospital, Ruth Abrams was a social work pioneer working with psychiatrist Jacob Finesinger, reporting on patient's guilt reactions related to the shame and sigma of a cancer diagnosis (Abrams & Fenesinger, 1953). She also collaborated with Finesinger on a description of the psychological mechanisms of patients (Shands, Finesinger, Cobb, & Abrams, 1951).

Another institution making early contributions to oncology through social work and psychiatry was Memorial Sloan Kettering Cancer Center (MSKCC), providing a collaborative model that continues almost 60 years later. Led by psychiatrist A. O. C. Sutherland, a crucial member of this clinical and research unit was social worker Ruth Dyk. The team wrote the classical papers on patients' response to mastectomy and colostomy and on mothers' reactions to their child's fatal illness (Sutherland, Orbach, Dyk, & Bard, 1952).

It has been an honor and privilege to continue the tradition of these two outstanding teams, with the added advantage today of greater attention to and understanding of the "science of care." This chapter builds on the potential implicit in the Memorial model and reflects our obligation and indebtedness to these strong, professional roots.

Introduction

Provision of health care along the continuum of illness and at the end of life requires effective collaboration among all clinical professionals, but especially social work and psychiatry. Regular conferences, clear patient plans, respect for the roles of other disciplines, and cross-training and education are components of this quality care (Mitchell & Crittenden, 2000).

Clinical interventions that involve medication management, psychological counselling, and practical services fall under the specific responsibility and are best served by a psychosocial team ideally mandated at the institutional and leadership level. Although an institutional mandate to set up specific collaborative structures is not always possible, the model for collaboration outlined in this chapter can be implemented into already existing structures within other institutions. At Memorial, social work and psychiatry have traditionally collaborated on an individual level. As with any relationship, there are struggles, conflicts, and a political history that carry the potential to impede forward motion. The solution from our standpoint is to identify the appropriate structure and place the provision of quality patient care as the core objective. Will this model eliminate all of potential problems and conflicts? Of course not: There are certain individuals and groups that will never be able to subsume their own needs for the sake of the larger objective, but attempting collaboration while holding on to past grievances and stereotypes tends to create the assumed outcome. In the course of development of this model at Memorial, there was doubt and cynicism about the efficacy of the effort, even though each department was aware of the benefits to patients and professional staff alike. And in truth this model has not worked equally well on every service. Collaboration will fail without a basic level of professional respect, openness to experiences beyond the stereotype of the other, and a dedication to the larger goal. But the success of this model on multiple Memorial services has demonstrated that even with initial mistrust, psychosocial collaboration maximizes our ability to provide the highest possible level of palliative care. We are grateful that the Memorial model described in this chapter was developed and nurtured by the leaders of social work and psychiatry with the enthusiastic sanction of the hospital's physician-in-chief.

Memorial Sloan Kettering Cancer Center Collaborative Model

The MSKCC model has four components: psychosocial care teams (PCTs); specialized clinical case conferences; research collaboration; and educational collaboration.

Psychosocial Care Teams

Psychosocial care teams were created to provide a structure that assumed productive collaboration among supportive care disciplines. The PCTs are comprised of social workers, a psychologist, a psychiatrist, a nurse, a chaplain, relevant ancillary staff, and physicians as appropriate. Regular conferences are held, depending on the needs of each service, to discuss clinical cases that demand close collaboration of team members. These teams target, most specifically, patients at the end of life and those with complex psychosocial circumstances or

difficult ethical dilemmas. The teams have been effective in focusing attention on important patient transitions by eliminating redundancies in care and creating a consistent, agreed-upon clinical approach to working with the patient and family. There are currently eight PCTs whose leaders meet at monthly to quarterly intervals for assessment of progress, assistance with barriers to care, or when there is need for attention to a crisis such as the death or illness of a member of the interdisciplinary team. Crisis and support meetings flow rapidly out of the PCT model, which provides an ongoing monitoring of the psychosocial environment of the unit.

Application

Our bias for creating a new structure is based on minimizing the past negative experiences with communication and collaboration. A new structure might provide a setting where no patterns have been established or power struggles have taken place. If it is not possible to create a new structure, working within an existing structure such as weekly interdisciplinary rounds may be a good alternative. If psychiatry has not had prior involvement, just the act of inviting them into the group can have a positive impact. If they have been involved in a less than effective way, then highlighting a case where both disciplines have contributed might be a helpful first step.

Specialized Clinical Case Conferences

Certain important issues can emerge that demand attention and specialized expertise. One such issue is that of suicidal ideation, and in the setting of life-threatening illness, differentiating actual suicidality from patient frustration with illness expressed as "I can't take this much longer" or "Sometimes I wish I were dead." The challenge for social work and psychiatry was to develop an assessment process and institutional guidelines. This involved establishing a clear evaluation criteria for suicidal ideation agreed to by both departments in a series of special conferences. In addition, the guidelines call for a joint patient conference with departmental leadership if conflicting opinions arise regarding the most appropriate treatment course. Mutual education, understanding, and role delineation are fostered through these discussions.

Application

The evaluation of suicidal ideation was an area of conflict between our two disciplines. A social worker would alert a psychiatrist to a "suicidal" patient, and the psychiatrist would disagree that psychiatric intervention was necessary. The social worker was left feeling the burden of responsibility for this patient's safety. An effective way to deal with this type of situation is to acknowledge another discipline's expertise. In this case, social work asked psychiatry to lead an educational session on the assessment of suicidal ideation, which started the process of putting in place the agreed-upon guidelines (see Box 44.1).

Mrs. M. is a 55-year-old woman diagnosed with ovarian cancer who had been involved in a domestic altercation. She reported to the team that she was very frustrated. "Maybe I should just kill myself and get it over with." The social worker was called to do an initial evaluation, which indicated a need for immediate psychiatric intervention. A psychiatrist came to the outpatient location, and the social worker and psychiatrist met with the patient together. Interventions were implemented to increase the level of safety in the home and to decrease patient's anxiety regarding diagnosis and environmental stressors through medication from the psychiatrist and follow-up counselling with the social worker.

Clinical Research Collaboration

Research collaboration between social work and psychiatry is an untapped resource in most institutions. An example of this in the Memorial model is the Geriatric Psychiatry Program in which research is often combined with shared clinical efforts.

Geriatric Psychiatry Program

Purpose. The Geriatric Psychiatry Program was developed in 2004 as an interdisciplinary effort within the newly formed MSKCC Geriatric Program. Its purpose was to address the clinical needs of the growing numbers of older patients and to undertake clinical research to explore the unique problems of older people facing aging and illness by devising interventions to address their specific needs. The mission is to ensure, through a collaborative, interdisciplinary effort, that all older cancer patients receive optimal psychosocial care as part of their quality cancer care and to advance psychiatric and psychosocial research in geriatric psycho-oncology.

Clinical Activities
Individual Sessions. Two psychiatrists and one psychologist meet patients individually at the Counseling Center focusing specifically on aging and cancer. Three social workers specialize in the emotional and practical issues of the older patient and their family by providing individual, group, couple, and family counseling as well as education and advice to staff on geriatric issues (see Box 44.2).

Group Sessions. Two psychiatrists and a social worker facilitate biweekly group psychoeducational sessions focusing on the combined issues of cancer and aging. A similar group, co-led by a social worker and psychiatrist, provides biweekly support for patients with advanced lung cancer.

Research Activities: Examples of the Joint Research within the Geriatric Psychiatry Program
Novel Psychotherapies for Older Cancer Patients. A group program is currently testing a therapeutic approach that brings together developmental theory of aging with meaning-based coping theory to help patients with distress related to aging and cancer. This therapy is being tested as a group-based format and in individual telephone sessions.

Geriatric Depression in Older Cancer Patients. A completed study addressed the need for a scale to measure depression in older cancer patients. Since results indicate no excellent option, the group is pursuing funding to develop a patient-reported measure that will better assess depression in this population.

The Impact of Cancer Treatments on Cognition in Older Adults. This current study is assessing the impact of hormone therapy on the cognitive functioning of older prostate cancer patients.

Application. Clinical research is an area where social work/psychiatry collaboration is a natural fit. Particularly in times of low staffing levels, developing and implementing protocols, applying for grants, and sharing the writing responsibilities can prove to be a productive use of resources that furthers the documentation and validation of our work. This in turn leads to more effective patient programs and increases our professionalism and status. This piece of the model does require social work departments to value and support research efforts. Struggling together to produce this research provides an insight and appreciation

Mr. S. is an 84-year-old retired business man and cancer survivor who had been treated for many years at the Counselling Center for hypochondriacal concerns and uncontrolled hostility, which were reasonably controlled through counselling and medication. Four years ago he began to develop cognitive deficits consistent with vascular dementia. Caring for him at home was his 82year-old wife who also had a history of cancer as well as depression. Over the 30 years of their marriage the patient had maintained tight control over finances and couple activities. At the time of intervention, Mrs. S. had become the focus of his paranoid delusions. Many aides had quit because of Mr. S.'s abusive behavior. As he moved toward the end stages of his disease, Mrs. S. was committed to keeping him at home regardless of this behavior. However, as his primary caregiver, she was beginning to experience the physical and emotional effects of this decision. Our collaborative efforts with this caregiver included individual in-person and telephone sessions focused on acknowledging her need to care for her husband while emphasizing the limits of her responsibility. She eventually was able to allow in-home case management consultation, seek additional support from the Alzheimer's Foundation, and consult with an elder law attorney regarding financial planning. To further decrease social isolation and share the responsibilities of decision making, Mrs. S. was encouraged to contact one of the husband's sons who supported her efforts to place Mr. S. in a facility appropriate to his needs. Support from both the authors continued through this transition so that Mrs. S. could increase self-care while still remaining connected to her husband.

of our different points of reference and potential contributions to the richness of each project.

Bereavement Program

This collaborative effort, under the leadership of the Department of Social Work, provides both time-limited support groups and educational lectures for families of deceased MSKCC patients. Psychiatrists participate as group co-leaders, as featured speakers at the quarterly lecture series, and as group consultants in the area of complicated grief, an issue that is being actively studied in a family therapy model to determine which factors most impact this severe reaction.

The Communication Skills Laboratory (COMSKIL). The COMSKIL Lab, conceived by the Chairman of the Psychiatry Department and developed by two psychologists, offers physician training with facilitation provided by attending physicians, psychiatrists, psychologists, and social workers. This program has focused a much needed emphasis on improving the skills of doctor–patient communication. Modules on termination of active treatment, palliative care, and end-of-life discussions have provided tools to young physicians while teaching them the patient benefit of interdisciplinary collaboration.

The Family Therapy Clinic. The Family Therapy Clinic is a collaborative effort in which psychiatrists and social workers act as co-therapists. Working with patients and their families approaching the end of life provides a truly collaborative means of increasing the quality of the patient's life and provides an excellent approach to anticipatory grief with continuing family contact after the patient's death.

Educational Collaboration

Grand Rounds

A social worker sits on a planning committee with two psychiatrists to develop an interdisciplinary educational program for the academic year. The goal is to create a multifaceted program that encompasses lectures on new research and clinical approaches related to the psychosocial care of the oncology patient.

Research Colloquia

Monthly research colloquia are held to discuss psychosocial research in progress from the earliest stages of idea development through the completion of an IRB protocol and grant submission. These sessions encourage individual and joint research projects through sharing of ideas, development of research skills, and necessary reinforcement of morale during the sometimes lengthy research process.

Application

All of the aforementioned programs were initially independent projects in the Department of Social Work or

Psychiatry. Through collaboration in other areas, both disciplines gradually developed a trust of the other's contributions and skills. We each opened our programs to the participation of members of the other's department. For example, in the Communication Skill Lab, social work has made a significant contribution in helping interns, residents, and fellows learn how to communicate with patients at the end of life. Although ours is a formalized program, the same result can be attained by a social worker and psychiatrist facilitating a group of young doctors struggling with communication at termination of disease-modifying treatment or as palliative care is integrated along the continuum of illness.

Challenges for Professionals

For maximal provision of care along the continuum of illness and at end of life, it is critical to understand what elements constitute and influence clinical collaboration. Challenges in collaboration can sometimes be compounded by the limitations of each discipline, incomplete understanding of the roles and expertise of other professionals, increased requirements for accountability and documentation, and complex diagnoses and treatment methods (Heinemann & Zeiss, 2002). Some of the elements necessary for collaboration are briefly discussed.

Institutional History

All institutions carry a history of collaboration or lack thereof, which has a direct impact on the quality of patient care. Any institution that is committed to providing the highest level of palliative care for their patients must also be committed to interdisciplinary collaboration as a means to attain it. In environments of distrust and past failures, departmental leadership must be committed to implementing a cultural change by creating new structures and fighting old stereotypes inherent in poor collaborative efforts.

Multiple Locations

With the locus of care continuing its shift to the ambulatory setting, collaboration becomes an even more challenging proposition. E-mail, electronic medical records, and conference calls compensate in some respects but cannot always make up for a lack of in-person contact with colleagues.

Time Factors

"Doing more with less" has become the reality of health and mental health care during economic downturns. Logically, collaboration in this environment would seem to be an imperative. However, with less time to see more patients, making an extra phone call or attending another meeting becomes difficult and at times collaboration is sacrificed.

Reimbursement Issues

The social work/psychiatry collaboration is hampered by different reimbursement patterns. In the inpatient setting, psychiatry is a fee-for-service department while social work services are financially bundled into a patient's other medical charges. Both systems are inadequate to meet patient's needs, and we propose that attention to this access-to-care issue should be made a priority at the national policy level.

Summary

Given the challenges of collaboration, it is important to question whether the time expended is valuable to our patients and families receiving palliative care along the continuum of illness and at the end of life. From clinical experience, both authors believe that working together with a consistent point of view provides the patient and family system the necessary time to focus on each other instead of having to deal with many disparate individual providers (Zeiss & Steffen, 1996). The most successful collaborations are committed to the idea that patients will be best served when their care is coordinated by a psychosocial team in which the members learn from each other, share the workload together, rely and trust each other, and challenge each other for the purpose of providing their patients with the highest possible quality of care.

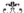
Conclusion

It is reassuring that almost 60 years after Sutherland established the first five-member psychosocial unit at Memorial we now have a significant number of professionals involved in interdisciplinary psychosocial care teams that cover the major clinical oncology services. Notably, research is now integrated into clinical care and a new era in the "science of care" is evolving. Social work and psychiatry contribute in large measure to this emerging science, but despite all these advances, the psychosocial needs of patients remain the same: compassionate care delivered by a competent team that addresses the patient as a whole person. Interestingly, today's concern about the level of humanism in medicine has been a concern over generations. The point raised by Francis Peabody in a 1927 *Journal of the American Medical Association* editorial has an important contemporary message for

those of us, whether social worker or psychiatrist, who focus on the supportive aspect of care:

> *The treatment of a disease may be entirely impersonal; the care of a patient must be completely personal…. One of the essential qualities of a clinician is interest in humanity, for the secret of care of the patient is in caring for the patient.*

LEARNING EXERCISE 1

- *Purpose:* To assess the need for closer social work/psychiatry collaboration in your setting.
- *Method:* Analyze the obstacles and barriers to past collaboration.
- *Goal:* Develop a strategic plan that includes two or three collaborative actions you can take to increase the potential for a closer working relationship between social work and psychiatry.
- *Evaluation:* At the end of 3 months, obtain feedback from those involved to determine the efficacy of this approach.

LEARNING EXERCISE 2

- *Purpose:* To develop one piece of a new collaborative structure within your setting.
- *Method:* Select one of the structures outlined in this chapter (i.e., psychosocial care team). Involve at least one social worker, one psychiatrist, and a nursing representative to discuss current palliative care patients on a semi-monthly or monthly basis.
- *Goal:* Implement the structure on one unit or within one physician's clinic.
- *Evaluation:* At the end of 3 months, obtain feedback from each team member on issues such as communication, role delineation, and the effect on patient care.

ADDITIONAL RESOURCES

National Academy of Elder Law Attorneys, Inc. (NAELA): http://www.naela.org
A nonprofit association that represents lawyers and bar organizations who are working with older clients and their families. Established in 1987, the Academy provides a resource of education, information, networking, and assistance to those who deal with the many specialized issues involved with legal services for seniors and people with special needs.
National Alzheimer's Association: http://www.alz.org
A nonprofit organization that offers education, caregiver support groups, patient day programs, and housing for the patient and family dealing with the challenge of Alzheimer's disease.

FILM

Iris: A 2001 biographical film about the Irish novelist Iris Murdoch who suffered from Alzheimer's disease, seen from the point of view of her husband, John Bayley. This is a moving take on the hopelessness and frustration of the caregiver. A Miramax film.

REFERENCES

Abrams, R. D., & Finesinger, J. E. (1953). Guilt reactions in patients with cancer. *Cancer, 6*, 474–482 .

Bard, M., & Sutherland, A. M. (1955). The psychological impact of cancer and its treatment. *Cancer, 8*, 656–672 .

Heinemann, G. D., & Zeiss, A. M. (2002). *Team performance in health care*. New York, NY: Springer Publishing.

Mitchell, P. H., & Crittenden, R. A. (2000). Interdisciplinary collaboration: Old ideas with new urgency. *Washington Public Health, Fall*, 1–3 .

Peabody, F.W. (1927). The care of the patient. *Journal of American Medical Association, 88*, 877–882 .

Shands, H. C., Finesinger, J. E., Cobb, S., & Abrams, R. D. (1951). Psychological mechanisms in patients with cancer. *Cancer, 4*, 1159–1170 .

Sutherland, A. M., Orbach, C. E., Dyk, R. B., & Bard, M. (1952). The psychological impact of cancer and cancer surgery. *Cancer, 5*, 857–872 .

Zeiss, A. M., & Steffen, A. M. (1996). Interdisciplinary health care teams: The basic unit of geriatric care. In L. L. Carstensen, B. A. Edelstein, & L. Dornbrand (Eds.), *The practical handbook of clinical gerontology* (pp. 423–450) Thousand Oaks, CA: Sage Publications, Inc.

45 *John Mondanaro and Stacey Needleman*

Social Work and Creative Arts Therapy Services

Our son ... has had two week-long hospitalizations in the past 2 years. Both times you have been there to help all of us get through them ... We want to thank you for easing a frightening and sometimes painful time.

—Patient's family

Key Concepts

- ◆ *Chronic illness can interfere with development in children and adolescents.*
- ◆ *Creative arts therapy and social work utilize a family-systems perspective.*
- ◆ *Loss, separation, and isolation impact coping.*
- ◆ *Patterns of family dysfunction may emerge in varying ways during times of crisis.*
- ◆ *Interdisciplinary collaboration is essential when providing family-centered care.*

Introduction

Approaching health care from a family-systems perspective has become a focus in pediatrics. When treating children with chronic medical conditions, our focus is not on the illness but rather on the ways in which the illness impacts both the child and the family unit. In this chapter we reflect on two narratives to illustrate the different ways that this can present.

Social Work in Collaboration with Creative Arts Therapy Services

Over the last several years, pediatric health care has moved in the direction of family-centered practice. Family-centered care highlights the important role that families play in ensuring the health and well-being of children, adolescents, and family members of all ages (Shields, Pratt, Davis, & Hunter, 2007). Family-centered care aims to integrate emotional and developmental needs into the practice of medicine. In doing so, clinicians not only see family involvement as essential to the child's care but also look to develop a treatment plan specific to each family (Kovacs, Bellin, & Fauri, 2006). Thus, we no longer look at the child or the illness in isolation but rather approach the two within the context of the various systems in which they both exist.

Psychosocial services at The Pediatric Neuroscience Institute and Comprehensive Epilepsy Center ensue from the collaborative effort of social work and creative arts therapy services. An institutional conviction to providing care within a family-systems model provides the context in which these two services can work cohesively, with social work focusing on the psychosocial assessment of the family unit and creative arts therapy services attending to the needs of the pediatric patient and his or her siblings.

Social workers place great emphasis on the initial assessment, and they approach this from a family-systems perspective. The identified client is best understood within the context of the systems they belong to; one of which is their family of origin. Cook (2000) proposes three roles for social workers in family-centered practice; these include assessment, support, and empowerment (Dewees, 2005). When approaching assessment, the social worker initially attempts to identify the biopsychosocial-spiritual aspects of the family's experience. Within this context, the social worker explores the culture and beliefs of the family, the strengths of each member of the family system, and the resources available (Dewees, 2005). In addition, patterns of communication and areas of conflict are identified as well as the degree to which the system has been disrupted by the presenting illness (Monroe, 1994). The social worker then utilizes the information gained to provide a forum for further exploration and support. Within the various relationships in the family system, ineffective means of coping are identified while strengths are highlighted. Drawing on this knowledge, the social worker seeks to empower the patient and/or family to create healthier patterns of communication and enhanced coping.

For creative arts therapy services, the assessment stage of treatment is approached creatively with emphasis placed upon the child's general understanding of the diagnosis and treatment plan (Gaynard et al., 1990; Klinzing, 1977; Leeuwenburgh et al., 2007; Levy, Kronenberger, & Carter, 2008; Orland, 1965; Petrillo, 1972; Plank, 1965; Thompson & Stanford, 1981). This approach highlights the child's "narrative" or version of the events that led to admission. Providing the child with a forum for both verbal and nonverbal expression through the arts is paramount to the planning of treatment that will truly optimize the patient's coping (Evans, 2000; Kennelly, 2000; Loewy, 1997; Mondanaro, 2005, 2008; Robb, 2003; Robbins, 1998). To this end, interventions in the form of psychoeducation, procedural support, and psychotherapeutic support are provided through the use of music, art, dance-movement, drama, and play therapies. These familiar and nonthreatening forums for expression allow a child's voice to be heard in a system that is all too often patriarchal in nature. Taking the time to elicit the child's comprehension of illness and hospitalization encourages the child to be an active participant in his or her care. Modeling this practice of inclusion can positively influence the culture of a pediatric unit and possibly the patient and family's perception of health care. The time spent with a child for these purposes creates an environment within which misconceptions are expressed, allowing the therapist immediate entry points into establishing a working therapeutic alliance that will serve not only the child but assist the interdisciplinary team in treatment planning as well.

Two contrasting narratives (see Boxes 45.1 and 45.2) involving the treatment of intractable epilepsy will be discussed in terms of the collaborative effort of these two disciplines. The optimal outcome for one 17-year-old female and her family contrasted significantly with the second narrative, which involved a 7-year-old female with whom the team had been providing care for over 6 years. While the two cases are markedly different, they both illustrate the concept of family-centered care and the clinical competence gained from utilizing a family-systems perspective.

Box 45.1
Patient/Family Narratives: Stephanie

Our introductions to Stephanie, a 17-year-old patient diagnosed with intractable epilepsy, occurred several days after phase one of a two-phase epilepsy surgery. Stephanie was initially diagnosed with epilepsy at 11 years of age and became a candidate for epilepsy surgery as a result of the focal origin of her seizure activity. Following our initial meeting with Stephanie and her family, the majority of our work focused on Stephanie and her mother. Paramount to this was the development of boundaries between Stephanie and her mother, who maintained a vigilant presence at the bedside throughout Stephanie's hospitalization.

During the initial assessment, the social worker identified that Stephanie demonstrated a lack of autonomy and sense of self-worth. The primary tasks of adolescence include achieving independence from parents and developing a strong sense of identity. The presence of a chronic condition can interfere with these developmental tasks (Austin, 2007). In addition, living with a chronic medical condition can diminish a child's self-worth, sense of competence, and emotional functioning (Evans, 2004). During our early work together, it was evident that Stephanie's development had been significantly impacted by the severity of her medical condition as well as her mother's need to protect her. As a result, Stephanie presented with anxiety and depression, which were often heightened during medical tests and procedures.

The social worker drew upon one of Stephanie's greatest strengths, which was a solid understanding of the way in which her body functions. Utilizing progressive muscle relaxation, the social worker empowered Stephanie to not only "self-soothe" during periods of increased distress but also enabled her to delineate the boundaries between herself and her mother. In doing so, Stephanie was able to be less dependent on her mother's support and instead draw support from her own internal resources. The social worker also provided a forum for Stephanie's mother to process her feelings surrounding Stephanie's condition. In doing so, she was better able to own her feelings and allow Stephanie the space in which to be autonomous.

Creative arts therapy services pursued parallel entry points to those assessed by social work by providing music therapy interventions that evolved through the vicissitudes of Stephanie's treatment. Initial sessions focused primarily on addressing pain through the use of music as a "soundbath" to provide comfort and aural recluse from the nontherapeutic sounds of a busy hospital unit (Dileo & Bradt, 1999; Eagle & Harsh, 1988; Loewy, 1997, 1999; Maslar, 1986; Mondanaro, 2008). Improvising music that would absorb and give aesthetic sense to the cacophony of beeps, overhead pages, ringing phones, and talking was the goal during the initial sessions. Later sessions broadened to include verbal discussion (Evans, 2002; Mondanaro, 2008; Nolan, 2005) in which loss and separation emerged as two prevailing themes that ensued from Stephanie's separation from school activities and peers during her senior year of high school. Unresolved conflict over interrupted goals, plans (Barry, 2006; Cushner-Weinstein et al., 2008; Prugh, 1978; Tosun et al., 2008), and specifically her inability to complete several music commitments contributed to her general state of anxiety and depression.

Given Stephanie's personal relationship to music as a means of self-expression, the direction of music therapy was chosen. Treatment goals were embedded in the creation of a recital that would encompass Stephanie's favorite songs from missed school concerts as well as an original incomplete piano composition that Stephanie had shared during sessions. Preparation for the recital provided structure and recluse from the medical regimen of her preparation for surgery, as she immersed herself in the self-actualizing motion of completing her piano composition and practicing her singing. Stephanie's recital occurred 6-1/2 weeks later—the day before her surgery. She sang and played through the program beautifully to the applause of family, nurses, doctors, dieticians, environmental services workers, social work staff, and child life staff, all of whom were present to show support. The video recording made of the recital along with the program she had designed would serve as important transitional objects upon discharge. Stephanie's surgery was successful and she emerged from the entire experience with a strengthened sense of self that would serve her well in the resumption of her life's dreams.

Box 45.2
Patient/Family Narratives: Kloye

Kloye is a 7-year-old female who was born prematurely. She presented with an intraventricular hemorrhage and subsequently developed hydrocephalus and intractable epilepsy. Hospitalized frequently since birth, her coping and adaptation during admissions reflected no sense of normalization or habituation to the environment. Over the years, the layers of traumatization either exacerbated an existing behavioral disorder or simply culminated into one. Reinforced by well-intentioned caregivers who were ineffective in setting appropriate limits, Kloye's behavior intensified between the ages of 3 and 7, resulting in a situation that was nearly unmanageable.

The social worker approached Kloye's presenting problem by exploring prevalent themes in the family unit. Since Kloye was raised in a single-parent family, an alliance was sought with her mother. Family factors frequently account for a child's responses to his or her illness or condition. A positive maternal adaptation often correlates with the child's ability to adapt to the situation as well (Shore, Austin, & Dunn, 2004). Maternal adjustment is also affected by the mother's ability to acknowledge and process her grief, which revolves around mourning the loss of the expected or healthy child (Brown & Mackenzie, 2005). When grief is complicated or interrupted, the child's developmental tasks may be disrupted along with the adaptation to illness. During early childhood, children rely on their attachment to a caregiver to develop trust and independence in their own environment. This independence is then generalized to other environments. When a caregiver is struggling with his or her own inability to cope, the caregiver is then unable to meet the developmental needs of his or her child (Austin, 2007). Thus, the child fails to master these tasks related to independence and trust and becomes immobilized by the fear of separation.

The social worker focused on providing a forum for Kloye's mother to process her loss. Central themes revolved around guilt and compensatory behaviors. In acknowledging and then processing these feelings, the social worker was able to open up a forum for healing and change. Intervention was initially geared toward delineating appropriate mother–child tasks and boundaries, and later behavioral modification was aimed toward creating opportunities to practice and maintain separation. While these tasks were met with much resistance on Kloye's part, the collaborative work of the creative arts therapist enabled them to be successful.

Because of the nature of the developmental and illness history, there had been limited work done with Kloye at the psychoeducational level. Intervention of this nature is something generally done as early as preschool age. Psychoeducation can provide developmentally appropriate medical information to a child so that a sense of mastery can be supported (Leeuwenburgh et al., 2007; Mondanaro, 2005, 2008). Before this work can be done, however, there must be trust and a therapeutic alliance in place. Toward this end, the creative arts therapist's interventions focused on supporting Kloye's sense of autonomy and encouraged integration of valuable learning opportunities while hospitalized. This work often felt futile, because family members misinterpreted the healthy display of projected emotions such as anger and anxiety as Kloye's rejection of the intervention. These episodes actually served as the basis for a working therapeutic relationship, from which an alliance could ensue. The therapist safely contained the anger, frustration, fear, and anxiety (Joseph & Heimlich, 1959; Loewy, 1997). Creating playful exchanges around Kloye's dramatic displays of opposition elicited verbal exchanges or laughter, both of which liberated her from the extended periods of stoic and nonverbal presentation for which she was known. Other than these intermittent displays of relatedness, however, there had been little room for more in-depth work. Only when Kloye's behavior had escalated to the point of being problematic at school and at home was there motivation and a concerted effort to commit to a psychosocial treatment plan.

Successfully meeting the mother's request for intervention was dependent upon an approach that was somewhat retrospective because Kloye was acting out years of unresolved conflict and anger pertaining to her medical history. A psychoeducational text was created in storybook form, to invite the reading and integration of her medical history. Such storybooks provide children with a safe and familiar structure in which to explore and organize potentially overwhelming information at a nonthreatening pace that is controlled by the child (Cattanach, 1997; Gersie, 1990; Leeuwenburgh et al., 2007; Mondanaro, 2005). Additionally, the inclusion of interactive activities such as coloring and using stickers provides intermittent recluse from verbal processing in exchange for direct portal into the nonverbal realm of creativity that is so innate to the learning processes of children (Gersie, 1990; Jennings, 1999). This book was introduced to Kloye in the setting of a safe therapeutic relationship several weeks before the first scheduled outpatient session.

Kloye began coming to weekly sessions as scheduled. Her ability to process issues of autonomy and control emerged during sessions in the form of teacher–pupil role play (Landy, 1993; Winnicott, 1971), in which she would play the stern "school marm" to the therapist's "misbehaved child." As planned, the completion of the agreed-upon 8-week treatment occurred simultaneous with Kloye's return to school. Although progress was made during treatment, her subsequent hospitalizations were no less traumatic. Her acting

Box 45.2 *(Contd.)*

out of pent-up aggression at home and at school lessened, but during hospitalizations, family members assumed familiar roles of reinforcing maladaptive patterns of behavior. Kloye denied having any understanding of her diagnosis, although it was reported by her mother that she had been reading her book in the privacy of her room, as well as to her younger sibling. Psychotherapeutic support in the form of expressive play opportunities continued to be offered during hospital admissions, and Kloye's caregivers demonstrated a growing diligence about honoring her time and space within the therapy sessions. Their efforts supported her growing recognition of her medical reality and her ensuing need to be seen not just as the child "too young to know," but as a young lady with the resilience to reconcile her physiological reality with her successes, disappointments, and dreams of being a princess.

Conclusion

The collaborative effort of social work and creative arts therapy services allows for effective implementation of family-centered care. When necessary, either discipline may transcend its modality in support of the patient and/or family facing the arduous journey of chronic illness. However, there are inherent challenges to this type of programming. For example, potential overlaps in service can make fertile the ground for staff and patient splitting. The resulting compromise to treatment effectiveness and efficiency can be minimized through regular discussion and negotiation. Additionally, the education of patients and staff about roles as well as mutually advocating for the inclusion of both disciplines can be cardinal to the success of such a model. Ultimately, family-centered care can best be approached through the use of a united psychosocial team. The therapeutic alliance achieved through such an approach can positively impact the course of treatment from the point of diagnosis through the transition back to the routines of daily life.

LEARNING EXERCISES

- What are three specific interventions utilized by creative arts therapy to optimize patient coping? How does the focus of each intervention specifically support this goal?
- What three elements do social workers incorporate when doing an assessment from a family-systems perspective? Consider how one of these elements can positively or negatively impact a family's ability to cope.
- Why is "narrative" an important form in working with pediatric patients during all phases of treatment? Discuss why the structure of a "storybook," can be effective in the provision of psychoeducation.

- In what ways might the presence of a medical condition impact a patient/family's level of functioning? Imagine a specific childhood medical condition and consider the adaptations required for both the child and the parents.

ADDITIONAL RECOMMENDED READINGS

Bradford, R. (1997). *Children, families, and chronic disease.* London, England: Routledge.

Dilieo, C. (Ed.) (1999). *Music therapy and medicine: Theoretical and clinical applications.* Silver Spring, MD: American Music Therapy Association, Inc.

Gaynard, L., Wolfer, J., Goldberger, J., Thompson, R., Redburn, L., & Laidley, L. (1998). *The psychosocial care of children in hospitals.* Rockville, MD: Child Life Council.

Hartman, A., & Laird, J. (1983). *Family centered social work practice.* New York, NY: Free Press.

Loewy, J. (1997). *Music therapy and pediatric pain.* Cherry Hill, NJ: Satchnote Press.

REFERENCES

Austin, J. (2007). Psychosocial aspects of pediatric epilepsy. In A. Ettinger & A. Kanner (Eds.), *Psychiatric issues in epilepsy* (pp. 514–525). Philadelphia, PA: Lippincott Williams & Wilkins.

Barry, J. (2006). *Public enemy no. 1: Depression and mood disorders in people with epilepsy.* Retrieved from http://www.epilepsyidaho.org/epilepsy-mood-disorder.ht

Brown, C., & Mackenzie, S. (2005). The role of the audiologist and family support worker in the Ontario infant hearing program: A team approach. *Journal of Speech-Language Pathology and Audiology, 29*(3), 106–111.

Cattanach, A. (1997). *Children's stories in play therapy.* London, England: Jessica Kingsley.

Cook, D. S. (2000). The role of social work with families that have young children with developmental disabilities. In M. Guralnick (Ed.), *Interdisciplinary assessments of young children with disabilities* (pp. 201–218). Baltimore, MD: Paul H. Brookes.

Cushner-Weinstein, S., Dassoulas, K., Salpekar, J. A., Henderson, S. E., Pearl, P. L., Gaillard, W. D., & Weinstein, S. L. (2008). Parenting stress and childhood epilepsy: The impact of depression, learning, and seizure-related factors. *Epilepsy and Behavior, 13*(1), 109–114.

Dewees, M. (2005). Postmodern social work in interdisciplinary contexts. *Social Work in Health Care, 39*(3), 343–360.

Dileo, C., & Bradt, J. (1999). Entrainment, resonance, and pain-related suffering. In C. Dileo (Ed.), *Music therapy and medicine: Theoretical and clinical applications* (pp. 181–188). Silver Spring, MD: The American Music Therapy Association, Inc.

Eagle, C., & Harsh, J. (1988). Elements of pain and music. *The Journal of the American Association of Music Therapy, 7*(1), 15–27.

Evans, D. (2002). The effectiveness of music as an intervention for hospital patients: A systematic review. *Evidence-Based Nursing, 5*(3), 86.

Evans, R. (2000). *Helping children to overcome fear: The healing power of play*. Stroud, Gloucestershire, UK: Hawthorn Press.

Evans, T. (2004). A multidimensional assessment of children with chronic physical conditions. *Health and Social Work*, 29(3), 245–248.

Gaynard, L., Wolfer, J., Goldberger, J., Thompson, R. H., Redburn, L., & Laidley, L. (1990). *Psychosocial care of children in hospitals: A clinical practice manual from the ACCH child life research project*. Rockville, MD: Child Life Council Inc.

Gersie, A. (1990). In N. King (Ed.), *Storymaking in education and therapy*. London, England: J. Kingsley.

Jennings, S. (1999). *Introduction to developmental play therapy: Playing and health*. London, England: Jessica Kingsley.

Joseph, E., & Heimlich, E. (1959). The therapeutic use of music with treatment resistant children. *American Journal of Mental Deficiency*, 63(7), 41–50.

Kennelly, J. (2000). The specialist role of the music therapist in developmental programs for hospitalized children. *Journal of Pediatric Health Care*, 14(2), 56–59.

Klinzing, D. (1977). *The hospitalized child: Communication techniques for health personnel*. Englewood Cliffs, NJ: Prentice-Hall.

Kovacs, P., Bellin, M. H., & Fauri, D. (2006). Family-centered care: A resource for social work in end-of-life and palliative care. *Journal of Social Work in End-of-Life and Palliative Care*, 2(1), 13–27.

Landy, R. (1993). *Persona and performance: The meaning of role in drama, therapy, and everyday life*. New York, NY: Guilford Press.

Leeuwenburgh, E., Mondanaro, J. E., Omens, S., Fogel, A., Kanazawa, M., Lynch,T., & Goldring, E. (2007). Creative arts therapies. In S. Chisolm (Ed.), *The health professions: Trends and opportunities in U.S. health care* (pp. 397–424). Sudbury, MA: Jones and Bartlett Publishers.

Levy, M. C., Kronenberger, W. G., & Carter, B. D. (2008). Brief report: Illness factors and child behavior before and during pediatric hospitalization. *Journal of Pediatric Psychology*, 33(8), 905–909.

Loewy, J. (1997). *Music therapy and pediatric pain*. Cherry Hill, NJ: Jeffrey Books.

Loewy, J. (1999). The use of music psychotherapy in the treatment of pediatric pain. In C. Dileo (Ed.), *Music therapy and medicine: Theoretical and clinical applications* (pp. 189–206). Silver Spring, MD: The American Music Therapy Association, Inc.

Maslar, P. (1986). The effect of music on the reduction of pain: A review of the literature. *Arts in Psychotherapy*, 13(3), 215–219.

Mondanaro, J. (2005). Interfacing music therapy with other creative arts modalities to address anticipatory grief and bereavements in pediatrics. In C. Dileo (Ed.), *Music therapy at the end of life* (pp. 25–32). Cherry Hill, NJ: Jeffrey Books.

Mondanaro, J. (2008). Music therapy in the psychosocial care of pediatric patients with epilepsy. *Music Therapy Perspectives*, 26(2), 99–26.

Monroe, B. (1994). Role of the social worker in palliative care. *Annals Academy of Medicine*, 23(2), 252–255.

Nolan, P. (2005). Verbal processing within the music therapy process. *Music Therapy Perspectives*, 23(1), 18–28.

Oremland, E. (1965). *Protecting the emotional development of the ill child: The essence of the child life profession*. Madison, CT: Psych Social Press.

Petrillo, M., & Sanger, S. (1972) *Emotional care of hospitalized children; An environmental approach*. Philadelphia, PA: Lippincott.

Plank, E. (1962). *Working with children in hospitals: A professional guide*. Cleveland, OH: The Child Life and Education Department at Metro-Health Medical Center.

Prugh, D. G. (1978). *The psychosocial aspects of pediatrics*. Philadelphia, PA: Lea & Febiger.

Robb, S. (2003). Designing music therapy interventions for hospitalized children and adolescents using a contextual model for music therapy. *Music Therapy Perspectives*, 21(1), 27–40.

Robbins, A. (1998). Dance/movement and art therapies as primary expressions of the self. In A. Robbins (Ed.), *Therapeutic presence: Bridging expression and form* (pp. 261–270). London, England: Jessica Kingsley Publishers.

Shields, L., Pratt, J., Davis, L., & Hunter, J. (2007). Family centered care for children in hospital. *Cochrane Database of Systemic Reviews*, 1. Art. No:CD004811.doi:10.1002/14651858. CD004811.pub2.

Shore, C. P., Austin, J. K., & Dunn, D. W. (2004). Maternal adaptation to a child's epilepsy. *Epilepsy and Behavior*, 5(4), 557–568.

Thompson, R. H., & Stanford, G. (1981). *Child life in hospitals: Theory and practice*. Springfield, IL: Charles C. Thomas.

Tosun, A., Gokcen, S., Ozbaran, B., Serdaroglu, G., Polat, M., Tekgul, H., & Gokben, S. (2008). The effect of depression on academic achievement in children with epilepsy. *Epilepsy and Behavior*, 13(3), 494–498.

Winnicott, D. (1971). *Playing and reality*. Harmondsworth, England: Penguin.

46 *J. J. Nadicksbernd, Kathryn Thornberry, and Charles F. von Gunten*

Social Work and Physician Collaboration in Palliative Care

Oh, I'm so glad you're here. The doctor just left and I don't understand.

—*Anonymous*

Key Concepts

- *Physicians and social workers have different training backgrounds.*
- *Communication styles for physicians and social workers are different.*
- *It is important to make conflicts explicit in order to promote teamwork.*

Introduction

Palliative care is done in teams. When there is not a team, well-meaning health professionals are doing something, but they are not doing palliative care (Loscalzo & von Gunten, 2008). While there is a paucity of research relating to interdisciplinary palliative care teams, the available data demonstrate positive effects (Higginson et al., 2003; Wagner, 2000). In addition, there is much older evidence to suggest that teams that include doctors and social workers lead to better outcomes (Curley, McEachern, & Speroff, 1998; Silver & Stiber, 1957; Sommers, Marton, Barbaccia, & Randolph, 2000). There has yet to be a controlled study comparing the effectiveness of different team models. There is minimal literature describing the relationship between physicians and social work in palliative care specifically, or in health care more generally.

In this chapter, we describe the relationship between the physician and the social worker in various settings where palliative care teams do their work. We describe the roles, the benefits, and the challenges of the relationship through the lenses of the authors, who have over 50 years of collective experience in working together in building interdisciplinary teams. We draw on examples from hospital, dedicated inpatient, and home palliative care services.

The Physician Role

The physician role in palliative care is to provide expertise in symptom control, understand and explain the illness, and provide a prognosis and treatment. Any licensed physician can play the physician role. With suitable training, a palliative medicine physician will have expertise that exceeds that of other physicians. This specialist expertise was recognized in 1987 in Great Britain and in 2006 in the United States. As a specialist consultant, the palliative medicine physician will engage with other physicians to debate the medical management of patients when decision making is complex.

471

The physician also helps clarify decision making with the referring team, patients, relatives, and sometimes with friends. In many settings, the specialist physician will also play a role in educating medical students, residents, nursing students, social work students, and other students in the health professions. Finally, the physician will play a political role in heightening awareness of palliative care among other doctors and those in hospital and other health care settings. In a few centers, the physician will also be involved in research, that is, the discovery of new knowledge so that improved treatment will be possible (Clark, 2003).

The physician role is an ancient one; there have been physicians for at least 5000 years. Consequently, the physician is a product of this history as well as the extensive training and socialization during the training period. In addition, patients, families, and other health care professionals react to the physician role based on the social role developed over those millennia.

A physician is trained to practice medicine. That training is overwhelmingly concerned with maintaining or restoring human health through the study, diagnosis, and treatment of disease and injury. For the past 150 years, the preparation is accomplished through a detailed application of the science of medicine to understand anatomy, physiology, disease, and treatment (Dunlop & Hockley, 1998). In principally applying the biological sciences in preference to the social sciences, the physician is trained to look less at the person than at the underlying disease. It is assumed that, if a patient seeks the care of a physician, the patient agrees to have the doctor diagnose and prescribe treatment. Increasingly, physicians rely on diagnostic testing to help with decisions. Doctors are trained to avoid long documentation. In contrast, they are trained to focus quickly and document incisively about what is wrong and what is to be done. In short, doctors are trained to fix. They assume authority in the doctor–patient relationship and are taught they are the leaders of any health care team on which they will serve. This role is reinforced by legal requirements that the physician write prescriptions and be responsible for the outcomes of health care for the patient. While physicians know about the roles of nurses, social workers, and others, physician training implies nonphysicians are subservient or ancillary to the physician role. Physicians are not explicitly trained to work with social workers, though they may serve on teams that include a social worker during their apprenticeship (residency or house officer) years. In all environments, doctors are taught to be fearless—particularly if they are uncertain.

The Social Work Role

The social work role on the palliative care team is to counsel and help patients and families use their own strengths and access resources available to them in their community. Their core competencies include navigating the medical and social systems; enhancing communication within the family system and between the family and health care system; assisting with advance care planning, establishing goals of care, clarifying resuscitation status, and identifying surrogate decision makers; identifying and ensuring that the emotional, practical, and spiritual needs of the patient and family are met; and assessing and intervening with the multidimensional aspects of pain and symptom management, including offering cognitive-behavioral interventions (Blacker, 2004). Social workers in specialty palliative care teams are often called on to apply these competencies in an environment of heightened emotion, conflict, and a compressed time frame.

Physicians, and other team members, frequently explain difficult patient or family behavior in terms of psycho-pathology (e.g., the patient is "borderline" or "narcissistic"). In contrast, social workers apply a systems approach, looking at a person in his or her environment, understanding the patient's functioning in the context of culture extending from the individual and family unit (micro system) out to the wider culture (macro system). This allows for a comprehensive view of clients who may be experiencing difficulties with their roles, self-perceptions, and expectations in their interactions with others in the context of their environments. Patients do not function in isolation from others nor from organizational systems. The possibilities to intervene multiply when they are responsive to the patient as well as any of the systems with which he or she comes in contact (family, religious, medical, transportation, social, financial, etc). This approach allows for less stigmatization of the patient and family and elicits more understanding and empathy from the treatment teams, which in turn facilitates healing on many levels.

Social workers collaborate with patients and families; they do not diagnose and treat pathology in the same sense that physicians do. Rather, social workers identify and work with inherent strengths or patterns of behavior. This creates an atmosphere where the patient and family are active members of the treatment team. The patient and family are supported to state their needs and problem solve solutions. This leads to better outcomes for all. The patient and family feel empowered, and the treatment team feels less frustrated.

The formal social work role is a recent one; it is no more than 150 years old. Social work is a profession that applies the social sciences rather than the biological sciences to improve the lives of people, groups, and societies (Loscalzo & von Gunten, 2008). Social work emerged in the nineteenth century in response to social problems arising from the Industrial Revolution. During the twentieth century, the profession began to rely more on research and evidence-based practice. In contrast with the training of physicians, the training of social work is more variable. Different schools have difference emphases or tracks; the tracks may include aging, child welfare, health, mental health, and social justice, to name a few. In contrast with the medical model, social workers are trained to observe the interaction and relationship between persons and their social surroundings and to intervene to mitigate obstacles to enhance functioning and the responsiveness of systems. Social workers are taught to honor patient self-determination; in reaching for the patient's strengths, blocks can be overcome. By joining a patient in his or her social system while being mindful of the patient's right to self-determination, the social worker can be the impetus of change.

The social worker relies heavily on abstractions, subtleties, environmental influences, and the process of interaction to form the database. There is no diagnostic testing, but there may be screening tools and formal assessment questionnaires in some settings. Generally, information is gathered through psychosocial assessments that are obtained from interviews and dialogues with a patient and family. These interviews and dialogues are not just the answers to questions. Rather, the social worker observes how the patient interacts with others and searches for meaning behind the words being used. The social worker watches for nonverbal cues such as eye contact and tone of voice.

The social worker is trained to look at and treat the patient as a whole, not just his or her disease. In addition, social workers look and treat a patient as part of a family unit, an element of a system versus just an individual. While social workers have expertise in understanding family systems and individual psychology, they are trained not to try to "fix" the patient or the family but instead to start with the patient's concerns, elicit the patient's strengths, build on those strengths (whether they be internal or external), and build consensus with the family and family system and treatment team to reach common goals.

In their training, health social workers do have practicums (internships) similar to physicians. Practicums are included within the 2-year course leading to the master of social work degree. Social workers with a master's degree who go on to achieve licensure must complete a residency of sorts where they are provided close clinical supervision for a specific amount of time (depending on their state regulations), usually between 2–4 years. Licensure is not always a requirement for working in a medical setting. In their training, social workers are aware of doctors, but they are not explicitly trained to collaborate with them. Their training in medical diagnosis and medical treatments is limited. Therefore, a social worker may never have collaborated with a physician before coming to a job on a palliative care team or working in an environment where physicians work. Consequently, they may be afraid of physicians.

Conflict or Collaboration

There is potential for conflict between physicians and social workers when they work together. Doctors are fixers; social workers are not. Physicians apply the biological sciences; social workers apply the social sciences. Doctors are taught that they lead teams, and they are the final authority for all decisions. This is reinforced by their unique and profound responsibility, which often involves life and death decisions and the real fear of liability for mishaps that might include malpractice, regulatory scrutiny, and in the extreme the loss of their right to practice. Social workers are taught they collaborate and build consensus on teams and that they are experts in communication and counseling; decisions are shared. Doctors value results; social workers value process. If all of this is true, how can the two disciplines work together?

There are several features of both physicians and social workers that influence the tendency to conflict or collaborate. The personality style of the person, particularly the need to be in control, is of paramount importance. Secondarily, the level of confidence and security in their own roles, as well as the understanding of each other's role is crucial. Those who do not have high control needs, and are confident, will collaborate well. Those who have high control needs, and are insecure, will not. Challenging one's own assumptions and having the willingness to learn is needed so that the other's role, background, and expertise are explored, shared, and respected. And thirdly the ability to communicate well is fundamental to a collaborative partnership. Physicians who define their role as team leader, the more traditional medical model use of hierarchy, will want good communication, but they often define good as "focused communication related to physicians' priorities" (Abramson & Mizrahi, 2003). The language of medicine is different from the language of social work. Consequently, when a social worker and physician must work together as part of a team, communication may be hampered.

In vignette 1 (Box 46.1), the behavior of the physician is likely explained by being nervous and feeling uncertain about her role. She knows she likes leading family meetings and goals of care discussions. The social worker, also a woman, is uncertain about how she will be treated by the physician. Both have high control needs. The solution to this situation is to make the conflict explicit and to invite discussion. The social worker might say, "*I need to know much more about what you mean. I consider myself expert in family meetings and goals of care discussions, too. Let's evaluate this together so we can come to a mutual understanding of how we will work together as part of this team.*" How the physician responds to this overture will be prognostic for their working relationship. In other words, for the physician and social worker to work

---

Box 46.1
Vignette 1: New Physician

A palliative medicine attending physician is rotating on a hospital-based palliative care team for a 1 month period. The team is composed of the attending physician, a physician fellow, a nurse practitioner, a social worker, and a pharmacist. During introductions, the attending physician announces, "I'm the expert on leading family conferences and goals of care discussions, so I will take the lead with them."

well together and in the interest of patient and family care, they must be able to give and receive feedback.

In vignette 2 (Box 46.2), it would be easy for the social worker and other team members to be upset and feel diminished. A passive-aggressive response to this upset resulted in another meeting being held without the doctor being invited. At a minimum, to prevent this from happening again, the social worker needs to provide the physician feedback about his behavior and its impact on the patient, family, and other team members. Looked at more deeply, it took both the social worker and the doctor to make this scenario happen. The social worker was silent when the doctor took over. When the meeting went awry, the social worker could have advocated on the patient's behalf during the initial family meeting. Even more, the social worker could have prepared for the family meeting in advance, negotiating with the doctor what his role would be. In our experience, physicians are delighted when they do not have to be in charge. In the absence of clear direction, they often assume they must be in charge. Even without such preparation, at the beginning of the encounter, the social worker could have welcomed the doctor, explaining what had transpired and what was happening now, and invited the doctor to sit down while maintaining and enhancing the role of meeting facilitator. In other words, the social worker must have the courage to behave as an equal member of the team. Vignette 3 (Box 46.3) illustrates a contrasting approach.

Box 46.2
Vignette 2: Physician Interruption

A social worker is facilitating a family meeting in a residential care facility for the elderly (RCFE). Barbara Thomas has become more ill and the nursing needs now exceed what can be provided in the RCFE. The doctor arrives with the meeting already in progress and takes over the leadership by disregarding the social worker's current question and interjects his opinion on what should happen, shifting the conversation with the result that the physician is doing most of the talking. The nurse and chaplain on the hospice team have been working with Ms. Thomas and her family for some time, preparing them for the inevitable clinical decline and consequent need for more nursing care. There are major financial implications for the family. Furthermore, Ms. Thomas' greatest fear is living in a skilled nursing facility. This part of the history is ignored or unknown to the doctor with the result that he prescribes the need to move Ms. Thomas to a skilled nursing facility without any recognition of the implications for her and her family. Ms. Thomas and her family are quiet; they nod in agreement because they and the team are intimidated by the physician's approach. After the meeting, it is apparent that Ms. Thomas and her family are not in agreement. Another family meeting is convened without the doctor. Ms. Thomas and her family are upset, stating they felt abandoned by the team's behaviors during the prior meeting and are considering disenrolling from hospice services. The team works to repair the relationship, clarifying the situation and deciding together what next steps are needed to insure Ms. Thomas will receive proper care.

Box 46.3
Vignette 3: Social Work Redirection

A family meeting is organized in the hospital with a patient, Chris Lear, who has progressive multiple myeloma; her daughter; the patient's sister from out of state; and the bone marrow transplant physician. The purpose of the meeting is to update Ms. Lear on her current medical status and to reevaluate goals of care. The palliative social worker leads the meeting, asking how she understood and assessed her condition. Ms. Lear knew she had pneumonia and is not surprised to get it "due to my medical condition." After some silence she states, "I'm tired" and then explains she is ready to die. She says that "when everything is in place" (meaning confirmation of whether she will reside at home or in a skilled nursing facility, a good treatment plan for care as she declines, and people she trusts to implement that care) she wants to stop coming to the cancer center. At this point the physician asks the patient, "So you don't want any more treatment?" The social worker intervenes and reframes the communication by stating that the patient would continue to get aggressive treatment for all her symptoms to keep her comfortable, confirming that she no longer wants to come to the cancer center nor to the emergency department. She clarifies for the physician that Ms. Lear stated she wants to die comfortably at her skilled nursing facility with hospice team support. The transplant physician responds by writing an order for hospice care, supporting her decision. A hospice representative meets with Ms. Lear and her family within the hour and she is discharged to hospice care in the nursing facility that day. She dies there 1 week later peacefully and pain free with her daughter at her side.

Using Conflict for Team Growth

In vignette 3, the social worker demonstrated leadership. In the presence of a bone marrow transplant physician, the social worker facilitated the meeting and assisted the physician to understand the patient's goals of care. She used a reframing intervention to correct the effect of a physician statement and validated for all that palliative and hospice care was not a choice for "no more treatment" but rather a choice for a different kind of treatment.

Since physicians and social workers bring such different skills to the bedside, conflict is expected and welcomed. The experience of conflict, if acknowledged, can be viewed as creative tension and as fuel for the engine of teamwork. The emotionally charged high-stress clinical environment, the endless demands of patient care, compulsiveness, the high need for control, the internal drive for excellence, and the natural competitiveness of health care professionals constitute the most fertile loam for deep roots of dissention. The social worker, trained in systems work, is probably most skilled at recognizing the elements of conflict and in helping the physician and others to recognize what it means, to avoid personalizing, and to use it for constructive benefit. Sometimes the social worker must lead the physicians. This is illustrated in the final vignette (Box 46.4).

This family is divided into two factions; the sisters on one side and the sons and father on another. Each faction communicates to the primary team concerns related to Ms. Hany's care at home. The sisters do not believe the husband was attentive enough to the patient and was withholding pain medication from her. The husband was keeping the sisters from his wife because he believed they were overreactive to her needs and wanted to keep her sedated.

The palliative medicine fellow takes the lead in an impromptu family meeting regarding goals of care and hospice. The meeting goes awry when the fellow is distracted by the intrafamily tension about "who is right" rather than focusing on the patient and her needs. Wanting to understand the root causes for the conflict and to discover the fears behind each side's concerns, the palliative social worker intervenes by asking the family to share their reactions to the suggestion of hospice care and eliciting what they believe to be Ms. Hany's needs. The oldest son says, "I want my mother to receive chemotherapy should she get stronger and that my

family's religious faith be honored." The family states that home hospice care had been presented as "additional help," which, from their perspective, is insulting. There is now agreement in the family on this one point: that they did not need additional help. They have sufficient money to hire help at home and there are many family members to provide care. What they need is the medical expertise to keep their loved one pain free at home and for their religious faith to be honored by whomever would provide that expertise. Another issue the social worker discovers is that Ms. Hany and her family are devout Chaldean Catholics. The family was told by a hospice worker that they would honor the patient's and family's need to pray five times a day facing Mecca, an Islamic practice. This is considered sacrilege to this family, who left their country of origin because of religious persecution.

Based on the agreed-upon goals of Ms. Hany and family, the palliative social worker suggests that Ms. Hany be admitted on home hospice care to obtain the palliative medicine expertise they need, with a clear stipulation that if her functional status improves, there will be a reassessment for further chemotherapy. Because of cultural considerations, it is inappropriate to address the role of antibiotics, artificial nutrition and/or hydration, or rehospitalizations in advance. The family finds it offensive to discuss the withholding of *future* curative or palliative treatment. They view this as a lack of faith because her life and death were "in God's hands." This family can only make those decisions when they present as issues in the context of Ms. Hany's overall functioning. The palliative physician makes recommendations about pain medications as one aspect of the medical expertise that is so important to this family.

Summary

Physicians and social workers are trained differently and apply different bodies of scientific knowledge. A productive collaboration on a palliative care team requires explicit acknowledgment of these differences and the potential strengths they bring to the care of patients and families. Conflict should be expected and welcomed.

LEARNING EXERCISES

- Compare and contrast the educational backgrounds of physicians and social workers. Identify why they might either collaborate or be in conflict as a result of this background.
- Play the role of the doctor and the social worker for each of the vignettes presented. Play the roles:
  a. To maximize conflict
  b. To minimize conflict
  c. To identify and resolve conflict

Box 46.4
Vignette 4: Social Work Clarification

Amira Hany, a married Middle Eastern woman, age 48, is admitted to an acute care hospital with neutropenic fever after treatment for multiple myeloma. Due to her ongoing fevers and infections and poor functional status (primarily bedbound), it is determined she is not a candidate for further chemotherapy. The hematology/oncology team recommend hospice.

Ms. Hany and her husband have three children, a daughter, age 31, who is severely physically handicapped and lives with them, and two sons, ages 26 and 22, both of whom are very successful in their careers. Ms. Hany and her husband, Chaldean Catholics, immigrated from the Middle East in 1977 due to persecution by the dominant religion, Islam. Prior to becoming ill, Ms. Hany was very active in her community in assisting other immigrants to assimilate. She is one of 12 siblings, all girls. One of her sisters recently took her vows as a nun and has come from out of state to be with her to assist in determining goals of care. The sisters present as a very tight knit group, very much confidantes of one another. Mr. Hany is a very successful and prominent businessman in the community.

Ms. Hany declines to participate in the decision making and defers to her husband. Her oldest son has assumed the role of the authority and decision maker in the family. Mr. Hany is having a difficult time dealing with the reality of his wife's poor prognosis, lack of treatment options, and his impotence to change the course of his wife's disease.

Hospice care is presented to the family by several staff members, including the inpatient case manager, the hematology/oncology attending physician and fellow, and a local hospice nurse representative. Hospice is repeatedly declined. Ms. Hany's and her family's goals are (1) for her to go home, (2) to have good symptom management, and(3) to get more treatment. The palliative care team is consulted by the hospital attending physician for symptom management and to get her enrolled in home hospice.

REFERENCES

Abramson, J. S., & Mizrahi, T. (2003). Understanding collaboration between social workers and physicians: Application of a typology. *Social Work in Health Care*, 37(2), 2003.

Blacker, S. (2004). Palliative care and social work. In J. Berzoff & P. R. Silverman (Eds.), *Living with dying: A handbook for end-of-life healthcare practitioners* (pp. 409–423). New York, NY: Columbia University Press.

Clark, D. (2003). *Cicely Saunders: Founder of the hospice movement: Selected letters 1959–1999*. Oxford, England: Oxford University Press.

Curley, C., McEachern, J. E., & Speroff, T. A. (1998). A firm trial of interdisciplinary rounds on the inpatient medical wards: An intervention designed using continuous quality improvement. *Medical Care*, 36, AS4–12.

Dunlop, R. J., & Hockley, J. M. (Eds.). (1998). *Hospital-based palliative care teams: the hospital-hospice interface* (p. 47). New York, NY: Oxford University Press.

Higginson, I. J., Finlay, I. G., Goodwin, D. M., Hood, K., Edwards, A. G. K., Cook, A.,... Normand, C. E. (2003). Is there evidence that palliative care teams alter end-of-life experiences of patients and their caregivers? *Journal of Pain and Symptom Management*, 25, 150–168.

Loscalzo, M. J., & von Gunten, C. F. (2008). Interdisciplinary teamwork in palliative care: Compassionate expertise for serious complex illness. In H. Chochinov & W. Breitbart (Eds.), *Oxford handbook of palliative psychiatry* (pp. 173–185). New York, NY: Oxford University Press.

Silver, G. A., & Stiber, C. (1957). The social worker and the physician: Daily practice of a health team. *Journal of Medical Education*, 32, 324–330.

Sommers, L. S., Marton, K. I., Barbaccia, D., & Randolph, J. (2000). Physician, nurse, and social worker collaboration in primary care for chronically ill seniors. *Archives of Internal Medicine*, 160, 1825–1833.

Wagner, E. H. (2000). The role of patient care teams in chronic disease management. *British Medical Journal*, 320, 569–572.

47

Holly Nelson-Becker and Betty R. Ferrell

Social Work and Nursing: Creating Effective Collaborations in Palliative Care

When my mother was dying in hospice, it felt like everyone was working together—like a team.
It made us feel secure and like they cared for me as much as they cared for my mother.
                                                                    —A bereaved daughter

Key Concepts

◆ *Opportunities abound for social work and nursing collaboration as nurses and social workers provide holistic integrative care for patients and their families informed by best practices from both professions.*

◆ *Specific strategies to enhance successful collaboration by nurses and social workers as members of interdisciplinary teams include role clarity, open communication, fluidity, collective ownership of goals, self and team reflection; and structural support.*

Introduction

At the most fundamental level, palliative care and hospice are interdisciplinary endeavors requiring collaboration by every profession involved in care. Social work and nursing professionals share a special role because they are often involved in the daily implementation of the interdisciplinary plan of care. In concert with their colleagues in medicine, spiritual care, rehabilitation, psychology, and other fields, they weave together comprehensive care that addresses physical, psychosocial, and spiritual needs. The narrative in Box 47.1 illustrates the intricacies of social work and nursing collaboration.

Discussion of Patient/Family Narrative

The care of the Hernandez family illustrates the clear need for interdisciplinary care and the unique collaboration of the nurse and social worker in a dynamic trajectory of care. Together, these professionals would assess, plan, and implement a plan of care that is revised in response to changing needs. Several strategies for successful collaboration have been identified in the literature. Among these is the essential role of interdisciplinary communication as well as mutual respect for the skills each professional brings to the team.

Strategies for Successful Social Work and Nursing Collaboration

The Context and Nature of Collaboration

Effective interdisciplinary collaboration is fundamental to provision of high-quality care and goal attainment in hospice settings (Atwall & Caldwell, 2006; Kearney, 2008; Netting & Williams, 1998; Parker-Oliver, Wittenberg-Lyles, & Day, 2006; Reese & Sontag, 2001). Identification of obstacles

Box 47.1
Patient/Family Narrative: Mrs. Hernandez and Family

Mrs. Juanita Hernandez, a 74-year-old widow, was seen in a hospital emergency room with complaints of severe nausea and abdominal pain. She was found to have stage IV ovarian cancer with extensive liver metastasis. After treatment of an acute bowel obstruction, she was discharged home to hospice care. Due to her extensive metastatic disease and significant cardiac and pulmonary coexisting diseases, her life expectancy was estimated to be 2–3 months.

Mrs. Hernandez lived with her recently divorced daughter, Eliza, and her four young grandchildren. She had been providing child care for these grandchildren so that Eliza could return to work as a secretary. Mrs. Hernandez' other daughter, Rosa, also lived nearby and was overwhelmed as a 20-year-old woman with two children (ages 4 months and 2 years). Rosa's husband was in the army and recently deployed to the Middle East.

The hospice social worker and nurse made a joint admission visit and completed a biopsychosocial-spiritual assessment of Mrs. Hernandez and her family. Her symptoms of nausea, pain, and constipation were poorly controlled, and both daughters were so emotionally distraught that they could only provide minimal help. Compounding the situation was the arrival of Mrs. Hernandez' son, Juan, who had come from out of state and accused his sisters of being responsible for their mother's terminal illness saying, "Mom has been so busy caring for your messed-up lives that she has neglected her own health—this is all your fault." Juan had been estranged from the family and reportedly had a history of alcohol abuse and gang activity.

Over the course of the next 2 weeks, the hospice team developed a comprehensive plan of care for this complex family focusing on intense symptom management. The social worker prioritized needs, paying special attention to addressing the complex family dynamics and practical concerns, including child care and house maintenance. Hospice volunteers were also called in to provide respite care. The hospice chaplain was immensely helpful in providing spiritual support for Mrs. Hernandez and her daughters. Unfortunately, Juan returned home but persisted in making threatening calls to his sisters. All further attempts by the team to reach out to Juan were unsuccessful.

Over the next several weeks, the hospice team met regularly to orchestrate care in support of Mrs. Hernandez and her family. Mrs. Hernandez' condition continued to decline, her symptoms escalated, and it appeared she would soon die. The nurse and social worker coordinated a family meeting to explore placement options. All agreed that she would receive optimum care in an inpatient setting where her daughters and grandchildren could be present during this critical time, but be relieved of the tasks of managing her worsening symptoms and providing her physical care. Mrs. Hernandez died 1 week later with her daughters and grandchildren present. The hospice team developed an individualized bereavement plan for each member of the family, recognizing their preexisting challenges as well as the impact of the quick decline of the family matriarch.

McCarthy, & Wells, 2004; Reese & Sontag, 2001; Salhani & Coulter, 2009). These include role overlap, status differences, and boundary blurring, but the focus of this chapter will be to identify areas of best practice in professional collaboration between social work and nursing. The complexity of care for the Hernandez family illustrates the need and the value of such collaborative care. Interprofessional collaboration both emerged from and became a normative standard of the modern hospice and palliative care models. Availability of different forms of expertise, experience, and ability within professional fields of practice led to holistic treatment of the individual and achievement of high quality of life within the dying experience (Saunders, 1999). Thus, the inherent value of collaboration and support among social workers and nurses who rank similarly on professional status scales within hospice teams is clear.

In multidisciplinary teams, members from several disciplines usually work independently within the bounds of their professions to assess patients and plan treatment. Care is often provided through layered interventions to meet multiple objectives. Interdisciplinary team (IDT) members collaborate in an integrative manner to solve problems synergistically and enhance life quality beyond the boundaries of a single discipline (Geriatric Interdisciplinary Team Training, 2001). Transdisciplinary teams are all this and more, including patient, family, and other stakeholders in their assessment, planning, and care processes. Furthermore, transdisciplinary teams are willing to transcend standard professional orientations to get the work done through novel methods or new kinds of solutions (Hermsen & ten Have, 2005). Within palliative care, IDT social workers and nurses cooperate at the level of a transdisciplinary team to ensure a range of biopsychosocial and (along with chaplains) spiritual needs are met.

Both social workers and nurses have been socialized according to the "grand narratives" of their professions. Social work emphasizes sensitivity to person-in-environment and biopsychosocial-spiritual perspectives. Nursing emphasizes holistic care, which includes physical, psychological, social, and spiritual well-being (American Nurses Association, 2001; Council on Social Work Education [CSWE], 2008; Netting & Williams, 1998). While professional preparation of each discipline shares these commonalities, they also have marked differences. Social workers are taught to consider the range of environmental influences on individual functioning and to operate fluidly in environments to help clients directly through therapeutic counseling approaches as well as by connecting clients to resources. Nurses hold expertise in medical areas with direct impact on pain management and maintaining the highest level of physical functioning possible within a specific disease course. Recognition of these combined and separate expertise domains can strengthen professional identity and lead to a strong consultative effect, where knowledge and advice are shared in peer meetings and enrich the completion of the tasks needed by palliative care institutions and patients alike.

and barriers to health care and hospice interprofessional teamwork abound in the literature (Atwall & Caldwell, 2006; Bliss, Cowley, & While, 2000; Lichtenstein, Alexander,

Strategies for Success

What is needed in successful social work–nursing interactions? Varying factors have been identified. Five elements of a successful interprofessional collaboration include interdependence, new professional activities, flexibility, collective ownership of goals, and reflection on process (Bronstein, 2003). Technical skill, clinical interaction skill, and social and emotional regulation skills are potentially accessible within a social work–nursing dyad (McCallin & Bamford, 2007). Knowledge of role differences, building trust and communication, and avoidance of fragmentation are also cited as key issues in optimally functioning health care teams (Arber, 2008; Parker-Oliver & Peck, 2006; Reese & Sontag, 2001; Sargeant, Loney, & Murphy, 2008; Suter et al., 2009). Based on the literature and our own understanding, we have identified several areas that assist in creation of optimal palliative care collaborations: achievement of role clarity; open communication; fluidity; collective ownership of goals; self and team reflection; and structural support.

Role Clarity
The ability of social workers and nurses to collaborate is enhanced by an understanding of the strengths, limits, and disciplinary approaches to treatment that provide measures of competency for each discipline. Competency is generally assessed according to access to specialized forms of knowledge, training that includes many forms of practice skill, and values or attitudes that are usually embodied in an ethical code. Both social work and nursing have codes that share some related and complementary concepts (Bronstein, 2003). Understanding one's relationship and access to professional knowledge can fortify professional identity and paradoxically permit appropriate (within code) role crossings in service to the client and family. Furthermore, creating a context of reciprocity can permit professionals to remain secure in their own value and identity while demonstrating respect for and supporting the work of colleagues. Learning with, from, and about each other's roles as work proceeds can strengthen the relationship (Sargeant et al., 2008). Collaboration functions well where allegiance is balanced between the profession and the interprofessional work.

Open Communication
The ability to communicate openly and well, without engendering confusion, is a fundamental skill. Similarly, the ability to resolve internal difficulties and tensions that emerge in the course of developing or adjusting treatment plans is important in interprofessional collaboration (Street & Blackford, 2001; Wittenberg-Lyles, 2005). Mediation skills are often part of professional social work courses, and nurses may also have some knowledge of these. It is helpful to encourage participation from all through pluralistic dialogue that includes sensitivity to emotional language and tone (McCallin & Bamford, 2007). Such pluralistic dialogue also recognizes diversity in worldviews, personality, preferred forms of information exchange, and interpersonal and leadership styles through understanding that communication occurs multilaterally across cognitive, social, emotional, and other domains. Communication is enhanced when there is emotional safety and trust within a larger climate that encourages discussion of the complexities of a case. Understanding discourse identities, or identity created through language, can assist teams in facilitating clear interactions (Arber, 2008). The use of questioning techniques is a low-risk behavior both professions can engage to collaborate fully with physicians to address their own and patient concerns (Arber, 2008).

Fluidity
In hospice care provided in community settings, when social workers and nurses visit patients together as in the case of Mrs. Hernandez, they can reinforce and learn from each other. Practicing within the bounds of their roles, they can each represent the thinking of the entire team when separate visits are made by responding to questions about care that they do not themselves provide. Fluidity is also shown when compromises are found even if there is initial disagreement about a goal for care. Negotiation, learning for oneself what perspective one is willing to release or adapt, is a valuable form of education in the moment between the two professional views. Furthermore, personal characteristics of individuals in the formal roles may vary. Individuals have different interests that lead to development of varying kinds of expertise within their disciplines. Facilitating professional growth means promoting creative expression of skills and interests. For example, a social worker with musical background may offer to play the guitar for a palliative care patient; a nurse with background in Zen Buddhism may offer to meditate with a client. Individual competency, as well as professional title, is considered in determining responsibility and functions.

Collective Ownership of Goals
Collective ownership of goals occurs when all persons believe they have added their perspectives to a discussion and their viewpoints have been heard. Being heard is a powerful mechanism to enable social workers, nurses, and other palliative care team members to mutually invest in both process and outcome goals. If viewpoints diverge by a large amount, it is often a result of greater diversity of thinking. Organizational studies report that greater diversity in thought may lead to greater conflict and discomfort, but if all parties can stay at the table, the *quality* of the decision-making process is usually better (Lichtenstein et al., 2004). Aiming for the same goal was cited by nurses as important in a study of multidisciplinary teamwork (Atwall & Caldwell, 2006). Social work–nursing collaboration can help build agreement with other team members about the aims, interventions, services, and hoped-for outcomes of care by ensuring all voices are heard.

Self and Team Reflection
A commitment to self-evaluation individually and as a team will enhance functioning (Bronstein, 2003). An evaluative process is part of assessing team functions and outcomes and

in determining what can be modified to improve functioning as goals change over time (Kapp & Nelson-Becker, 2007; Wittenberg-Lyles, Parker-Oliver, Demiris, Baldwin, & Regehr, 2008). However this self-reflection process is enhanced when self-care issues are addressed. Processing difficult deaths together and exploring experiences with dying patients can help nurses and social workers better understand their contributions to care and restore their capacity to give. Sometimes this is best accomplished in the presence of an outside facilitator, so all team members have the opportunity to work through difficult feelings without being overburdened by the role of facilitating for others. Furthermore, palliative care treatment decisions are often made when circumstances are ambiguous (Hermsen & ten Have, 2005). Nurses and social workers can join with other team members to reflect upon ethical decisions both as they are crafted and after the situation has fully unfolded.

Structural Supports

Good collaboration occurs when institutional supports for that collaboration are strong. Such administrative factors as a manageable workload and regular time and space for collaboration to take place are important features. Organizations that do what they can to flatten hierarchies while supporting professional autonomy in a work culture that values participation and minimizes competition also assist social workers and nurses to do their best work. At the request of a hospice director, the first author facilitated hospice staff support groups for two teams over five years in Kansas, leading to outcomes that included greater appreciation and valuing of role differences. In this type of palliative care institution, work is designed to provide invitation to explore possibility, authentic self-reflection, and inspiration to staff and patients as it also fulfills necessary functions (Brown, 2008).

Summary

While interprofessional *competition* does exist in some settings, it damages the effectiveness of collaborations. A best practices approach to social work and nursing clinical interaction recognizes the distinct and similar role functions and places value on each. Optimal palliative care collaborations identified here include achievement of role clarity; open communication; fluidity; collective ownership of goals; self and team reflection; and structural support. These optimal practices are best begun in professional practice schools, where social workers and nurses can have some joint training to gain greater role knowledge of allied professions. Interventional research in clinical palliative settings will be enriched with the engagement of both social work and nursing skills. Working together, social workers and nurses can provide stability to a team and enhance quality of life for patients and families who are living with life-threatening illnesses as well as those who are dying.

The intent of these exercises is to create an opportunity for nurses and social workers to learn from each other. These exercises may be done in an educational setting with social work and nursing students or in a professional workplace to cultivate greater interprofessional knowledge and skills as part of a continuing education format. Twenty to thirty minutes may be allowed for each task.

- Ask social workers and nurses to separately develop a short list of questions designed to elicit information about their sister profession. Questions may include specific job-related tasks or educational training processes. They may also include a comparison of ethical code similarities and differences. Invite the social workers and nurses to form pairs and ask each other their list of questions, being willing to also pursue other questions that may arise. This information may also then be shared in a larger group format as the small groups report back. The objective is for both professionals to come away from the encounter with increased appreciation for the work of their colleague, and greater knowledge about areas of commonality and difference in both their work and points of view.

- Compare suggestions for difficult cases. Either in pairs or in a larger group format, social workers and nurses may take turns presenting a difficult patient or client situation. The social worker or nurse summarizes the narrative in 5–10 minutes. Each responding professional then draws on his or her own body of knowledge to share alternative viewpoints in 3–5 minutes. The social worker or nurse who presented the patient/client case can then respond back in 1–3 minutes about what he or she learned from his or her colleague. This consultative type session may enhance either real or theoretical decision-making options.

ADDITIONAL SUGGESTED READINGS

Whyte, D. (1992). *The house of belonging*. Langley, WA: Many Rivers Press.
Whyte, D. (2001). *Crossing the unknown sea: Work as a pilgrimage of identity*. New York, NY: Riverhead Books.

ADDITIONAL RESOURCES AND WEB SITES

American Nurses Association: http://www.nursingworld.org/ MainMenuCategories/EthicsStandards/CodeofEthicsforNurses. aspx
Code of ethics for nurses. This code may be used to compare with the National Association of Social Workers Code of Ethics.
The End-of-Life Nursing Education Consortium (ELNEC): http:// www.aacn.nche.edu/ELNEC/

A national education initiative to improve palliative care by training palliative care nurses so they can teach this essential information to nursing students and practicing nurses.

Hartford Institute for Geriatric Nursing: http://www.hartfordign.org/trythis

Many of these articles and videos on this Web site may serve as excellent resources for social workers. From the Web site: "Newest in our resource base is the *How to Try This series*, a John A. Hartford Foundation–funded project provided to the Hartford Institute for Geriatric Nursing at New York University's College of Nursing in collaboration with the *American Journal of Nursing*. This initiative will translate the evidence-based geriatric assessment tools in the *Try This* assessment series into cost-free, web-based resources including demonstration videos, and a corresponding print series featured in the *AJN*, developed to build geriatric assessment skills the foundation for appropriate care of older adults."

Lippincott's Nursing Center. *How to try this: Assessments and best practices in care of older adults*: http://www.nursingcenter.com/library/static.asp?pageid=730390

Pain and Palliative Care Resource Center (PRC): http://prc.coh.org

Serves as a clearinghouse to disseminate information and resources to assist others in improving the quality of pain management and end-of-life care.

Southern California Cancer Pain Initiative (SCCPI): http://sccpi.coh.org/

A nonprofit volunteer interdisciplinary organization composed of physicians, nurses, pharmacists, social workers, and many other professionals dedicated to the relief of cancer pain.

REFERENCES

American Nurses Association. (2001). *2001 approved provisions*. Retrieved from http://www.nursingworld.org/MainMenu Categories/EthicsStandards/CodeofEthicsforNurses/2110 Provisions.aspx

Arber, A. (2008). Team meetings in specialist palliative care: Asking questions as a strategy within interprofessional interaction. *Qualitative Health Research, 18*(10), 1323–1335.

Atwall, A., & Caldwell, K. (2006). Nurses' perceptions of multidisciplinary team work in acute care. *International Journal of Nursing Practice, 12*(6), 359–365.

Bliss, J., Cowley, S., & While, A. (2000). Interprofessional working in palliative care in the community: A review of the literature. *Journal of Interprofessional Care, 14*(3), 281–290.

Bronstein, L. R. (2003). A model for interdisciplinary collaboration. *Social Work, 48*(3), 297–306.

Brown, T. (2008). Design thinking. *Harvard Business Review, 86*(6), 84–92.

Council on Social Work Education. (2008). *Educational policy and accreditation standards (EPAS)*. Retrieved from http://www.cswe.org/File.aspx?id=13780

Geriatric Interdisciplinary Team Training (GITT). (2001). *Teams and teamwork*. Retrieved from http://www.jhartfound.org/pdf%20files/GITT.pdf

Hermsen, M. A., & ten Have, H. A. (2005). Palliative care teams: Effective through moral reflection. *Journal of Interprofessional Care, 19*(6), 561–568.

Kapp, S. A., & Nelson-Becker, H. B. (2007). Evaluating hospice services for improvement: A manageable approach. *The Journal of Pain and Palliative Care Pharmacotherapy, 21*(2), 17–26.

Kearney A. (2008). Facilitating interprofessional education and practice. *The Canadian Nurse, 104*(3), 22.

Lichtenstein, R., Alexander, J. A., McCarthy, J. F., & Wells, R. (2004). Status differences in cross-functional teas: Effects on individual member participation, job satisfaction, and intent to quit. *Journal of Health and Social Behavior, 45*(3), 322–335.

McCallin, A., & Bamford, A. (2007). Interdisciplinary teamwork: Is the influence of emotional intelligence fully appreciated? *Journal of Nursing Management, 15*(4), 386–391.

Netting, F. E., & Williams, F. G. (1998). Can we prepare geriatric social workers to collaborate in primary care practices. *Journal of Social Work Education, 34*(2), 195–210.

Parker-Oliver, D., Bronstein L. R., & Kurzejeski, L. (2005). Examining variables related to successful collaboration on the hospice team. *Health Social Work, 30*(4), 279–286.

Parker-Oliver, D., & Peck, M. (2006). Inside the interdisciplinary team: Experiences of hospice social workers. *Journal of Social Work in End of Life and Palliative Care, 2*(3), 7–21.

Parker-Oliver, D., Wittenberg-Lyles, E., & Day, M. (2006). Variances in perceptions of interdisciplinary collaboration by hospice staff. *Journal of Palliative Care, 22*(4), 274–280.

Reese, D. J., & Sontag, M. A. (2001). Successful interprofessional collaboration on the hospice team. *Health Social Work, 26*(3), 167–175.

Salhani, D., & Coulter, I. (2009). The politics of interprofessional working and the struggle for professional autonomy in nursing. *Social Science and Medicine, 68*(7), 1221–1228.

Sargeant, J., Loney, E., & Murphy, G. (2008). Effective interprofessional teams: "Contact is not enough" to build a team. *Journal of Continuing Education in the Health Professions, 28*(4), 228–234.

Saunders, C. (1999). Origins: International perspectives, then and now. In I. B. Corless & Z. Foster (Eds.), *The hospice heritage: Celebrating our future* (pp. 1–8). New York, NY: Haworth Press.

Street, A., & Blackford, J. (2001). Communication issues for the interdisciplinary community palliative care team. *Journal of Clinical Nursing, 10*(5), 643–650.

Suter, E., Arndt, J., Arthur, N., Parboosingh, J., Taylor, E., & Deutschlander, S. (2009). Role understanding and effective communication as core competencies for collaborative practice. *Journal of Interprofessional Care, 23*(1), 41–51.

Wittenberg-Lyles, E. (2005). Information sharing in interdisciplinary team meetings: An evaluation of hospice goals. *Qualitative Health Research, 15*(10), 1377–1391.

Wittenberg-Lyles, E., Parker-Oliver, D., Demiris, G., Baldwin, P., & Regehr, K. (2008). Communication dynamics in hospice teams: Understanding the role of the chaplain in interdisciplinary team collaboration. *Journal of Palliative Medicine, 11*(10), 1330–1335.

48 *Robin Pollens and Marie C. Lynn*

Social Work and Speech Pathology: Supporting Communication in Palliative Care

Everybody is talking about me, but nobody is talking to me.
    —*Patient who was unable to talk but could type out her concerns on a device*

Key Concepts

- *Speech-language pathologists and social workers can collaborate to support communication and self-determination for individuals with communication impairments.*
- *Speech pathology and social work bring a unique synergy to counseling that focuses on adjustment to illness and medical decision making.*
- *Rehabilitation therapists may collaborate with social workers to provide specific expertise to support palliative care goals.*

Introduction

The goals of palliative care include enhancing quality of life for patients and families and optimizing function (National Consensus Project, 2009). This chapter will demonstrate clinical outcomes for palliative care patients who received care through the collaboration of a speech-language pathologist and health social worker. This collaboration resulted in the support of communication, self-determination, and quality of life for patients and families. The interdisciplinary relationship and the care provided by the speech-language pathologist and the health social worker can serve as a model for other rehabilitation therapists in palliative care.

Facilitating Communication

Communication is a key component of palliative care and an expected skill for all members of the palliative care team. Much of the literature in palliative care describes how the team can better communicate with the patient or family (von Gunten, Ferris, & Emanuel, 2000). Skillful communication by the health social worker is vital both to establish and to maintain effective relationships between the patient, the family, and the team (Farrelly, 2009). However, what happens to the palliative care process when the patient himself or herself has a serious communication deficit?

Individuals with head and neck cancer, stroke, traumatic brain injury, or various degenerative neurologic diseases may have severe communication impairments. Achieving quality goals of palliative care may then be compromised (Salt & Roberson, 1998). In addition, a patient's agitation and anxiety may increase due to the patient's frustration and fear of not being able to communicate (Garrett, Happ, Costello, & Fried-Oken, 2007).

Certain patients may need to be supported communicatively so that they can participate in establishing goals of care with the social worker, their family, and other members of the team. The social worker may request consultation by the speech-language pathologist. The speech-language pathologist can assess the patient's communication and cognitive status in the context of the family or team interaction. If possible, appropriate strategies will be developed to assist the *patient* to provide input for care decisions, *the family* to advocate based on the patient's wishes and to maintain social closeness, and the *palliative care team* to provide effective symptom management and engage the patient in psychosocial discussions (Pollens, 2004).

In our first patient and family narrative (Box 48.1), the speech-language pathologist is consulted for the purpose of reducing caregiver stress and facilitating the health social worker's ability to do reminiscence therapy with a patient with severe aphasia.

Many complexities can develop within family systems during times of crisis (Farrelly, 2009). The speech-language pathologist or other rehabilitation professionals may need to consult with the health social worker to provide guidance and support to the patient (see Box 48.2). The social worker may initiate or lead a family meeting to develop care strategies. At times, patients, family members, and team members may use different communication modalities, which can impact the social worker's ability to facilitate the family meeting (Powazski, 2009). The speech-language pathologist

---

Box 48.1
Patient/Family Narrative: Mr. Hendricks

Mr. Hendricks, a 63-year-old gentleman with glioblastoma and resulting aphasia, was receiving care at home with his wife as primary caregiver. The patient's verbal communication was very limited, and he had additional cognitive impairments. When the social worker met with his wife, she was tearful and overwhelmed. Her husband was becoming increasingly angry and aggressive toward her when she could not understand his attempted communication. The health social worker requested a speech-language pathologist consult to assess the patient's communication abilities and the family's communication interaction.

After the initial assessment, the speech-language pathologist demonstrated the use of strategies that could help Mrs. Hendricks to shape the communication interaction more effectively. For example, she learned to write down key words during a conversation to help her husband to understand what she was saying. She also wrote short lists for him to indicate his choice when he could not verbalize his ideas (Lasker, Garrett, & Fox, 2007).

Mrs. Hendricks learned to more effectively determine the main topic or direction of her husband's communication attempt. She gained a sense of competence because she now had tools to help her to understand his concerns. The communication deficit remained, but the wife had gained an appreciation of her husband's disease-related challenges and limitations. The social worker noted that the couple was better able to function as a unit to meet daily care needs, and the patient appeared to have reduced frustration.

The health social worker was also able to use these communication strategies to engage the patient in reminiscence therapy, and she determined that the patient had fond memories of listening to gospel music as a child. The social worker informed the nurse that gospel music may be a tool to relieve pain and distress, and a referral was initiated to the music therapist.

Box 48.2
Patient/Family Narrative: Mrs. Smith

Our second narrative begins with a nursing request for the speech-language pathologist and occupational therapist (OT) to assess the status of Mrs. Smith, a 76-year-old woman with advanced renal disease and diabetes. She recently had a stroke, seemed somewhat confused, and was having physical difficulties due to new hemiparesis. The speech-language pathologist determined that she was having language and memory difficulties; reasoning and judgment skills appeared intact. The OT recommended a commode near the patient's hospital bed and a raised toilet seat. All team members believed that it was not safe for her to be alone.

During the next home visit, the patient informed the speech-language pathologist that she had a son, Craig, who was deaf and lived in her basement apartment. The speech-language pathologist interviewed Craig via writing, because he appeared to have difficulty lip reading. Craig's written language used the syntax of American Sign Language (ASL), and the speech-language pathologist was concerned about the potential for errors in interpretation (Allen, Meyers, Sullivan, & Sullivan, 2002). The speech-language pathologist made a referral for a health social worker on staff who was fluent in ASL.

The health social worker met with the patient and son to do a psychosocial assessment. Using ASL, the son stated that the hospital staff had not communicated with him because he was deaf. The social worker was aware that many people in the Deaf community are often isolated within the medical system without access to information (Allen et al., 2002). The son wanted to be included in the care of his mother and Mrs. Smith agreed. The health social worker coordinated a family meeting that included the care team and a certified interpreter. Even though the health social worker signed, she knew that the "wearing of two hats" could cause an overlap in roles and that the quality of medical care could be compromised if an interpreter was not involved (Flores, 2005).

Craig now had a voice and he took an active part in the meeting, brainstorming solutions to problems. The patient requested that he be her representative payee, that his name be put on her checkbook, and that he become her patient advocate. The registered nurse taught Craig how to monitor his mother's blood sugar levels. He also agreed to provide 24-hour basic care for his mother. The team agreed that this plan would enable the patient to remain at home in a safe and caring environment

---

and health social worker may then collaborate for optimal care on behalf of the patient and family.

Supporting Self-Determination

One of the tenets of palliative and end-of-life care is that a competent adult has the right to make treatment decisions. Patients with communication challenges can participate in this process with support. At times, the speech-language pathologist may help to determine whether a patient with a communication impairment has decision-making capacity and whether the patient needs augmentative strategies to express his or her preferences (Sharp & Payne, 1999). Certain tools may be helpful, such as pictorial communication booklets that enable patients to point to preferences regarding life-sustaining treatment options (Kagan & Shumway, 2003). The scope and accuracy of information conveyed by the patient can be significantly enhanced through appropriate use of augmentative strategies or materials (see Box 48.3).

Intervening with Dysphagia

Speech-language pathologists are also consulted to assess and provide education for patients with difficulty swallowing (dysphagia). Dysphagia commonly occurs in head and neck cancer, stroke, progressive neurologic disease, and dementia, and it may be a primary factor prompting the referral to a palliative care team (Pollens, Hillenbrand, & Sharp, 2009).

Both the speech-language pathologist and health social worker can assist the patient with dysphagia and their family in exploring long-term care decisions or preparing for end-of-life care. Often, there is a need for the health social worker to counsel patients and family members as they adjust to the illness, terminal status, or changes in lifestyle and grieve the many losses implicit in these processes. The patient and family may then be better able to make treatment decisions and long-term care plans (see Box 48.4).

Box 48.3
Patient/Family Narrative: Mr. Chevalier

Mr. Chevalier, a 62-year-old gentleman with severe bulbar amyotrophic lateral sclerosis (ALS), was no longer able to produce any intelligible words. The speech-language pathologist had instructed this gentleman on the use of other nonverbal means to communicate, including a device in which he could type his message using a text-to-voice output to generate expression of his ideas.

Mr. Chevalier's long-time partner had recently died, and he was living alone in his home with intermittent support of close friends. Realizing the severity of his disease progression, Mr. Chevalier contacted a hospice organization and requested the speech-language pathologist to attend the initial intake meeting. The intake nurse asked the patient: "Is it your preference to continue living in your own home?" The patient nodded, "Yes." The nurse began to ask a second, unrelated question. The speech-language pathologist intervened and suggested that the patient use his augmentative communication device to further explain his perspective. The patient then typed and generated the following auditory output message: "I would like to stay at home, but I realize that under certain conditions I may need to go to a nursing home." This prompted the social worker to probe several key factors. When he became more debilitated, would he have a large enough support system to remain at home? Does he have adequate financial resources to continue home care? The speech-language pathologist guided the health social worker in optimal strategies for conducting a conversation using the augmentative device, and the patient was able to discuss these important issues with the social worker.

Box 48.4
Patient/Family Narrative: Mrs. Conway

Mrs. Conway, an 88-year-old woman with a progressive neurologic disease, could no longer produce intelligible speech. She also had cardiac disease and severe arthritis with chronic pain. Her adult children lived in other states.

The speech-language pathologist initial assessment determined that the client could communicate effectively through writing and she appeared cognitively competent to make decisions. Mrs. Conway was currently only drinking oral supplements and losing weight. Assessment of her swallowing ability revealed profound oral-pharyngeal dysphagia as described in a recent swallowing videoflouroscopy report. Due to her severe muscle weakness, she coughed uncomfortably following most swallows. It was clear that she would not be able to maintain nutrition and hydration through her oral intake. The patient stated that her daughter, Suzanne, was encouraging her to have gastrostomy tube surgery to supplement her oral intake.

Both the speech-language pathologist and the social worker provided counseling pertinent to their disciplines. The social worker explored Mrs. Conway's feelings regarding tube feeding and her beliefs and values. She determined that the patient was considering the gastrostomy tube only to "appease" her daughter. She felt that she had lived a long life and currently was uncomfortable due to her severe medical problems.

The speech-language pathologist explained that even with the gastrostomy tube placement, she would still be at risk for aspiration or pneumonia. She also informed Mrs. Conway of research which indicates that at the end of life many people eat or drink minimal amounts or may stop oral intake without discomfort (Fromme, 2004). The speech-language pathologist also instructed her in strategies that enabled her to sip the supplement to enjoy the taste with reduced coughing.

Ultimately, the patient decided not to have a gastrostomy tube. With the patient's permission, the social worker contacted Suzanne to explore her feelings and opinions about her mother's decision. At the conclusion of the conversation, the daughter expressed, "Well, Mom always wanted to make her own decisions, so I'll need to respect her decision on this one too."

The patient's strength declined and she remained in bed. Writing became an effort. The speech-language pathologist created a communication board with key items chosen by Mrs. Conway. One of the messages stated "I am ready to be with God." After the patient died, the social worker provided bereavement counseling to Suzanne, who stated that she was comforted knowing that her mother was able to communicate this message of peace and acceptance as she came to the end of her life.

Additional Collaborations

The expertise of other rehabilitation therapists may also assist the social worker, patient, and family to understand the level of care that is needed and the implications for long-term care decisions. For example, if an individual with a life-threatening illness and hemiparesis is deciding whether he or she wants to remain at home, a physical therapy consult focused on transfer evaluation and skill building may help to alleviate the caregiver's fear of injuring his or her loved one while transferring him or her into bed (Frost, 2001). The occupational therapist may be able to suggest resources and equipment that can assist a patient to do self-care (dressing, bathing) in a safe manner which can serve to support the patient's sense of competence (Rahman, 2000).

At other times rehabilitation therapists may assist the patient in adaptive strategies to maintain a sense of purpose in the patient's life. For example, the speech-language pathologist may develop a written prompt sheet so that a patient with aphasia is able to access her computer and organize her life photography into a book. A physical therapist may teach a caregiver how to safely transfer a patient into the family rowboat so he can enjoy his favorite pastime of fishing. A social work interview may identify activities that are most meaningful to the individual or reveal important goals that contribute to closure at the end of life. Consultation with the rehabilitation professional can then facilitate the realization of these life goals.

Conclusion

Speech-language pathologists and other rehabilitation therapists provide care in palliative care settings to improve the quality of life for patients and families. Speech pathology and social work collaboration can be a key factor in provision of quality care for individuals with communication impairments and for facilitating care decisions for individuals with severe dysphagia. Self-determination can best be supported by enabling patients to use supported communication techniques if communication barriers preclude full participation. Speech pathology consults can provide important expertise in this area. Positive outcomes can be achieved when all members of the palliative care work synergistically on behalf of patients and family members.

LEARNING EXERCISES

- Give two reasons why a social worker on a palliative care team may request a speech pathology consult.
- If a patient or caregiver has a communication challenge, name two ways the speech-language pathologist can facilitate the team's ability to meet palliative care goals.
- What may be the counseling roles of the speech-language pathologist and social worker for a patient with severe dysphagia (difficulty swallowing)? What cultural or spiritual beliefs may factor into decisions about feeding tubes?
- State an example illustrating why a social worker may collaborate with a physical therapist or occupational therapist to enhance the quality of life for a patient receiving palliative care.

- An experience of aphasia

    a) Students or participants should first view the initial 20 minutes of an instructional DVD. This DVD illustrates tools for effectively communicating with an individual with aphasia. The DVD, *Supported Conversation for Adults with Aphasia*, can be ordered through the Web site of the Aphasia Institute of Toronto, Canada: http://www.aphasia.ca/resources.html
    Question probe: *What are some ways to support a person with aphasia in his or her communication?*

    b) All participants should then be divided into dyads to participate in a simulation exercise. The instructor informs the group that the first member of the dyad has aphasia. This individual cannot speak any words but can understand basic conversation. The individual cannot write words but can draw and can read single words. The second member of the dyad is then given a paper with a series of questions. The member is instructed to have a conversation with the "person with aphasia" using these questions. (10 minutes)

    c) The instructor interrupts the conversation and announces a change. The second member of the dyad now has aphasia, and the first member of the dyad is given paper with a different series of questions. The same instructions are provided as above. (10 minutes).

    d) The instructor then leads a discussion.
    - What was it like to have aphasia?
    - What was it like to be a person communicating with someone with aphasia?
    (10 minutes)

    Group 1 Questions
    1) Do you have any pets?
    2) What is your favorite season?
    3) What kind of music do you like?
    4) What can we do about the problem of homelessness?

    Group 2 Questions
    1) Do you have any brothers or sisters?
    2) What is your favorite food?
    3) What kind of sports do you like?
    4) How can we help the environment?

This exercise was developed for training students in the Aphasia Communication Enhancement Program, Western Michigan University (Glista & Pollens, 2007).

ADDITIONAL RESOURCES

Gooden, J-F., Jones, C., Mann, A., McDowall, M. & Shugg, J. (2005). *Care and communication: The role of the speech pathologist in palliative care*. Melbourne, AU: La Trobe University. Retrieved from http://www.latrobe.edu.au/careandcommunication

Hinkley, J. J. (2000). *What is like to have trouble communicating? A series of simulation activities to educate family, friends and caregivers.* Stow, OH: Interactive Therapeutics Inc.

Schnabel, J. (Director). (2007). *The diving bell and the butterfly.* Hollywood, CA: DreamWorks & Miramax Films.

REFERENCES

Allen, B., Meyers, N., Sullivan, J., & Sullivan, M. (2002). American Sign Language and end-of-life care: Research in the deaf community. *HEC Forum, 14*(3), *197–208.*

Farrelly, M. (2009). Families in distress. In D. Walsh (Ed.), *Palliative medicine* (pp. 63–69). Philadelphia, PA: Saunders Elsevier.

Flores, G. (2005). The impact of medical interpreter services on the quality of health care: A systematic review. *Medical Care Research and Review, 62*(3), 255–299.

Fromme, E. (2004). Should my loved one get a feeding tube? *Journal of Palliative Medicine, 7*(4), 735.

Frost, M. (2001). The role of physical, occupational, and speech therapy in hospice: Patient empowerment. *American Journal of Hospice Palliative Care, 18*(6), 397–401.

Garrett, K., Happ, B., Costello, J., & Fried-Oken, M. (2007). AAC in the intensive care unit. In G. K. Buekelman & K. Yorkston (Eds.), *Augmentative communication strategies for adults with acute or chronic medical conditions,* (pp. 17–59). Baltimore, MD: Brookes.

Glista, S., & Pollens, R. (2007). Educating clinicians for meaningful, relevant, and purposeful aphasia group therapy. *Topics in Language Disorders, 27*(4), 351–371.

Kagan, A., & Shumway, E. (2003). *Talking to your counsellor or chaplain.* Toronto, Canada: Aphasia Institute.

Lasker, J. P., Garrett, K., & Fox, L. E. (2007). Severe aphasia. In G. K. Buekelman & K. Yorkston (Eds.), *Augmentative communication strategies for adults with acute or chronic medical conditions,* (pp. 163–207). Baltimore, MD: Brookes.

National Consensus Project for Quality Palliative Care. (2009). *Clinical practice guidelines for quality palliative care, second edition.* Retrieved from http://www.nationalconsensusproject. org/guideline.pdf

Pollens, R. (2004). Role of the speech-language pathologist in palliative hospice care. *Journal of Palliative Medicine, 7*(5), 694–702.

Pollens, R., Hillenbrand, K., & Sharp, H. (2009). Dysphagia. In D. Walsh (Ed), *Palliative medicine* (pp. 871–877). Philadelphia, PA: Saunders Elsevier.

Powazski, R. D. (2009). The social worker. In D. Walsh (Ed), *Palliative medicine* (pp. 269–273). Philadelphia, PA: Saunders Elsevier.

Rahman, H. (2000). Journey of providing care in hospice: Perspectives of occupational therapists. *Qualitative Health Research, 10*(6), 806–818.

Salt, N., & Roberson, S. (1998). Communication: The contribution of speech and language therapy to palliative care. *European Journal of Palliative Care, 10,* 806–818.

Sharp, H. M., & Payne, S. K. (1999). Caring for patients at the end of life. In P. A. Sullivan & A. M. Guilford (Eds.), *Swallowing intervention in oncology* (pp. 329–341). San Diego. CA: Singular.

von Gunten, C. F., Ferris, F. D., & Emanuel, L. L. (2000). Ensuring competency in end-of-life care: Communication and relational skills. *Journal of the American Medical Association, 284,* 3051–3057.

49

John M. Quillin, Jaclyn Miller, and Joann N. Bodurtha

Social Work and Genetics

Putting up bird feeders was the sort of thing her mother used to do but would never have occurred to Janice when they were younger and old Bessie was still alive. Our genes keep unfolding as long as we live.

— Rabbit at Rest, John Updike

Key Concepts

◆ *Genetics contributes to the etiology and expression of significant health conditions and well-being at all stages of the life span, including genetic legacy issues at the end of life.*

◆ *The conceptualization of family includes social, psychological, environmental, and genetic interactions.*

◆ *Interdisciplinary teamwork with medical geneticists and genetic counselors becomes an increasingly important component of social work practice as genetic information, a complex subject open to misinterpretations, ethical debate, and highly personal decision making, continues to evolve rapidly.*

Introduction: Genetic Practice across the Life Span

Some genetic understanding, especially the importance of family history, has been around since recorded history began. The current rapid pace of technology advancement, however, has contributed to headlines about test tube designer babies, cloning, total gene screen, and others that emphasize the "slippery slope" toward the science fiction side of genetics. In contrast, the day-to-day reality of genetic practice includes newborn screening, interdisciplinary clinics for individuals with Down syndrome, cancer and heart disease prevention strategies for those identified at highest risk, DNA banking, and an appreciation that our DNA does matter.

Medical geneticists, who are physicians with specialty board certification, began to use the emerging understanding of chromosomes and Mendelian conditions in health care in the 1960s. Genetic counselors, who are master's prepared, established their own board for certification in 1993. Their professional organization, the National Society of Genetic Counselors, approved the following definition of genetic counseling in 2006:

> *Genetic counseling is the process of helping people understand and adapt to the medical, psychological and familial implications of genetic contributions to disease. This process integrates the following: interpretation of family and medical histories to assess the chance of disease occurrence or recurrence; education about inheritance, testing, management, prevention, resources, and research; counseling to promote informed choices and adaptation to the risk or condition. (Resta et al., 2006, p. 77)*

While some programs were initially integrated into Masters of Social Work (MSW) programs, today accredited Masters of Genetic Counseling programs are separate, though they include courses that overlap with social work curricula and may have MSW students attend. The National Society of Genetic Counselors' Code of Ethics (http://www.nsgc.org/about/codeEthics.cfm) outlines the discipline's professional perspectives and standards. Genetic counseling training, accredited by the American Board of Genetic Counseling, emphasizes competence in communication skills; critical-thinking skills; interpersonal counseling, and psychosocial assessment skills; and professional ethics and values (http://www.abgc.net/english/View.asp?x=1529).

Genetic Historical Perspective

In the past 100 years, there have been devastating challenges to public appreciation of genetics, from the eugenic movement, including the killing of persons with disabilities and those of Jewish background in the Holocaust, to discrimination against those who are sickle cell carriers or have "preexisting" conditions or genetic susceptibilities. In recognition that we all have genetic susceptibilities, the U.S. federal government passed the Genetic Information Nondiscrimination Act in 2008. This legislation represented an important step forward for integrating genetics into medical care, and it has relieved concerns of many prospective genetic counseling patients. However, many social and psychological aspects of genetic disease can remain a challenge (e.g., discovering mis-attributed paternity, "survival guilt" of siblings unaffected by a genetic condition, and "transmission guilt" of parents of children with an inherited condition). Social workers may be particular attuned to identify and address these social aspects of genetic diseases.

The Human Genome Project (1990–2003) accelerated the pace at which genetic tests have become available (see http://GeneTests.org), but given the slower pace of effective treatments, health care practitioner knowledge, the challenges of health care financing, the varied public demand for scientific explanations, health disparities, and the complexities of macro- vs. micro-management of health and disease in the twenty-first century, the clinical utility of such testing has not been fully realized. The salience of genetic information can vary over time for individuals and families and is always embedded in multifaceted diverse cultural traditions. While genetic information can have impact from "womb to tomb" (i.e., preconception to postmortem), the majority of genetic counselors currently have jobs in settings where the emphasis is on prenatal or cancer genetics.

Our social worker (see Box 49.1) is in familiar territory. The presenting problem is medical and genetically determined, but she will assess Ms. B. "in situ" from the same biopsychosocial-spiritual perspective undergirding all social work practice. She will support Ms. B. and her daughter during their diagnosis and treatments and will provide as much education about what they are experiencing as they desire. But first she will listen to where they are emotionally and what personally and culturally based meaning they ascribe to their experience. She will reach out to the extended family to do the same. She will assist with basic resources such as housing, transportation, and entitlements and will learn about their resources and strengths: social, spiritual,

---

| Box 49.1 |
| Patient/Family Narrative: Ms. B. and Family |

After she was diagnosed with colon cancer in 2002, then with Familial Adenomatous Polyposis (a dominant genetic condition with nearly 100% chance of developing colon cancer from hundreds of polyps before middle age), 35-year-old Ms. B. told others, "It's in the family, the genes." Although the first to be diagnosed, her father, two brothers, a twin sister, and her teenage daughter have now been diagnosed as well. The hospital social worker was there from the beginning to work with both Ms. B. and N., her daughter, who were not only facing the challenges of the disease and its treatment but also basic survival issues. Moving from a homeless shelter to a basement apartment with the help of funds from the Department of Homeless Services, their environment was insecure and financial support from federal programs such as SSI were not available because Ms. B. is not a U.S. citizen (NY Times, Neediest Cases: January, 27, 2007).

---

psychological, and so forth. She may advocate for them with local and state agencies and in the hospital/medical system. She will ensure that confidentiality, self-determination, and other ethical principles are followed. She will collaborate actively with the interdisciplinary team, perhaps adding other experts and resources as her client's needs indicate. This is but one practice situation in which it is clear that a social worker will be effective to the degree she knows what "it's in the family, the genes" means, both literally and figuratively: Her knowledge of genetic conditions; ability to collaborate with genetic counselors and geneticists; understanding of how the family copes and makes sense of reality and "risk"; and knowledge of resources will be essential to assisting Mrs. B. and her family.

Social Work and Genetic Practice

Although in 1917 Mary Richmond recognized the importance of family history and the concept of heritability in good casework practice, formal Standards for Integrating Genetics into Social Work Practice were not published until 2003 by the National Association of Social Workers (NASW). These guidelines were based on the work of the Human Genome Education Model (HuGEM) project funded by the National Institutes of Health (Lapham, Kozma, Weiss, Benkendorf, & Wilson, 2000) and on genetics core competencies established by The National Coalition of Health Professionals in Genetic Education (NCHPEG), and they validate the basic elements of practice noted in the narrative in Box 49.1. The objectives of the NASW Standards (2009) include all social workers having "basic understanding about genetics ... including its biological, psychosocial, ethical and legal aspects" (p. 8); improving the quality of social work services to clients with genetic disorders; ensuring the NASW Code of Ethics guides all services; advocating for clients' rights; and participating in relevant public policy discourse and development (p. 5). Interdisciplinary practice, a collaborative practice approach with clients, self-awareness, and engagement in research, is highlighted.

These common themes have appeared in the social work literature. For example, Sammons (1978), focusing on amniocentesis and selective abortion, analyzed the ethical issues involved, citing work in the 1970s on genetics and genetic counseling. Seeing the social worker as part of the health care team, Sammons highlighted psychosocial implications of rapidly developing genetic technology, noting "yesterday's heroics are today's routine procedures" (p. 238). Her discussion of the right "not to know," "to ignore," and the potential conflict between a client's right to privacy and her relatives' right to genetic information that may be relevant to their or their child's health (p. 240) is just as pertinent to the issue of DNA banking in palliative care and other more contemporary arenas of genetics-related practice. In 1981, Weiss brought the psychosocial aspects of diagnosed genetic diseases to the center of social work role in health care settings in her study of personal, marital, parental, family, group and community levels of "costs" of genetic disease diagnoses, with an emphasis on the emotional impact of stress over time. In 1980, Dils and Smith looked at genetic counseling and prenatal testing from a psychoanalytic perspective and raised practice questions about affective and interpersonal dynamics that might be stirred by those processes. In 1997, Richards tackled the practice challenges in predictive testing, especially for "untreatable, late onset conditions" (p. 61), insisting on the centrality of professional ethics, along with principles of bioethics such as autonomy, beneficence, non-malfeasance, and justice, in such situations where there is no easy solution to the dilemma. Critical and analytical thinking is paramount in such practice arenas.

More recently, McCutcheon (2006) wrote about the genetic components of mental illnesses and stressed the relevance of knowledge of gene–environment interactions in social work practice. Three interactive models used in mental health research, the biopsychosocial, diathesis/stress, and phenotypic vulnerability models, are described. Based on research demonstrating that early negative life experiences such as abuse and other traumas can have lasting adverse physiological effects impacting psychological functioning, the phenotypic vulnerability model takes a conceptual step forward by including those experiences as diatheses/vulnerability while continuing to assess recent stressors on the stress side. For example, the stressors of living in poverty and exposure to extreme life conditions (Keinan-Baker, Vin-Ravis, Lipshitz, Linn, & Barcana, 2009) do seem to negatively impact the immune system, opening the way for expression of genetic predispositions that might otherwise remain dormant.

While social work practice on site in genetics clinics may be limited, a facility with genetics content is required for all health care practice and increasingly so for most other areas of interdisciplinary social work practice. For example, our

work with individuals and families around pregnancy and pregnancy loss (e.g., amniocentesis, elective abortion); fertility/infertility (e.g., surrogacy, methods for having a "genetic child"); adoption (e.g., local or international, "special needs"); understanding and managing emotional and behavioral challenges in children and adolescents (e.g., attention-deficit hyperactivity disorder, bipolar disorder, obsessive-compulsive disorder, and eating disorders); developmental disabilities; substance abuse and addictions; and chronic health conditions in family members and in communities (e.g., diabetes, heart disease) where collaboration across disciplines is critical.

Social Work, Genetics, and Palliative Care

A great challenge of the new millennium for the hospice and palliative care movement will be its capacity to employ an ethnographic sensibility that is responsive to the great diversity of meaning-making practices engaged in by individuals and families with serious illness at the end of life (Browning, 2004).

While this challenge certainly applies to all of social work practice and to care along the continuum of illness, end of life carries unique meanings in almost all cultures and religions that range in expression from total denial to active celebration. And there is no dearth of protocols, assessment formats, or social work strategies that can be modified to include family conversations, in general, about what one passes on to those we leave and more specific conversations about heritability, genetic testing, and DNA banking. For example, both the protocol for a culturally sensitive approach to exploring the meaning of a respectful death in palliative care (Farber, Egnew, & Farber, 2004) and Blacker and Jordan's (2004) outline for a comprehensive family assessment in palliative care can be enhanced by including relevant inquiry about genetics and heritability. With such content included, the conversation with the family is opened at the beginning and can be revisited throughout our work with them.

Reith and Payne (2009) set out a number of roles for social workers working with families in palliative care, one of which is helping them "fulfill important life tasks and plan important life decisions …" (p. 90). Their examples focus on young children who will be left and how to plan for their futures. Yet many of the parents in these examples were dying of cancers with known genetic determinants, including a young mother with colon cancer and a 40-year-old mother with advanced breast cancer. In situations such as these, the challenges of the imminent are infinitely more real in their immediacy than those of the future, yet if current family needs are being addressed and a relationship has been established with a social worker who has a beginning understanding of this family's dynamics, referral for genetic testing and/or banking DNA can be introduced as one of this family's important life decisions. One might even suggest there is an ethical obligation to raise the issue. Ethical dilemmas inherent in such positions as a person's "right to know" or "right not to know," and the responsibility practitioners have "to inform" and to educate have all been raised in palliative care and end-of-life practice. They are also relevant in the ethical dilemma social workers may face when an individual chooses not to inform other family members of their potential genetic inheritance.

DNA is clearly part of the common discourse today, particularly in North America (Tanenhaus, 2010.) According to Lebner (2000), medicalization, which is the expansion of the medical into our way of thinking about conditions, concerns, or life circumstances, has moved to geneticization, an explanatory paradigm that leads us to see human strengths and weaknesses in genetic terms and to talk about "genetic risk" as something to be managed actuarially. Once again, as the knowledge pendulum and dominant discourse shift, we must remind ourselves that our humanness is "embedded in and influenced by the complex of biological reactions, and social and economic relationships" (p. 373) or, in social work terms, the micro, mezzo, and macro elements of, and interactions with, our environment.

Genetics and Perinatal Death

One often thinks of medical genetics as serving expectant parents, providing risk assessment for individuals, or treating an individual with a genetic condition. The familial nature of many genetic conditions, however, means that genetic understanding of an individual's disease can also benefit the extended family. In the case of Julia (Box 49.2), the finding of a chromosome abnormality did not change Julia's life course, but it did provide insight that could be useful to her surviving relatives. Genetic services can be helpful throughout the life trajectory, including end-of-life (Quillin, Bodurtha, & Smith, 2008).

Genetic conditions account for a significant proportion of infant and early childhood illness and death. One study found that more than one-third of pediatric admissions involved clear genetic diagnoses (McCandless, Brunger, & Cassidy, 2004). Perinatal hospice is a growing but relatively new service for children diagnosed with life-limiting diseases such as Trisomy 13 (an extra chromosome condition with multiple congenital anomalies) identified in the pre- and perinatal periods (Ramer-Chastek & Thygeson, 2005; Romesberg, 2007); however, these infants, children, and their families have been and will continue to be seen in the neonatal intensive care unit and pediatric services by hospital staff nurses and social workers on a daily basis. The services that are needed include psychosocial support, resources, and information for families in anticipation of a child's birth and death, and this requires coordination among multiple disciplines. Team members often include social workers,

nurses, geneticists, genetic counselors, and chaplains, among others. The team needs to be prepared to help this family deal with the present, assimilate a good deal of new information while under stress, involve other family members, and consider the future. And, as we can see with the Iglesia family, the team needs to be responsive to family and cultural dynamics as well as potential religious, spiritual, and generational sensitivities.

Julia's diagnosis prompted targeted genetic studies of her parents. This information, in turn, could be helpful for the Iglesias and Mr. Iglesia's relatives if they plan to have more children. The key to Julia's case, and others like hers, is that genetics services were consulted *before* she died, and a blood sample was obtained. Without Julia's diagnosis other family members may never have learned about the familial nature of her disease. Having a tissue sample from Julia was critical to making the diagnosis. Even if a diagnosis was not possible by current genetic tests, having DNA-containing tissue stored keeps the option of future testing available, as genetic science advances. Several centers offer *DNA* banking services to store tissue of a dying person for later genetic diagnosis or research. (For more information and a listing of centers offering DNA banking, see the GeneReviews Web site at http://www.genereviews.org.)

Genetics and Family Communication

Mr. Iglesia ran into a roadblock when trying to discuss family health history with his mother. The familial nature of genetic testing distinguishes it from other medical tests. Scientists can calculate and communicate objective risks. Understanding and communication of lived risks within families, however, can be psychosocially loaded. Feelings of responsibility and guilt can drive or hinder communication. Discussing illness or miscarriages might be taboo in families and can inhibit family knowledge.

Box 49.2
Patient/Family Narrative: Julia and Family

Julia was Mr. and Mrs. Iglesia's first child. She was born in December, and everyone was concerned when she did not cry. Julia's doctors determined that she had a complex heart defect, and she might not survive. While working through the best way to treat Julia, Dr. Brown consulted the medical genetics service and arranged for the Iglesias to meet with their hospital's perinatal hospice service. The geneticist obtained a blood sample for genetics studies. Julia died the next day, and her parents agreed to an autopsy. Later the Iglesias met with the geneticist and learned that Julia was born with a chromosome abnormality that could be related to an inherited chromosome rearrangement from a parent. Both parents were tested, and Mr. Iglesia was found to have a chromosome rearrangement. When Mr. Iglesia asked his mother about any family history of other birth defects, miscarriages, or stillbirths, she became tearful and said she did not want to discuss it.

A recent systematic review of genetic communication in families depicts a deliberative process that includes making sense of personal risk, assessing the vulnerability or receptivity of family members to genetic information, and deciding what and when to share information (Gaff et al., 2007). Yet no universal "right" approach for family communication of genetic information exists. When working with parents like the Iglesias, it is often the social workers and other direct health providers who have a relationship with the family and/or the frontline opportunities to inform them of the possibility of a genetic diagnosis, to convey the potential familial nature of the disease, and to provide anticipatory guidance about family communication. Who in the family is most open to gathering and communicating family health history information (i.e., a "kin keeper")? How do relatives work though serious illnesses? At what point in the grieving process should one broach the topic of inherited risk? Who might benefit medically from knowing the information? Hospice and palliative care have traditionally had a family focus, yet the genetic aspect of disease adds a new dimension to this service.

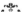

Conclusion: The Future

The Human Genome Project has brought media attention and public interest to genetics. Recent proposals in the United States for universal health insurance have included attempts to translate genetic research into individualized health care practices. Risk assessment and individualized health care through genetic testing have been most broadly applied in cancer medicine with the use of *BRCA1* and *BRCA2* gene testing (for breast and ovarian cancer genetic susceptibility) and other genetic risk testing. It is not clear how many years away "individualized," "personalized" precision medicine is. It is also debated how much genetic profiling will improve health care. Health and disease are the result of complex interactions of genes, environment, and nurture. Nonetheless, as scientific understanding advances, the public uses genetic information in family planning in its broadest sense and potentially in more individual health choices. Notably the cost and complexity of genetic health information may add to growing health disparities unless the ethical challenges are addressed. New genetic information and evidence from social work research will continue to need to be woven into the wisdom of the lives of families, social work experience and practice, and genetic counseling.

Read Box 49.3 and consider the following questions, which may help initiate discussion:

1. What are the social worker's responsibilities to Mrs. Hughes and her relatives regarding the sharing of this family genetic information?
2. What are the potential clinical and ethical challenges for the social worker in this situation and how might she address them?

Box 49.3
Patient/Family Narrative: Mrs. Hughes: A Learning Exercise

Mrs. Hughes arranged for her mother who had developed dementia in her mid-50s to have genetic susceptibility testing. The test was positive, thus indicating that Mrs. Hughes and her full siblings had a 50% chance of developing early dementia. Mrs. Hughes decided that she did not want to tell her own adult children, her siblings, nor her nieces and nephews. She did, however, tell her mother's social worker, who had provided counsel and support to the family when her mother received palliative care and then hospice support prior to her death.

---

3. How would the interdisciplinary team work together to meet the needs of this patient and her family?

ADDITIONAL RESOURCES

Association of University Centers on Disabilities: http://www.aucd.org/template/news.cfm?news_id=3436&parent=6&parent_title=LENDs
LEND modules on genetic awareness, family history, and newborn screening.
Edwards, K. (2005). *The memory keeper's daughter.* New York: Penguin Books.
Genetic awareness checklist: http://www.aucd.org/docs/lend/genetics/checklist_genetics_vcu121106.pdf
"Information for Genetic Professionals": http://www.kumc.edu/gec/geneinfo.html
Educational resources from Kansas University
March of Dimes "Genetics & Your Practice": http://www.marchofdimes.com/gyponline/index.bm2
Educational modules about genetics.
National Coalition of Health Professional Education in Genetics: http://www.nchpeg.org/
Core competencies about genetics for health professionals and targeted educational programs.
National Human Genome Research Institute: http://www.genome.gov/Education/
"Secrets of the Sequence" : http://www.pubinfo.vcu.edu/secretsofthesequence/
Brief videos and lesson plans about genetics
U. S. Department of Health and Human Services: http://www.hhs.gov/familyhistory/
Since 2004, the US Surgeon General has annually publicized Thanksgiving as family health history day, encouraging communication about health and disease factors within families, and providing an excellent web tool that is available in Spanish and print.

PRACTICAL TIPS

Nine things you can encourage clients/patients to do to use genetic health information constructively:
1. No matter what your genetic makeup, exercise daily, eat a healthy diet, and do not smoke.

2. If you are a potentially pregnant women, follow the Centers for Disease Control and Prevention's recommendation to have a diet rich in folate (naturally green foods) and take 0.4 mg of folic acid (in most multivitamins) daily in order to reduce the chance of congenital anomalies, such as spina bifida and anencephaly (open spine and brain). See http://www.cdc.gov/ncbddd/folicacid/index.html.

3. Talk with your relatives about their health conditions. The Surgeon General has a Web-based tool that prints out a family tree and gives some general health recommendations: http://www.hhs.gov/familyhistory/.

4. Stay tuned. Some genetic tests may not be ready for prime time. If it sounds too good to be true, a healthy dose of skepticism may be in order.

5. Use reliable Web tools to increase your genetic health literacy. Genetics home reference (http://ghr.nlm.nih.gov/) and GeneTests (http://www.ncbi.nlm.nih.gov/sites/GeneTests/?db=GeneTests) are reliable Web resources with many helpful links.

6. Advocacy groups (accessible under the umbrella of http://www.geneticalliance.org) and research networks such as ClinicalTrials.gov are gateways to more condition-specific information, support networks, and research.

7. Feel comfortable discussing second opinions with your health care provider, particularly if there is not a clear-cut organizing cause for a variety of your symptoms and findings.

8. For all of us, illness is a risk of being alive in the first place. Some of us may have genetic dispositions that place us at higher risk. The challenge is to appreciate individual and family strengths, while understanding what aspects of your genetic makeup place you at higher risk and to stay up to date about any improved prevention and management for those conditions.

9. Talk with your health care provider about family history and ask others in your family to share a positive family history of similar findings, rare conditions, early deaths, and extraordinary lab tests (especially genetic tests) from both sides of the family, all of which can be clues to more specific diagnoses.

REFERENCES

Blacker, S., & Jordan, A. R. (2004). Working with families facing life-threatening illness in the medical setting. In J. Berzoff & P.R. Silverman (Eds.) *Living with dying* (pp. 548–570). New York:Columbia University Press.

Browning, D. (2004). Fragments of love: Explorations in the ethnography of suffering and professional care giving. In J. Berzoff & P. R. Silverman (Eds.), *Living with dying* (pp. 21–42). New York, NY: Columbia University Press.

Dils, S. M., & Smith, L. L. (1980). Genetic counseling: Implications for social work practice. *Clinical Social Work Journal, 8*(2), 99–107.

Farber, S., Egnew, T., & Farber, A. (2004). What is a respectful death? In J. Berzoff & P. R. Silverman (Eds.), *Living with dying* (pp. 102–107). New York, NY: Columbia University Press.

Gaff, C. L., Clarke, A. J., Atkinson, P., Sivell, S., Elwyn, G., Iredale, R., & Edwards, A. (2007). Process and outcome in communication of genetic information within families: A systematic review. *European Journal of Human Genetics, 15*, 999–1011.

Keinan-Baker, L., Vin-Ravis, N., Lipshitz, I., Linn, S., & Barcana, M. (2009). Cancer incidence in Israeli Jewish survivors of World War II. *Journal National Cancer Institute, 101*(21), 1489–1500.

Lapham, E. V., Kozma, C., Weiss, J. O., Benkendorf, J. L., & Wilson, M. A. (2000). The gap between practice and genetics education of health professionals: HuGEM survey results. *Genetics in Medicine, 2*, 226–231.

Lebner, A. (2000). Genetic "mysteries" and international adoption: The cultural impact of biomedical technologies on the adoptive family experience. *Family Relations, 49*(4), 371–377.

McCandless, S. E., Brunger, J. W., & Cassidy, S. B. (2004). The burden of genetic disease on inpatient care in a children's hospital. *American Journal of Human Genetics, 74*, 121–127.

McCutcheon, V. V. (2006). Toward integration of social and biological research. *Social Service Review, 80*(1), 159–178.

National Association of Social Workers (NASW). (2003). *NASW standards for integrating genetics into social work practice.* Retrieved from http://www.naswpress.org/publications

National Association of Social Workers (NASW). (2009). *NASW standards for social work practice in palliative and end of life care.* Retrieved from http://socialworkers.org/practice/bereavement/standards/default.asp

Quillin, J. M., Bodurtha, J. N., & Smith, T. J. (2008). Genetics assessment at the end of life: Suggestions for implementation in clinic and future research. *Journal of Palliative Medicine, 11*(3), 451–458.

Ramer-Chrastek, J., & Thygeson, M. V. (2005). A perinatal hospice for an unborn child with a life-limiting condition. *International Journal of Palliative Nursing, 11*(6), 274–277.

Reith, M., & Payne, M. (2009). *Social work in end-of-life and palliative care.* Chicago, IL: Lyceum Books.

Resta, R., Biesecker, B. B., Bennett, R. L., Blum, S., Hahn, S. E., Strecker, M. N., & Williams, J. L. (2006). A new definition of genetic counseling: National Society of Genetic Counselors' Task Force report. *Journal of Genetic Counseling, 15*(2), 77–83.

Richards, F. (1997). Social work and genetic testing: Ethical issues encountered in predictive testing for Huntington disease. *Australian Social Work, 50*(4), 61–67.

Romesberg, T. L. (2007). Building a case for neonatal palliative care. *Neonatal Network, 26*(2), 111–115.

Sammons, C. C. (1978). Ethical issues in genetic interventions. *Social Work, 22*(3), 237–242.

Weiss, J. O. (1981). Psychosocial stress in genetic disorders: A guide for social workers. *Social Work in Health Care, 6*(4), 17–31.

50 *Donna L. Soltura and Linda F. Piotrowski*

Teamwork in Palliative Care: Social Work Role with Spiritual Care Professionals

I dream of a collaboration that would finally be total, in which the librettist would often think as a composer and the composer as a librettist.

—Jacques Ibert, French composer (1890–1962)

Key Concepts

- ◆ *Collaboration between social workers and spiritual care professionals can enrich the care of patients and families.*
- ◆ *There are similarities and differences in each discipline's values, roles, and tasks.*
- ◆ *Challenges and opportunities abound in the collaboration between social work and spiritual care.*

Introduction

This chapter assists social workers in enhancing their collaborative practice with spiritual care providers on a palliative care team. Similarities and differences in training and perspective, as well as challenges and opportunities in the care of patients and the achievement of an interdisciplinary, rather than multidisciplinary team, are discussed.

Social Work Role with Spiritual Care Professional

You are on this team because you have all been, in your prior organizations, the one to take the tough shot and successfully sink the basket. You wouldn't be here if you hadn't. Your challenge now is to trust each other enough to hand off the ball to the person best-positioned to take the shot, to work as a team instead of as a group of individuals ... (personal communication, February 30, 2010)

With these words, Dr. Ira Byock, director of the palliative care service at Dartmouth-Hitchcock Medical Center (DHMC) in Lebanon, New Hampshire, began a 2006 team retreat. Dr. Byock had just added the most recent discipline, social work, to the medical center's palliative care team. Three months previously he had brought on the team's first chaplain and a volunteer coordinator. He had transformed the formerly physician and nursing-only team into a multidisciplinary team, but these words stated his goal of creating a truly *interdisciplinary* team. Both collaborative approaches encompass the varied fields of expertise needed to adequately respond to the biopsychosocial-spiritual needs of palliative care patients and their families, but the charge to be "interdisciplinary" reflected not only the variety of players but also the *process* by which they met their objective: to provide whole-person, family-centered care to persons living with serious illness, addressing each as a whole person, including physical comfort, confidence, emotional well-being, spirituality, and dignity.

The "process" of being an interdisciplinary team is reflected in how patients and families are presented and discussed—"those for whom it matters" (Byock, 2009, p. 111). Optimally, the patient's initial palliative care service (PCS) visit is attended by both a medical and a psychosocial or spiritual care clinician. Prior to meeting the patient, medical records are reviewed to help make the clinicians aware of the patient's diagnosis and prognosis as well as the patient's functional, emotional, financial, and spiritual well-being. The clinicians decide which of them will "lead" the visit, which involves introducing the service by describing palliative care; noting the disciplines that are members of the team; and facilitating a discussion regarding the patient's goals, needs, and concerns. If a social worker or spiritual care provider cannot accommodate every new patient admission visit, he or she reviews patient information and screens for higher risk needs, prioritizing those visits in his or her limited schedule or providing the admitting clinicians with helpful resources and strategies for addressing those needs. Additionally, unanticipated needs identified by doctors and nurse practitioners during the initial visit are referred to their social work and spiritual care colleagues for immediate telephone follow-up or with a scheduled visit. This requires that psychosocial and spiritual care education be provided to our medically trained teammates. Initial screening tools can be made up of a few key questions such as the following:

- "Is this medication affordable for you at this time, given all your regular expenses?"
- "Where do you pull your strength from as you go through this difficult experience?"
- "Are you, as a family, able to talk about your health and what you think the future holds?"

Ideally case discussions include all team disciplines, from the clinicians to volunteers. New patient presentations can begin with the patient's psychosocial or spiritual information rather than the traditional medical model. For instance, "A 30-year-old woman with newly diagnosed metastatic colorectal cancer admitted to the Emergency Department following fulminate hepatic failure, now in room 302" becomes the following:

> Joan Smith is a 30-year-old mother of twin 2 year olds. She is married to Bob, an independent carpenter, in Cornish, NH. Joan, a dress designer and seamstress, is an independent small business woman. She describes herself as deeply spiritual. Joan engages in daily meditation. This practice is now challenged due to the intensity of her disease symptoms and caring for her twins.

Joan and her family are introduced as a whole person/family with health care issues rather than a disease with a person attached.

Having the social worker or spiritual care provider make a case presentation, or share in it, also helps educate the team regarding biopsychosocial-spiritual issues and the language used by our professions, as well as insuring our input into the assessment, clinical conceptualization, treatment planning, and goals. It also challenges social workers and spiritual care providers to familiarize ourselves with the language of medicine, a seemingly daunting yet vital skill.

To check your team's interdisciplinary pulse, ask yourselves these questions:

- How are decisions made?
- Does each discipline have a voice?
- Who presents?
- What dimension of care is presented first?
- What language is used?
- How are decisions made?
- How are disagreements processed and resolved?
- Does each discipline have a voice as well as an equal role in decision making? Are each discipline's assessment, interventions, and other recommendations taken into account in care planning?
- Is there a blend of expertise, a shared base of knowledge that is carried within and used by all members, or does each discipline act independently and simply report back to the team?

A good interdisciplinary team shares the wealth. They learn skills and perspectives from each other and utilize those tools in their own interactions with patients and families, knowing when referral to a specialized discipline is needed for greater depth and breadth in the work (Otis-Green et al., 2009).

For the purpose of this chapter we will focus on the collaborative relationship between spiritual care professionals and social work. These two disciplines have much in common, the greatest of which is that they are both, as our clinical director, Dr. Sharona Sachs, says, "connectionologists." We study the connections that are meaningful in the lives of the people that we serve. Spirituality has connection at its core. The 2009 Consensus Conference defined spirituality as "the aspect of humanity that refers to the way individuals seek and express meaning and purpose and the way they experience their connectedness to the moment, to self, to others, to nature, and to the significant or sacred" (Puchalski et al., 2009). It is natural that social work and chaplaincy meet around this inherent part of what it means to be human. There are other similarities, as well as some differences, in the training, values, and roles of social workers and spiritual care professionals.

Social workers receive training in psychology, sociology, biology, history, and philosophy of social work, theory and practice, human behavior and the social environment, social welfare policy, program development, legal aspects of social work, communications, research, human diversity, ethics, and professional standards and practices. They may also receive training in the fields of elder issues, juvenile delinquency, death and dying, child welfare, addictions, trauma, school practice, and spiritual dimensions of social work practice. They incorporate these fields of study in their work with individuals, families, institutions, communities, and society at large. Social work practice is self-reflective as well as peer supervised. Social work core values, as stated in the National Association of Social Workers (NASW) Code of Ethics, include service, social justice, dignity and worth of the person, importance of human relationships, integrity, and competence.

Professional (board-certified) chaplains offer spiritual care to all who are in need and have specialized education to help patients cope more effectively by mobilizing spiritual resources. Professional chaplains are trained in sociological and psychological disciplines, ethnic and religious cultures, human development, group dynamics, organizational behavior, religious beliefs and practices, death and dying, grief and bereavement, and ethics appropriate to the pastoral context. The expertise acquired through this training is utilized in service of the individuals, families, faith communities, caregivers, intuitional members, and the larger medical community. Board-certified chaplains are trained in formulating and utilizing spiritual assessment in the development of care plans, to inform outcomes, and to advocate for persons in their care. Like their social work counterparts, their practice is self-reflective and peer reviewed. Chaplaincy core values are discipleship, integrity, stewardship, compassion, inclusivity, professionalism, leadership, and empowerment (Council on Collaboration, 2004).

Not all spiritual care providers possess the same training, knowledge, and expertise. For example, ordained clergy are certainly spiritual care providers. However, most do not receive the same level of training or possess the skills and competencies related to ministry in a health care setting as the board-certified chaplain (see definitions in Table 50.1). This can contribute to confusion. Hospices and small community hospitals often hire "spiritual care professionals," that is, retired clergy, seminary students, and so on, to provide chaplaincy services rather than board-certified chaplains. The variations in training, code of ethics, board certification, professional accountability, ongoing education, and continuing education responsibilities make a difference in how spiritual care is provided.

Challenges

Professions that have significant similarities in their training are likely to experience an intersection of their roles and tasks. Who "owns" family meeting facilitation, hospice referrals, or bereavement counseling? Is pain management strictly a medical intervention, or can the chaplain and social worker assist in treatment planning and intervention in a significant way? Does spiritual angst belong wholly to the chaplain, or

---

Table 50.1.
Definitions

Chaplains (board certified): Spiritual care specialists who have extended education in pastoral care, spirituality, and ethics. The requirements for board certification are 1600 hours of clinical pastoral education, demonstrated skills in required competencies, ongoing continuing education, peer review, and renewal of certification every 5 years. Certification is granted by a number of professional chaplaincy organizations.

Collaboration: The process by which two or more people work together to accomplish a goal.

Culture: The sum total of a way of living. It involves the values, beliefs, standards, and language of a people. It influences our thinking patterns, communication style, and what we consider "normal" behavior. It guides our decisions and creates our expectations. When living with life-threatening illness, culture determines how we find meaning in our experience, in suffering and dying. It explains cause and effect. In health care, it defines the role of "healers" in both physical and spiritual realms.

Interdisciplinary: Collaborative process that creates a more integrative and comprehensive plan of care than simply a composite of individual recommendations.

Multidisciplinary: A variety of professionals from different disciplines working together in a coordinated team.

Spirituality: The aspect of humanity that refers to the way individuals seek and express meaning and purpose and the way they experience their connectedness to the moment, to self, to others, to nature, and to the significant or sacred.

Source: Puchalski et al., 2009.

---

can a social worker skillfully explore "making meaning" with a client who feels abandoned by God?

In fact, a well-skilled, interdisciplinary palliative care team provides an abundance of opportunity for clients to receive comprehensive biopsychosocial-spiritual care from all members of the team. How then, does one determine who is needed for specific assessments and interventions? There can be several factors, both practical (such as staffing constraints) and emotional (such as territoriality), which challenge us when determining role or task assignments.

Staffing

An obstacle for social work and spiritual care program staffing in most medical settings is that they are nonbillable services. Many palliative care teams do not have full-time social workers or chaplains who are easily identified by others in their institutions as palliative care team members. They may be allocated a few hours to attend team meetings and see patients. They are not immersed in the day-to-day relationships, decision making, and process of a fully integrated team. In settings in which social work or chaplaincy are not full-time, dedicated roles, tasks may be assigned more broadly to these similar disciplines (see Table 50.2) when the preferred discipline is not available. Redistributable tasks may include, but are not limited to, assisting patients and families in coping with bad news; the initial psychosocial or spiritual assessment; being present for or immediately after a death; introducing palliative care as a service; and deescalating high-anxiety situations.

Territoriality

While we all strive to avoid being territorial, we may not always share the same viewpoint on what kind of expertise or practice style is best suited to a particular task. Specialists may feel unappreciated and underused if their team sees social workers and chaplains as fully interchangeable. Individual practitioners may hold fast to their traditional domain, fearing loss of their place on the team.

Social workers and chaplains must be able to articulate, in the language of the environment in which they work, their unique skills and perspectives. They must also be willing to share their knowledge and tools and learn from others. On our palliative care team the social worker and chaplain identified a need to redistribute tasks. Each covered both inpatient and outpatient environments daily, leaving both feeling ineffective and inadequate in service to their clients. They recommended to their administration that the chaplain cover the inpatient units while the social worker covered the outpatient units. This adjustment in work responsibilities meant that the social worker left the work she enjoyed in the intensive care unit while the chaplain lost the visible presence in the outpatient clinics that often lead to spontaneous spiritual care referrals by non–palliative care staff. Both of them felt they were giving up something important with the expectation that patients would ultimately be better served. To minimize that loss, they agreed to meet regularly to discuss cases in detail so that each would learn from the other the skills needed to make an initial assessment in the other's absence. They reviewed assessment tools, discussed various scenarios, cross-practiced new language and phrasing, and developed creative ideas that might help a patient and his or her family in the immediate while arranging a visit for specialized support from their counterpart.

Similarities

The statements in Box 50.1 illustrate a similarity in values and tasks with a difference in language that demonstrates the subtle nuances that differentiate the professions. For example,

chaplaincy utilizes the notion of hospitality in patient interactions. Hospitality makes space for the other. When meeting a new patient, the chaplain reflects on how to invite the other to share, and on how the chaplain's own faith might impact the relationship. Henri Nouwen defines this: "Hospitality … means primarily the creation of a free space where the stranger can enter and become a friend instead of an enemy. The goal is not to change people, but to offer them space where change can take place" (Nouwen, 1998, p. 71). The provision of spiritual care entails accompanying, linking, discerning, and ritualizing (Hayes & Van der Poel, 1990). Relationship development is key to the pastoral relationship.

Table 50.2.
Social Work and Chaplaincy Where Roles Overlap

- Utilizing knowledge of illnesses and disease processes and their effect on emotional, social, psychological, and spiritual wholeness

- Intensive skilled listening to the spirit/spirituality in the body, mind, and spirit of a person

- Engaging the length, breadth, and depth of an individual's life in review

- Assessing resources and stressors

- Initiating, building, and sustaining helping relationships

- Providing support

- Working with the interdisciplinary care teams to ensure that patient needs are met

- Supporting the mobilization of both religious and nonreligious spiritual resources in response to the stresses of illnesses, hospitalization, and treatment

- Providing supportive care and counseling to patients, families, and staff on a non-fee basis

- Crisis care and counseling, especially related to trauma, "bad news," or sudden death

- Support and counseling related to end-of-life decisions

- Facilitation of grief and anticipatory grief

- Utilizing integrative interventions to reduce acute anxiety and pain

- Sensitivity and respect for the diversity of culture, religious faiths, spiritual traditions, and those with no spiritual or religious traditions

- Assisting with understanding bioethical issues

- Utilizing psychological and behavioral models as they relate to illness responses

In social work terms, one "starts where the client is at." Another social work premise is "It's all about relationship." Social workers utilize peer supervision to understand complex patients and families and to discuss transference and countertransference, in cases where they may have conflicted feelings or be overly identified with their client. The common ground with chaplaincy is in creating a safe space for the client to expose vulnerability and other feelings; and in attention to the clinician's own assumptions, values, and biases.

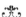

Opportunities

Social workers can learn much from their collaboration with chaplains. Chaplains teach about the diversity of spiritual beliefs and supports, effective spiritual assessment and intervention, and a language for the exploration of existential issues such as meaning and purpose. In addition to assisting patients in spiritual distress, chaplains are available to their social work colleagues as a self-care resource. Tending to the needs of persons with chronic, serious, and life-threatening illness requires equal attention to the psychosocial-spiritual needs of the professional doing the caring. In the midst of tending to patient needs through personal encounters, social workers can become drained and in spiritual anguish themselves. Chaplain colleagues can serve as a listening ear, an understanding heart, and a place of rest and companionship in the midst of stress, loss, and death.

Social workers can offer chaplains a skilled ear to discuss clinical care and psychosocial and family systems issues; they can also be a resource for self-care, a partner on the journey, and an advocate for chaplaincy services. Social workers, trained in organizational change and policy development, can assist chaplains in professional empowerment to insure that every patient and family has access to a source of advocacy from a spiritual perspective. Collaboration between our similar, yet different, disciplines enhances our abilities to respond to both spiritual and psychosocial needs as they present themselves, with specialized expertise only a referral away.

Box 50.1.
Patient/Family Narrative: Eric

Eric is a 44-year-old gay Latino man, originally from New York City, now living alone in rural Vermont, after moving here with his partner, Peter, who unexpectedly died of pancreatic cancer 7 years ago. Eric is a waiter and is currently unable to work due to debilitating pain from shingles. He has been HIV positive for 18 years. He is referred to the palliative care service by infectious disease for uncontrolled pain.

The patient's family history includes severe alcohol use by his mother (deceased at age 41, Eric was 12 at the time) and current cocaine addiction by his only sister. He has four brothers and a father in New York. When Eric disclosed his sexual orientation to

them 19 years ago, they beat him so badly that he had to be hospitalized. He has had no contact with them since he disclosed his HIV-positive status a year later. Eric is close to his sister's three daughters, who live near him. He sees himself as the stable person in their lives and enjoys cooking for them and "just fooling around and being silly." One of his nieces, Angela, works as a secretary in a local hospital. Their two younger sisters live with her and are in high school.

Eric is an active alcoholic, consuming "two or three large cocktails" upon waking each morning and before going to bed at night. He has been seen by infectious disease here for 6 years, and his medical record reflects several discussions with clinicians encouraging him to access alcohol treatment. He has been open about his alcohol use and about his decision not to seek treatment for that. In our discussion today the patient initially declined assistance, stating that his alcohol use was not a problem. He further states that drinking is the only way he can sleep at night. He is overwhelmed with grief regarding Peter's death. He has not seen a therapist for grief work. He feels God is punishing him for being gay.

The nurse practitioner (NP) works with Eric to assess his symptoms and make pain management recommendations. They have agreed on a plan and will meet again in 1 week to reassess. The NP must leave to see another patient, but the social worker has scheduled extended time with the patient to address his psychosocial needs.

The social worker noted, out loud, his loss history (mother/ mothering; sister; brothers; father; his partner; the family of his partner; many friends to AIDS; his gay community in New York City; employment/income; his car; a sense of safety in a sexual relationship; his expectation that Peter would be his caregiver when his HIV symptoms debilitated him; and his faith in a loving God), Eric began to cry. He did not think people in a predominately heterosexual, Caucasian, rural community would understand his losses and the depth of his grief. He admits to being angry that Peter died before he did. He had deeply feared that talking about it all would be so painful that he would never recover from it. He was surprised to find that this conversation gave him a sense of relief, rather than desolation.

They also discussed his financial situation. He has enough reserves to live on for a while. He is hopeful his pain will be managed well enough for him to return to work, and he has transportation (his niece drives him). They also discussed his alcohol use. Eric and the social worker set goals for their next meeting. He would consider going into alcohol treatment, she would research gay-oriented supports, including grief counseling, for him. Eric was offered a visit with the palliative care chaplain to talk about his feelings regarding God and how to make meaning of all he had experienced. He adamantly declined this support.

Two days later, Eric called the social worker and stated that he was willing to enter a residential, 30-day alcohol treatment facility. "I think you're right," he said, "My drinking is keeping me from letting my wounds heal. I am just ripping them open again every night when I hurt so bad I have to get drunk." The social worker made the arrangements and Eric's niece transported him to treatment.

The social worker and NP presented Eric's case to the palliative care team. While the patient declined chaplaincy support, the

Box 50.1 *(Contd.)*

social worker and chaplain agreed to meet regularly so that the chaplain could offer expertise regarding Catholic philosophies and teachings to help her understand the culture of his religion. The collaborative goal was to assist Eric in discovering ways to begin to work toward a different understanding and potential for peace in his relationship with God.

Over the next several months the social worker continued to see Eric for grief work, exploration of his goals regarding familial relationships, and financial and resource issues. He continued to decline chaplaincy supports. The social worker did inform him that she was accessing the chaplain as a spiritual care consultant regarding his needs. In the meantime, the social worker and chaplain were also mindful of Eric choosing a comfortable replacement for the deeper spiritual work a chaplain is trained to do.

One day Eric called the social worker and stated that he was feeling suicidal. He was admitted to this hospital that night. The next day, the social worker and chaplain visited Eric. They felt that he might finally work with the chaplain if he could meet her and feel her loving and accepting presence. The social worker recognized the risk of bringing the chaplain to meet Eric, given that he had declined chaplaincy referrals in the past. He might feel that the social worker was taking control of his choices, which could negatively impact the trust he had in her. Before making the decision to have the chaplain go to his room, the interdisciplinary team had debated the potential risks and benefits. The social worker and NP who had been working closely with Eric felt certain that he would be able to decline the chaplain's visit, without feeling resentment or that he was disappointing his providers, if he did not want to talk with her. Their opinions were based on Eric's consistent ease with discussion and decision making regarding several other issues in their therapeutic relationships. The social worker was sensitive to how she presented Eric the option of having the chaplain stay or leave, emphasizing that it was completely up to him and that he would not hurt anyone's feelings if he did not care to have the visit. While no longer suicidal, he is very depressed and his speech is slow. After introductions, Eric declines the chaplain's invitation to speak privately but asks that both the social worker and chaplain remain with him. As they sit together, the chaplain quietly talks with him about his feelings of despair. She asks if he, in any way, finds a source of comfort in any kind of relationship with God. She helps him identify where he has felt unconditional love in his life. Eric asks her to pray for him. He weeps while she prays aloud. Afterward he admits that he has not been able to pray since Peter died. He comments on the beauty of her words. He states that it makes him hopeful that God might still want to be a part of his life.

The chaplain continues to visit Eric while he is hospitalized. With Eric's agreement, the social worker intentionally stays away so that he can also build a trusting relationship with the chaplain. The chaplain discusses Eric at morning rounds so the social worker is kept up to date and can offer expert advice on psychosocial issues. After discharge, Eric meets with the chaplain and social worker on an alternating basis. The chaplain focuses on his spiritual struggles as well as his relationship with God. The social worker focuses on his ongoing familial and psychosocial needs and goals.

ADDITIONAL RESOURCES AND WEB SITES

Bakitas, M., Stevens, M., Ahles, T., Kirn, M., Skalla, K., Kane, N.,... The Project ENABLE Co-investigators. (2004). Project ENABLE: A palliative care demonstration project for advanced cancer patients in three settings. *Journal of Palliative Medicine, 7*(2), 363–372.

Berlin, E. A., & Fowkes, W. C. (1983). Teaching framework for cross-cultural care: Application in family practice. *Western Journal of Medicine, 139*(6), 934–938.

Byock, I. (1997). *Dying well: The prospect of growth at the end-of-life.* Washington, DC: Georgetown University Press.

Byock, I. (1998). Hospice and palliative care: A parting of the ways or a path to the future? *Journal of Palliative Medicine, 1*(2), 165–176.

Byock, I. (2007). To life! Reflections on spirituality, palliative practice and politics. *Journal of Hospice and Palliative Medicine, 23*(6), 136–138.

Fitchett G. (2002). *Assessing spiritual needs: A guide for caregivers.* Lima, OH: Academic Renewal Press.

Gordon, S. (2009). Spiritual needs rank high as death from cancer nears. *Health Day.*

Gordon, T., & Mitchell, D. (2004). A competency model for the assessment and delivery of spiritual care. *Journal of Palliative Medicine, 18,* 646–651.

Hanks, G., Cherny, N., Christakis, N, Fallon, M., Kaasa, S., & Portenoy, R. (2010). *Oxford textbook of palliative medicine* (4th ed.). New York, NY: Oxford University Press.

Kleinman, A.(1978). *Explanatory models in healthcare relationships, National Council for International Health: Health of the family.* Washington, DC: National Council for International Health.

National Association of Catholic Chaplains. (2007). Standards for certification. Milwaukee, WI: Author.

National Association of Social Workers (NASW). (2008). Code of ethics. Retrieved from http://www.naswdc.org/pubs/code/default.asp

Piotrowski, L. (2007). Setting the Palliative Care Record Straight. *Plainviews, 4*(29). Retrieved from http://www.plainviews.org

Piotrowski, L., & Soltura, D. (2008). A journey with Eric: Reaching out with cultures, subcultures in mind. *Vision, 18*(8).

Pruyser, P. W. (1976). *The minister as diagnostician.* Philadelphia, PA: Westminster Press.

Steinhauser, K., Clipp, E. C., McNeilly, M., Christakis, N. A., McIntyre, L. M., & Tulsky, J. A. (2000). In search of a good death: Observations of patients, families, and providers. *Annals of Internal Medicine, 132*(10), 825–832.

Walter, T. (2000). Spirituality in palliative care: Opportunity or burden? *Journal of Palliative Medicine, 16,* 133–139.

Wintz, S., & Cooper, E. (2003). Developing learning modules to address cultural and spiritual sensitivity. *Chaplaincy Today, 19*(2), 3–6.

WEB SITES

Dying Well: http://www.dyingwell.org

Dr. Ira Byock's Web site, defining wellness through the end of life. Resources for people facing life-limiting illness, their families, and their professional caregivers.

The Healthcare Chaplaincy: http://healthcarechaplaincy.org/ pastoral-care-management/cultural-and-spiritual-values-tutorials.html

Cultural and spiritual values tutorials.

REFERENCES

Byock, I. (2009). Dying well in corrections: Why should we care? *Journal of Correctional Health Care, 9*(2), 107–116.

Council on Collaboration-Spiritual Care Collaborative, Portland, Maine. (2004). *Common code of ethics for chaplains, pastoral counselors, pastoral educators, and students.* Retrieved from http://www.spiritualcarecollaborative.org/standards.asp

Hayes, E., & van der Poel, S. (1990). *Handbook for chaplains.* Mahwah, NJ: Paulist Press.

Nouwen, H. (1998). *Reaching out: Three movements of the spiritual life.* Minneapolis, MN: Zondervan.

Otis-Green, S., Ferrell, B., Spolum, M., Uman, G., Mullan, P., Baird, P., & Grant, M. (2009). An overview of the ACE project—Advocating for Clinical Excellence: Transdisciplinary palliative care education. *Journal of Cancer Education, 24*(2), 120–126.

Puchalski, C., Ferrell, B., Virani, R., Otis-Green, S., Baird, P., Bull, J., Nelson-Becker, H.,… Sulmasy, D. (2009). Improving the quality of spiritual care as a dimension of palliative care: The report of the consensus conference. *Journal of Palliative Medicine, 12*(10), 887.

51 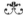 *Gary L. Stein and Jeanne Kerwin*

Social Work and Bioethics: Enhanced Resolution of Ethical Dilemmas and the Challenges along the Way

With thorough grounding in ethical principles, complex ethical dilemmas, and mediation skills, social workers can strive towards equal footing with other members of the health care team in ethics consultation, staff development, and institutional policy formation.
                                                            —Stein and Kerwin

Key Concepts

- *Collaboration among ethics consultants and the social workers involved in patient and family care is the key to successful resolution of ethical dilemmas.*
- *Effective partnerships among social workers and bioethics consultants require social workers who are both informed about and skilled in applying the principles of bioethical analysis and recognizing the parameters of current ethical concerns.*
- *For social workers, collaboration aids in a better understanding of the clinical and ethical issues involved in patient care, thereby leading to improved "translation" of these matters to patients and families.*
- *Social workers require leadership skills to enhance their roles, active participation, and visibility on interdisciplinary hospital care teams, including ethics committees.*

Introduction

More than two decades ago, social work ethics leader Frederic Reamer observed that "there is no limit to the number of ethical issues that now touch the lives of social workers in the health field" (Reamer, 1985, p. 271). These ethical issues currently include, but are not limited to, rationing of care, emphasis on reducing lengths of stay and costs, increasing high-volume case loads, family concerns about financial resources for long-term and home care, complex medical needs of patients, uncertainty in prognosis and life expectancy, fragmented and poor communications among multiple caregivers, and the extraordinary burden of decision-making about the provision or limitation of life-sustaining treatments. Health care social workers are most effective in addressing these issues when collaborating with bioethics consultants in patient and family care and through the institutional ethics committee. Such effective partnership requires social workers who are both informed about and skilled in applying the principles of bioethical analysis and recognizing the parameters of current ethical concerns.

The Practice Environment

The role of the social worker in an acute care hospital is driven by multiple priorities and simultaneously constrained by system demands (Bendor, 1987). The first professional priority for a social worker is to provide psychosocial support to patients and their families and to assist them in coping with chronic or life-threatening illness. A second major priority is guiding the patient and family to develop a safe and appropriate discharge plan in the community. These straight-forward patient-centered tasks have far greater complexity in the acute care hospital environment when the twenty-first-century hospital pressures of discharge planning—reducing lengths of stay and the costs of care—are factored in (Beder, 2006).

In a more perfect world, the physician, nurse, and social worker caring for these patients would have the time and expertise to meet and discuss all of the issues, thereby promoting a safe and appropriate discharge plan for the patient. The reality in today's highly specialized medical centers, however, is quite different. The immense pressure on social workers to plan and implement discharge plans during a rapid short-term hospital stay often deprives them of the time they might choose to spend with patients and families discussing values and wishes and negotiating a consensus among conflicted members of the family.

Time and heavy case loads are not the only demands that interfere with the traditional role of the social worker. Recall that the first hospital social workers were frequently trained as nurses and were able to manage the medical aspects of illness trajectory and expected outcomes in the context of early 1900 medicine (Nacman, 1977). Today's patients are far more complex in terms of medical needs and treatment options. Detailed discussions about the appropriateness of gastric feeding tubes, chemotherapy, radiation, surgery, ventilators, tracheostomies, resuscitation, intensive care, and the extensive list of options patients and families are offered require specialized medical knowledge about the treatments proposed, their potential benefits and burdens, and the appropriateness of treatments for a particular illness or condition. This imperative has fostered the integration and collaboration of social work into bioethics and palliative care teams, encouraging the enhancement of the social work role through training and participation in the field of bioethics.

At the heart of many of these issues lies the moral compass, and the examination and study of that compass, known as bioethics. The principles of bioethics—respect for patient autonomy, acting in the best interests of the patient (beneficence), doing no harm (nonmaleficence), and the fair allocation of scarce resources (justice)—play a significant role in the ability of a social worker to execute the tasks assigned (Beauchamp & Childress, 2008). There is an increasing need for the expertise and counsel of bioethics consultants in many of the complex cases in which conflicted values and divergent understandings of the patients' best interests are barriers to creating an appropriate plan. These ethical dilemmas are illustrated by the highly publicized cases of Karen Ann Quinlan, Nancy Beth Cruzan, and Terri Schiavo, but they are routinely found in cases of hospitalized patients without the drama of courtrooms and the media. Many serious dilemmas arise at the bedside of seriously ill and dying patients: questions about who should make decisions among estranged and conflicted family members, differences between a patient's written wishes and the family's or physician's interpretation of those wishes, issues concerning the withholding of diagnostic information from dying patients, families demanding treatments deemed futile by physicians, and every possible scenario one might imagine. These are the complexities that drive hospital social workers to interact and collaborate with multidisciplinary expertise in the hospital setting. A bioethics consultant or team may be required on cases involving ethical concerns to facilitate and guide decisions based on ethical principles and mediation of disputes.

Palliative care teams, comprised of physicians, nurses, social workers, chaplains, and others now exist in many hospitals. While these teams assist patients and families along the continuum of illness and with end-of-life clinical issues such as pain and symptom management, they also address psychosocial issues and guide families through end-of-life decision-making. Social workers play a vital role by participating either as a standing member of a bioethics or palliative care "team" or as the "ad hoc" social worker brought in on a case because she had been working with that patient and family. Collaboration between the consultants and the social worker involved with that patient and family is key to the ultimate success of the case.

Background Literature

As noted by Reamer in 1985, health care social workers will be more effective with a specialized knowledge base in values and ethics generally, and particularly in bioethics (Reamer, 1985). Although policy statements of the National Association of Social Workers (NASW) advocate the integration of principle of bioethics into professional practice (NASW, 2004, 2009), very limited research literature suggests that this standard is frequently unmet.

In a survey of health care social workers from Texas, Csikai and Bass (2000) found that an overwhelming majority had little or no formal training in ethics in spite of the extremely complex ethical dilemmas they encounter. Common issues included confusion because of the lack of an advance directive or the interpretation of an existing directive, questions of competency, uncertainty of patient wishes, and disagreements between patients and their families. However, because "such knowledge is essential if social workers are to be active participants in resolving complex ethical dilemmas," they suggested that social workers should be trained in bioethics during their master's or post-master's-level training (Csikai & Bass, 2000, p. 19).

In a multistate study of ethical dilemmas in hospice care, Csikai (2004) reported that hospice social workers, like their hospital-based colleagues, were ill prepared to assume a leadership role in their interdisciplinary care teams. Just over half of the survey respondents said they had been exposed to ethical theories during their professional training, and even fewer had been exposed to current ethical issues in general or to biomedical ethics in particular. She concluded that "education on ethical issues in end-of-life care is an unclaimed area that social workers have an opportunity to seize and to develop expertise that can be shared" (Csikai, 2004, p. 75). Similarly, in a South Carolina study of social workers' attitudes toward physician-assisted suicide, Manetta and Wells (2001) found that many social workers employed in hospital settings received little grounding in ethics during their professional training or from NASW's policies.

There have been significant advancements in social work practice, continuing education, and research on palliative and end-of-life care during the past decade. Not reflected by the aforementioned studies are the development of social work post-master's certificate programs by Smith College, New York University, and Kean University (Stein, Sherman, & Bullock, 2009); diverse practice and research models promoted by the Social Work Leadership Development Awards Program of the Project on Death in America; the formation of leadership networks, such as the Social Work Hospice and Palliative Care Network; numerous professional symposia; fellowships and important publications (Berzoff & Silverman, 2004). However, these advancements need to be integrated more widely into master's-level and post-graduate education and assure greater attention to bioethical concerns.

Box 51.1
Patient/Family Narrative: Mr. Smith and Family

Mr. Smith was 72 years old when he and his wife executed their advance directives for health care, stating their wishes for end-of-life care. Mrs. Smith succumbed to Alzheimer's disease 5 years later, while Mr. Smith remained robust and active. Mr. Smith cared for his wife for 5 years until he reached age 83. He then considered an offer from his son, one of two children, to come and live with his family. His son and daughter-in-law would build an addition onto their home to accommodate Mr. and Mrs. Smith and would help in the care of Mrs. Smith. Mr. Smith agreed to pay for the building of the addition out of the proceeds from the sale of his existing home. Mr. Smith suffered a massive hemorrhagic stroke 2 days following this verbal agreement with his son. He was now unresponsive on a ventilator in the intensive care unit. The doctors told the family that the prognosis was not encouraging due to the extent of brain damage. Mr. Smith's living will was discussed with the family and the conflict began. Mr. Smith wrote: "If I am unable to interact with my family, I do not want my life prolonged by any artificial means." At this point, he had been ventilator dependent for 12 days and unable to breathe on his own. If someone shouted his name, he became startled and opened his eyes, but he was unable to follow any simple commands. His son maintained that his father was "interacting with his family" because he opened his eyes when they called his name. Mr. Smith's daughter stated that her father's living will described this situation as "exactly what he did not want."

A bioethics consultation was called to facilitate a resolution to this conflict. The team met with the two children and the social worker in the intensive care unit where Mr. Smith received care. The team listened carefully as family members expressed their feelings about what had happened to their father and what should be done in accordance with his wishes. The team then explained the patient's medical condition in great detail, including his limited prognosis for any cognitive recovery beyond his current status. The burdens of further life-sustaining treatment were described and, most important, his expressed written wishes were discussed. The son and daughter remained unable to agree, but the daughter

ultimately deferred to her brother, who had been named as her father's health care proxy. The bioethics team advised the son of their opinion that it was ethically appropriate to follow the wishes stated in the living will and to withdraw the ventilator, allowing Mr. Smith to die naturally. The son acknowledged the opinion, but he would not agree to the withdrawal at that time.

The anger between the adult children of this patient was deeply rooted in long-standing family dynamics. Concerns about financial gains as a result of the promised home addition, a long history of role conflict between the children, grief about the loss of one parent to Alzheimer's and now the other to death, guilt, and other issues complicated the decisions about the appropriate care plan for this patient. The patient's wishes, as clearly expressed, caused moral distress for the doctors and nurses caring for him through the many days before he was allowed to die.

The integration of the social worker into the bioethics consult in this case was critical to developing Mr. Smith's plan of care. She played a key role in explaining to both children what kind of long-term care Mr. Smith would require, as well as the cost of that care, both financially and emotionally for the family. It was the social worker who remained in close daily contact with the conflicted family, recognizing that the son and daughter's unique emotional processes needed to be acknowledged and respected. Because she had been part of the bioethics consultation, she had an appreciation of the anger and the conflicted opinions of the two children, as well as an understanding of the medical prognosis and the ethical opinion to honor the patient's written wishes. Through this knowledge, she was able to follow the patient and family through to an appropriate ending, in which the son agreed to remove the ventilator and allow his father to die peacefully in a hospice unit.

The family narrative in Box 51.1 illustrates the benefits of social work participation in ethics consults. In this case, the social worker assists the family by translating medical information, discussing the psychosocial impact of the patient's prognosis, and mediating family conflict regarding whether or not to follow their ailing father's wishes not to be maintained on life-sustaining medical treatment.

Box 51.2.
Patient/Family Narrative: Mr. and Mrs. G.

Mr. and Mrs. G. arrived in the United States 2 weeks ago from India to visit their daughter, her American husband, and their newborn grandson. Mr. G. suffered a severe headache after dinner on the second night of their visit. After several hours of no relief from Tylenol, he became unresponsive and was rushed to the hospital where he was diagnosed with an intracerebral bleed. He was taken to the operating room by the on-call neurosurgeon, where he underwent evacuation of the bleed, which was very large and extended into both ventricles of the brain. The doctors told the family that the prognosis after such a large hemorrhage into the brain was very poor. Mr. G. was placed on a ventilator in the intensive care unit, where he remained for 10 days without improvement. He remained unresponsive and ventilator

Box 51.2 (Contd.)

dependent, with little chance of any meaningful recovery. The daughter was on the phone each day with her older brother, who was a doctor in India. The family insisted that all aggressive life supports be continued as they waited for signs of improvement. They made inquiries about medical information as relayed from the doctor-son in India. The wife refused to make any decisions to limit aggressive care and was found weeping in the room each day. The bioethics team was requested to help with this case.

The social worker on the bioethics team was well versed in the cultural variations that influence how families deal with serious life-threatening situations. She was also trained in bioethics and had a clear understanding of where this family needed help. As part of the team, the social worker was able to clarify the issues for discussion. Initially, she met with the family to hear their version of what had happened. Before setting up the bioethics family meeting, she already understood that in this culture, the wife may not be the decision-maker and the eldest son, who was a doctor, might assume this important role. The fact that the eldest son advised the couple not to travel to America because of Mr. G's hypertension and advanced age had left the wife with extraordinary feelings of guilt for wanting to come to visit her new grandchild. The social worker also spoke to the daughter to find out more about her relationship with her brother and mother. She learned that the brother was not pleased with his sister's marriage to a man of another culture and religion. Because of this estrangement, the cultural influences, and the sister's feelings of guilt for inviting her parents to come for a visit, she deferred to her brother's medical opinion about what was best. The social worker realized that the meeting with the bioethics consult team would be fruitless unless the doctor-son was part of the meeting. Since he could not leave his practice and his family in India, she arranged a conference call to include the son at a time that worked for all parties. She also realized that the doctor-son would have to hear directly from the neurosurgeons about his father's prognosis.

The meeting occurred and the son in India had all of his medical questions answered directly from the neurosurgeon caring for his father. As a result, he felt that he had enough control of the situation to advise his mother and sister that it was appropriate to remove his father from the ventilator and to allow a natural death. The family seemed relieved to be unburdened from the pressure of medical decision-making. Although saddened by the anticipated death of their loved one, the family was able to resolve the impasse and move forward in their grief as a family.

The family narrative in Box 51.2 illustrates the professional knowledge and skills base that social workers bring to the bioethics team. In this case, the social worker on the team integrates her expertise in family dynamics with cultural proficiency skills to facilitate a long-distance family meeting to make difficult end-of-life decisions.

Benefits and Challenges

There is a dual benefit to the inclusion of social workers in bioethics consultations, in addition to palliative care consultations. Knowledge of one's area of expertise in the complex environment of an acute care hospital is most effectively shared in the context of individual cases, both demonstrating the unique social work skill set while enhancing the knowledge of all specialists on the team. No one expects each professional to have expertise in all areas needed to manage the complex issues of today's patients and families. However, a collaborative team approach to complex issues enhances the performance of all professionals involved. For social workers, collaboration aids in a better understanding of the clinical and ethical issues involved in patient care, thereby leading to improved "translation" of these matters to patients and families. Most important, team approaches prevent the patient and family from receiving fragmented, contradictory, and confusing information during this stressful time in their lives.

To promote social work effectiveness in collaboration with bioethics consultants and institutional ethics committees, significant training gaps should be addressed (Stein & Sherman, 2005). The need for thorough grounding in ethical principles, complex ethical dilemmas, and mediation skills cannot be overemphasized. With this background, social workers can obtain more equal footing with other members of the health care team in patient consults, staff development, and institutional policy formation. Social workers also require better education on medical issues to better understand the benefits and risks of medical interventions (such as resuscitation, breathing tubes, and artificial nutrition and hydration), and to enhance proficiency in translating medical information into language patients and families can understand.

Finally, social workers require leadership skills to enhance their roles on interdisciplinary care teams. Working in hospital and other medical settings most often led by doctors and nurses, and compromised by a challenging economic environment, social workers can be overlooked in ethics deliberations, whether in case consults or ethics committees. Social workers can be leaders on the bioethics team—they have the understanding of family dynamics, communications skills, and community resources that are necessary for effective resolution of ethical dilemmas, development of advance care plans, and formulation of care plans generally. Collaborative approaches in bioethics and palliative care present important opportunities to enhance social worker roles and responsibilities in health care settings, as well as reinforcing their vital presence and demonstrated skill set in patient and family care.

LEARNING EXERCISE

- *Role play:* Assign roles of family members and health care professionals in the narratives in Boxes 51.1 and 51.2 with scripted perspectives of each. Role play participants are only given their perspective in a script. After role play enactment of the narrative scenario, each participant describes how it "feels" to be in that role, what was helpful to each of them, and what was confusing or frustrating. Feedback from each participant is elicited about each role. Faculty provides positive reinforcement and feedback on the role play.

- *Note:* It is educational and instructive for social workers to experience the role of doctor, nurse, patient, and family member, as well as playing the role of social worker in these scenarios.

ADDITIONAL RESOURCES AND WEB SITES

Brody, J. (2009). *Jane Brody's guide to the great beyond: A practical primer to help you and your loved ones prepare medically, legally, and emotionally for the end-of-life.* New York, NY: Random House.

Dubler, N. N., & Liebman, C. B. (2004). *Bioethics mediation: A guide to shaping shared solutions.* New York, NY: United Hospital Fund of New York.

Fins, J. J. (2006). *A palliative ethic of care: Clinical wisdom at life's end.* Sudbury, MA: Jones and Bartlett Publishers, Inc.

Post, L. F., Bluestein, J., & Dubler, N. N. (2006). *Handbook for health care ethics committees.* Baltimore, MD: Johns Hopkins University Press.

Moyers, B. (2000). *On our own terms: Bill Moyers on dying.* New York, NY: Educational Broadcasting Corporation/Public Affairs Television, Inc. For more information, see http://www.pbs.org/wnet/onourownterms

Nichols, M. (Director). (2001). *Wit.* New York, NY: HBO Home Video.

WEB SITES

The American Society for Bioethics and Humanities: http://www.asbh.org
Promotes the exchange of ideas and fosters multidisciplinary, interdisciplinary, and interprofessional scholarship, research, teaching, policy development, professional development, and collegiality among people engaged in clinical and academic bioethics and the medical humanities.

The Center to Advance Palliative Care (CAPC): http://www.capc.org
Provides health care professionals with the tools, training, and technical assistance necessary to start and sustain successful palliative care programs in hospitals and other health care settings.

The Hastings Center: http://www.thehastingscenter.org
An independent, nonpartisan, and nonprofit bioethics research institute. The Center addresses fundamental ethical issues in the areas of health, medicine, and the environment as they affect individuals, communities, and societies.

The National Hospice and Palliative Care Organization–Caring Connections: http://www.caringinfo.org
Contains a comprehensive consumer education about advance care planning, including state-specific advance directives.

The Social Work Hospice and Palliative Care Network: http://www.swhpn.org
An emerging network of social work organizations and leaders who seek to further the field of end-of-life and hospice/palliative care.

REFERENCES

Beauchamp, T. L., & Childress, J. F. (2008). *Principles of biomedical ethics* (6th ed.). New York, NY: Oxford University Press.

Beder, J. (2006). *Hospital social work: The interface of medicine and caring.* New York, NY: Routledge.

Bendor, S. (1987). The clinical challenge of hospital-based social work practice. *Social Work in Health Care, 13*(2), 25–33.

Berzoff, J., & Silverman, P. R. (2004). *Living with dying: A handbook for end-of-life healthcare practitioners.* New York, NY: Columbia University Press.

Csikai, E. L. (2004). Social workers' participation in the resolution of ethical dilemmas in hospice care. *Health and Social Work, 29*(1), 67–76.

Csikai, E. L., & Bass, K. (2000). Health care social workers' views of ethical issues, practice, and policy in end-of-life care. *Social Work and Health Care, 32*(2), 1–22.

Manetta, A., & Wells, J. G. (2001). Ethical issues in the social worker's role in physician-assisted suicide. *Health and Social Work, 26*(3), 160–166.

Nacman, M. (1977). Social work in health settings: A historical review. *Social Work in Health Care, 2*(4), 7–23.

National Association of Social Workers (NASW). (2004). *NASW standards for palliative and end of life care.* Washington, DC: Author.

National Association of Social Workers (NASW). (2009). End-of-life care. In S. Lowman & L. O'Hearn (Eds.). *Social Work Speaks, Eighth Edition, NASW Policy Statements, 2009–2012* (pp. 114–120). Washington, DC: NASW Press.

Reamer, F. G. (1985). The emergence of bioethics in social work. *Health and Social Work, 10*(4), 271–281.

Stein, G. L., & Sherman, P. A. (2005). Promoting effective social work policy in end-of-life and palliative care. *Journal of Palliative Medicine, 8*(6), 1271–1281.

Stein, G. L., Sherman, P. A., & Bullock, K. (2009). Educating gerontologists for cultural proficiency in end-of-life care practice. *Educational Gerontology, 35*, 1008–1025.

52 Wendy Walters and Dennis E. Watts

Social Work and Volunteers

The principle of compassion lies at the heart of all religious, ethical, and spiritual traditions, calling us always to treat all others as we wish to be treated ourselves.

— Excerpt from the "Charter for Compassion, 2009"

We can do no great things, only small things with great love.

— Mother Theresa

Key Concepts

- ◆ *Volunteer roles, which encompass a wide spectrum of services, require diverse support from the social worker.*
- ◆ *Ethical issues faced by volunteers should be addressed by the social worker through ongoing, informal communication and through continuing education and care planning with the volunteer.*
- ◆ *Led by the social worker, volunteer recruitment, training, and retention can improve patient care by enabling a more complete understanding of how the unique dynamics of each family may benefit from different levels of support from various members of the interdisciplinary team.*

Introduction

Palliative care involves the use of an interdisciplinary team to provide comprehensive care to patients and their families, and in many settings, the volunteer is an intrinsic member of that team. Volunteers provide a rich dimension to the overall support system that improves the ability of both patient and family to live their lives with the best possible quality.

Professional social workers often serve as the primary coordinators of volunteer services, providing ongoing continuing supervision and education for volunteers about such topics as interpersonal and service boundaries, communication skills, family systems, self-care, and grief responses.

In the United States, the first modern hospices were community-based programs run solely by volunteers; it was not until the creation of the Medicare Hospice Benefit in 1982 that hospice programs with paid professional staff became more widespread, with more than 4580 programs in 2008 (National Hospice & Palliative Care Organization [NHPCO], 2009). However, the federal government, recognizing that the role of the volunteer remains crucial to the overall delivery of care, requires Medicare-certified programs to document evidence that administrative or direct patient care delivered by volunteers equals a minimum of 5% of the total patient care hours provided by the paid staff (Department of Health and Human Services, 2008). Today, many palliative care programs have not yet integrated volunteers. While guidelines provided by the National Consensus Project for Quality Palliative Care (National Consensus Project, 2009) encourage palliative care programs to include volunteers as part of the interdisciplinary team, there is no federal mandate for volunteer assistance as there is for hospice programs that are Medicare certified.

Volunteer Roles

Be the change you want to see in the world.
—*Mahatma Gandhi*

A wide spectrum of services are provided by volunteers in a variety of settings, including private homes, hospitals, nursing homes, retirement homes, and hospices. In many settings, the social worker serves as the primary "matchmaker" to ensure that the support provided by individual volunteers is appropriately suited to each patient's unique needs and each volunteer's unique abilities. For example, the social worker, working with the volunteer, may find that the optimal role for a particular volunteer may be to sit or read with the patient, run errands, provide child care, or perform household chores. Volunteers can also be of significant help in other ways, for example, revisiting the patient's favorite memories, accompanying patients to their favorite haunts, facilitating patient visits with pets, or offering the patient's primary caregiver a much needed physical break. Many specialized services, such as art, music, and massage therapy, are delivered by appropriately trained and licensed volunteers. Administrative volunteers can provide substantial cost savings to programs by filing, answering the telephone, supporting data entry, handling bereavement mailings, and organizing supplies. Additional roles that professional social workers may identify and support include volunteer service in fundraising efforts, for example, helping to prepare mailings, sending thank-you letters, organizing fundraising events, and assisting with the program's appeals to prospective major donors. Some volunteers may also be well suited to help increase awareness of the importance of palliative care by making presentations at community events or at public hearings focused on health policy issues. Other volunteers might assist with the program's bereavement program by helping with patient support groups, memorial services, and mailing programs. In brief, matching patients' and families' needs with available and appropriate volunteer expertise is a vital function of the professional palliative social worker.

A number of national programs provide structured opportunities for volunteers to contribute directly to patient and family care. *No One Dies Alone* is a program that began in 2001 at Sacred Heart Medical Center in Eugene, Oregon, by Sandra Clarke, an intensive care nurse. This nurse's personal experience in caring for the dying led her to form a volunteer program composed of both health care professionals and community members to provide companionship for those patients without friends or family with whom to share the end of their life (Sacred Heart Medical Center, 2009). Similarly, "doula" programs have emerged around the country, providing care to persons living with life-threatening illness through trained volunteers who offer companionship, advocacy, spiritual, social, and emotional support (Shira Ruskay Center, 2009).

Another national program, *Project Storykeeper*, provides structured ways to help volunteers capture the life stories of the patients with whom they work through the use of music, scrapbooking, photos, videos, and other ways to create legacies (Project Storykeeper, 2008). This type of program enables patients to create their own "ethical will," a concept rooted in both Hebrew and Christian traditions. As compared to a traditional will that bequeaths valuables, the ethical will is a tool that can be used to pass on morals, values, important family stories, traditions, advice, and reflections (Baines, 2002).

While the "modern" relationship between health professionals and patients can sometimes dehumanize both, good communication and coordination between a program's clinical team and its volunteers, with the social worker as primary liaison, can help to personalize the experiences of living with life-threatening illness and dying and thereby provide individual patients and their families more complete and humane care. Indeed, volunteers may create an environment of empathy and reassurance by their mere, silent "presence." Presence is defined as a mode of being, a sense of intuitiveness and connectedness, being comfortable with oneself, and accepting vulnerability (Stanley, 2002). By simply "being there," volunteers may also inspire others, including the patient's family and friends, to bolster their efforts to support the patient's need for companionship.

Ethical Issues Faced by Volunteers

In the end-of-life setting, volunteers maintain a unique relationship with the patient and family. Social workers can be invaluable in providing ongoing support and education to the volunteer in role clarification and service boundaries. One study conducted with hospice volunteers found that their most common ethical dilemmas revolved around receiving gifts, patient care and family concerns, roles and boundaries, and suicide or hastening death (Berry & Planalp, 2009). An earlier Canadian study found other ethical challenges for volunteers, including issues surrounding communication (i.e., who should know about the patient's prognosis), confidentiality, conflicts of interest, and concerns about adequate pain control (Rothstein, 1994).

Each of these issues should be addressed by the social worker as part of ongoing continuing education and care planning. The social worker can thereby remain instrumental and engaged in helping volunteers discuss and work through challenging situations. The social worker's training in family-systems theory, crisis intervention, and communication skills provides a sounding board for the volunteer's experience with the patient and family, and it should empower volunteers to remain thoughtful, sensitive, and vigilant. The trained professional social worker is receptive to volunteers' questions, creating a safe, comfortable relationship within which disagreements can be aired and any ethical concerns can be discussed. Keeping this relationship open and authentic involves creating both formal and informal opportunities for communication and dialog between the volunteer and the social worker. General group discussions of ethical issues can create the context for directly addressing patient-specific issues with the social worker on other occasions. In response to the volunteer's questions, the social worker may share with the volunteer how they have personally resolved or approached similar dilemmas in the past. Gaining the respect and trust of the volunteer also requires follow-up communication by the social worker to include every reasonable effort to reach closure on the specific ethical concerns that are brought to the social worker's attention.

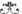

Volunteer Recruitment, Training, and Retention

The volunteer, working in conjunction with the interdisciplinary team, helps strengthen not only the individual patient and family system but also contributes to the overall health of society. Wuthnow's study of volunteering in the United States found that Americans value taking care of each other and identify volunteering as a "way of envisioning a better society" (Wuthnow, 1991, p. 266). Individuals choose to volunteer for many different reasons; some may have had a personal experience with the hospice or palliative care program and want to give back as a sign of gratitude. The social worker, whether functioning as the volunteer coordinator or as part of the screening/training team, should be involved in the assessment of each volunteer's own grieving process. Many programs choose to set a time parameter, typically a year after the death, before family members of former patients can become volunteers.

To ensure that each volunteer is prepared for the unique demands of working with seriously ill patients, most palliative care programs and hospices require volunteers to complete a general training program and agree to a background evaluation. Additional training may be organized by the social worker to enable volunteers to meet special program and patient needs.

Volunteers also need ongoing training and support, especially as they encounter difficult situations. Social workers can help the volunteer to understand family systems and communication styles, to use reflective listening skills when patients ask difficult questions, and to understand developmental expectations when working with children. Social workers can also help to process the volunteer's own emotions when working with complex patients and families or those with acute stress and grief. The volunteer, through a unique relationship not realized by the rest of the team, contributes to understanding the complexity of the family dynamics and how each unique family requires different levels of support from various team members. While palliative care organizations, through their social workers' efforts, often appropriately recognize the contribution of their volunteers, it is also common for expressions of gratitude to come from patients

and their families. Reciprocally, volunteers often express their gratitude to their social worker colleagues for the opportunity to serve patients and families along the continuum of illness and at end of life with the respectful, kind, and personalized companionship that we each hope for ourselves.

The professional social worker serving as the volunteer coordinator is responsible for keeping volunteers engaged, appreciated, and supported to enhance the meaning of their contributions and to retain the volunteers for the future benefit of the program's patients and their families. Hospice and palliative care programs invest a considerable amount of money and time in each volunteer (Silbert, 1985), and this investment can strengthen the program's ability to support patients and their families. In efforts to recruit, train, and retain volunteers, existing volunteers may also collaborate with the social worker in volunteer program planning, participating in volunteer training, and/or recruiting other volunteers. Volunteer involvement in these activities can thereby optimize program understanding among volunteers and bolster other prospective and current volunteers' personal commitments.

Summary

Volunteerism is, by its very nature, altruistic, and making a decision to work with seriously ill patients and their families is to choose to witness suffering. The process of living with illness and anticipating the end of life is a unique time for each individual and is essential to the meaning of our humanity. Volunteers can make a powerful impact by providing services to organizations and contributing their skills and talents and a compassionate presence to patients who may be coming to the end of their lives. The volunteer who contributes to the organization through non-patient-related care is equally valuable to the overall effectiveness of the program. Honoring the various individuals and organizations who contribute in different ways to the humane care of patients who have a terminal illness or injury should always be considered important. Volunteers may offer an especially significant service by contributing their personal skills, talents, and a compassionate presence to patients. Indeed, the volunteer is in a unique position and often may devote more time to the patient and family than other members of the palliative care team. Consequently, volunteers may provide useful observations and other information that impacts and enriches the overall care plan. Volunteers may also make key contributions in interdisciplinary efforts to educate the public about thoughtful end-of-life choices that benefit not only patients and their families but also the health care system that delivers care. Working partnerships between the volunteer and the professional social worker can enhance the psychosocial functioning of patients and their families, just as the social worker's collaborations with nurses and chaplains improve the physical and spiritual aspects of patient care. Volunteers remain a vital force on the palliative care team and deserve appropriate continuing recognition.

In summary, volunteers frequently find their experience in palliative care to be a unique opportunity to give and receive personalized messages of love, compassion, joy, and peace. With adequate preparation, good communication, and close collaboration between the social worker and the volunteer, their common efforts can lead to new and endearing lifelong friendships and memories. In addition, volunteers may learn that if one gives patients and their families the freedom to be who they are, they (more frequently than not) respond with expressions of hope, kindness, humor, and courage. Indeed, people living with serious illness and entering the last days and weeks of their lives remain individuals with distinct personalities and varied physical, social, emotional, and spiritual needs. Our experience with them, whether we serve them as volunteers or as paid health professionals, should never be treated as obvious or routine. Each individual deserves our entire humanity (the application of our abilities to reason and empathize) and a unique compassionate response.

LEARNING EXERCISES

- Develop a legacy building exercise with a patient and family or within your classroom with a fellow student. This exercise might be a letter, video, or artwork. Assist in the actual process of developing the particular exercise. Share the results with each other, working to understand the creative experience itself and also the history and meaning implicit in the legacy as reflected in the letter, video, or artwork. The goal of the exercise is to help volunteers appreciate the impact that legacy work can make with a family.
- Poetry reading: Volunteers and social workers read and discuss the following poems in relation to motivation for volunteering and for clinical work: *in time of daffodils* (e.e. Cummings, 1958) and *Kindness* by Naomi Shabib Nye below and available in *Words Under the Words* (1995, p. 42).

Kindness

Before you know what kindness really is
You must lose things,
Feel the future dissolve in a moment
Like salt in a weakened broth.
What you held in your hand,
What you counted and carefully saved,
All this must go so you know
How desolate the landscape can be
between the regions of kindness.

How you ride and ride
Thinking the bus will never stop,
The passengers eating maize and chicken
Will stare out the window forever.

Before you learn the tender gravity of kindness,
You must travel where the Indian in a white poncho
Lies dead by the side of the road.
You must see how this could be you,
How he too was someone
Who journeyed through the night with plans
And the simple breath that kept him alive.

Before you know kindness as the deepest thing inside,
You must know sorrow as the other deepest thing.
You must wake up with sorrow.
You must speak to it till your voice
Catches the thread of all sorrows
And you see the size of the cloth.

Then it is only kindness that makes sense anymore,
Only kindness that ties your shoes
And sends you out into the day to mail letters and
purchase bread,
Only kindness that raises its head
From the crowd of the world to say
It is I you have been looking for,
And then goes with you everywhere
Like a shadow or a friend

—*Naomi Shabib Nye, 1995*
(reprinted with permission of the author)

ADDITIONAL RESOURCES

BOOKS

Baines, B. (2002). *Ethical wills: Putting your values on paper.* Cambridge, MA: Perseus Publishing.

Callanan, M. (2008). *Final journeys: A practical guide for bringing care and comfort at the end of life.* New York, NY: Bantam Dell.

Callanan, M., & Kelley, P. (1992). *Final gifts.* New York, NY: Poseidon Press.

Faulkner, A., & Maguire, P. (1996). *Talking to cancer patients and their relatives.* New York, NY: Oxford University Press.

Frankl, V. (1959). *Man's search for meaning.* Boston, MA: Beacon Press.

Remen, R. N. (1996). *Kitchen table wisdom.* New York, NY: Riverhead Books.

Sheikh, A. A. (2002). *Handbook of therapeutic imagery techniques.* Amityville, NY: Baywood Publishing Company.

Wooten-Green, R. (2001). *When the dying speak: How to listen to and learn from those facing death.* Chicago, IL: Loyola Press.

WEB SITES

The American Academy of Hospice and Palliative Medicine (AAHPM): http://www.aahpm.org
Professional organization for physicians specializing in hospice and palliative medicine. Membership is also open to social workers, nurses, and other health care providers who are committed to improving the quality of life of patients and families facing life-threatening or serious conditions.
Chapters of Life: http://www.chaptersoflife.com
Helps individuals preserve their memories with memoirs and personal histories, family memory books, oral and spiritual histories, and corporate histories.
The Charter for Compassion: http://www.charterforcompassion.org
The result of Karen Armstrong's 2008 TED Prize wish and made possible by the generous support of the Fetzer Institute. The Charter of Compassion is a cooperative effort to restore not only compassionate thinking but, more important, compassionate action to the center of religious, moral, and political life.
Ethical Wills: http://www.Ethicalwill.com
Provides resources to help people write and preserve their legacy of values at any stage of life.
Hospice Foundation of America: http://www.hospicefoun dation.org
A not-for-profit organization that provides leadership in the development and application of hospice and its philosophy of care.
The Legacy Center: http://www.Thelegacycenter.net
Dedicated to preserving personal stories, values, and meaning. They provide workshops and resources for all people interested in preserving their legacy in some way.
The National Hospice and Palliative Care Organization (NHPCO): http://www.NHPCO.org
Dedicated to promoting and maintaining quality care for terminally ill persons and their families, and to making hospice an integral part of the U.S. health care system.
National Institutes of Health (NIH): http://bioethics.od.nih.gov
A catalogue of bioethics resources within the NIH.

REFERENCES

Baines, B. (2002). *Ethical wills: Putting your values on paper.* Cambridge, MA: Perseus Publishing.
Berry, P., & Planalp, S. (2009). Ethical issues for hospice volunteers. *American Journal of Hospice and Palliative Care, 25,* 458.
Cummings, E. (1958). *95 poems.* New York, NY: Liveright Publishing Corporation / W. W. Norton & Company, Inc.
Department of Health and Human Services, Centers for Medicare and Medicaid Services. (2008). The Medicare conditions of participation for hospice care. *Federal Register, 73*(109), 32202.
National Consensus Project for Quality Palliative Care. (2009). *Clinical practice guidelines for quality palliative care, second edition.* Retrieved from http://www.nationalconsensusproject. org/AboutGuidelines.asp
National Hospice & Palliative Care Organization (NHPCO). (2009). *NHPCO facts and figures: Hospice care in America.* Retrieved from http://www.nhpco.org/files/public/Statistics_ Research/NHPCO_facts_and_figures.pdf
Nye, R. (1995). *Words Under the Words.* Portland, OR: Far Corner Books.
Project Storykeeper. (2009). Retrieved from http://www. storykeeper.org/hospice-project/
Rothstein, J. M. (1994). Ethical challenges to the palliative care volunteer. *Journal of Palliative Care, 10,* 79–82.
Sacred Heart Medical Center. (2009). *No one dies alone.* Retrieved from http://www.peacehealth.org/Oregon/ NoOneDiesAlone.htm
Shira Ruskay Center. (2009). *Doula to accompany and comfort.* Retrieved from http://www.shiraruskay.org/doula.html
Silbert, D. (1985). Assessing volunteer satisfaction in hospice work: Protection of an investment. *American Journal of Hospital Care, 2,* 36–40.
Stanley, K. (2002). The healing power of presence: Respite from the fear of abandonment. *Oncology Nursing Forum, 29*(6), 935–940.
Wuthnow, R. (1991). *Acts of Compassion: Caring for Others and Helping Ourselves.* Princeton, NJ: Princeton University Press.

VI

Regional Voices from a Global Perspective

"I am proud when I think about my work and honored to be in the group of professionals doing this work all over our country and world. They inspire me to do the best work I possibly can and my patients spur my passion for expanding our field. This is the job I have worked the hardest at and loved the most."

Kelly C. Markham LCSW
Palliative Care Coordinator
Baptist Hospital
Pensacola, FL

Medical Spanish: To Donald

In East Harlem as a new doctor, my brother mastered medical Spanish translating loss and worry to the dream of health and healing. His elegant medical tools provided clues but not solutions. His years of education on a memory grid were not complete. He explained carefully, slowly each symptom and possible cause. Each patient was different, each solution unique. He used the vital signs of his senses: to touch, to see, to hear. Listening is the important verb: dolor, dolor, dolor, pain, pain a haiku with a different text.

Constance H. Gemson LMSW
New York, NY

53 *Rebecca S. Myers and Elizabeth J. Clark*

The Need for Global Capacity Building in Palliative Social Work

The good we seek for ourselves is precarious and uncertain until it is secure for all of us.
—Jane Addams (as cited in Bush, 1993)

Key Concepts

- *Palliative care is a human right.*
- *The need for palliative care is growing.*
- *Nations and communities have not fully met the needs for palliative care.*
- *Social workers must provide leadership to build capacity for palliative care around the world.*
- *Strategies and plans to increase capacity for palliative care will differ with each community and nation.*

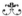

Introduction

This quote by social work founder Jane Addams (Bettis, n.d. expresses an essential facet of social work practice: the need to advocate for systemic change at the institutional, community, national, and global levels. Palliative care is an indispensable contribution to care along the continuum of illness, yet it is unevenly acknowledged and included as such around the world. This chapter provides a foundation for the necessary integration of palliative care in health care systems worldwide, as well as a framework for advocating for and strengthening the provision of palliative social work.

The Growing Need for Palliative Care

By 2050, the number of people worldwide over age 60 is predicted to grow from 600 million to 2 billion. Globally, incidences of cancer will more than double by 2050. Both of these statistics point to a growing need for palliative care. Pain control and palliative care have proven to increase treatment adherence in cancer and HIV/AIDS. Yet, according to the World Health Organization (WHO), few countries have incorporated palliative care in their cancer control programs (Open Society Institute & Equitas, 2007).

Palliative Care Is a Human Right

According to the United Nations Office of the High Commissioner for Human Rights (OHCHR), human rights are defined as follows:

> [R]ights inherent to all human beings, whatever our nationality, place of residence, sex, national or ethnic origin, colour, religion, language, or any other status. We are all equally entitled to our human rights without discrimination. These rights are all interrelated, interdependent and indivisible. (UNOHCHR, 2009)

Many international documents, including those of the United Nations and World Health Organization, imply that palliative care is a human right. To emphasize this point, international pain and palliative care organizations, as well as individuals, have signed on to the "Joint Declaration and Statement of Commitment on Palliative Care and Pain Treatment as Human Rights," coordinated by the International Association for Hospice and Palliative Care (IAHPC) and the Worldwide Palliative Care Alliance (WPCA).

In a November 2006 report prepared by the International Observatory on End-of-Life Care (IOELC), *Mapping Levels of Palliative Care Development: A Global View*, the authors conclude in the Executive Summary that "despite increasing calls for palliative care to be recognized as a human right, there is a long way to go before palliation is within reach of the global community" (Wright, Wood, Lynch, & Clark, 2006, p. 8).

Building Capacity for Palliative Care

With a demonstrated growing need—coupled with a belief that palliative care is an inherent human right—social workers must use our leadership and advocacy skills to ensure it is available around the world. To do so, we must answer the following questions:

- What is the ideal?
- What is the assessment of palliative care now?
- What strategies can move the community or nation toward the ideal?

Ideal Standards for Palliative Care

To date, there is no internationally recognized standard for palliative care. There are, however, several documents and resources that may be helpful in guiding these efforts to strengthen palliative care.

The National Consensus Project for Quality Palliative Care (NCP), a consortium of four national palliative care organizations in the United States—the American Academy of Hospice and Palliative Medicine, the Center to Advance Palliative Care, the Hospice and Palliative Nurses Association, and the National Hospice and Palliative Care Organization—developed the *Clinical Practice Guidelines for Quality Palliative Care* in 2004 "to describe the core precepts and structures of palliative care programs" (NCP, 2009, p. iv). A second edition was released in August 2009 that revises and updates Guideline definitions and references as well as incorporates revisions "to reflect the growing practice and evidence of palliative care as it moves into mainstream healthcare" (NCP, 2009, p. iv). The Guidelines consist of eight domains:

1. Structure and processes of care
2. Physical aspects of care
3. Psychological and psychiatric aspects of care
4. Social aspects of care
5. Spiritual, religious, and existential aspects of care
6. Cultural aspects of care
7. Care of the imminently dying patient
8. Ethical and legal aspects of care (NCP, 2009, p. 4).

Using the NCP *Guidelines*, the National Quality Forum (NQF) developed a framework for quality care with 12 structural and programmatic elements essential to palliative care programs:

1. Interdisciplinary teams
2. Diverse models of delivery
3. Bereavement programs
4. Educational programs
5. Patient and family education
6. Volunteer programs
7. Quality assessment/performance improvement
8. Community outreach programs
9. Administrative policies
10 Information technology and data gathering
11. Methods for resolving ethical dilemmas
12. Personnel self-care initiatives (NQF, 2006, p. vi).

These elements, along with the eight domains of quality palliative care developed by the National Consensus Project, led to the creation of 38 preferred practices, outlined in NQF's report, *A National Framework and Preferred Practices for Palliative and Hospice Care Quality: A Consensus Report.* These are listed in the Appendix (NQF, 2006).

The *Guidelines* have also been used by The Joint Commission, who accredits health care organizations in the United States as underlying principles for palliative care certification. For information on standards in countries other than the United States, visit the National Hospice and Palliative Care Organization Web site that contains a chart of international standards and guidelines of practice, with links to the standards and guidelines of palliative care practice in various countries around the world.

Palliative Care Assessment

In the IOELC's *Mapping Levels of Palliative Care Development* report, the project aimed to assess the state of palliative care in each of the United Nations' list of 234 countries in 2006 (see Fig. 53.1). While about 50% of the countries had at least one or more palliative care services, only 15% achieved a major integration with mainstream service providers, and in 33% of the countries, no palliative care activity could be identified (Wright et al., 2006).

In addition to contrasts in hospice and palliative care among nations, there are vast differences within regions and settings. Recently, we had the opportunity to travel to Cape Town, South Africa, where we visited St. Luke's Hospice and met with the social work staff there. The St. Luke's Hospice is a beautiful facility. It is reminiscent of the well-known St. Christopher's Hospice in London. The main building is an impressive structure, a well-maintained, old mansion with beautiful gardens. During our visit, the social workers described their work and what a typical workday entailed. One social worker noted that the most difficult thing for her was splitting her time between visiting patients with financial means in the morning and later visiting persons who were dying in the nearby shantytown. Shantytowns are makeshift communities of people who are impoverished. In some cases in South Africa, people have fled their home country due to war or famine and have created or reside in the shantytowns. In Cape Town, the majority of persons who lived in the shantytown near Cape Town were black.

The hospice social worker described the overwhelming conditions of her work in the shantytown: the small, temporary housing structures of wood or cardboard house many family members or even multiple families. There is no running water, limited electricity, and few family or individual resources. There are no options for special diets, or oxygen, or privacy. Cleanliness and pain control are major concerns. Yet the social worker visits on a regular basis to offer comfort, support, and what palliative care she can. The needs are great. The challenges for palliative social work are even greater (Clark, Myers, & Snell, 2008).

The WHO report, *A Community Health Approach to Palliative Care for HIV/AIDS and Cancer Patients in Sub-Saharan Africa*, details a project to strengthen palliative care in five countries in sub-Saharan Africa. The report provides a model for national capacity building, including the following:

- Common standards for care
- Elements of a situation analysis or current assessment
- Methods to collect information on the current situation
- Analysis of situation
- Elements of plans of action.

Appendices in this report detail a variety of instruments used in this project, including a situational analysis guide, needs assessment tools, questionnaires, and team development directives, to name a few (WHO, 2004).

When conducting an assessment, the following are some areas to consider:

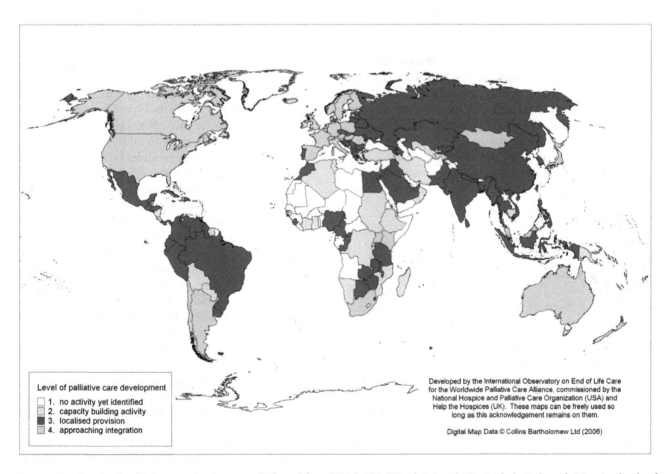

Figure 53.1. Levels of palliative care development. (Adapted from Wright, M., Wood, J., Lynch, T., & Clark, D. [2008]. Mapping levels of palliative care development: A global view. *Journal of Pain and Symptom Management, 35* [5], 469–489.)

- *Stigma*—Are there diseases that carry shame or disgrace within the community or that are seen as socially unacceptable? Stigma can make it difficult for communities to provide palliative care services and for people to request the palliative care services needed for a particular disease.
- *Pain control*—access to opioids and nonopioid pain relievers. What are the laws and rules related to medications used for pain control? Various international conventions list pain control as a human right; yet most nations of the world unreasonably restrict access to necessary analgesic medications. (Visit the Medicines section, *Access to Analgesics and to Other Controlled Substances*, on WHO's Web site for more information about global programs and strategies to increase access to necessary pain medications.)
- *Political context*—How does the current political context shape the provision of palliative care? Some governments may be supportive of the need for palliative care, while some may deny its necessity.
- *History*—Has the history of the country shaped its inclination for palliative care? In some countries health care, including palliative care, has long been provided. In other countries, wars and oppression have caused an upheaval in the health care system overall. There may be certain groups or geographic areas in a country that have historically been neglected from a health care perspective.
- *Chronic disease*—What are the major chronic diseases in the country, and what are the trends for chronic disease? As countries develop, there is less infectious disease and more chronic disease. Chronic disease often indicates a longer trajectory of palliative care from diagnosis through death.
- *Culture*—What are the cultural norms, values, and beliefs about disease, dying, caretaking, and healing?
- *Health care system*—What is the structure of the health care system?

Strategies for Change

There are many ways to approach capacity building, and listed here are some examples and possibilities:

Participate in the World Hospice and Palliative Care Day. World Hospice and Palliative Care Day is a global observance, led by the Worldwide Palliative Care Alliance and held annually on the second Saturday in October, to celebrate and support hospice and palliative care around the world. According to the World Day Web site, one of the major barriers to the availability of palliative care is the lack of understanding about this type of care and of its benefits to people. This coordinated, yearly event can provide support to local and national efforts to increase the provision of palliative care.

Advocate for changes in laws and regulations. In many countries, laws regarding pain control and controlled substances are in need of change. In addition to offering strategies to increase access to necessary pain medications, the WHO Web site on *Access to Analgesics and to Other Controlled Medicines* also offers background tools to guide such legal changes. There may be changes required in the regulatory arena, health care system, or in the payment of health care benefits that will support palliative care.

Using human rights mechanisms. In a special article in the *Journal of Pain and Symptom Management* (Gwyther, Brannan, Obs, & Harding, 2009) the authors detail a number of methods from the human rights arena that can advance access to palliative care. Among those suggested are corresponding with the special Rapporteur to the UN Human Rights Commission on the Right to Health or making a complaint to the Commission.

Increase education and training. Often, more training is required for caregivers, health care providers, and the public in the scope and practice of palliative care. The *3 by 5 Initiative* was a project of WHO with a goal to treat 3 million people living with HIV/AIDS by 2005. The project Web site has many resources for providers to use to educate patients, caregivers, and families regarding symptom management and end-of-life care. The National Coalition for Cancer Survivorship (NCCS) in the United States offers a free audio program in three languages to help people develop important skills to address their diagnosis and illness. One of the modules is "Dying Well—the Final Stage of Survivorship." An example of an international collaboration to increase training and education of providers is detailed in Box 53.1.

Political advocacy and organizing. Social workers are privileged to see the full range of need for palliative care in their communities and nations. Because they see a variety of clients, social workers can often discern policy and regulatory changes that are needed to enhance the provision of palliative care. Leading and/or collaborating with like-minded agencies, organizations, or individuals for policies that strengthen palliative care can be important in ensuring care is provided. Activities could include actions to enforce current laws or regulations that may support palliative care but are currently being ignored, as well as new efforts to obtain additional resources.

Financial support. International collaborations can be helpful in matching financial resources to the need. An illustration of this strategy is provided in Box 53.2.

As part of its Social Workers Across Nations (SWAN) initiative, the National Association of Social Workers (NASW) partnered with CancerCare, Inc. of New York City and the University of Debrecen, Faculty of Health in Nyiregyhaza, to assist with capacity building for oncology social work in Hungary. Hungary was chosen as the first venue because it has the highest cancer rates of any country in Europe and because social work as a modern profession began here in 1989 with the change in the political structure of the country. Additionally, there was a U.S. oncology social worker in residence through a Fulbright Scholar Lecturer Award, and the University was in the beginning stages of developing a health care–social work focus.

The initiative included hosting an exchange summit on psychosocial oncology in Hungary, the development of 10 imperatives for psychosocial care, and an online training course for health care professionals. More important, seed grants were awarded to six individuals and groups to extend their current programming to include palliative care, family support, and bereavement care (Walsh, Csikai, Patyan, Allen, & Walsh, 2009).

Box 53.2
National Narrative—Foundation for Hospices in Sub-Saharan Africa (FHSSA): An International Model for Matching Resources between Organizations in the United States and Sub-Saharan Africa

FHSSA is an example of international collaboration. Founded in 1999, FHSSA is an affiliate of the U.S.-based National Hospice and Palliative Care Organization (NHPCO), whose mission is to support organizations in their development and provision of hospice and palliative care initiatives in sub-Saharan Africa. Hospice and palliative care organizations in the United States are partnered with similar organizations in sub-Saharan Africa to generate resources and to provide technical support. FHSSA was launched as the result of visits by hospice professionals in the United States to hospice professionals on the continent of Africa who witnessed African hospice programs struggling and unable to meet the needs of their HIV-positive patients. Due to the HIV/AIDS virus, there were great demands on the hospice organizations of Africa, and talks between the groups resulted in the ongoing partnership matching resources in the United States to assist with the needs of the hospices in Africa. As of its tenth anniversary in October 2009, there were 83 partnerships in 16 African countries and 28 states in the United States.

Box 53.3
National Narrative—Cambodia: Providing Palliative Care with Limited Resources and Continuing to Build Capacity

During the reign of the despot Pol Pot in Cambodia from 1975 to 1979, much of the professional class was annihilated. It is estimated that 21% of the population was killed. That meant that many young children were left without parents and that the older population was left without adult children to support them in their old age. The health care system was decimated without professional health care workers. The needs for daily survival still take precedence today. There are tens of thousands of homeless children who live on the streets of Phnom Penh, and few places exist to care for the sick and the elderly. Nongovernmental organizations (NGOs) and humanitarians are the best hope. One such place is run by a priest. His agency is a residence that he runs for the elderly who have no one to care for them and nowhere else to go. It consists of open buildings. Each person has a pallet and a blanket. Every day the priest has to raise enough money to feed those he is trying to help.

In the midst of these overwhelming conditions, the profession of social work is growing. Many NGOs are run and staffed by social workers from around the world. Ellen Minotti, a social worker from the United States, has spent almost 20 years teaching social work theory, practice, and ethics to young students. She has had almost 3000 students finish her program. The University of Washington partnered with the Royal University of Phnom Penh in creating a social work program. The Department of Social Work opened in the fall of 2008. Development of bachelor of social work (BSW) and master of social work (MSW) programs is continuing in the next phases of the project.

It will be probably be decades before standard palliative or hospice care is available to those needing it in Cambodia, but social workers are at the forefront trying to build the needed capacity.

of illness and some focused on end of life—all situated within a specific context, unique to the area. This chapter, coupled with these models, will expand your thinking about what can be done to strengthen the provision of palliative care around the world.

LEARNING EXERCISES

- Are there diseases and chronic conditions in your community that are stigmatized? How does this stigma affect the need for and provision of palliative care? What strategies could address the effects of the stigma or eradicate it?
- What trends do you see that will affect the need for and provision of palliative care in your region? For instance, are there changes to how health care is delivered, or are there new prevention efforts? Are there diseases that are now considered or will soon be considered chronic? Are there new treatments for diseases that change the experience of the disease?

Doing what you can, where you are. Sometimes you need to start with small steps and programs, providing what you can right where you are. One model of this approach is given in Box 53.3.

The subsequent chapters in this section will provide information about social work and palliative care in specific countries and regions of the world. You will see a diversity of models—some reflective of palliative care along the continuum

- Who are the primary caregivers of palliative care in your community? What are the challenges they face in providing this care? What types of support are available for them?
- What are the palliative care "gaps" in your community? What strategies do you suggest to close those gaps and strengthen palliative care?

APPENDIX

Preferred Practices for Palliative and Hospice Care Quality developed by the National Quality Forum. National Quality Forum. (2006). *A national framework and preferred practices for palliative and hospice care quality: A consensus report* (Monograph). Retrieved from http://qualityforum.org/ Publications/2006/12/Executive_Summary_for_Hospice_ Report.aspx

1. Provide palliative and hospice care by an interdisciplinary team of skilled palliative care professionals, including, for example, physicians, nurses, social workers, pharmacists, spiritual care counselors, and others who collaborate with primary health care professional(s).
2. Provide access to palliative and hospice care that is responsive to the patient and family 24 hours a day, 7 days a week.
3. Provide continuing education to all health care professionals on the domains of palliative care and hospice care.
4. Provide adequate training and clinical support to assure that professional staff is confident in their ability to provide palliative care for patients.
5. Hospice care and specialized palliative care professionals should be appropriately trained, credentialed, and/or certified in their area of expertise.
6. Formulate, utilize, and regularly review a timely care plan based on a comprehensive interdisciplinary assessment of the values, preferences, goals, and needs of the patient and family and, to the extent that existing privacy laws permit, ensure that the plan is broadly disseminated, both internally and externally, to all professionals involved in the patient's care.
7. Ensure that upon transfer between health care settings, there is timely and thorough communication of the patient's goals, preferences, values, and clinical information so that continuity of care and seamless follow-up are assured.
8. Health care professionals should present hospice as an option to all patients and families when death within a year would not be surprising and should reintroduce the hospice option as the patient declines.
9. Patients and caregivers should be asked by palliative and hospice care programs to assess physicians'/health care professionals' ability to discuss hospice as an option.
10. Enable patients to make informed decisions about their care by educating them on the process of their disease, prognosis, and the benefits and burdens of potential interventions.
11. Provide education and support to families and unlicensed caregivers based on the patient's individualized care plan to assure safe and appropriate care for the patient.
12. Measure and document pain, dyspnea, constipation, and other symptoms using available standardized scales.
13. Assess and manage symptoms and side effects in a timely, safe, and effective manner to a level that is acceptable to the patient and family.
14. Measure and document anxiety, depression, delirium, behavioral disturbances, and other common psychological symptoms using available standardized scales.
15. Manage anxiety, depression, delirium, behavioral disturbances, and other common psychological symptoms in a timely, safe, and effective manner to a level that is acceptable to the patient and family.
16. Assess and manage the psychological reactions of patients and families (including stress, anticipatory grief, and coping) in a regular, ongoing fashion in order to address emotional and functional impairment and loss.
17. Develop and offer a grief and bereavement care plan to provide services to patients and families prior to and for at least 13 months after the death of the patient.
18. Conduct regular patient and family care conferences with physicians and other appropriate members of the interdisciplinary team to provide information, to discuss goals of care, disease prognosis, and advance care planning, and to offer support.
19. Develop and implement a comprehensive social care plan that addresses the social, practical, and legal needs of the patient and caregivers, including but not limited to relationships, communication, existing social and cultural networks, decision making, work and school settings, finances, sexuality/intimacy, caregiver availability/stress, and access to medicines and equipment.
20. Develop and document a plan based on an assessment of religious, spiritual, and existential concerns using a structured instrument and integrate the information obtained from the assessment into the palliative care plan.
21. Provide information about the availability of spiritual care services and make spiritual care available either

through organizational spiritual care counseling or through the patient's own clergy relationships.

22. Specialized palliative and hospice care teams should include spiritual care professionals appropriately trained and certified in palliative care.

23. Specialized palliative and hospice spiritual care professionals should build partnerships with community clergy and provide education and counseling related to end-of-life care.

24. Incorporate cultural assessment as a component of comprehensive palliative and hospice care assessment, including but not limited to locus of decision making; preferences regarding disclosure of information; truth telling and decision making; dietary preferences; language; family communication; desire for support measures such as palliative therapies and complementary and alternative medicine; perspectives on death, suffering, and grieving; and funeral/burial rituals.

25. Provide professional interpreter services and culturally sensitive materials in the patient's and family's preferred language.

26. Recognize and document the transition to the active dying phase and communicate to the patient, family, and staff the expectation of imminent death.

27. Educate the family on a timely basis regarding the signs and symptoms of imminent death in an age-appropriate, developmentally appropriate, and culturally appropriate manner.

28. As part of the ongoing care planning process, routinely ascertain and document patient and family wishes about the care setting for the site of death and fulfill patient and family preferences when possible.

29. Provide adequate dosage of analgesics and sedatives as appropriate to achieve patient comfort during the active dying phase and address concerns and fears about using narcotics and of analgesics hastening death.

30. Treat the body after death with respect according to the cultural and religious practices of the family and in accordance with local law.

31. Facilitate effective grieving by implementing in a timely manner a bereavement care plan after the patient's death, when the family remains the focus of care.

32. Document the designated surrogate/decision maker in accordance with state law for every patient in primary, acute, and long-term care and in palliative and hospice care.

33. Document the patient/surrogate preferences for goals of care, treatment options, and setting of care at first assessment and at frequent intervals as conditions change.

34. Convert the patient treatment goals into medical orders and ensure that the information is transferable and applicable across care settings, including long-term care, emergency medical services, and hospital care, through a program such as the Physician Orders for Life-Sustaining Treatment (POLST) program.

35. Make advance directives and surrogacy designations available across care settings, while protecting patient privacy and adherence to HIPAA regulations, for example, by using Internet-based registries or electronic personal health records.

36. Develop health care and community collaborations to promote advance care planning and the completion of advance directives for all individuals, for example, the Respecting Choices and Community Conversations on Compassionate Care programs.

37. Establish or have access to ethics committees or ethics consultation across care settings to address ethical conflicts at the end of life.

38. For minors with decision-making capacity, document the child's views and preferences for medical care, including assent for treatment, and give them appropriate weight in decision making. Make appropriate professional staff members available to both the child and the adult decision maker for consultation and intervention when the child's wishes differ from those of the adult decision maker.

ADDITIONAL RESOURCES

Abegunde, D., & Stanicole, A. (2006). *An estimation of the economic impact of chronic noncommunicable diseases in selected countries.* Retrieved from World Health Organization Web site: http://www.who.int/chp/working_paper_growth%20model29may.pdf
Working paper regarding chronic disease and its economic impact, including the growth of the incidence of chronic disease.
The Capacity Project: http://www.capacityproject.org/
An innovative global initiative funded by the U.S. Agency for International Development (USAID), the Capacity Project strengthened human resources to implement quality health programming in developing countries. This was a 5-year project from 2004 to 2009. Resources on the site include an action framework.
Chacko, S. (2009, June 3). The worldwide rise of chronic diseases and potential nutritional solutions [Web log message]. Retrieved from http://www.huffingtonpost.com/sunil-chacko/the-worldwide-rise-of-chr_b_207418.html
Blog post by Sunil Chacko, medical doctor, public health and finance specialist, and university professor, regarding the growth of chronic disease and the decline of infectious disease.
Foundation for Hospices in Sub-Saharan Africa (FHSSA): http://www.fhssa.org/i4a/pages/index.cfm?pageid=1
Web site providing information, resources, partnerships, and programs on FHSSA, an affiliate of the U.S.-based National Hospice and Palliative Care Organization and the National Hospice Foundation, created to help generate resources and technical support for hospice organizations in sub-Saharan Africa.
Furst, C. J., Lima, L. D., Praill, D., & Radbruch, L. (2009, May 9). *The Budapest commitments—a framework for palliative care*

development. Retrieved from European Association for Palliative Care Web site: http://www.eapcnet.org/congresses/Budapest2007/Budapest2007Commitments.htm

Emanating from the 10th Congress of EAPC in 2007, this initiative is based on a strategy which includes using a framework that will help identify and establish development goals in five major areas: drug availability; policy; education; quality and research. Within this framework, national associations for palliative care will be invited to choose commitments from a list of proposals or draft their own among these five areas. The commitments should be based on measurable indicators.

Help the Hospices. (2007). *Access to pain relief—an essential human right* [PowerPoint slides]. Retrieved from Worldwide Palliative Care Alliance Web site: http://www.hospicecare.com/resources/pain_pallcare_hr/docs/access_to_pain_relief_a_human_right_world_day.pdf

Comprehensive review addressing access to analgesics and opioids worldwide, as well as solutions.

HRH Global Resource Center: http://www.hrhresourcecenter.org/

A global library of human resources for health (HRH) resources focused on developing countries.

International Association for Hospice and Palliative Care, & Worldwide Palliative Care.

Alliance. (2009). *IAHPC–WPCA joint declaration and statement of commitment*. Retrieved November 19, 2009 from http://www.hospicecare.com/resources/pain_pallcare_hr/jd.html

The statement is available in four languages; a list of signatories is also provided.

Murray, S. (2010). The quality of death: ranking end-of-life care across the world (D. Line, Ed.). Retrieved from:http://www.lifebeforedeath.com/pdf/Quality_of_Death_Index_Report.pdf

Commissioned by the Lien Foundation, this report provides a Quality of Death Index and ranks 40 countries according to their provision of end-of-life care. The report also identifies major areas of focus needed to improve palliative and end-of-life care.

National Association of Social Workers: http://www.socialworkers.org/practice/intl/hungary2008/default.asp

A variety of materials in Hungarian and English used in the "Best Practices in Psychosocial Oncology Exchange between Hungary and the United States of America" summit held November 7–9, 2008, in Nyiregyhaza, Hungary.

National Coalition for Cancer Survivorship: http://www.canceradvocacy.org/toolbox

A free, self-learning audio program developed by leading cancer organizations that contains a myriad of resources for both cancer patients and health care professionals to help them develop important skills to better meet and understand the challenges of cancer.

National Hospice and Palliative Care Organization, *International standards/Guidelines of practice*: http://www.nhpco.org/i4a/pages/Index.cfm?pageID=5261

Information on the international standards and guidelines of practice of palliative care in various countries around the world.

National Hospice and Palliative Care Organization, *U.S.-African partnership initiative*: http://www.nhpco.org/files/public/FHSSA/US_Africa_Partnerships.pdf

A current list of partnerships between United States and sub-Saharan African hospice and palliative care organizations.

World Health Organization, *Achieving balance in national opioids control*

Information regarding the guidelines, as well as a self-assessment checklist.

World Health Organization, *The 3 by 5 initiative*: http://www.who.int/3by5/capacity/palliative/en/

Information about WHO's *3 by 5 initiative*, as well as resources for providers to use to educate patients, caregivers, and families regarding symptom management and end-of-life care.

World Health Organization, *Access to controlled medications programme* [Briefing note]: http://www.who.int/medicines/areas/quality_safety/ACMP_BrNoteGenrl_EN_Feb09.pdf

Fact sheet for program to increase access to medications controlled under international drug conventions.

World Health Organization, *Access to analgesics and other controlled medications*: http://www.who.int/medicines/areas/quality_safety/access_Contr_Med/en/

Information regarding global programs and strategies to increase access to necessary pain medications.

World Health Organization, *Facts related to chronic diseases*: http://www.who.int/dietphysicalactivity/publications/facts/chronic/en/index.html

Facts about chronic disease and prevention efforts especially related to the global strategy on diet, physical activity, and health.

World Health Organization, *World health statistics reports*: http://www.who.int/whosis/whostat/en/

WHO's annual World Health Statistics reports present the most recent health statistics for WHO's 193 Member States. All reports are available for download in Adobe PDF and Excel, when applicable.

World Hospice and Palliative Care Day, *Hospice and palliative care: Discovering your voice*: http://www.worldday.org/about/

Web site dedicated to World Hospice and Palliative Care Day that includes background information about World Day, event details, news, materials, archives, and more.

REFERENCES

Bush, M. (1993). Jane Addams: No Easy Heroine. *Free Inquiry*, *13*(4), Fall 48–49.

Bettis, N. (n. d.). *Jane Addams 1860-1935*. In *Women's intellectual contributions to the study of mind and society*. Retrieved from Webster University Web site: http://www.webster.edu/~woolflm/janeadams.html

Clark, E. J., Myers, R. S., & Snell, C. (2008). *Delegation leaders' combined journals of professional activities: Social work delegation to the Republic of South Africa, Cape Town and Johannesburg, October 14-22, 2008*. Retrieved from National Association of Social Workers Web site: http://www.socialworkers.org/practice/intl/southAfrica2008/documents/South%20Africa%20Report.pdf

Gwyther, L., Brennan, F., Obs, D., & Harding, R. (2009, November). Advancing palliative care as a human right. *Journal of Pain and Symptom Management*, *38*(5), 767–774.

National Consensus Project for Quality Palliative Care (NCP). (2009). *Clinical practice guidelines for quality palliative care, second edition*. Retrieved from http://www.nationalconsensusproject.org/guideline.pdf

National Quality Forum (NQF). (2006). *A national framework and preferred practices for palliative and hospice care quality: A consensus report.* Retrieved from http://qualityforum.org/Publications/2006/12/Executive_Summary_for_Hospice_Report.aspx

Open Society Institute & Equitas - International Center for Human Rights Education. (2007). *Palliative care and human rights: A resource guide.* Retrieved from http://www.hospicecare.com/resources/pain_pallcare_hr/docs/draft_resource_guide_palliative_care_human_rights_english.pdf

United Nations Office of the High Commissioner for Human Rights. (2009). *What are human rights?* Retrieved from http://www.ohchr.org/EN/Issues/Pages/WhatareHumanRights.aspx

Walsh, K., Csikai, E., Patyan, L., Allen, F., & Walsh, K. (2009). *Best practices in psychosocial oncology exchange between Hungary and the United States of America.* Retrieved from National Association of Social Workers Web site: http://www.socialworkers.org/practice/intl/hungary2008/english/HungaryReport.pdf

World Health Organization (WHO). (2004). *A community health approach to palliative care for HIV/AIDS and cancer patients in sub-Saharan Africa.* Retrieved from http://www.who.int/hiv/pub/prev_care/en/palliative.pdf

Wright, M., Wood, J., Lynch, T., & Clark, D. (2006). *Mapping levels of palliative care development: A global view.* Retrieved from International Observatory on End of Life Care Web site: http://www.eolc-observatory.net/global/pdf/world_map.pdf

54 *Linda Anngela-Cole, Lana Sue Ka'opua, and Yvonne Yim*

Palliative Care, Culture, and the Pacific Basin

Kakou—it's not about me, it's about us. Cancer happens to one person and affects their person-hood, their lives. Family members become victims, too. What allows me to go beyond the cusp is the kakou.

—Cancer survivor and family member of a cancer survivor
(Kakou means "we" or "ours")

Key Concepts

♦ *The concept of "collectivism" offers an important framework for understanding palliative care in the Pacific.*

♦ *A deep sensitivity to subtle culturally based communication styles is vital.*

♦ *It is important to understand how systemic barriers may present challenges to obtaining quality palliative care for this population.*

♦ *The role of the social worker in palliative care in the Pacific is unique and challenging due to the considerable diversity in end-of-life beliefs and practices as well as the wide diversity in language.*

Introduction

This chapter highlights issues crucial to consider in social work intervention with culturally diverse Asian and Pacific Islander (A/PI) patients living in the Pacific Basin who are in need of palliative care. Diverse groups of Polynesian, Micronesian, East Asian, and Southeast Asian peoples live in the Pacific Basin (U.S. Census, 2000). For the purpose of this chapter, A/PI patients of the Pacific Basin include those who are permanent residents of the State of Hawaii, as well as those who are migrants or U.S. nationals originating from the U.S. Affiliated Pacific Islands (USAPI).

Hawai'i is a state of great ethnic/racial diversity and provides a rich context for viewing social work intervention and palliative care at their intersection with culture. The state's major A/PI groups include Native Hawaiians, the indigenous people of the Hawaiian Islands, as well as Chinese, Japanese, and Filipinos. Samoans, primarily originating from American Samoa, comprise the state's second largest Polynesian group (U.S. Census, 2000). Interestingly, culturally based healing traditions may be perpetuated within a specific ethnic group, as well as accepted, learned, or diffused in the state's broader multiethnic population. For example, *lomilomi* or therapeutic Hawaiian massage is used by patients of all ethnocultural backgrounds to alleviate distressing physical symptoms related to biomedical treatments (Bushnell, 1993).

As a center of advanced medical treatments and technologies, the state continually attracts those from the USAPI who seek care unavailable in their homelands. The USAPI is comprised of the Freely Associated States (FAS) or sovereign nations that include the Federated States of Micronesia (FSM), the Republic of the Marshall Islands (RMI), and the Republic of Palau (ROP), as well as the U.S. territories of American Samoa, Guam, and the Commonwealth of the Northern Mariana Islands. Since the mid-1980s, an estimated 8000 migrants have left the FSM, RMI, and ROP to live, at least temporarily, in Hawai'i. Notably, migration is frequently precipitated by serious illness and the need to obtain medical treatments not available in the homelands

(Pobutsky, Buenconsejo-Lum, Chow, Palafox, & Maskarinec, 2005). The cost of "offshore care" (care provided outside of the homeland) may be subsidized by USAPI governmental entities and/or by patients and their families. Common offshore referrals are for treatments such as hemodialysis and chemotherapy. Patients with conditions such as renal failure and cancer may also receive palliative treatments, the latter of which may be unfamiliar or even culturally dystonic to Pacific Islander healing traditions.

The USAPI is a region characterized by great cultural and linguistic diversity. Importantly, many of the indigenous cultures have well-developed traditions of indigenous medicine, which include methods for palliation of distressing conditions (Bushnell, 1993; Kiste & Marshall, 1999; Whistler, 1992). Conflict and misunderstanding in Western biomedical health care settings may occur when patients are introduced to unfamiliar treatments. Such misunderstandings may be further exacerbated by linguistic diversity and the lack of native speakers trained in medical interpretation. Linguistic diversity may be considerable. For example, in the FSM there are eight official languages and seven other spoken languages (FSM Government, Department of Economic Affairs, Division of Statistics, 2000).

Collectivism as a Framework for Understanding Palliative Care Work in the Pacific

Despite great diversity among A/PI peoples living in the Pacific Basin, cultural values and practices tend to be undergirded by collectivism; that is, the individual is viewed in relation to others, usually members of the extended family of blood relations and fictive kin (McLaughlin & Braun, 1998). Thus, decisions about treatments, including palliative care, involve the family. Decision making relies on what best benefits the collective as well as the individual (Braun, Mokuau, & Tsark, 1997). For example, in *fa'aSamoa* (Samoan cultural worldview), collectivism permeates every aspect of life. Leadership is provided by village *matai* (titled heads or chiefs of the *aiga* or extended family) through a centuries-old family governance system. Collective well-being and reciprocity between family members are prized, as motivated by values such as *osi aiga* (take care of the family) and *ola mo isi* (support that benefits the collective or family) (Mulitalo-Lauta, 2000). Given the pervasive influence of collectivism, the individual patient may be highly discomforted when asked to make a decision about treatment and/or the addition of palliative care.

Important considerations for social work assessment and intervention are as follows: *(1)* who in the patient's family needs to be involved in decision making, *(2)* what roles do individual members have in times of illness and crisis, *(3)* do some family members (e.g., elders, titled leaders, ministers) exert greater influence than others, and *(4)* is there a traditional process (e.g., Hawaiian *ho'oponopono*) used to

reach family agreement on the treatment course and the use of palliation (Ka'opua, 1994, 2003).

Communicating Sensitive Issues

Collectivist cultures are characterized by high levels of sensitivity to nonverbal and indirect communications (Kagawa-Singer & Blackhall, 2001; Matsumura et al., 2002). Silence, posture manipulation, and sentence pauses are examples of nonverbal forms of communication. Providers should not dismiss these as random or idiosyncratic behaviors. Inattention to these types of communication could result in misunderstanding the treatment preferences of collectivist-oriented patients and their family members. Indirect verbal communication may also be normative to those socialized in collectivist cultures. Within Japanese culture a fatal diagnosis may be communicated to and among family members, but not directly addressed with the patient. This behavior is understood as a means for shielding the patient from the burden of diagnosis and treatment decision making. By protecting the patient from burden and possible embarrassment, the patient is allowed to maintain his or her honor; in turn, this maintains the family's well-being (Kagawa-Singer & Blackhall, 2001).

Systemic Barriers to Quality Palliative Care

Many people living in Hawai'i are not U.S. citizens; therefore, they are not eligible for Medicare or Medicaid (Pobutsky et al., 2005), which are critical to obtaining medical care in the United States. People come from all over the Pacific Basin to stay with relatives who are U.S. citizens, but they themselves are not able to obtain the Western health care provided to others. For newcomers, access to Medicare and/or Medicaid is not an immediate option. In addition, there are many island nations in the Pacific that are not U.S. Affiliates and have very little medical care of any kind. In such places, palliative measures may be handled very much the same as it has been for generations. Hospitals may be difficult to access for those living on islands or atolls remote from municipal centers; when hospitals are accessible, services provided may be limited. Those who are severely or chronically ill are cared for at home, by family members, with traditional indigenous medicines and traditional healers from within their communities.

Even for individuals who are eligible for Medicare or Medicaid (or other insurance benefits) in Hawai'i, though, barriers still exist for some. Under the current Medicare Hospice Benefit, the plan requires patients to sign informed consent forms before they can be admitted (Ngo-Metzger, Phillips, & McCarthy, 2008). To be able to sign an informed consent form, a patient must understand and accept a terminal prognosis. This presents a major barrier for native cultures due to their collectivist practices of utilizing a family-centered model of decision making. This practice often involves not sharing the ill person's prognosis with the person, as a means of preventing the ill person from "giving up" and thus enabling the person to remain hopeful (McLaughlin & Braun, 1998).

Palliative Care and the Social Worker Role in the Pacific

Asian and Pacific Islanders create a unique and challenging clientele for palliative social workers due to their considerable diversity in end-of-life beliefs and practices as well as their wide diversity in language (Browne & Broderick, 1994). Opportunities for cross-cultural misconceptions and misunderstandings are presenting themselves more frequently. For this reason it is vital for social workers to understand their client's beliefs and needs through a culturally competent framework. One way to gain this understanding is to find a cultural resource, meaning someone in a local community-based organization or church who is willing to help you gain this level of understanding. Social workers who work to gain this level of cultural understanding can respectfully acknowledge cultural differences and work with the clients and their families' attitudes, beliefs, family structure, and hierarchy. Gathering such information helps to recognize potential cultural conflicts and assess possible solutions to such conflicts. Creating a familiarity of differing perspectives between the social worker, the client, and their family will also help to create mutual ground in which a meaningful discussion of differences can take place in a respectful manner.

People of the Pacific Basin face many barriers to palliative care across the illness trajectory, including geographical barriers, eligibility barriers, communication barriers, and systemic barriers. To address these barriers, palliative care social workers must ask open-ended questions, in respectful ways, and provide culturally sensitive care that acknowledges and regards deeply held cultural values and beliefs, particularly in palliative care situations. Now let's consider the patient/family narrative in Box 54.1 as a means of applying the concepts described in this chapter about working with families in the Pacific Basin.

Box 54.1
Patient/Family Narrative: Mrs. I. and Her Family

Mrs. I and family, age 65, from American Samoa, visiting family in Hawai'i; Clinical focus: Cultural differences explored in two ways: (1) family conflict regarding treatment decision making; and (2) health care workers' conflict with family members regarding desire for 24 hr support of patient while hospitalized.

Mrs. I. is a 65-year-old, U.S. national (American Samoa). While visiting family members in Hawai'i, she complains of chronic pain to her neck and arm. She is brought to clinic by Mr. I., her adult son who is a resident of Hawai'i. Mr. I. was raised in American Samoa

and is the eldest of nine children. Educated at a well-known American university, he is a practicing attorney in Honolulu, but makes frequent trips to the territory in order to ensure that family members are well. Results of Mrs. I.'s physical examination and subsequent, diagnostic testing reveal that she has stage IV breast cancer with metastasis to the brain. Aggressive chemotherapy and radiation are strongly recommended. She is told that her treatment will take 4 months. During her treatment, she must stay in Hawai'i because neither radiation nor chemotherapy is currently available in American Samoa. She is told that she will die in 3–6 months if treatment is not taken. Upon learning of his mother's diagnosis, Mr. I. contacts his college friends who now are physicians at a well-known university medical center located in the continental United States. They inform him that the university medical center has an effective cancer trial with outstanding results. However, his mother would need immediate admission to join the program. Subsequently, Mr. I. makes travel arrangements for his mother and himself. At the advice of his law partner, Mr. I. sets up an advance health care directive and an estate plan.

Mrs. I. is referred to you for a biopsychosocial-spiritual assessment. She shares that her relationship with her son is a close one. She is proud of his career accomplishments and reflects with gratitude that his education was generously supported by the aiga or family members, most of whom continue to reside in the Samoan village of their ancestors. As you are interviewing Mrs. I., her son arrives at the clinic and shares the details of the treatment recommended by his friends, travel plans, and legal work done on behalf of his mother. Mrs. I. thanks him, but states that she will telephone the village matai [titled leaders or chiefs] to discuss what she should do. Mr. I. states that he does not understand why "others" need to make this decision or even get involved when it is a decision that his mother should make. In the midst of this conversation, the nurse manager informs you that a small crowd of Mrs. I.'s family is in the waiting room with blankets, pillows, and coolers. They plan on staying overnight or until Mrs. I. is discharged. She requests that you have them leave because "camping" is not allowed. As you leave to talk with other family members, you hear Mr. I. expressing frustration. He leaves the hospital without speaking to family members "camping" in the hospital waiting area.

Application of Learning: Patient/Family Narrative and Exercise

We observe fa'alavelave. In English, the word translates to something like "family entanglement" which sounds bad from a Western perspective. But to us—it gathers the family together, keeps us connected with each other, and preserves the fa'a Samoa.

—a patient from American Samoa

fa'alavelave—family entanglement, any event such as birth, death, or illness that gathers the family together.
fa'a Samoa—traditional Samoan cultural worldview, or Samoan culture.

LEARNING EXERCISE

- If you were a social worker involved with this family, how might you handle the following situations, keeping in mind issues of communication sensitivity and collectivism as guiding principles?
- It is apparent that collective decision making is highly valued by Mrs. I. Using open-ended questions, what might you ask Mr. I. to assess his understanding of his mother's preferences; his concerns; his orientation to decision making that includes members of the extended family comprised of intergenerational blood relations and fictive kin? It is possible that Mr. I.'s concerns are driven by his need to handle arrangements for his mother in a timely fashion. Would it be appropriate to explore ways of communicating with "off-island" relatives so that they could offer their input?
- How will you approach Mrs. I.'s relatives who are "camping" out in the waiting room and anxious to provide support and learn of her condition?
- In discussions with Mrs. I. and her family members, would it be appropriate to seek the assistance of a family elder or spiritual leader? Are there culturally grounded processes that might facilitate resolution of Mrs. I's care?

ADDITIONAL SUGGESTED RESOURCES

AUTHOR'S RECOMMENDATIONS

The authors recommend talking with a cultural resource, someone in a local community-based organization or church. Should no local resource be readily available, the authors recommend contacting the Asian & Pacific Islander American Health Forum (APIAHF), which is available at: http://www.apiahf.org. Phone: (415) 954-9988.

BOOK

The authors encourage Fadiman's use of A. Kleinman's eight questions for eliciting a cultural explanatory model for working with culturally diverse patients and families.

Fadiman, A. (1997). *The spirit catches you and you fall down: A Hmong child, her American doctors, and the collision of two cultures*. New York, NY: Farrar, Straus, & Giroux.

JOURNAL ARTICLES

Little, V. (2009). Palliative care needs in American Samoa. *Journal of Palliative Medicine, 12*(5), 411–413.

McLaughlin, L., & Braun, K. (1998). Asian and Pacific Islander cultural values: Considerations for health care decision making. *Health and Social Work, 2*(23), 116–126.

REFERENCES

Braun, K. L., Mokuau, N. K., & Tsark, J. U. (1997). Cultural themes in health, illness, and rehabilitation for Native Hawaiians: Observations of rehabilitation staff and physicians. *Top Geriatric Rehabilitation, 12*(3), 19–37.

Browne, C., & Broderick, A. (1994). Asian and Pacific Island elders: Issues for social work practice and education. *Social Work, 39*(3), 252–259.

Bushnell, O. A. (1993). *The gifts of civilization. Germs and genocide in Hawaii*. Honolulu, HI: University of Hawai'i.

FSM Government, Department of Economic Affairs, Division of Statistics. (2000). *2000 population and housing census report*. Palikir, Pohnpei: Author. Retrieved from http://www.spc.int/prism/Country/FM/stats/Publications/Census_Survey/2000_Census/FSM/Analytical%20Report/00NatlCenRept.pdf

Kagawa-Singer, M., & Blackhall, L. J. (2001). Negotiating cross-cultural issues at the end of life: "You got to go where he lives." *Journal of the American Medical Association, 286*(23), 2993–3001.

Ka'opua, L. S. (1994). Cultural competency in the HIV epidemic. *1994 national HIV frontline forum multimedia self-study kit* (pp. 18–23). New York, NY: NCM Publishers.

Ka'opua, L. S. (2003). Training community practitioners in a research intervention: Practice examples at the intersection of cancer, western science, and Native Hawaiian Healing. *Cancer, Culture, and Literacy, supplement to Cancer Control: Journal of the Moffitt Cancer Center, 10*, 5–12.

Kiste, R. C., & Marshall, M. (1999). *American anthropology in Micronesia. An assessment*. Honolulu, HI: University of Hawai'i.

Mulitalo-Lauta, P. (2000) *Fa'a Samoa and social work within the New Zealand context*. Palmerston North, New Zealand: Dunmore.

Matsumura, S., Bito, S., Liu, H., Kahn, K., Fukuhara, S., Kagawa-Singer, M., & Wenger, N. (2002). Acculturation of attitudes toward end-of-life care: A cross-cultural survey of Japanese Americans and Japanese. *Journal of General Internal Medicine, 17*, 531–539.

McLaughlin, L., & Braun, K. (1998). Asian and Pacific Islander cultural values: Considerations for health care decision making. *Health and Social Work, 2*(23), 116–126.

Ngo-Metzger, Q., Phillips, R. S., & McCarthy, E. P. (2008). Ethnic disparities in hospice use among Asian-American and Pacific Islander patients dying with cancer. *Journal of the American Geriatrics Society, 56*, 139–144.

Pobutsky, A. M., Buenconsejo-Lum, L., Chow, C., Palafox, N., & Maskarinec, G. G. (2005). Micronesian migrants in Hawaii: Health issues and culturally appropriate, community-based solutions. *Californian Journal of Health Promotion, 3*, 59–72.

U.S. Census Bureau. (2000). *2000 census of population*. Retrieved from http://quickfacts.Census.gov/qrfd/meta/long_68182.htm

Whistler, W. A. (1992). *Tongan medicine*. Honolulu, HI: University of Hawai'i.

55 *Susan Cadell and Harvey Bosma*

Palliative Social Work in Canada

[The palliative social worker] was respectful to our culture. You know, she helped us so much, because your culture is part of your healing process. [She knew you can] simply ask them— look, is there anything I should know about your cultural aspects that would help me to help you without offending you, because of my lack of understanding of your social and cultural background?

—*A family member of an oncology patient (Kelley, 2009)*

Key Concepts

♦ *Canada is a large but sparsely populated country with cultural, linguistic, and geographic variability that affects palliative social work practice.*

♦ *Advances in research, interprofessional education, and establishing competencies have been successes of the Canadian professionals.*

Introduction

Geographically, Canada is the second largest country in the world. For its size it is sparsely populated. It is currently ranked 36th in the world with a population of just under 34,000,000 (United Nations, 2007, as cited in Public Health Agency of Canada, 2008). It is a country comprised of ten provinces and three territories with two official languages, French and English. In addition, Canada opens its doors to large numbers of immigrants and refugees each year. In 2006 foreign-born individuals comprised one-fifth of the population (Statistics Canada, 2009b). It has had a system of universal Medicare since the mid-1960s. While many aspects of the country are governed by the federal government, health care is managed separately by each province or territory. All this makes for a large variation across the country in the implementation of palliative care and the role of social work within this field.

Palliative Care: An Overview

There is a friendly rivalry in the Canadian context in terms of where palliative care began in Canada. In 1974, the first palliative care unit in the country officially opened in St. Boniface in Winnipeg, Manitoba, just days before a similar unit in Montréal, Québec. Balfour Mount, the physician who facilitated the opening of the Montréal unit, is anecdotally credited with coining the term *palliative care* in the English language. This term was chosen because the word *hospice* has negative connotations in the French language that are associated with care of the poor and marginalized.

The national association, the Canadian Hospice Palliative Care Association (CHPCA), began in 1991. The organization was originally the Canadian Palliative Care Association, but the name was changed in 2001 to include hospice (CHPCA, 2009). The change reflects the notion that "hospice care" and "palliative care" are not distinct areas of practice. Social workers represent one of the interest groups that make up the CHPCA with representatives from across the county. No other national group currently exists for social workers who work specifically in palliative care.

While Canada has a national strategy on palliative and end-of-life care that emphasizes care across the continuum of illness (Health Canada, 2007), there is no national policy concerning the delivery of services. In some places, palliative services can be accessed at several locations that include palliative care units in hospitals, free-standing hospices, and home care programs. However, this range of services can vary in a single province and not be equally available throughout, let alone from one province to another.

There is one national policy specific to end of life care, which is the Compassionate Care Benefits program that falls under the national employment programs (Service Canada, 2009). Under this program, eligible family members of individuals considered to be at the end of life can take a leave from work and receive financial compensation for up to 6 weeks. Some provinces have additional programs that cover costs of caring for a family member at home, such as those related to hospital equipment, medical supplies, and medications (British Columbia Ministry of Health, 2006).

Palliative Social Work

The profession of social work varies throughout Canada. For example, social services workers can have community college diplomas while social workers variously have bachelor's and master's degrees. Doctoral degrees in social work emphasize research training more than preparation for advanced practice. Regulatory bodies exist in some provinces but not in others. The Canadian Association of Social Workers (http://www.casw-acts.ca) has a code of ethics, though the provincial organizations have not all opted into the latest version. For instance, British Columbia has opted to stay with the former variation of the code. Consequently, the framework for social work delivery may vary in different regions of the country. However, education and training programs are similar because schools of social work are accredited by one national body comprised of member schools.

Palliative services are delivered by teams that frequently include social workers in various practice settings in both adult and pediatric care. Programs exist in free-standing hospices, hospital units, and home care. There are a number of social realities that make the delivery of palliative care, and social work practice within it, unique in Canada. One of these is the large numbers of languages and cultures in the country. Canada has a rich history of immigration, and large numbers of immigrants and refugees call this country home each year. Historically, the majority of new Canadians arrived from the United Kingdom and Europe. However, during the past decade, most new immigrants are East and Southeast

Asian, South Asian, and Chinese (Statistics Canada, 2009c). Specifically, they are arriving from the Philippines, India, and mainland China (Statistics Canada, 2009a).

Canada has a long-standing tradition of multiculturalism. This has implications for the practice of palliative care throughout the country because the role of culture is significant as persons live with life-threatening illness and come to the end of life. Cultural meanings of illness, suffering, and dying influence interactions between individuals, families, and health care professionals and shape the subsequent experience of care. Social work is sensitive to issues of diversity and the importance of cultural awareness in health care. In a recent survey, Canadian palliative social workers recommended that cultural competency be included as an essential component of practice (Bosma et al., 2009).

A second Canadian cultural aspect of care relates to the large number of First Nations, Inuit, and Metis peoples. Long before Europeans arrived, there were already people who populated this land. Many injustices have been committed against these peoples who are the first citizens. Our governmental and educational systems are making progress in the provision of culturally specific services that are designed to right some of these historical wrongs. Because social work as a profession is firmly committed to advancing social justice, social workers often promote this goal in palliative care by advocating for the provision of culturally safe care to these individuals and communities. This reflects the call of Aboriginal physicians for health care providers to acknowledge the social, political, linguistic, economic, and spiritual dimensions of First Nations clients in their interactions with them (Indigenous Physicians Association of Canada–The Royal College of Physicians of Canada [IPAC-RCPSC] Core Curriculum Development Working Group, 2009).

In addition, Canada has a wide split between urban and rural communities. Because the majority of the population lives in the south of the country, where it is warmer, urban centers and most services are located there. In addition to the aforementioned variability in the provincial health care systems, the absence of a national model of palliative care service delivery means that variation can be great. For instance, in one large city, one hospital might operate on a model of a separate team of professionals who become involved when someone is considered to be at the end of life, whereas another institution might not have this practice. In contrast, individuals in small communities and geographically remote areas have various needs that may not be met in their immediate regions. In some cases, palliative care, if it is practiced at all, is provided by only one physician. This has implications for social work as well as other disciplines that would make up an interprofessional team. Often social workers are expected to wear many hats and provide a range of services because they are the only practitioners in the area. Consequently, they may be expected to provide palliative services as part of their generalist practice.

There are a number of ways that social workers in palliative care in Canada have made their mark and are forging new paths in the profession. These include research, interprofessional education, and establishing clinical competencies.

Social Work Research in Palliative Care

The national health research body, the Canadian Institutes of Health Research, funded 10 palliative care research teams in 2004. The teams of five to seven researchers were encouraged to be interdisciplinary because this is one of the pillars of the agency. This initiative created a unique opportunity for social workers to become important members of major research infrastructure and to promote their points of view within various interdisciplinary teams. Not every team has a social worker, but the psychosocial perspective is enshrined in each, and in many cases this is highlighted through the presence of a social worker. These infrastructure grants also allowed the funded teams to provide scholarships for students in various disciplines, including social work, in order to mentor the next generation of palliative care researchers.

The holistic nature of social work practice ensures that research poses questions that advance our understanding of what clients and families in palliative care are experiencing and then translates that resulting knowledge back into practice. Social workers may undertake research alone (Kelley, 2007), in teams with other social workers (Cairns, Thompson, & Wainwright, 2003; Jones, Christ, & Blacker, 2006), and in interprofessional teams (Steele et al., 2008a; Steele et al., 2008b; Straatman, Cadell, Davies, Siden, & Steele, 2008).

Interprofessional Education in Palliative Care

Interprofessional education in health care has been established as a priority in Canada, and social work plays an important role in this movement. One example of interprofessional education in palliative care is a course that has been offered at the University of British Columbia in Western Canada for 8 years (Cadell et al., 2007). The course is offered in an intensive format over 4 weeks with social work, pharmacy, medicine, and nursing students. The students work in interprofessional teams from the first day of the course as well as learn within their professional groups. The emphasis of the course is on collaborative teamwork and how it addresses whole-person care along the continuum of illness and at end of life. There are other interprofessional opportunities that involve social work that have become available online such as the Interprofessional Psychosocial Oncology Distance Education project (http://www.ipode.ca) and the Interdisciplinary Palliative Care Program at Lakehead University in Northern Ontario (cedl.lakeheadu.ca). McMaster University in Ontario has a continuing education program in interprofessional palliative care that has been in existence for many years (Latimer, Kiehl, Lennox, & Studd, 1998).

The Canadian Partnership against Cancer (http://www.partnershipagainstcancer.ca) has recently launched an online directory of educational opportunities in palliative care and psychosocial oncology. Many of the resources involve and are available to social workers. Educational opportunities take the form of practicum placements, university courses, and continuing education programs.

Social Work Competencies in Palliative Care

Perhaps the most significant accomplishment of palliative social workers in Canada is the recent establishment of practice competencies. A small group of social workers began meeting under the auspices of the national Secretariat on Palliative and End-of-Life Care. The need for clinical competencies specific to social work was identified as other professions developed their own. A process of national consultation was undertaken, and 11 competencies were developed (see Table 55.1; Bosma et al., 2009).

Each competency was initially developed by the working group and then a national Delphi process was used to establish consensus. Embedded in each are the applicable attitudes/values, knowledge, and skills. The competencies can be downloaded from the CHPCA Web site (http://www.chpca.net). The establishment of the clinical competencies was the first phase.

The second phase involved an additional national consultation process to validate the competencies and to create a plan for implementation into education and practice settings. Focus groups were held with four clusters of people. *Family members of oncology patients* who received palliative care services from a social worker were interviewed about the competencies based on their lived experience. *Representatives from social work associations* were consulted as were *social work educators*. In addition, *practitioners from various palliative care settings* were asked about the validity and strategies for implementation of the competencies.

All those consulted agreed that the 11 competencies are well founded and useful. The family members of oncology

Table 55.1.
List of Competencies

Advocacy	Assessment
Care delivery	Care planning
Community capacity building	Evaluation
Decision making	Education and research
Information sharing	Interdisciplinary team
Self-reflective practice	

Source: Bosma et al., 2009

patients identified the value of social work in cancer care. They expressed that social workers helped them to deal with the illness, as well as dying, death, and bereavement. Social workers' skills in relationship building and their knowledge base of relevant palliative care processes were of importance to the patient and families interviewed. The representatives from social work associations viewed the competencies as a great benefit to social workers practicing in remote or rural areas and suggested that they be used as a resource by other social workers who are not working in palliative care as well as the general public.

The social work educators recognized the value of the clinical competencies for field education and suggested that they be used to promote palliative care education in the schools of social work nationally. The link between theory and practice was underlined as a benefit. The social work practitioners who were consulted also agreed that the competencies are useful, particularly for staff development, supervision, evaluation, hiring, and the creation of job descriptions. They made additional suggestions for making the competencies more accessible to social workers and family members. For example, an article was written connecting the competencies to clinical scenarios in order to demonstrate the potential process and outcomes involved with actualizing each of the 11 competencies (Cadell, Johnston, Bosma, & Wainwright, 2010). It is anticipated that the article will be useful to incorporate into teaching modules and as a guide for clinicians.

Overall, the two phases of the work have confirmed the value of the clinical competencies for social workers in palliative care. The competencies have been widely promoted through the national consultation processes and at national and international conferences. The next phase is to build on the partnerships established through the first two steps to implement the competencies into national social work education curricula. This third phase has recently been funded by Canada's national health agency in partnership with the Canadian Hospice Palliative Care Association.

Conclusion

As a large country with a relatively small population, Canada has much diversity in its peoples and its systems. Despite the lack of national palliative social work representation, important national advances have been made in research, education, and competencies. Like elsewhere in the world, palliative social work in Canada focuses on the people and families throughout the trajectory of serious illness and at the end of life. In maintaining and building upon the progress already made, the practice of social work will continue to advance excellent palliative care.

The Canadian Association of Psychosocial Oncology: http://www.capo.ca
Comprised of professionals trained to assist patients and families dealing with cancer on an emotional, psychological, and spiritual level.
The Canadian Association of Social Work: http://www.casw-acts.ca
A coalition of 10 social work organizations that strive to progress the field of social work in Canada.
The Canadian Association for Social Work Education: http://www.caswe-acfts.ca
A voluntary organization made up of university faculties, schools, and departments that offers professional education in social work.
The Canadian Hospice Palliative Care Association: http://www.chpca.net
Offers leadership in hospice palliative care in Canada.
The Canadian Interprofessional Health Collaborative: http://www.cihc.ca
Advocates for a better health care system by working together with health and education.
The Canadian Partnership Against Cancer: http://www.partnershipagainstcancer.ca
An organization that explores and implements new research to manage cancer for Canadians.
The Interdisciplinary Palliative Care Program at Lakehead University: http://www.cedl.lakeheadu.ca
Offers the Palliative Care Certificate for students and professionals in disciplines related to the field of palliative care.
The Interprofessional Psychosocial Oncology Distance Education: http://www.ipode.ca
Provides graduate-level electives and continuing education credits through courses on the Web. These courses focus on the education gap in psychosocial oncology.

REFERENCES

Bosma, H., Johnston, M., Cadell, S., Wainwright, W., Abernethy, N., Feron, A., ... Nelson, F. (2009). Creating social work competencies for practice in hospice palliative care. *Palliative Medicine, 23*, 1–9. doi:10.1177/0269216309346596.

British Columbia Ministry of Health. (2006, July 17). *BC palliative care benefits program application: Pharmacare BC palliative care drug program and health authority palliative care medical supply and equipment program.* Retrieved from https://www.health.gov.bc.ca/exforms/pharmacare/349.pdf

Cadell, S., Bosma, H., Johnston, M., Porterfield, P., Cline, L., da Silva, J., ... Boston, P. (2007). Practicing interprofessional teamwork from the first day of class: A model for an interprofessional palliative care course. *Journal of Palliative Care, 23*(4), 273–279.

Cadell, S., Johnston, M., Bosma, H., & Wainwright, W. (2010). An overview of contemporary social work practice. *Progress in Palliative Care, 18*(4), 205–211.

Cairns M., Thompson M., & Wainwright W. (2003). *Transitions in dying and bereavement: A psychosocial handbook for hospice and palliative care.* Baltimore, MD: Health Professions Press.

Canadian Hospice Palliative Care Association (CHPCA). (2009). *The Canadian Hospice Palliative Care Association... A history.* Retrieved from http://www.chpca.net/about_us/history.html

Health Canada. (2007). *Canadian strategy on palliative and end-of-life care: Final report.* Retrieved from http://www.hc-sc. gc.ca/hcs-sss/alt_formats/hpb-dgps/pdf/pubs/2007-soin_fin-end_life/2007-soin-fin-end_life-eng.pdf

Indigenous Physicians Association of Canada - The Royal College of Physicians of Canada (IPAC-RCPSC) Core Curriculum Development Working Group. (2009). *Promoting culturally safe care for First Nations, Inuit and Métis patients: A core curriculum for residents and physicians.* Retrieved from http://www.ipac-amic.org/docs/21118_RCPSC_CoreCurriculum_Binder.pdf?PHPSESSID=facb7cd3936c7c7db9ce77301152ba8b

Jones, B. L., Christ, G., & Blacker, S. (2006). Companionship, control, and compassion: A social work perspective on the needs of children with cancer and their families at the end of life. *Journal of Palliative Medicine, 9*(3), 774–788.

Kelley, M. L. (2007). Developing rural communities' capacity for palliative care: A conceptual model. *Journal of Palliative Care, 23*(3), 143–153.

Kelley, M. L., Kortes-Miller, K., Kerbashian, J., Cadell, S., Feron, A., Wainwright, W.,... Thompson, M. (2009, May). *Palliative end-of-life care: A dialogue about social work practice competencies and educational strategies for implementation.* Panel presentation at the meeting of Canadian Association of Social Work Educators Annual Conference 2009, Ottawa, ON.

Latimer, E. J., Kiehl, K., Lennox, S., & Studd, S. (1998). An interdisciplinary palliative care course for practicing health professionals: Ten years' experience. *Journal of Palliative Care, 14*(4), 27–33.

Public Health Agency of Canada. (2008, June 6). *The chief public health officer's report on the state of public health in Canada 2008: Chapter Three—Our population, our health and the distribution of our health.* Retrieved from http://www.phac-aspc.gc.ca/publicat/2008/cphorsphc-respcacsp/cphorsphc-respcacsp06a-eng.php

Service Canada. (2009). *Employment insurance (EI) compassionate care benefits.* Retrieved from http://www.servicecanada.gc.ca/eng/ei/types/compassionate_care.shtml#receive

Statistics Canada. (2009a). Immigrant population by place of birth and period of immigration (2006 Census). Retrieved from http://www40.statcan.gc.ca/l01/cst01/demo24a-eng.htm

Statistics Canada. (2009b). *2006 census: Immigration in Canada: A portrait of the foreign-born population, 2006 census: Highlights.* Retrieved from http://www12.statcan.ca/census-recensement/2006/as-sa/97-557/p1-eng.cfm

Statistics Canada. (2009c). *Population by selected ethnic origins, by province and territory (2006 census) (Canada).* http://www40.statcan.gc.ca/l01/cst01/demo26a-eng.htm

Steele, R., Bosma, H., Johnston, M.F., Cadell, S., Davies, B., Siden, H., & Straatman, L. (2008). Research priorities in pediatric palliative care: A delphi study. *Journal of Palliative Care, 24*(4), 229–240.

Steele, R., Derman, S., Cadell, S., Davies, B., Siden, H., & Straatman, L. (2008). Families' transition to a Canadian paediatric hospice. Part two: Results of a pilot study. *International Journal of Palliative Nursing, 14*(6), 287–295.

Straatman, L., Cadell, S., Davies, B., Siden, H., & Steele, R. (2008). Pediatric palliative care research in Canada: Development and progress of a new emerging team. *Paediatrics and Child Health, 13*(7), 591–594.

56 Csaba L. Dégi

Palliative Social Work in Central-Eastern Europe: The Emerging Experience of Romania

In Romanian culture everything connected to death is taboo. At first it was difficult for patients and families to accept my services because they were used to solving problems themselves and they also didn't understand what my role was. Since then we have made good progress and manage to make meaningful connections.

—*B. Mild, palliative social worker*

Key Concepts

◆ *Palliative care is new, unrecognized, and still in development in Romania.*

◆ *Cancer and HIV/AIDS-related needs are prevalent in Romania.*

◆ *Social work in palliative care is limited in Romania, with few training opportunities.*

◆ *Traditional, family-based culture of care is central to palliative practice.*

Introduction

Two decades ago communism collapsed in Romania, the second largest country of the former East communist block. From 1990 to 2005 Romania experienced a long and painful transition period filled with economic, social, and political change. During that time, cancer incidence rates in Romania for all types of cancer have rapidly increased, from 119.44 per 100,000 in 1990 to 240.66 in 2005 (World Health Organization [WHO], 2009a). More than two-thirds of cancer patients are diagnosed with advanced stages of disease (Mosoiu, 2002). Thus, the absolute number of persons dying from cancer in Romania is 45,383—higher than Hungary, with 32,057 cancer deaths, which has the highest rate of cancer deaths in Europe (WHO, 2009b). Although cancer is the second leading cause of death in Romania, one out of every five hospitalized cancer patients are not informed about their cancer diagnosis (Dégi, 2009).

Furthermore, Romania has the largest group of children living with HIV/AIDS in Europe, over 7000 (United Nations General Assembly Special Session [UNGASS], 2008). They were infected between 1987 and 1991 when needles for vaccination were reused and transfusions were done using unscreened blood. Eighty percent of children living with HIV/AIDS in Romania have not been told about their medical status (Ionescu, 2006).

Palliative social work in Romania inevitably needs to address the increasing burden of cancer diseases and HIV/AIDS, but recognition of the social work profession is low level and there is lack of public and professional awareness about issues of palliative care. More than 90% of the population does not understand the meaning of the term "hospice" and is not aware of the services provided by palliative medicine or social work (Hospice Romania, 2008). Currently, there is no national plan for palliative care in effect in Romania.

Development of Social Work and Palliative Care in Romania: Milestones

The social work profession's training and services were completely abolished in Romania under 50 years of totalitarian communist rule. In 1969 social work as an autonomous profession was legally eliminated, university departments of social sciences were closed down, and the national communist propaganda banished social problems and the need for social services or formal social welfare. After the fall of the Ceausecu communist regime in 1989–1990, the social work profession reemerged, social work training and education reappeared, and social services were gradually reestablished in Romania, mainly due to transnational-Western funding and support (Crawford, Walker, & Granescu, 2006; Dümling, 2004).

At the same time palliative care started to develop in Romania, mostly as a parallel service, avoiding any permanent or valuable partnership or collaboration with social work. Landmarks of palliative care development in Romania are summarized as follows (Dumitrescu, 2006; European Association of Palliative Care [EAPC], 2006; Martin-Moreno et al., 2008):

> **1992**—Hospice Casa Sperantei (HCS) was established in Brasov, at the initiative of Graham Perolls, and supported with financial and educational means by The Ellenor Foundation from the United Kingdom. Perolls is the executive director of Hospices of Hope, the leading palliative care charity in South-Eastern Europe. Based on the model of St Christopher's Hospice, the first modern hospice founded by Dame Cicely Saunders, Daniela Mosoiu and colleagues developed a hospice best-practice example adaptable to other developing countries. Because of their outstanding work, HCS was identified as a palliative care "beacon" in South-Eastern Europe.
>
> **1997**—The Princess Diana Hospice Education Center was opened by HCS in Brasov. This center is accredited by Ministry of Public Health (MPH) as the National Study and Resource Center for Palliative Care. In 2000 it became the Regional Palliative Care Training Center for South-Eastern Europe.
>
> **1998**—National Association for Palliative Care (ANIP) was formed to promote palliative care in Romania. It is affiliated with EAPC.
>
> **2000**—Palliative care was recognized as a medical subspecialty or specialty competence. Physicians are required to take a 12-week course to acquire subspecialty competence.
>
> **2002**—Standards and basic requirements for palliative care services were established, based on the collaboration of HCS and ANIP with the National Hospice and Palliative Care Organization (NHPCO) from the United States.
>
> **2003**—Law on patients' rights was passed. The Patients' Rights Act legally recognized the right to palliative care in any illness circumstance.
>
> **2005**—The National Health Insurance House (NHIH) included funding of inpatient palliative care in the framing of contracts. This means that institutions that signed the frame or financing contract on the provision of palliative care as a medical service receive reimbursements and co-financing from NHIH. Amount of subvention for each patient per day is about U.S.$35–50, up to 56 days yearly. Although funding of home-based palliative care was not included in this framework, through the social insurance fund some home care services can be reimbursed, including symptom management, rehabilitation, and psychosocial assessment.
>
> **2005**—World Health Organization (WHO) guideline-based reform of drug control policy for palliative care took place in Romania. Law No. 339 replaced a 35-year-old restrictive legislation concerning medical use of opioids and embodied the principle of balance, which represents a dual imperative of governments to establish a system of control to prevent diversion and misuse of opioid analgesics while, at the same time, ensuring their adequate availability for medical and scientific purposes.
>
> **2008**—National Palliative Care Plan was formulated by HCS, MPH, and the Federation of Associations for Cancer Patients, under auspices of the National Cancer Plan.

Palliative Care Development in the European Context

Palliative care development in the countries of Central and Eastern Europe (CEE), including Romania, is still limited, inconsistent, uncoordinated, and poorly integrated. There is continued risk of inadequate availability, which produces persistent disparity in access to care (Clark & Centeno, 2006; Mosoiu, Ryan, Joranson, & Garthwaite, 2006) despite vital and major financial support since the late 1990s from the Open Society Institute (OSI). As opposed to the national hospice and palliative care movements in Western Europe, which have been developing since the late 1960s, in the former communist countries of CEE palliative care initiatives generally started only in the 1990s (Clark & Centeno, 2006).

Needs, Actual Situation, and Key Challenges: The Role of Social Workers in Palliative Care

The need for palliative care is high in Romania. Using a WHO (2007) assessment template based on deaths per year, we estimate that in Romania more than 4,200,000 individuals with cancer or HIV/AIDS and their families need palliative care services. Although almost 20% of the population in Romania is affected by cancer and incurable diseases, per year only an estimated 3900 (less than 5%) adults and children with life-limiting and terminal illnesses are cared for by palliative care services in Romania (EAPC, 2006; Mosoiu, 2002).

Wright, Wood, Lynch, and Clark (2008) have recently mapped levels of palliative care development in Europe and worldwide. This comparative study of palliative care systems classifies all countries in four categories: (1) no identified hospice-palliative care activity, (2) capacity building, (3) localized hospice-palliative care provision, and (4) palliative care approaching integration with wider health and social care delivery and policies. Authors based evaluation on two criteria: available palliative care resources and vitality of the field. Globally, hospice palliative care services are reaching a measure of integration with mainstream service providers in only 35 countries, one of them being Romania. The United States and almost all countries in Western Europe are approaching integration, whereas all CEE countries are involved in capacity building, with the exception of Poland, Hungary, Romania, and Slovenia. In regard to palliative care resources, Romania is one of the least developed European countries, like Greece, Malta, Portugal, Slovakia, and Estonia, but its palliative care vitality is as high as that of Belgium or Spain (Wright et al., 2008). Therefore, Romania has been included in the "approaching integration" category, due to the successful initiatives that have been taken by palliative care activists in developing services, changing policies, education, and legislation and not due to broad awareness of palliative care services or their extensive number (Mosoiu, Mungiu, Gigore, & Landon, 2007).

Romania has a total of 80 palliative care services. Besides Romania in CEE, only Poland (362) and Russia (124) have 50 or more palliative care services. However, in terms of palliative care coverage Romania is underdeveloped compared to other European countries. In Romania the ratio of hospice palliative care services per million people is 0.59, whereas in Hungary it is 4.3; in Poland, 9.5; and in the United Kingdom, 16.0 (Centeno et al., 2006).

Hospice and palliative care provision for adults and children in Romania includes 24 home care teams, 23 day care facilities, 14 inpatient palliative care units with at least 150 beds, 9 free-standing hospices, 7 bereavement support teams, 2 consultant teams, and 1 mobile team in hospitals (Dumitrescu, 2006a; EAPC, 2006; Martin-Moreno et al., 2008). The hospital palliative care mobile team is a multidisciplinary team that supports acute care teams in the management of patients with palliative care needs mainly through advice, consulting, support, and training. There is a great absence of hospice mobile teams and palliative services in nursing homes. Most service provision is home care, day care, and inpatient care, mainly directed toward cancer patients and children with HIV/AIDS. It is estimated that 90% of the Romanian patients receiving palliative care die at home, whereas in Poland this percentage is 48% and in the United Kingdom or Denmark is 24% (Dumitrescu, van den Heuvel-Olaroiu, & van de Heuvel, 2007). Mosoiu explains: "Romanian society has traditionally been one in which family ties are very strong. For this reason, home care seems to be more appropriate [even if] a very stressed family has to undertake all the care, with no support" (EAPC, 2006, p. 20).

The palliative care workforce capacity is insufficient in Romania. The EAPC (2006) reported that an estimated 38 nurses, 17 physicians, 10 spiritual/faith leaders, 5 social workers, 2 psychologists, 2 physiotherapists, and 2 occupational therapists are working full time in palliative care services in Romania, together with the help of about 160 volunteers. Although palliative workforce capacity figures are small, at least 272 physicians and 697 nurses have undertaken advanced, specialty training in palliative care and over 2000 other professionals (mostly pharmacists and volunteers) participated at the introductory palliative care courses sponsored by the European Union's PHARE program, OSI, and USAID/World Learning. Still 60% of the Romanian general practitioners report having insufficient medical knowledge for provision of home-based palliative care and 77% assess the opportunities for provision of palliative care in Romania as poor or very poor (Dumitrescu, van den Heuvel, & van den Heuvel-Olaroiu, 2006).

The number of social workers in palliative care in Romania is staggeringly small. Ideally, according to the Romanian national standards in palliative care, social workers are members of the hospice palliative multidisciplinary team and provide a broad range of multilevel social services encompassing the client, the family, and larger environment (HCS, ANIP, & NHPCO, 2002). The reality of palliative social work in Romania, however, proves to be different. Collaboration in palliative multidisciplinary teams is not yet recognized as a professional value or good practice, and the role of social workers in the teams is not clearly established. Social workers' expertise in palliative care in Romania is limited to dealing with administrative and financial difficulties, resource gathering, referrals, patient and family advocacy, and family mediation. Emotional support to incurable patients is provided mainly by priests and rarely by social workers or psychologists. Moreover, in practice the minimum ratio of one social worker to 25–30 patients, which is intended to prevent burnout, is not implemented.

Finally, to work in palliative care services in Romania, social workers are basically required to have a college or university degree in social work, 1 year experience under supervision, and participation in an introductory course in palliative care. However, the existing undergraduate and postgraduate social work education does not include courses on palliative, end-of-life care, and grief (PEG) work. It is encouraging to have national standards for palliative care, but we have to admit that they do not necessarily change detrimental attitudes and practices nor have they infused the education and training of social workers. Despite appallingly low involvement of social workers in palliative care, we contend that discovering the joy and rewards of shared human experience, the promising initiatives in palliative care at the start of this century, and hope in the prospective developments will sustain social workers in palliative practice in Romania.

Although in the last years palliative care in Romania has made considerable progress, there are significant barriers to further development, most of them being present in other CEE countries as well (Lynch et al., 2009):

- There is a lack of integration of medical care and social care.
- The number of, access to, and availability of PEG services are less than adequate.
- There is low awareness and priority given to palliative care and its applicability.
- Sustainability is an unsolved and challenging issue because of limited financial, material, and human resources.
- The lack of resources tends to translate into a more evident focus on the biomedical worldview, that is, on curative medicine.
- There is a lack of comprehensive PEG training, education, and research.
- Social work practitioners have a powerless perception about influencing and shaping social work practice.

Conclusions

In Romania there is an undeniable need for palliative social work, especially with cancer patients and children with HIV/AIDS, but practice, experience, training, and resources in this area are scarce. Scarcities in palliative social work in Romania are mainly explained by historical, developmental, cultural, and financial aspects. In Romania both social work and palliative care were almost nonexistent under communism; their development started recently after the political upheaval in the 1990s and was strongly supported by international expertise and grants. Unfortunately social work and palliative care developed mostly without common initiatives and interests, and there continues to be little cooperation between health care and social care sectors, which would be imperative for high-quality palliative care. Hence, we are now struggling with some of the most challenging problems, such as diminished governmental commitment and significant lack of finances. Moreover, because social work and palliative care are relatively new services that are still in development in Romania, professionals and the general public are not familiar with their services and benefits.

Romanian culture of care also plays an important role. Traditionally in Romania problems are solved by families, informal networks, and religious and/or ethnic groups, not by formal services. Thus, care for people with life-limiting and terminal illnesses is usually provided at home by family members, without professional help and support. Palliative social work can be one of the comprehensive support sources in Romania, which can lessen patient and family distress and burdens by empowering the existing family networks to provide better care to enrich quality of life while ensuring that families in need of counseling and/or entitlements and benefits have unrestricted access to them. By providing psychosocial and practical support to families, we address a part of the psychological and social problems. Palliative social work in Romania can also advocate for the development of new palliative care services.

LEARNING EXERCISES

- How would you empower palliative social work development in CEE countries? What kind of knowledge, skills, experiences, and resources would you use for empowerment and development?
- Please make a short analysis of palliative care in Romania from your point of view.
- How would you build on the family-centered culture of care specific to Romania?

ADDITIONAL RESOURCES

SUGGESTED READINGS

Centeno, C., Clark, D., Lynch, T., Rocafort, J., Flores, L. A., Greenwood, A., … DeLima, L. (2007). *EAPC atlas of palliative care in Europe*. Milan, Italy: IAHPC Press.

Clark, D., Wright, M., Łuczak, J., Fürst, C. J., & Sauter, S. (2002). *Transitions in end-of-life care. Hospice and related developments in Eastern Europe and Central Asia*. Sheffield, England: OSI.

WEB SITE

Palliative Care in CEE e-mail newsletter in English: http://www.hospice.hu/newsletter

REFERENCES

Centeno, C., Clark, D., Rocafort, J., Flores, L. A., Lynch, T., Praill, D., … Pons, J. J. (2006). *A map of palliative care specific resources in Europe: 4th Research Forum of EAPC*. Venice, Italy: European Association of Palliative Care.

Clark, D., & Centeno, C. (2006). Palliative care in Europe: An emerging approach to comparative analysis. *Clinical Medicine, 6*, 197–201.

Crawford, K., Walker, J., & Granescu, M. (2006). Perspectives on social care practice in Romania: Supporting the development of professional learning and practice. *British Journal of Social Work, 36*, 485–498.

Dégi, C. (2009). Non-disclosure of cancer diagnosis: An examination of personal, medical, and psychosocial factors. *Supportive Care in Cancer, 17*(8), 1101–1107.

Dumitrescu, L. (2006). *Palliative care in Romania* (Doctoral dissertation, Rijksuniversiteit Groningen, 2006). Retrieved from http://dissertations.ub.rug.nl/faculties/medicine/2006/l.dumitrescu/

Dumitrescu, L., van den Heuvel, W. J. A., & van den Heuvel-Olaroiu, M. (2006). Experiences, knowledge, and opinions on palliative care among Romanian general practitioners. *Croatian Medical Journal, 47*(1), 142–147.

Dumitrescu, L., van den Heuvel-Olaroiu, M., & van de Heuvel, W. J. A. (2007). Changes in symptoms and pain intensity of cancer patients after enrollment in palliative care at home. *Journal of Pain and Symptom Management, 34*(5), 488–496.

Dümling, B. (2004). Country notes: The impact of Western social workers in Romania - A fine line between empowerment and disempowerment. *Social Work and Society, 2*(2), 270–278.

European Association of Palliative Care (EAPC). (2006). *EAPC task force on the development of palliative care in Europe. County Report: Romania.* Retrieved from http://www.eapcnet.org/download/forPolicy/CountriesRep/Romania.pdf

Hospice Casa Sperantei (HCS), National Association for Palliative Care (ANIP), & National Hospice and Palliative Care Organization (NHPCO). (2002). *National standards in palliative care.* Retrieved from http://www.nhpco.org/files/public/national_standards.doc

Hospice Romania. (2008). *National awareness campaign on problems faced by patients with incurable diseases.* Retrieved from http://web.ubbcluj.ro/ro/pr-acad/rezumate/2010/sociologie/Gorog_ileana_ro.pdf

Ionescu, C. (2006). Romanian parents keep HIV a secret from infected children. *Lancet, 367*(9522), 1566–1566.

Lynch, T., Clark, D., Centeno, C., Rocafort, J., Flores, L. A., Greenwood, A., … DeLima, L. (2009). Barriers to the development of palliative care in the countries of Central and Eastern Europe and the Commonwealth of Independent States. *Journal of Pain and Symptom Management, 37*(3), 305–315.

Martin-Moreno, J. M., Harris, M., Gorgojo, L., Clark, D., Normand, C., & Centeno, C. (2008). *Palliative care in the European Union* (Ref. IP/A/ENVI/IC/2007-123). Brussels, Belgium: European Parliament.

Mosoiu, D. (2002). Romania 2002: Cancer pain and palliative care. *Journal of Pain and Symptom Management, 24*(2), 225–227.

Mosoiu, D., Mungiu, O. C., Gigore, B., & Landon, A. (2007). Romania: Changing the regulatory environment. *Journal of Pain and Symptom Management, 33*(5), 610–614.

Mosoiu, D., Ryan, K. M., Joranson, D. E., & Garthwaite, J. P. (2006). Reform of drug control policy for palliative care in Romania. *Lancet, 367*(9528), 2110–2117.

United Nations General Assembly Special Session (UNGASS). (2008). *UNGASS country progress report. Romania.* New York, NY: Author.

World Health Organization (WHO). (2007). *Cancer control—knowledge into action. WHO guide for effective programmes: Palliative care.* Geneva, Switzerland: Author.

World Health Organization (WHO). (2009a). *Health for all database.* Retrieved from http://data.euro.who.int/hfadb/

World Health Organization (WHO). (2009b). *European Mortality Database.* Retrieved from http://data.euro.who.int/hfamdb/

Wright, M., Wood, J., Lynch, T., & Clark, D. (2008). Mapping levels of palliative care development: A global view. *Journal of Pain and Symptom Management, 35*(5), 469–485.

57 Elena D'Urbano

Palliative Social Work in Buenos Aires, Argentina

How to add a beautiful dimension in ill people's lives

—Hostal de Malta

Key Concepts

- Patients with advanced stages of oncologic disease received services at the day center Hostal de Malta.
- The program is based on a social model designed to minimize social isolation and redefine identity in the setting of incurable illness.

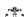

A Theoretical Basis for Social Intervention

Integrated palliative care addresses not only physical symptoms but also involves the emotional, spiritual, and social needs of patients and their families. It is possible that physicians and other health care professionals may avoid or control physical symptoms and even unpleasant deaths, but it is less probable that they can avoid the isolation often experienced by patients during the disease process. The disease and the incurable prognosis affect people's identity and restrict everyday projects, usually interrupting work activities or interfering in previous family roles.

In a parallel development with palliative care, advances in science allow people with life-threatening diseases to live sometimes for years with a concurrent fracture of the integrated social self. Patients may gradually experience some sort of "social death." Integration of the prolonged illness and its consequences involves shaping a different identity, and neglecting this aspect of the person's experience means that we may minimize some aspects of suffering. For many, living with ongoing disease involves defining a new identity.

Dr. Pablo Rispo, in his book *Cáncer Diálogo de Intimidades*, refers to his own experience as an oncology patient:

> *That component or added value that we attribute to plain objects and people, to family and social events, that human warmth of historic and cultural sharing fades away, snaps and breaks as a result of a flashing collision that ends up in a load of rubble and all experienced contents... locked up in the existential collapse. (Rispo & Rafti, 2004, p. 261)*

In a society that avoids death and mandates confronting the disease with every possible treatment approach, even when these may be futile, the family experience of this process is often expressed by the following supporting argument: "We have to feel we did every possible thing." The societal mandate complemented by this family response can increase patient isolation as their disease progresses and "every possible treatment" proves unsuccessful. The patient begins to give up on communication. Downhearted, with less strength, he or she is asked to keep up the fight. Patients will gradually refrain from responding and distance themselves from feelings of failure, emptiness, and nonexistence. It is this isolation and fractured social self that is at the heart of the program at Hostal de Malta. The day center is based on a social model, the objective of which is to rebuild that every-day space that has become so determined by the disease. It is then necessary that our professional focus include a search for transformation and understanding while creating and redefining significant aspects of social life within the framework of an advanced disease.

The Family Perspective

The patient is part of a family with a past and future, in a social and cultural context. During the terminal disease period, the patient's context may become restricted to the home and the medical treatment center. The Argentinean proposal for palliative intervention, in a social and health care system that lacks proper hospitalization facilities for patients with advanced and incurable diseases, focuses on home care that involves active family participation. But the family model in our country of Argentina, as in other Latin American countries, is in constant transformation, searching for new ways to survive. The family has also suffered the impact of economic crisis and tightening public policies, with an increasing rise in unemployment, subemployment, fear of losing work activities, the worsening of working conditions, the absence of projects, and the frustration of not being able to achieve a successful social profile of stability, sustainability, and financial achievements.

Today's family has lost its traditional supporting features. Relatives and close friends experience the same or similar worries and needs. Their concerns focus on these social and survival issues that require their attention. Similar to the patient, they formulate the question, "Why?" as they struggle to understand the social and economic challenges that they face. They have to sort out practical daily needs, requiring at least a couple of hours respite from their usual all-day care of the patient. Attending to the respite needs of caregivers not only helps their current circumstances but also avoids the potential negative impact on their health and ability to continue in their role as caregiver. These are actions of assistance and of a preventive nature.

The Social Work Perspective

As far as the social worker is concerned, the patient is not a person with problems; rather, he is part of a social network. He is someone who owns a variety of forces and resources within himself and who needs to rediscover or define his possible life quality in the framework of an advanced disease (Monroe, 2005; Sheldon, 1999). Day treatment care as an assistance method is focused on the construction of a social

and therapeutic space that favors rebuilding social integration in an interpersonal relationship framework and offers family relatives and friends the opportunity to take a breath in the active process of providing care. Our program has a holistic vision that integrates patient and family values in each step of the disease process. Conceptual framework for interventions is based upon the following values:

- Defense of patients' rights
- Acknowledgement of quality of life as a treatment objective
- Acceptance of the treatment unit as being the patient and family
- Relevance of biopsychosocial-spiritual aspects in treatment selection
- Holistic vision as an integrating concept toward patients and families
- Beliefs and values that infuse the experience of the disease process

The model depicted in Figure 57.1 captures the assessment and intervention conceptualization for the program at Hostal de Malta.

Day Center Background

Pallium Latinoamérica is a nonprofit organization, head-quartered in the city of Buenos Aires, Argentina, with three fundamental axes: teaching, palliative care clinical research, and the palliative home care program and day center. Thanks to the financial support of the Asociación de Caballeros

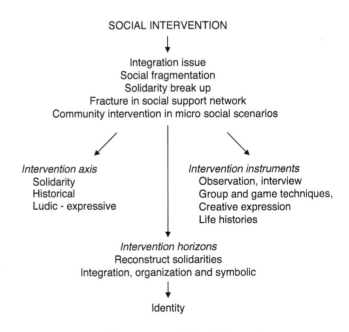

Figure 57.1. Social intervention (Carballeda 2005).

Argentinos de la Soberana y Militar Orden de la Malta, the Palliative Care Program of "Hostal de Malta" was born, including the start of a day center, the first of its kind, specifically focused on palliative care in South America.

Scope

The day center Hostal de Malta is designed to address the needs of adult patients, both male and female, with diagnosed advanced oncology disease, who are not bedridden. The overall aim of the center is to create new significance and strengthen dignity in patients' lives, while giving relatives a short rest in the daily provision of care, sometimes for long periods. In short, the activity can be defined as "reasserting life without denying the disease process" (Pallium Latino-america retrieved from http://www.pallium.org.ar). The activities are provided in an old remodeled house. The architecture, the warm and functional atmosphere, and adapted facilities for weakened patients enable a very comfortable stay. The center keeps a home-like profile and is situated in a quiet, easily accessible and traditional zone in Buenos Aires, Argentina. The specific purposes of the day center can be summarized as follows:

- Strengthen dignity in the setting of an evolving disease process
- Boost creativity through different techniques linked to art: painting, sculpture, music, writing workshops, and so forth
- Develop complementary pain relief treatments such as massage, reiki, reflexology, shiatsu, yoga, Bach flower therapy activities, and so forth
- Generate opportunities to actualize unfulfilled wishes
- Favor self-care as well as caring for others
- Encourage decision making
- Facilitate the transition toward death and acknowledge the grief related to the death of fellow patients
- Prevent family from *claudicating*, that is, becoming incapable of adequately meeting the patient's needs, making it more difficult to maintain a positive interaction with the patient
- Provide family respite when the patient attends the day center's activities
- Contribute to community with a specific resource that satisfies needs through a nonprofit organization.

Professional Staff

The emotional atmosphere of the day center is crucial; therefore, special attention is given to the selection of personnel. The staff must show particular sensitivity, listening abilities, and a conciliating will. It is coordinated by a social worker supported by a secretary and qualified volunteers. The day center is not staffed with a doctor or nurse in the house but has specialists available for any phone questions that might arise during daily activities. Most day centers in Anglo Saxon countries provide medical and health care. We have chosen this model for Hostal de Malta to reinforce the fact that throughout years of experience, even working with patients having severe physical damage, the activities do not require medical resources.

The Setting

The activities take place in a setting where the patient can express his or her emotions and get in touch with innate internal potential. The working team is simply a facilitator to develop the creativity, reflecting and exchanging worries and questions. Adopting a nonjudgmental posture, the facilitator encourages self-made decisions and assists patients to carry out their activities. A calm, inviting, pleasant atmosphere is ensured, so the patient can feel "at home."

The Death of Others

The space where activities of the day care center take place generates emotional attitudes of care and respect between patients who meet through their disease. This creates an incentive to drift away from the daily routine and isolation and drift toward others. The setting and activities encourage sharing and expand the patient's emotional world, but they also force the patient to face new losses: the deaths of others. From our experience, when a patient stops attending it is because he or she is experiencing worsened symptoms, is going through a stage of illness that restricts the ability to move independently, or is approaching death. It is necessary to work with "the loss," using activities that usually include farewell rituals such as letters and drawings that a volunteer will take to the dying person's house. The deaths represent the concrete presence of life's ending, and a reflecting and holding space is provided for patients to help them express both the loss of the "partner" as well as the anguish or fear of their own death. This space must be respected and is useful in a therapeutic sense because it provides an opportunity for ambivalent feelings and unmentionable fears to appear. We live in a society determined to deny death (Levine, 1997). The day center invites patients to reflect on life or death in a unique setting.

The Program

Comparing our experience with those in other countries, we discovered that during 2000, research conducted at St Christopher's Hospice in London found that taking part in a creative arts project can feed hope in a day center. The analysis at St Christopher's Hospice identified the main feelings associated with participation in a creative arts project: enjoyment, enthusiasm, pride, achievement, satisfaction, sense of purpose, mutual support, and permanence. These aspects were interpreted as positive experiences of self-esteem, autonomy, social integration, and hope (Kennett, 2000). There are some similarities with our experience. In their paint workshop, as well as in ours, while the group was not working with the goal of an exhibition, every member wanted his or her work to be displayed. In our setting, the same interest came up and several expositions were held in prestigious art centers in the city of Buenos Aires. Our patients also sold paintings for amounts that in Latin America are equal to their monthly incomes received from a social benefit. We were able to combine the transcendence of an artwork that will survive them with the opportunity for economic help, which is so necessary given the situation that patients and families are experiencing.

Visual arts are one of the best tools in the day center, since they historically re-create a person's most essential way of communicating, allowing expression through images, feelings, and experiences that may be impossible to transmit in a verbal way and, once shared, become less threatening to patients. According to Daley (1987), the artistic activity becomes therapeutic and contributes to terminally ill persons because they can express ambivalent and contradictory emotions that would be more difficult to express with words. In our work we found that the possibility of capturing images is a significant tool to deepen the spiritual field of patients, since it connects them to their pending, unsolved issues, the most terrifying zones, and simultaneously to the most luminous zone of healing (see Box 57.1).

Music is another tool of essential importance in the creative process; it encourages the expression of inner feelings, beliefs, and thoughts, connecting patients to their most intimate emotions. Music is not only an ideal way of communicating for weakened people, but it also is found in every culture, thus universalizing feelings and emotions. Experience shows that music is an important option for all patients in palliative care. In our program, we developed a tango workshop, an activity in which patients sing, dance, and even dramatize. In Argentinean culture, tango is a way of expressing emotion. With a strong melancholic content, it frequently refers to death. In a society that avoids the subject of death, tango is a facilitator that makes possible the expression of the less acceptable feelings of fear and anger (see Boxes 57.2 and 57.3).

Central Goals of the Interventions: Resilience and Spiritual Transformation

The different activities developed are directed toward two central pillars in the social-therapeutic work processes with seriously ill patients: resilience and spiritual transformation. As humans, we are the only living beings that grow and develop in contact with an *other*. A dog is a dog, even if it

> **Box 57.1**
> **Patient Narrative: Yolanda**
>
> *Yolanda, a 53-year-old woman, enters the day center by referral from her medical oncologist, who notices that she is going through her illness with symptoms of excessive isolation and withdrawal. She has breast cancer with bone metastases and is currently living with her sister and her family in a very small apartment, sharing the room with three family members. During the day she stays in bed in order to "not disturb" other members of the group. She never married nor had children and started working when she was very young, age 14, as a maid and was highly appreciated by her employers for her responsibility and commitment to her work. Because of her disease, she decided to give up her work and requested a disability pension. She is quiet and submissive and attends the day center to comply with her doctor's recommendation. In response to her personal inclinations, we stimulate her to paint, focusing the intervention on the years of her life she most remembers. She began making very basic drawings of the countryside where she grew up; her connection with nature and her childhood memories filled her with peace. She had parents and numerous siblings, to whom she had never said goodbye, not even at the time of their deaths. Three years passed until her death and she attended three times a week. Yolanda was able to share her history and get in touch with both her frustrations and her achievements. Before she died, she painted her childhood country fields full of sunflowers, with intense color and images that were used in different events and exhibitions. It gave her great comfort to feel that place so strongly through her work. She was able to get angry, get in contact with her deepest fears, and make decisions about her disease. She died hospitalized and in peace.*

never meets a match. A person does not reach one's full dimension until going through a process away from the mother's reach, in which he or she learns to reach his or her human potential, in contact with other social networks that are perceived as significant and help make up his or her identity. As social beings we usually live in networks, and these structures come to constitute the antidote to alienation. Existing evidence states that a well-fed social network is healthy, meaning it may prevent diseases and favors the recovering of health (Dabas & Perrone, 1999). Social relationships contribute to giving sense to our lives, reflecting identity through the gaze of others.

The concept of resilience is therefore a useful resource when undertaking a life project during the disease process. Being resilient does not mean recovering in the strict sense of the word or adapting to the illness situation, but growing toward something new. Returning to the initial state is now impossible; instead a new process has to be built without denying the past and the painful present, but overcoming it. Resilience is more than resistance itself and wider than adaptability, which is only one of its elements (Melillo, Suárez Ojeda, & Rodriquez, 2004). But the disease does not arrive only to be fought back; instead it can be the door that leads toward a spiritual transformation (Grun, 1997). If we work in this internal process, a path can be initiated, at the end of

---

Box 57.2
Patient/Family Narrative: Juan

Juan, a 43-year-old man, attends the day center by suggestion of a patient he met at the hospital where he has been cared for. He has colon cancer with multiples metastasis. Physically, he is really damaged and close to his death and attends the interview in search for help. Married with three young children, he reports a detailed and accurate account of his illness and prognosis. He talks about his death in a highly rational and objective manner. He has always worked in computers and could not easily get in touch with his emotions, but his request for help made us think that there were issues that he needed to share. He shared with us just 2 months of his life. While he maintained a substantially formal posture, Juan had another posture that reflected his most creative and cheerful personality. For several years he had been part of a street band, a typical Buenos Aires neighborhood activity, where people dress up and dance rhythms, similar to Brazilian carnival. He had never shared this activity with his family, and what he most wanted was his wife and children to see him in costumes and accompanied by other members of the group. We enabled this meeting in the patio of the house and in the presence of his family. Juan found no other way to show his emotions. After this activity we worked regularly with him and his family, centered on making it possible for them to share those aspects of him that had been so repressed, and that he wanted so much for his children to notice. In addition, Juan and his wife were helped to learn how to manage information with the children, communicating and orienting them as the disease process evolved. Juan died at home, accompanied by his relatives, and we are currently working with his family to help them throughout the mourning process.

Box 57.3
Patient/Family Narrative: German

German, a 70-year-old man, is referred to day center by his psychologist for presumed symptoms of depression. He has pancreatic cancer. He is a successful engineer, husband, and father of three, with excellent economic stability. Now facing death and with a limited prognosis, he became irritable and very sad, with a feeling of existential emptiness that he attributes to different choices made during his life. In the first interview he relates that his greatest suffering is not having pursued his dream vocation: tango music. While still young and a good pianist and composer, he chose to leave this vocation in order to pursue a more financially prosperous one.

For a year, German participated in a tango workshop, which was attended by many patients and leading figures of tango in Argentina. German took on a different spirit and taught us the poetic value of our popular music. We were also able to share his feeling of frustration, which was more related to the proximity of his finitude than to the choices made during his life. It is quite common for patients to grieve for the unrealized as a way to sidestep the real pain of the incurability.

His wife and children were involved in reconciliation interviews. These were intended to repair the bad moments experienced by them since the time of his diagnosis, during which German had become aggressive and somewhat ruthless. He died at his home accompanied by his family.

which, there will be a healed and peaceful person. For a person's suffering to have a transforming force, he or she must be set free from isolation and separation and be heard by people willing to share their deepest pain. Solidarity during pain becomes essential on the road toward transformation.

Conclusions

Throughout years of work, people with diagnosed terminal diseases have been offered worthy answers through a non-profit organization. To the community, it means counting on an innovative resource that complements the existing. Bioethics was implemented with competence and compassion as the main pillars of the labor (Manzini, 1997). Being a witness to the process and the benefits obtained by patients and families helped minimize the inconveniences that appeared which increased in geometrical progression our motivation toward action. To undertake this road, the desire to provide a different work model was complemented by a search for knowledge. The patients validated the proposal in their daily life.

ACKNOWLEDGMENTS

My gratitude goes to my coworkers and team at Pallium Latinamerica, who trusted my project and fed the daily job. A very special thanks to the patients who gave me the privilege of sharing such a precious time of their lives,if we refer to people who have diseases, and not diseases that have people, we should not forget we are people developing our professional role and not professionals who do not look inside our own selves. I celebrate life that fulfills us with opportunities, and I appreciate my own losses, which have added so much to my professional growth.

LEARNING EXERCISES

- Identify at least three factors that fragment social integration in the process of illness in a terminal patient.
- Identify at least three sociotherapeutic benefits for a patient who develops activities in a day center. Consider how you might integrate these activities into the care that you are currently providing to patients and their families.

ADDITIONAL SUGGESTED READINGS

Frankl, V. E. (2001). *El hombre en busca de sentido.* 152. Editorial Herder. 21°. Edición.
Rilova Salazar, F. (2001). *Cuando el cuerpo solicita la palabra.* Grupo Editorial Lohlé Lumen.

REFERENCES

Carballeda, A. J. (2002). *La intervención en lo social: Exclusión e integración en los nuevos escenarios sociales.* Buenos Aires, Argentina: Paidós.

Dabas E., & Perrone, N. (1999). *Redes en Salud.* Retrieved from http://www.baemprende.gov.ar/areas/salud/dircap/mat/matbiblio/redes.pdf

Daley, T. (1987). *El arte como terapia.* Barcelona, Spain: Editorial Herder.

Grun, A. (1997). *Transformación. Una dimensión olvidada de la vida espiritual.* Ed Lumen. Buenos Aires, Argentina.

Kennett, C. E. (2000). La participación en un proyecto de artes creativas puede nutrir la esperanza en un centro de día. *Palliative Medicine.* (14). pp. 419–425.

Levine, S. (1997). *¿Quién muere? In E. Naciente (Ed Errepar),* Buenos Aires, Argentina.

Manzini, J. L. (1997) *Bioética paliativa.* La Plata, Argentina: Quirón.

Melillo, A. Suarez Ojeda, E. N., & Rodriguez, D. (2004) *Resiliencia y subjetividad: Los ciclos de la vida.* Buenos Aires Argentina: Paidós.

Monroe, B. (2005). Social work in palliative medicine. In D. Doyle, G. W. C. Hanks, N. Cherny, & K. Calmen (Eds.), *Oxford textbook of palliative medicine* (3rd ed., pp. 1005–1017). New York, NY: Oxford University Press.

Rispo, P., & Rafti, V. (2004). *Cáncer, diálogo de intimidades.* Buenos Aires, Argentina: Fundación CAPAC.

58

Julie Garrard, Julie Greathouse, Sue Hearn, and Patricia McKinnon

Australian Palliative Social Work

She [the palliative social worker] made something which could have been an absolute nightmare very, very acceptable.
— *Daughter reflecting on her mother's last weeks of life in a nursing home*

Key Concepts

◆ *Historical and geographic issues have an essential impact on the provision of palliative social work in Australia.*
◆ *System changes and challenges impact the palliative social work role; and social work profile, education, research, and interventions develop in response to changes.*
◆ *Palliative social work focus on the needs of minority groups*
◆ *Models of bereavement services vary significantly across Australia.*

Introduction

While each state and territory of Australia has palliative social workers, there is no national network. As social workers from the most populous eastern state of New South Wales (NSW), we aim to provide a snapshot of palliative social work in Australia and some insights into key innovations where social work has taken a leading role. The NSW Palliative Care Social Work Practice Group operates under the auspice of the Australian Association of Social Workers. Members meet 3 times per year and communicate regularly to share professional development, educational initiatives, conference opportunities, knowledge, resources, and to raise ethical and practice issues.

Demographics

Australia is a vast and ancient land, occupied by Aborigines and Torres Strait Islander peoples for tens of thousands of years. It was settled by Great Britain initially as a penal colony in 1788. It became a federation of six states and two territories in 1901. Australia increasingly became a multicultural society during the twentieth century and now has an older migrant group mainly from the United Kingdom and Europe, with more recent immigrants from Asia, South Africa, South America, and the Middle East. In 2008, 25% of the Australian population was born overseas. The population is concentrated in large cities, mainly around the eastern and southern coastlines. Others, including many indigenous people, live in and around large rural towns, with a smaller but significant number living in the remote desert inland and coastal areas. Palliative care services tend to mirror this population distribution pattern, challenging the capacity to deliver palliative care to all Australians.

The Changing Face of Palliative Care and Challenges for Social Work

The Australian hospice-based palliative care movement parallels the British model. In the 1960s, Australian services, mainly run by religious groups, offered long stay options for cancer patients until their death. A shift to government funding of hospices and the development of community palliative care services has accompanied the rise of palliative care as a medical specialty in the last 20 or so years. Inpatient hospice care was mainly provided by nurses and nuns before these changes. The organization of palliative care services varies considerably across the states, but it is mostly funded through the public health system and therefore free to patients. Many inpatient hospices have been renamed specialist palliative care units (PCUs), providing symptom control for patients with life-threatening illness and terminal care, offering shorter stays and providing specialist care only to patients and families with complex needs. Many frail elderly patients, contrary to their expectations of dying in the inpatient hospice, are transferred to residential aged care facilities when assessed as medically stable. During the first 20 or more years of the hospice movement here, long stays were normal, so community expectations were formed then and have not changed to reflect the shorter stay policies. There is an increasing focus on providing palliative care in the community and developing consultative services in acute hospitals. The home death rates vary across Australia according to availability of adequate home-based nursing services and access to PCUs. Palliative patients in Australia commonly express a desire for a home death, but the reality shows us that as death approaches, they are more likely to be admitted to an inpatient hospice when there is one nearby. Our domiciliary care services are frequently not adequate in Australia, especially for overnight nursing care in the terminal stage. Other influences include the patient's perception of caregiver burden.

The National Strategy is a needs-based model with a focus on most end-of-life care being delivered by primary care services with specialist palliative care services (SPCS) providing consultation if required. Only the most complex cases will be managed by SPSC (Palliative Care Australia, 2005). The majority of patients using SPCS have a cancer diagnosis, though there are an increasing proportion of patients with nonmalignant diseases. Social work interventions to assist patients with end-stage nonmalignant diseases and dual diagnoses of terminal and psychiatric illness focus on advocacy for more appropriate accommodation and psychosocial care. The palliative social worker provides all the psychosocial care for nonmalignant patients in the same way as for cancer patients and will liaise with specialist mental health services if required, but commonly these services are no longer involved at this late stage in the patients' lives. Access to specialist palliative care psychology and psychiatry is very limited.

Models of outreach from SPCS to residential aged care facilities (Garrard, 2009; Lake, Broadbent & Hearn, 2009) show partnerships and education can improve end-of-life care in facilities. Garrard (2006, 2009) has demonstrated the value of palliative social work interventions that enhance the transition process from palliative care settings to residential aged care.

Interdisciplinary care is the hallmark of modern Australian palliative care. Social workers are the main providers of psychosocial care in urban and regional settings. However, specialist palliative social workers are rarely available outside major cities. Outreach programs link urban and rural services, with social workers participating in tele- and videoconferences.

As advocates for choice in place of care and equity of access, social workers are challenged by the predictions of longer life expectancy, a disproportionate number of aged people, the increase in patients being cared for at home with limited community services, and insufficient numbers of palliative social workers. Also the new focus on admitting cancer patients to inpatient hospice units for pain and symptom management while undergoing curative chemotherapies and radiation may further expand the traditional role of SPCS beyond those patients living with incurable life-threatening illness and at end of life.

Education and Research

Increasingly, Australian universities are providing palliative care postgraduate education, including a social work–specific postgraduate certificate in "Dying, Death, and Palliative Care" in the Faculty of Education and Social Work at University of Sydney. Undergraduate social work student practicums are widely offered by palliative social workers and many are undertaking doctoral research in palliative care. Funding incentives from national and state governments, which have focused on patients living with life-threatening illness and at end of life, have fostered an enhanced social work research culture. The Program for Education in the Palliative Approach is a national scheme that allows generalist social workers to gain 2 weeks of specialist palliative care experience and education. It provides workshops, distance education, clinical placements, and mentoring (http://www.pepaeducation.com).

Description of the Palliative Social Work Role

A recent study shows the primary focus of Australian palliative social work is psychological adjustment to illness and anticipated death, including crisis intervention; anticipatory grief and bereavement counseling; and exploration of existential, spiritual, and meaning-of-life issues. Frequent additional interventions are focused on preparing children for loss and change, supporting caregivers, relationship and work concerns, processing prognosis, advocacy for preferred place of care and death, effects of social isolation, estrangement, migration and trauma, and financial and legal impacts of illness (McKinnon, Garrard, Graham, Myhill, & Bateman, 2007).

Palliative social workers are committed to a comprehensive psychosocial assessment of the relevant history, present, and future needs of patients, families, and caregivers. We are frequently involved at critical points of change in the illness trajectory (Christ & Blacker, 2005), working therapeutically to create a trusting, safe environment in which to hold and/or explore difficult thoughts and emotions. Key social work interventions focus on the containment of distress and uncertainty for patients, families, and caregivers (Douglas, 2007) and the maintenance of hope while working with emerging and evolving reality. We are also using a range of creative therapeutic strategies at the end of life, including reminiscence, recording life stories, memory boxes, letters, audiotapes, and videotapes (McKinnon, 2005; Pynn, 2008). Major clinical challenges arise in situations of family violence or abuse, where the social worker plays a pivotal role in assessment and protective interventions (Garrard & McIlwain, 2007; Wright, 2003).

The First Australians: Aboriginal and Torres Strait Islanders

In writing this segment we would like to acknowledge the original custodians on whose land we are living today. We would also like to pay our respects to Elders past and present. As non-Aboriginal or Torres Strait Islander social workers, we look forward to this segment being written by an Aboriginal or Torres Strait Islander social worker in the future.

Box 58.1
Patient/Family Narrative: Ivan—Disconnection and Reconnecting, Social Work with the Socially Marginalized

Ivan, aged 76, was admitted to the hospice with terminal lung cancer but stated he had a cold. He became agitated in hospital, requiring a dedicated nurse to be with him full time due to his disturbed behavior. Ivan had a diagnosis of schizophrenia as a younger man. He had come to Australia at age 16 from the former Czechoslovakia and was sent to an immigration camp. Ivan then worked as a skilled tradesman, maintained steady employment, and managed his own affairs. Following a brief marriage, his wife left with their baby daughter. Despite efforts to locate his daughter, he had never seen her again.

Interventions: Ivan shared his life story with the social worker, who searched widely and finally located his daughter. She had made sporadic attempts to find her father and was emotionally overwhelmed at the social worker's call. The social worker carefully prepared and facilitated their reunion and provided containment in the journey leading to Ivan's peaceful death some weeks later.

Extended family, kinship, and cultural obligations among indigenous peoples require culturally appropriate approaches and interventions. Indigenous people have significantly lower life expectancy than other Australians, a reality often compounded by late diagnosis. Other barriers to accessing health services include language, distance, and past government policies, which included forced relocation from traditional lands and the removal of "mixed" race children (Australian Department of Health and Aging, 2004). Specialist care is most often only available in major towns and cities. This requires moving away from community and being cared for in an alien hospital environment. Many prefer not to access care rather than risk dying away from country. Statistics show very few Aboriginal and Torres Strait Islanders are accessing palliative care services. Most are cared for by family, community, or Aboriginal and Torres Strait Islander primary health services (Australian Department of Health and Aging, 2004, p. 6).

Palliative care is provided within a complex background of unresolved and cumulative grief (Swan, 1998). Complex kinship and extended family ties can mean that a whole community is grieving (Australian Department of Health and Aging, 2004). Many communities are still grieving one death while caring for other family who are living with life-threatening illness and coming to the end of life. Grief is frequently prolonged and complicated. Access to culturally appropriate services is limited.

Models of social work practice need to be flexible, consultative, and collaborative and utilize partnerships with indigenous health and welfare staff (Read, 2006). There is a need to provide palliative care in more culturally appropriate settings than the hospital or hospice (Belfrage, 2007). Getting to one's ancestral home to die can be the ultimate goal. We need to understand family values and beliefs around illness, death, and grieving, which may diverge from Western norms. For example, the death of an elder may be grieved significantly more by a community than the death of a child.

Cultural Diversity

Our Western cultural norms have been challenged in palliative care to ensure we meet the needs of diverse populations, who hold beliefs that differ from the Western values of "open disclosure" or "truth telling" and a "good death." A variety of spiritual beliefs, resistance to opioid use, the desire for curative treatments, and the importance of maintaining hope and protecting the dying patient until the end are common in non-Western cultures. These beliefs, coupled with the grief and loss of the migration story or the traumas of refugee and war experiences, require the palliative social worker to develop sophisticated cultural competencies (McKinnon, 2005). Social workers frequently become the advocates for culturally sensitive care in our interdisciplinary teams as a result of our psychosocial assessments (Box 58.2).

Box 58.2
Patient/Family Narrative: Mrs. K—Cultural Issues and Long-Term Care

Mrs. K. was a 65-year-old Chinese-speaking woman with a brain tumor who had been cared for by her daughter at home. She was transferred to the palliative care unit (PCU) from an acute hospital, with an uncertain prognosis. Mrs. K.'s daughter advocated for continuing active treatment, resisted the plan for nursing home transfer, and refused to "give up" on her mother's potential for recovery. Her responses resulted in conflict with the team. After an extended stay, Mrs. K. was transferred to a Chinese nursing home. She improved unexpectedly after several months and enjoyed weekly visits home. She died at the nursing home peacefully, and Mrs. K.'s daughter felt they had all adjusted well to the experience.

Interventions: Social work assessment revealed Mrs. K.'s daughter's severe caregiver stress. Ongoing liaison, mediation, education, and compromise were required in the PCU and the nursing home. For example, in the PCU there were regular arguments about the value and meaning of taking Mrs. K.'s blood pressure daily, and in the nursing home, the general practitioner and care staff allowed the daughter to give her mother Chinese herbs. The act of taking Mrs. K.'s blood pressure and providing herbal treatments comforted her daughter. The social worker provided cultural advice to the team, support and advocacy for Mrs. K. and her daughter throughout the transition, assistance with a visa for Mrs. K.'s son, and access to a caregiver massage program. A trusting relationship developed between the social worker and Mrs. K.'s daughter, allowing anticipatory grief counseling to begin after earlier attempts had been rejected. Counseling also assisted her daughter to resolve the tensions between her strong sense of family duty and her experience of caregiver burden.

Pediatric Palliative Care

Approximately 5300 children in Australia required palliative care in 2009, using a population formula (Royal College of Paediatrics and Child Health, 1997). Less than half have a malignancy (Hynson, Gillis, Collins, Irving, & Trethewie, 2003). The challenges of delivering pediatric palliative care include a growing cultural diversity, large geographical areas, and lack of access to specialist pediatric palliative care. The majority of care is provided in the home with support of community clinicians. Two pediatric hospices in Sydney and Melbourne provide respite and end-of-life care. The few pediatric social workers in Australia play a crucial role in providing ongoing specialist palliative care education, consultation to community clinicians, individual counseling, and group programs (Royal Children's Hospital, 2009).

Innovations include communication workshops for health care professionals (Camden, 2009), forming a partnership with the NSW Ambulance Services to provide continuity of care to children in their home when an ambulance is called, appointing a coordinator to recruit and train home family

support volunteers, developing an "Allow Natural Death" form (Jones et al., 2008), and Web-based resources for families and health professionals in Victoria (Royal Children's Hospital Melbourne, 2009).

Bereavement

Diverse models of bereavement support have developed across Australia. The Palliative Care Australia Standards require that "formal mechanisms are in place to ensure that caregiver/s and family have access to bereavement care, information and support services" (Palliative Care Australia, 2005). Social workers in SPCS provide follow-up to the bereaved, including children, send bereavement letters, organize memorial services, and provide education to community groups and health professionals. They may be employed as bereavement counselors or coordinate volunteer bereavement services. Voluntary organizations run peer support group programs and provide telephone counseling services and some teleconferencing services to remote areas.

Debate continues about the ethics and appropriateness of bereavement risk assessment. Within the Australian medicolegal framework, including medical documentation and privacy laws, assessing and documenting the bereavement risk for relatives requires open contracting with grieving families. This is complicated because, legally speaking, the family is not the identified patient despite palliative care focusing on both the patient and family as the unit of care.

Concerns also exist about reliance on volunteer bereavement counselors in many areas and the inability to ensure standards. These issues highlight the difference between bereavement care and bereavement counseling. Bereavement services are not well or equitably funded in Australia, making access to support and counseling difficult.

Conclusion

Palliative social work in Australia has a strong identity and often a stable, highly experienced workforce. Our professional identity is separate from oncology social work in the more populous states, but it is usually integrated in the other states. Psychosocial care in specialist palliative care services has traditionally been the domain of social workers, but not all services employ social workers, particularly in rural Australia. Future challenges for us include the expansion of our role as the palliative population diversifies, as inpatient hospice stays reduce in length, as demands for outcome measures grow, and as the debate continues about the best way to assess bereavement risk and provide bereavement services. These are exciting times to be a palliative social worker!

LEARNING EXERCISES

- *Disconnection and reconnecting, social work with the socially marginalized: Review Narrative of Ivan*
  - To what extent is the social worker responsible to explore patients' unresolved issues as they come to the end of life?
  - What risks may be associated with assisting patients to reconnect with estranged family and friends?
- *Cultural issues and long-term care: Review Narrative of Mrs. K.*
  - How does your service ensure ongoing care for patients who no longer require specialist palliative care and are transferred to a residential aged care facility?
  - How do you as a social worker ensure support is respectful of the values and beliefs of the culturally diverse groups who access your service? What cross-cultural services, resources and training are available in your community?

ADDITIONAL RESOURCES

Australian Association of Social Workers. (2003). *Working with Aboriginal people and communities: A practice resource. Practice standards for social workers: Achieving outcomes: (2).* Retrieved from http://www.aasw.asn.au/document/item/16

Australian Government. Department of Health and Aging. (2005). *Journeys: Palliative care for children and teenagers.* Canberra, Australia: Palliative Care Australia.

Kellehear, A. (1999). *Health promoting palliative care.* Melbourne, Australia: Oxford University Press.

Kristjanson, J., Lobb, E., Aoun, S., & Monterosso, L. (2006). *A systematic review of the literature on complicated grief.* Perth, Australia: WA Centre for Cancer and Palliative Care, Department of Health and Ageing.

Mitchell, M., & Hussey, L. M., (2006). The Aboriginal health worker. *Medical Journal of Australia, 184*(10), 529–530.

The National Palliative Care Program. (2006). *Guidelines for a palliative approach in residential aged care.* Retrieved from http://www.nhmrc.gov.au/_files_nhmrc/file/publications/synopses/pc29.pdf

Palliative Care Australia. (2009). *End of life: Towards quality care at the end of life.* Retrieved from http://www.palliativecare.org.au

WEB SITES

Australian Bureau of Statistics: http://www.abs.gov.au
Assists and encourages informed decision making, research, and discussion within government and the community by leading a high-quality, objective, and responsive national statistical service.

The Australian Centre for Grief and Bereavement: http://www.grief.org.au
An independent, not-for-profit organization, it is the largest provider of grief and bereavement education in Australia.

The Bereavement Care Centre: http://www.bereavementcare.com.au
Provides comprehensive and accessible counseling and support services for the terminally ill and their families, and for those recently bereaved.

Beyond Blue: http://www.beyondblue.org.au
A national, independent, not-for-profit organization working to address issues associated with depression, anxiety, and related substance misuse disorders in Australia.

CareSearch: http://www.caresearch.com.au
An online resource of palliative care information and evidence.

Grief Link: http://www.grieflink.asn.au
An information resource on death-related grief for the community and professionals. Because the site is based in South Australia, some information about support services and educational activities is specific to that state.

The National Association for Loss and Grief: http://www.nalag.org.au
One of the leading providers of bereavement education in New South Wales, Australia, whose objective is to enhance the well-being of individuals, organizations, and communities following loss, grief, bereavement, and trauma.

The National Centre for Childhood Grief: http://www.childhoodgrief.org.au
Provides loving support in a safe place where children grieving a death can share their experience as they learn to live with its impact on their lives.

Palliative Care Australia: http://www.pallcare.org.au
The peak national organization representing the interests and aspirations of all who share the ideal of quality care at the end of life.

Program of Experience in the Palliative Approach: http://www.pepaeducation.com/
A site to improve the quality and accessibility of palliative care services to all people with life-limiting conditions and their families.

Solace: http://www.solace.org.au
A not-for-profit volunteer organization offering grief support for those grieving over the death of their partner.

REFERENCES

Australian Department of Health and Ageing. (2004). *Providing culturally appropriate palliative care to Indigenous Australians.* Retrieved from http://www.caresearch.com.au

Belfrage, M. (2007). Why "culturally safe" healthcare? *Medical Journal Australia, 186*(10), 537–538.

Camden, C. (2009). The journey from nought: Developing communication workshops for professionals experiencing difficult conversations regarding child life-limiting illness. *Pallium, Autumn,* 8–11.

Christ, G., & Blacker, S. (2005). Enhancing our understanding of the impact of transition to end of life caregiving. *Journal of Palliative Medicine, 8*(3), 622.

Douglas, H., (2007). *Containment and reciprocity.* New York, NY: Routledge.

Garrard, J. (2006). *Transferring the trust: Improving the experience of transition from palliative care units to nursing homes.* Paper presented at 5th Annual Kaleidoscope Conference, Dublin.

Garrard, J. (2009). Making a difference in the transition experience from palliative care to residential aged care. Paper presented at

Caring Together: 10th Australian Palliative Care Conference, Perth, Western Australia.

Garrard, J., & McIlwain, M. (2007). *Domestic violence and elder abuse in palliative care: What have we learnt from a series of case studies?* Paper presented at the NSW Palliative Care Conference, Orange, NSW.

Hynson, J. L., Gillis, J., Collins, J. J., Irving, H., & Trethewie, S. J. (2003). The dying child: How is care different? *Medical Journal of Australia.* Retrieved from http://www.mja.com.au/public/issues/179_06_150903/hyn10360_fm.pdf

Jones, B. P., Parker-Raley, J., Higgerson, R., Christie, L. A., Leggett, S., & Greathouse, J. (2008). Finding the right words: Using Allow Natural Death (AND) and Do Not Resuscitate (DNR) in paediatric palliative care. *Journal of Healthcare Quality, 30*(5), 55–63.

Lake, G., Broadbent, A., & Hearn, S. (2009). *A collaborative project between a specialist palliative care service and residential aged care facilities.* Poster presented at Caring Together: 10th Australian Palliative Care Conference, Perth, Western Australia.

McKinnon, P. (2005). *The use of the narrative in psychosocial palliative care.* Paper presented at the Mind, Body, Spirit Palliative Care Conference, Capetown, South Africa.

McKinnon, P., Garrard, J., Graham, C., Myhill, B., & Bateman, M. (2007). *Initiative in developing KPI's: Evaluating palliative care*

social work. Poster presented at the 9th Australian Palliative Care Conference, Melbourne, Victoria.

Palliative Care Australia. (2005a). *A guide to palliative care service development: A population based approach.* Retrieved from http://www.pallcare.org.au

Palliative Care Australia. (2005b). *Standards for providing quality palliative care for all Australians.* Retrieved from http://www.pallcare.org.au

Pynn, P. (2008). *Last wishes; Lasting effects.* Paper presented at 17th International Congress on Palliative Care, Montreal, Quebec.

Read, C. M. (2006). Working with an Aboriginal community liaison worker. *Rural and Remote Health, 6,* 381.

Royal Children's Hospital Melbourne. (2009). Retrieved from http://www.rch.org.au/rch

Royal College of Paediatrics and Child Health. (1997). *A guide to the development of children's palliative care services.* Report of a joint working party of the Association for Children with Life-threatening or Terminal Conditions and their Families and the Royal College of Paediatrics and Child Health, London, England.

Swan, P., (1998). Grief and health: The indigenous legacy. *Grief Matters, 1*(2), 9–11.

Wright, J. (2003). *Considering issues of domestic violence and abuse in palliative care and bereavement situations.* Retrieved from http://www.dulwichcentre.com.au

59 *Jennifer Jane Hunt and Valerie Maasdorp*

Palliative Social Work: An African Perspective

Palliative social worker Elgar arrives at the home of a recently bereaved, ill widow who cares for four children of her own and three belonging to her deceased sister who died recently from AIDS. When Elgar enquires about her loss and grief, she replies, "I am too hungry to grieve and my children are starving."

— *recently bereaved, widowed mother*

Key Concepts

♦ *Palliative social work in Africa is, and needs to be, an adaptation of traditional Western palliative social work.*

♦ *Poverty and practical needs dominate palliative social work and leave little time for emotional care.*

♦ *Palliative social work training and resultant human resource constraints continue to limit expansion of palliative social work in Africa.*

Introduction

Although the continent of Africa comprises 50 diverse countries with multiple cultures, tribes, races, and faith systems that defy homogeneity, the introduction of palliative care in 1979 (in Zimbabwe) and its rapid expansion into at least 20 countries (African Palliative Care Association [APCA], 2009) brings an adapted, yet recognizable practice of palliative care throughout the continent. Specific issues facing the continent impact on the need for, and provision and character of, palliative care.

A common feature of many sub-Saharan countries in particular is the role of the human immunodeficiency virus/ acquired immune deficiency syndrome (HIV/AIDS) epidemic in shaping the development of palliative care. Several countries in the region (Swaziland, Botswana, Lesotho, and Zimbabwe) have some of the highest HIV/ AIDS rates in the world with limited infrastructures to manage seriously ill and dying patients within mainstream health systems. Cancer prevalence is high and rising in several countries, and in the absence of any national strategies to counter cancer incidence, health systems in many countries fall woefully short of adequately supporting patients living with life-limiting illnesses (Hunt, 2009).

Home-based care (HBC) is one of the models that have been promoted to deliver cost-effective and comprehensive palliative care since the beginning of the HIV/AIDS epidemic across Africa. HBC has rapidly been adopted by many communities in Sub-Saharan Africa due to health facilities being overburdened by the demand for HIV/AIDS care and support services. With its reliance on family and volunteer caregivers attending to the patient in the home, HBC is a model that optimizes scarce human and financial resources and transfers many key aspects of palliative care to nonprofessionals. Bringing palliative care so directly into the home has an impact on relationships, roles, and attitudes toward death and dying, and this necessarily impacts on the role of the palliative social worker.

A lack of national palliative care policies, including those pertaining to community and home-based care (HBC), leaves a guidance vacuum in the field. Effective treatments for pain control, symptom management, and antiretroviral treatments (ARVs) are compromised by lack of medical insurance, unaffordable cost, sporadic medication supplies, and inaccessibility. Moreover, the prescriber–patient ratio for morphine in most African countries is so low as to render effective pain control virtually unachievable. Some elements of palliative care in Africa may seem unfamiliar to those familiar with the traditional view of palliative care. Household chores (collecting firewood and drawing water); income generation activities; financial support for food, shelter, funeral costs, and school fees; and orphan care are add-ons in a world where care for the dying is far down the priority list of health needs. All this presents serious challenges to the implementation and scale up of palliative care in general, and to palliative social work in particular. On the other hand, the fragile legislature and absence of any meaningful bureaucracy that exists in many African states results in some surprising benefits for palliative social workers eager to assist across a broad spectrum of palliative care needs and unrestricted by red tape.

This chapter will begin with an overview of palliative social work training and education leading to a discussion of the role of the social worker on a palliative care team in an African setting. Conclusions concerning palliative social work in Africa will then be analyzed with a view to recommending a way forward to enhance practice across the continent.

Training and Education

The beginnings of palliative care in Africa were built by dedicated and generically qualified nurses, physicians, and social workers who benefited from the instruction and experience of Dame Cecily Saunders and her team at St Christopher's Hospice in London. Individual physicians and nurses independently undertook training abroad (albeit largely Eurocentric and not always appropriate for Africa), often at their own expense, and contributed to the growing wealth of knowledge at their own institutions. This set the initial tone for training in Africa, and self-styled in-service training of staff and volunteers based upon literature from the West continues to characterize many palliative care and hospice organizations. Despite a lack of academic accreditation, this approach has accounted for the knowledge of the majority of palliative care practitioners in Africa (see Table 59.1). The need for international recognition and standardized quality has been pressing, however, and the Department of Medicine at the University of Cape Town in South Africa was the first African University to offer specialist palliative care training when it enrolled its first cohort of 23 medical students in January 2001. The course began as a diploma in palliative medicine and has developed into a degree in palliative medicine with a research component and remains strongly medical in focus. Hospice Uganda followed in 2002 with an 18-month distance-learning diploma in conjunction with Makerere University. Twenty participants (physicians and

Table 59.1.
Range of Island Hospice in House Palliative Care Training since 1982

Module/Meeting	Content	Who attends
1 and 2 50 hours	All aspects of terminal illnesses, their treatment, holistic approach, counseling skills, family systems, roles of team players, working with children	Nurses, social workers, volunteers
3 25 hours	Bereavement training: grief and loss models and working approaches; different grief reactions and deaths	Nurses, social workers, volunteers
Interdisciplinary meeting: Weekly	Holistic palliative care issues	Nurses and social workers
Medical meeting: Weekly	New referral presentations, complex cases, death reports	Nurses and social workers; Medical director leads
Clinical social workers meetings: Monthly	Case presentation for discussion with enhanced learning on specific issues	Social workers and voluntary attendance by nurses
Supervision: Monthly	Identified problem areas with patients and families as well as personal issues impacting work. Focus is on increasing self-awareness	All social workers have individual time with a clinically experienced senior social worker

Source: Jennifer Hunt and Valerie Maasdorp obtained information concerning training at Island Hospice and put it in tabular form.

nurses only) enrolled in the first course, including nine from outside of Uganda. University-accredited courses are now run in Uganda (Makerere University), Kenya (Oxford Brookes University United Kingdom), and South Africa, but they continue to be overwhelmingly subscribed to by physicians and nurses. Palliative care training in Africa is especially challenged by the residual taboo against talking of death and illness, with witchcraft often still viewed as the reason for an incurable illness. Many patients routinely visit traditional healers before consulting staff trained in Western methods. In the context of care at the end of life, there is a growing appreciation that collaboration with traditional healers brings benefits for the patient in that they represent indigenous traditions that form a link between past, present, and future (Wright & Clark, 2006).

Although education is identified by the World Health Organization (WHO) as a key component in the development of palliative care (Powell, Mwangi-Powell, Ddungu, & Downing, 2007), the number of formally trained practitioners remains low (Hunt, 2008). In June 2004 the African Palliative Care Association (APCA) was formally established to support scale-up of affordable palliative care provision across Africa through a culturally appropriate public health approach. One of its main objectives is to promote adapted palliative care training programs suitable for African countries. It achieves this by assisting Ministries of Health in developing core curricula as well as providing support for technical assistance, including lecture faculty drawn from other African countries. This goal is a long-term investment in the education of palliative care practitioners, but it will be several years before palliative care education, especially for social work, can be said to be comprehensive. To date there is no palliative social work credentialing body as there is in the United States (National Hospice and Palliative Care Organization). Neither is there specialist palliative social work registration such as The Association for Death Education and Counselling (ADEC) in the United States, which offers a certification in thanatology to those in a relevant field such as social work.

Palliative Social Work in Africa: What Is the Role?

Because social workers are low in numbers over most of the continent and in the face of no specific palliative care training, there are few opportunities for palliative care organizations to employ social workers. A notable exception is Island Hospice and Bereavement Service in Harare, Zimbabwe, where the ratio of social workers to medical staff is 1:2, which is significantly more than anywhere else in the world (Williams, 2000). Global surveys that focus on the value of social workers to a palliative care team conclude that their underrepresentation leads to some weaknesses in the organization (Johnson, 1999; Parry, 2001; Reese & Raymer, 2004).

Too often, palliative social workers tend to be seen as a "luxury" rather than an integral part of the team. Consequently much of palliative care across Africa is undertaken by HBC groups that utilize primarily nurses and volunteers (Maasdorp & Martin, 2003). As such, the role of the social worker when one is included in the interdisciplinary team may be misunderstood and underutilized. Referrals are often for practical issues such as assisting with housing, school fees, nutritional support, linking resources and families, community networking, and income-generating projects. Attention to the "psychosocial" component in African palliative care means in reality attending to the social rather than the emotional needs of patients and families. The value of good counseling skills in situations where there is limited ability to provide effective pain control, symptom assessment, and treatment is unacknowledged, yet it is precisely in these circumstances of limited medical support that good counseling may be the single most helpful intervention that can be offered.

A traditional medical hierarchy still exists in Africa, where physicians are revered and nurses pay homage to physicians and senior nurses. Social workers are seldom recognized as allied health professionals because their training is strongly focused on welfare and development issues. Lobbying for an equal place on the team remains difficult. The unrealized potential of palliative social work is highlighted by a study in the United States that identified six areas of concern in which social work assessment and intervention could have impacted on dying patients' quality of life and that of their carers: loss and dependency, family-centered issues, carers' needs, practical tasks, emotional and spiritual struggles, and finally, support needs of staff (Clausen, Kendall, Murray, Worth, & Boyd, 2005). Few of these beyond the practical tasks are undertaken by palliative social work in Africa.

In the generalized African context described earlier, the palliative social worker is asked to operate within both Western medical structures and local culturally defined settings. In the absence of a comprehensive national health system and private medical insurance schemes, the social worker becomes intimately and directly involved with patients and families in the quest for improved dying conditions. Their training equips them with unique, in-depth knowledge of and expertise in working with ethnic, cultural, and economic diversity; family and support networks; multidimensional symptom management; bereavement; trauma and disaster relief; interdisciplinary practice; interventions across the life cycle; and systems interventions that address the fragmentation, gaps, and insufficiency in health care (National Association of Social Workers [NASW], 2009). As such, they are well placed to support and intervene with families who can never hope to receive mainstream health and psychological services.

Specific issues facing palliative social workers in Africa help define their role on the team. Palliative care has never attracted as much funding and interest as it does now in Africa due to the HIV/AIDS burden that threatens to undermine years of health progress. Working with HIV/ AIDS brings an intrinsic dynamic to palliative care beyond other life-limiting illnesses such as cancer. The sexual transmission of the virus exposes the possibility that staff may themselves be positive, their partners may be unfaithful, and their children may be affected by the virus. Alongside the usual personal confrontation with mortality that the palliative care practitioner must process, come issues of stigma, discrimination, blame, and guilt.

Additionally, the majority of organizations delivering elements of palliative care at the local community level are almost entirely dependent on donor support from foreign governments and nongovernmental organizations. Proposals and projects inevitably guarantee maximum numbers of recipients of care to justify funding, attaching strings and conditions to palliative care delivery. Psychosocial care, the domain of the social worker, may attract equal funding to physical care in a project. In reality, however, large numbers of patients will seldom be attended to by trained social workers but will rely heavily on volunteers with often minimal psychosocial training in the era of donor dependency. Clearly there is a risk of diluted quality, especially in relation to time available for in-depth emotional support for patients and families.

Poverty characterizes much of the continent. In 2004, the then U. K. Prime Minister, Tony Blair, described Africa as "the only continent to become poorer in the last 25 years," where world trade has halved in recent years and where direct foreign investment has diminished to less than 1% (Wright & Clark, 2006, p. 5). This is reflected most obviously in health care where food, medical supplies, human resources, and health services are all underfunded and in short supply. Consequently, African palliative care operates within resource-constrained settings, and palliative social work in particular needs to attend to the psychosocial impact of poverty on the health of patients. Such communities have limited access to the basics of accommodation and shelter, potable water supply, transport, clothing, and food. The patient narrative in Box 59.1 exemplifies these challenges.

African governments seldom prioritize the social welfare, education, and health of their citizens. Extreme underfunding of these departments renders them helpless to provide a safety net for those living in poverty and unable to provide for their own needs. Palliative social workers are usually unable to refer clients to the appropriate department for state support because the systems are inadequately funded. Inevitably the task to seek support and resources falls to the palliative social worker.

Rapid changes in family and social structures characterize modern Africa. Emigration to Europe, the United States, and elsewhere in the West is common due to local economic and political instability. It is estimated that 10% of Zimbabweans are living in the diaspora (Maasdorp & Martin, 2003), seeking employment and better living conditions for their families once outside their country of origin. A change in the dynamic of family hierarchy and power seems to reflect a

---

Box 59.1
Palliative Care in Africa: The Reality

When palliative social worker Chipo visited newly referred Mrs. D. and her three children in an iron and plastic shack in an overcrowded area, she discovered that Mrs. D.'s husband had died 3 years previously of AIDS-related cancer, and a child had died 4 years ago of AIDS. The oldest child, her daughter Rudo (13 years), was the primary caregiver, attempting to make a little income by selling vegetables at the roadside, and was not attending school. Her son Chenjerai (10 years) was attending school courtesy of a benefactor from the church, while the youngest boy Esnat (6 years) was also sickly and being cared for by Rudo. The local clinic had no medications. The palliative care nurse was attempting to access medications for both Mrs. D. and Esnat from a donor program. It became clear that Mrs. D. had not had the opportunity or support to process the losses of her husband and child. In the course of the interview, Chipo discovered that Mrs. D. had also lost three sisters and two brothers to AIDS. Her mother was living in a rural area hours away and caring for eight orphaned grandchildren. The extended family was decimated and unable to offer financial or emotional support.

---

shift from elders to those who are economically empowered. Families are fragmented; traditional values and support systems have been eroded; and the sick, the elderly, and grieving orphans can no longer rely on immediate family members to provide for them. The intimate personal care and emotional support required when living with a life-threatening illness has been transferred to neighbors and community caregivers (Hunt, 2009). Burial attendance and rituals, once so ingrained in African society, are sporadic and dependent on transport, money, and geographical distance rather than bound by kin and clan.

Conclusion

This chapter has offered a brief insight into some of the challenges faced by palliative social work in the African context. While on balance this may present a negative face, there are salient lessons to be learned by palliative social workers in the developed West. An approach has been described that demands a truly holistic understanding, paying considerable attention to the social, educational, and economic issues that are so often consequent to life-threatening illness but perhaps not prioritized in the developed world. The African perspective offers a concept of palliative care that works with and in the community, rather than apart from it, visiting, treating, and supporting patients and their families in their familiar home setting. Such a community-based approach integrates, supports, and educates local government employees, community leaders, and informal carers and is advocated as a best practice approach to palliative care (APCA, 2009; Chowns, 2007 Chowns, G. (2007). *Draft report on travelling fellowship, Winston Churchill Memorial Award.* Unpublished). However, to improve the provision of palliative social work, there is an urgent need to address the many constraints that have been mentioned. Issues around poverty need to take priority to enable patients to access resources and to redress the emphasis on "fixing" practical problems while omitting skilled emotional care. The isolation of social workers, often working singly, could be alleviated by intense scaling up of education and training to increase numbers of palliative social work practitioners. Quality of care can be enhanced by attending to supervision and mentoring skills, utilizing the few existing specialists on the continent to model, inform, and guide professional and lay counselors. Palliative social work in Africa is and indeed needs to be different than other parts of the world, but there is no reason to accept any inferior quality of care. Patients and families living in resource-poor countries on the continent deserve more than bare necessities. They too require a quality of life that can be achieved through provision of good palliative care that is affordable and culturally appropriate.

REFERENCES

African Palliative Care Association (APCA). (2009). *Annual report 2008/9.* Kampala, Uganda: Author. Retrieved from http://www.apca.co.ug/education/index.htm

Clausen, H., Kendall, M., Murray, S., Worth, A., & Boyd, K. (2005). Would palliative care patients benefit from social workers' retaining the traditional "casework" role rather than working as care managers? A prospective serial qualitative interview Study. *British Journal of Social Work, 35*(2), 277–285.

Hunt, J. (2008). Palliative care in resource-poor countries. In S. Payne, J. Seymour, & C. Ingleton (Eds.), *Palliative care nursing* (pp. 680–694). Maidenhead, England: Open University Press.

Hunt, J. (2009). Family carers in resource-poor countries. In P. Hudson & S. Payne (Eds.), *Family carers in palliative care* (pp. 73–92). Oxford, England: Oxford University Press.

Johnson, M. (1999). Governing hospice projects: A review of governance, leadership and management as seen in the foundation of the modern hospice movement. *Corporate Governance: An International Review, 7*(1), 21–30.

Maasdorp, V., & Martin, R. (2004). Grief and bereavement in the developing world. In E. Bruera, L. De Lima, R. Wenk & W. Farr, (Eds.), In *Palliative care in the developing world: Principles and practice* (pp. 33–66). Houston, TX Texas: IAHPC Press.

National Association of Social Workers (NASW). (2009). *Standards for social work practice in palliative and end of life care.* Retrieved from http://www.socialworkers.org/practice/bereavement/standards/default.asp

Parry, J. (2001). *Social work theory and practice with the terminally ill* (2nd ed). New York, NY: The Haworth Press Inc.

Powell, R., Mwangi-Powell, F., Ddungu, H., & Downing, J. (2007). *Pain assessment and management in sub-Saharan Africa: An overview and way forward.* Paper prepared for PEPFAR implementers meeting in Kigali in 2007. Kampala, Uganda: African Palliative Care Association.

Reese, D., & Raymer, M. (2004). Relationships between social work involvement and hospice outcomes: Results of the National Hospice Social Work Survey. *Social Work, 49*, 415–422.

Sheldon, F. (1995). Education for palliative care professionals: The future. *European Journal of Palliative Care, 2*(1), 36.

Williams, S. (2000). Global perspective: Zimbabwe. *Palliative Medicine, 14*, 225–226.

Wright, M., & Clark, D. (2006). *Hospice and palliative care in Africa.* Oxford, England: Oxford University Press.

60

Aarti Jagannathan and Srilatha Juvva

Palliative Care: An Indian Perspective

My family members and my local doctor did not tell me that I was suffering from a terminal illness like cancer. When I was shifted to the cancer hospital, I realized that I could be suffering from this illness. Initially I could not believe that I was afflicted with this illness. Slowly as reality began to dawn, I began to accept—maybe it was an outcome of the sins (Karma) that I have committed in my past life, that I am suffering today.

—Mr. RM, 40-year-old man from rural India, diagnosed with cancer of larynx

Key Concepts

- *It is important to assess and understand the coping strategies used by palliative care patients and their families to develop culturally appropriate interventions.*
- *Family is an integral part of the patient's treatment process and family members are the primary caregivers of the patients; thus assessment includes considering relevant biopsychosocial-spiritual and family factors.*
- *Interventions commonly provided in India for palliative care are casework (supportive therapy, psychoeducation, and individual counseling), group work (family therapy and support groups), and psychosocial rehabilitation (home/hospice care, referrals, resource counseling, welfare measures).*
- *It is essential to identify barriers to effective palliative care at the macro level to ensure that all individuals experience the highest quality of life throughout the continuum of illness.*

Introduction

In India, the understanding of palliative condition varies according to the treatment facility. For example, in hospice facilities palliative care is viewed along the continuum of illness, whereas in hospital-based care, it is synonymous with end of life. This dichotomy is present because of lack of appropriate and accessible infrastructure facilities and the presence of a supportive family and community system. Especially for patients along the continuum of illness, rehabilitation (i.e., enabling the patient to resume his or her activities in the community), including home/hospice care available in the community, welfare measures by the government, and resource counseling for community rehabilitation, is preferred.

Coping with Palliative Conditions

Whether sudden or expected, living with life-threatening illness and coming to the end of a person's life is a unique experience that has a great impact on the person and his or her family. A patient's responses are modulated by medical (disease symptoms and predicted course), psychological (preexisting character style, resilience, coping ability, ego strength, developmental stage of life, and impact and meaning of the disease at that stage), and interpersonal (family, social support, and input of health team) factors. It is extremely important to assess and understand the patient's customary coping mechanisms before conducting any assessments and interventions specific to cater to palliative care needs. Coping strategies may focus on problems, solutions, or emotions (Lazarus, 1974). Furthermore, social support is also an important determinant of coping. We shall now look briefly at how patients suffering from cancer, renal failure, neurological disorder, HIV, and chronic heart condition cope with their illness in India and how professional clinicians perceive their needs and adaptation:

- *Cancer*: Acceptance of cancer involves the recognition of the medical reality and the initiation of a strategy for coping with the challenge (Lala, 1999). Advanced stage cancer patients in India seem to use spiritual methods of coping (such as prayer and meditation, adopting a positive attitude) more frequently than mainstream coping strategies (such as taking medications, indulging in exercise and activities to divert one's attention) (Jagannathan & Juvva, 2009).

Some patients are in denial about their illness and hope that everything will be fine. Thus, we professionals do not insist on breaking the bad news to them.

— Dr. Saraswati Devi, physician

- *Chronic heart disease*: Patients suffering from chronic heart disorders often experience intense pain and fatigue. Their mobility is affected and thus they have increasing dependency on others for activities of daily living. As they become bedridden, complete trust in the treating doctor and God (prayer) are two methods in which these patients cope with their illness.

A number of them deify their doctor to the position of God who can save or heal them. This acts as a positive coping mechanism for them where they feel that they are supported by someone in their crisis.

— Radhika Gopakumar, health social worker

- *Neurological disorders*: Patients suffering from neurodegenerative disorders often do not realize the severity of their illness, unless educated. It is not uncommon for some of them to lose the will to live after the diagnosis and outcome are stated to the patient.

Most of these patients do not know how to adjust to the new life situation or how to accept their disability. Thus, a professional may tell the diagnosis to the family members first and based on the coping capacity of the patient, the family members are asked to reveal the prognosis of the illness to the patient.

—Dr. Prakashi Rajaram,
neuropsychiatric social worker

- *Renal disorders*: Patients are offered palliative care in renal disorders only when they do not have any finances for dialysis, the dialysis has failed to help, or when the family has difficulty meeting the dietary requirements. In such cases the patients go through intense reactions such as anger (why does it have to happen to them), guilt (that they are a burden to the family), and helplessness.

Whenever there is a medical emergency for the patient, there is a psychosocial emergency for the family, which

in turn, also has an effect on the emotional reaction and coping of the patient.

—Dr. Usha Bapat, medical social worker

- *HIV/AIDS*: HIV patients at the end of life are most often unable to function on their own. They may also need to deal with the stigma of having contracted HIV. The coping mechanisms of the patient thus depend on the patient and community's understanding of the HIV infection. If the understanding is that one has a terrible disease and may die, one may indulge in negative coping.

Once they have accepted the outcome of HIV, in words or through action, some patients are ready to move on in life and believe philosophically that contracting the disease was their "Karma" due to their misdeeds either in the present or previous life.

—Father Mathew Perumpil,
Director of rehabilitation centre

As the family system is an integral part of the Indian culture, besides patients, family members who are most often also the primary caregivers are an important part of the patient's treatment process. As caregivers they face challenges such as financial and emotional burden, lack of adequate support systems. They also face stress due to repeated and long-term hospitalizations and a sense of impending doom and fear of losing a loved one. Thus, at the palliative stage, assessments and interventions need to be targeted both toward the patients and family members to help them to cope with the situation.

Assessment

Comprehensive and culturally sensitive social work assessment in the context of palliative care includes considering relevant biopsychosocial-spiritual factors and the needs of the individual client and the family (Bailey, 2009). In India, a comprehensive assessment will need to include both patient and family and the following areas:

- *Biological factors*: Process of disease progression, symptoms, past history, or comorbid illness and current health situation (including the impact of problems such as pain, depression, anxiety, delirium, and decreased mobility)
- *Psychological factors*: Patient's/caregiver's understanding about the disease, how they deal with life— their coping strategies/reactions to various crisis situations, risk of suicide/homicide, and client's/ family's goals in palliative treatment
- *Social factors*: India is a welfare state and hence health care is the responsibility of the government. Health care insurance is just starting to take root in the country.

Thus, the majority of the patients cannot afford expensive private hospitals/hospice services. Hospital/hospice services run by nongovernmental organizations and the government are the main health care resources for the poor. Hence, an assessment of globalization, privatization, and its impact on health care can help us understand whether these factors have led to lack of affordable palliative care services for the needy in the country. Thus, it is important to assess the following:

- Social support, resources available, societal structures, and barriers to accessing societal resources
- Cultural values and beliefs
- Macro-level factors influencing current living situations, such as the influence of globalization, inadequate public health facilities, privatization, and changing and rising economic costs of health care
- Structural inequities such as poverty and gender and caste-based exclusion, especially to health care services; women and some caste groups in India are marginalized and are largely excluded from health care services; poverty and other societal influences in these groups not only makes health care services unaffordable but also inaccessible for them.

- *Family factors*: Caregivers', patients', and children's needs; family structure; psychosocial dynamics in the family (roles, leadership, communication, and decision-making styles, coping strategies); socio-economic factors and family support; family life-cycle stage; and relevant developmental issues
- *Spiritual factors:* In India, people have a strong spiritual orientation, which is linked to their religion. They have a philosophical understanding of life/death and other experiences. Hence, it is important to understand patient and caregiver's spiritual orientation, guiding spiritual/religious philosophies, spiritual metaphors that aid coping and preparation for end of life, resilience emanating from one's spirituality, coming to terms with the life situation and reality, all of which influence palliative care planning.

Intervention

Social workers plan interventions with their clients based on these assessment parameters and constantly reassess and revise their treatment plans in response to newly identified needs and goals of care (Bailey, 2009). These interventions are guided by theoretical grounding which is drawn from a range of perspectives such as systems perspective; medical model of a chronic illness; problem-solving approach; strengths perspective; anti-discriminatory practice perspectives (Payne, 1997); rights-based approach; and a partnership practice perspective. Thus, when confronting palliative care needs, social workers play a multidimensional role: as clinicians, educators, researchers, advocates, and community leaders (Bailey, 2009). Interventions commonly provided in India for palliative care include the following:

1. *Working with individuals—Casework:*

   - *Information giving* about resources and linking clients to resources outside of their home, helping them access appropriate treatment and care facilities, besides identifying donors for funding of treatment where necessary
   - *Psychoeducation* to improve patients' and family members' understanding of the disease and to reinforce patients' strengths, resources, and coping skills
   - *Individual counseling* using cognitive-behavioral interventions, crisis counseling, symptom/disability management, planning for future, and breaking the "bad news." (In India, the task of breaking the bad news is usually allocated to the social worker. In some degenerative disorders, clinicians do not have the time to sit and break the bad news to the family members as: 1) the doctor-patient ratio in India is disproportionate and the clinician finds it challenging to spend extra time with each patient and family 2) it involves taking out extra time to manage their emotions after they hear the news.)
   - *Supportive therapy*: Ventilation of emotions and feelings, like guilt, fear, and associated distress. Actively listening to their concerns; helping them to prioritize their issues.

2. *Working with groups/group therapy:*

   - *Family therapy:* Collusion (withholding of information) is very common in India, where family members make most of the decisions and insist on not telling the patient anything about the disease or its likely progression. Family therapy or cognitive reframing helps to bring behavioral, attitudinal change; reduces interpersonal barriers; and helps to deal with collusion.
   - *Support groups:* Patient and family self-help and bereavement groups help the family think of ways to take care of themselves and to cope with loss/grief, and they also provide support to caregivers. Indian Cancer Society (ICS), Cancer Patient Aid Association (CPAA), and V Care are some of the family and patient support groups available to cancer patients in India.

3. *Community interventions:*

   - *Community palliative care services,* which include all services based in, owned, and managed by the community and in which patients are partners in palliative care, community mobilization, organization, and participation in palliative care programs

- Sensitizing and creating awareness about palliative care to ensure smooth functioning of the programs
- *Home/hospice care services* with doctor, nurse, social worker, and volunteer for patients who are unable to follow up with their physicians regularly. Karunalaya in Bhopal, Karunashraya in Bangalore, and Shanti Avedna Sadan in Mumbai are some of the hospice centers for cancer patients in India.
- *Welfare measures* to support family caregivers in becoming independent after the loss of an earning family member by providing vocational training, jobs, monetary help to start their own small business, and educational support (fees, uniforms, books, shoes, writing material) for siblings or children of the patients. Activities include fund-raising and administration of the palliative programs.

4. *Research and advocacy:*

- Undertaking *action research* for evidence-based good practices, identifying issues through research that need to be addressed in palliation of differing population groups
- Documentation and dissemination of good practices, which then serve as models to be emulated
- *Advocacy* for palliation does not exist in a significant way. Therefore, using research findings for the purpose of establishing effective programs and informing practice is crucial.

5. *Spirituality:*

- *For coping:* In the Eastern part of the world, most of the religious scriptures reiterate that it is easier for people to cope when there is a grounded sense of God because it helps them to surrender to the Supreme/Unknown and feel secure. Some of the alternate therapies such as Pranic healing, Reiki, Art of Living, and Yoga use aspects of prayer and meditation, which the person can practice alone as a process of healing. Thus, the spiritual component in a person's life acts as a calming force, which in turn enables him or her to have a more positive understanding about life and death, reinforcing spirituality as a coping mechanism.

Conclusion

There a few distinguishing factors in palliative care in India as compared to the West that have been highlighted throughout this chapter:

- The importance of including the family in the palliative care process because the family members are the primary caregivers of the patients in India. The trend in end-of-life care in India is toward family care in one's own home rather than toward hospice care. The trend of working with community/family rather than working with individuals is one of the reasons for fewer hospice centers for palliative care patients in India as compared to the West.
- Integrating spirituality as a way of life to help in coping and understanding the palliative process is seen in all patients. Thus, once they have accepted their condition, death is seen as a natural progression of the outcome. Men and women in India differ in their coping styles. Men tend not to express (are emotionally quiet) during the process of closure; however, women seem to go through the closure stage by engaging in excessive caring (because they suddenly may realize that their loved one may die and their motherly instincts come forth to care for them, especially during their end-of-life stage).
- Palliative care in India is a specialized care facility provided at the tertiary health centers. Barriers to effective palliative care at the macro level include stigma associated with approaching a palliative treatment center and a lack of available, affordable, and accessible palliative care services to the rural poor people in India (most palliative/hospice centers are located in the urban cities of India). Only if these issues are addressed effectively can all individuals experience the highest quality of life during the palliative stage of their illness.

LEARNING EXERCISES

- In small groups brainstorm the coping strategies adopted by palliative care patients in India (cancer, neurological disorders, chronic heart disease, HIV/AIDS, renal disorder). What are your feelings and thoughts about each experience?
- Form a group of interested citizens who wish to offer a community palliative care service. How would you go about this process of setting up a program, offering interventions, and sustaining quality? Role play. What are the techniques of intervention you would use at the individual, family, and community levels? Class follows the fish bowl method of participation. (A small group is formed and each student answers the question. A student who is not part of the small group replaces any one member by indicating so—either by gesture, touching the shoulder, or going up to the chair of the person he or she intends to replace—to add a new dimension to the answer. This technique enables all the students in the class to give their responses and add their dimensions to the questions posed.)

- Points for discussion:
  - What relevant biopsychosocial-spiritual and family assessment needs to be considered in the context of palliative care? How does this influence intervention?
  - What are the theoretical frameworks that are most suited for interventions commonly provided in India for palliative care?
  - How important is culture in influencing response to palliative care?

ADDITIONAL RESOURCES

RECOMMENDED INDIAN MOVIES

- *Shwas (Breath of Life)*. Language: Marathi. Directed by Sandeep Sawant, this film focuses on the experiences of a grandfather hailing from a small village in the Konkan region in Maharashtra, who travels to Pune to get his grandchild's eyes treated (diagnosed with retino blastoma).
- *Phir Milenge (We'll Meet Again)*. Language: Hindi. Director Revathy depicts how a cynical lawyer fights against an AIDS victim's professional persecution, which includes issues that go beyond physical disorders (e.g., stigma, victim's emotional turmoil of knowing her diagnosis of AIDS).

ACKNOWLEDGMENTS

The authors would like to acknowledge the contributions of the following individuals for preparing this chapter: Dr. Savita Goswami, clinical psychologist, Psychiatric Unit, Tata Memorial Cancer Hospital, Mumbai, India; Dr. Saraswati Devi, professor and head, Department of Anesthesia, Pain Relief and Palliative Care, Kidwai Memorial Cancer Hospital, Bangalore, India; Radhika Gopakumar, former medical social worker, Centre for Heart Diseases, Amrita Institute of Medical Sciences, Kochi, India; Dr. Prakashi Rajaram, associate professor of psychiatric social work, Neurology Unit, National Institute of Mental Health and Neurosciences (NIMHANS), Bangalore, India; Dr. Usha Bapat, lecturer and medical social worker, Department of Renal Medicine, St. John's Medical College, Bangalore, India; Dr. Deepthi Varma, former social worker, HIV clinic, National Institute of Mental Health and Neurosciences (NIMHANS), Bangalore, India; Father Mathew Perumpil, director of Snehadan: Care, Support and Treatment Centre for people living with HIV, Bangalore, India; and Dr. Krishna Vaddiparti, assistant professor, Department of Psychiatric Social Work, Institute of Human Behaviour and Allied Sciences (IHBAS), Delhi.

REFERENCES

Bailey, G. (2009). *NASW standards for social work practice in palliative and end of life care*. Retrieved from http://www.socialworkers.org/practice/bereavement/standards/default.asp

Jagannathan, A., & Juvva, S. (2009). Life after cancer in India: Coping with side effects and cancer pain. *Journal of Psychosocial Oncology, 27*, 344–360.

Lala, R. M. (2001). *Celebration of cells: Letter from a cancer survivor*. New Delhi, India: Penguin Books Ltd.

Lazarus, R. S. (1974). Psychological stress and coping in adaptation and illness. *International Journal of Psychiatry in Medicine, 5*, 321–333.

Payne, M. (1997). *Modern social work theory* (2nd ed.) Chicago, Ill: Lyceum Books.

61 *Yukie Kurihara*

Palliative Social Work in Japan

Please don't tell my mother that the chemotherapy has stopped working, she is worried enough already, and that will just make everything worse.
    —*Daughter of a 78 year old woman with advanced lung cancer*

Key Concepts

◆ *Staff education at both the generalist and specialty level and the public promotion of the early introduction of palliative care have been a national effort supported by the enactment of the Cancer Control Act.*

◆ *The scope of social workers' roles in palliative care range from direct clinical practice to the development of a community network across care-settings for the seamless provision of quality palliative care.*

◆ *Although challenged by limited staffing, social workers play a vital role in interdisciplinary collaboration through their skillful engagement with people of various backgrounds, comprehensive assessment, and connecting necessary resources.*

The Hospice and Palliative Care Movement in Japan

The hospice care concept reached Japan in the late 1970s to the early 1980s, with the first Japanese Hospice, Seirei Mikatahara Hospice, founded in Shizuoka in 1981. Since then, three types of specialized palliative care services have been developed in Japan, i.e., palliative care units, hospital palliative care teams, and specialized home-care clinics (Yamagishi, Morita, Miyashita, 2008). In 1990, a reimbursement system was established for the admission to the palliative care unit (PCU), which provides specialty care for the terminally ill (with the prognosis of less than 6 months). The number of PCUs has grown steadily since then; as of June 2009, the number of accredited hospice/PCUs is 195 with 3850 beds available for patients (Tsuneto & Uchinuno, 2010). Also in the 1990s, consultation-liaison services for palliative care, as in the form of a palliative care team (PCT), started in the general hospitals and cancer centers. The reimbursement system for PCTs was established in 2002, which helped promote PCTs; as of May 2009, the number of facilities with accredited PCTs is 99 (Tsuneto & Uchinuno, 2010). As for the home care clinics, they can obtain additional remuneration for the specialized care (including 24-hour service for terminally ill patients) since the designation of "Specialized home care support clinics" in 2006 (*Office for Cancer Control, Health Services Bureau, Ministry of Health, Labour and Welfare, 2010*).

As the World Health Organization (WHO) modified the definition of palliative care in 2002, Japan has also been observing the paradigm shift from "hospice/terminal care" to "palliative care" emphasizing earlier intervention in the disease course. However, the term "palliative care" is still relatively new to the general public in Japan, and those who are familiar with the term associate "hospice" with scary images of "the last resort" or "doing nothing and just letting patients die." The Japanese Society for Palliative Medicine, the leading association with over 9000 multidisciplinary members, has been actively promoting the concept of palliative care as "specialty care for those patients with distress wherever in their disease course" through pamphlets and media broadcasting.

What Does "Respect" Look Like to You?

JK (Box 61.1) is 76 years old and was diagnosed with colon cancer 4 years ago. She had surgery followed by a number of chemotherapy treatments, which gradually became ineffective. JK's cancer metastasized to the bones, liver, and lung, and she was admitted to the PCU 3 days ago for severe pain in her back and mild dyspnea. SK, 50 years old, is the youngest daughter who has the role of primary caregiver. Since admission, SK appears guarded and avoids eye contact with the nursing staff in the unit; she just sits quietly at her mother's bedside watching her intensely. At the interdisciplinary team meeting, a nurse voiced a concern that several nurses were feeling nervous when entering the patient's room because they felt that their every move was being monitored while they provided care to JK. They also felt helpless not knowing what to say to the daughter. The social worker went in and joined SK, sitting at the bedside. SK tearfully expressed the story of her mother's illness. She also explained how frightening it was to see her mother change over such a short time. She shared ambivalence about her decision to bring her mother into the PCU. The social worker gently reviewed the content of the family meeting, which was held on the day of admission, going over SK's understanding of the patient's overall condition and the treatment/care plan. She was realizing her mother's deterioration, yet it was difficult for her to accept it on an emotional level. She also felt inadequate and powerless to provide sufficient care to her mother. The social worker observed that SK was attentive to her mother's need for subtleness in personal contacts, and perhaps she could show the staff "the respectful way to touch."

"Being respected as an individual" is one of the 10 core domains of the Good Death Inventory (GDI), based on the population-based study of the Japanese people (see Table 61.1). The GDI provides clinicians a framework for assessment and care planning by identifying aspects of care that are important to the patient and/or can become a source of the patient's distress if these same aspects are threatened. However, one needs to be cautious because it is a frame of reference and requires clinicians to conduct a careful assessment to identify the perceptions and feelings of the individual patient.

For instance, the "touch," which is usually an expression of caring and kindness, can be interpreted, as SK did, as "rather

---

Box 61.1
Patient/Family Narrative: JK

"She has been drowsy and unable to talk since she came here…the pain medicine may have been too strong for her…My mother is a vibrant woman who had been the head of the family business, and I cannot stand watching her like this! And I don't feel comfortable with the way the staff is touching her. She isn't like one of those "touchy-feely" type women, and I don't think she would like to be treated like one. But she cannot say that, you know."

---

invasive and not respecting JK's personal space." It is important to note that how people perceive "respect" is unique; thus, health care staff need to be sensitive to each person's individual needs and perceptions. Perhaps observing SK's attentiveness to her mother and to the environment would provide staff hints about her interpretation of respectful care.

Also, attuning to SK's helplessness over the "sudden change" in her mother's physical status may help staff more effectively approach SK's anticipatory grief and her dismay over her inability to provide care. The assessment of SK's perceptions as well as other family members', their communication style, and the level of mutual support among family provide clinical clues as to how best to address the support needs of JK's family. Respecting SK's role as a primary caregiver and validating that she was doing her best to address her mother's care needs can be a starting point to build rapport with SK. Perhaps through the rapport, the staff may collaborate with SK in providing care to her mother and alleviate SK's sense of helplessness. Through the engagement and assessment, the social worker can become a bridge between the JK's family and the health care team.

Social Work's Role in the Team Approach

The aforementioned narrative is a snapshot of a social work intervention in the palliative care unit. There are various ways that social workers are involved in palliative care in Japan: direct practice through PCU and on palliative care teams (PCTs), which can be based in acute care settings; long-term care facilities; and/or home care settings. For instance, social workers may be the first staff member who responds to a patient and/or a family member who has an inquiry about admission to the PCU. The social worker may conduct an assessment of the psychosocial-spiritual aspects of the patient and family and plan the care accordingly. They may also be involved in the discharge planning. Because of the nature of PCU, where patients and families admitted are most likely to face end-of-life issues, social workers often get involved in the variety of themes surrounding death and dying. For instance, patients may express fear and anxiety over the approaching death or grief over the loss of function, various roles, identity, and/or autonomy, which may also alter personal relationships. Through close interaction, social workers may assist patients to find meaning in the midst of suffering, providing a place to review lives that were well lived, and/or finding the connecting link with their own spirituality. As described in the narrative, social workers also work closely with family members as they are also going through the ups and downs, grieving over multiple losses, and fearing the uncertainty, together with patients through the trajectory of the illness.

However, the number of social workers who are involved in the PCU exclusively is rather small. In a 2000 survey (Ayumi Corporation, 2001) of 78 facilities with a PCU, only

Table 61.1.
Good Death Inventory (GDI) (2008)

Core Ten Domains	Optional Eight Domains

1. Physical and psychological comfort
   Patient was free from pain.
   Patient was free from physical distress.
   Patient was free from emotional distress.
	1. Receiving enough treatment
	   Patient received enough treatment.
	   Patient believed that all available treatments were used.
	   Patient fought against disease until the last moment.

2. Dying in a favorite place
   Patient was able to stay at his or her favorite place.
   Patient was able to die at his or her favorite place.
   The place of death met the preference of the patient.
	2. Natural death
	   Patient was not connected to medical instruments or tubes.
	   Patient did not receive excessive treatment.
	   Patient died a natural death.

3. Maintaining hope and pleasure
   Patient lived positively.
   Patient had some pleasure in daily life.
   Patient lived in hope.
	3. Preparation for death
	   Patient met people whom he or she wanted to see.
	   Patient felt thankful to people.
	   Patient was able to say what he or she wanted to dear people.

4. Good relationship with medical staff
   Patient trusted the physician.
   Patient had a professional nurse with whom he or she felt comfortable.
   Patient had people who listened.
	4. Control over the future
	   Patient knew how long he or she was expected to live.
	   Patient knew what to expect about his or her condition in the future.
	   Patient participated in decisions about treatment strategy.

5. Not being a burden to others
   Patient was not being a burden to others (*)
   Patient was not being a burden to family members (*)
   Patient had no financial worries (*)
	5. Unawareness of death
	   Patient died without awareness that he or she was dying.
	   Patient lived as usual without thinking about death.
	   Patient was not informed of bad news.

6. Good relationship with family
   Patient had family support.
   Patient spent enough time with his or her family.
   Patient had family to whom he or she could express feelings.
	6. Pride and beauty
	   Patient felt burden of a change in his or her appearance (*).
	   Patient felt burden of receiving pity from others (*).
	   Patient felt burden of exposing his or her physical and mental weakness to family (*).

7. Independence
   Patient was independent in moving or walking up.
   Patient was independent in daily activities.
   Patient was not troubled with excretion.
	7. Feeling that one's life is worth living
	   Patient felt that he or she could contribute to others.
	   Patient felt that his or her life is worth living.
	   Patient maintained his or her role in family or occupation.

8. Environmental comfort
   Patient lived in quiet circumstances.
   Patient was independent in daily activities.
   Patient was not troubled by other people.
	8. Religious and spiritual comfort
	   Patient was supported by religion.
	   Patient had faith.
	   Patient felt that he or she was protected by a higher power.

9. Being respected as an individual
   Patient was not treated as an object or a child.
   Patient was respected for his or her values.
   Patient was valued as a person.	

10. Life completion
   Patient had no regrets.
   Patient felt that his or her life was completed.
   Patient felt that his or her life was fulfilling.	

*Inverse items.

Source: Miyashita, M., Morita, T., Sato, K., et al. (2008). Good Death Inventory: A Measure for Evaluating Good Death from the Bereaved Family Member's Perspective. *Journal of Pain and Symptom Management, 35*(5): 486–498.

24% had social workers. It is more common to see only a handful of social workers employed in a major hospital with 500–600 beds; thus, devoting their time exclusively to palliative care can be unrealistic. Many social workers in health care settings are involved in the "patient/family support division," which is also called "general consultation division" or for those facilities with an accredited cancer center and hospital, the "cancer care support center." These are independent divisions, where anyone can stop by regarding a wide variety of issues and/or concerns. As for the involvement in the PCT, some facilities have social workers as exclusive members of the team, whereas others may be on an individual case basis following a referral.

Recent Shift in Palliative Care in Japan: The Influence of Cancer Control Act

As a result of rigorous advocacy activities by many patient support organizations, together with the collaboration with politicians who are also cancer patients, the Cancer Control Act was enacted in April 2007. It has the following basic principles: (1) promotion of cancer research; (2) equalization of medical services for cancer treatments; and (3) development of cancer-related medical services reflecting patients'

needs. Based on the Cancer Control Act, the Basic Plan to Promote Cancer Control Programs was launched in June 2007. It has three focus areas: (1) promotion of training of oncologists and radiation oncologists; (2) palliative care from the early phase of cancer treatment; and (3) promotion of cancer registry. All of those focus areas together aim for the relief of all cancer patients and their families from distress of cancer as well as caregiving burden (Fig. 61.1).

Upon the enactment of Cancer Control Act in 2007, 375 hospitals were designated as accredited regional cancer centers and hospitals by the Ministry of Health and Labor (http://hospdb.ganjoho.jp/kyotendb.nsf/fKyoten ByoinIchiran? OpenForm). These facilities are equipped with a PCT and cancer care support center, and they are staffed with trained consultants with social work and/or nursing backgrounds who provide information, consultation, and counseling.

The Impact of Cancer Control Act on Palliative Social Work

The enactment of the Cancer Control Act has increased national interest in palliative care. There are newly formed PCTs and cancer care support centers throughout the country that are still in progress. There is a strong demand for skill

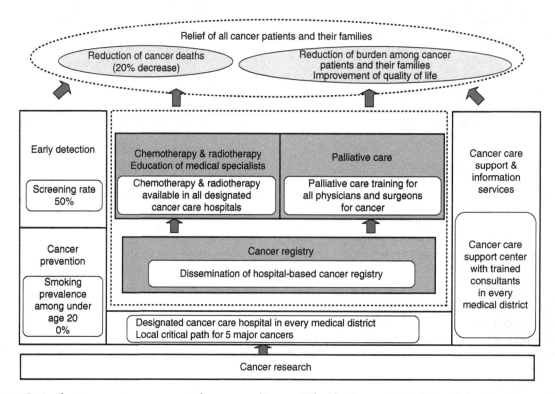

Figure 61.1. Basic plan to promote cancer control programs. (Source: Office for Cancer Control, Health Services Bureau, Ministry of Health, Labor and Welfare, 2006; available at: http://www.mhlw.go.jp/english/wp/wp-hw2/part2/p3_0026.pdf)

training and education to train palliative care specialists in medicine, nursing, pharmacy, social work, and other disciplines. Those more seasoned social workers in the country have been forming a group to provide skills training on a regular basis.

Those trends have encouraged hiring more social workers, whose knowledge and skills are recognized as vital for the service provision at cancer care support centers. Also, as a consequence of the recent revision of National Health Insurance reimbursement system, social work involvement in the discharge planning (i.e., family meetings) became a reimbursable service.

Decreasing "Cancer Refugees": Future Tasks and Challenges

TA (see Box 61.2), 58 years old, was one of those "cancer refugees" who was unable to receive sufficient care at T hospital due to the absence of a palliative care–trained physician but was denied care at M hospital due to their "hospital policy" that PCU only accepts patients with advanced stage cancer. TA had a reasonable understanding that palliative care is applicable for patients in distress irrespective of treatment status. Disappointed and depressed, she returned to T hospital to see a social worker at the cancer care support center. Through the discussion, it turned out that there were two issues: (1) TA was not able to tell her oncologist that the pain medication was not effective, and (2) she thought that palliative care was only provided at PCU. In fact, there was a newly formed PCT at T hospital, which was not yet recognized throughout the facility. The social worker encouraged TA to speak to her oncologist first regarding her pain, and the social worker also gave information on PCT. TA did speak to her oncologist, who then consulted PCT for pain management and changed her pain medication accordingly, which finally alleviated the pain to a manageable level.

Box 61.2
Patient/Family Narrative: TA

"I was admitted to T hospital with severe abdominal pain and was told that I have stage IV interhepatic bile duct cancer. Way too advanced to operate, and chemo was the only way, the oncologist told me. Sure I had no choice but to do it. I was devastated and confused, and in pain, which was far from being controlled. The pain medicine my oncologist prescribed was not easing my pain, which made me really depressed—who wants to live like this! My family heard about "palliative care" and took me to M hospital for a second opinion; we learned that the hospital has a PCU providing both inpatient and outpatient services. However, when I went there hoping for my pain to be under control, I could not believe what the doctor told me. He told me that I had to stop chemo if I want to receive palliative care there!"

Cancer has been the leading cause of death in Japan since 1981; about 344,000 people died of cancer in 2009. It is assumed that nearly 900,000 people will be newly diagnosed with cancer in 2015, which is translated as one out of two men and one out of three women. Palliative care can be applicable for those in distress while receiving active cancer treatments. The social worker's role involves listening to the voice of patients and families, being an advocate for them, and empowering them; this continues to be essential for promoting equal access to good cancer care with integrated palliative care.

CREATIVE TEACHING TECHNIQUES AND LEARNING EXERCISES

In small groups, discuss the following:

1. What things would be important to you if you were to approach the end of life?

   a. What would you want to do during that time (1 year, 6 months, 3 months, 1 months, 2 weeks, 1 week)?

   b. What are the things that you would like your family and friends to remember about you?

   c. What things might be important when being cared for by health care professionals during that time?

Use the trigger film: *Zo no senaka* (Back of the elephant) (2007) directed by Satoshi Isaka. A man who was diagnosed with lung cancer with a prognosis of 6 months declined anticancer treatment and spent the time completing "unfinished business."

2. What are the things that are important for your culture/religion at the funeral rituals?

   a. Are there any taboos that people should be aware of?

   b. Are there any anniversary/commemoration rituals/events to acknowledge the deceased after funeral (e.g. the following year and after)?

Use the trigger film: *Okuribito* (Departures) (2008) directed by Yojiro Takita. A cellist becomes a "Nokanshi" (encoffineer), who prepares deceased bodies for the funeral.

3. What are the things that are important to you in maintaining your dignity, i.e., what are the things that make you feel you are respected?

REFERENCES

Yamagishi, A., Morita, T., Miyashita, M., Akizuki, N., Kizawa, Y., Shirahige, Y., Akiyama, & M., Eguchi, K. (2008). Palliative Care in Japan: Current Status and a Nationwide Challenge to Improve Palliative Care by the Cancer Control Act and the Outreach Palliative Care Trial of Integrated Regional Model (OPTIM) Study. *American Journal of Hospice & Palliative Medicine, 25*(5), 412–418.

Tsuneto, A. & Uchinuno, A. (2010). History and Current Situation of Palliative Care. In Tsuneto & Uchinuno (Eds.), *Palliative Care: Systematic Nursing Forum* (2nd ed.). Tokyo, Japan: Igaku-shoin.

Ayumi Corporation. (2001). Health and Labor Scientific Research Team on "Development of the Service Provision of Palliative Medicine" : Current Situation and Future Vision of Hospice and Palliative Care Unit. In Tsuneto & Uchinuno (Eds.), *Palliative Care: Systematic Nursing Forum* (2nd ed.)(pp. 2–68). Tokyo, Japan: Igaku-shoin,

Office for Cancer Control, Health Services Bureau, Ministry of Health, Labour and Welfare. (2010). Retrieved September 10, 2010 from http://ganjoho.ncc.go.jp/data/public/statistics/backnumber/odjrh3000000vdf1-att/cancer_control_e.pdf

Ministry of Health, Labour and Welfare. Population Survey Report (2009). Retrieved September 10, 2010 from http://www.mhlw.go.jp/english/database/db-hw/populate/pop1-t1.html.

Tobias, K. (2006). Epidemiology and Pathology, In Tsuji, Riu & Kimura (Eds), *Cancer Rehabilitation* (p. 3.). Tokyo, Japan: Kimbara Shuppan.

ADDITIONAL REFERENCES

Cancer Control Act:
Available from http://www.mhlw.go.jp/english/wp/wp-hw2/part2/p3_0026.pdf
Cancer Statistics:
Available from http://ganjoho.ncc.go.jp/public/statistics/backnumber/2008_en.html

Hirai, K., Miyashita, M., Morita, T., Sanjo, M., & Uchitomo, Y. (2006). Good death in Japanese cancer care: A qualitative study. *Journal of Pain and Symptom Management, 31*(2), 140–147.

Miyashita, M., Morita, T., Sato, K., Hirai, K., Shima, Y., & Uchitomi, Y. (2008). Good death inventory: A measure for evaluating good death from the bereaved family member's perspective. *Journal of Pain and Symptom Management, 35*(5), 486–498.

Miyashita, M., Shiozaki, M., Morita, T., Hirai, K., & Uchitomo, Y. (2007). Good death in cancer care: A nationwide quantitative study. *Annals of Oncology, 18*, 1090–1097.

EXISTENTIAL CONCERNS OF JAPANESE PEOPLE

Morita, T., Kawa, M., Honke, Y., Kohara, H., Maeyama, E., Kizawa, Y., …Uchitomi, Y. (2004). Existential concerns of terminally ill cancer patients receiving specialized palliative care in Japan. *Support Care Cancer, 12*(2), 137–140.

Murata, H., Morita, T., & Japanese Task Force. (2006). Conceptualization of psycho-existential suffering by the Japanese Task Force: The first step of a nationwide project. *Palliative and Support Care, 4*(3), 279–285.

FAMILY CARE AT END OF LIFE

Morita, T., Hirai, K., Sakaguchi, Y., Maeyama, E., Tsuneto, S., Shima, Y., & Japanese Association of Hospice and Palliative Care Units. (2004). Measuring the quality of structure and process in end-of-life care from the bereaved family perspective. *Journal of Pain and Symptom Management, 27*(6), 492–501.

Morita, T., Chihara, S., Kashiwagi, T, & Quality Audit Committee of the Japanese Association of Hospice and Palliative Care Units. (2002). A scale to measure satisfaction of bereaved family receiving inpatient palliative care. *Journal of Palliative Medicine, 16*(2), 141–150.

Shiozaki, M., Morita, T., Hirai, K., Sakaguchi, Y., Tsuneto, S., & Shima, Y. (2005). Why are bereaved family members dissatisfied with specialized inpatient palliative care service? A nationwide qualitative study. *Journal of Palliative Medicine, 19*(4), 319–327.

62

Pamela Pui Yu Leung and Cecilia Lai Wan Chan

Palliative Care in the Chinese Context: An Integrated Framework for Culturally Respectful Practice

Coming to the end of my life, I have my son and daughter-in-law walking with me, accompanying me on this last journey. I feel very grateful.
—Mr. Liang, age 70, a Chinese patient with end-stage lung cancer

Key Concepts

- *There are important values and behaviors that are integral to the palliative care of patients and families in a different culture. Social workers need to respect patients' and family's values while offering opportunities to consider alternate ideas and values that might help patients and families living with serious illness and coming to the end of life.*
- *Culturally respectful palliative social work practice for Chinese patients empowers and supports them and their families in ways they consider appropriate. A practice model called SET & GO, which contains the themes of surviving the stress of impending death, empowering individuals, transforming the experience of loss into personal and spiritual growth, and setting goals in life for bereaved people to go on with life, is proposed.*

Introduction

One-fifth of the world's population is ethnic Chinese. As one of the key migrant groups in different parts of the world, it is unhelpful to assume that these people share one single mode of "Chinese culture." Cultures change as levels of education increase, as gender equality becomes a goal, as individuals become more aware that cultures other than their own make different choices. We work mainly in Hong Kong, and our examples are taken from our perspective of Chinese culture (Chan & Chow, 2006). The following are important values and behaviors that are integral to the palliative care of our patients and families, which in Hong Kong is currently focused on patients facing end of life.

- Family orientation, filial obligations, and respect for elders remain core components of Chinese culture, and this chapter focuses on how these beliefs interact with the experience of dying inform palliative social work at end of life.
- Family members assume responsibility for making decisions on behalf of patients who are seriously ill and are involved at levels that may be considered inappropriate in other cultures. For example, it is not uncommon for family members to insist that a dying patient not be informed of the severity of his or her condition, in an attempt to protect the patient from distress.
- With strong beliefs in family obligations and the expectation to conform to societal norms, social workers need to appreciate the role of family hierarchy and self-imposed sanctions on what people "ought to do" and "ought not to do." For instance, being at your parents' bed-side to witness the moment of death is part of a child's filial responsibility.
- Fear of ghosts, unquiet spirits, and their malevolent interest in the living is still strong in Hong Kong and not limited to only the elderly or less educated. This affects decisions about where people should die. Death

in a hospital is often preferred because it obviates two problems: the chance of a ghost remaining in residence and the reduction in the value of an apartment in which there has been a recent death. The recently bereaved are believed to carry bad luck and traditionally were unwelcome to visit the homes of family and friends for a period of months (Chan, 2009a; Reese, Chan, Perry, Wiersgalla, & Schlinger, 2005).

- The strong taboos associated with death make it very difficult for terminally ill patients and their relatives to have the conversations that they need to have in relation to practical issues like wills, funerals, and burial arrangements (Ho & Chan, in press). Even more difficult are discussions about feelings, such as expressing love and concern, asking for forgiveness, or apologizing. Chinese culture does not encourage open sharing of feelings; instead, affection tends to be expressed by small acts of kindness. For instance, preparing a favorite or nutritious soup is heavily laden with positive symbolism.

- As death nears, there are some things that may need to be said. Facilitating these sorts of conversations and helping family members to find resolution and closure are probably the most important contribution that a palliative social worker can make (Lee, Ng, Leung, & Chan, 2009).

- Social workers need to respect the patient's and family's values while offering opportunities to consider alternate ideas and values that might help patients and

families living with serious illness and coming to the end of life (Chan & Palley, 2005).

Integrative Intervention: The SET & GO Model

Culturally respectful palliative social work practice for Chinese patients empowers and supports them and their families in ways they consider appropriate. In our practice, we developed a model called SET & GO (see Fig. 62.1), which contains four major themes (Chan, Chan, Tin, Chan, & Ng, 2009; Chan, 2010):

S: Surviving the stress of impending death
E: Empowering individuals—living life to the fullest
T: Transforming the experience of loss into personal and spiritual growth
GO: Setting goals in life for bereaved people to *go on* with life

Chinese families feel no less than families from other cultures, but tradition does not encourage the expression of emotion. Chinese families may benefit from palliative social workers to sensitively assist them in determining how and whether they wish to address unfinished business, articulate interpersonal regrets, facilitate relational reconciliation, and leave a meaningful legacy for family members (Chan, 2009b; Chan, Chan et al., 2009).

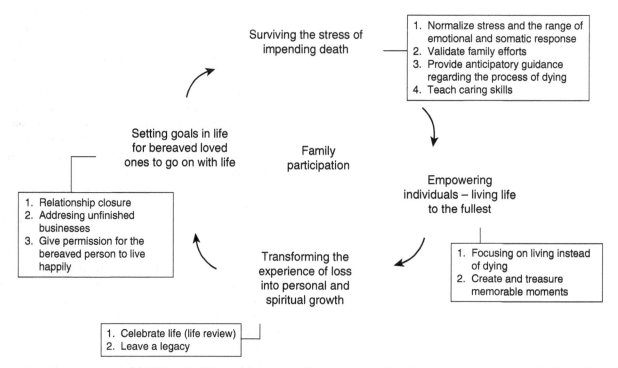

Figure 62.1. Intervention model: SET & GO. This model was created by the authors of this chapter. It can also be found in Chan, Chan, Tin, Chan, & Ng, 2009; Chan, 2010.

Surviving the Stress of Impending Death

Dying patients and their family caregivers may be overwhelmed by the demands of end-of-life decisions and anticipatory grief. Family members can harass patients with inappropriate offers of support, while patients struggle with the paradox of not wanting to be a burden yet desiring family help (Chan, Epstein, Reese, & Chan, 2009). Both sides typically want to do their best for the other without necessarily knowing how.

Social Work Interventions

Normalize stress and the range of emotional and somatic responses. It is not unusual for Chinese people to manifest stress through physical symptoms (somatization) like poor appetite, weight loss, and sleeping difficulties. They may be very accepting of traditional Chinese medical practices; therefore, discussions about using complementary and alternative medicine is often helpful (Ng, 2006). Palliative social workers should familiarize themselves with cultural common practices. For instance, ice cold drinks are considered harmful, so if a drink is offered at a clinic it shows sensitivity to produce a cup of hot water or milk-free tea.

Validate family efforts. Guilt is common among family caregivers if they cannot ease the patient's suffering. Recognizing that they have done all that is possible brings them comfort.

Providing anticipatory guidance regarding the process of dying. It is vital to educate the patients and their family about the usual trajectory of the illness and the emotional, behavioral, and physiological responses involved in both dying and watching a loved one die. Patients and family members can be invited to discuss where the patients would like to die, at home or in the hospital, as well as the advanced care plan. Yet these discussions should be carried out after considering the readiness of patients and family. By asking for patients' and family members' perception of the condition of the patients and their hopes and wishes, social workers can get an idea about how ready the patients and family members are to discuss death and dying. Discussion of dying may need to be introduced in a gradual way and with sensitivity. Chinese patients may want to fight to stay alive for as long as possible to fulfill their filial obligations. Advanced directives, such as no resuscitation, may be seen as "giving up," which is in conflict with an expected filial obligation to fight and to live as long as possible. Social workers need to discuss with the patient and the patient's family their concept of a good death and good comfort care and invite them to consider alternative ideas of fulfilling filial obligations, such as avoiding prolonged suffering. Respecting patients and their family's choices and offering opportunities to explore alternative values are very important before discussing advance care planning.

Teaching caring skills. Practical guidance on coping with physical symptoms such as constipation, breathlessness, pain, and fatigue is usually well received by Chinese patients who lean toward the practical, rather than the emotional. Direct teaching of caring skills such as turning, cleaning, dressing, simple massage, and exercises are typically welcomed by patients and their family members.

Empowering Individuals: Living Life to the Fullest

Terminally ill people may experience intense frustration and disappointment when they feel their life goals are unachievable. It is potentially more devastating to their well-being than the physical deterioration when a patient stops engaging in meaningful daily activities and gives up on enjoying life due to life goals being unachievable. Palliative social workers can ask the patient whether she or he would like to hear how other patients in a similar situation have found ways to make their last days fulfilling; social workers can also share testimonies of others who have fulfilled their aspirations in alternative and creative ways. Video stories of Chinese patients' experiences of death preparation, end-of-life decisions, and bereavement support can be found at the interactive platform on death education and bereavement adjustment of ENABLE (Empowerment Network of Adjustment to Bereavement and Loss in End-of-life): http://www.enable.hk/tch/main/index.aspx.

Social Work Intervention

Focus on living instead of dying. Living well is the objective. Actively look for meaningful and enjoyable things to do, like eating or tasting favorite foods (see Box 62.1). Eating is central to a good life in Chinese society, even when you are dying.

Create and treasure memorable moments. The filial obligation to be present at the moment of death of family members is significant, but tradition does not provide guidance about what to say or do. Remind family members that patients can still appreciate a warm and positive atmosphere, and that memorable moments from these last days will be important for them later. Activities around the sick bed can help patients and families, for example, playing cards and games, looking at old photograph albums, or watching favorite movies.

Transforming the Experience of Loss into Personal and Spiritual Growth

Confronting death often prompts a reappraisal of the meaning and value of life that may involve spiritual growth,

---

Box 62.1

Patient/Family Narrative: Mr. Ma, Age 59, with Terminal Lung Cancer–Living Life to the Fullest

Mr. Ma, with end-stage lung cancer, was an active member of a cancer patients' support group. He believed that a good death came with accepting one's death and living life fully. He enjoyed life every day and remained active socially even as his illness progressed. He went to daily qigong practice and actively participated in the patient support group's activities. The weekend before he died, he went lawn bowling with his group. Although too weak to play, Mr. Ma watched and chatted. The next day he went to eat roast goose with his friends, enjoying the taste despite his limited appetite. The day before his final hospital admission, he went to breakfast with his family. He died peacefully 2 days after the admission. Before his death, Mr. Ma was interviewed by the local media and asked to share what he had learned about living while dying, including maintaining social life, keeping daily exercise, and enjoying every moment Mr. Ma created many fond memories for those he left behind and was an inspiration for others.

Box 62.2

Patient/Family Narrative: Thomas and His Father, Age 70, with End-Stage Lung Cancer—Life Review and Leaving a Legacy

Thomas was away on a missionary trip when his father was diagnosed with terminal lung cancer. His father deliberately did not tell him the news. Upon his return, Thomas was shocked to learn his father was dying and decided to take a year's leave. He accompanied his father to Macau, his father's childhood home, sharing fond memories of the good old days and "spoiling" his father with his favorite food. Thomas produced a video of his fathers' life. His father was able to discuss the funeral arrangements with Thomas as well as asking him to look after his mother. Thomas' father died from heart failure in the hospital and maintained a good physical condition until the end. The video became a treasured legacy for Thomas and a testimonial to a well-lived life.

---

finding or building a stronger faith, or recognizing nature as a source of spiritual peace and comfort.

Social Work Intervention

Celebrating life (life review). Encourage visiting childhood haunts, reviewing photo albums, or producing a life-story book, family video, or Web page. All of these ways of reviewing and celebrating life can involve both patients and family members (Chan & Chan et al., 2009).

Leaving a legacy. Invite patients to share what they have learned about life with younger family members (Chan, 2009b). This act is part of the Chinese cultural imperative to transmit values and inculcate virtue in the next generation. Family members can also share their appreciation of how the patient will be a living legacy in their life. The story of Thomas and his father (Box 62.2) is an effective demonstration of how patients and family members can develop a sense of satisfaction through explicit appreciation of each other performing their filial duty.

Setting Goals in Life for Bereaved Loved Ones to Go on with Life

For many dying persons and their loved ones, a sense of proper closure and consensus about a continuing bond after death are important. It is helpful for palliative social workers to assess whether there is unfinished business that is related to expression of thanks, showing gratitude and appreciation, apologizing, or seeking reconciliation.

Social Work Intervention

Relationship closure. Chinese, especially elderly men, may find it especially hard to seek pardon and express appreciation. Yet articulation of love, forgiveness, and reconciliation may be essential to a satisfactory closure of intimate relationships before dying. When listening to patients' stories, social workers have to explore the meaning patients ascribe to significant events and important people in their lives. This helps social workers to assess whether relationship closure is an important issue to the patient and his or her family. Relationship closure can be verbal, symbolic, or through metaphor. Chinese people may use symbolic or nonverbal means such as passing on a special gift, a drawing/painting, or a letter. When the person is unavailable, patients can express themselves through writing, prayer, meditation, ritual, storytelling, or artwork. Palliative social workers are in the best position to encourage mutual appreciation and to facilitate communication and reconciliation to achieve relationship closure in culturally respectful ways (Box 62.3).

Addressing unfinished business. Fulfilling previous promises and discussing wills and funeral arrangements can help eliminate possible sources of regret, guilt, and self-blame. We find it helpful to share stories where family members found great relief, after discussing with patients their wishes regarding funeral arrangement before the death. Very often, patients find it helpful to hear and learn from others' experience. It is important that such sharing is used to offer alternative perspectives, while always respecting patients' decisions.

Giving permission for the bereaved person to live happily. Chinese widows may perceive life after bereavement as prolonged black widowhood. Ideally, the social worker needs to facilitate a conversation between the dying and the about-to-be-bereaved that gives permission to the former to die peacefully without struggling to extend life in ways that are painful and undignified; and permission to the latter to grieve for a seemly length of time and then move on with a happy and satisfying life. If open discussion of dying is not acceptable, the social worker needs to discuss with the bereaved person, after the patient's death, about giving oneself the permission to resume normal living. There is a common myth among bereaved persons that living a happy life after the death of a loved one means forgetting the deceased. It is important to let the bereaved person know that he or she can live a happy life while maintaining a continuing bond with the deceased.

Conclusion

Chinese cultural practices change, but the deep-seated values of filial obligations and family responsibilities have remained durable. Understanding these beliefs, priorities, and rituals can ensure that palliative social workers work with their Chinese families more effectively.

ACKNOWLEDGMENTS

This work was supported by funding from the Hong Kong Jockey Club Charities Trust; the Si Yuen Professorship in Social Work and Social Administration; and the General Research Fund, Research Grant Council, Hong Kong SAR Government (reference no.: 740909), and the CRGC Seed Funding Program for Basic Research, the University of Hong Kong (reference no.: 200902159002). We would also like to acknowledge Professor Veronica Pearson for her invaluable advice and all of the ENABLE team members (Dr. Amy Chow, Dr. Siuman Ng, Miss Celia Chan, Miss Agnes Tin, Dr. Wallace Chan, Miss Pandora Ng, Mr. Eric Leung, Miss Venus Wong, Miss Tonia Chan, and Mr. Andy Ho) for their support. Last, but not least, we are grateful to the patients and service users who granted permission for us to share their stories.

LEARNING EXERCISES

- *Breathing.* A simple technique that integrates breathing and chanting to generate a sense of calmness. Breathe in, smile, and slowly take the air deep down through the lungs and abdomen. When breathing out, let the air escape with a "ha" sound (or whatever sound feels comfortable). Do this 10 times, or as many times as you find soothing.
- *Forgiveness imagery.* Close your eyes and focus on your breathing. When it becomes steady and calm, visualize a soft, warm light cast over your whole body, filling you with love. Then imagine the light as a healing energy that nurtures acceptance and forgiveness from yourself or a person from whom you seek forgiveness.

Box 62.3
Patient Narrative: Mr. Shek, Age 64, Seeking Pardon and Relationship Closure

*Mr. Shek was diagnosed with lung cancer with brain metastasis. Except for a few friends, nobody visited him in the palliative care ward. In a conversation with the social worker, Mr. Shek shared some unfinished business—his desire to seek pardon from his wife and children whom he had abandoned 20 years previously to escape huge gambling debts. Knowing that he was dying, Mr. Shek's last wish was to seek forgiveness from his wife, despite having had no contact for 20 years. The social worker helped Mr. Shek in his search and simultaneously facilitated a process of relationship closure through guided imagery. Mr. Shek was asked to imagine that his wife and his two sons were present and to speak directly to them expressing his deep regret, his sincere apologies, his wish for them to lead **happy** lives, and to visualize sending them loving energy. This was tape-recorded so that the tape could be given to his wife when she was located. After this, Mr. Shek said that even though his wife was absent, he still felt better and had a great sense of relief at having done what he could.*

- *Create a "legacy" life-story book or video (e.g., for a parent or grandparent).* Ask the patient about his or her parents and grandparents, childhood, school, favorite toys or places to visit as a child, working life, memorable events, influential people, lessons learned from past failures and successes, and his or her life wisdom. This could become a treasured legacy for the family.

ADDITIONAL RECOMMENDED RESOURCES

ENABLE: http://www.enable.hk/tch/main/index.aspx
Interactive online platform in both English and Chinese on life and death education, with professionals, patients, and families sharing their stories regarding death bereavement.

ADDITIONAL SUGGESTED READING

Chan, C. L. W., Chan, C. H. Y., Tin, A. F., Chan, W. C. H., & Ng, P.O.K. (2009). *In celebration of life: A self-help journey on preparing a good death and living with loss and bereavement.* Hong Kong: Centre on Behavioral Health, the University of Hong Kong.

REFERENCES

Chan, C. L. W. (2009a). Chinese death taboos. In C. D. Bryant & D. L. Peck (Eds.) *Encyclopedia of death and the human experience* (Vol. 1, pp. 190–192). Thousand Oaks, CA: Sage.

Chan, C. L. W. (2009b). Living legacy. In D. L. Peck & C. D. Bryant (Eds.), *Encyclopedia of death and the human experience* (Vol. 2, pp. 666–668). Thousand Oaks, CA: Sage.

Chan, C. L. W. (2010). GET SET & GO in bereavement. In S. Keys (Ed.), *Where would you like your dishwasher? My story of life, love and loss* (pp. 226–242). Hong Kong: Haven Books.

Chan, C. L. W., Chan, C. H. Y., Tin, A. F., Chan, W. C. H., & Ng, P. O. K. (2009). *In celebration of life: A self-help journey on preparing a good death and living with loss and bereavement.* Hong Kong: Centre on Behavioral Health, the University of Hong Kong.

Chan, C. L. W., & Chow, A. Y. M. (Eds.). (2006). *Death, dying and bereavement: A Hong Kong Chinese experience.* Hong Kong: Hong Kong University Press.

Chan, C. L. W., & Palley, H. A. (2005). The use of traditional Chinese culture and values in social work health care related interventions in Hong Kong. *Health and Social Work, 30*(1), 76–79.

Chan, W. C. H., Epstein, I., Reese, D., & Chan, C. L. W. (2009). Family predictors of psychosocial outcomes among Hong Kong Chinese cancer patients in palliative care: Living and dying with the "support paradox." *Social Work in Health Care, 48*(5), 519–532.

Ho, A. H. Y., & Chan, C. L. W. (in press). Liberating bereaved persons from the oppression of death and loss in Chinese societies: Examples of public health approaches. In S. Conway (Ed.), *Governing death and loss: Empowerment, involvement and participation.* Oxford, England: Oxford University Press.

Lee, M. Y., Ng, S. M., Leung, P. P. Y., & Chan, C. L. W. (2009). *Integrative body-mind-spirit social work: An empirically based approach to assessment and treatment.* New York, NY: Oxford University Press.

Ng, S. M. (2006). The role of Chinese medicine in cancer palliative care. In C. L. W. Chan & A. Y. M. Chow (Eds.), *Death, dying and bereavement: A Hong Kong Chinese experience* (pp. 195–208). Hong Kong: Hong Kong University Press.

Reese, D., Chan, C. L. W., Perry, D., Wiersgalla, D., & Schlinger, J. (2005). Beliefs, death anxiety, denial, and treatment preferences in end-of-life care: A comparison of social work students, community residents and medical students. *Journal of Social Work in End-of-Life and Palliative Care, 1*(1), 23–47.

63

Cheng Wan Peh and Tzer Wee Ng

Palliative Social Work in Singapore

Other things may change us, but we start and end with the family.
—Anthony Brandt (as quoted in Thinkexist, 2009)

Key Concepts

♦ *Palliative care service delivery is based on the primary value of family as the unit of care.*
♦ *Culturally appropriate assessment is integral and essential.*
♦ *Culturally sensitive intervention tools enhance the clinical relationship and outcomes.*
♦ *Decision making and truth telling are collaborative processes that begin with family.*

Introduction

In Singapore, palliative social workers developed their unique set of culturally sensitive and appropriate assessment and intervention tools through their clinical experiences and use them to guide their practice in a multiracial and multicultural society. Their success in the formulation of assessment includes the important consideration of family taking precedence to patients in the context of decision making and truth telling. Their assessment process is also built on establishing a social worker–patient relationship that creates a nurturing platform for eliciting emotions through expressions that are often associated with cultural-specified language usages. In Singapore society, where family forms the basic unit of care, the intervention with patients has to be done within the context of families. The approaches also include creative ways of engaging patients and their families to do things together, both showing respect for the patient family bond and nurturing a patient–worker relationship on an informal platform that leads to therapeutic outcomes. Such creative interventions include the use of food and metaphors. The palliative social workers in Singapore continuously seek to develop a set of clinical competencies to grow the speciality and guide their service delivery.

Palliative Social Work in Singapore

Singapore is a multiethnic and multicultural Asian society. Our population of 5 million people is made up of 74.1% Chinese, 13.4% Malays, 9.2% Indians, and 3.3% from other ethnic groups (Statistics Singapore, 2010). With an aging population, Singapore is actively advocating for greater awareness and utilization of palliative care in order to better support individuals nearing the end of life. Currently, palliative care in Singapore is provided through palliative care consultation teams in acute hospitals as well as hospices. As of September 2009, five of Singapore's seven restructured hospitals have an established palliative care consultation team. The hospices provide three types of services, namely inpatient hospice care, home hospice care, and hospice day care. Singapore has eight hospice care providers of which only four provide inpatient hospice care. All hospices are run by nongovernmental organizations and are freestanding facilities in the community.

Palliative social work in Singapore is a relatively new and evolving area of specialty. Our core team in palliative care mainly consists of the physician, nurse, and medical social worker (MSW). It is the norm not to have a chaplain, psychologist, psychiatrist, music therapist, palliative care counselor, or bereavement care counselor as an integral part of the team. As such, MSWs are expected to identify and work on all issues of concern apart from medical and nursing care. A palliative MSW looks into financial, emotional, psychosocial, and spiritual aspects of care. In Singapore, where varied racial and cultural beliefs and practices exist, it is essential for MSWs to be culturally sensitive, versatile, and skillful workers with a good grasp of the subculture differences in the populations we serve.

Given the uniqueness of our population's makeup and culture, the remaining sections in this chapter will provide readers with some common issues that we encounter during assessment as well as culturally relevant intervention tools that were developed from our clinical practice.

Culturally Appropriate Assessment

Family-Oriented Society

In Singapore, the emphasis is on family as a basic unit of care. Family values and cultures, such as the responsibility of the family and kinship ties, are being emphasized in our social policies. Thus, our family-oriented society is an important factor to consider during our assessment.

Our patients have to be assessed within the context of their families. In Singapore, the family is made up of various groups of significant others such as a patient's parents, grandparents, children, siblings, nieces, nephews, and the in-laws (parents-in-law, siblings-in-law, grandparents-in-law, and children-in-law). As individuals in a family-oriented society, we are raised to stay close to or within the family. We are socialized to be interdependent within the family unit, to make decisions that benefit the family unit, and to make choices for, and in support of, the family unit. Often, family members' preferences are respected and prioritized over an individual's preferences. The needs of our family are placed above the needs of the self in our cultural context. The decision-making process is usually a collective one within the family, sometimes without consulting the patient.

In general, the most elderly person in the family hierarchy holds the authority and is treated with respect. These elderly figures are often looked upon as the decision makers, and their decisions are seldom challenged. In their absence or if they are the patients, the males in the families tend to take on this role.

Decision Making

It is culturally appropriate for health care professionals to approach family members to provide information and to assist with making decisions for patients. It is considered insensitive and inappropriate for any health care professional to go to a patient directly when the patient has a next of kin. When the patients are involved in the discussion, the decisions made by patients tend to be influenced by family members, even if the decision is against the patient's wish. Patients choose the path that maintains peace and harmony among family members. This is illustrated in Box 63.1, which is accompanied by a genogram, a clinical tool integrated into our routine practice.

Box 63.1
Patient/Family Narrative: Mr. R.

Mr. R., a 60-year-old Indian, was diagnosed with end-stage cancer. His wife and daughter were the only persons in his life. His wife is more than 30 years younger than he and came from India, spoke only Tamil, and had no friends or relatives in Singapore. Mr. R. was known to both the hospital and hospice palliative medical social workers (MSWs). In all the assessments conducted by the MSWs with Mr. R., it was clear that he wanted to die at home because he would like to be cared for by his wife and 5-year-old daughter.

In the course of working with Mr. R. and his wife, we found out that this was his third marriage. He was no longer in contact with his two ex-wives and children from previous marriages. He had cut off ties with his family of origin because they did not acknowledge his current marriage. They felt the marriage was inappropriate because Mr. R. and his third wife had vast differences in their economic status.

One day, Mr. R.'s siblings and cousins found out that Mr. R. was terminally ill and started to visit him in the hospital. Mr. R. shared with the palliative care team his resentment toward their sudden reappearance in his life. Shortly after, Mr. R.'s symptoms limited him in his expressions of his wishes and his siblings conveniently took over the decision-making power from his wife. They disregarded Mr. R.'s rights as the decision maker of his own care and his wife's position as the closest next of kin.

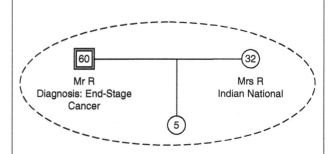

Figure 63.1. Genogram (immediate family I) of Mr. R

Box 63.1 *(Contd.)*

Although Mr. R. was very upset with his siblings' involvement, he decided not to confront or oppose them because he felt it was more important to maintain peace and harmony between those who would remain after his death: his siblings and his wife. He believed that attempts to placate his siblings would help ensure that his wife and child would continue to receive some form of support upon his death. Mr. R. eventually died in the hospital.

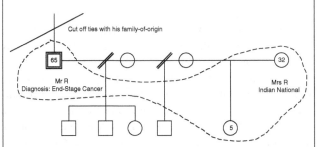

Figure 63.2. Genogram (immediate family II) of Mr. R

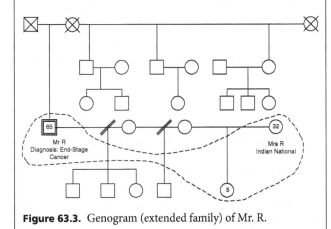

Figure 63.3. Genogram (extended family) of Mr. R.

Truth Telling

In a culture where truth telling involves not just the health care practitioners and patients but also the family members, the palliative care team members are often confronted with the challenge of dealing with collusion. It is common to find family members expressing discomfort about revealing the patient's diagnosis and/or prognosis to another family member, as illustrated in the patient/family narrative in Box 63.2.

We have also encountered family members who have expressed discomfort revealing the diagnosis and/or prognosis to the patient. This is illustrated by the patient/family narrative in Box 63.3.

Box 63.2
Patient/Family Narrative: Guan

Guan, a 48-year-old Chinese man, was diagnosed with cancer of the tongue. In view of his elderly mother's heart condition, his siblings made a collective decision not to tell her about Guan's illness despite objection from his wife. Guan went along with his siblings' decision, believing that it was in the best interest of his mother. To this day, Guan's death remains unknown to his mother.

Box 63.3
Patient/Family Narrative: Madame Lee

Madame Lee was a 58-year-old Chinese lady, who was diagnosed with lung cancer and presented with breathlessness and one-sided weakness. She verbalized concerns over her inability to get better and inquired about her illness. Upon admission, her three children instructed the hospice team not to reveal her diagnosis and prognosis to her because she was known to be a pessimistic person and would not be able to handle the bad news. They feared that she would give up hope and die sooner. The hospice team acknowledged their struggles and respected their special instructions. In the course of her stay, Madame Lee's condition quickly deteriorated and she started asking why she was not getting better. The hospice social worker attended to her feelings that resulted from the uncertainty and anxiety created by her unanswered questions. The conversations provided her the opportunity to explore and verbalize her thoughts and feelings surrounding her perception and intuitive understanding of why her family members were evasive in answering her questions. She also share that she thinks they were trying to hide bad news from her in attempt to protect her.

The Social Worker–Patient Relationship

We purposefully establish the social worker–patient relationship on an informal platform, bringing our skills and expertise in assessment and intervention into the relationship. Due to the intensity of the work involved at a stage where a patient and family members are being confronted with a crisis, we tend to become an integral part of the family system while dealing with the challenges. We reveal the vulnerable side of ourselves in front of patients and their family members. In the same way, they also put themselves in a vulnerable position as they allow us to walk into their lives, sharing their stories, thoughts, and feelings. The patient/family narrative in Box 63.4 illustrates a hospice social worker–patient relationship and its therapeutic effects.

Expression of Emotions

Expression of emotions among patients in Singapore may change with time. Greater exposure to Western culture

---

Box 63.4
Patient/Family Narrative: Mr. M.

Mr. M. was a 50-year-old Indian gentleman who was transferred from a destitute home to an inpatient hospice care for care of his terminal mouth cancer. He said he was not afraid of dying because he had no family members. Knowing his interests, the hospice social worker managed to place a fish tank next to his bed and set aside a plot of land for him to plant his favorite flowers in the hospice garden. One night, he had an episode of massive bleeding. The hospice team thought they were going to lose him. The hospice social worker asked whether he was afraid of seeing so much blood. He said he was not afraid. But he was sure that she was. They had a good laugh together. He added that he was sad to die because he now had a family—the hospice team. Mr. M. celebrated his fiftieth birthday with the hospice family before he passed away peacefully. The hospice social worker followed up with his funeral in accordance with his wishes for Hindu rituals.

---

among our younger generation may mean that future patients are more comfortable with expression of emotions. However, in the past three decades, we see a more conservative expression of emotions in our cultural context. Phrases like "I love you" and "Please forgive me" are seldom heard, and types of touch such as hugging are also less common than more distanced types of touch such as handshakes. An action like making sure the child has enough food and money to spend signifies parental love and concern. Screening questions for depression such as "Are you depressed?" may not be effective in eliciting an answer. Emotions are more commonly expressed through behaviors. Mood state and behavioral indicators of depression may be better psychological screens. For example, refusal of medication and food, becoming more quiet and withdrawn, and loss of interest in activities are good indicators to screen for depression.

Language

The expression of emotions is closely tied to language usage. Language forms the basis of transmitting cultural beliefs and practices. A culturally specific term could have a very different meaning in the context of another culture. Understanding the meaning and interpretation of different languages are crucial elements in the formulation of a thorough and objective assessment.

The ways we greet and address the elders are significant in conveying our respect for them. Hence, we often greet our elderly patients and their family members using culturally appropriate languages such as "popo," "ah em," "makcik," and "pathi" (for Cantonese-speaking, Hokkien-speaking, Malay-speaking, and Indian-speaking elderly ladies, respectively). Our patients and family members in turn

address us by our first name in their respective languages. For patients or family members who are much younger than the social workers, they often address us as "jie jie," "Kakak," and "akah" ("elder sister" in Chinese, Malay, and Tamil, respectively).

Culturally, across the various ethnic groups and their subcultures, there are similarities in the choice of words patients and families use to discuss issues surrounding death and dying. The words "die" and "death" are seldom used in conversations. Instead, we use culturally specific descriptions that require fairly in-depth understanding and appreciation. Among the Hokkien-speaking Chinese community, for instance, it is very common to use descriptions such as "aged away" and "hand in identification card." This is directly meaningful in the sense that upon death, we need to surrender our country identification card to the police as part of the procedures required when reporting a death. Our Cantonese-speaking community typically uses "passed away at a hundred years old" as a respectful way of communicating about the death or impending death of an elderly person. Similarly, it is culturally more common for our Malay and Indian communities to use phrases such as "Jika saya tiada lagi" (If I am no longer around) and "Go up" or "It's time already," respectively, when having conversations surrounding death and dying. Having a good knowledge and grasp of the language usage in the various cultures are powerful tools in engaging and assessing patients and families in their respective culture and context.

Culturally Sensitive Intervention Tools

Working within the Context of Families

It is culturally imperative for us to formulate our assessment and intervention within the context of families. We often have to work with patients through their families, and this forms part of the challenge of our intervention. The follow-up on the earlier patient and family narrative about Madame Lee (see Box 63.5) illustrates this point.

Doing versus Being

In the eyes of the older generations, social workers are more commonly perceived as the "Welfare Department" in which our roles are limited to financial and practical aspects of care. And in the eyes of the younger generations, social workers are often mistaken for volunteers. With the evolvement of social work in Singapore, unspoken expectations from our patients and their families regarding our assessment and intervention plans have also developed with time. Social workers are perceived as helpful only when we help the people we serve secure some tangible benefits. In some

---

Box 63.5
Patient/Family Narrative: Madame Lee (continued)

Not long after, the medical social worker initiated a family conference with Madame Lee's three children to talk about concerns surrounding truth telling. This meeting provided a platform for the hospice team to help address family members' concerns and fears, which led to the family's consent for the team to be present to provide support and facilitation when the eldest daughter shared the diagnosis and prognosis with their mother. Although there was expression of emotions through crying and exchange of words, they also expressed feelings of relief in not having to carry the burden of hiding the truth anymore. Subsequently, Madame Lee was able to share her own treatment preferences and wishes for her funeral and last rites.

Box 63.6
Patient/Family Narrative: Madame Daisy

Madame Daisy, a 78-year-old Indian, was referred to the social worker for psychoemotional support in dealing with her end-of-life issues. She shared that she could not bear to leave her family because she has a wonderful family, but at the same time understood that death is inevitable. The social worker suggested leaving behind something for her family to remember. After sharing more about her life, Madame Daisy decided to leave behind a "family recipe." Using food as a tool, the social worker worked with Madame Daisy on her choice of dishes to be included in the family recipe, the significance and meaning of the dishes, and eventually her hopes for the family. After the death of Madame Daisy, the family was presented with the booklet, and it contributed to the family's healthy adaptation in bereavement.

---

ways, the tangible benefits secured by social workers tend to hold similar meanings as those given by family members. However, tangible benefits given by social workers are not perceived as acts of love, but more as acts of concern. In our cultural context, benefits from counseling and emotional support are perceived as intangible and thus are given lower priorities. Performing simple tasks like filling out an application form, escorting the patient to the hospital, or helping the patient run errands are considered social work interventions. Perhaps such tasks may not fall within the professional scope of the social worker in some other culture and are perceived as unnecessary or unskilled manual tasks. However, in our context, performance of such tasks would allow the patient to experience the personal touch and genuineness of the social worker. It is a therapeutic and powerful strategy to build bonds and deepen professional ties with the patients to pave the way for further therapeutic intervention.

Food

In many cultures, people "eat to live." In Singapore, people often "live to eat," with food having an additional significance and meaning. Being able to share a meal together is a very powerful way of bringing two parties together. Our patients and families feel less comfortable and more restrained when communicating in formal settings. It is common for us to inject flexibility and creativity in our engagement with them over meals or coffee. Interventions of such a nature are often therapeutic. Food serves as a very good entry point and platform for relationship building. We also purposefully integrate it as a tool for patients and families to tell their story, and in the process (see Box 63.6), life review takes place. Food often becomes a form of attachment for us and is a powerful intervention tool throughout the continuum of one's life and intensifies toward end of life.

Use of Metaphors

We highlighted the importance of using culturally specific language in our assessment. It is common for our patients to be indirect in conveying what is on their mind by either dropping hints or using metaphors. The palliative social worker needs to listen, think critically, and be culturally sensitive to understand, elicit, or surface the underlying issues of concern, which would in turn inform the intervention (see Box 63.7).

The following brief dialogue between a palliative social worker and Mandarin-speaking patient, Mr. Tan, illustrates a conversation about death and dying using culturally unique words (translated from Mandarin to English) that are used as an intervention tool:

Social worker: Can you tell me what is going on in your mind?
Mr. Tan: Look at me. My legs are swelling and I have no appetite at all.
I think it will not be long before I go and sell preserved duck eggs.
Social worker: Can you share more about your thoughts surrounding your time being close to selling preserved duck eggs?
(Note: To "sell preserved duck eggs" is a common cultural euphemism for death.)

Conclusion

Palliative social workers in Singapore need a unique set of clinical competencies to guide their work in a multiethnic and multicultural society. The need to conduct culturally appropriate assessment and intervention, coupled with the expectation to apply basic knowledge and skills from psychology to spirituality counseling, calls for great flexibility and creativity. Yet no competencies or practice standards exist for delineating the

Box 63.7
Patient/Family Narrative: Mr. Ng

Mr. Ng, 78 years old, was single and worked as a trishaw rider. He was referred to the palliative social worker for care issues after he was diagnosed with advanced cancer. Mr. Ng described himself as a "sparrow." There is a Chinese idiom that describes a sparrow as small but having all it needs for survival. He described that even though a sparrow is small, we cannot underestimate its ability to lead a simple, but fulfilling and carefree life. He then emphasized that it was important for the sparrow to find a home. That was actually his way of conveying to the social worker about his needs: His top priority was finding a place of care for himself because he was no longer able to manage self-care.

skills and appropriate flexibility and creativity necessary in the practice of palliative social work in Singapore. Palliative social work is a young but growing specialty in health care social work in Singapore. We see leadership, mentoring, creativity in assessment, and interventions as crucial elements in the development of a set of clinical competencies in palliative social work service delivery that would guide future directions for palliative social work in Singapore.

ACKNOWLEDGMENT

The authors would like to thank Ivan Mun Hong Woo, senior research executive with Lien Centre for Palliative Care, Duke-NUS Graduate Medical School Singapore, for his assistance in the completion of this manuscript.

LEARNING EXERCISES

- *Use of food as intervention tool.* Bring to class a type of food that has a symbolic meaning to you or your family. Share with the class the significance and meaning of it within your culture and within the history of your family.
  Reflection: What is it like for you as you processed a decision about the food item? What does the food item remind you of? How comfortable are you in talking about food? What was it like to talk to someone about food? What was easy or difficult?
- *Truth telling and working within the context of families.* The family genogram presented in Figure 63.4 is a graphic illustration of a new patient, Mr. Soh, assigned to you.

Mr. Soh has just been recently admitted through the emergency department. After thorough investigations, doctors diagnose pancreatic cancer with a prognosis of less than 3 months. Prior to his admission, he had no signs of being ill, not to mention having a terminal illness. The doctor spoke with Lawrence, his son, who told him not to reveal the truth to Mr. Soh because he is worried that he "might not be able to take it" at his advanced age and might deteriorate faster.

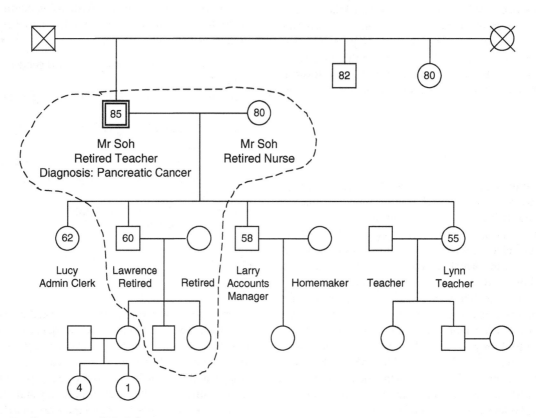

Figure 63.4. Family genogram of Mr. Soh

You are the palliative social worker assigned to work with Mr. Soh and his family members.

Questions:

(i) How would you formulate your assessment of the issues you are dealing with while bearing in mind the importance of the family as a unit?

(ii) How would you engage Mr. Soh in conversations surrounding his awareness and coping with his serious illness? What would be the considerations in guiding your interventions in truth telling?

(iii) How would you manage the challenges of respecting the patient's wishes and the family's request to keep the diagnosis from Mr. Soh?

ADDITIONAL RESOURCES

READINGS

Beng, A. K. L., Fong, C. W., Shum, E., Goh, C. R., Goh, K. T., & Chew, S. K. (2009). Where the elderly die: The influence of socio-demographic factors and cause of death on people dying at home. *Annals Academy of Medicine, 38*(8), 676–683.

Goh, C. R. (2008). Challenges of cultural diversity. In J. Beattles & S. Goodlin (Eds.), *Supportive care in heart failure* (pp. 451–461). New York, NY: Oxford University Press.

Goh, C. R. (2008). Culture, ethnicity and illness. In T. D. Walsh, A. T. Caraceni, R. Fainsinger, K. M. Foley, P. Glare, C. Goh, M. Lloyd-Williams, J. N. Olarte, & L. Redbruch (Eds.), *Palliative medicine* (pp. 51–54). Philadelphia, PA: Saunders Elsevier.

Tong, C. K. (2004). *Chinese death rituals in Singapore*. London, England: RoutledgeCurzon.

Woo, I. M. H., & Ow, R. (2007). Hope among terminally ill patients in Singapore: An exploratory study. *Social Work in Health Care, 45*(3), 85–106. doi:10.1300/J010v45n03_05.

WEB SITES

COMMUNITY PALLIATIVE CARE SERVICE PROVIDERS

Agape Methodist Hospice: http://www.mws.org.sg/
Assisi Hospice: http://www.assisihospice.org.sg/

Bright Vision Hospital: http://www.bvh.org.sg/
Dover Park Hospice: http://www.doverpark.org.sg/
HCA Hospice Care: http://www.hca.org.sg/
Metta Hospice Care: http://metta.org.sg/
Singapore Cancer Society: http://www.singaporecancersociety.org.sg/
St. Joseph's Home and Hospice: http://www.stjh.org.sg/

SOCIAL WORK PROGRAMS IN SINGAPORE

Monash University: http://www.med.monash.edu.au/bsw/bsw-singapore.html
National University of Singapore: http://www.fas.nus.edu.sg/swk
SIM University: http://www.unisim.edu.sg

PROFESSIONAL SOCIAL WORK ASSOCIATION IN SINGAPORE

Singapore Association of Social Workers: http://www.sasw.org.sg/site/

OTHERS

Lien Foundation: http://lienfoundation.org/PalliativeCare.htm
Ministry of Community Development, Youth and Sports: http://www.mcys.gov.sg
Ministry of Health: http://www.moh.gov.sg
Singapore Hospice Council: http://singaporehospic.org.sg/

REFERENCES

Statistics Singapore. (2010). *Census of population 2010: advance census release*. Retrieved from http://www.singstat.gov.sg/pubn/popn/C2010acr.pdf

Thinkexist. (2009). *Anthony Brandt quotes*. Retrieved from http://thinkexist.com/quotes/anthony_brandt/

64 *Malcolm Payne and Margaret Reith*

Palliative Social Work in the United Kingdom

She's made me value my own life, value the importance of my life and made me feel important as an individual which was lacking and which was very important to me...
— *Beresford, Adshead, & Croft (2007, p. 122)*

Key Concepts

- *Palliative care in the United Kingdom is integrated with the U.K. National Health Service.*
- *Government policy is to transfer expertise drawn from palliative care services for people with advanced illness into end-of-life care for all citizens approaching the end of life.*
- *Palliative social work in the United Kingdom is centered on a network of in-patient hospices, most of which also provide community palliative care.*
- *Palliative care teams in hospitals may also include social workers.*
- *The palliative social work emphasis on interpersonal practice contrasts with the mainly administrative care management role of most social workers in adult social care services in the United Kingdom.*

Introduction

Palliative care services in the United Kingdom are integrated within the National Health Service (NHS), an executive agency of the U.K. governments. Policy, law, and administration differ slightly between the U.K. constituent nations: England, Northern Ireland, Scotland, and Wales, following the policies of the separate parliaments or legislative assemblies in each. The largest country with the greatest resources, England, and its Department of Health (DH), has strong policy and professional influence. The patient narrative in Box 64.1 provides a picture of the typical organization of palliative care services as part of the NHS, with which social work and social care services are connected. It shows a system in which most palliative care is provided in independent not-for-profit hospices, which connect with generalist palliative care provided by community health services and provide support and advice to medical teams working with sick people in hospitals.

The National Institute for Health and Clinical Excellence (NICE) is an independent agency funded by the DH to provide advice on professional standards in health care. Primary care trusts (PCTs) use it to determine appropriate standards of service for the NHS. In 2004, after extensive multiprofessional consultation, it published a manual of guidance (NICE, 2004) and associated costing and research reviews, available on the World Wide Web http://www.nice.org.uk/nicemedia/pdf/csgspmanual.pdf, which provides the basis for financing and organizing palliative care services.

Palliative Social Work and Social Care

Most of the approximately 100,000 registered social workers in the United Kingdom are employed in local government "social care" services. Social workers are also employed in a variety of private and not-for-profit agencies offering residential, day, and domiciliary services for various client groups, although most hands-on care is provided by less highly qualified practitioners called social care workers.

Box 64.1
Patient/Family Narrative: Shirina

Shirina, a 36-year-old Indian woman living in south London, is concerned that she may have a recurrence of cervical cancer. Like nearly all U.K. residents, she is registered with an independent family doctor (a general practitioner, or GP) who contracts with the National Health Service (NHS) to provide most health treatment and care for people registered with him and to organize access to other NHS care. He and his team will retain coordinating responsibility for Shirina's care throughout treatment by any other part of the NHS. She telephones the surgery (the doctor's workbase) that he shares with a group of other GPs in a health center provided by the local administration of the NHS, in England a primary care trust (PCT). As required by government NHS policy, she receives an appointment at he surgery within 48 hours. Her GP refers her for tests at the local hospital. NHS policy dictates that patients who may have cancer get an appointment for tests within 2 weeks; the results are e-mailed to her GP. When he sees her again the next day, he confirms that her cancer has returned and offers referral to a specialist oncology team. Through the Internet, he books an appointment at the local hospital of her choice.

A course of treatment, which includes a combination of radiotherapy and chemotherapy, is unsuccessful, and her oncology team refers her to the south London site of the Royal Marsden Hospital, a specialist cancer hospital, where she has greater opportunity to benefit from experimental treatments. These are unsuccessful, and her local hospital again provides outpatient treatment. This time, however, alongside attempts to limit the progress of disease, she is referred to the hospital palliative care team, one of 345 hospital support services nationally (Help the Hospices, 2009) for help in managing what is likely to be a dying process. They get in touch with the GP, who will be providing nonspecialist palliative care, including home visits along with the PCT's team of district nurses. After a period, Shirina's worsening condition leads him to refer her to the home care team of the local hospice, one of 217 hospices and palliative care inpatient units in the United Kingdom providing specialist palliative care and offering a total of 3194 beds. The hospice's community nurse specialist (CNS) assesses and then visits regularly, providing advice on pain and symptom management. This is the usual approach to basic care in the 308 home care services nationally. The hospice's multiprofessional team in turn supports her, including specialist palliative care physicians, nurses (the majority staff group), social workers, physical and other specialist therapists, and a spiritual care practitioner. For a while, Shirina attends the hospice day center, one of 279 nationally, which provides a range of artistic and social opportunities (Hartley & Payne, 2008); this also facilitates nurse, physician, and treatment appointments.

Eventually, on a further admission to the hospital for symptom management, Shirina is considered to be within a few days of death. Although many people are cared for in their own home by hospice home care teams and GPs and their teams, due to her worsening symptoms she is referred to the hospice inpatient unit, where 3 days later she is placed on the Liverpool Care Pathway. This is a care program that helps staff manage the last 48 hours of life effectively, and it is widely used in both hospitals and hospices (Ellershaw & Ward, 2003). She dies 36 hours later.

All these services and medications provided by the hospital are free of charge, paid from general taxation, and administered by the NHS. When her GP prescribes medication, Shirina pays a per-item subsidized charge at the local pharmacy. In south London, as in most of the United Kingdom, hospice care is provided free of charge by a network of not-for-profit organizations, administered by independent charitable companies. Hospices receive contributions from their local PCTs in return for contracting to provide palliative care services for their area; about 32% of hospice funding is provided in this way; the rest of the £730 million of hospice annual expenditure is provided through charitable donations and fund-raising. A few large hospices are major specialist centers, while many are smaller in scale, providing local community service; some only provide home care. Since most palliative care services are independent, the pattern of administrative arrangements varies across the country, but there are usually close links between GP and community nonspecialist palliative care clinicians and hospital and hospice palliative care services.

These services are either provided directly by local government "councils" or on contract by private or not-for-profit organizations.

Palliative social work is among a number of professional specialties in U.K. social work. Most practitioners are employed by hospices or hospital palliative care teams and move into the specialty after experience in local government or hospital social work. A majority of palliative social workers, about 400, are members of the Association of Palliative Care Social Workers. The NICE (2004) guidance manual reviews positive research support for incorporating social work within specialist palliative care multiprofessional teams, and it confirms the importance of incorporating psychological, social, spiritual, family, and bereavement support within palliative care services. This manual provided an authoritative basis for including social work in palliative care.

Most people in the United Kingdom would understand social work as a function of their local government council, which provides what are called social care services for people with chronic sickness, physical, or intellectual disabilities; mentally ill people; and older people. Adult social care departments of the council covering the locality are the usual providers. Most older and disabled people using palliative care services would already be receiving or would be referred for social care services from palliative care. Social care services include social work help, residential and day care, adaptations to the home, and assistive technology to help with managing disability or frailty. Domiciliary care services provide for visits by caregivers to assist with everyday practical tasks such as washing, dressing, and shopping. Meals may be delivered or prepared by domiciliary caregivers. See Payne (2009) for more extensive discussion of adult social care. Palliative social workers, by contrast, focus more on psychosocial reactions to illness among patients and their families, and the needs of family and other informal caregivers.

The main role of social workers in the adult social care system is "care management," carrying out assessments of people's needs and arranging packages of care for adults, who are usually called "service users" rather than "clients"; palliative social workers would call on care managers to organize the provision of social care services for people that they work with. Local government adult social care practitioners also assist people with the practical and emotional effects of disabilities or illnesses and consequent changes in their lives, but assessment is the main role. "Personalization" has developed, where service users receive cash payments for their care; here, social workers may act as advisers and "brokers" to service users and their families in deciding on their care arrangements.

Most hospices have a palliative social work team, whose members are also attached to inpatient, day care, and community multiprofessional teams responsible for complex psychosocial care needs that cannot be met by physicians and nursing staff. It is a particularly important role where families experience severe deprivation and family conflict. They often provide access to information, advice, and support in applying for social security and other practical benefits. A few larger hospices have welfare rights departments employing specialist staff to undertake this role; other hospital or hospice palliative care services may have an arrangement for support in this task by Citizens Advice, a not-for-profit agency specializing in legal and general advice (Levy & Payne, 2006). Social work teams usually also organize a bereavement service, often by recruiting, training, and supervising volunteer bereavement support workers. Social workers may take responsibility for more complex bereavement needs. In addition to individual social work help to patients and families, many social work teams offer groups for patients, family caregivers, and bereaved family members (Firth, 2005).

Palliative social work focuses first on facilitating communication among family members affected by the patient's illness and quite often on helping children come to an understanding of the approaching death of a family member who is important to them. Members of the family may find clinical work that focuses on interpersonal tasks at the end of life useful. For example, Saunders (Earnshaw Smith, 1990) emphasized working on the tasks of saying "goodbye," "I love you," "thank you" for care and support, and "sorry" for real or imagined difficulties in their relationships. A second focus is help in deciding how to manage care and responsibilities within the family and integrating this with formal care services. An aspect of this may be arranging social care packages in patients' homes as they become increasingly frail or disabled, or planning and arranging admission to a care or nursing home. A third issue may be anticipating family life and care arrangements after the death of the patient; this may include concerns for child care or the care of other vulnerable adults such as older relatives or people with intellectual disabilities. This is especially important where difficult family relationships or social deprivation are having an impact on the patient's care. As part of the multiprofessional team, social workers make a particular contribution in responding to social issues, such as concerns about abuse or neglect of

vulnerable adults where a recent U.K. prevalence study shows that up to 4% of older people experience physical neglect or financial abuse in any given year (Payne, 2008). Social workers may also help with issues arising from cultural difference and discrimination because of race, gender, or other prejudices. Research shows that the responsiveness, flexibility, and focus on family and personal issues in palliative social work are appreciated by patients and their families (Beresford et al., 2007; Clausen et al, 2005).

Some hospices also employ clinical psychologists, counselors, or psychiatrists to treat mental illness among patients or family members, but the majority of staff providing specialist psychosocial care are social workers (Price, Hotopf, Higginson, Monroe, & Henderson, 2006). A few hospices have a care manager seconded from the local council to facilitate arrangements for social care.

General practitioners (GPs) providing nonspecialist palliative care and hospital palliative care teams usually do not have access to a social worker on their own team. General practitioners refer patients needing social care services to their local council, and there may be formal liaison arrangements. Hospitals often have local council care managers working on site, and palliative care teams refer patients needing services to them. Some hospital palliative care teams include a social worker, whose role is similar to that of hospice social work. The following case study (Box 64.2) illustrates the role of specialist palliative social workers in hospice and hospital settings.

End-of-Life Care Developments

Palliative care developed mainly for cancer patients, although services for people with other conditions such as the end stages of chronic obstructive pulmonary disease, heart disease, and neurological conditions have increased recently (Addington-Hall & Higginson, 2001). Government policy has recently moved to transfer specialist palliative care expertise with patients who have a diagnosed advanced illness to focus on end-of-life care for the whole population, particularly older people who are becoming frail or who have long-term disabling conditions. This move recognizes that specialist palliative care is only provided for a small proportion of persons living with life-threatening illness and imminent death, and most people who do not have a diagnosed major illness do not receive an equal level or quality of care. The End-of-life Care Strategy for England has been influential (DH, 2008). This aims for practitioners in nonspecialist palliative care and in social care to have training in communication and care planning to help people achieve a satisfactory end-of-life experience. Another objective is to reduce the emergency admission of people dying at home or in care homes to hospital for end-of-life care, since a busy acute care environment is often inappropriate for their needs. Therefore, important elements of the end-of-life care strategy are

---

Box 64.2
Patient/Family Narrative: Fay and Family

Fay, age 45, was diagnosed with secondary breast cancer 2 years ago. She is married to Harry, with two children, Robert, 10, and Chloe, 12. Until 2 weeks ago, Fay was receiving a new trial drug to arrest progression of her disease. Although the children had lived with their mother's illness for some time, they did not know how serious her disease was and believed that the new drug would work.

Fay was admitted to hospital with pain and vomiting. She was also incontinent and very weak. The hospital palliative care team was asked to review Fay's symptom management. The team could see that Fay was dying and needed to help the whole family face this. First, it was essential to talk with both Fay and Harry. The palliative social worker explained her role and asked how things were going for Fay and her family. Fay was finding it hard to talk but indicated that she would like Harry and the social worker to talk at her bedside. The main focus of this discussion was to understand what Fay thought was happening, how Harry was coping with her deterioration, and how much and what the children had been told.

Harry was taking time off work to visit Fay during school hours; the children were reluctant to visit their mother in hospital. Both children were about to go on a week's holiday with their aunts and cousins, and the family had decided it would be better if the children went away as planned. Although adults in the family knew that Fay might die quite soon, no one could be open about it, so it is not surprising that the children were not being prepared for their mother's death. Harry had been waiting for the children to ask questions because he did not want to "upset" them by telling them that the drug did not seem to be working, especially just before their holiday. Well-meaning family members were encouraging him to delay telling the children, thus supporting his belief that he would achieve nothing by talking about their mother's death before they left. It also became clear that Fay's recently widowed and isolated mother was struggling with her daughter's illness and needed to be offered support. Fay's brother was not visiting her at all, leading other family members to judge him as uncaring and selfish, thereby creating additional tension in the family.

By actively discussing these issues, the social worker was able to help Harry to see that ultimately he could not protect the children from losing their mother but could engage them in the family process of caring and planning for the future together. By not talking with his children, he was risking their trust and ability to count on him, the one remaining parent in their lives. There would never be "a right time." He felt burdened by having to make decisions on their behalf. While troubled about the holiday plans, he was carried along with family encouragement. Exploring these decisions, Harry could see that his reasoning was flawed, and he said he would go home and talk honestly to the children that evening. The social worker suggested that the children could be asked to make their own choices about the holiday and that the burden that Harry felt could be shared. The dynamics in the family changed dramatically once this block was removed. Support was offered and accepted by Fay's mother and brother, and all family members were able to support each other, share their sadness openly, and say their goodbyes.

---

developing appropriate support to people dying in care homes. For example, the Gold Standards Framework (GSF) (http://www.goldstandardsframework.nhs.uk/) provides training and management support to GP practices and care homes, permitting them to register and promote their expertise in nonspecialist support for dying people (GSF, 2009).

Creative Arts

Because enabling creativity to achieve personal fulfillment is an important part of helping older people, social workers and others intervene to assist elders to develop skills and interests in later life. Through education and program planning, this has become an important objective of social care services. Increasingly, therefore, creative arts are used in palliative care services, and this may be extended to social work, which can help clients record life histories, undertake creative writing, and use memory boxes to build interpersonal relationships with relatives that will maintain continuing bonds after bereavement (Reith & Payne, 2009).

Advance Care Planning

The development of advance care planning has emerged from a number of initiatives. Palliative care services have considerable experience with advance directives (see chapter 69), which allow patients to give instructions for limiting medical intervention near the end of life, if they became unable to communicate their wishes. The Mental Capacity Act 2005 takes this further by requiring all health and social care services to facilitate and enhance the mental capacity of all patients and clients to give informed consent for their care and treatment. People may authorize, in advance of losing mental capacity, a relative, friend, or official to act on their behalf either in health and welfare or in finance and property matters by conferring "lasting powers of attorney" (Department for Constitutional Affairs, 2007). The preferred priorities for care (PPC) program enables health and social care service users to specify in advance the care arrangements that best suit their needs. In the long term, the intention is for people to carry with them constantly updated documents that express their wishes and preferences in personal and health care decisions and authorize action to meet their needs (Henry & Seymour, 2007). Social work interventions can enable people to think through their life objectives using these processes, as the narrative in Box 64.3 shows.

Bereavement Services

Bereavement services are an important role of social work in palliative care. Experience in this field has led to palliative

Box 64.3
Patient Narrative: Annie

Annie, age 88, lived alone with no surviving relatives. She was diagnosed with a glioma, an aggressive brain tumor, but declined treatment, believing that this might prolong her life without necessarily improving its quality. She was not afraid of dying but feared losing control over her life, by losing her independence, mobility, speech, and other faculties. At her request she was referred to the local hospice palliative care team and the social worker helped her to arrange her affairs so that if or when she lost capacity, her wishes would be documented and known by all services and agencies caring for her. With the social worker's help, she sought admission to the care home of her choice, taking with her an advance care plan documenting her wish to have no life-prolonging interventions, but to be kept comfortable and to die with peace and dignity. The social worker visited her weekly, and when Annie could no longer talk, she found it possible to communicate with her through using preprepared cue cards. With her knowledge of Annie's life story, she was able to develop ways of communicating using narrative, photographs, and other artefacts and closed questions to maintain contact. It was also important to acknowledge with Annie her huge sense of frustration and anger once she had lost her speech. The social worker was also able to liaise with staff in the home and ensure that her wishes were implemented at the end of her life.

social work influencing wider bereavement initiatives in health care and community bereavement services both for children and for adults. Bereavement clinicians have increasingly expanded their role to provide wider public education and support when public disasters, combined with social and cultural isolation, require interventions designed to prevent posttraumatic stress disorders among people affected by untoward events in today's increasingly complex social life. Among examples of this were bereavement support services in football stadium disasters in the 1980s and 1990s and in railway and natural disasters in the 1990s and early 2000s (Reid, Field, Payne, & Relf, 2006).

Conclusion

Social work and social services have been an important aspect of palliative care in the United Kingdom. The three major areas of practice have been help with practical and social security benefits, development of bereavement services, and psychosocial help to patients and families, strengthening family relationships through interpersonal practice. Social work has cemented a role in palliative care because of this family and social focus, in contrast to the primarily individualistic practice of health care services and other psychosocial helping professions (Reith & Payne, 2009). The family and interpersonal focus of palliative social work has had an important role in maintaining expertise in

interpersonal psychological help as part of social work (Payne, 2006).

Thus, palliative social work in the United Kingdom has established a valuable role in U.K. health care. Alongside a number of other social work specialties, it has maintained a wide conception of the psychosocial role of social work within care provision. This contrasts with the more limited, care management focus of social work within local government adult social care. In this way, palliative social work makes a specific contribution to palliative care, and by doing so enhances and develops the understanding of social work as a profession in the United Kingdom.

ADDITIONAL RESOURCES

WEB SITES

Association of Palliative Care Social Workers: http://www.apcsw.org.uk/welcome/
British Association of Social Workers: http://www.basw.co.uk/
The professional association for social workers in the United Kingdom has little involvement in palliative care.
Department of Health: http://www.dh.gov.uk/en/Healthcare/IntegratedCare/Endoflifecare/index.htm
The Web site of the main government department, this is a large and constantly changing but searchable Web site. A good place to start is the end-of-life care strategy page.
Help the Hospices: http://www.helpthehospices.org.uk/
Represents not-for-profit palliative care organizations.
Hospice Information: http://www.helpthehospices.org.uk/hospiceinformation/
This is a joint project of the national organization Help the Hospices and St Christopher's Hospice. Readers can sign up for a print bulletin and e-mail newsletters covering the United Kingdom, international issues, and education and training courses.
National Council for Palliative Care: http://www.ncpc.org.uk/
Covers not-for-profit and state palliative care.
NHS Evidence: Palliative and Supportive Care: http://www.library.nhs.uk/PALLIATIVE/ViewResource.aspx?resID=70692
This is a database of practice evidence in palliative care, supplied by the NHS for its staff.
Social Care Online: http://www.scie-socialcareonline.org.uk/default.asp
This is the search Web site of the Social Care Institute for Excellence, which offers a database covering the international literature on social work and social care topics, with an emphasis on U.K. interests; you can sign up for a regular update.

SUGGESTED READINGS

NICE. (2004). *Palliative and supportive care: The manual.* London, England: National Institute for Health and Clinical Excellence.
The manual of U.K. standards in palliative and supportive care, including the role of social work.

Reith, M., & Payne, M. (2009). *Social work in end-of-life and palliative care*. Chicago, IL: Lyceum.
Text on practice by the present authors, based on U.K. experience.

REFERENCES

Addington-Hall, J. M., & Higginson, I. J. (Eds.). (2001). *Palliative care for non-cancer patients*. Oxford, England: Oxford University Press.

Beresford, P., Adshead, L., & Croft, S. (2007). *Social work, palliative care and service users: Making life possible*. Philadelphia, PA: Jessica Kingsley.

Clausen, H., Kendall, M., Murray, S., Worth, A., Boyd, K., & Benton, F. (2005). Would palliative care patients benefit from social workers' retaining the traditional "casework" role rather than working as care managers? A prospective serial interview study. *British Journal of Social Work, 35*, 277–285.

Department of Constitutional Affairs. (2007). *Mental Capacity Act 2005: Code of Guidance*. London, England: TSO.

Department of Health. (2008). *End of life care strategy: Promoting high quality care for all adults at the end of life*. London, England: Department of Health. Retrieved from http://www.dh.gov.uk/prod_consum_dh/groups/dh_digitalassets/@dh/@en/documents/digitalasset/dh_086345.pdf

Earnshaw Smith, E. (1990). Editorial: The hospice social worker in the multiprofessional team. *Palliative Medicine, 4*(2), i–iii.

Ellershaw, J., & Ward, C. (2003). Care of the dying patient: The last hours or days of life. *British Medical Journal, 326*(7379), 30–34.

Firth, P. (2005). Groupwork in Palliative Care. In P. Firth, G. Luff, & D. Oliviere (Eds.), *Loss, change and bereavement in palliative care* (pp. 167–184). Maidenhead, England: Open University Press.

Gold Standards Framework. (2009). *About GSF*. Retrieved from http://www.goldstandardsframework.nhs.uk/about_GSF

Hartley, N., & Payne, M. (Eds.). (2008). *Creative arts in palliative care*. Philadelphia, PA: Jessica Kingsley.

Help the Hospices. (2009). *Facts and figures*. Retrieved from http://www.helpthehospices.org.uk/about-hospice-care/facts-figures/

Henry, C., & Seymour, J. (2007). *Advance care planning: A guide for health and social care staff*. London, England: Department of Health.

Levy, J., & Payne, M. (2006). Welfare rights advocacy in a specialist health and social care setting: A service audit. *British Journal of Social Work, 36*(2), 323–331.

National Institute for Clinical Excellence (NICE). (2004). *Improving supportive and palliative care for adults with cancer: The manual*. London, England: National Institute for Clinical Excellence.

Payne, M. (2006). Identity politics in multiprofessional teams: Palliative care social work. *Journal of Social Work, 6*(2), 137–150.

Payne, M. (2008). Safeguarding adults at end of life: Audit and case analysis in a palliative care setting. *Journal of Social Work in End-of-Life and Palliative Care, 3*(4), 31–46.

Payne, M. (2009). *Social care practice in context*. Basingstoke, England: Palgrave Macmillan.

Price, A., Hotopf, M., Higginson, I. J., Monroe, B., & Henderson, M. (2006). Psychological services in hospices in the UK and Republic of Ireland. *Journal of the Royal Society of Medicine, 99*, 637–639.

Reid, D., Field, D., Payne, S., & Relf, M. (2006). Adult bereavement in five English hospices: Types of support. *International Journal of Palliative Nursing, 12*(9), 430–437.

Reith, M., & Payne, M. (2009). *Social work in end-of-life and palliative care*. Chicago, IL: Lyceum.

65

Shlomit Perry

Palliative Social Work in Israel

The State of Israel will foster the development of the country for the benefit of all its inhabitants… it will ensure complete equality of social and political rights irrespective of religion, race, or sex.

—The Israeli Declaration of Independence (May 14, 1948)

Key Concepts

◆ *The importance of interdisciplinary care.*
◆ *Finding the balance between secular and religious end-of-life ethics.*
◆ *The impact of government legislation on end-of-life care.*
◆ *The role of the social worker in implementing public health care.*

Introduction

The Jewish people have an ancient history and deep-rooted traditions, although the state of Israel was reestablished only in 1948 following the gathering of Jews from the Diaspora. Israel continues to have a heterogeneous immigration from around the world. Israel's population stands at 7.4 million people. Of these, 76% identify themselves as Jewish. The balance represents a variety of nationalities, the majority of which are of Arab descent. Among the Jewish population, more than 40% define themselves as secular, and less than 20% define themselves as being religious. Most of the Jewish inhabitants were born in Israel (68%), although the proportion of native Israelis among the elderly is much less so (Central Bureau of Statistics, 2009).

Structure of the Health Care

Western attitudes have a major impact on the nature of Israel's medical system: the doctor–patient relationship, emphasis on patient rights and autonomy, and the use of modern drugs. Israel's health care system is, in principle, a public system that combines community- and hospital-based medicine which is funded by taxes and government budgets. Medical care is supplied by four *public health funds*, which are nonprofit medical organizations (Rosen & MerKur, 2009). In 1995, the Israeli parliament passed the National Health Insurance Law, with a view toward providing equitable medical care for all of Israel's residents (Hart, 2001). According to the law, a *basket of health services* is defined and updated annually. Social work services are included as part of the basket.

Alongside the equitable state health care system, private medical care has also developed, which is supported by increasing the premiums paid to the *public health funds* and through private insurance. The balance and dialogue between the private and public health care systems is a challenge for Israeli society as a whole and for the social work profession in particular, in its attempts to treat and represent society's vulnerable populations.

Social Work in the Health Care System

The first social workers in the medical sphere cared mainly for patients who had contracted contagious and chronic illnesses. This was due the fact that most of the population were Holocaust survivors from Europe, refugees, or immigrants from Arab countries (Auslander, 2001). The National Health Insurance Law, passed in 1995, states that social work is a mandatory and integral part of the "basket of health services." The law defines the following goals: psychosocial services for medical purposes in severe cases and for chronic illnesses, and treatment for the patient and his or her family as an alternative to or to prevent hospitalization. Social services within the health care system operate in accordance with social work principles and are subject to several specific laws and procedures, such as those dealing with domestic violence, adoption, command centers in the event of terrorist attacks and multivictim incidents, planned discharge, appointing guardians for the purpose of taking medical action, abortions, perinatal death, and others. Social workers in the health care system integrate their treatment with individual psychotherapy, couples therapy, family therapy, and group therapy, which are mainly provided as short-term interventions. They also assist with social and economic resources, advocate on behalf of patients, and work with multidisciplinary teams. Social workers are expected to function in cooperation with the psychological and psychiatric services.

Palliative Care and the "Dying Patient Law"

Palliative care in Israel began to take shape in the early 1980s. The first hospice was founded in 1983, and since that time additional home-care units and inpatient hospices have been established. In 2005, the Parliament passed the Dying Patient Law (Steinberg & Sprung, 2006), which was an additional catalyst for the development of palliative care. The law aimed to regulate the care of dying patients, who are defined as those who will die within 6 months despite medical therapy. The last 2 weeks of expected life is defined as the terminal stage. Although the law does not apply to the entire population of patients requiring palliative care (e.g., the chronically ill), it did place the importance of palliative care on the public agenda and helped to raise consciousness of end-of-life care and questions regarding communication between the health care system, the patient, and his or her family.

A public committee was established to formulate the proposed Dying Patients Law, which included providers from all the relevant professions: doctors, nurses, social workers, psychologists, lawyers, and experts in religious and ethical issues. It should be noted that the unique "stamp" of the social work representatives is evident primarily in establishing that the health care system must treat the patient's family as an integral part of the patient's overall care, thus removing the need to appoint a legal guardian for dying patients. The purpose of this change was to reinforce and encourage the treatment dialogue between the health care system and the patient and his or her family. The law provides several significant innovations:

- For the first time in Israel, legislation was passed that requires the health care system to provide palliative care for the dying patient and his or her family.
- The doctor in charge must do everything possible to relieve the pain and suffering of the dying patient, even if this involves a *reasonable* risk to the patient's life.
- The law establishes detailed mechanisms for advance directives or a surrogate decision maker in the event the patient is not competent to make medical decisions.
- Jewish traditional religious law, the *Halacha,* maintains a distinction between withholding and withdrawing treatment at the end of life; therefore, it considers human intervention to end the life of dying patients unethical. According to the *Halacha,* actively stopping mechanical ventilation could be understood as the cause of death (i.e., active euthanasia). However, if the ventilator works intermittently (for example, run by a timer), then the patient can be assessed each time the ventilator stops, and a decision can be made afresh whether to reintubate. A timer on ventilators offers a unique solution that attempts to respect the Jewish religious while finding a practical solution that respects the wishes of patients and families (Ravitsky, 2005). The law requires the health care system to develop technologies that would help turn every continuous medical treatment into an intermittent form.
- The law states that the health care system must act in accordance with advance directives or the patient's legal representative. In the absence of either of these, the family should be involved in discussion and a decision reached together. Following the Dying Patients Law, it became unnecessary to appoint a legal guardian for terminal patients, which had often caused undue burden for the family. Cases of disagreement are addressed by a special ethics committee established to deal with dying patients.
- The Patients Rights Law of 1996 was influenced by liberal/Western philosophy and bioethics, and it emphasizes patient autonomy and discussing the patient's rights. The law stated that the doctor must provide the patient with information concerning his diagnosis, treatment, and prognosis and that concealing information from a patient must be discussed with the hospital's ethics committee. The Dying Patients Law involves the family in the decision process, but it places the onus on the doctor to inform the patient that he or she is "dying" so as to enable the patient to talk about how he or she wishes to live out the remainder of his or her days/life. In reality, however, ethics committees almost never meet, and these cases usually are decided

at the patient's bedside (Wenger, Golan, Shalev, & Glick, 2002).

Palliative Social Work

Developments in palliative care in Israel and all over the world, along with the passing of the Dying Patients Law, have given Israel a unique opportunity to shape the direction in which palliative care can advance. This includes palliative social work as an essential component.

Palliative care has grown in Israel in recent years in both the medical and nursing spheres. The palliative care nurse practitioners were recently recognized by the Israeli Ministry of Health. However, for physicians there is still no official training or residency program. In the wake of the law, this year the Ministry of Health adopted the recommendations of an advisory committee (including senior personnel from various Israeli palliative care settings) on the application and deployment of palliative care in Israel. According to the Israeli Ministry of Health, hospitals and *public health funds* are now required to provide palliative care services, to establish palliative care units in the relevant settings (hospitals, communities, and nursing homes), and to ensure that the necessary personnel are trained. Palliative care teams must include a doctor, nurse, social worker, or/and a psychologist.

Since 2004, about 130 social workers have taken part in a national training program established by Ben-Gurion University. A course evaluation study captured a complicated picture of the social work profession and its unique problems (Pesach Shwartzman, personal communication, 2009). Social workers, more than the other professions, felt that the course did not address their needs and that some of the material covered in the course was not relevant to their work. The findings emphasized the need to more clearly define the unique roles of the palliative social worker, the body of knowledge required, and the need to characterize the unique aspects of palliative social work. In light of these findings, it was decided that the first palliative care course for social workers would begin in 2009. The course is supported by the Ben-Gurion University, Ministry of Health, the Israel Cancer Association, and several other organizations interested in promoting this issue.

Challenges and Dilemmas Faced by Palliative Social Workers

Is Palliative Social Work the Same as Health Social Work?
The principles underlying both social work and palliative care are similar. There is an emphasis on the patient's quality of life within society, a respect for culture, and a moral obligation to treat the patient and his family until the end of life. The similarity between the two spheres raises questions regarding the uniqueness of palliative social work versus general health social work, and it requires that particular working guidelines be defined among social workers. In oncology and nephrology departments, the work model focuses on the continuity of care, quality of life, and survival. The social worker is part of the preliminary team that accompanies the patient and his family through the trajectory of the disease and continues treatment even after the goal has changed and the emphasis shifts to palliation. The development of palliative care units in hospitals offers other options whereby palliative social workers can enter the picture during the final stages along with the staff of the palliative care unit. It is still too early to predict the future directions, but the impression is that all of the social workers currently active in hospital departments that care for patients suffering from life-threatening illnesses or those suffering from multiple symptoms and severe damage to their quality of life should include palliative care as an essential part of their training. Whether they are working in oncology as an "oncology social worker" or as a "palliative social worker" may ultimately be merely a question of semantics.

The similarity between the principles underlying social work and palliative care also raises questions regarding role differentiation of social work within the palliative care team. There is definitely a consensus regarding the central role of social work with regard to the family, the relationship with the community, and its ability to contribute toward enlisting resources. The unique skills of the social workers, which are also recognized, include their ability to work within a network of complex systems; to see the patient within the context of the family, society, and community; and to be present for the team as they care for patients, family members, and caregivers.

The Role of Palliative Social Workers: Providing Information and Discussing the Prognosis

Social workers' responses to an evaluation study about the multidisciplinary palliative care course in Israel reflect their dilemma regarding the definitions and boundaries of their role (personal communication, Pesach Shwartzman, 2009). The social workers were not sure about their ability and their authority in treating patients suffering from depression or anxiety, nor were they certain of their role in the process of offering information, discussing prognosis, defining the goals of treatment, and assisting in medical decision making. In contrast with what the multidisciplinary organizers of the palliative course had expected, the social workers themselves were unclear about their role in the process of providing and processing information. While the organizers of the course believed that the social workers needed to be involved in the process of providing information and the clinical work implicit in this task, the social workers themselves were unsure of their role. This disparity requires serious attention by social workers in Israel. We must remember that providing information is not a one-time episode, especially when it comes to painful information, to which patients and families may respond with denial or feelings of being overwhelmed and confused. Social workers are expected to aid the physicians, medical staff, and ultimately the patients and families to integrate information, which is as much an emotional issue as a cognitive one for both patients and their families.

Literature and clinical experience teaches us that the information becomes a "conscious knowledge" in a cautious reciprocal process in which the social workers listen, clarify, and interpret. Giving information is not just the moment when the doctor tells facts to the patient and family. It also includes the process during which the knowledge is translated into the patient's narrative and is given new meaning. Undoubtedly, social work's ability to fulfill our role of supporting and assisting the patient and families depends upon the information that we have and they have about the disease. We cannot help patients and families integrate their reality, organize treatment at home, or, alternatively, plan a transfer to a hospice without discussing the prognosis. It is impossible to guide the ill or healthy parent on how to relate to their children without first discussing questions about the seriousness of the illness and the possibility of death (Deja, 2006).

Social Work: Autonomy and Talking about Death

Sociological literature describes Israeli society as a family-oriented society (Bar Yosef & Lieblich, 1983), a land where the Diaspora has been gathered; a land of multiple nationalities. With this social complexity, it is interesting to note that in practice Israeli society is a mixture of both strong family involvement values and the importance of the autonomy of the individual. However, the Patients' Rights Law emphasizes the centrality of the individual's autonomy to exclusion of the family's traditional role. On the other hand, the Dying Patients Law attempts to correct the situation by emphasizing the importance of the family, and to see the terminal illness as a family affair. Both laws lead to greater openness about impending death and involvement in the death process, despite fears and the tendency to deny death. Yet it is not sufficiently clear to us what is best for the dying patient, and oftentimes denial should be protected. The patient narratives in Box 65.1 will illustrate this difficulty.

These narratives illustrate the difficulty in applying the law when the simple interpretation of *the right* to know is translated into the doctor's *obligation* to inform and could lead to a situation in which the patient *is required* to be aware of his impending death, and when the right to denial *is revoked* (Perry & Wein, 2008). It would appear that social workers have the tools to help implement the laws while offering a more complex interpretation that respects the patient and his family and takes into consideration various cultural, psychological, and social differences.

Box 65.1
Patient/Family Narratives

One patient, a sociology professor with whom I was in contact for quite some time, said to me during the last weeks of his life, "During the illness, when I was receiving chemotherapy, I was able to talk freely about death. Now it is as if my personality has totally changed and I cannot talk about it." When I asked him, "Do you want me to help you talk about death or help you close the subject?" he responded, "Help me not talk about death."

Another patient wanted to ask the doctor about her prognosis, noting that according to the Patients Right Law, it was the doctor's obligation to provide her with this information. I suggested that we call the doctor and talk with him. She panicked and said, "Maybe not… I don't want the answer to be heard in the universe."

Bereavement Counseling

Despite the investment in and advanced treatment of families that have lost sons and daughters in the line of duty (army) or terrorist attacks (sudden death), Israel has no formal framework for treating families who have lost loved ones as a result of illness. Bereavement counseling is not part of the role of the hospital social workers and is not sufficiently dealt with at the community level. Palliative social workers will apparently have to pick up the gauntlet and undertake the task of developing interventions that integrate the treatment of families coping with advanced illness, the process of dying and death, and the treatment of grief at a later stage. This need is particularly vital with regard to young families with small children. At this stage the research and the clinical data regarding how children cope with the expected death of a parent are ambiguous. We are not sure whether and how much we can prepare children for their parent's death and whether such advance preparation is beneficial (Saldinger, Porterfield, & Cain, 2004). Clinical experience teaches us that the encounter with an anticipated death is experienced differently by each family member and coping with one's own death is not the same as coping with the death of someone else. Awareness of an impending death may provoke an intense dissonance; on the one hand, a desire to become closer and more connected in order to take advantage of the time you have left together; and on the other hand, it also initiates processes of separation that may be reflected in one's imagination, thoughts, or behavior (Grassi, 2007). Social workers, as part of their training in palliative care and as a members of the caregiving team, should develop interventions that will help the patient and family create the therapeutic space and ease the tension between preparations for death and the continuity of life, between highlighting the awareness of death and maintaining hope, in order to enable the patient to have a "good death" and to prevent complicated grief in the future among the family members.

Palliative Social Work in Different Settings

In Israel, palliative social work has developed mainly in the psycho-oncology setting, to a large extent through the initiative of the Israel Cancer Association, which founded the first hospice and which funds social work positions within oncology wards, trains social workers, and aids in the activity of the Israel Psycho-oncology Association. Concomitantly, Israel's *public health funds* have opened home-care units for the treatment of terminally ill patients who are confined to home as an alternative to hospitalization. At present we need to develop leadership among palliative social workers in various spheres and institutions with a view toward expanding, enhancing, and strengthening palliative social workers all over the country, in various frameworks, particularly in nursing homes.

Conclusion

In Israel, social workers, along with other health care professionals, are currently dealing with the task of applying the Dying Patients Law in clinics, at the patient's bedside, in research, and in developing policies. The law provides us with new opportunities, but we cannot ignore the fact that it reflects a specific cultural approach, influenced by Western norms, that encourages direct dialogue about the impending death; a dialogue that is apparently not appropriate or desired by a large number of patients. The palliative social worker is encouraged to take a more active role at both the clinical and policy level. It is further important for palliative social workers to raise awareness regarding the advantages of preparing advance directives or appointing a proxy. Training and psychosocial interventions for the families of dying patients as well as preparation for death and bereavement counseling are integral to the palliative social work role. Social work leaders in the area of palliative care are being called upon to develop the palliative social work field, to expand it to include other settings such as nursing homes and population groups where talking about death is not a norm and dying at home is a preferred choice. Palliative care is leading the way toward

a shift in the treatment paradigm that goes beyond the "doctor–patient relationship" toward a "health care unit–patient/family relationship." This shift must be accompanied by new definitions for the role, authority, and responsibility of the social worker. We must endeavor to achieve a "patient-focused and family-centered" approach, in which information is viewed as a process and social workers are an integral member of the treatment team.

REFERENCES

Auslander, G. (2001). Social work in health care: What have we achieved? *Journal of Social Work, 1*, 201–222.

Bar Yosef, R., & Lieblich, A. (1983). Comments on Brandow's ideology, myth and reality: Sex equality in Israel. *Sex roles, 12*, 561–570.

Central Bureau of Statistics. (2009). Retrieved from Population, p.10 http://www.cbs.gov.il/publications/isr_in_no8h.pdf

Declaration of Independence of the State of Israel. (May 15, 1948). *Official Gazette.*

Deja, K. (2006). Social workers breaking bad news: The essential role of an interdisciplinary team when communicating prognosis. *Journal of Palliative Medicine, 9*, 807–809.

Hart, J. (2001). Reform of the health care service system in Israel 1995–2000. *World Hospital Health Services, 37*, 9–11.

Grassi, L. (2007). Bereavement in families with relatives dying of cancer. *Current Opinion in Supportive and Palliative Care, 1*, 43–49.

Perry, S., & Wein S. (2008). The dying patient: The right to know versus the duty to be aware. *Palliative and Supportive Care, 6*, 397–401.

Ravitsky, V. (2005). Timers on ventilators. *British Medical Journal, 330*, 415–417.

Rosen, B., & Merkur, S. (2009). Israel: Health system review. *Health Systems in Transition, 11*(2), 1–226.

Saldinger, A., Porterfield, K., & Cain, A. (2004). Meeting the need of parental bereaved children: A framework for child-centered parenting. *Psychiatry, 67*, 331–352.

Steinberg, A., & Sprung, C. L. (2006). The dying patient: New Israeli legislation. *Intensive Care Medicine, 32*, 1234–1237.

Wenger, N. S., Golan, O., Shalev, C., & Glick S. (2002). Hospital ethics committees in Israel: Structure, function and heterogeneity in the setting of statutory ethics committees. *Journal of Medical Ethics, 28*, 177–182.

66 Hanan Qasim

Selected Issues in Palliative Care among East Jerusalem Arab Residents

This is God's will and one mustn't protest. A person who believes accepts all that God gives.
—Anonymous patient

Key Concepts
- *Understanding cultural context is important when working with Palestinian patients, particularly in Israeli hospitals.*
- *Cultural competence includes individual assessment of communication needs and preferences.*

Introduction

The Oncology Institute of Shaare Zedek Hospital is located in Jerusalem and treats patients from all sectors of the Israeli society. Twenty-four percent of Israel's population is Arab, 82% of which is Muslim. The majority of Arab patients receiving care at Shaare Zedek are East Jerusalem residents. There are 250,000 East Jerusalem Arabs in the city. They are "permanent residents," rather than citizens, a status that entitles them to many social rights, such as social security and health care.

Although the general Arab population in Israel is very diverse and is composed of a variety of groups such as Muslims, Christians, and Druze, as well as subgroups belonging to different geographical locations, it does share some common cultural features. Successful treatment of an Arab cancer patient requires a culturally sensitive professional intervention that addresses the significance of his or her cultural identity. In view of this, the Hospital's administration appointed an Arab social worker to assist the treatment of Arab patients in a targeted manner.

The East Jerusalem Arab population is distinguished from other Arabs in Israel in their legal status and insofar as they are less integrated into Israeli society. Their school curriculum is Palestinian or Jordanian rather than Israeli, many cannot speak Hebrew, and they reside in separate Arab neighborhoods. This chapter reflects experience derived from working with this population. By understanding and attending to the culture, beliefs, and perceptions of the East Jerusalem Arab community, the social worker can better understand the Arab cancer patient and his or her family's preferred coping paths. Such insight is the first step toward adequate clinical intervention. Culturally sensitive intervention is the key concept here. A caregiver working with the Arab population needs to possess cultural knowledge, sensitivity, and the ability to mediate between the majority culture (which is often Western) and Arab culture. This chapter focuses on the following central topics: the structure of the Arab society, cultural aspects shaping attitudes toward cancer (shame, secrecy), attitudes toward pain, women's status, dealing with death and preferences at life's end, and patterns of caregiving and receiving.

The Structure of Arab Culture and Family

Haj-Yahia (1994) sees value orientation as a structured, general framework that shapes a person's perception of time, nature, place in nature, desired and undesired qualities, and interpersonal interactions. By being attuned to the value orientation of the East Jerusalem Arab population, the social worker can better understand the coping mechanisms preferred by the Arab patient and his or her family, and can structure intervention accordingly.

Arab society is composed of the following central units: the *hamula* (a large kin network), the extended family, and the nuclear family. The society is stable, and strong emotional, social, and economic ties exist between its members. Men hold the primary authority within each of these units. The father is the head of the family and has legitimate authority to make decisions regarding all aspects of family members' lives. The father is subordinate to the male head of the extended family, who is in turn subordinate to the head of the *hamula*. The status of women in the Arab family is usually lower than that of men. "The Arab woman is expected to be dependent on her husband, to submit to his will and needs and to be a source of support for him and for his family" (Haj-Yahia, 1994).

While modern, Western values and behavioral codes are widespread among the Jewish Israeli majority, the Arab Israeli population in general, and East Jerusalem Arabs in particular, still adhere to traditional customs and norms governing family life, gender roles, childrearing, and everyday conduct.

> *The expression of conflict, whether internal or external, and the expression of negative feelings are not well accepted in the Arab culture. The anxious self-absorption that often accompanies a depressed mood is viewed negatively as "thinking too much," which is in turn viewed as a narcissistic preoccupation. Physical symptoms, however, are accepted as legitimate and morally acceptable expressions of pain.*
> *(Al-Krenawi & Graham, 2000, p. 16)*

Attitudes toward Cancer and Expressions of Emotional Pain

Among the East Jerusalem Arab population, cancer is accompanied by a sense of shame and fear of genetic transmittance. Secrecy prevails because knowledge of the patient's sickness among the wider society might harm family members' marriage prospects. Keeping the secret is related to society's expectation of the individual to remain calm, suffer quietly, not show signs of weakness, and protect the family's interests. Concealment makes it difficult for patients to seek and receive external help, especially through participation in support groups.

Many Muslim families believe that those who suffer more will receive a greater reward in the afterlife. Protesting one's fate is not accepted because fate is considered to be God's will. Patients are expected to accept their disease. Interventions that encourage the expression of emotions or normalize feelings of anger or protest often elicit reactions such as "This is God's will and one mustn't protest. A person who believes accepts all that God gives." Faisal Azaiza and Miri Cohen in their study of Israeli Arab women's attitudes toward breast and cervical cancer also find that some still perceive cancer "as either a punishment or as a test devised by God" (Azaiza & Cohen, 2008, p. 34).

Patients perceive the expression of physical pain as more legitimate in comparison with emotional pain. This is illustrated in the narrative in Box 66.1.

Coping with Death and End of Life

The main support networks of the Arab family are often informal ones, including neighbors, friends, and kin. Most Arab families see hospitalization at a hospice in end-of-life situations as disrespectful and believe that the family owes it to the patient to enable him or her to spend the last days at home. Many see the transfer of the patient to a hospice or to any other palliative framework as a failure. In everyday speech they refer to such institutions as "death institutions," and they do not regard them as places that might improve a patient's quality of life. The narrative in Box 66.2 illustrates the impact of these beliefs.

In contrast, the society is more accepting of home care or home hospice, because it combines the tradition of caring for the patient at home and modern medicine. While home care might be the best way to maintain respect for family values and enhance patient care, it is not easily accessible for East Jerusalem Arabs. Today, home care is provided for people

---

Box 66.1
Patient Narrative: Yusra

Yusra, a 48-year-old female patient with metastatic cancer, suffered from stomach aches every time she dined with her family. This symptom did not appear, however, when she dined with other people. One of the conclusions she reached as a result of counseling was that her expression of emotional pain was not acceptable in her family and that she found it difficult to meet her family's expectations to be strong and to continue functioning as usual within the family. As she developed skill in expressing her emotional distress, the stomach aches disappeared and she no longer needed to find alternative outlets for her emotional pain.

Box 66.2
Patient Narrative: Ahmad

In an attempt to admit Ahmad, a 54-year-old terminal patient, to a hospice, his extended family became very angry with his wife, claiming that she was shirking her natural role as his caretaker and accusing her of being disrespectful. The wife was hospitalized that same day suffering from a nervous breakdown due to the stress generated by the reaction of the family. The family was not sympathetic to the wife's condition. In response, my professional intervention entailed gathering the family and explaining to them the complexity of Ahmad's medical situation. I reached out to the head of the family and engaged the physicians on the medical team to add their authority to a discussion about the severity of Ahmad's condition. Following a difficult and painful conversation, he agreed to transfer Ahmad to a hospice in collaboration with Ahmad's wife.

residing near the city center while physical and political conditions make East Jerusalem Arab neighborhoods less accessible to such arrangements.

Seeking Help

Haj Yahia (1994) argues that everyday behavioral orientation among Arabs imposes self-discipline and the notion that a person can attain complete self-control, including control of one's emotions and meeting one's responsibilities in various areas of life. The Arab individual is expected to be composed, patient, not to protest at times of distress, and to endure painful moments quietly. In many cases, Arab patients find it difficult to share personal problems and feelings with a person who is not a family member or a member of the community. A person who does share such issues with an outsider is perceived as weak and disloyal (Al-Krenawi & Graham, 2000).

Furthermore, the special political and legal status of East Jerusalem Arabs makes it even more difficult for them to seek help from Israeli state institutions or their representatives. Meetings of Arab patients, their partners or companions, with the social worker are often very charged and characterized by substantial suspicion. Since many members of the Arab population see social workers as representatives of the establishment, they may not seek assistance. It is critical then, that social workers explain their role and assert their readiness to work with the family, partner, or children as well as with the patient. Commonly, the social worker's outreach initiatives will be rebuffed until trust is developed, thus underscoring the importance of relationship building and perseverance.

Some patients and family members are apprehensive about the idea of emotional support and about discussing one's feelings, and others are apprehensive about receiving help from a professional external to the family system. The role of the social worker as part of the medical team is not self-evident to many Arab patients. This understanding starts to develop when the medical team uses the services of the Arabic-speaking social worker as an interpreter, because most patients do not speak Hebrew and the medical staff often does not speak Arabic. The sensitivity to cultural issues and familiarity of language helps establish trust between patients and the medical team.

Arab men tend to disclose and interact less with the psychosocial staff than do women. They often prefer to suffer quietly and focus on practical assistance. It is unclear whether this is affected by the gender of the social worker or mental health clinician or due to the cultural requisite of being reserved. This is a question meriting further inquiry.

To address the difficulty that East Jerusalem Arabs have in seeking formal help, we take the following steps:

- Raise awareness and educate about the role and work of the social worker
- Initiate referral of the patient, as part of the routine work of the medical staff, to the psychosocial staff, since a society that has much respect for authority tends to follow the recommendations of the medical staff
- Insist on transmitting information in the patient's native language.

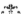

Conclusion

The treatment of cancer patients, along the continuum of illness, requires attention to culture, values, and traditions. The East Jerusalem Arab population has a special status and their unique needs must be addressed accordingly. Several issues require deeper attention. It is important to understand that cancer is still accompanied by a sense of social shame among the Arab population and causes some patients and their families to keep it secret, a practice that often leads to feelings of isolation and loneliness. There is still a lack of awareness and information about the disease in the Arab population, and efforts must be made to disseminate knowledge about cancer, about treatment options, and about attitudes toward those who suffer from cancer. The available support systems must be adjusted to address tradition and culture, especially the cultural inhibition, which make it difficult to speak about painful feelings.

It is important to stress that this population suffers from limited access to medical and paramedical care, and that the home care staff that are trained to care for terminal patients cannot access East Jerusalem Arab neighborhoods due to physical and political conditions. This problem becomes even more acute in cases of immobile patients who cannot travel to receive medical care.

The value of accepting one's fate does not contradict the need to provide patients with emotional and medical palliative care. There is an urgent need for a system of home care teams to be established inside East Jerusalem Arab neighborhoods to accommodate the culturally mandated practice of spending one's last days at home. The challenge in treating Arab patients is in creating conditions in which Arab cultural reality and medical services would supplement, rather than contradict, each other. The skills of staff members attending to the Arab population should include, alongside conventional medical knowledge, awareness of and sensitivity to cultural issues, as well as an ability to mediate between the majority culture, which is often Western, and the minority Arab culture.

ADDITIONAL RESOURCES

READINGS

Al-Krenawi, A. (1998). Contribution of the constructivist approach to professional practice in a multicultural society [In Hebrew]. *Society and Welfare, 18,* 253–267.

Al-Krenawi, A. (1999a). Explanations of mental health symptoms by the Bedouin-Arab of the Negev. *International Journal of Social Psychiatry, 45*(1), 56–64.

Al-Krenawi, A. (1999b). Culturally sensitive mental health therapy with Arabs [In Hebrew]. In C. Rabin (Ed.), *Being different in Israel: Ethnicity, gender and therapy* (pp. 65–82). Tel-Aviv, Israel: Ramot, Tel-Aviv University Press.

Al-Krenawi, A., & Graham, J. R. (1999). Social work and Koranic mental health healers. *International Social Work, 42,* 53–65.

Al-Krenawi, A., Maoz, B., & Reicher, B. (1994). Familial and cultural issues in the brief strategic treatment of Israeli Bedouin. *Family Systems Medicine, 12,* 415–425.

Cohen, M., & Azaiza, F. (2005). Early breast cancer detection practices, health beliefs, and cancer worries in Jewish and Arab women. *Preventive Medicine, 41,* 852–858.

Haj-Yahia, M. (1995). Toward culturally sensitive intervention with Arab families in Israel. *Journal of Contemporary Family Therapy, 17*(4), 429–447.

Haj-Yahia, M. (1997). Culturally sensitive supervision of Arab social work students in western universities. *Social Work, 42,* 166–174.

WEB SITES

The Israel Cancer Association: http://www.cancer.org.il
More than 50 years of involvement and a proud record of achievement have earned the ICA widespread recognition, both nationally and internationally, as a prime leader in the fight against cancer.

The Middle East Cancer Consortium: http://mecc.cancer.gov
The MECC's objective is to reduce the incidence and impact of cancer in the Middle East through the solicitation and support of collaborative research.

REFERENCES

Al-Krenawi, A., & Graham, J. R. (2000). Culturally sensitive social work practice with Arab clients in mental health settings. *Health and Social Work, 25*(1), 9–22.

Azaiza, F., & Cohen, M. (2008). Between traditional and modern perceptions of breast and cervical cancer screenings: A qualitative study of Arab women in Israel. *Journal of Psycho-Oncology, 17,* 34–41.

Haj-Yahia, M. (1994). The Arab family in Israel, its cultural values and their relevance to social work [In Hebrew]. *Society and Welfare, 14,* 249–264.

VII
Ethics

"We often experience the honor of being invited into sacred spaces with our patients and families. In these spaces, we are given the opportunity to practice social work in its truest form – allowing the self-determination of each patient and family to guide the process toward unique and evolving definitions of quality of life and comfort."

Jennifer Christophel Lichti MSW, LCSW
Clinical Social Worker
Adult Palliative Care Team
St. Vincent Hospital

Do not ask me
*Do Not Ask Me
if I have given up.
I am still breathing
Aren't I?*

*If and when
I am ready
I will not give up
I will let go.*

*It will not be
your way
or your timing.
God and I will decide.*

*This is my time.
Though it may be
limited it is
still mine.*

*Tomorrow
I may die
but today
I am going to live.*

Deb Kosmer MSW, CSW, CT
Bereavement Coordinator
Affinity Visiting Nurses Hospice

67 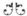 *Patricia O'Donnell*

Ethical Considerations in Palliative Care: An Overview

Can I trust you?

—Libby, a 36-year-old patient with metastatic cervical cancer

Key Concepts

- *The National Association of Social Workers (NASW) Code of Ethics includes a statement of mission and values that are actualized in ethical principles that inform social work practice standards.*
- *Social work practice standards include ethical responsibilities to clients, colleagues, practice settings, the profession, and society.*
- *An ethical dilemma occurs when a social worker must make a choice between two or more ethically justified directives or obligations that cannot be equally met at the same time.*
- *The ethically competent social worker recognizes ethical problems, proactively responds to ethical challenges to practice, participates in improving the ethical environment in his or her practice setting, and works to assure that patients and families have equal and fair access to needed services.*

Introduction

Social workers in health care bring a wealth of interventions to their work beginning with a proficiency in improving the interactions between patients and their environment. This may include modifying the environment that encompasses the patient's relationships with family and care team, and modifying the treatment settings to make them more responsive to the patient's health care–related needs and preferences (Germain, 1984). Additionally, social workers and other psychosocial professionals are valued team members because their skills in listening and communication are particularly useful in enhancing the relationships within which health care is negotiated and provided (Block, 2007). Equally valued is their commitment and ability to advocate for comprehensive services. Advocacy is a key social work professional obligation both to individuals and to the common good of society (Christ, 2005; Rose & Shelton, 2006; Saunders, 2001).

The social work profession is grounded in a set of core values that serve as the foundation for the ethical principles which mandate social work ethical obligations and practice standards to our patients and their families, our colleagues and practice settings, our profession, and society as a whole (National Association of Social Workers [NASW], 1999). These values include service, the dignity and worth of the individual, integrity, the importance of human relationships, social justice, and competence as delineated in the introduction to the NASW Code of Ethics. In addition, the NASW has developed a set of practice standards to inform the service to patients at the end of life (NASW, 2004). These standards define ethical practice in end-of-life care and require the social worker to acquire necessary skills to recognize and analyze ethical issues related to value conflicts common in palliative and end-of-life care. To accomplish this, the social worker develops competence in addressing bioethics-based issues, including the right to refuse treatment, the parameters of surrogate decision making, and decisions about the withholding and withdrawing of treatment. Additionally, the palliative social worker is expected to be able to apply a model of ethical problem solving in concert with the patient, family, and other professionals toward resolution of ethical conflicts. This process includes the ability to consider the contextual aspects of the dilemma, the relevant ethical perspectives and principles, any applicable laws and regulations, the ethical obligations derived from professional Codes of Ethics, and the range of personal, professional, and societal values influencing the perspectives of the patient, family, and team members in moving toward a thorough exposition and eventual resolution of the ethical dilemma (Agency for Healthcare Research and Quality, 2009; Joseph, 1985).

Practice in interdisciplinary settings is characterized by a team model in which key disciplines use their individual professional expertise in collaboration with each other to provide for the care needs of the patient and family. However, this approach can give rise to ethical issues of collective responsibility in team work and concerns about how conflicts are resolved (Abramson, 1984). Across the professions in a palliative care team, the bioethical principles of autonomy, beneficence, nonmaleficence, and justice provide guidance in determining professional practice at the bedside and in the organization (Beauchamp & Childress, 2001). The principle of autonomy supports the patient's right to participate in all aspects of, and decisions related to, their treatment and mandates informed consent, confidentiality, privacy, and truth telling in the professional relationship. The principle of beneficence directs that the professional place the interests of the patient first in making any recommendations for intervention and care. The principle of nonmaleficence guides the professional to actions that will prevent or avoid harm coming to the patient, and to assess the potential burden associated with recommended treatments in terms of pain, cost, suffering, and discomfort. The principle of justice directs that the professional treat all patients equitably and be attentive to the just allocation of resources. At their source, ethical issues arise in clinical practice when there is an apparent conflict with patients, families, and team members of values and ethical principles or when weighing the potential benefits over possible burdens associated with recommended interventions (Lo, 2000). While values and principles may be commonly held by health care professionals, variation in the hierarchy of those same values and principles, and differences in opinion about what is legal versus what is ethical may generate ethical conflict (Calman, 2004; Meisel, 2000). These conflicts may be internal for an individual team member or couched in the relationship and collaborations among the patient, family members, and team members or health care professionals external to the team but intimately involved in the care of a mutual patient.

Randall and Downie (1999) support the team approach to palliative care as the ideal service delivery system to meet the total needs and interests of the patients and their families. Social workers are integral members of the palliative care team particularly because they are clinically trained to consider and support the concept of the patient and the family as the unit of care, a hallmark of palliative care (King & Quill, 2006). Practice in interdisciplinary settings and on care teams often gives rise to ethical issues of collective responsibility in team work, and it generates questions related to how best to resolve ethical conflicts among individual team members (Abramson, 1984). It is imperative that the team have a sense of individual as well as group accountability in service provision and accept when compromise may be the best thing for the patient but not for the individual team member. For example, a team member may disagree with the team recommendation that a patient be placed because the patient has stated she wants to remain home at all costs. However, the team feels the family is exhausted and the patient's safety is at stake; thus, they believe the principle of beneficence trumps the principle of autonomy in this recommendation for the patient's best interests. Cohesiveness in a palliative care team promotes effectiveness and support for members (Meier & Beresford, 2008). However, Pellegrino (1998) expressed a concern that on some palliative care teams that same cohesiveness can lead members to shun or discourage dissent to avoid offending colleagues; assume team wisdom over the patient's expression of his or her needs; and focus on the care needs of team members over patient's care needs. Corley (2002) notes that moral distress for the professional can arise when the team member recognizes and voices an ethical issue but is unable to take action to resolve the issue due to constraints from within the team or the organization. Other team members threatened by an individual team member's dissent to a recommendation may pressure the dissenting team member to conform to a recommendation to preserve the cohesiveness of the team. Holland and Kilpatrick (1991) identify social work's interpersonal approach to ethical problems as one focused on the mutual and common goal of promoting client autonomy and independence, which may not be the team's priority. The authors recommend a strong base in ethical reflection and judgment for social workers working on teams especially because other team members may have differing approaches to ethical problems based on their unique professional codes of ethics and their perspectives as specialist clinicians.

This chapter will explore a number of common ethical issues that challenge social workers in palliative care in their everyday clinical relationships with patients, families, team members, and others health professionals within the care setting. These issues include truth telling; confidentiality and privacy; competence; and boundary relationships and potential conflicts of interest (Calman, 2004; Ulrich et al., 2007). The components of ethical decision making will serve as a template for the discussion of these issues. Subsequent chapters will address more extensively issues related to advance directives; decision making and surrogacy; and questions of assisted suicide and euthanasia. This chapter will conclude with recommendations for social work education and ongoing support in managing ethical issues associated with palliative care.

Ethical Issues

Truth Telling

Millstein's (2000) report on a study of confidentiality found ethical practice related to confidentiality issues was the greatest source of conflict for social workers working collaboratively within and outside agencies. McMahon (2003) notes that in health social work, the social worker's holistic perspective may be in conflict with the medical model of patient care, where authority resides in the team, not the patient. The social worker may be asked to withhold information from a patient and family for a range of ethically justifiable reasons arising from altruistic intentions, including the concern about how the patient will react to difficult information. Team members may worry that the patient will, in reaction, give up hope or even withdraw from the professional relationship. Team members may be uncomfortable sharing information or have difficulty dealing with uncertainty. Information may be directed to only positives or otherwise be not as inclusive as required for the patient to make an informed decision. In addition, some health care professionals' training has not prepared them on the best approach in sharing uncertain or ambiguous information.

Box 67.1A
Patient/Family Narrative: Libby

Libby is a 36-year-old divorced woman with metastatic cervical cancer. The team finds her "difficult" in that she is never satisfied with care; double checks information from team members; is nonadherent with treatment regimens; manipulates the staff by suggesting one member contradicts another; and never says thank you even for extra effort. Libby lives alone. She has close friends who are available to her evenings and weekends. She is estranged from her mother. Her father died when she was 7, and she was sexually abused by her stepfather from ages 11 to 14. The accusation led to her placement in foster care and the eventual breakup of her mother's marriage. Libby has made attempts in the past to reconcile with her mother but with no success. She is generally suspicious of health care, because she feels she was misdiagnosed and misled by her family physician and oncologist. She feels she must be vigilant to prevent further errors and adverse events. She asks that you help remove a new RN staff member from her team because she is concerned about the nurse's technique and seeming unfamiliarity with her overall condition. Libby is depressed and being followed by a psychiatrist in addition to the palliative care team. She has asked that you not reveal nor document in her medical record her history of sexual abuse. With time, Libby developed a trusting relationship with the social worker who was able to convey her concerns and promote her sense of safety with the staff. However, she was upset when the social worker refused to stay for dinner and to accept a gift she had specially selected. The social worker was able to work through that rift. Libby never became the team's favorite patient but was able to negotiate for her preferences and died at home with her mother at her bedside.

While there may be agreement that the truth should be shared with patients and their families, questions arise in deciding when to tell, how much to tell, and who to tell (Weir, 1986). The ethical principle of respect for autonomy requires respectful actions based on the patient's right to determine what is best for him or her in response to the information provided about his or her diagnosis, prognosis, and current status. In some families and cultures this same right to determine what is best may mean that the patient chooses not to be informed or delegates decision making to others, which is acceptable if the patient requests this approach. In general, however, it is believed that patients need timely, complete, and direct information to make their decisions. There may also be some pressure at times for the social worker to share information with the team either verbally or in the medical record that the social worker believes is not germane to the patient's care or cannot be protected if documented in the medical record. The social worker may consider her options in consultation with a social work colleague or supervisor to determine how and with whom confidential information should be shared.

The principle of beneficence supports truth telling in the sense of promoting patient well-being, that is, if the patient has the essential information he or she can make needed decisions. This principle also directs the professional to place his or her own interests (avoiding discomfort) secondary to the best interests of the patient to receive needed information. The principle of nonmaleficence can be utilized to justify sharing information to avoid harm to the patient, and it can also be used to justify withholding information to prevent causing the patient distress. However, when considering the vulnerability of the patient in relationship to the more knowledgeable professional, there would be no justification for a professional to use information to mislead a patient even if the professional's intent is to protect the patient (Weir, 1986). Emanuel and Emanuel's (1992) review of the patient and physician relationship reinforces that the relationship is more effective for both when the professional provides information, offers guidance on recommendations, and then reflects with the patient on how the treatment recommendations are informed by and congruous with the patient's values.

The NASW Code of Ethics (1999), Standards 1.01 and 1.02, support truth telling as a professional obligation to promote the patient's well-being and self-determination; thus, these standards ethically justify sharing the truth with the patient. The clinical question remains in the nuances of how the information will be shared. The social worker's assessment of the patient's level of understanding and preferences; the supports available to the patient to help with decision making; and their cultural beliefs around sharing information will help the team establish a clinical plan to meet the individual needs of the patient in truth telling. This approach may also help to relieve the team's anxiety and uncertainty about how and when to share information. Social workers are also mandated by their code of ethics to be respectful of their colleagues' concerns and to promote understanding of the patient's point of view in collaborative relationships (NASW, 1999).

At the organizational level, health care settings have instituted policies to disclose outcomes and adverse events to patients and families. The policy may be mandated by state law and regulatory agencies such as The Joint Commission but is grounded in the ethical principles of autonomy, beneficence, and nonmaleficence as are other truth-telling encounters with the patient. This applies to all patients but can be particularly difficult in cases where a patient's death was caused or hastened by the adverse event. In fact, providing the family with known details of the event; offering a statement of regret or an apology; and sharing actions taken to prevent future events have decreased the number of lawsuits in these cases and increased overall satisfaction with the disclosure process (Gallagher, Studdert, & Levinson, 2007). Institutional leadership may accept the mandate but be reluctant to fully implement the process for many of the same reasons that clinicians avoid truth telling. Social work participation in the development of the policy and procedure as well as a distinct role on the disclosure support team can promote the patient's perspective in the process. In summary, truth telling promotes trust in professional relationships with patients, accountability in sharing among team members, and integrity and transparency in the organization as a whole.

Patients identified as "difficult" because of unacceptable behaviors can be easily marginalized by the team (Degnin, 2009). It is the responsibility of the team members to adjust their expectations, set limits, and discuss their concerns with the patient when difficult provider–patient relationships threaten the care of the patient (Potter & Reynolds, 2000). It is also the responsibility of the team to become conscious of the language and descriptors that may reinforce any negative perceptions that foster the marginalization rather than the expectation that staff, as skilled professional caregivers, work together to create a plan that maximizes patient care. Glajchen

and Zuckerman (2001) offer a model utilizing a stepwise process to resolve conflict and facilitate decision making that focuses on the patient's needs and interests. The steps in the process begin with establishing diagnosis and prognosis, eliciting the perspectives of the patient and family, and presenting the views of the treatment team via mediation to promote communication and to achieve a resolution of the conflict.

Confidentiality and Privacy

Whatever I see or hear in the lives of my patients, whether in connection with my professional practice or not, which ought not to be spoken of outside, I will keep secret, as considering all such things to be private. (Hippocratic Oath, translated by M. North; retrieved from the United States National Library of Medicine, https://www.nlm.nih.gov/hmd/greek/greek_oath.html)

The intimacy of the relationships between patients and professional caregivers often results in the sharing of information that is considered private by the patient. Beyond the patient's expectation that the professional will place the interests of the patient secondary to the professional's interests is the expectation that the professional will respect the privacy of the patient and maintain confidentiality with respect to information shared in the professional relationship. This obligation requires that information is shared only with the consent of the patient, and that the information shared is relevant and essential to promoting the well-being of the patient. The professional must balance the use of psychosocial information for the patient's good and the casual distribution of privileged information with consequent loss of respect and dignity for the patient (MacDonald, 2004; McMahon, 2003). Exceptions to this obligation include the duty to prevent harm to the patient and others and the legal mandate to report criminal activity, certain public health concerns such as communicable diseases, and suspected abuse (Beauchamp & Childress, 2001).

The professional must consider what information to share, how to share it, with whom to share it, and the purpose of sharing it. This obligation is grounded in the principle of autonomy, the right of patients to decide what to share about themselves with others. The principle of fidelity, the obligation to keep promises, mandates that professionals respect their duty to the patient by not revealing information shared by the patient to others without the patient's permission. Beneficence directs that information be shared to promote the interests of the patient, while nonmaleficence cautions that the information should not bring harm to the patient.

The NASW Code of Ethics has since its inception evolved in concert with the changes in social work service provision and practice (Reamer, 2009). Reamer identifies the current stage of the Code of Ethics as the Ethical Standards and Risk Management Period, because the code not only provides

---

Box 67.1B
Patient/Family Narrative: Libby (continued)

In response to Libby's concerns, the social worker received permission from the patient to speak with her psychiatrist. The social worker and the psychiatrist were able to negotiate with Libby an agreement to disclose of Libby's past to the team that enabled them to understand how best to care for Libby while maintaining her privacy about the history of sexual abuse. Concise, factual, and accurate information settled the patient's suspicious behavior. In addition, the psychiatrist and the social worker met with key team members to identify team responses to Libby that Libby might perceive as rejection and abandonment. Team members were reluctant at first to make changes in their interactions with Libby but were pleased with the positive results when they tried.

practice standards but also offers guidance in how to avoid risk to the client, the practitioner, and the practice setting of the practitioner. Standard 1.07 of the Code of Ethics (NASW, 1999) requires that information gained in a professional encounter be shared only with the client's consent and only divulged without patient consent to prevent serious, foreseeable, and imminent harm to the patient or other parties. An important role for the social worker on many teams is to be the holder of the patient's story. The social worker's discretion directs what information will be documented in the medical record; what will be shared in team meetings and rounds; and what will be used in supervision and education. The patient should be advised on exactly what will be shared with whom and why, and then be asked for his or her consent. The consent may be verbal or written, but it should be documented.

At times, to obtain needed services or protect the patient, team members may ask the social worker to inflate symptoms or omit information from the record. The social worker cannot be complicit with any activity that could be interpreted as fraud because this could result in the risk of penalties to the patient, practitioners, and the care setting. It also threatens the integrity of the professionals and the institution's status in the community.

Competence

Social workers under Section 1.04 of the Code of Ethics (NASW, 1999) are directed to practice within their scope of practice, to pursue new skills via continuing education and training, and to be accountable for their own practice standards. While this applies to the individual social worker, managing a concern about the competency of other practitioners in either social work or other professions can be a difficult challenge. Social workers expend time and energy building rapport and trust within the team, and they may be reluctant to report incompetency because it may threaten the cohesion of the team, their place on the team, or result in retaliation. The social worker's initial evaluation should begin with self-examination of his or her own motives about why he or she believes that the issue of competency of a colleague needs to be addressed. This should be followed by a careful consideration of the issue and include a review of how the incompetence is negatively affecting the patient, the team, and the care setting (Reamer, 2009). Standard 2.11 of the Code of Ethics (NASW, 1999) suggests first speaking with the colleague or supervisor, and it requires that the social worker be familiar and comply with the formal processes and procedures involved in reporting ethical concerns within his or her setting. This minimizes risk to any patients who may be involved in the situation as well as risk to the practitioner and the care setting. If the social worker has heard colleagues question the competence of others, the social worker must encourage those colleagues to comply with further investigation and reporting procedures. The standard also mandates that the social worker speak up on behalf of colleagues wrongly accused of incompetence.

The Ethics of Care perspective focuses on the practitioner's relationships with the patient and with team members. The perspective enhances rules-based morality by considering the impact of ethical decisions on the maintenance or restoration of relationships among individuals (Lo, 2000). The Ethics of Care would ask how will the decision restore family harmony or ensure the patient that the care team is respectful of the patient's values in considering options for the patient. All parties in a caring relationship are treated with compassion, fidelity, accountability, trust, and sensibility (Beauchamp & Childress, 2001). This would justify measured consideration and response in evaluating the level of potential harm to a patient if the practitioner's incompetence is not addressed but also maintain focus on the outcome to the practitioner whether questions of competence are reported or not. Attention to maintaining positive relationships underscores the process. The ethical principle of justice would also support an assessment based on equity of response and a consideration of the level of burden placed on both the patient and practitioner in addressing questions of competence.

Conflicts of Interest

A conflict of interest is defined as a circumstance that interferes with professional discretion and impartial judgment leading to potential harm to patients, colleagues, and the care setting. Standard 1.06 of the Code of Ethics (NASW, 1999) directs social workers to avoid dual relationships that may exploit patients to further the social worker's personal, religious, or business interests. This mandate is based on the concern for patients in crisis who may be very vulnerable and unable to protect themselves from possible exploitation. Patients and family members may interpret professional interest as friendship, especially in the setting of the level of intimacy that exists in the professional relationship when the patient and family are stressed by the threat of and actuality of cumulative losses. The professional relationship may be misread as more personal than the practitioner intends. It is

---

Box 67.1C
Patient/Family Narrative: Libby (continued)

Libby brings mistrust to her current relationships with health care staff based both on her early history and her suspicion that she has been misdiagnosed. Her fear of potential adverse events and her lack of understanding of standard nursing practice results in her asking to have a new nurse removed from her team. She has misinterpreted the new nurse's questions as incompetence rather than understanding that this is the usual procedure for an initial interview, where review of the care plan is an essential part of establishing a collaborative relationship with patients.

the duty of the social worker to establish, maintain, and monitor clearly the appropriate boundaries of the relationship and to share them both with the patient and family (see Box 67.1D).

These same parameters ought to be established and universalized to all members of the care team. Establishing personal friendships with patients; giving and accepting gifts; and extending favors can be misinterpreted within the team and by outside observers of team practice. Team members need to be even more vigilant when recruiting patients and family members for needed research in palliative care (Casarett, 2005). Potential subjects should clearly understand the purpose of the study and the potential benefits for themselves and future patients, the extent of short-term and long-term risks, and that they have the right to refuse to participate without that refusal affecting the level of care that will be provided to them now and in the future. The researcher should not be primarily involved in the patient's care because there may be a perceived pressure felt by the patient to join the study to please the researcher or to maintain the professional relationship. Conversely, the researcher's judgment may be clouded by the care relationship with the patient. Patients generally volunteer for studies for altruistic reasons, to find meaning or have some good come from their illness, understanding that the protocol results may not directly benefit them (Appelbaum, Lidz, & Klitzman, 2009). Casarett (2005) also suggests that at the end of the study, results that could benefit the patient be shared with the patients and provided to the subjects in the research. The ethics of care and the ethical principles of beneficence and nonmaleficence would support this outreach in that patients would benefit from the information derived from the study that could positively impact their health.

An unanticipated outcome of the social worker being identified as a nonjudgmental helper, problem solver, and caring colleague is that members of the team may turn to him or her for help with personal problems. While this might by perceived by the social worker as a show of confidence and a compliment to their skills, it holds potential boundary violations for both the social worker and colleague. The social worker may listen to their colleagues' concern and offer support and referrals for service but should avoid providing therapeutic interventions. If therapy is offered, the professional relationship has irrevocably changed, and this altered relationship may adversely impact patient care. The same

---

Box 67.1D
Patient/Family Narrative: Libby (continued)

The social worker reminded Libby of their mutual understanding of the limits of the professional relationship and explained that accepting a personal gift would be considered a violation of the social worker's professional ethics. Libby reluctantly agreed and decided to donate the gift to the hospital's fundraiser as a silent auction item at the social worker's suggestion.

---

potential occurs when the social worker seeks out personal clinical advice from team members.

The care setting can facilitate avoidance of conflicts of interest by establishing policies that identify expected standards in professional relationships and by providing a supportive culture that promotes professional care and compassion in the setting. Organizational ethical issues such as monitoring professional self-referral patterns, implementing cost savings equitably, and maintaining fidelity to mission are the responsibility of institutional leadership. The principles of beneficence and justice support the initiatives to maintain the patient perspective first in organizational planning.

Recommendations

Ethical considerations permeate all aspects of the practice of social work in responding to questions of moral choice, social justice, and personal accountability in all professional activities (Goldstein, 1998; Manning, 1997). It is essential that social workers have ethics education in their graduate studies, orientation, and continuing education. Ethics education not only helps social workers determine the extent to which problems they encounter in practice are related to ethics but can also help them clarify their own values and beliefs and develop the skills needed to manage ethical problems (Grady et al., 2008; Landau, 1999). Christ and Blacker (2005) add that since the members of the team are expected to work together, ethics training should be a shared experience among team members. The content of the training critical to palliative care includes curriculum specific to bioethics which would include, at a minimum, ethical perspectives, principles, and models for ethical decision making (Csikai & Bass, 2000; Csikai & Raymer, 2005). Social workers who develop skills to recognize and present an ethical issue, ask relevant questions, and seek resolution within the team or care setting represent the interests of the patients and families, team, and setting in which they practice (Csikai, 2004).

Social workers should have access to additional ethical resources such as consultation services to support an ethical approach to practice (O'Donnell et al., 2008). Social workers are generally included in the rosters of their setting's ethics committee but need to define their role and contribution to the committee on an ongoing basis. The social work focus on the patient and family in the context of the patient's illness and dying is a unique perspective from which other professionals on the committee can learn. The effective social work committee member not only initiates discussion of ethical conflict but suggests solutions that promote ethical awareness in the setting, revises policy that reflects and improves the patient and family experience, and offers means for all committee members to ensure ethical practice.

The NASW Code of Ethics directs social workers to be particularly attentive to the needs of vulnerable populations, which would encompass advocacy at a macro level for patients and their families at the end of life. Mizrahi (1992) noted the strong tradition of social work advocacy that expands from the bedside to addressing how society as a whole meets the needs of patients. Wesley (1996) suggests that social workers can influence their institution's level of compassion and benevolence for patients by helping individuals determine what is their own best quality of life and, in addition, advocating for better societal supports for all patients. Stein and Sherman (2005) recommend that social workers, consequent to their direct experience and knowledge, assume a leadership role in advocating for changes in policies at the institutional, regulatory, state, and federal levels that affect palliative care and end-of-life care and services. This would be operationalized by the social worker's active participation in research, utilization of techniques that empower patient and families to present their perspectives in a variety of media, and leadership to assess and meet community needs. These interventions not only serve our patients and families but actualize our profession's ethical obligations to the common welfare, a goal true to our tradition of advocacy for those who are suffering and in need.

LEARNING EXERCISES

- Investigate the laws in your state (or neighbouring states if your practice area expands beyond your state) concerning confidentiality, privileged communications, and the duty to protect, as they apply to social workers.
- Determine what distinguishes boundary relationship crossings from violations. Make a list of acceptable boundary crossings in professional relationships. Are there cultural influences and settings such as home care that determine acceptable boundary crossings?
- Describe team models of problem solving. Decide which are the most effective and why? Would this model work in addressing a colleague's clinical incompetence?

ADDITIONAL SUGGESTED RESOURCES

WEB SITES

The American Society for Bioethics and Humanities: http://www.asbh.org
Promotes the exchange of ideas and fosters multidisciplinary, interdisciplinary, and interprofessional scholarship, research, teaching, policy development, professional development, and collegiality among people engaged in clinical and academic bioethics and the medical humanities.
Bioethics.net: http://www.bioethics.net

Founded in 1993 as the first bioethics Web site, bioethics.net and *The American Journal of Bioethics* (AJOB) have grown to become the most read source of information about bioethics. AJOB is published in print and online by Taylor & Francis Group and housed at bioethics.net.
Cleveland Clinic, The Department of Bioethics: http://my.clevelandclinic.org/bioethics/
Established in 1983 and is administratively located in the Chief of Staff's Office. The Department's mission includes clinical consultation, research ethics, institutional ethics support, education, and research.
The Emory Center for Ethics: http://ethics.emory.edu/
Dedicated to exploring how ethical issues underlie the decisions that shape our minds, lives, and society. To do so, scholars from across the university gather at the Center to collaborate and study.
EthicShare: http://www.ethicshare.org
A research and collaboration Web site for scholars working in the field of ethics. Developed with an initial focus on bioethics, the EthicShare collection features scholarly articles, books, archival and digital objects, popular press literature, dissertations, and commission reports, as well as blogs and other sources.
Ethics Updates: http://ethics.sandiego.edu
Founded in 1994 by Lawrence M. Hinman, a professor of philosophy at the University of San Diego. Originally, it was intended to update the bibliographical essays in two of his books, *Ethics: A Pluralistic Approach to Moral Theory* and *Contemporary Moral Issues*. The site still reflects its origins: the structure of the two principal components of the site reflects the tables of contents of those two books.
The Hastings Center: http://www.thehastingscenter.org
An independent, nonpartisan, and nonprofit bioethics research institute founded in 1969. The Center's mission is to address fundamental ethical issues in the areas of health, medicine, and the environment as they affect individuals, communities, and societies.
Kenan Institute for Ethics: http://kenan.ethics.duke.edu/
Works across the university as one of Duke's signature initiatives rather than being housed in any specific school or department. The institute is an interdisciplinary "think and do" tank committed to understanding and addressing real-world ethical challenges facing individuals, organizations, and societies worldwide.
The MS-PCE Project: http://www.mcw.edu/eperc
Supports individuals involved in the design, implementation, and/or evaluation of End-of-Life/Palliative education for physicians, nurses, and other health care professionals.
The National Center for Ethics in Health Care: http://www.ethics.va.gov
Utilizes a multidisciplinary staff representing various fields, including medicine, nursing, philosophy, law, policy making, education, theology, social work, and health care administration. Center activities and initiatives support clinical ethics, organizational ethics, and research ethics throughout VHA. Under the Center's auspices VHA's National Ethics Committee provides analysis and guidance on controversial ethics issues affecting patients, providers, health care managers, and health policy makers in concise, practical reports.
The National Reference Center for Bioethics Literature (NRCBL): http://bioethics.georgetown.edu

A specialized collection of books, journals, newspaper articles, legal materials, regulations, codes, government publications, and other relevant documents concerned with issues in biomedical and professional ethics. The library holdings represent the world's largest collection related to ethical issues in medicine and biomedical research. This collection functions both as a reference library for the public and as an in-depth research resource for scholars from the United States and abroad.

The Neiswanger Institute for Bioethics and Health Policy: http://www.bioethics.lumc.edu

Dedicated to the three-fold mission of research, education, and service. The Institute serves the students and faculty of the Stritch School of Medicine, health care professionals and patients of Loyola University Health System, and professionals from the regional community and across the nation.

The Office of Human Subjects Research (OHSR): http://ohsr.od.nih.gov

Established to help National Institute of Health's Intramural Research Program (IRP) investigators understand and comply with the ethical guidelines and regulatory requirements for research involving human subjects. OHSR's overall goal is to promote and support the IRP's efforts to conduct innovative research that protects the rights and promotes the welfare of human subjects.

Silence Kills: http://www.silencekills.com/

Past studies have indicated that nearly three in four medical errors are caused by mistakes in interpersonal communication. This study builds on these findings by exploring the specific concerns people have a hard time communicating that may contribute to avoidable errors and other chronic problems in health care.

The Stanford Encyclopedia of Philosophy (SEP): http://www.plato.stanford.edu

Designed so that each entry is maintained and kept up to date by an expert or group of experts in the field. All entries and substantive updates are refereed by the members of a distinguished Editorial Board before they are made public. The Table of Contents lists entries that are published or assigned.

The University of Toronto Joint Centre for Bioethics (JCB): http://www.jointcentreforbioethics.ca/

A partnership between the University of Toronto and affiliated health care organizations. The JCB studies important ethical, health-related topics through research and clinical activities.

BOOKS

Cooper, D. E. (2004). *Ethics for professionals in a multicultural world.* Englewood Cliffs, NJ: Pearson/Prentice Hall.

Lowenberg, F. M., Dolgoff, R., & Harrington, D. (2009). *Ethical decisions for social work practice* (8th ed.). Monterey, CA: Books/Cole Cengage Learning.

Manning, S. (2003). *Ethical leadership in human services: A multi-dimensional approach.* Boston, MA: Pearson Education, Inc.

Reamer, F. G. (2001). *Tangled relationships: Managing boundary issues in the human services.* New York, NY: Columbia University Press.

ARTICLES

Freud, S., & Krug, S. (2002). Beyond the code of ethics, Part I. Complexities of ethical decision making in social work practice. *Families in Society, 83*(5), 474–483.

Greene, A. D., & Latting, J. K. (2004). Whistle-blowing as a form of advocacy: Guidelines for the practitioner and organization. *Social Work, 49*(2), 219–231.

Jennings, B. (1987). The public duties of the professions. *The Hastings Center Report,* Special Supplement, 1–20.

Manning, S. S., & Gaul, C. E. (1997). The ethics of informed consent: A critical variable in the self-determination of health and mental health clients. *Social Work in Health Care, 25*(3), 103–117.

Mattison, M. (2000). Ethical decision making: The person in the process. *Social Work, 45*(3), 201–212.

Mayer, L. (2005). Professional boundaries in dual relationships. *Journal of Social Work Values and Ethics, 5*(5). Retrieved from http://www.socialworker.com/jswve/content/view/25/37/

Ozar, D.T. (1982). Three models of group choice. *Journal of Medicine and Philosophy, 7*(1), 23–34. doi:10.1093/jmp/7.1.23.

Reamer, R. G. (2005). Ethical and legal standards in social work: Consistency and conflict. *Families in Society, 86*(2), 163–169.

Reeves, R., Douglas, S. P., Garner, R. T., Reynolds, M. D., & Silvers, A. (2007). The individual rights of the difficult patient. *The Hastings Center Report, 37*(2), 13–18.

REFERENCES

Abramson, M. (1984). Collective responsibility in interdisciplinary collaboration. *Social Work in Heath Care, 10*(1), 35–43.

Agency for Healthcare Research and Quality (2009). National Consensus Project for Quality Palliative Care. Clinical practice guidelines for quality palliative care. Retrieved from http://www.guidelines.gov/content.aspx?id=14423

Appelbaum, P. S., Lidz, C. W., & Klitzman, R. (2009). Voluntariness of consent to research: A conceptual model. *Hastings Center Report, 39*(1), 30–39.

Beauchamp, T. L., & Childress, J. F. (2001). *Principles of biomedical ethics* (5th ed.). New York, NY: Oxford University Press.

Block, S. D. (2007). Clinical and ethical issues in palliative care. *Focus, The Journal of Lifelong Learning in Psychiatry, 5*(4), 393–397.

Calman, K. (2004). Ethical issues–Introduction. In D. Doyle, G. Hanks, N. I. Cherny, & K. Calman (Eds), *Oxford textbook of palliative medicine,* (3rd ed., pp. 55–57). New York, NY: Oxford University Press.

Cassarett, D. (2005). Ethical considerations in end-of-life care and research. *Journal of Palliative Medicine, 8*(Suppl.), S148–S160.

Christ, G. (2005). End-of-life and palliative care policy: Social work's perspective and contributions. *Journal of Palliative Medicine, 8*(6), 1269–1270.

Christ, G., & Blacker, S. (2005). Improving interdisciplinary communication skills with families. *Journal of Palliative Medicine, 8*(4), 855–856.

Corley, M. (2002). Moral distress: A proposed theory and research agenda. *Nursing Ethics, 9*, 636–650.

Csikai, E. L. (2004). Social worker's participation in the resolution of ethical dilemmas in hospice care. *Health and Social Work, 29*(1), 67–76.

Csikai, E. L., & Bass, K. (2000). Health care social worker's views of ethical issues, practice, and policy in end-of-life care. *Social Work in Health Care, 32*(2), 1–22.

Csikai, E. L., & Raymer, M. (2005). Social workers' educational needs in end-of-life care. *Social Work in Health Care, 41*(1), 53–72.

Degnin, F. D. (2009). Difficult patients, overmedication, and groupthink. *Journal of Clinical Ethics, 20*(1), 64–74.

Emanuel, L., & Emanuel, E. (1992). Four models of the physician-patient relationship. *Journal of the American Medical Association, 267*(16), 2221–2226.

Gallagher, T. H., Studdert, D., & Levinson, W. (2007). Disclosing harmful medical errors to patients. *New England Journal of Medicine, 356*, 2713–2719.

Germain, C. B. (1984). *Social work practice in health care: An ecological perspective.* New York, NY: The Free Press.

Glacjchen, M., & Zuckerman, C. (2001). Resolving conflict and making decisions. *Journal of Palliative Medicine, 4*(2), 221–225.

Goldstein, H. (1998). Education for ethical dilemmas in social work practice. *Families in Society: The Journal of Contemporary Human Services, 79*(5/6), 241–253.

Grady, C., Danis, M., Soeken, K., O'Donnell, P., Taylor, C., Farrar, A., & Ulrich, C. (2008). Does ethics education influence the moral action of practicing nurses and social workers? *American Journal of Bioethics, 8*(4), 4–11.

Hippocrates (4th Century, BCE). *Hippocratic Oath.* (M. North, Trans.) Retrieved from United States National Library of Medicine Web site: https://www.nlm.nih.gov/hmd/greek/greek_oath.html.

Holland, T. P., & Kilpatrick, A. C. (1991). Ethical issues in social work: Toward a grounded theory of professional ethics. *Social Work, 36*(2), 138–144.

Joseph, M.V. (1985). A model for ethical decision making in clinical practice. In C. B. Germain (Ed.), *Advances in clinical practice* (pp. 207–217). Silver Spring, MD: National Association of Social Workers.

King, D. A., & Quill, T. (2006). Working with families in palliative care: One size does not fit all. *Journal of Palliative Medicine, 9*(3), 704–715.

Landau, R. (1999). Professional socialization, ethical judgment, and decision making orientation in social work. *Journal of Social Service Research, 25*(4), 57–75.

Lo, B. (2000). *Resolving ethical dilemmas: A guide for clinicians* (5th ed.). Philadelphia, PA: Lippincott, Williams, & Wilkins.

Manning, S. S. (1997). The social worker as moral citizen: Ethics in action. *Social Work, 42*(3), 223–230.

McDonald, N. (2004). Confidentiality. In D. Doyle, G. Hanks, N. I. Cherny, & K. Calman (Eds.), *Oxford textbook of palliative medicine* (3rd ed., pp. 17–43). New York, NY: Oxford University Press.

McMahon, R. L. (2003). An ethical dilemma in a hospice setting. *Palliative and Supportive Care, 1*, 79–87. doi:10.1017/S1478951503030013.

Meier, D. E., & Beresford, L. (2008). The palliative care team. *Journal of Palliative Medicine, 11*(5), 677–681. doi:10-1089/jpm.2009.9907.

Meisel, A., Snyder, L., & Quill, T. (2000). Seven legal myths to end-of-life care: Myths, realities, and grains of truth. *Journal of the American Medical Association, 284*, 2495–2501.

Millstein, K. (2000). Confidentiality in direct social work practice: Inevitable challenges and ethical dilemmas. *Families in Society: The Contemporary Human Services, 81*(3), 270–282.

Mizrahi, T. (1992). The direction of patient's rights in the 1990s: Proceed with caution. *Health and Social Work, 17*(4), 247–252.

National Association of Social Workers (NASW). (1999). *Code of ethics.* Washington, DC: Author.

National Association of Social Workers (NASW). (2004). *NASW standards for social work practice in palliative and end of life care.* Retrieved from http://www.socialworkers.org/practice/bereavement/standards/standards0504New.pdf

O'Donnell, P., Farrar, A., Brintzenhofe-Szoc, K., Conrad, A. P., Danis, M., Grady, C., … Ulrich, C. (2008). Predictors of ethical stress, moral action and job satisfaction in health care social workers. *Health and Social Work, 46*(3), 29–51.

Pellegrino, E. D. (1998). Emerging ethical issues in palliative care. *Journal of the American Medical Association, 279*(19), 1521–1522.

Potter, R. L., & Reynolds, D. F. (2000). *Guidelines for providing ethical care in difficult provider-patient relationships.* Kansas City, MO: Midwest Bioethics Center.

Randall, F., & Downie, R. S. (1999). *Palliative care ethics: A companion for all specialities* (2nd ed.). Oxford, England: Oxford University Press.

Reamer, F. G. (2009). *The social work ethics casebook: Cases and commentary.* Washington, DC: NASW Press.

Rose, S. L., & Shelton, W. (2006). The role of social work in the ICU. *Journal of Social Work in End-of-Life and Palliative Care, 2*(2), 3–23. doi:10.1300/J457v02n02_02.

Saunders, C. (2001). Social work and palliative care-the early history. *British Journal of Social Work, 31*, 791–799.

Ulrich, C. M., O'Donnell, P., Taylor, C., Farrar, A., Danis, M., & Grady, C. (2007). Ethical climate, ethics stress, and the job satisfaction of nurses and social workers in the United States. *Social Science and Medicine, 65*(8), 1708–1719.

Weir, R. F. (1986). Truth telling in medicine. In R. F. Weir (Ed.), *Ethical issues in death and dying* (pp. 25–47). New York, NY: Columbia University Press.

Wesley, C. A. (1996). Social work and end-of-life decisions: Self-determination and the common good. *Health and Social Work, 21*(2), 115–121.

68 *Tracy Borgmeyer*

The Social Work Role in Decision Making: Ethical, Psychosocial, and Cultural Perspectives

When I have a major illness requiring highly specialized treatment, I will seek out a doctor skilled in its provision. But I will not expect of him that he will understand my values, my expectations for myself and those I love, my spiritual nature, or my philosophy of life. That is not what he is trained for and that is not what he will be good at.
— Sherwin B. Nuland, from How We Die: Reflections on Life's Final Chapter, p. 266

Key Concepts

- ◆ *The role of palliative social workers in the health care decision-making process is multifaceted.*
- ◆ *Various psychosocial and spiritual circumstances influence decisions made by patients and their families.*
- ◆ *Cultural backgrounds and beliefs influence the illness experience as well as the social work role and response in serving patients and families of diverse cultures.*
- ◆ *Advance directives have value and limitations in the process of medical decision making.*
- ◆ *Conversations about personal preferences, values, and beliefs are essential to the decision-making process.*
- ◆ *Social work skills in palliative care include the application of ethical principles and an understanding of the competing ethical principles often encountered in the decision-making process.*
- ◆ *Knowledge of ethical principles leads to the responsibility to advocate and educate within the health care teams and the institution.*

Introduction

Social workers in palliative care assist those with chronic and progressive illness and coming to the end of life to evolve a plan of care that best reflects and responds to their unique needs. Through careful assessment of the person-in-environment, we attend to psychosocial factors that will impact patients' coping, family responses, and ultimately the decisions made in the setting of advanced illness. We also acknowledge that health care outcomes depend in part upon providing care that is culturally relevant and respects diverse values, beliefs, and practices. Black (2004, 2005, 2006) has identified the social work roles of initiator, educator, facilitator, advocate, and liaison in work with patients, families, and the health care team. Additionally, palliative social workers are observant and inquisitive participants in the helping process, demonstrating both a knowledge of ethical principles as well as skills that help to identify and integrate the cultural and spiritual beliefs, practices, and needs of individual patients, families, and intimate networks into the decision-making process.

Infusing Psychosocial-Spiritual Considerations

It is important for social workers to understand the many psychosocial factors influencing the choices our patients make about medical care. Family roles and dynamics, socio-economic factors, prior history with illness and/or treatment, and many other psychosocial issues may influence decision making. Spiritual or religious beliefs and practices may guide decisions, particularly at the end of life. Established family roles and patterns of interaction may apply in health care decision making, just as they do in other aspects of life. However, those roles may be strained and challenged by the new stress of a serious illness. For example, a patient whose family consults a male head of household (such as a father, uncle, or grandfather) for decisions involving financial expense may adhere to this same pattern about expenses related to treatments, not realizing that these decisions not only take financial acumen but also an ability to integrate and synthesize medical concepts to weigh the benefits and risks of treatments as well as the cost.

Patients and families may also develop their unique process for handling medical issues, such as relying on the guidance of a family member who is a physician or nurse. Thus, even decisions such as the scheduling of an office visit may be determined by the availability of that trusted family member.

Socioeconomic factors such as poverty, financial dependence, and access to transportation may influence what medical care is pursued and whether adherence to treatment schedules is possible. Missed appointments may be interpreted as non-adherence or ambivalence about treatment when they truly reflect an absence of resources or practical services like transportation. A patient's personal or family history can also have a significant influence on receptiveness to treatment recommendations. A patient whose parent died on the operating table may have an exceptionally fearful attitude toward surgery, tending to overemphasize risks; a patient who faced a very difficult postoperative course after a surgery may decline to undergo another procedure.

Social workers are trained to help patients identify their concerns, and to address them with a variety of interventions, toward a goal of empowering the patient. By clarifying values and goals, and exploring options, social workers aim to help patients achieve best outcomes as defined by the patient. Social workers may also identify systemic and environmental obstacles impacting decision making and advocate for services that better respond to or accommodate patient needs.

Based on the ethical principle of autonomy, the profession of social work upholds the value of client self-determination. Social workers foster a belief that, in the majority of situations, the most appropriate outcomes derive from patient-directed decision making (National Association of Social Workers [NASW], 2004). The core values embraced by the social work profession, in particular the values of social justice and dignity and worth of the person, are congruent with patient-centered approaches to care (NASW, 1999).

Yet autonomous decision making is not an absolute. Some patients, even those able to articulate their wishes, defer decision making to a family member, a whole family, or a community. Recognizing that the nuclear family may or may not be the most immediate support for patients, social workers regularly tailor interventions to meet the needs of the patient. Family patterns, power structures within a community, and cultural values may influence the patient's approach to illness. This can be a challenge for many disciplines on the medical team, because most have training that emphasizes independent decision making and often signed consents by the patient, with a focus on individual best interests. Those cultures that embrace family decision making can be of some concern in medical settings that are structured around the value of individual autonomy. Those persons or family members who are uncomfortable signing papers require additional time and sometimes accommodation. Social workers collaborate with the health care team to lend understanding to the social, spiritual, and historical context that is the basis for the patient's and family's responses to medical care and to facilitate optimal approaches to care.

The narrative in Box 68.1 embodies work that weaves ethics and legal variables and bio-psychosocial-spiritual aspects of the person's experience and demonstrates how one can reconstruct some semblance of a person's life and values by respecting and understanding history and integrating the extended family or kin network. As well as acknowledging the importance of history, the clinical and decision-making process for George created an opportunity for his son Paul, perhaps, to begin a process of healing related to his father. This demonstrates that this essential work which respects the past and validates the present also has the potential to inform the future of the patients and families whom we serve.

Advanced Medical Technology, Bioethics, and the Role of Social Work

Social workers have been talking with patients and their families about preferences for treatment and care in the setting of chronic and progressive illness for a long time (Csikai, 2004.) From the early twentieth century to the present, in hospitals, hospices, cancer centers, dialysis centers, and nursing facilities, to name only a few settings, social workers have been actively engaged in discussions about patients' needs in times of illness and at the end of life.

Modern medical technology has made it possible for patients and surrogates to choose life-prolonging interventions, even in the setting of irreversible medical conditions, far beyond a point when the patient's cognitive capacity allows him or her to still understand options and participate in treatment decisions. The same technologies that may make recovery possible for some illnesses or injuries may complicate medical prognostication, as well as the decision-making process for the surrogates or families of patients. The question of how long a patient may survive becomes answerable in part by matters of access to life-prolonging interventions, the willingness of medical professionals to employ them, and the personal, cultural, and spiritual values and beliefs guiding patients or surrogates in decision making. Social workers on palliative care services often assist patients and families to cope with the stress of the decisions they face, as well as the loss and grief common in the experience of progressive illness.

The use of advanced medical technologies and medications also presents ethical challenges for members of the health care team, in considering when life-sustaining treatment may be withdrawn, as well as in instances when it is continued beyond any expectation of benefit to the patient.

Box 68.1
Patient/Family Narrative: George

George, a man in his late 60s, was a recovering alcoholic who collapsed after an Alcoholics Anonymous (AA) meeting. He was intubated by paramedics due to concerns about airway management, and at the hospital it was discovered that he had sustained an intracranial bleed. He was admitted to the intensive care unit, on a mechanical ventilator. In the emergency department, a chaplain had attempted to identify the legal next of kin. George's AA friends, who had followed the ambulance to the hospital, reported that George had no family. The palliative social worker was consulted and met with several men close to George's age who identified themselves. "We're the closest thing to a family George has." It was clear none were related to him. They inquired about whether he would have to "stay on the vent" and all agreed he would not have wanted that. It was too early in the medical course to make that determination, and confidentiality and privacy laws limited what information could be revealed. George's network could be helpful in locating anyone who might be the legal next of kin. His friend Phil, offered, "George has a son, but they haven't spoken in years." He had no idea how the son might be contacted.

The social worker emphasized the importance of any assistance they might provide in locating family and Phil, who had a key to George's apartment, agreed to search for names and phone numbers and any advance directive that George may have completed. Inquiry about advance directives, such as a living will or power of attorney, provoked a response that invited a beginning understanding of George, his values, and beliefs. "George lived one day at a time."

For days a stream of visitors came to see George, sharing information about their beloved friend which continued to inform the staff's understanding of the person: "George has been in recovery for 20 years. Some of the guys you see coming in here, George helped them get sober. He was hardcore, did some bad things, spent a lot of time in jail, a lot of time on the streets. His family gave up on him, and he gave up on himself. After he sobered up, it was too late—his family had already moved on. He was all alone. If he'd wanted an excuse to keep drinking, he'd have had one."

The social worker assisted the staff in their responses to the cohort of friends. While they could provide no medical information directly, their attitudes and care of George symbolized how they too might be cared for; the staff's behaviors and words went beyond the care of George and had the power to reassure all these men who had struggled with substance abuse that perhaps they too would be cared for in an expert and compassionate manner.

After a number of days, Phil and another friend, Dave, provided the name and phone number of George's son, Paul. They reported that George had been in phone contact with Paul in recent years. There had been a brief visit; it had not been a warm or joyful reunion but rather reflective of the turmoil and suffering that had been a part of their history when George was actively drinking.

The social worker consulted with Risk Management regarding the family relationship issues. In accord with state statutes, which required contact with the legal next of kin, regardless of the estrangement, Paul was contacted. The attending physician informed Paul about his father's current medical condition and expected clinical course, as well as the options for further management and comfort measures. The social worker inquired

about the existence of additional children, assessed Paul's willingness to make decisions, his knowledge of his father's wishes, and whether his current feelings and attitudes about his father would allow him to make thoughtful decisions. The social worker also advised Paul about the alternative if he felt unable to assume the decision-making role; the hospital would petition the court for guardianship. A judge would typically appoint a public administrator or legal advocate to make decisions. According to George's doctors, he would probably not survive long enough to complete the guardianship process. The social worker invited Paul, who lived two states away, to visit if being present would help him to better comprehend the medical condition and inform his decisions. Though he declined, Paul gave consent for George's friends to have information and to visit. He intended to contact them to gain additional understanding of his father beyond his early experiences.

The following week, Paul notified the social worker that he had been speaking by phone with Phil, Dave, and other AA friends. He felt comfortable that he understood his father's values and beliefs well enough to consent to withdraw ventilator support and to provide medical care aimed at the goal of comfort, which included psychological and spiritual support to George, Paul, and the network of friends. His father's reliance on a higher power was of significance to Paul, himself a "person of faith." In collaboration with the clinical team the social worker explored the factors and process that surrounded Paul's decision and all agreed that his process and decision seemed congruent with his father's values as known, medically appropriate, and not primarily driven by the complex feelings that pervaded their relationship.

After the decisions had been reviewed and accepted, Paul commented that his conversations with his dad's friends had brought him peace about the man his father had become. He had seen this in his visit some time ago, but he had been reluctant to trust that the change was real or sustainable. Hearing the impact his father had on others helped redeem him somewhat in Paul's eyes. He said, "I admit, when you called, I wanted to decline to get involved, and let the hospital just work with the courts on the matter. But I'm glad I got to know about him, and I really thank you for looking for me."

Palliative social workers often encounter opportunities to inform ethical deliberations and lend support to the professional caregivers who may find it difficult to understand the choices being made by patients, physicians, and families. Social workers can also advocate for staff education on topics such as ethics, patient rights, and caregiver wellness.

The conversation between a nurse and social worker in Box 68.2 also provided an opportunity to acknowledge the importance of a work environment that encourages discourse on ethical issues, and ethics education for all disciplines. The social worker commended the nurse for speaking up about a statement that raised ethical concerns for her, and she emphasized the importance of staff paying attention to their internal struggles with ethical issues, both to initiate dialogue with other staff for further exploration or to refer to ethics committees for resolution of unsettled ethical questions. While this patient and his wife had a well-established

Box 68.2
Patient/Family Narrative: Donald

Donald, a patient in his early 70s with non-Hodgkins lymphoma, had undergone numerous rounds of chemotherapy over the course of 3 years. The disease was no longer responding to treatment, and his symptoms and side effects had become intolerable. However, Donald, determined and optimistic throughout his life, declined hospice despite his oncologist's assurance that all chemotherapies had been exhausted and that symptom management and continued attention to his needs and those of his family was the appropriate plan of care. When Donald's wife, Ann, brought him to the emergency room, he was minimally responsive, with extensive lymphadenopathy and labored respirations. Though Donald could not communicate, his wife agreed with the oncologist that a do not resuscitate (DNR) order was appropriate. The doctor prepared Ann and one of the couple's daughters that Donald would not likely survive beyond a few hours to a few days, and Donald was admitted for end-of-life care.

On the day after admission, the social worker was approached by a nurse who was confused and uncomfortable with a conversation she had at Donald's bedside with Ann. The nurse had commented to Ann that "the important thing is that you are honoring his wishes." Ann and her daughter had exchanged glances and smiled, responding "Oh, no, this is not his "wish" at all! He refused hospice, and he would have refused the DNR order if he thought there was any chance he could come through this." The nurse, suddenly at a loss for words, excused herself from the bedside. In questioning the social worker about the remarks, she recalled, "in our training, we were told that the family should try to make the same decision the patient would make. So how is this okay? Are they admitting that they are going against his wishes?"

The social worker reviewed the medical record and met with Ann to establish rapport and begin to understand what factors informed and influenced the current approach to care. In discussing the days leading up to Donald's hospitalization, as well as the couple's recent office visits with the oncologist, the social worker gathered a sense of the patient and family's approach to the progression of the illness. "Don always felt he had to be hopeful—for us, I think. He never talked to me about dying. He would just say "You will know what to do, and you'll have the kids to help you." But his friend, John, is a funeral director, and they've been meeting for coffee with a group of guys for years. Don would never go to the funeral home, but last month he gave John all his instructions. I think he knew he didn't have a lot of time."

Ann continued, "In the emergency room, his doctor told us that trying to resuscitate him would be futile, that it would cause him harm, and would not help him, not change anything. I called the kids, and they said, 'Mom, we have to let go. He's fought this as long as he can.'"

This situation provided an opportunity for the social worker and the nurse to discuss the principle of autonomy, as well as the limits of autonomy, and the principles of beneficence and nonmaleficence. Ann's comments had not been intended as an indication of disregard for what her husband wanted, but an acknowledgement of her husband's perpetual hope and his reluctance to verbally acknowledge dying. Ann's request to the doctor had been "please don't hurt him." Nonmaleficence, the duty to avoid harm, had been the guiding principle. The ethical concept of "benefit vs. burden" applied, with the assessment that the burden of further interventions would be greater than any benefit. The nurse expressed a better understanding of the decision-making process, but she acknowledged that her training had emphasized that families and surrogates should try to "honor the patient's wishes." In reframing this scenario, the social worker noted that the family had, in fact, honored Donald's wishes for as long as possible. They supported his choice to continue with therapy despite a difficult course, and Ann had cared for him at home, without the support of hospice, out of respect for his choices. His comment to her: "You will know what to do" had implied a time when he could not decide for himself. Furthermore, through the act of making funeral arrangements with his friend, Donald had given some indication that he knew he would die soon, even though he did not communicate about it with his family.

relationship and history with the treating physician, there are times when we care for patients whose histories and families are not known to the physician or team. Providing good care may involve paying attention to circumstances that seem incongruent or signal conflict.

O'Donnell et al. (2008) explored ethical stress, moral action, and job satisfaction among social workers in health care. The availability of ethics resources, positive support for ethical reflection and decision making from team members, and an organizational climate that permits and encourages open discussion of ethical concerns were identified as important to social workers for management of ethical stress and job satisfaction. The lack of support for ethical stress and moral action was a factor in the decision of some social workers to leave the field.

The Patient Self-Determination Act of 1991 (PSDA) was an initiative to ensure that a patient's preferences would be honored in the event that he or she became unable to communicate his or her decisions about medical care (Patient Self-Determination Act, 1990). The PSDA was the result of a focused national effort following the Cruzan decision by the Supreme Court in 1990 (Cruzan v. Director, 1990). Nancy Cruzan's family faced opposition when they requested to discontinue artificial tube feeding tube for Nancy, who had been in a persistent vegetative state for several years, a result of anoxic brain injury after a car accident (Colby, 2002.) From this public discussion, a consensus developed that patients should have a mechanism to express their wishes in advance of a catastrophic injury or illness. Congress passed the PSDA, which became law in December 1991 (Patient Self-Determination Act, 1990). Health care providers receiving federal funding are required to inform patients, upon admission, of their rights and hospital policies and procedures regarding advance directives. In hospitals nationwide, this mandate has had implications for social workers, who have often been the designated staff responding to requests for patient education and assistance in completing advance directives. (For more information, see Chapter 69)

Yet nearly two decades since the enactment of the PSDA, there are many challenges to decision making along the continuum of illness and at end of life (SUPPORT, 1995). The mere existence of an advance directive does not ensure the quality of discussions, that surrogates have been involved, or that the decisions of surrogates will reflect patient preferences. Ongoing conversations between patients, their surrogates, families and intimate network, and between patients and physicians are essential in the endeavor to provide appropriate care (SUPPORT, 1995). However, not all patients will have these kinds of crucial conversations for a variety of complex individual, family, cultural, spiritual, and systemic reasons. Consider the following examples:

- A divorced mother of teenagers delays discussions about the seriousness of her illness, anticipating that the children's father and grandparents will argue about who will be the better primary custodian.
- A married man with end-stage chronic obstructive pulmonary disease (COPD) declines hospice, fearing that hospice caregivers will discover how much he struggles to care for his wife with dementia, and the two will have to enter a nursing home.
- The wife of a patient with end-stage lung cancer rescinds her husband's do not resuscitate/do not intubate (DNR/DNI)) order, believing that if intubation is not provided her husband will die in acute respiratory distress.
- An 80-year-old Mandarin-speaking grandmother appoints her grandson as health care agent, simply because he speaks English. He is not the decision maker in the family, and if he is expected by staff to act, the family structure and his place within the family may be seriously impacted.

Social workers are often called to assist when these scenarios result in the crisis of an emergent hospitalization. Just as social workers provide an effective response to the patient in crisis, social workers are uniquely prepared to address these issues early in the continuum of illness and may develop screening tools and referral processes that identify those patients who may benefit from services. When palliative care is introduced early in the continuum of illness, there is opportunity to assist the person whose needs may reasonably be expected to change in the future, even if the timeline is elusive. Knowledge of community resources and processes, along with skills for initiating and communicating about difficult subjects, complements a professional principle of empowering the client to examine options and make choices. Using a strengths-based perspective, a social worker may use conflict resolution skills to prepare a mother to address the issue of custody with her former spouse and her parents. Grief counseling and knowledge of community resources for caregivers, adult day care, legal resources, guardianship, and hospice may assist a married man to explore possibilities for addressing the needs of his wife, while optimizing his own health and quality of life in order to be a caregiver as long as possible. A social worker who is

comfortable with complexities of medical language can translate that information in lay terms to provide clarifications that facilitate decision making by the man with lung cancer while he is able to speak for himself. Including his wife in discussions prepares her for the expected progression of end-stage disease, validates her fear and anxiety as normal in the anticipation of loss, and provides needed emotional support. Joining with medical colleagues to openly discuss effective symptom management or palliative sedation to manage a possible crisis of acute or intractable dyspnea provides a framework for patients and families to know what will be provided if they chose a DNR/DNI order.

Social workers who understand the cultural aspects of Chinese family structure, the potential consequences of disrupting that structure, and the importance of having an advocate who speaks the language of the institution are in a pivotal position to mediate these variables to ensure that the decision-making processes do not inadvertently harm the grandson. It is important to consider that our ethical obligations to beneficence (to do what is good) and nonmaleficence (do no harm) extend beyond the patients to their families and intimate network and beyond the present to the future well-being of the family system.

In most medical settings, physicians make determinations about whether a patient has the capacity to make decisions. Social workers in palliative care need excellent assessment and listening skills to identify possible signs that decision-making capacity is compromised. A medical evaluation is essential both to determine whether there is impaired capacity and to determine the etiology in an effort to treat symptoms that are correctable with the goal of restoring capacity. When the patient's ability to give medical consent is questionable, such as with a patient who is heavily medicated or intermittently delirious, it becomes a priority to assist the patient to appoint a surrogate for medical decision making because compromised capacity for complex medical decisions does not automatically extend to the capacity to appoint a surrogate (Arnold, 2006).

Palliative social workers familiar with common symptoms, signs, and indicators for a variety of conditions and/or social issues, such as dementia, depression, substance abuse, physical abuse and/or neglect, or exploitation can identify problems that may impair or impede the patient's ability to make informed, independent choices about medical care. Social workers gain information from observation, interviewing, collaborating with past providers, and reviewing documentation in the medical record. In interdisciplinary team collaboration, it is the shared responsibility to assess all available information, including the potential to enhance capacity for decision making and when appropriate to enlist the agent, surrogate, or legal next of kin to speak for the patient. Where there are ethical conflicts, lack of clarity, or an absence of consensus, social workers need to know how ethical dilemmas are managed within a specific practice setting and suggest an ethics consult to assist clinicians.

Cultural Considerations

Social workers have a rich history of working with diverse groups, and the health care setting places social workers in a helping relationship with people of many different cultures. Racial, ethnic, religious, and lifestyle diversity in our communities necessitates that palliative care clinicians become familiar with various cultural beliefs and practices, as well as common stereotypes and myths. Hospice chaplain and educator Kenneth Doka outlines characteristics of culturally effective counselors, including intellectual curiosity and a willingness to learn about the people and groups they serve (Doka, 2009). While it may not be possible to acquire thorough knowledge of all cultures a clinician may encounter, it is essential to a social work skill set to learn about those most often encountered within a community or workplace (Crawley, Marshall, Lo, & Koenig, 2002). There are readily accessible tools and references that can enhance knowledge of additional cultures. In addition, care and relationships are enriched by the ability to place ourselves in the position of humble learner, asking patients and families about aspects of their culture that may influence their experience and our ability to be helpful.

Learning about the group traits of a culture allows us to have a hypothesis, a place to start. The unique individuals and families we meet test, inform, and correct the hypothesis as long as we are humble, open, and available to learning. In addition to the NASW Code of Ethics, which sets a standard of cultural sensitivity and knowledge for social workers (NASW, 1999), a number of regulatory bodies for health care now set standards for cultural respect among health care staff, in order to provide care that is both sensitive and appropriate. Understanding the person-in-environment (the cultural context) and advocating for culturally responsive care, social workers can be bridge builders between patients, families, and health care systems.

Culture is a significant influence on one's view of illness, coping style, and beliefs about family roles, as well as one's own approach to his or her death. Understanding cultural variables and factors that mediate these influences such as acculturation, assimilation, and education, is essential to understanding how best to serve patients and families who are asked to make decisions at a time of crisis within a health care system that is unfamiliar and at times intimidating. A lack of understanding can create a barrier, leading to breakdown in relationships between patients and clinicians, and among members of the team, thwarting the helping process and leading to poor outcomes (Crawley, et al., 2002; Doka, 2009). A person's culture or community will often provide comfort, familiarity, and constancy, particularly when the patient may be cared for within a setting where the culture of his or her caregivers and the primary language spoken is different. Familiarity with cultural beliefs about illness, medical care, and culture-based health care practices, along with a comfort in communicating with patients and families about beliefs and practices, are essential to the skill set of palliative social work and integral to the health care setting's response to persons from diverse backgrounds.

Social workers must also be prepared to recognize when dominant cultural and religious beliefs of staff or clinicians are imposed in a way that causes suffering or conflict or compromises patients' decision making. For example, a physician repeatedly approaches a woman who is a Jehovah's Witness, attempting to persuade her to receive blood transfusions, even after she has been counseled about the benefit, risks, and expected outcome if she declines blood products. Initiating a professional dialogue, with candor and respect, about a clinician's beliefs, may enable social workers to learn about the values that inform a physician's approach when asked to provide care the physician views as inappropriate, or when prevented from providing care that might be beneficial. In situations where concerns persist about a clinician's ability to respect patients' wishes when they differ from cultural or spiritual beliefs of the clinician, social workers follow the established institutional procedure for consultation to resolve and mediate these complex, often emotional dilemmas. Most health care settings and professional codes of ethics utilize conscience clauses, whereby clinicians may refrain from participating in care that violates personally held beliefs. In these scenarios, clinicians are typically obligated to refer to another practitioner or facility.

Race, ethnicity, and religion are common types of cultural identity, and there are unique cultures of other groups, such as deaf persons, lesbian, gay, bisexual, and transgender (LGBT) persons, and persons with developmental disabilities—each having its own community, with norms, resources, and accepted practices, existing within the larger community. Persons who are homeless as a lifestyle may follow "street culture" with its own popular places and customs. Persons in recovery from substance abuse often refer to the recovery community. (For more information see Chapters 35 and 34) Veterans may come from diverse racial, ethnic, religious, and socioeconomic groups but may identify with other veterans from the same branch of service (such as Army or Marines) or from the same era (such as World War II or Gulf War) (For more information see Chapter 12). Palliative care considers the patient and family as the unit of care; and social workers when engaging the family, friends, and intimate network of the patient move beyond the traditional definition of family both to understand and to respect the external and preexisting networks created by the patient. It is also important to recognize that cultural networks and social supports are not available in all communities, and for some persons, such as lesbians and gay men, access to a supportive community may be very limited. Factors such as nondisclosure to the family of origin or fear of repercussions such as discrimination may limit the extent to which a community may be a supportive network for some persons with advanced illness. Technology, however, offers some an opportunity to create a virtual experience that has the potential to diminish isolation and provide a network of support.

Box 68.3
Patient/Family Narrative: Danielle

Danielle was in her early 30s and had undergone extensive treatment for metastatic breast cancer. As her pain and dyspnea increased, Danielle was encouraged by her oncologist to "put her affairs in order" and to consider hospice. Presenting to the social worker, she announced, "I have to make some decisions, and they're going to have to be in writing somewhere. So what do I do?"

The social worker provided a private office for discussion. In an effort to understand the context in which Danielle was operating and her perception of her prognosis and options for treatment, the social worker explored the medical and treatment history. As Danielle considered who she might name as durable power of attorney (DPOA), she shared her personal and family circumstances, which moved the context from the medical to the person and her history, all of which inform the process of decision making.

A couple of years ago Danielle had come out to her parents as a lesbian, and a short time later introduced her partner, Megan. Danielle's parents, particularly her father, still struggled a great deal with her sexual orientation. Later that year, Danielle's parents separated. Their marital problems had been long term. Their attempts to avoid each other complicated their ability to organize schedules and be present to help care for Danielle. They were supportive of Danielle throughout treatment, but they seemed to resent Megan's presence. At the same time they were critical of Megan for occasionally leaving Danielle, even when Megan's leaving was to give the parents time and privacy with their daughter.

The social worker acknowledged Danielle's distress because of her parents' lack of comfort with her same-sex partner but also normalized the tension, common for young adults with cancer, between parents and a spouse or significant other. Danielle's mother and father, unable to be around each other without arguing, would only come to the house after verifying that the other parent was not there. Danielle questioned her parents' ability to agree on anything, especially the complex and profoundly emotional treatment decisions about their only daughter. She described her father, a veteran, to have a philosophy of "never giving up" and her mother to be a woman of deep faith who prayed for a miracle. "They're both so unrealistic," Danielle said, "and I am their only daughter." Clinical intervention included efforts to assist Danielle to question whether these two sets of expectations, "never give up" and praying for a miracle, had any commonality, exploring their meaning beyond the words her parents articulated. Was hoping for a miracle unrealistic in her mothers' context? Did it imply that she understood that Danielle's medical condition was beyond the ability of her physicians? What did "never give up" mean to her father? Did he truly believe that her disease progression was a matter of will and strength? Had either parent had any assistance in integrating the serious life-threatening illness of their only daughter? Was it possible that parents could choose to allow their daughter to die?

Danielle was aware that her parents would be legally entitled to make decisions about her care, should she become unable to make or communicate her wishes, and she knew she could place that authority with Megan by naming her DPOA. However, Megan was uncomfortable with conflict. Danielle was reluctant to place

Megan between her mother and father. In examining who she might trust to make decisions for her, only her older brother Dennis came to mind. Because of the age difference between them, Danielle and Dennis had not been close in childhood. He was married, with children of his own, living in another state, so it had not been easy for them to be close. However, their relationship had grown since Danielle had come out; she recalled how he reached out with support by calling her often, something he had never done before. When she was diagnosed with cancer, he dropped everything to come home and see her—again, something he had not done before—and he visited several times during her treatment. Their parents' separation united them as siblings even more.

As the social worker inquired about their ability to communicate honestly, and Dennis's dependability as a person of support, as well as his neutrality in relationship to both their parents and Megan, Danielle expressed regret only that Dennis lived too far away to serve as her DPOA. Based on an understanding of the medical realities and after discussion with the oncologist, the social worker was able to reassure her that she may very well be able to communicate and make decisions for herself either prior to or during her final hours and that, when and if a DPOA takes effect, most of the obligations of a DPOA can be carried out by phone, as long as they can be contacted. Dennis had already demonstrated that he could come to be with her when he perceived she was in need. Danielle felt very comfortable that he was the right choice to be her surrogate.

The social worker encouraged Danielle to have a very thorough conversation about her wishes and to assess for herself Dennis's comfort with this role. She included specific values and choices on the health care directive and shared these same thoughts with her health care team. As the discussion turned to Danielle's particular wishes for end-of-life care, the written health care directive helped guide her thoughts and considerations. She recalled a conversation she had weeks ago with a hospice nurse and remembered the death of a grandfather, in a critical care unit, connected to tubes and monitors. Through this process of reflection, Danielle concluded that hospice services might now be the best way to continue to have her pain and symptoms addressed as her condition changed. Danielle was encouraged to speak with her parents and Megan frankly about her wishes, as soon as possible. By exploring the unique ways each was describing his or her hopes and expressing his or her helplessness, Danielle became less responsive to their emotions and focused on sharing her decisions and creating time with each family member. She was encouraged to consider the possibility of enhancing their common goals, which might at the very least ensure comfort and care for all at the end of life.

Medically, there was no further disease-modifying treatment because there was no additional chemotherapy that would prove beneficial. This information was essential to helping her parents and partner to understand that she was not refusing treatments but rather there were none to be considered. The social worker also framed the experience of all as infused with loss—through illness, now terminal; through separation and divorce; through unfulfilled goals and dreams. Time was spent identifying what was most important to Danielle, and what new goals and hopes she might have in light of this limited time. As this process evolved, Danielle recognized the many ways in which putting her affairs in order were not about "just getting something in writing." It was a time to communicate her wishes clearly with her family, her partner, and her physician and to consider their responses and behaviors in a

Box 68.3 *(Contd.)*

different light. It was about protecting her family from choices that could be hers, putting in place services and a plan of care that would provide care for herself and her family and ensure that her preferences would be honored as her condition changed.

Decision Making beyond the Western Model

Cultural considerations in decision making about care may include how and by whom decisions are made, and even how much information is disclosed to the patient. For example, in Japanese and Chinese cultures the family may express a wish that the patient not be informed of a diagnosis or prognosis (Lapine et al., 2001). The family rather than the individual may direct care. Withholding information may be viewed as beneficent, protecting from harm or maintaining dignity, rather than as an act of deception. This presents a challenge in a U.S. health care setting, where informing the patient about a diagnosis is integral to medical practice, both legally and ethically. The obligation to inform the patient, and the "good" of autonomous decision making by the individual, must be weighed against the obligation to do no harm (non-maleficence) and the dignity of the person. A social worker may inquire about the knowledge and preferences of the patient. What are her needs? What does she want to know or understand? With whom would she like the physicians and staff to speak? Similarly, the ethical principle of proportionality may be applicable. If there are no options for curative treatment, autonomous decision making by the patient may be less imperative than when several options are available and consent for a treatment protocol must be obtained (van Bogaert & Ogunbanio, 2005). When there are medically appropriate treatment options, it becomes necessary to establish the patient's preferences concerning the process of decision making, within the context of the family. A social worker may elicit from the family their beliefs about the possible impact of disclosure to the patient and explain the boundaries of informed consent. Social workers can assist with projecting anticipated reactions and creating an opportunity for the conversation to occur in a supportive and responsive environment with skilled clinicians presenting information and responding to the dynamics of the patient and family.

Culture may also influence numerous aspects of care, such as symptom management, completion of advance directives, and decisions about post-hospital care, including home health or hospice. In some cultures, such as traditional Cambodian culture, it is important to be a "good patient" by not complaining or requesting anything. The social worker may encounter a patient who appears to be in significant pain and find that the patient has not informed the nurse by using the call button as instructed. Understanding cultural beliefs may enable us to alter our approaches to provide responsive and respectful palliative care.

The narrative in Box 68.4 illustrates several facets of work with a patient and his support network that differ from the medical and social work "cultures." The blend of the patient's biological and religious "families," the all-male demographic

Box 68.4
Patient/Family Narrative: Father William

Father William was a priest, age 88, who was brought by ambulance to the emergency department with sepsis and respiratory failure. He was unresponsive and was accompanied by a member of his biological family, as well as a brother from his religious order. Both men affirmed that Father William had been ill for many months and had required total care due to multiple comorbid conditions. They attested that no aggressive or invasive life-prolonging measures were desired, and that comfort was the only goal, but neither man was the durable power of attorney. The social worker and the physician (both of whom were female) examined the patient's advance directive. It was too nonspecific to fit the current medical context and to guide treatment decisions, but it did identify the provincial of the order as Father William's durable power of attorney (DPOA). It was becoming clear that the patient would not breathe on his own much longer. The social worker and the physician attempted to contact the DPOA at the monastery, leaving many messages with a member of the order who verified that the DPOA was on the premises. The doctor characterized the urgency of the call as "a matter of life and death" for Father William, yet the calls went unreturned. The physician, social worker, and nurse questioned whether, given the inability to make contact with the DPOA, the patient's family member, as the legal next of kin, could make decisions about care. Ultimately, after 2 hours and numerous attempts, the physician made contact with the DPOA. After listening to the physician discuss the patient's condition and the options for treatment, the DPOA indicated that, if it were possible for Father William's condition to improve with antibiotics and intravenous hydration, then the DPOA believed this should be attempted. However, the DPOA requested no further acceleration in the level of care. The interventions requested by the DPOA, including transfer to a critical care unit for close monitoring, were more than the care requested by the two men who accompanied Father William to the hospital. This circumstance underscored for the team that, despite the obvious closeness and concern shown by the men present in the emergency department, it did not follow that they would make the same decisions about care as the DPOA.

The following morning, the social worker consulted a chaplain who was familiar with the order. The chaplain asked, "Did you try having a male place the call to the DPOA?" The chaplain described that the men of the order are primarily from countries in Southeast Asia. Considering the traditional roles related to gender, as well as the culture of an all-male religious order, he said, "It has been our experience that having a male communicate makes a difference." The social worker later reviewed the circumstances with the physician, and both agreed that in the urgency to make contact, it had not occurred to them to ask a male colleague to assist with communication. Throughout the patient's hospitalization, both the social worker and the physician often worked with male chaplains and nurses to facilitate contact with the provincial.

of the religious order, and the implicit bias in favor of communication with males from the hospital setting were all factors requiring the team to draw on the knowledge of their chaplain colleagues who were most familiar with the order. The practitioner must develop awareness of the resources, both internal to the organization and in the larger community, who may assist and educate us with regard to various groups, toward a goal of promoting understanding and improving the process of health care decision making.

Conclusion

Social workers in palliative care offer essential knowledge and skills that can facilitate the process of decision making. Advanced and progressive illness and coming to the end of life present significant challenges to patients and caregivers, as well as numerous intersections where options and outcomes are not always clear. Social workers collaborate with other health care clinicians to provide care that is sensitive to the unique psychosocial, spiritual concerns and cultural values of patients and infuses ethical principles that are key to the process. Health care and end-of-life care choices involve much more than simple documents to convey wishes; medical, legal, and ethical knowledge is invaluable and conversations are an essential part of the process. Social workers can facilitate and promote the kinds of conversations that help us to discover the values and beliefs of our patients, the sociocultural context within which they occur, how they experience illness and healing, and the patterns of interaction with the health care system. It is with this knowledge and skill set that we can become effective facilitators of decision-making processes that promote respect and ensure patients' rights in a complex and ever-changing health care system.

ADDITIONAL RESOURCES

WEB-BASED TOOLS: A SAMPLE OF WEB RESOURCES TO FACILITATE DISCUSSION AND DECISION MAKING

Aging with Dignity: http://www.agingwithdignity.org
A national nonprofit, inspired by the life and work of Mother Teresa of Calcutta, with a mission to "affirm and safeguard the human dignity of individuals as they age and to promote better care for those near the end of life." Site users can access and order the Five Wishes document, a tool for recording one's wishes for end-of-life care and communicating with family members and health care providers.
Caring Connections: http://www.caringinfo.org
A site sponsored by the National Hospice and Palliative Care Organization (NHPCO) providing resources, information, state-specific advance directives, and publications about care at the end of life and expressing one's wishes.

Center to Advance Palliative Care (CAPC): http://www.getpalliativecare.org
A site sponsored by and edited by palliative medicine physicians. The site provides information about palliative care and includes a directory of hospitals with palliative care programs.
Center for Practical Bioethics: http://www.practicalbioethics.org
Offers Caring Conversations, a free publication and consumer education initiative, that helps individuals and their families share meaningful conversations while making practical preparations for end-of-life decisions. Workbooks are available in English and Spanish, for young adults, and for veterans.
The Community Health Improvement Clerkship: http://www.doyourproxy.org
Developed by two fourth-year medical students as a project, with a goal of increasing the numbers of people completing advance directives and making it easier to legally document one's wishes.
The Cultural Competence Resources for Health Care Providers: http://www.hrsa.gov/culturalcompetence
Published by the Health Resources and Services Administration (HRSA) of the U. S. Department of Health and Human Services.
Hard Choices: http://www.hardchoices.com
A Web-based tool of A&A Publishers, Inc., provides several documents to educate and stimulate discussion and decision making about end-of-life care. Documents include *Hard Choices for Loving People*, in English and Spanish, and *Light in the Shadows: Meditations While Living with a Life-Threatening Illness*.
Jamarda Resources: http://www.jamardaresources.com
A commercially available program where print manuals, assessment tools, and a single-user licensed Web-based reference tool can be purchased (*Culture, Ethnic, and Religious Manual for Health Care Providers*, 3rd edition).
Robert Wood Johnson Foundation: http://www.rwjf.org
Provides numerous publications and research on hospice and palliative care.

REFERENCES

Arnold, R. (2006). *Decision making capacity, second edition. Fast facts and concepts.* Retrieved from http://www.eperc.mcw.edu/fastFact/ff_55.htm
Black, K. (2004). Advance directive communication with hospitalized elderly patients: Social workers roles and practices. *Journal of Gerontological Social Work, 43*(2/3), 131–145.
Black, K. (2005). Advance directive communication practices: Social workers' contributions to the interdisciplinary health care team. *Social Work in Health Care, 40*(3), 39–55.
Black, K. (2006). Advance directive communication: Nurses' and social workers' perceptions of roles. *American Journal of Hospice and Palliative Medicine, 23*(3), 175–184.
Colby, W. (2002). *Long goodbye: The deaths of Nancy Cruzan.* Carlsbad, CA: Hay House.
Crawley, L. M., Marshall, P. A., Lo, B., & Koenig, B. A. (2002). Strategies for culturally effective end-of-life care. *Annals of Internal Medicine, 136*(9), 673–679.
Cruzan v. Director, Missouri Department of Health. 497 U.S. 261 (1990).

Csikai, E. L., & Raymer, M. (2005). Social workers' educational needs in end-of-life care. *Social Work in Health Care, 41*(1), 53–72.

Csikai, E. L. (2004). Social workers' participation in the resolution of ethical dilemmas in hospice care. *Health and Social Work, 29*(1), 67–76.

Doka, K. J. (2009). Cultural capsule: Characteristics of culturally effective counselors. In K. J. Doka & A. S. Tucci (Eds.), *Diversity and end-of-life care* (pp. 33–34). Washington, DC: Hospice Foundation of America.

Lapine, A., Wang-Cheng, R., Goldstein, M., Nooney, A., Lamb, G., & Derse, A., (2001). When cultures clash: Physician, patient, and family wishes in truth disclosure for dying patients. *Journal of Palliative Medicine, 4*(4), 475–480.

National Association of Social Workers (NASW). (1999). *Code of ethics of the National Association of Social Workers*. Retrieved from http://www.socialworkers.org/pubs/code/default.asp/

National Association of Social Workers (NASW). (2004). *NASW standards for social work practice in palliative and end of life care*. Washington, DC: Author.

O'Donnell, P., Farrar, A., BrintzenhofeSzoc, K., Conrad, A. P., Danis, M., Grady, C., Taylor, C., & Ulrich, C. M. (2008). Predictors of ethical stress, moral action and job satisfaction in health care social workers. *Social Work in Health Care, 46*(3), 29–51.

Patient Self-Determination Act. Public Law No. 101-508. (1990).

SUPPORT Principal Investigators. (1995). A controlled trial to improve care for seriously ill hospitalized patients: The study to understand prognoses and preferences for outcomes and risks of treatment (SUPPORT). *The Journal of the American Medical Association, 274,* 1591–1598.

van Bogaert, G. A., & Ogunbanio, G. A. (2005). The principle of proportionality: Foregoing withdrawing life support. *South African Family Practice, 47*(8), 66–67.

69 *Karen Bullock*

Advance Directives from a Social Work Perspective: Influence of Culture and Family Dynamics

When it's my time to go, please don't keep me hanging on. There is a better life for me on the other side; my daughter understands my wishes, she will do the right thing when it is time.
—*Annie Mae, a 65-year-old African-American woman who chose not to consent to a "do not resuscitate" order*

Key Concepts

- *Advances in medical technology have raised complex practice issues for social workers in palliative and end-of-life care.*
- *It is important to understand the ethical, moral, and legal aspects of caring for patients with serious and terminal illnesses.*
- *Advance care planning is a process in which treatment preferences are made known through the use of advance directives.*
- *Advance directives are oral or written instructions that are invoked when patients lack the capacity to make their own decisions about medical care.*
- *Understanding culture and family dynamics as the cornerstone of effective advance care planning allows practitioners to provide care infused with dignity and respect and consistent with patient and family wishes.*

Introduction

Increasingly, advances in medical technology make it possible for people to live longer, and with more debilitating chronic illnesses. Furthermore, physicians are able to offer patients a plethora of life-sustaining options depending on their diagnoses and preferences for treatment (Pendergrast, Claessens, & Luce, 1998). Many of these interventions are considered expensive, aggressive, painful, and invasive (Emanuel & Emanuel, 1998; Meisel, 1995); some produce effects but not necessarily benefits. Moreover, previous research has suggested that these treatments are received at points along the illness trajectory when they are not likely to benefit the patient over a period of time (Bradley, Fried, Kasl, & Idler, 2001). Because of the myriad of treatment options available, patients may find themselves confronted with overwhelming decisions about care when faced with serious and/or terminal illnesses.

Historically, patients tended to be passive consumers of medical services with physicians making unilateral decisions about the degree and intensity of treatment in acute care settings based solely on their clinical judgment (Reith & Payne, 2009). What we have learned from a decade of data gleaned primarily from Caucasian patients with serious and terminal illnesses and their family members is that most would prefer to die at home, free from pain and with their loved ones (Dunlop, Davies, & Hockley, 1989; Emanuel & Emanuel, 1998; Flory, Young-Xu, Gurol, Levinsky, Ash, & Emanuel, 2004; Grande, Addington-Hall, & Todd, 1998; Pritchard et al., 1998; Steinhauser et al., 2000). While race can be a proxy for culture and the available data on relatively homogeneous racial groups may be useful for generalizing to diverse patient populations, it behooves us as social work practitioners to consider differences in decision making across groups in our efforts to encourage and support patients and families in advance care planning.

The worldview, health behaviors, and attitudes shared by a group of individuals (Bullock, McGraw, Blank, & Bradley,

2005) tend to shape one's culture. More broadly, we think of people as belonging to the same cultural group if they share identity such as racial/ethnic group, religious orientation, first language, sexual orientation, or family type. In the United States, the philosophies and practices of Western-based medicine may be inconsistent with the cultural norms and practices of patients and families of diverse background and experiences (Betancourt, Green, Carrillo, & Ananeh-Firempong, 2003). Understanding cultural differences and family perspectives in advance care planning is important.

Advance care planning is a process in which individuals engage in thoughtful preparation and communication about their health care preferences, prior to a medical crisis, to address issues about how they would want to be cared for should they find themselves in a noncommunicative state (Blacker & Jordan, 2004; Galambos, 1998; Teno, Stevens, Spernak, & Lynn, 1998). Advance directives (ADs) are tools that allow capacitated individuals to communicate specific instructions about their values and wishes for and against medical treatment at a time when they are competent to provide such guidance so that in the event they become incapacitated and there is a need for surrogate decision making, the patient's wishes are known (Kelly, Lipson, Daly, & Douglas, 2009; Knox & Vereb, 2005; Samanta & Samanta, 2006).

These tools are important for health care practitioners who care for patients along the continuum of life-threatening illness, across differing settings and diagnoses, because they assist practitioners in providing quality care for the patient. Health care researchers argue that quality palliative and end-of-life care is consistent with patient preferences, well-managed pain, and minimal burden to loved ones (Bradley, Fried, Kasl, & Idler, 2001; Emanuel & Emanuel, 1998; Steinhauser et al., 2000; Tong et al., 2003). Providing optimal care may be complicated by disagreements between physicians and patients and families (Hanson, Danis, & Garrett, 1997; Hanson & Rodgman, (1996), reliance on surrogate decision making (Berger, DeRenzo, & Schwartz, 2008) or preferences for and decisions about care that are culturally distinct (Crawley, Marshall, Lo, & Koenig, 2002; Galanti, 1997. Moreover, it is necessary to think critically about the influence of race, gender, and religion on one's personality and value structure (Csikai & Chaitin, 2006) as these decisions are made.

To be effective in promoting advance care planning, practitioners need to (1) acquire knowledge about the culture(s) of the patient and family; (2) review her/his own cultural norms, values, and expectations in comparison and contrast to that of the patient; and (3) utilize a social work skill set that includes culturally specific problem-solving strategies, culturally congruent communication styles, and respect for divergent views and perspectives. In accordance with the patient's wishes, this is an important time to engage family members because they may be the practitioner's most valuable asset when caring for a patient who is faced with evolving illness and death and dying. It is typically family members who serve as surrogate decision makers for incapacitated patients; thus, their perspectives on end-of-life preferences and outcomes are valuable (Teno et al., 2004).

This chapter discusses advance directives from a social work perspective with an emphasis on cultural influence and family dynamics. To this end, we begin with a look at the impetus for advance directives and the various types. Next, the social context in which advance directives can be effectively constructed is highlighted in addition to a review of practice skills and competencies necessary for promoting advance directives. The perspective provided in this chapter is relevant to social work practice across the spectrum of palliative care from clinicians and educators to researchers and policy makers. The role of the social worker is to ensure that care supports dignity and respect for patient's autonomy and self-determination (NASW, 2004), which in actual practice may involve remaining autonomous by delegating decision making to others.

Legal and Ethical Background

Currently, in the United States, individuals have an inherent and legal right to make their own decisions regarding their medical treatment. Before the 1970s, health care ethics were based on professional authority and beneficence (Pellegrino & Thomasma, 1987; Porter & Warren, 2005; Reamer, 1999). Physicians made decisions on behalf of patients and family members with a medicalized perspective focused on preserving life and heavily dependent upon clinical judgment (Beauchamp, 2001; Devettere, 2000). With technological advances in life-saving procedures and mechanical devices that make it possible to keep patients alive artificially, comes a growing concern about assisting patients to come to the end of life with dignity and coherence with their values and beliefs (Gessert & Reynolds, 2010; Younger, Arnold, & Schapiro, 1999). These advances can complicate decision making for patients, family members, and health care providers. Ethical conflicts and dilemmas abound both for those involved in offering treatment options and for those deciding which to choose. Therefore, the importance of helping individuals to understand the process of advance care planning as it relates to anticipated medical crises and the potential interventions should not be underestimated. Now, more than ever, competency-based practice and indelible policy that protects patients' autonomy are needed to guide and direct those who engage in end-of-life decision making (Camhi et al., 2009; Galambos, 1998).

Furthermore, a growing interest and commitment to ethical principles and beneficent, informed medical and psychosocial care in U.S. hospitals (Beauchamp, 2001; Devettere, 2000; Pellegrino & Thomasma, 1987; Reamer, 1999) led to the passage of legislation to provide some assurance that individuals are helped to actualize their moral, legal, and ethical rights to care. This Patient Self-Determination

Act (PSDA) (Public Law No. 101–508, 1990) was a part of the Omnibus Budget Reconciliation Act of 1990 and was intended to support patient autonomy and improve end-of-life care. A patient's right to self-determination is a major ethical and legal principle guiding health care in the United States, not only for social work but for all health care providers (Csikai & Bass, 2000; Garrett, Baillie, & Garrett, 1993; Joffe, Manocchia, Weeks, & Cleary, 2003; Reamer, 1999). This federal law provides an option for patients to inform decisions about their own health when they no longer have the capacity to communicate their health care wishes through a mechanism known as advance directive. Noteworthy is the fact that the PSDA is essentially based in Western values (Ulrich, 1994), which may be culturally incongruent with other worldviews, especially those cultures that are collective in nature and for whom present rather than future orientation is of primary value. Furthermore, taking as its premise autonomy and informed consent, the PSDA expresses the fundamental right of all competent individuals to have information and to control their fate as it relates to the course of illness, death, and dying. This includes but is not limited to decisions about the continuation, withholding, or withdrawal of medical and/or surgical interventions. Within this legislation, provisions were made for the use of an advance directive to guide care if and when a person became unable to make decisions for himself or herself.

Advance Directives

Advance directives are informed by two basic principles: the individual's right to influence how he or she comes to the end of life and a person's right to die with dignity, which may be uniquely defined by each individual. It can be challenging and distressing to integrate complex medical information and make decisions about when and in what context a loved one might want to cease interventions that serve to prolong life. This requires an effort to identify and quantify the attributes that contribute to dignity as defined by the unique person. In addition, it requires sound medical judgment to ensure that the nature of the medical condition meets the criteria as set forth in the advance directive. For example, while a patient may choose not to be resuscitated if coming to the end of his or her life consequent to progressive cancer, the patient may choose resuscitation in the setting of a pneumonia from which he or she is expected to recover and return to baseline function.

The benefits of advance directives as reported in the health care literature include autonomy in decision making regarding wishes and preferences for care (Csikai & Chaitin, 2006), congruence between personal values and end-of-life choices (Steinhauser et al., 2009), increased likelihood that the patient's wishes will be honored (Dawson, 1991), less burden on family and health care providers as wishes are known,

potential to improve overall quality of end-of-life care (Teno, Gruneir, Schwartz, Nanda, & Wetle, 2007), and possible decrease in costs (Bradley et al., 2001).

Most experts in the field of palliative and end-of-life care would argue that there are two types of advance directives, instruction directives and proxy directives. The proxy directive or durable power of attorney (DPOA) for health care agent names a patient advocate to speak on the patient's behalf and in accordance with the patient's beliefs and values, in the event she or he becomes unable to do so. The living will is an instruction directive in which the individual's wishes are expressed in a written document, but a patient advocate is not named (Muller, 2008). The health care agent's ability to use appropriate substituted judgment is important, because it may not be possible to anticipate the full range of medical situations that can arise as illness evolves and patients are in a medical crisis and/or coming to the end of life. This once again assumes that the agent is provided the best medical and prognostic information upon which to think through decisions.

The promotion of advance care planning may be one way to increase the likelihood that racial and ethnic minority groups will benefit from hospice and palliative care. Practitioners, who work closely with racial and ethnic minorities, may find it useful to frame the discussion around the two types of advance directives (written and oral), with emphasis on the oral directive. Latino and African Americans, in particular, may be less inclined than Anglo/European Americans to complete a written directive, because both groups tend to value and rely on oral traditions (Crawley et al., 2002). Because ethnicity has been linked to end-of-life decisions and the completion rates of advance directives (Blackhall et al., 1999; Caralis, Davis, Wright, & Marcial, 1993; Dupree, 2000; Garrett, Harris, Norburn, & Danis, 1993) with African Americans reporting the lowest completion rate and whites the highest (Kelly et al., 2009; Salmond & David, 2005), it is essential to understand the culturally bound behaviors and attitudes that may contribute to racial disparities in advance care planning.

It can be argued that higher completion rates among white individuals in contrast to racial minorities is an indication of the culturally bound philosophy of care that puts the individual at the center of the care paradigm as opposed to a more collective decision-making approach that is family centered and inclusive of other members of the patient's social support network and might be more consistent with the values and behaviors of Hispanics, Asians, and African Americans. In addition, in some cultures, it is unacceptable to talk about death because the belief is that the discussion of death hastens its occurrence (Blackhall, Murphy, Frank, & Azen, 1995; Carrese & Rhodes, 1995) or presumes knowledge of the future, which ultimately rests with God. The Western worldview of autonomy and self-determination is a reflection of one's desire to control his or her destiny and possibly his or her fate. This value has translated into moral imperatives for quality care at end of life. However, the expectation that people will want to have control over their life and death may be culturally induced. In some religious cultures, it is believed that God is the master of your fate and *He* will control your destiny, including your death and dying (Yasmeen, 1991). Furthermore, the belief in miracles identified among some Asian groups (Hirayama, 1990; Lang, 1990), Hispanic (Rael & Korte, 1988), and African Americans (Reese, Ahern, Nair, O'Faire, & Warren, (1999) can lead patients and family members to request what might seem to providers to be unnecessary or inappropriate care. Open-ended questions that build on and explore culturally specific health practices, values, beliefs, and behaviors, while addressing associated affect and emotion, may help facilitate discussions about goals of care and medical decision making along the continuum of illness. Crawley and colleagues (2000) argue for strategies for culturally respectful end-of-life care. Implicit in this clinical goal is the need for further research and exploration to discern the influences of culture on end-of-life preferences, advance care planning, and the completion of advance directives. It has been suggested that in addition to addressing physical suffering, the conversation around these concerns should be extended beyond the physical self to acknowledge and explore psychosocial, existential, or spiritual suffering (Lo, Quill, & Tulsky, 1999). This is consistent with the social work value of respect for personhood and the National Consensus Project Guidelines for Quality Palliative Care (National Consensus Project, 2009).

The Patient's Self-Determination Act (PSDA) obligates health care facilities to inform patients about their rights to use advance directives, to inquire whether patients have advance directives upon admission to hospital, and to facilitate their completion if the patient so desires. While the intent of such legislation is often framed as the promotion of less aggressive, less invasive interventions at end of life so that patients might die comfortably, at home, surrounded by loved ones (Joffe et al., 2003; Pellegrino & Thomasma, 1987; Porter & Warren, 2005; Steinhauser et al., 2000), the reality for many patients is that they do experience pain and symptoms (Steinhauser et al., 2000) and/or may wish to have medical treatments and surgical interventions that are offered while living with a terminal illness. Furthermore, there are patients for whom dying at home is not preferred, as documented in some of the palliative care literature (Crawley et al., 2000; Flory et al., 2004; Hanchate, Kronman, Young-Xu, Ash, & Emanuel, 2009) For some cultural groups, the withdrawal of treatment is viewed as "giving up" and the withholding of hydration and nutrition is considered "starving" the patient (Bullock et al., 2005; Galanti, 1997). These cultural beliefs and others (Bullock, 2006) may influence the completion of advance directives and contribute to the low utilization rate of hospice and palliative care among racial and ethnic minority patients. Recent data show that less than 20% of hospice patients are people of color (7.2% blacks; 7.8% other) in contrast to white patients (81.9%), for which there has been a decrease between 2007 and 2008 (National Hospice and Palliative Care Organization, 2009). This speaks

to the need to reinforce palliative care as a specialty that joins with patients and families along the continuum of illness regardless of prognosis or treatments that are chosen.

In an effort to systematically examine the use of advance directives, a landmark Study to Understand Prognoses and Preference for Outcomes and Risks of Treatment (SUPPORT) was undertaken to understand the impact of advance directives on the care of hospitalized patients (Support Principal Investigators, 1995). Two years of prospective observational study revealed that the completion of advance directives did little to improve communication between physicians and patients at end of life. The study documented advance care planning discussions noted in patients' medical records, DNR orders written, available living wills, and other identifiable evidence of instruction directives. While the study did emphasize the importance of knowledge and effective communication between nurses and their patients, it did not shed light on the role of social workers who are essential to the palliative and end-of-life care teams.

The Social and Cultural Context

Several studies have helped define key components of what some describe as a "good death" (Bradley et al., 2001; Clark & Seymour, 1999; Emanuel & Emanuel, 1998; Steinhauser et al., 2000). The implementation of state and federal policy is not enough to guarantee that all patients will seek and/or receive optimal care at end of life. The Schiavo case (*Bush v Schiavo*, 885 So 2d 321) made this apparent in 2005 when Terri Schiavo's private family conflict about withdrawing life-sustaining treatment became public. Terri had suffered a cardiac arrest and, according to the autopsy reports, was in a persistent vegetative state for the 15-year duration of her illness. Schiavo experienced an unanticipated medical crisis at a young age and had not established advance directive or an appointed health care agent. This example of moral legal controversy points to one reason why it is important to understand culture and family dynamics. Furthermore, a review of the case suggests that having both an advance directive and a surrogate decision maker *may* prevent a death surrounded by controversy, distress, and family trauma.

In situations where members of the patient's family vehemently disagree about the approach to care, such as in the Schiavo family, most states purport to have policies and procedures in place to solve these unfortunate dilemmas. The court appoints one person among the disputing family to serve as surrogate decision maker. However, this forced resolution provides no guarantee that the patient's values will be reflected in the decision of the representative nor does it safeguard against further family conflict and suffering related to the end-of-life care for the seriously ill or dying patient (Burt, 2006).

Family and members of the patient's social support networks are typically appointed or become the surrogate decision maker. Engaging the social network and/or the surrogate in the process of medical explanation and advance care planning can assist social workers and health care providers to avoid many of the complications that can arise when a person is faced with a serious or terminal illness. While hesitancy to discuss death makes it extremely difficult to explore a plan of care for emergent medical or end-of-life situations, a discussion of values, spiritual and philosophical beliefs, and metaphoric communication can be helpful and inform the thoughtfulness that needs to be brought to these conversations. For some patients and family members, advance care planning may not be acceptable because their belief is that merely speaking of death can hasten it (Blackhall et al., 1995). Others may believe that dying at home is unacceptable because it leaves behind spirits, which linger and compromise the living environment (Burr, 1995; Rael & Korte, 1988; Yasmeen, 1991). It behooves us as social work clinicians to evaluate our knowledge, attitude, and competence in understanding and respecting the cultural variables that infuse the subject of advance directives. For example, some Asian patients and families "may oppose acceptance that death is coming and focus on prayer for a miracle or may see the experience of illness as a test of religious commitment or death as a release to a better existence (Reith & Payne, 2009, p. 100)," and this may impact their participation in advance care planning, if the only focus of the conversation relates to death and dying. In a study conducted by Caralis and colleagues (1993), the majority of Hispanic patients expressed preferences for being kept alive using life-prolonging interventions. Noteworthy is the fact that these research participants were not likely to complete a written directive, but most reported that they would entrust decision making to family members in the event that they could not speak for themselves.

Practice Skills and Competencies

While practice skills and competencies have been developed by social work leaders, training of practitioners has been cited as a major barrier to improving the system of care for patients with life-threatening illnesses and for the bereaved (Black, 2006; Christ & Sormanti, 1999). It is necessary to validate and evaluate tools and measures of practice competencies. Similar to physicians and nurses, the learning challenges in our profession are being clarified through research and practice initiatives. Christ and Sormanti (1999) utilized a practitioner survey, focus groups, and a survey of social work school faculty to understand gaps in education and training so that interventions could be designed to respond to needs and educate academics and practitioners about advance care planning and other palliative care and end-of-life practice issues. Results suggested that, not unlike the professions of medicine and nursing, social work knowledge and skill development in the care of the dying was uneven

and not integrated sufficiently with theoretical concepts and research. Social workers felt ill prepared for this work by their master's-level training and inadequately supported by continuing education programs. Participants were able to identify only a few social work scholars who were role models in comprehensive training, knowledge building, innovation, and advocacy. An outgrowth of this research was a program for leadership development sponsored by the Soros Foundation to test new approaches to professional development in the care of the dying and the bereaved.

Recognizing that role models, mentors, and peer support are essential to the educational process, the Open Society Institute established the Project on Death in America (PDIA). Its mission was to understand and transform both the culture and experience of dying and bereavement in the United States through funding activities in professional and public education, research, clinical care, the arts and humanities, and public policy (Open Society Institute, 2004, p. 2). The Social Work Leadership Development Award was one such initiative, which supported emerging leaders by funding projects and creating collegial networks of practitioners working in practice settings caring for seriously ill patients and their families. In addition, a national Social Work Leadership Summit on Palliative and End-of-Life Care held in 2002 recommended the development of a document to describe the knowledge, skills, and values that are requisite for the unique, essential, and appropriate role of social work (Gwyther et al., 2005).

Once we understand the skill set necessary to provide quality care, it is imperative that the effect of social work intervention to enhance advance care planning in various settings be evaluated. To this end, Morrison and colleagues (2005) assessed the effect of a multicomponent advance care planning intervention that focused on identification and documentation of preferences for medical treatments and on patient outcomes. The intervention consisted of advance care planning education at baseline. They incorporated small-group workshops and role play/practice sessions for social workers who were a part of the intervention. This included structured advance care planning discussions with residents and their agents at admission, after changes in clinical status, and at yearly follow-ups; formal structured review of residents' goals of care at regular team meetings; the identification of advance directives on nursing home charts; and feedback to individual health care providers related to the congruence of care they provided with the preferences specified in the advance care planning process. Those social workers who were not a part of the structured, multicomponent intervention received an educational training session on New York State law regarding advance directives, but they did not receive the full complement of training or interventions.

The researchers (Morrison et al., 2005) found that those residents who did not receive the advance care planning intervention were significantly more likely than those who did receive the intervention to experience treatments discordant with their prior stated wishes. Moreover, it was argued that the generalizable intervention directed at nursing home social workers significantly improved the documentation and identification of patients' wishes regarding common life-sustaining treatments and resulted in a higher concordance between patients' prior stated wishes and treatments received (p. 292).

Failure to address advance directives in social work practice may lead to various adverse consequences, including disregard for the patient's autonomy, increased psychosocial distress for family members, and moral duress for the health care provider (Csikai & Chaitin, 2006; Reith & Payne, 2009). Ethical and value issues surrounding the social work role and responsibility to help the patient and family members are moral imperatives. Dealing with such issues in a way that allows the practitioner to meet the needs of diverse patient populations may require ongoing dialogue with colleagues to discern the unique variables, continuing education to achieve cultural competence, and recognizing when to balance practice advocated by rules (Payne, 2006) with an openness and flexibility that integrates patient and family cultural differences.

Social workers are often called upon and see themselves as change agents; they are trained in a discipline that holds as core values social justice and the right of the individual to self-determine the care she or he receives. Furthermore, the social worker's skill often includes creating a safe, accepting environment within which individuals feel able to share the questions, struggles, and conflicts they may be experiencing in making decisions for and/or about the care of a dying family member or friend; and to be self-reflective in the therapeutic relationships when considering the impact of decisions on future bereavement. In many cultural groups, decisions made about the care of a dying relative have long-lasting consequences and infuse the family system and family legacy, as was the case with Annie M.'s relatives (see Box 69.1). Her family members worried about how they would "get along" once the elder matriarch and loved one had died. They struggled during the dying process to come to terms with decisions that would not tear the family apart or impede communication during a period of time when closeness of family members may serve as a buffer to complicated grief and feelings of loss.

professionals. Annie Mae is unmarried and has lived alone for the past 10 years since her youngest son left home for the Navy. She lives in the community she grew up in, surrounded by extended family and friends.

Principles: Annie Mae does not wish to complete a written advance directive. She states her daughter will make decisions about her care. Annie Mae explains that she is not ready to "give up" and wants to talk to the oncologist about whether she can take one more round of chemotherapy. She delegates: "The family can make whatever decisions they would like [about her care]." She expressed no interest in going to an inpatient hospice unit even if there is no further chemotherapy because she is "not going to give up the fight."

Patient autonomy (self-determination), beneficence (benefit), nonmaleficence (to do no harm), truth telling (honest details), confidentiality, and equitability are the principles of interest in providing optimal care for Annie Mae.

Clinical focus: The challenge for the social worker is that this family has a mistrust of formal providers. There is no written advance directive because, culturally, the family does not believe in planning for death and dying. Furthermore, decision making is a collective effort among family members, with each being an active participant in the process.

Intervention: This family believes in "miracles." The Lord was going to "take care of the rest." Like many African American families, this family has strong religious and spiritual beliefs about death and dying. Neither the patient nor her family members want to "give up" because perseverance is a core cultural value. There was no written advance directive, but the patient had verbalized her consent to have family members make decisions about her care without having appointed a surrogate decision maker. Knowing that there is a tendency for African Americans to mistrust the medical system, it was important to build trust. This was accomplished through ongoing interactions with the social worker and palliative care team, who maximized opportunities for family members to receive information and work through the disputes, conflicts, and decisions by drawing upon the strengths of their family bond and supportive network. This was one way to respect their autonomy and minimize potential ethical challenges that can arise when there is disagreement between the patient and family or between the family and the provider.

Outcome: Annie Mae's daughter, Katie, eventually agreed to take her mother home after Annie Mae was evaluated in the emergency department and it was determined that she was actively dying. Annie Mae died at home 2 days later with hospice care.

Box 69.1
Patient Narrative: Annie Mae

Annie Mae is a 65-year-old African American woman of Southern Baptist religious faith. She has one adult daughter, Katie; two adult sons, John and Orlando; one sister, Febbie; one adult nephew, Charles; and one adult niece, Darlene, who are involved in her care.

Annie Mae has a long employment history as a textile worker. A diligent and responsible employee of the company, she has not been absent from work in 20 years. She is proud of her work ethic and is an inspiration to her adult children who are aspiring career

When working in end-of-life care, whether in research or clinical practice, critical thinking about the goals and focus of our interventions needs to include a contextual perspective so we may adapt to the unique individuals we serve. For example, older adults who have historically deferred to the medical professional to make the care decision and who may be living with chronic or serious illnesses in the later stage of the life course may be very different than a younger person who has been raised to question and challenge. Autonomous decision making for some elders may feel like abandonment by the respected physicians whom they expect and assume will provide the best care. It is this individualized perspective that complicates and enriches the work of advance care planning.

Of particular concern is how we understand and address cultural issues with underserved racial and ethnic minorities. In targeted interventions, research has reported moderately successful results in promoting the completion of advance directives among African Americans (Bullock, 2006; Crawley et al., 2000; Dupree, 2000) and the utilization of palliative care services among Hispanic/Latino patients (Braun, Beyth, Ford, & McCullough, 2008; Smith, Sudore, & Perez-Stable, 2009). To gain more insight about what influences African Americans' decisions about completion of advance directives, a faith-based promotion model was used to recruit 102 African Americans aged 55 years or older through local churches and community-based agencies to participate in a pilot study to promote advance care planning. Data were gathered through focus group discussions about preferences for care, desire to make personal choices, values and attitudes, beliefs about death and dying, and advance directives. Three-fourths of the participants refused to complete advance directives. Nonetheless, this research (Bullock, 2006) offered insight into influential factors, which included spirituality, making sense of suffering, cultural meanings associated with death and dying, as well as the involvement of members of social support networks. Barriers to engaging in advance care planning included the lack of trust in the health care system. Other research (Bullock et al., 2005) identified mistrust of formal providers and the need for family involvement as important factors to be considered when promoting advance directives among African Americans (Dula, 1994).

The influence of race/ethnicity on end-of-life decision making and the completion of advance directives had been documented in a number of studies (Caralis et al., 1993; Fried, Bullock, Iannone, & O'Leary, 2009; Garrett et al., 1993; Tulsky, Cassileth, & Bennett, 1997; Tong et al., 2003). Specifically, it has been reported (McKinley, Garrett, Evans, & Danis, 1996) that ambulatory African American patients with a terminal diagnosis were more likely than Caucasians to want the benefit of life-sustaining technology when death was imminent. More recently, Givens and colleagues (2010) found racial differences in hospice use among patients with heart failure, with Hispanic and African Americans being far less likely than whites to receive this care. Of particular relevance to the discussion of ethical issues that surround the completion of advance directives is the finding by Dupree (2000) that African Americans prefer to rely on family members to voice a patient's wishes, more so than using written documentation and legal directives. Furthermore, when minority and nonminority individuals participated in a qualitative study to understand attributes of a "good death," differences were noted in the area of spiritual concerns, cultural concerns, and individualization. Those who identified themselves as minority were more expressive about religion and spiritual care needs at end of life and said they felt

providers would not understand or respect their cultural traditions (Tong et al., 2003). The completion of an advance directive may be viewed as one way to ensure autonomy and to have some control over decision making. However, for some people who place a certain cultural value on familial relationships and shared decision making, designating one person to serve as the sole decision maker and to sign a written document that expresses wishes may be a symbol of implicit mistrust and offensive to those trusted loved ones. Trying to understand advance care planning as a process of health behavior change may offer a different perspective on what is needed to develop effective interventions with advance directives. Variability in individuals' readiness, barriers and benefits, as well as perceptions must be understood (Fried et al., 2009) through appropriate assessments if we are to increase the depth of communication and collaboration needed to assist patients and families in a compassionate and individualized process of decision making.

It is important to go beyond the advance directive and focus more on the clinical relationship and process as the tool which elicits and responds to patients' and family members' emotions, with less attention to specific treatments, but more on the values, beliefs, and goals of patient and family care. Tulsky (2005) argues that patients and family members are so overwhelmed by the plethora of choice that bombard them when it has been determined that a patient has a noncurable illness that often the critical factors that affect clear decision making get overlooked. Through the use of a patient's narrative, issues of trust, uncertainty, emotion, hope, and the influence of multiple medical providers surface and frame the perspective on care. For example, Gamble (1993) argues that African Americans have a legacy of distrust of the institution of medicine due to decades of discrimination and denial of access to care in the United States. When one's lived experiences have not been infused with fairness and equity, it is especially difficult to convince those individuals and families to believe the messages they receive about quality and optimal care at end of life. This sentiment is captured in the comments of an older African American in rural southeastern United States:

> We have seen too many people be mistreated by doctors and nurses and just don't believe all this stuff they are telling us about a good death. If they don't treat you good when you are getting around well, why would they honor and respect you when you are on your last leg and dying. It just don't make sense to us old black people. (Bullock, 2006, p. 191)

The approach that we take to discussing palliative and end-of-life concerns may have an impact on the quality of communication among and between patients, families, and the social worker and can ultimately enhance the quality of care provided by the entire palliative and end-of-life care team (Black, 2007; Galambos, 1998; NASW, 2004). Social work's foundation values and core principles of self-determination, common good, and respect for the dying person and those who matter to them guide our practice (Brandsen, 2005). These values also inform effective practice interventions that emanate from an assessment of psychological, social, spiritual, cultural, medical, physical, and financial aspects of the patient and family experience. However, attention to increasing cultural proficiency (Stein, Sherman, & Bullock, 2009) through the understanding of attitudes, behaviors, and values that are influenced by life experiences and histories of discrimination and oppression will enable practitioners to engage patients and families in meaningful discussions about illness, goals of care, and decision making that are culturally appropriate and respectful of their unique history and experience.

Most attempts to improve the use of advance directives have focused directly on patients with a limited view of family involvement. To achieve culturally sensitive assessment, interventions and outcomes, practitioners work to (1) understand the impact of cultural identity of the patient and family; (2) acquire assessment skills through role playing and review of culturally specific practice models; (3) understand meaning and impact of illness, symptoms, treatments, grief, and loss; (4) encourage the use of community representatives and resources; (5) understand the definition and structures of families using such tools as genograms and ecomaps; and (6) incorporate a framework of culturally respectful interventions. Genograms (McGoldrick, Gerson, & Petri, 2008) are useful tools for identifying and describing kinship relationships (Bullock, 2004). When used in a flexible method that allows for the inclusion of fictive kin (non–blood relatives/non–marriage connected) and intergenerational relationships, this tool can shed insight on social order and cultural norms. (For more information on Social Work Practice: Screening, Assessment & Intervention, see Chapters 16–29.) Ecomaps (Hartman, 1995) begin with the patient and draw in environmental factors and physical connection/distance between and among family members and formal service providers (Bullock, 2004). These recommendations are evidenced through social work training and education programs (Stein et al., 2009). The crucial point is to seek consent of the patient to include family members along the continuum of illness and in decision making.

Conclusion

Key social work skills such as empathic inquiry and active listening can be invaluable in the advance care planning process. While patients may have very different attitudes, beliefs, and expectations about palliative and end-of-life care than the providers, conversations about pain, suffering, and treatment options need to occur if patients are to receive optimal care. Creating a safe, respectful, and welcoming environment for people to feel comfortable to share their individual and

unique cultural ideals can help to facilitate discussions about sensitive topics such as death and dying. Because there is diversity within cultural groups and most people have more than one level of culture (i.e., race, gender, sexual orientation, religion, and geographic location/place of birth, social class, level of education, and more), each patient and family should be approached as individuals and assessed for social supports and network as well as cultural assets that can be valuable in problem solving around palliative and end-of-life care issues.

LEARNING EXERCISES

- Describe three innovative approaches that can be applied to the various populations you serve who are living with life-threatening illness or who are at the end of life.
- Make a cultural assessment of your own background using an ecomap to identify relationships and environmental influences that encompass you. Apply the knowledge gained to develop your understanding of the cultural and systems factors that might affect your unique approach to decisions related to illness and end of life.

REFERENCES

Beauchamp, T. L. (2001). *Principles of biomedical ethics* (5th ed.). New York, NY: Oxford University Press.

Betancourt, J. R., Green, A. R., Carrillo, J. E., & Ananeh-Firempong, O. (2003). Defining cultural competence: A practical framework for addressing racial/ethnic disparities in health and health care. *Public Health Report, 118*(4), 293–302.

Berger, J. T., DeRenzo, E. G., & Schwartz, J. (2008). Surrogate decision making: Reconciling ethical theory and clinical practice. *Annals of Internal Medicine, 149*(1), 48–53.

Black, K. (2006). Advance directive communication: Nurses' and social workers' perceptions of roles. *American Journal of Hospice and Palliative Medicine, 23*(3), 175–184.

Black, K. (2007). Advance care planning throughout the end-of-life: Focusing the lens on social work practice. *Journal of Social Work in End-of-Life and Palliative Care, 3*(2), 39–58.

Blacker, S., & Jordan, A. R. (2004). Working with families facing life-threatening illness in medical settings. In J. Berzoff & P. R. Silverman (Eds.), *Living with dying: A handbook for end-of-life healthcare practitioners* (pp. 548–570). New York, NY: Columbia University Press.

Blackhall, L. J., Frank, G., Murphy, S. T., Michel, V., Palmer, J. M., & Azen, S. P. (1999). Ethnicity and attitude toward life sustaining technology. *Social Science and Medicine, 48*(12), 1779–1789.

Blackhall, L. J., Murphy, S. T., Frank, G., Michel, V., & Azen, S. P. (1995). Ethnicity and attitude toward patient autonomy. *Journal of the American Medical Association, 274*(3), 820–825.

Bradley, E. H., Fried, T. R., Kasl, S. V., & Idler, E. (2001). Quality-of-life trajectories of elders in the end of life.

In M. P. Lawton (Ed.), *Annual Review of Gerontology and Geriatrics* (Vol. 20, pp. 64–96). New York, NY: Springer Publishing.

Brandsen, C. K. (2005). Social work and end-of-life care: Reviewing the past and moving forward. *Journal of Social Work in End-of-Life and Palliative Care, 1*(2), 45–70.

Braun, U. K., Beyth, R. J., Ford, M. E., & McCullough, L. B. (2008). Voices of African American, Caucasian, and Hispanic surrogates on the burdens of end-of-life. *Journal of General Internal Medicine, 23*(3), 267–274.

Bullock, K. (2004). Family social support. In P. J. Bomar (Ed.), *Promoting health in families: Applying family research and theory to nursing practice* (3rd ed., pp. 142–161). Philadelphia, PA: Saunders/Elsevier Publisher.

Bullock, K. (2006). Promoting advance directive among African Americans: A faith-based model. *Journal of Palliative Medicine, 9*(1), 183–195.

Bullock, K., McGraw, S. A., Blank, K., & Bradley, E. H. (2005). What matters to older African Americans facing end-of-life decisions? A focus group study. *Journal of Social Work in End-of-Life and Palliative Care, 1*(3), 3–19.

Burr, F. A. (1995). The African American experience: Breaking the barriers to hospice. *Hospice Journal, 19*(2), 15–18.

Burt, R. (2006). Law's effect on the quality of end-of-life care: Lessons from the Schiavo case. *Critical Care Medicine, 34*(11), 5348–5354.

Bush v Schiavo, 885 So 2d 321 (Fla 2004), Schiavo ex rel Schindler v Schiavo, 403 F 3 d 12223 (11th Cir 2005).

Camhi, S. L., Mercado, A. F., Morrison, R. S., Qingling, D., Platt, D. M., August, G. I., & Nelson, J. E. (2009). Deciding in the dark: Advance directives and continuation of treatment in chronic critical illness. *Critical Care Medicine, 37*(3), 919–925.

Caralis, P. V., Davis, B., Wright, K., & Marcial, E. (1993). The influence of ethnicity and race on attitudes toward advance directives, life-prolonging treatments, and euthanasia. *The Journal of Clinical Ethics, 4*, 155–165.

Carrese, J. A., & Rhodes, L. A. (1995). Western bioethics on the Navajo reservation. *Journal of American Medical Association, 274*(3), 826–829.

Ceccarelli, C., Castner, D., & Haras, M. (2008). Advance care planning for patients with chronic kidney disease-Why aren't nurses more involved. *Nephrology Nursing Journal, 35*(6), 553–557.

Christ, G. H., & Sormanti, M. (1999). Advancing social work practice in end-of-life care. *Social Work in Health Care, 30*(2), 81–99.

Clark, D. & Seymour, J. 1999. Refelctions on palliative care. Buckingham, UK: Open University Press.

Crawley, L., Payne, R., Bolden, J., Payne, T., Washington, P., & Williams, S. (2000). Palliative and end-of-life care in the African American community. *Journal of American Medical Association, 284*, 2518–2521.

Crawley, L. M., Marshall, P. A., Lo, B., & Koenig, B. A. (2002). Strategies for culturally effective end-of-life care. *Annals of Internal Medicine, 136*, 673–679.

Csikai, E., & Bass, K. (2000). Health care social workers' views of ethical issues, practice, and policy in end-of-life care. *Social Work in Health Care, 32*(2), 1–22.

Csikai, E., & Chaitin, E. (2006). *Ethics in end-of-life decisions of social work practice*. Chicago, IL: Lyceum Books.

Dawson, N. (1991). Need satisfaction in terminal care settings. *Social Science and Medicine, 32*, 83–87.

Devettere, R. J. (2000). *Practical decision making in health care ethics: Cases and concepts* (2nd ed.). Washington, DC: Georgetown University Press.

Dula, A. (1994). African American suspicion of the healthcare system is justified: What do we do about it? *Cambridge Quarterly of Healthcare Ethics, 3*, 347–357.

Dunlop, R. J., Davies, R. J., & Hockley, J. M. (1989). Preferred versus actual place of death: A hospital palliative care support team experience. *Journal of Palliative Medicine, 3*(3), 197–201.

Dupree, C. Y. (2000). The attitudes of Black Americans toward advance directives. *Journal of Transcultural Nursing, 11*(2), 12–18.

Emanuael, E. J., & Emanuel, L. L. (1998). The promise of a good death. *The Lancet, 351*, S21–S29.

Flory, J., Young-Xi, Y., Gurol, I., Levinsky, N., Ash, A., & Emanuel, E. (2004). Place of death: US trends since 1980. *Health Affairs, 23*(3), 194–200.

Fried, T. R., Bullock, K., Iannone, L., & O'Leary, J. R. (2009). Understanding advance care planning as a process of health behavior change. *Journal of the American Geriatric Society, 57*(9), 1547–1555.

Galambos, C. M. (1998). Preserving end-of-life autonomy: The Patient Self-Determination Act and the Uniform Health Care Decisions Act. *Health and Social Work, 23*(4), 275–281.

Galanti, G. A. (1997). *Caring for patients from different cultures*. Philadelphia, PA: University of Pennsylvania Press.

Gamble, V. N. (1993). A legacy of distrust: African Americans and medical research. *American Journal of Preventive Medicine, 9*(Suppl. 6), 35–38.

Garrett, J., Harris, R., Norburn, J., & Danis, M. (1993). Life sustaining treatments during terminal illness: Who wants? *Journal General Internal Medicine, 8*, 361–368.

Garrett, T. M., Baillie, H. W., & Garrett, R. M. (1993). *Health care ethics: Principles and problems* (2nd ed.). Englewood Cliffs, NJ: Prentice Hall.

Gessert, C.E., & Reynolds, D. F. (2010). Identifying and addressing ethical issues in advanced chronic illness and at the end of life. In, Bern-Klug, M. (Ed.). *Transforming palliative care in nursing homes: The social work role*. New York, NY: Columbia University Press.

Givens, J. L., Tjia, J., Chao, Z., Emanuel, E., & Ash, A. S. (2010). Racial and ethnic differences in hospice use among patients with heart failure. *Archives of Internal Medicine, 170*(5), 427–432.

Grande, G. E, Addington-Hall, J. M, & Todd, C. J. (1998). Place of death and access to home care services: Are certain patient groups at a disadvantage? *Social Science and Medicine, 47*(5), 565–579.

Gwyther, L. P., Altilio, T., Blacker, S., Christ, G., Csikai, E. L., Hooyman, N., Linton, J., Raymer, M. & Howe, J. (2005). Social work competencies in palliative and end-of-life care. *Journal of Social Work in End-of-Life and Palliative Care, 1*(1), 87–120.

Hanchate, A., Kronman, A. C., Young-Xu, Y., Ashy, A. S., & Emanuel, E. (2009). Racial and ethnic differences in end-of-life costs: Why do minorities cost more than whites? *Archives of Internal Medicine, 165*(5), 493–501.

Hanson, L. C., Danis, M., & Garrett, J. (1997). What is wrong with end-of-life care? Opinions of bereaved family members. *Journal of the American Geriatrics Society, 45*(11), 1339–1344.

Hanson, L.C., & Rodgman, E. (1996). The use of living wills at the end-of-life. A national study. *Archives of Internal Medicine, 156*(9), 1018–1022.

Hartman, A. (1995). Diagrammatic assessment of family relationships. *Journal of Contemporary Human Services, 762*(2), 111–122.

Hirayama, K. K. (1990). Death and dying in Japanese culture. In J. K. Parry (Ed.), *Social work practice with the terminally ill: A transcultural perspective* (pp. 159–174). Springfield, IL: Charles C. Thomas.

Heyman, J. C., & Gutheil, I. A. (2006). Social work involvement in end of life planning. *Journal of Gerontological Social Work, 47*(3–4), 47–61.

Joffe, S., Manocchia, M., Weeks, J. C., & Cleary, P. D. (2003). What do patients value in their hospital care? An empirical perspective on autonomy centered bioethics. *Journal of Medical Ethics, 29*(2), 103–108.

Kelly, C., Lipson, A., Daly, B., & Douglas, S. (2009). Advance directive use and psychosocial characteristics: An analysis of patients enrolled in a psychosocial cancer registry. *Cancer Nursing, 32*(4), 335–341.

Knox, C., & Vereb, H. (2005). Allow natural death: A more humane approach to discussing end-of-life directives. *Journal of Emergency Nursing, 31*(6), 560–561.

Lang, L. T. (1990). Aspects of the Cambodian death and dying process. In J. K. Parry (Ed.), *Social work practice with the terminally ill: A transcultural perspective* (pp. 205–211). Springfield, IL: Charles C. Thomas.

Lacey, D. (2005). Nursing home social worker skills and end-of-life planning. *Social work in Health Care, 40*(4), 19–40.

Lo, B., Quill, T., & Tulsky, J. (1999). Discussing palliative care with patients. *Annals of Internal Medicine, 130*(9), 774–749.

McGoldrick, M., Gerson, R., & Petri, S. (2008). *Genograms: Assessment and intervention* (3rd ed.). New York, NY: W. W. Norton & Company.

McKinley, E. D., Garrett, J. M., Evans, A. T., & Danis, M. (1996). Differences in end-of-life decision making among African American and Caucasian ambulatory cancer patients. *Journal of General Internal Medicine, 11*(11), 651–656.

Meisel, A. (1995). *The right to die: The law of end-of-life decision making* (2nd ed.). New York, NY: Aspen Publishers.

Morrison, R. S., Chichin, E., Carter, J., Burack, O., Lantz, M., & Meier, D. E. (2005). The effect of a social work intervention to enhance advance care planning documentation in the nursing home. *Journal of the American Geriatrics Society, 53* (2), 290–294.

Muller, L. (2008). Power of attorney and guardianship. *Professional Case Management, 13*(3), 169–172.

National Association of Social Workers (NASW). (2004). *Standards for social work practice in palliative and end of life care.* Washington, DC: NASW Press.

National Consensus Project Guidelines for Quality Palliative Care. (2009). *Clinical practice guidelines for quality palliative care.* Retrieved from http://www.nationalconsensusproject.org/Guidelines_Download.asp

National Hospice and Palliative Care Organization (NHPCO). (2009). *NHPCO facts and figures: Hospice care in America.*

Retrieved from http://www.nhpco.org/files/public/Statistics_Research/NHPCO_facts_and_figures.pdf

Omnibus Budget Reconciliation Act. (1990). Title IV, Section 4206, Congressional Record, 1263–1264.

Open Society Institute. (2004). *Project on death in America.* Report of Activities January 2001-December 2003. Retrieved from http://www.soros.org/resources/articles_publications/publications/report_20041122/a_complete.pdf

Payne, M. (2006). Identity politics in multiprofessional teams: Palliative care social work. *Journal of Social Work, 6*(2), 137–150.

Pellegrino, E. D., & Thomasma, D. C. (1987). The conflict between autonomy and beneficence in medical ethics: Proposal for a resolution. *Journal of Contemporary Health Law and Policy, 3*(23), 23–46.

Pendergrast, T. J., Claessens, M. T., & Luce, J. M. (1998). A national survey of end-of-life care for critically ill patients. *Journal of Respiratory and Critical Care Medicine, 158*(4), 1163–1167.

Porter, T., & Warren, N. (2005). Bioethical issues concerning death: Death, dying, and end-of-life rights. *Critical Care Nurse Quarterly, 28*(1), 85–92.

Pritchard, R. S., Fisher, E. S., Teno, J. M., Sharp, S. M., Reding, D. J., Knaus, W. A., … & Lynn, J. (1998). Influence of patient preferences and local health system characteristics on the place of death. *Journal of the American Geriatric Society, 46*(10), 1242–1250.

Rael, R., & Korte, A. O. (1988). El ciclo de la vida y muerte: An analysis of death and dying in a selected Hispanic enclave. In S. R. Applewhite (Ed.), *Hispanic elderly in transition: Theory, research, policy, and practice* (pp. 189–202). New York, NY: Greenwood Press.

Reamer, F. G. (1999). *Social work values and ethics* (2nd ed.). New York, NY: Columbia University Press.

Reese, D. J., Ahern, R. E., Nair, S., O'Faire, J. D., & Warren, C. (1999). Hospice access and use by African Americans: Addressing cultural and institutional barriers through participatory action research. *Social Work, 44*(6), 549–559.

Reith, M., & Payne, M. (2009). *Social work in end-of-life and palliative care.* Chicago, IL: Lyceum Books Inc.

Salmond, S., & David, E. (2005). Attitudes toward advance directives and advance directive completion rates. *Orthopedic Nursing, 24*(2), 117–127.

Samanta, A., & Samanta J. (2006). Advance directives. Best interests and clinical judgment: Shifting sands at the end of life. *Clinical Medicine, 6*(3), 274–278.

Smith, A. K., Sudore, R. L., & Pérez-Stable, E. J. (2009). Palliative care for Latino patients and their families: Whenever we prayed, she wept. *Journal of American Medical Association, 301*(10), 1047–1057.

Stein, G. L., Sherman, P. A., & Bullock, K. (2009). Educating gerontologists for cultural proficiency in end-of-life care practice. *Journal of Educational Gerontology, 35*(11), 1008–1025.

Steinhauser, K. E., Clipp, E. C., McNeilly, M., Christakis, N. A., McIntyre, L. M., & Tulsky, J. A. (2000). In search of a good death: Observations of patients, families, and providers. *Annals of Internal Medicine, 132*, 825–832.

Support Principal Investigators. (1995). A controlled trial to improve care for seriously ill hospitalized patients (SUPPORT). *Journal of American Medical Association, 274*, 1591–1598.

Teno, J. M., Clarridge, B. R., Casey, V., Welch, L. C., Wetle, T., Shield, R., & Mor, V. (2004). Family perspectives on end-of-life care at the last place of care. *Journal of American Medical Association, 291*(1), 88–93.

Teno, J. M., Gruneir, A., Schwartz, Z., Nanda, A., & Wetle, T. (2007). Association between advance directives and quality of end-of-life care: A national study. *Journal of the American Geriatric Society, 55*(2), 189–194.

Teno, J. M., & Lynn, J. (1994). Putting advance-care planning into action. *Journal of Clinical Ethics, 7*(3), 205–213.

Teno, J. M., Stevens, M., Spernak, S., & Lynn, J. (1998). Role of written advance directives in decision making. *Journal of the American Geriatric Society, 13*, 439–446.

Tong, E., McGraw, S. A., Dobihal, E., Baggish, R., Cherlin, E., & Bradley, E. H. (2003). What is a good death? Minority and non-minority perspectives. *Journal of Palliative Care, 19*(3), 168–175.

Tulsky, J.A. (2005). Beyond advance directives: Importance of communication skills at the end of life. *American Medical Association, 294*(3), 359–364.

Tulsky, J.A. Cassileth, B.R., & Bennett, C.L. 1997. The effect of ethnicity on ICU use and DNR orders in hospitalized AIDS patients. *Journal of Clinical Ethics, 8*(2), 150–157 .

Ulrich, L. P. (1994). The Patient Self-Determination Act and cultural diversity. *Cambridge Quarterly of Healthcare Ethics, 3*(3), 410–413.

Volker, D. (2005). Control and end-of-life care: Does ethnicity matter? *American Journal of Hospice and Palliative Medicine, 22*(6), 442–446.

Yasmeen, M. N. (1991). The end of human life in light of the opinion of Muslim scholars and medical science. *Journal of the Islamic Medical Association, 23*(2), 74–81.

Younger, S., Arnold, R. M., & Schapiro, R. (1999). *The definition of death: Contemporary controversies.* Baltimore, MD: Johns Hopkins University Press.

70

Hollye Harrington Jacobs

Pediatric Palliative Care Ethics and Decision Making

We can and must reduce the number of those who fail to receive consistent, competent care that meets not only their physical needs but their emotional, spiritual, and cultural ones as well.

—Institute of Medicine (IOM) Report, "When Children Die: Improving Palliative and End-of-Life Care for Children and Families," 2003, p. xv

Key Concepts

- *Pediatric palliative social workers can improve the care that children and their families receive by providing information and emotional support throughout the decision-making process.*

- *Ethical issues are inherent in the care of children facing potentially life-limiting illness. To prevent an ethical issue from becoming an emotionally laden ethical dilemma, social workers engage in rational discernment and effective communication.*

- *When working with children and their families, sensitivity to cultural and language differences is key to effective communication and decision making.*

- *Because children are in the developmental process with varying abilities to participate in the decisions about their own care, pediatric palliative social workers need competencies in child development, bioethics, and conflict resolution.*

Introduction

The death of an infant, child, or adolescent is a unique sorrow—an event that is contrary to the laws of nature. Pediatric death contradicts conventional assumptions about what constitutes normal or acceptable life order. Pediatric social workers care for families with infants, children, and adolescents at the end of life with startling frequency. Many children who are born dying or who in previous years would have died immediately are now being kept alive due in part to the technological advances in the neonatal intensive care unit (NICU) (Catlin, 2005). Prenatal diagnosis and treatment is a rapidly evolving specialty. Parents and families require specialized support as they anticipate birth while knowing that their baby will be born with a potentially life-threatening congenital condition.

As a result of these changes, social workers in pediatric palliative care serve a wide variety of clients facing potentially life-limiting illnesses, including fetuses who die in utero; die shortly after birth from congenital defects or prematurity; live with chronic illnesses, such as cystic fibrosis, cancer, or congenital anomalies; and those who die suddenly, such as from accidents, murder, or suicide. The majority of children who die in the United States do so in institutions, primarily hospitals (Davies et al., 2008; Field & Behrman, 2002). In addition to the infants, children, and adolescents who die, there are an estimated 1 million children living in the United States with a potentially life-limiting condition who could benefit from pediatric palliative care services (Children's Hospice International [CHI], 2003; Levetown, 2000).

Pediatric palliative care is a medical specialty and philosophy of care that aims to provide physical, psychosocial, emotional, developmental, and spiritual care to children and their families facing life-threatening and serious illness that may result in death. The ultimate goal of pediatric palliative care is the best quality of life for children and their families, throughout the trajectory of an illness, or injury, regardless of the outcome (Rushton & Catlin, 2002). Because of the unique sadness associated with the illness, dying, and death of a child, caring for these patients is incredibly challenging for families and health care providers.

Families benefit from the presence of a trusted interdisciplinary health care team that includes social workers, physicians, nurses, chaplains, child life specialists, music therapists, and volunteers (Dickens, 2009). Palliative care services include assistance in decision making throughout the illness, advance care planning, psychosocial and spiritual support, pain and symptom management, care at the time of death, financial counseling, funeral planning, respite, and bereavement. Additionally, emotional support, often spearheaded by the team social worker, plays a significant role in helping families cope with the tragic effect of a child's looming death (Steele, Davies, Collins, & Cook, 2005).

Pediatric palliative care is distinctly unique from adult palliative care for a number of reasons (Field & Behrman, 2003; Freyer, 2004; Hilden,et al., 2001; Himelstein, Hilden, Boldt, & Weissman, 2004):

- In modern Western Societies, the death of a child may be perceived to be "untimely" and "unnatural".
- Children die of rarer conditions.
- Children are in a unique developmental process.
- Prognostication is more difficult.
- There is less reimbursement for services.
- There may be a higher emotional intensity when death occurs at the beginning of life.
- Caregivers often feel a sense of failure when a child dies.
- Less research exists.
- There is a lack of education and training for staff.

Children, therefore, are not "little adults." Pediatric patients have unique needs that require distinctive services. It is the moral and ethical obligation of social workers and the entire health care team to acknowledge these differences and advocate for the unique needs of children and their families facing life-threatening illnesses.

Basics of Pediatric Ethics and Decision Making

Pediatric palliative care is a naturally occurring iteration of delivering ethically sound, comprehensive care to infants, children, and adolescents. Ethical issues are inherent in virtually every clinical interaction. For example, decisions are made daily regarding the following:

- Whether to initiate or discontinue an intervention
- Disclosure to patients
- Patient access to therapies
- Patient preferences
- Engaging hospice care consultation.

The key, however, is preventing an ethical issue from becoming an emotionally laden ethical dilemma by engaging in a process of rational discernment and decision making. The process of decision making in pediatric palliative care is founded on core ethical values and principles that include the following:

- Beneficence: "doing good" by using treatments based on the benefits they provide
- Nonmaleficence: "doing no harm" by considering the potential harm as well as benefits to patients
- Autonomy: respect for life and persons by accepting that individuals may judge benefits, burdens, and risks differently
- Justice: giving fair and equitable access to all patients (Beauchamp & Childress, 2001; Becker & Grunwald, 2000; Frankel et al., 2005; Jonsen, Siegler, & Winslade, 2006; Kunin, 1997).

Informed consent, capacity, and assent, a concept unique to pediatrics, are core components inherent in the pediatric palliative care decision-making process. Because infants, children, and adolescents below the age of 18 are considered "incompetent" under the law, they are legally unable to make decisions about their health care. Parents assume the legal right and obligation to make medical decisions for their children.

The ability to participate in the informed consent process is predicated on a requisite decisional capacity to comprehend information, weigh options, evaluate benefits and burdens of treatments, and communicate decisions. In the process of obtaining informed consent, there are circumstances when the relevance and weight of parental preferences conflict with the recommendations of health care providers or when failure to provide the fundamental needs of a child represents incompetence (Jonsen et al., 2006). An example of a conflict is a Jehovah Witness parent who, against the recommendation of the health care team, refuses a blood transfusion for a child based on religious convictions. Social workers serve as experts in evaluating and creating social, psychological, and environmental conditions that either interfere or contribute to a parent's ability to give informed consent.

In some states, exceptions to parental consent exist. The emancipated minor and mature minor doctrines are two such exceptions. An emancipated minor is a person under the age of 18 years who demonstrates clear patterns of independent living, including being married, serving in the armed forces, managing personal financial affairs, or living apart from their parents and, as such, may be treated without parental consent (Blustein, 1996; Hinds et al., 2006; Jonsen et al., 2006). A mature minor is an adolescent who, though below the statutory age of 18 years and usually over the age of 15 years, is judged to possess the capacity for giving informed consent. This capacity is assessed by intelligence, maturity, and an ability to make reasoned decisions (Blustein, 1996; Jonsen et al., 2006). Determination of emancipation or maturity of minors may be done by the interdisciplinary team and, when there is question, through an ethics consultation.

The social worker must be knowledgeable of state laws regarding when, and in what situation, a minor can consent to or refuse treatment.

Decisional capacity is another component of ethical decision making that refers to the ability of a patient, or surrogate, to consent to or refuse medical interventions. Decisional capacity is a clinical judgment about the ability of the decision maker to understand the medical situation, weigh the benefits and burdens of actions, and communicate choice (Jonsen et al., 2006).

Determining true decisional capacity can be a challenging process. All too often communication falters when the health care team becomes trapped in technical language or worries about harming the patient. Patients and families, on the other hand, may not fully understand the medical terminology; may be overwhelmed by fear and anxiety, which inteferes in integrating information; and/or may possibly be unable, for a myriad of reasons, to ask questions. Therefore, the social worker and team members must ascertain specifically what the parents understand by talking as simply and clearly as possible. Additionally, some cultures and religions have certain customs and beliefs about health care that may be unfamiliar to the pediatric palliative care team. Differences in communication styles may delay or even adversely affect the way decisions are made. For example, lapses in cultural sensitivity have the potential to irreversibly sever the ability to build trust that is crucial to engaging and fostering the communication process. Even though decisional capacity is usually only questioned when parents refuse or discontinue medically indicated interventions (Jonsen et al., 2006), it is imperative that the interdisciplinary team work to assure that the family has a full understanding of all aspects involved in making decisions about treatments and goals of care.

Despite the fact that children and adolescents are not legally able to provide consent, they often have either developing capacity or full capacity to participate in decisions about their care and provide assent. Developing capacity refers to the acquired ability to express personal preferences based on the knowledge and experience a child gains from being in treatment for long periods of time. For example, a 9-year-old child diagnosed with cancer at age 4 is likely to have a better understanding of disease processes, pain and symptom management, and communication styles than an adult who has never been exposed to a hospital system. In addition to giving informed consent for their child's medical interventions, parents have another important role to play. They are the people who guide their child through the encounter with health care professionals and show how capable their child is in the decision-making process (Tycross, Gibson, & Coad, 2008).

In determining pediatric capacity, the social worker and health care team evaluate using the same standards of adult capacity. They ensure that the young person understands the nature, purpose, and implications of treatment; can weigh benefits, burdens, and consequences; and can anticipate outcomes of interventions and communicate preferences. Although children may not be able to verbally articulate treatment options, benefits and burdens, and outcomes, there are a myriad of communication techniques that can be employed when working with children, including the following (Hockenberry et al., 2003):

- Storytelling
- Bibliotherapy
- Word association game
- Sentence completion
- Writing
- Drawing
- Play
- Painting
- Magic
- Music

The health care team, therefore, must be flexible in respecting the communication styles and unique ways that children might demonstrate comprehension and understanding.

The concept of assent emerged in the 1970s as a way to delineate a *legally valid consent* from a child's *willingness* to participate or not participate in treatment (Kunin, 1997). This concept assumes that children have insight into their disease process and their body's responses to treatment interventions and therefore should be included in the decision-making process. Ideally, children and parents are able to come to the same conclusions about treatments. Child assent is best paired with parental consent. Many child advocates believe that children as young as 7 years old can and should be allowed to give assent (Hinds, 2006). Therefore, this requires the health care team to communicate directly with children in a developmentally appropriate manner. Whenever possible, encouraging children to openly discuss their feelings, concerns, and desires will contribute to the process of decision making (Liben, Papadatou, & Wolfe, 2008).

Decision making in pediatric palliative care is a process of ethical discernment that is affected by access and delivery of information, beliefs and values, cognitive function, and societal norms. Communication with children and families requires an understanding of child development and practical skills, including the following (Kurz, Gill, & Mjones, 2006):

- Empathic attitude
- Credibility and honesty
- Respect
- Attentive listening and talking
- Simplicity of speech.

The pediatric palliative social worker serves a pivotal role in understanding the unique imperatives of communication with children and families and in assisting them through the decision-making process.

❧
Challenges in Pediatric Palliative Care Decision Making

Communication is fundamental to the patient–interdisciplinary team relationship and is associated with patient satisfaction (Kersun, Gyi, & Morrison, 2009). However, despite the best efforts and intentions of team members, breakdown in communications happens with alarming frequency. All too often, parents experience the absence of staff training and competence in sensitive conversations at difficult transitions in the disease process, either during treatment or in later stages of illness (Sumner, 2003). A single incident of miscommunication can cause parents profound and lasting psychological distress (Contro, Larson, Scofield, Sourkes, & Cohen, 2002).

There are many challenges associated with decision making in pediatric palliative care. For example, there is tremendous variation in duration, type, and intensity of care required by individual patients across the trajectory of a disease process (McConnell, Frager, & Levetown, 2004). Additionally, prognostic uncertainty adds to the complicating factors associated with decision making in pediatric palliative care (McConnell et al., 2004). Thanks to technological advances, children are living longer with diseases that historically would certainly have led to death; this fortunate circumstance, however, results in heightened levels of uncertainty during the care and treatment process.

Emotional considerations also contribute to challenges in decision making. For example, the fact that pediatric death is contrary to the natural order, combined with the health care provider's sense of failure and incalculable parental distress, often results in an avoidance of decision making about pediatric palliative care (Liben et al., 2008). This avoidance makes a bad situation worse. By incorporating cultural norms, spiritual beliefs, and family dynamics, the social worker can advocate for the child and family by serving as both an educator and supporter of the team to promote culturally sensitive participation and disclosure in the decision-making process.

Language and cultural differences between families and interdisciplinary teams add another variable to the process of effective communication and decision making. These differences may infuse every aspect of a family's experience, resulting in a potentially compromised ability to integrate complete information, to feel understood, and to fully grasp the scope of the medical condition, treatment, and prognosis (Contro et al., 2002). The social worker and team observe and assess how a child and family communicate and the role of culture in decision making to ensure respectful and effective interactions.

It is the role of the health care team, specifically the social worker, to ensure that communication is adapted to assist children and their families in understanding the disease process, treatment options, benefits, burdens, and consequences of treatments. When this happens, the already burdensome process of decision making becomes more tenable.

Participants in the Decision-Making Process

Patient

Regardless of whether they are judged to have capacity, nearly all children have thoughts and feelings about treatment (Wright, 2009). In the last decade, there has been a positive, increased emphasis on the active involvement of children (Coad & Shaw, 2008). In fact, the American Academy of Pediatrics (AAP) and the Institute of Medicine recommend that children and adolescents be engaged in the decision-making process as much as possible in a developmentally appropriate manner (AAP, 2000; Field & Behrman, 2003).

One of the unique aspects of working with children is that they are in a developmental process with different levels of understanding, awareness, and behaviors. In addition to verbal communication, children use nontraditional, nonverbal modes of communication to ask questions and voice concerns to parents, family members, health care providers, and peers suffering from the same disease (Liben et al., 2008). These include art, dramatic play, dance, puppetry, music, and medical play. Guidelines for verbal communication with children include (Faulkner, 2009) the following:

- Optimize the setting by offering privacy and support.
- Ascertain what the child already knows and understands using simple questions.
- Find out what the child wants to know. Children have a right to *not* know.
- Provide information in small amounts, at the level of the child's understanding.
- Respond to a child's feelings.
- At the end of the discussion, invite children to continue the dialogue at any time.

A social worker or other team member must always obtain the permission of the parent or guardian before talking with a child. In instances when parents are hesitant to disclose information to a child, assessment includes understanding the history and the reasoning that inform this concern. Often, the hesitation stems from an ill-informed or culturally embedded assumption that children do not understand the information or will be hurt by it. Although children may not understand the medical terminology or pathophysiology of a disease process, children as young as 18 months can participate in the decision-making process provided developmentally appropriate and engaging methods are used. While parents' wishes need to be respected, health care providers trained to explain the benefits of involving children in the decision-making process may help parents to agree to an open dialogue and disclosure. This collaboration and respect for parental judgment go a long way toward maintaining the integrity of the family unit; the same unit that will have to continue to function long after the palliative care team has left their lives.

Communication with and care of an adolescent requires special considerations. The balance between independence and autonomy with the requirements of their care is delicate

(McConnell et al., 2006). Cognitive and psychological maturation, together with an increased need for autonomy, have an impact on the involvement of adolescents in the decision-making processes. The adolescent has the capability to take a more active and engaged role in his or her personal care. Stellar communication is considered the most important component of care for an adolescent because it presumes an attitude of respect, candor, and collaboration (Freyer, 2004). Despite the fact that adolescents may express a fervent desire to participate in medical decision making, team members often report discomfort in having end-of-life discussions with them (Wiener et al., 2008). Discomfort can be reduced or alleviated through education and psychosocial support.

The importance of giving young people the opportunity to participate in decisions about their care cannot be overemphasized. This inclusion demonstrates a clear respect for persons that will consequently help to engage them as active participants rather than passive recipients of care. It is the shared responsibility of the team and the social worker to ensure that adults and young people participate in developmentally appropriate decision making. By communicating more effectively, having a policy of inclusion, and actively assessing capacity, an environment is created that encourages a child or adolescent to assume an active role in the treatment. It is important to build on the strengths of children and adolescents and for the health care team to work in tandem with them rather than operating from a position of authority.

Family

Health care professionals must be intimately aware of the emotional, spiritual, financial, and physical impact of an illness, both at the individual level as well as on the family unit as a whole. Pediatric palliative care requires a highly skilled team that attends to the needs of each member of the family, in addition to the patient. The palliative care team, therefore, must give attention to parents, grandparents, siblings, aunts, uncles, and cousins.

Family structures also come in a variety of different forms. For example, with high divorce rates, step-parents and biological parents may share physical custody of a child, including a shared decision-making process. These diverse family structures have ramifications on family dynamics and the decision-making process. Not only must the social worker be sensitive to these often-complicated dynamics, he or she must also identify accurate information recorded from relevant legal documents.

Similarly, despite everything that is known about the needs of the siblings of pediatric patients, evidence shows that they do not receive the psychosocial support that they need (Contro et al., 2002). Siblings may have a number of issues, including the following:

- Erroneous beliefs about the nature of the illness because of the lack of a visible focus of disease (e.g., in leukemia compared to an amputation)

- His or her own private version of the causation of the patient's illness
- Misconceptions about the hospital clinic and the treatment program
- Fear of developing the same illness
- Guilt relating to relief for not developing the illness, ambivalent feelings about the patient (envy, resentment over family's preoccupation with patient)
- Shame over the patient's disfigurement as marking the family as different
- Compromised academic and social functioning because of preoccupation with the stress of illness.

Working with parents to include siblings in decision making may create a valuable opportunity to engage and support siblings and to explore some of the feelings, thoughts, and misconceptions just described.

Team

The delivery of pediatric palliative care and the ethical deliberations that evolve usually happen within the context of a team. The social worker maintains a critical role on the pediatric palliative care team by providing emotional support and information to families. Pediatric palliative care is a specialty that requires a distinct knowledge and skill set that is integral to providing family-level care, facilitating the decision-making process, and discussing feelings, reactions, and psychosocial concerns (Steele et al., 2005). Social workers provide much-needed emotional and spiritual support to children and their families through supportive counseling and developmentally appropriate interventions (Jones, 2006). Additionally, social workers assess mental health needs of all family members. It is the team social worker who frequently helps the family navigate the often daunting world of insurance reimbursement and assists with practical and necessary needs such as obtaining durable medical equipment (DME). As an experienced listener, the social worker prioritizes the problems and concerns of all involved parties and seeks to expedite solutions for them.

The value of the interdisciplinary team meeting is to weave together unique contributions of each team member and to complement different disciplinary perspectives, thereby creating a safety net for children and their families that enhances their ability to live with illness over time and, at times, survive the death of their child (Sumner, 2009). Social workers also play a valuable role in linking patients and families to appropriate community-based psychosocial and mental health resources.

Guardians

In the rare circumstances when parents are judged to be incompetent to make decisions for their child, a social service surrogate or guardian assumes that responsibility. In such circumstances, the surrogate will become intimately involved in the decision-making process (Wright, Frager, & Levetown, 2009). Legal guardians have a challenging job because they must try to understand and respond to situations that they themselves have never faced (McConnell et al., 2006). The social worker can ease this burden by ensuring access to the best medical information and providing support, guidance, and reassurance during the decision-making process.

Decisions That Need to Be Made

There are many decisions that are made throughout the trajectory of a child's illness. Some of these decisions follow a logical, systematic process, while others are fraught with emotion. At each point in a child's illness, decisions include seeking a cure, slowing the progression of disease, handling remission, making contributions to research, prolonging life, achieving life goals, maximizing comfort and periods of lucidity and minimizing symptoms. When end of life is expected, the child and the family may have to decide the best place for the child to come to the end of life (McConnell et al., 2004).

Advance care planning and advance directives are mechanisms for considering in advance the extent of medical interventions desired by patients (Catlin, 2005). When congruous with cultural and spiritual beliefs and values, they help facilitate discussion of potential decisions that may have to be made in pediatric palliative care by allowing patients and families to consider and discuss medical interventions in a calm and composed environment rather than under duress. While these tools are generally reserved for adult palliative care, they can be helpful in perinatal and pediatric palliative care (Catlin, 2005; Hammes, Klevan, Kempf, & Williams, 2005; Wiener et al., 2008; Zinner, 2009). Most advance care plans are composed in a letter format that describes the child's diagnoses and prognosis, the types of treatment determined to be helpful or harmful, and the ethical and personal justification for the plan (Hammes et al., 2005). These tools are incredibly helpful in providing a sense of empowerment, control, and hope as well as helping patients and families to create legacies and find meaning as they anticipate and imagine the end-of-life experience they may create for their child and their family (Zinner, 2009).

When formulating an advance care plan, the topic of withholding and withdrawing nonbeneficial medical interventions is usually included. Advancements in technology force patients and health care providers to face the serious challenge of keeping a neonate or child alive when treatment is futile and will not result in a cure, restoration of function, or improved quality of life. This challenge subsequently raises questions about whether to start or discontinue nonbeneficial medical therapies (Pinter, 2008) and whether treatments that were once beneficial evolve to having no effect or causing harm. While there is no ethical distinction between withholding or withdrawing interventions, they often feel different to the clinicians, patients, and their families (Akpinar, Senses, & Er, 2009; Crawford & Way, 2009; Jonsen et al., 2006). There is evidence that parents are sometimes more comfortable with withholding interventions because this process seems less guilt laden than stopping an intervention that is extending life (Akpinar et al., 2009; Tan, Balagangadhar, Torbati, & Wolfsdorf, 2006). In other words, withholding treatment is more passive in comparison to withdrawing a nonbeneficial treatment, which is more active (Akpinar et al., 2009). For example, the discontinuation of mechanical ventilation is frequently difficult and emotionally disturbing for families and health care teams. Thoughtful discussions and meticulous care planning eases anxiety and may afford a family the opportunity to spend their child's last hours or days wherever and however they wish (Sine et al., 2001).

An excellent tool to bridge differences of opinions, hopes, and expectations is to trial an intervention for an agreed-upon amount of time to measurably identify whether an intervention produces a positive benefit. Trialing an intervention can help focus decision making around an observable or measureable outcome and has the potential to help clinicians, patients, and families replace assumptions and projections with a joint process of observation and evaluation.

Pain management is a fundamental component of pediatric palliative care that is directly related to the ethical principle of beneficence and is a primary concern for parents (Contro et al., 2002). At times decisions about pain and symptom management are agonizing. Witnessing suffering is incredibly difficult, and treatment decisions often involve the weighing of benefits and burdens. For example, medications may cause drowsiness or mental clouding, but when weighed against a child in uncontrolled pain, these side effects become more tolerable. The measurement and management of pain in children needs to be done in a proficient, proactive, and timely manner (Frager & Collins, 2006).

However, there are different types of pain: physical, spiritual, and emotional. The spiritual needs of children often receive less attention than physical and emotional pain. Just as beneficence and respect for persons drive the mandate to manage physical symptoms, so do these principles require that we consider and respect the spiritual aspects of the child or adolescent's experience. This is a shared responsibility of the palliative care team—assisting children, adolescents, and parents with the spiritual and existential aspects of life-threatening illness and death (Davies, Brenner, Orloff, Sumner, & Worden, 2002).

Medically provided hydration and nutrition are options in pediatric palliative care, ideally addressed early in the care planning process. Adults have an instinctual need to feed children. Consequently the decision to withhold or withdraw food and water can be very painful and among the most difficult decisions to make (McConnell et al., 2004). Social workers and palliative care colleagues work together to validate the difficulty of the decision-making process, incorporate and respect cultural and religious influences informing the discussion, and remain available for ongoing exploration and dialogue because the processes surrounding these subjects often occur over time, are revisited, and elicit intense emotions.

The decisions related to resuscitation are difficult for parents and health care providers. The process for discussing resuscitation occurs in the context of a knowledge and respect for the unique family dynamics, their culture and spiritual beliefs and values, and generally includes a description of what cardiopulmonary resuscitation (CPR) involves, for example, chest compressions, intubation, and medication administration. Additionally, the team conveys the likely outcomes for attempting CPR, including whether restoration to the child's current condition is possible or whether there will be complications that could significantly alter his or her quality of life (Rushton, 2009). It is important to reassure parents that "do not resuscitate" does not equate to "do nothing" or "do not treat." An order "not to resuscitate" is a discrete decision particular to CPR. It may signify a change in goals of care, but it does not equate with cessation of other life-sustaining therapies. It is often reassuring to explain that no matter what treatment decisions are made, the clinical team will not abandon the patient and family.

There is a trend in pediatric palliative care to change the terminology from "do no resuscitate" to "allow natural death" ("AND") (Sulmasy, 1998). Rationale for this movement is that "allow natural death" is gentler language and shifts the burden from "not doing" to "allowing." By using the term "AND," parents and clinicians acknowledge that the child is dying and that everything that is being done will allow the dying process to occur as comfortably as possible.

Location for death is another topic for discussion in the decision-making process with parents and families. Some people fervently feel that they want their child to be home in his or her own bed surrounded by the smells, sounds, and feelings of home. Other families cannot bear the thought of having their child die at home because the anticipated burden of the memory is too much to handle. The interdisciplinary team, often spearheaded by the social worker, assists the child and family to identify their preferences and potential resources as well as any fears associated with a child dying at home, which may include worries about pain and symptom management and the processes for death pronouncement and removal of the body, to name a few. Informed consent and respect for autonomy requires that the specialists help the family predict possible outcomes for the patient as well as other family members, problem solve, educate, and support the family to empower them to care for their dying child, if that is their wish. It is essential to reassure the family that whatever they decide to do is fine and that a team will be present to support them, wherever they are.

When dealing with the death of a child, no decision is an easy one. However, engaging in a thoughtful, sensitive, and systematic process of decision making can lessen the burdens.

Communication and the Decision-Making Process

The process for decision making begins with a foundation of good communication, considered the most important factor in avoiding conflicts (Stenson & McIntosh, 1999). There is,

therefore, a premium placed on communication skills in pediatric palliative care (Field & Behrman, 2003). Because communication is both verbal and nonverbal, it is an art and a science that is not static but rather an ongoing and dynamic process requiring robust collaboration among the interdisciplinary team.

All too often, health care providers and families harbor concerns that sharing prognostic information will cause harm and violate the ethical principle of nonmaleficence by causing distress and loss of hope. This may lead some clinicians to avoid the topic of death and to disclose vague or overly optimistic information (Mack, Wolf, Grief, Cleary, & Weeks , 2006). Despite these beliefs, studies have shown that parents have specific needs when making decisions about palliative and end-of-life care. These include (Heller & Solomon, 2005; Meyer, Ritholz, Burns, & Truog, 2006) the following:

- Honest and complete information
- Access to staff
- Communication
- Care coordination and continuity
- Presence
- Emotional expression
- Support by staff
- Preservation of the integrity of the parent–child relationship
- Faith
- Cultural sensitivity.

A common and practical approach used by some to enhance the decision-making process and incidentally prevent ethical issues from becoming ethical dilemmas is by using the Four-Box Method (Table 70.1). The Four-Box method provides a straightforward approach to facilitate good communication and understanding, to identify the pertinent facts and values of any clinical situation, and to facilitate the discussion and resolution of ethical issues. With the Four-Box Method, every clinical case can be analyzed by means of the following four topics: clinical indications, patient preferences, quality of life, and contextual features (Jonsen et al., 2006).

Four-Box Method

The narrative in Box 70.1 demonstrates some of the decision-making challenges faced by parents and the health care team. The concept of autonomy in neonatology involves questions about who should determine the best interest of a neonate: parents, health care professionals, or society. By utilizing the Four-Box method, a team can navigate these taxing circumstances (Table 70.1).

The first topic to analyze is the medical indications for or against diagnostic and therapeutic interventions (Jonsen, 2006). The goals of all medical interventions include saving

Box 70.1
Patient/Family Narrative: Agnes

Agnes is a 3-week-old infant who has been in the neonatal intensive care unit (NICU) since birth. She was born at 36 weeks gestation with severe holoprosencephaly. She also has a cleft lip and palate and severe seizures. She is on anti-seizure medication, in addition to artificial hydration and nutrition. She has had three cardiopulmonary arrests and been resuscitated each time. Agnes's mother, Mrs. S., had no prenatal care. Her parents are married. Agnes has a 7-year-old sister and Mrs S. does not know how to speak with her about Agnes's condition. Mrs. S. is unemployed and the family's livelihood depends on Agnes's father's modest income working part time as a plumber. Their only health insurance comes from their state Medicaid program. Mr. S. is a Catholic Latino and her mother is a Baptist African American; both are active participants in their respective churches. The NICU team has told Agnes's parents that her prognosis is grim, and it is likely that Agnes will die within days or weeks. Mrs. S. wants her daughter to be discharged home with hospice. Mr. S. insists that "everything" be done for Agnes.

life, restoration of health and function, prevention of death, or assisting in a peaceful death (Jonsen, 2006). Prior to talking with the Agnes's parents, the team acquires a full understanding of the medical diagnosis, treatment options, and prognosis in order to ascertain whether Agnes's problems are acute, critical, chronic, or reversible. They consider the following: What are the goals of Agnes's treatment? What are the probabilities of success and the plans in case of therapeutic failure? A team meeting is a forum for exploring these questions, working through disagreements, and building consensus before meeting with Agnes's parents.

In addition to a full understanding of the medical indications of a clinical situation, patient preferences are considered. Infants at the beginning of life have no capacity for preferences; therefore, parents and guardians have the moral and legal authority to make decisions for and act in the best interest of children (Jonsen et al., 2006). The team considers whether Agnes's parents have been fully informed of the benefits and risks of therapeutic interventions and, just as important, ascertain whether they fully understand the information given to them. For example, Agnes's father states that he wants "everything" done. By exploring thoughtfully and delicately the meaning of "everything," the team can begin to understand the values, beliefs, and fears that underlie his words. Some parents think that if they choose to stop disease-modifying treatment or life support interventions and choose comfort care they will be viewed as no longer caring for their child (Beargen, 2006) or that there will be no care provided. The social worker and interdisciplinary team can help Agnes's parents understand that there is no cure for Agnes and that they may be doing "everything" that may benefit Agnes by ensuring the relief of pain and suffering,

Table 70.1.
Four-Box Method

Medical Indications	Patient Preferences
• What is the child's medical problem? History? Diagnosis? Prognosis? • Is the problem acute? Chronic? Critical? Emergent? Reversible? • What are the probabilities of success? • What are the plans in case of therapeutic failure?	• Assess knowledge of current situation, then ask: • Have prior preferences been expressed by either child or family? • Who is the designated decision maker for the child? • Is the child unwilling or unable to cooperate with the medical treatment? • What are the child and family hoping for? • What would the child/family find to be helpful right now?
Qualitative	**Contextual Features**
• What are the prospects, with or without treatment, for a return to normal life? • What physical, mental, and social deficits is the child likely to experience if treatment succeeds? • Are there biases that might prejudice the provider's evaluation of the child's quality of life? • Is the child's present or future condition such that his or her continued life might be judged undesirable? • Is there any plan and rationale to forego treatment? Are there plans for comfort and palliative care?	• Are there family or provider issues that might influence treatment decisions? • Are there financial and economic factors? • Are there religious or cultural factors? • Are there problems of allocation of resources? • How does the law affect treatment decisions? • Is there any conflict of interest on the part of the providers or the institution?

Source: Clinical ethics: A practical approach to ethical decisions in clinical medicine (6th ed.). New York: McGraw-Hill, 2006. Reprinted with permission.

responding to the request for help with Agnes's siblings, and creating an environment of support and comfort.

Attention to culture and spirituality plays a significant role in supporting patients and families through changing goals of care. Studies demonstrate that spiritual support is significantly associated with starting an end-of-life conversation (Tan et al., 2006). The concept of adherence to religious laws plays a significant role for Agnes's parents, and these values and beliefs are essential aspects of their experience. It would be important to offer the parents the assistance of a Baptist minister and/or a Catholic priest.

Medical interventions aim to restore, maintain, or improve quality of life. Therefore, the third issue, *quality of life*, is considered in clinical situations (Jonsen et al., 2006). The team might decide to ask Agnes's parents what "quality of life" means to them, explore their beliefs about her prospects for a normal life, and consider how to best explain what her physical, social, and mental deficits are expected to be. Most important in Agnes's care, the team and family need to examine whether her present or future condition is such that the quality of her continued life would be judged as unacceptable to her parents (Jonsen et al., 2006). Finally, the team needs to clearly articulate the rationale and plan to achieve the agreed-upon goals, minimize her pain and suffering, and maximize the quality of Agnes's life and that of her family. In addition to understanding what interventions are considered harmful or no longer beneficial, families need to hear clearly the medical, psychosocial, and spiritual care that will be available.

Because every clinical case is embedded in a larger context of families, communities, institutions, and financial and social arrangements, the fourth topic, *contextual features*, must also be considered (Jonsen et al., 2006). Contextual features address the ethical principles of loyalty, fairness, and justice. Due to the complexity of physical and psychosocial care, the potential for discord between and among health care providers and with families is very high. Conflict between parents and among health care team members most often occurs in situations of poor prognosis involving treatments, which may cause discomfort, suffering, and unknown outcome (Kopelman, 2006). Agnes's parents have already articulated a difference of opinion regarding the plan of care. Resolution of conflict necessitates a consideration of the social, legal, economic, and institutional circumstances in which a particular case occurs. For example, because personal, family, and provider issues have the potential to influence treatment decision, these topics are assessed (Jonsen et al., 2006). The team has a responsibility to consider, respect, and support Agnes's parents both individually and as a married couple and also to consider the ethical struggles of clinicians who are asked to do things that they do not believe in or that they perceive will cause harm.

Financial and economic factors and cultural and religious influences must also be considered in *contextual features*. The family's finances and insurance limitations may preclude caring for Agnes at home. Agnes's parents' different religious and cultural backgrounds may also influence their beliefs and values and inform their decision making. In this aspect of care the team is often led by the social worker in a shared effort to respectfully reconcile these differences into a unified treatment plan that is in the best interest of Agnes first and then her family.

Managing Conflict

As demonstrated in the illustrative narrative in pediatric palliative care, there are often different points of view about an appropriate course of action (Isaacs et al., 2006; Wright, Aldridge, Wurr, Tomlinson, & Miller, 2009). Ideally, it is best if parents and clinicians agree on the plan of care for a child, whether intensive treatment, palliative interventions, or a combination of both. However, due to multiple and complex ethical issues inherent in palliative care, for example, futility, resuscitation, withholding, and/or withdrawing nonbeneficial interventions, the health care team and parents may not always be aligned in determining the best treatment approach.

Conflict is a circumstance in which there is disagreement in the opinions of two or more people (Dahlin & Giansiracusa, 2006). It may occur among a variety of constituents, for example, between parents, between parents and children, parents and the interdisciplinary team, or among team members, to name a few. Conflicts in pediatric palliative care cannot be avoided and have the potential to be beneficial. For example, when parents move forward in disagreement rather than simply agreeing to recommendations, they more thoroughly evaluate all options and thereby have the potential to avoid regret later (Field & Behrman, 2003). Additionally, dialogue and disagreement among team members can create a healthy opportunity to examine all options and can serve to develop sensitivity in overly confident or assertive clinicians (Field & Behrman, 2003). Often, especially when parents are young and/or unmarried, the older generations are strong influences or even assume the role of decision makers, which may or may not provoke conflict and needs to be explored.

In the often emotionally distressing circumstances of decision making in pediatric palliative care, extended or severe conflicts can be detrimental to and potentially derail the creation of a care plan. Social workers are trained in group and family dynamics and develop competence in conflict resolution. A systematic approach that recognizes different rationales and perspectives can be very helpful to resolve disagreements (McConnell et al., 2006). Conflict prevention and/or consensus building are two effective ways of handling decision making. There are strategies at the individual, team, and organizational levels to prevent or resolve conflict.

Some conflicts are about facts or values, while others are about emotional issues related to loss of power, guilt, anger, or fear (Field & Behrman, 2003). In such circumstances psychosocial counseling, often spearheaded by the team social worker, can help diffuse emotions and therefore conflict.

Acknowledging the source and nature of conflict is a very important part of the resolution process. Conflict resolution training can be a valuable preventative tool that provides staff with strategies to address concerns and to create a shared responsibility (Sumner, 2009). Strengthening an individual's knowledge base for decision making is also effective in conflict resolution. Though more scientific information will not prevent or resolve all disputes, when clinical practice is guided by research that demonstrates what works and what does not, social workers are better equipped to handle potentially distressing circumstances (Field & Behrman, 2003).

Continued discussion and involvement of new parties may help (Field & Behrman, 2003) bring objectivity as well as new information. The introduction of an ethicist, for example, can assist the team to recognize that despite best efforts communication is hampered.

Interdisciplinary team meetings are another mechanism for conflict resolution and may also serve to provide staff support. A safe, trusting work environment that is established over time and has a common value and mission fosters an environment in which staff is encouraged to articulate and debate thoughts and opinions (Sumner, 2009). Consensus-building techniques implemented in a team meeting can also work to resolve conflicts. Examples of consensus-building techniques are (Field & Behrman, 2003) as follows:

- Avoiding personalization of issues
- Engaging in consultation to proffer new and different ways of looking at a situation
- Avoiding all-or-nothing decisions whenever possible by implementing time-limited trials of medical interventions
- Delaying decision making to take time to reflect on goals of care.

Organizationally, the engagement and utilization of ethics committees is useful (Field & Behrman, 2003). An ethics consultation should not be seen as a pejorative or punitive experience. Rather, they intend to improve the process and outcome of care by identifying, analyzing, and working to directly resolve conflict (Jonsen et al., 2006) or to develop professional consensus on institutional policies, thereby providing a mechanism for conflict resolution. It is important to remember that the decision of an ethics committee is not legally binding. However, it can serve to facilitate the decision-making process. Litigation is considered a last resort in resolving conflicts because of the emotional and financial burden for all involved (Field & Behrman, 2003). Conflict resolution has the potential to increase or decrease the possible harm to all involved parties. It is the role of the social worker to utilize any and all strategies to resolve conflict by working to improve teamwork and communication with families and team members.

Training and Support

Moral distress (Austin, Kelecevic, Goble, & Mekechuk, 2009; Davies, 1996; Klein, 2009) is often encountered when conflicts about goals of care are unresolved and when a clinician believes he or she knows the right thing to do but is unable to do it for various reasons. As a consequence, the clinician's integrity is threatened. For example, a social worker may feel that his or her ethical and moral principles are compromised when a patient continues to receive treatments that they perceive not to be in the child's best interest (Janiver, Nadeau, Deschenes, Couture, & Barrington, 2007). Moral distress can be encountered anywhere, from the NICU to the home.

There are, however, ways to address moral distress. For example, increasing trust and communication among team members and enhancing education and discussing the dilemmas with supervisors or peers are suggested ways to manage and perhaps resolve experiences of moral distress (Austin et al., 2009).

Despite the emotional and ethical challenges of working in pediatric palliative care, comprehensive education on pain and symptom management, child development, psychosocial issues, ethics, and grief and bereavement provides a solid foundation to enable social workers to deliver effective pediatric palliative care. Pediatric palliative care can be taught in an organized and systematic fashion (Kersun et al., 2009), and there are numerous national pediatric palliative care training programs (Table 70.2).

Staff support is another key component to mitigating the impact of painful decision making, ethical dilemmas, and sustained long-term care of children and their families facing potentially life-limiting illness. The following resources are potential sources of support for staff who wish to ameliorate or prevent caregiver suffering (Sumner, 2009):

- Employee assistant programs (EAPs) that provide confidential counseling
- Bereavement support with trained bereavement professionals, both immediately after a death and on an ongoing basis
- Interdisciplinary team support, formal and informal
- Supervision, consultation, and peer support, including shared learning experiences.

It is not enough to simply offer services to staff and team members. It is important to assess the efficacy of the staff support and education by including it in an organization's annual internal review, conducting an employee satisfaction survey, and possibly doing one-on-one interviews (Sumner, 2009). Utilizing these resources and promoting staff education and training, both formal and informal, will serve individuals, teams, and most important, children and their families whose lives are faced with unimaginable sorrow.

Table 70.2.
Educational Programs in Pediatric Palliative Care

Education Program	Program Description
ACE Project	The ACE Project at the City of Hope National Medical Center is one education program whose goal is to enhance the leadership and advocacy skills of psychologists, social workers, and spiritual care professionals through a transdisciplinary educational experience (http://www.cityofhope.org/education/health-professional-education/nursing-education/ACE-project/Pages/default.aspx).
PCEP	Harvard Medical School Center for Palliative Care offers the Program in Palliative Care Education and Practice. This offers intensive learning experiences for physician and nurse educators who wish to become expert in the clinical practice and teaching of comprehensive, interdisciplinary palliative care, as well as to gain expertise in leading and managing improvements in palliative care education and practice at their own institutions http://www.hms.harvard.edu/pallcare/pcep.htm). While this course is geared toward physicians and nurses, social workers are invited to participate.
ELNEC	The End-of-Life Nursing Education Consortium (ELNEC) project is a national education initiative to improve palliative care. Although this training is geared toward nursing, social workers are invited and encouraged to attend (http://www.aacn.nche.edu/ELNEC).
IPPC	The Initiative for Pediatric Palliative Care (IPPC) is an education and a quality improvement effort whose goal is to enhance family-centered care for children and their families facing life-threatening conditions. The IPPC interdisciplinary curriculum addresses knowledge, attitudes, and skills necessary to serve children and their families (http://www.ippcweb.org/index.asp).

Conclusion

Caring for infants, children, and adolescents and their families facing life-limiting illness is a profound honor and a truly sacred experience. There are tremendous opportunities for hope and for growth. However, it is also a process fraught with ethical issues and challenges in decision making. Ethical decision making must take place within the context of a moral framework, with sound knowledge of the issues and respect for cultural concerns. As active participants in pediatric palliative decision making, children and their families deserve comprehensive information about medical interventions and procedures at a pace and cognitive level that they can understand (Dill et al., 2006).

Social workers need to work closely with other disciplines to understand and utilize the ethical process for seeking balance by addressing values and understanding the needs of all involved. Working together to maintain integrity, to pursue clinical excellence, and to practice with compassion, palliative care clinicians share a responsibility to children and families who struggle to weigh choices and make the most profound decisions. Engaging in ethical discernment, discourse, and decision making is a way for social workers to maintain the integrity of children and to show respect for their lives.

ADDITIONAL RESOURCES

The American Academy of Pediatrics: http://www.medicalhomeinfo.org/publications/palliative_pro.html

The American Academy of Pediatrics' Palliative Care in the Medical Home's goal is to ensure that children and youth with special needs have a medical home where health care services are accessible, family-centered, continuous, comprehensive, coordinated, compassionate, and culturally competent. Physicians, parents, administrators, and other health care professionals have access to educational, resource, and advocacy materials, guidelines for care, evaluation tools, and technical assistance.

Caring Connections: http://www.caringinfo.org/index.cfm?page=610

Caring Connections' Pediatric Outreach has resources that are available to educate and engage the community around pediatric end-of-life care and support for families with a seriously ill child.

Children's Hospice International (CHI): http://www.chionline.org

Provides education, training, and technical assistance to those who care for children with life-threatening conditions and their families.

Children's Hospice and Palliative Care Coalition (CHPCC): http://www.childrenshospice.org

A social movement led by children's hospitals, hospices, home health and grassroots agencies, and individuals to improve care for children with life-threatening conditions and their families. The Children's Hospice & Palliative Care Providers' Network promotes best practices in family-centered palliative care by sharing up-to-date information and resources for providers caring for children with serious illnesses.

Decision-Making Tool: http://www.promotingexcellence.org/downloads/grantee_tools/chrmc2.pdf

Decision-Making Tool tutorial is available at: http://www.cshcn.org/palliativecare/DMT_Tutorial_files/frame.htp

Duke Institute on Care at the End of Life: http://www.iceol.duke.edu

Facilitates and engages in important dialogue with diverse religious, spiritual, patient, and advocacy communities concerned about access to and quality of palliative and end-of-life care.

The Multidisciplinary Order Sheet/Advance Care Plan for the Child with Life Limiting Conditions: http://www.mywhatever.com/cifwriter/content/41/pe3745.html

Tools and materials to assist family-centered care planning and coordination of care developed by the FOOTPRINTS program staff of Cardinal Glennon Children's Hospital.

The National Consensus Project for Quality Palliative Care (NCP): http://www.nationalconsensusproject.org/

A major objective of the NCP is to heighten awareness of palliative care as an option in treating those with a life-limiting or chronic debilitating illness, condition, or injury and to raise public understanding of the growing need for such care.

National Hospice & Palliative Care Organization (NHPCO): http://www.nhpco.org/i4a/pages/index.cfm?pageid=3351

Partnering for Children: http://www.partneringforchildren.org

National awareness campaign led by the Children's Hospice and Palliative Care Coalition to promote compassionate, family-centered health care for children with life-threatening conditions. Many families do not have access to the pain and symptom management, emotional, social, and spiritual support offered by palliative care and hospice.

Pediatric Palliative Care Project at Children's Hospital and Regional Medical Center, Seattle, Washington: http://www.promotingexcellence.org/childrens

For tools and materials to assist coordination and continuity of palliative care delivery.

The Sesame Street Project: http://www.sharethecare.org

A video resource intended to organize and sustain a team that connects the helpers with the "helpees."

Starlight Starbright Children's Foundation: http://www.starlight.org

Health Professionals section is a resource for nurses, physicians, doctors, pediatricians, and others seeking information on behalf of patients. Starlight Starbright has dedicated itself to improving the quality of life for children with serious medical conditions by providing entertainment, education, and family activities that help them cope with the pain, fear, and isolation of prolonged illness.

The Toolkit of Instruments to Measure End-of-Life Care (TIME): http://www.chcr.brown.edu/pcoc/toolkit.htm

Although not specific to pediatrics, four instruments for measuring interpersonal (relational) aspects of continuity are reviewed. There is also a general discussion of the multiple dimensions of continuity based on a review of the literature and the challenges of measuring these dimensions

REFERENCES

American Academy of Pediatrics. (2000). Palliative care for children. *Pediatrics, 106*, 351–357.

Akpinar, A., Senses, M. O., & Er, R. A. (2009). Attitudes to end-of-life decisions in pediatric intensive care. *Nursing Ethics, 16*(1), 83–92.

Austin, W., Kelecevic, J., Goble, E., & Mekechuk, J. (2009). An overview of moral distress and the pediatric intensive care team. *Nursing Ethics, 16*(1), 57–68.

Beargen, R. (2006). How hopeful is too hopeful? Responding to unreasonably optimistic parents. *Pediatric Nursing, 32*(5), 482–486.

Beauchamp, T. L., & Childress J. F. (2001). *Principles of biomedical ethics.* New York, NY: Oxford University Press.

Blustein, J. (1996). Confidentiality and the adolescent: An ethical analysis. In R. C. Cassidy & A. R. Fleischman (Eds.), *Pediatric ethics–From principles to practice* (pp. 83–96). Amsterdam, The Netherlands: Harwood Academic Publishers GmbH.

Brook, L., & Hain, R. (2008). Predicting death in children. *Archives of Disease in Childhood, 93*(12), 1067–1070.

Catlin, A. & Carter, B. (2002). Creation of a neonatal end-of-life palliative care protocol. *Journal of Perinatology, 22*(3), 184–195.

Catlin, A. (2005). Thinking outside the box: Prenatal care and the call for a prenatal advance directive. *Journal of Perinatal Nursing, 19*(2), 169–176.

Children's Hospice International (CHI). (2003). *About children's hospice, palliative & end-of-life care. An unmet need.* Retrieved May 20, 2008 from www.chionline.org/resources/about.php

Coad, J. E., & Shaw, K. L. (2008). Is children's choice in health care rhetoric or reality? A coping review. *Journal of Advanced Nursing, 64*(4), 318–327.

Contro, N., Larson, J., Scofield, S., Sourkes, B., & Cohen, H. (2002). Family perspectives on the quality of pediatric palliative care. *Archives of Pediatric and Adolescent Medicine, 156*, 14–19.

Crawford, D., & Way, C. (2009). Just because we can, should we? A discussion of treatment withdrawal. *Pediatric Nursing, 21*(1), 22–25.

Dahlin, C. M., & Giansiracusa, D. F. (2006). Communication in palliative care. In B. R. Ferrell & N. Coyle (Eds.), *Textbook of palliative nursing* (pp. 67–90). New York, NY: Oxford University Press.

Davies, B., Brenner, P., Orloff, S., Sumner, L., & Worden, W. (2002). Addressing spirituality in pediatric hospice and palliative care. *Journal of Palliative Care, 18*(1), 59–67.

Davies, B., Clarke, D., & Connaughty, S. (1996). Caring for dying children: Nurses experiences. *Pediatric Nursing, 22*, 500–507.

Davies, B., Sehring, S. A., Partridge, J. C., Cooper, B. A., Hughes, A., Philip, J. C., & Kramer, R. K. (2008). Barriers to palliative care for children: Perceptions of pediatric health care providers. *Pediatrics, 121*(2), 282–288.

Davies, D. (2004). *Child development: A practitioner's guide.* New York, NY: The Guilford Press.

Faulkner, K. (2009). Children's understanding of death. In A. Armstrong-Dailey & S. Zarbock (Eds.), *Hospice care for children* (3rd ed., pp. 9–23). New York, NY: Oxford University Press.

Field, M. J., & Behrman, R. E. (Eds.). (2003). *When children die: Improving palliative and end-of-life care for children and their families.* (Report of the Institute of Medicine Task Force). Washington, DC: National Academies Press.

Frader, J., Morgan, E., Levinson, T., Morrow, J., & Saroyan, J. M. (2004). Barriers, education, and advocacy in palliative care. In B. S. Carter & M. Levetown (Eds.), *Palliative care for infants, children and adolescents: A practical handbook* (pp. 44–66). Baltimore, MD: The Johns Hopkins University Press.

Frager, G., & Collins, J. J. (2006). Symptoms in life-threatening illness: Overview and assessment. In A. Goldman, R. Hain, & S. Liben (Eds.), *Oxford textbook of palliative care for children* (pp. 231–245). New York, NY: The Oxford University Press.

Freyer, D. R. (2004). Care of the dying adolescent: Special considerations. *Pediatrics, 113,* 381–388.

Hammes, B. J., Klevan, J., Kempf, M., & Williams, M. S. (2005). Pediatric advance care planning. *Journal of Palliative Medicine, 8*(4), 766–774.

Heller, K. S., & Solomon, M. Z. (2005). Continuity of care and caring: What matters to parents of children with life-threatening conditions. *Journal of Pediatric Nursing, 20*(5), 335–346).

Hilden, J. M., Himelstein, B. P., Freyer, D. R., Feiebert, S., & Kane, J. R. (2001). End-of-life care: Special issues in pediatric oncology. In K. Foley (Ed.), *Improving palliative care for cancer* (pp. 161–198). Washington, DC: National Academies Press.

Himelstein, B. P., Hilden, J. M., Boldt, A. M., & Weissman, D. (2004). Pediatric palliative care. *New England Journal of Medicine, 350,* 1752–1762.

Hockenberry, M., Wilson, D., Winkelstein, M. L., & Kline, N. (2003). *Wong's nursing care of infants and children* (pp. 150–153). St. Louis, MO: Mosby.

Isaacs, D., Kilham, H., Gordon, A., Jeffery, H., Tarnow-Mordi, W., Woolnough, J., … Tobin, B. (2006). Withdrawal of neonatal mechanical ventilation against parents wishes. *Journal of Pediatrics and Child Health, 42,* 311–315.

Janiver, A., Nadeau, S., Deschenes, M., Couture, E., & Barrington, K. J. (2007). Moral distress in the neonatal intensive care unit: Caregiver's experience. *Journal of Perinataology, 27,* 203–208.

Jones, B. L. (2006). Companionship, control, and compassion: A social work perspective on the needs of children with cancer and their families at the end of life. *Journal of Palliative Medicine, 9*(3), 774–788.

Jonsen, A., Siegler, M., & Winslade, W. (2006). *Clinical ethics: A practical approach to ethical decisions in clinical medicine* (6th ed.). New York, NY: McGraw-Hill.

Kersun, L., Gyi, L., & Morrison, W. E. (2009). Training in difficult conversations: A national survey of pediatric hematology-oncology and pediatric critical care physicians. *Journal of Palliative Medicine, 12*(6), 525–530.

Klein, S. M. (2009). Moral distress in pediatric palliative care: A case study. *Journal of Pain and Symptom Management, 38*(1), 157–160.

Kopelman, A. (2006). Understanding, avoiding, and resolving end-of-life conflicts in the NICU. *The Mount Sinai Journal of Medicine, 73*(3), 580–586.

Kunin, H. (1997). Ethical issues in pediatric life-threatening illness: Dilemmas of consent, assent, and communication. *Ethics and Behavior, 7*(1), 43–57.

Kurz, R., Gill, D., & Mjones, S. (2006). Ethical issues in the daily medical care of children. *European Journal of Pediatrics, 165,* 83–86.

Levetown, M. (Ed). (2000). *Compendium of pediatric palliative care.* Alexandria, VA: National Hospice and Palliative Care Organization.

Levetown, M. (2006). Pediatric care: Transitioning goals of care in the emergency department, intensive care unit and in between. In B. R. Ferrell & N. Coyle, N. (Eds.), *Textbook of palliative nursing* (pp. 925–943). New York, NY: Oxford University Press.

Liben S., Papadatou, D., & Wolfe, J. (2008). Paediatric palliative care: Challenges and emerging ideas. *The Lancet, 371,* 852–864.

Mack, J. W., Wolfe, J., Grier, H. E., Cleary, P. D., & Weeks, J. C. (2006). Communication about prognosis between parents and physicians of children with cancer: Parent preferences and the impact of prognostic information. *Journal of Clinical Oncology, 24*(33), 5265–5270.

McConnell Y., Frager, G., & Levetown, M. (2004). Decision making in pediatric palliative care. In B. S. Carter & M. Levetown (Eds.), *Palliative care for infants, children and adolescents: A practical handbook* (pp. 69–111). Baltimore, MD: The Johns Hopkins University Press.

Meyer, E. C., Ritholz, M. D., Burns, J. P., & Truog, R. D. (2006). Improving the quality of end-of-life care in the pediatric intensive care unit: Parents' priorities and recommendations. *Pediatrics, 117,* 649–657.

Pinter, A. B. (2008). End-of-life decision before and after birth: Changing ethical considerations. *Journal of Pediatric Surgery, 43,* 430–436.

Rushton, C. H. (2009). Ethical decision making at the end of life. In A. Armstrong-Dailey & S. Zarbock (Eds.), *Hospice care for children* (3rd ed., pp. 457–485). New York, NY: Oxford University Press.

Rushton, C. H., & Catlin, A. (2002). Pediatric palliative care: The time is now! *Pediatric Nursing, 28*(1), 57–60.

Sine, D., Sumner, L., Gracy, D., & von Gunten, C. F. (2001). Pediatric extubation: "pulling the tube." *Journal of Palliative Medicine, 4*(4), 519–524.

Steele, R., Davies, B., Collins, J. B., & Cook, K. (2005). End-of-life care in a children's hospice program. *Journal of Palliative Care, 21*(1), 5–11.

Stenson, B., & McIntosh, N. (1999). Some ethical considerations in the neonatal intensive care area. *European Journal of Pediatrics, 158,* S13–S17.

Sulmasy, D. P. (1998). Killing and allowing to die: Another look. *Journal of Law, Medicine and Ethics, 26,* 55–64.

Sumner, L. (2003). Lighting the way: Improving the way children die in America. *CARING Magazine, 14,* 14–17.

Sumner, L. (2009). Staff support in pediatric hospice care. In A. Armstrong-Dailey & S. Zarbock (Eds.), *Hospice care for children* (3rd ed., pp. 240–265). New York, NY: Oxford University Press.

Tan, G. H., Balagangadhar, R. T., Torbati, D., & Wolfsdorf, J. (2006). End-of-life decisions and palliative care in a children's hospital. *Journal of Palliative Medicine, 9*(2), 332–342.

Tycross, A., Gibson, F., & Coad, J. (2008). Guidance on seeking agreement to participate in research from young children. *Pediatric Nursing, 20*(6), 14–18.

Wiener, L., Ballard, E., Brennan, T., Battles, H., Martinez, P., & Pao, M. (2008). How I wish to be remembered: The use of an advanced care planning document in adolescent and young adult populations. *Journal of Palliative Care, 11*(10), 1309–1313.

Wright, B., Aldridge, J., Wurr, K., Tomlinson, H., & Miller, M. (2009). Clinical dilemmas in children with life-limiting illnesses: Decision making and the law. *Palliative Medicine, 23,* 238–247.

Zinner, S. E. (2009). The use of pediatric advance directives: A tool for palliative care physicians. *American Journal of Hospice and Palliative Medicine, 25*(6), 427–430.

71

Tracy A. Schroepfer, John F. Linder, and Pamela J. Miller

Social Work's Ethical Challenge: Supporting the Terminally Ill Who Consider a Hastened Death

We can't make judgments...everybody who gets involved in this (discussion of hastened death)...use it as an opportunity. It is not just an opportunity for the patients, to look inside themselves, but it is an opportunity for all of the team, the family, and the caregivers to do it...to walk with someone down the path, that they really do take some time to look inside their hearts.

—*Miller, Mesler, & Eggman (2002)*

Key Concepts

♦ *The options for hastening death at the end of life have increased the ethical issues and uncertainties faced by social workers who work with patients with life-threatening illness and their families.*

♦ *Research findings indicate that the factors motivating the consideration of a hastened death by individuals with life-threatening illness are most often psychosocial and spiritual in nature, issues that fall within the realm of social work practice.*

♦ *The social work profession has formulated guidance for practitioners and advocates alike in dealing with the consideration to hasten death.*

♦ *Although the legal option to end life by a prescription is available in only a few places, political, ethical, and clinical ramifications exist that infuse clinical work. Social workers need to be prepared to work with the complex conversations and emotions that arise as patients consider the end of life.*

Introduction

In recent years, social workers practicing in end-of-life care have found themselves faced with terminally ill clients (a prognosis of less than 6 months to live) and their families who want to discuss options for a hastened death or, in particular, physician assisted-suicide, two terms that have become firmly entrenched in the landscape of end-of-life health care policy and practice. Although these actual practices and conversations about them with patients and families remain controversial, it is difficult for social workers to ignore the ever-growing role these concepts and options play in the lives of their clients and families. Research has shown that compared with physical factors, the unmet psychosocial and/or spiritual needs of terminally ill individuals are more often the motivating factors behind the consideration of, or request for, a hastened death (Arnold, 2004; Breitbart, Rosenfeld, & Passik, 1996; Chochinov et al., 1995; Emanuel, Fairclough, & Emanuel, 2000; Schroepfer, 2006, 2008). Since a role of social workers practicing in palliative care is to address the psychosocial and existential needs of individuals and their families, it is not surprising that social workers may find themselves involved in discussions about hastening death (Arnold, 2004; Ogden & Young, 2003). The probability of such discussions occurring has also increased due to the potential of individuals experiencing a lengthier dying process.

As advances in medical technology and public health (e.g., improved sanitation and clean water) have rapidly increased, so have the ethical issues and uncertainties faced by social workers striving to assist patients who are facing a lengthier, but not always quality, dying process. The creation of clear guidelines for dealing with such situations has failed to keep pace, as has the dissemination of information regarding hastening death and the role social workers might play. Is it ethical for a social worker to participate in a discussion of a client's desire to hasten death? How do the guidelines for participation differ based on whether the form of hastening

651

death being discussed is or is not legal in the state where the social worker is practicing? Furnishing social workers with knowledge about the methods used to hasten death, the guidelines and legalities associated with each, the relevance of the social work profession's code of ethics, and the role social workers are expected to play is crucial if they are to meet their clients' psychosocial needs and do so in both an ethical and legal manner.

This chapter seeks to inform social work practice in palliative care by directly addressing the social worker's role in discussions with clients who consider hastening their death, both in states where some form of hastening death is legal and where it is not legal. We will first provide background information on the forms that a hastened death can take and the factors motivating individuals to consider hastening their death. Next, we will discuss guidelines concerning the role of social workers in states where physician-assisted suicide is legal and illegal, as well as the ethical issues and the role of advocacy. Finally, we will report on the experiences of Oregon social workers where physician-assisted suicide has been practiced legally since 1997.

Options for Hastening Death

As lives have been extended consequent to advances in medical technology, the various options for hastening one's death have grown in number. Although *physician-assisted death*, *physician-assisted euthanasia*, and *physician-assisted suicide* are the terms most often heard and discussed, many more options exist that social workers need to understand in order to be prepared for discussions with patients, families, and professional staff.

The term *hastened death* refers to a number of end-of-life options, including, but not limited to, withholding and withdrawal of life-sustaining treatment, voluntary cessation of eating and drinking, palliative sedation, and physician-assisted death. In the United States, the least controversial of these options is the refusal of life-sustaining treatment via withholding or withdrawal, an option both legally and ethically accepted (Quill, Lee, & Nunn, 2000). In most states, patients with capacity or the designated agents of those who are without decisional capacity can decide not to start a treatment or to stop a treatment at any time, even if doing so will result in death. The role of health care professionals in these situations is to determine the patient's mental capacity to make the decision and then insure that the patient, family member, or agent making the decision is fully informed of the risks and benefits, as well as each option's impact on family and family caregivers. Voluntary cessation of food and drink is a choice that can be made exclusively by the individual without permission from or participation of a physician. Some health care professionals may struggle with this choice and want to insure that the patient has capacity and is not suffering from major depression or being quietly coerced to end

his or her life. Professional staff and family must determine whether and how they can be supportive of the patient throughout a process that leads to death within 1 to 3 weeks.

Another treatment that may hasten death is palliative sedation, sometimes referred to as terminal sedation, which, while accepted in the United States, remains controversial. The preferred term by healthcare professionals is *palliative sedation* because the intent of this treatment is not to hasten the patient's death; rather, the intent is to sedate an imminently dying patient only to the level of unconsciousness necessary to relieve his or her uncontrollable pain or other symptoms (Carr & Mohr, 2008). Since palliative sedation can hasten death because the patient neither eats nor drinks and the medication is ordered by the physician, some comparisons have been made to physician-assisted euthanasia. Differences do exist between palliative sedation and physician-assisted euthanasia, however, particularly in regard to the role of health care professionals. The decision to administer a sedative, while ultimately ordered by a physician, is made within the context of an informed consent discussion with the team, the patient, if she or he is deemed mentally competent, and family. The medicine is administered by professional staff and, once the patient is sedated, the dosage is increased only to maintain the level of sedation. These actions are very different from those taken when physician-assisted euthanasia is involved, wherein the intent is to medicate until death occurs. Furthermore, when death does occur in the case of palliative sedation, those involved recognize that the primary intent was to manage intractable symptoms, not to hasten death (Carr & Mohr, 2008).

Physician-assisted death (PAD) is by far the most controversial of the options to hasten death, and it is a term used to encompass both physician-assisted euthanasia (PAE) and physician-assisted suicide (PAS). As the ethical and legal debates continue to grow regarding PAE and PAS, so does the need for the use of consistent terminology in order to insure informed debates and decisions, as well as the comparability of research results. Physician-assisted euthanasia refers to the situation in which a physician gives a mentally competent, terminally ill patient a lethal injection at the request of the patient. This method of hastening death is not legal anywhere in the United States but has been legal in the Netherlands and Belgium since 2002. Physician-assisted suicide refers to situations in which a physician provides a mentally competent, terminally ill patient with a prescription for a lethal medication at the patient's request, which the patient then ingests. The practice of PAS has been legal in Oregon since 1997, and in Washington and Montana since 2008. Montana's decision differed from that of Oregon and Washington, however, because in these latter two states the law on PAS was approved by voters in a statewide referendum and in Montana ruled a legal right by a state district judge. In January 2009, the judge's ruling was supported when the Montana State Supreme Court ruled that state criminal law does not forbid PAS and so physicians cannot be prosecuted for assisting terminally ill residents (O'Reilly, 2010). As the number of states legalizing PAS grows, so does the need to understand why someone would choose to hasten his or her death, particularly via physician-assisted suicide. Researchers conducting studies on this topic are providing insight into such a choice.

Factors Motivating the Consideration to Hasten Death

Two approaches have been taken to determine the factors that motivate an individual's consideration to hasten his or her own death: retrospective and prospective. Researchers using the retrospective approach review case studies written by health care professionals whose patients either considered hastening their death or did so, as well as interview family and friends of the deceased. Researchers employing a prospective approach focus on interviewing individuals with a terminal illness (an illness likely to result in death) or who have been defined as terminally ill (less than 6 months to live) about whether they have considered hastening their death and, if so, the factors that motivated them to do so. Both approaches have garnered a deeper understanding of the factors that motivate the consideration of a hastened death—knowledge that serves to inform the provision of palliative care at end of life.

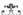

Retrospective Studies

The retrospective research approach has found that compared to physical factors, psychosocial factors are more often reported as motivators of a hastened death. These psychosocial factors include a loss of autonomy and a decreased ability to participate in activities that make life enjoyable (Oregon Department of Human Services, 2008), loss of control over bodily functions (Back, Wallace, Starks, & Pearlman, 1996: Oregon Department of Human Services, 2008), loss of dignity and feeling one is a burden (Back et al., 1996; Meier et al., 1998; Oregon Department of Human Services, 2008), loss of meaning in life (Meirer et al., 1998), and loss of control over the manner of death (Oregon Department of Human Services, 2000; Volker, 2001). Although two studies reported the role of current pain as a motivator for hastening death (Back et al., 1996; Meier et al., 1998), the *fear* of uncontrollable symptoms (Meier et al., 1998) or uncontrollable pain (Oregon Department of Human Services, 2008; Volker, 2001) was more often reported.

Ganzini et al. (2002) and Jacobson et al. (1995) conducted two quantitative retrospective studies of health care professionals and caregivers, respectively, and neither found pain to be a significant predictor of the consideration to hasten death. Ganzini et al. (2002) interviewed hospice nurses and social workers who reported that a desire to control the circumstances of death, the wish to die at home, feeling that living was pointless, and loss of dignity were most often discussed by patients desiring a hastened death. Jacobson et al. (1995) interviewed decedents and asked about satisfaction with comfort care. Survivors reported that most deceased individuals who were believed to have wanted PAE or PAS (90%) were satisfied with their comfort (palliative) care. Clearly, both qualitative and quantitative retrospective studies provide evidence of the important role that psychosocial factors play in the dying process and the consideration to hasten one's death.

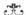

Prospective Studies

Quantitative prospective studies provide additional support regarding the role of psychosocial factors in the consideration to hasten death, as well as evidence of the role physical factors play. Both terminally ill patients or patients with a terminal illness who were considering a hastened death reported few social supports (Breibart et al., 1996), experienced a low quality of social support (Arnold, 2004; Breibart et al., 1996; Chochinov et al., 1995; Schroepfer, 2007, 2008), and perceived their caregiving needs as high (Emanuel et al., 2000). In addition, these individuals reported a lack of enjoyment in life, feelings of uselessness, and being a burden (Schroepfer, 2006), a higher level of anxiety, a lower level of hope (Arnold, 2004), and a higher level of depression (Arnold, 2004; Breibart et al., 1996; Chochinov et al., 1995; Emanuel, Fairclough, Daniels, & Clarridge, 1996; Emanuel et al., 2000) than those individuals not considering a hastened death. Prospective quantitative results regarding the role of pain have remained mixed. In four cross-sectional studies (Breitbart et al., 1996; Chochinov et al., 1995; Emanuel et al., 1996; Schroepfer, 2008), pain was not found to be a significant predictor of the consideration to hasten death, but it was found to be significant in two other such studies (Arnold, 2004; Emanuel et al., 2000). One of the few studies that involved interviewing terminally ill patients diagnosed with cancer at two different time points found that a decline in the severity of pain did not serve to reduce patients' desire to hasten death (O'Mahony et al., 2005).

Several qualitative prospective studies have also been conducted. Lavery, Boyle, Dickens, Maclean, and Singer (2001) interviewed patients with HIV-1 or AIDS and found that loss of control over bodily functions, a loss of dignity, and a lack of social support were reported by patients considering a hastened death. In another qualitative study (Schroepfer, 2006), terminally ill elders revealed that psychosocial factors, including loneliness, not enjoying life, lack of hope, boredom, uselessness, being a burden, and a desire for control over the manner of death, were factors in their considering a hastened death, as well as current pain and the fear of future pain. Clearly, the importance of psychosocial factors in the consideration to hasten death is well supported in the literature.

For social workers involved in providing psychosocial support to people along the continuum of life-threatening illness and at the end of their lives, the desire to hasten death is likely to emerge either directly or indirectly in conversations with them. Furthermore, although one study (Ganzini, Goy, Dobscha, & Prigerson, 2009) found that hastening death does not necessarily have negative mental health effects on survivors and may actually assist with greater preparation for and acceptance of death, the role of family members in these conversations still cannot be ignored. When patients express a desire to hasten death or request assistance with hastening death, many important ethical issues emerge for social workers. Having a fundamental knowledge of the profession's guidelines and code of ethics is essential for social workers employed in the complex systems that provide care to those living with life-threatening illness and those who are dying. The next section of this chapter delves into the area of ethics and advocacy, and the role they play in clients' requests to hasten their death.

Ethics and Advocacy

Self-determination is one of the social work profession's core principles. One implication of this is that social workers tend to be inclined to support an individual's autonomy and freedom of choice, provided the choice is fully informed, freely made, and untainted by depression or other mental health factors. This support of an individual's right to freedom of choice is present even when it may be at odds with a given social worker's own beliefs, such as in the case of social workers' attitudes toward a hastened death. Research has shown that social workers demonstrate this commitment to autonomy by either not opposing a client's choice or right to choose a hastened death where legal, or by being supportive of a client's desire to discuss hastening his or her death (Csikai, 1999; Ganzini et al, 2002; Harvath et al., 2006; Miller, Mesler, & Eggman, 2002; Ogden & Young, 2003). The issue of physician-assisted dying is complex, however, with unique, interwoven medical, ethical, relational, spiritual, cultural, and social factors influencing its consideration by a client.

In the United States, two documents particularly guide social work practice vis-à-vis requests for hastened death. The first document is the position statement of the Association of Oncology Social Work (AOSW, 2008), which cogently articulates the complexity of the issue. The organization's position is that it does not support the legalization of physician-assisted euthanasia or physician-assisted suicide, but it does support improved access to affordable palliative and hospice care for all patients and families. These two distinct aspects of the AOSW's position statement cannot be separated and must be parsed carefully within the context of the whole document, because a policy of nonsupport is different from a position of opposition. The document recognizes that the issue of hastened death cannot be extracted from its context and considered in a vacuum. The position statement goes into detail regarding the context in which a discussion arises or a request is made, acknowledging that such requests are often expressions of "existential suffering and inadequate symptom management," and that these concerns must be assessed and addressed in a thorough, just and equitable manner (p. 1). The two aspects of AOSW's position statement are further evidence of the intersection of practice and advocacy that is at the center of the social work profession.

The second document is the National Association of Social Workers (NASW) position statement on end-of-life care (NASW, 2006), which delineates social work responsibilities to clients and families at the end of life (practice), and social work's role in the larger society (advocacy). Using the NASW Code of Ethics, *Standards for Social Work Practice in Palliative & End of Life Care* (NASW, 2004), and prevailing law as the foundation, the NASW position statement offers social workers specific guidance regarding hastened death. Advance care planning, thorough knowledge of end-of-life options, excellent symptom management, a focus on quality of life, cultural sensitivity, and worker self-awareness cannot be separated from either the choice to be present at a client's death (hastened or otherwise) at the client's request or a conscience-driven exception to opt out (with appropriate transfer of care) for social work professionals. This document provides a balanced discussion of the complexity of the issue and the potential for conflict among various social work and bioethics principles.

Self-reflection and self-knowledge are important enough to the social work profession to be included in the Code of Ethics. Several articles (Csikai, 1999, 2004; Mackelprang & Mackelprang, 2005; Manetta & Wells, 2001) articulate this process of reflection and offer various social work views on policy and practice related to hastened death. Many areas of potential conflict can arise, including but not limited to competing sequelae of hastened death on patients and their survivors; unequal access to care resulting in poor symptom management and burden on caregivers; concerns about the coercion of those who are poor, homeless, of limited decisional capacity, elderly, or who have disabilities; decisions based on inadequate resources; values conflicts regarding hastened death; care teams divided on a patient's mental status or depressive symptoms; and autonomy and self-determination versus the ethical and social imperative to protect the vulnerable from undue external influences.

Social work professionals are particularly well suited to deal with the complex relationships and value-laden discussions and decisions encountered when delivering end-of-life care (Linder & Meyers, 2009). These professionals have been recognized as integral components of hospice and palliative care teams since the beginnings of the modern hospice movement (Clark, 1998, NHPCO, 2000). Indeed, Dame Cecily

Box 71.1
Patient/Family Narrative: Robert

Robert is a 59-year-old Caucasian male with stage IV non-small cell lung cancer. He is married, though Janet, his wife of 34 years, does not join him in his counseling sessions. For weeks, he has been talking about "wanting this to be over." He complains of being a burden to Janet, his family, and friends. He is increasingly short of breath and able to engage in fewer and fewer of the activities that he enjoys such as hiking, biking, or playing golf. Robert is an attorney, but he has been forced to give up his practice. He and Janet have three adult children, five grandchildren, and a very supportive network of friends, particularly from the church he and "Jan" had joined before they were married. Robert has stated on several occasions that his Catholic faith prevents him from killing himself, but he feels his diminished state is "a waste" and "only causes all of us to suffer." Despite this, he reluctantly continues to receive disease-directed treatment and accepts palliative interventions, including oxygen and liquid morphine for shortness of breath. When he again asks why this has to go on, the therapist, a social worker, suggests that there are a number of choices he could make that would be legal and might hasten his demise such as discontinuing treatment, choosing to discontinue taking food and fluids, refusing antibiotics if he gets an infection, and so forth. Surprisingly, Robert recoils from these suggestions with a look of terror distorting his features. What should the social worker do next?

Saunders, the founder of the modern hospice movement, was first a social worker.

Clinical Response

Social work practice involves "starting where the client is." In the case presented in Box 71.1, acknowledging the visceral reaction elicited by the social worker's comment is the starting point. Providing emotional validation and support for the reaction holds opportunities for exploring its nature and roots, and for asking the client's help in correctly interpreting the repeated references to prolonged and seemingly futile survival made now and in earlier sessions. In addition, an apology for failing to clarify these references earlier may also be appropriate.

Returning to those earlier references re-presents the chance to discern the feelings and day-to-day experiences that prompted the client to comment about "wanting this to be over." Remarks containing an element of the desire to die may have several meanings. Indeed, in this case, it will only become clear which of these meanings was intended by exploring them with the client. The client may be overwhelmed with feelings of being a burden and so a joint session or family conference including those he fears he is burdening may be an appropriate intervention. Perhaps the client has physical symptoms degrading his quality of life

that are not fully addressed; advocacy with the medical team would then be appropriate. He may be giving voice to psychological or spiritual distress and so assessing for underlying depression or helping the client mobilize more involvement by his faith leaders or faith community may be helpful. He may be practicing an idea, bringing it to the light of day, not expecting it to be repeated but perhaps observed and shared in the setting of a trusted, relatively benign relationship where he might experiment with a thought. The client may simply never have followed his desire-for-death statements through to their logical conclusion. After overcoming his initial revulsion, he may actually want to talk about alternatives that would hasten death, making psycho-educational interventions appropriate. Any response by the social worker that communicates acceptance of his emotions and promotes a more complete understanding of the statements and the client's reaction would be appropriate.

Oregon's Experience

Oregon's Death with Dignity Act (ODDA) was first approved by Oregon voters in 1994 and reaffirmed in 1997. Over 11 years, 460 terminally ill citizens of the state have met the requirements to receive a prescription for a lethal dose of drugs to end life. Almost 82% had cancer, and 98% were white, 1.5% Asian, 0.2% American Indian or African American, and 0.4% Hispanic. Oregon is less diverse than other states, but that is changing. Over 90% of Oregon is white, 1.9% is African American, 1.4% American Indian, 10% Hispanic, and 3.9% is Asian/Pacific Islander. Eighty-eight percent of those who used the law were enrolled in hospice at the time of death. The most striking and significant difference between those who ended their lives through use of the law and all other persons who died in Oregon is the high level of educational achievement. Of those who used the Act, 44% had a baccalaureate degree or higher and another 23% had some college. The three main reasons given for choosing to use the Act have remained constant over the years: loss of autonomy, less able to engage in activities that make life enjoyable, and loss of dignity. The Oregon Public Health Division is required to keep information about the Act, and the 12 years of data and the requirements of the law are available at their Web site (Oregon Department of Human Services, 2010).

Social Workers' Experiences

Arnold, Artin, Person, and Griffith (2004) surveyed hospice social workers in the southeast region of the United States. The authors found that "consideration of hastening death among hospice patients does not appear to be a rare event, as most social workers had experienced one or more cases in the past year" (p. 529). Although these results may not be generalized to other hospice patients and social workers, the findings are not so different from studies conducted in Oregon where the practice is legal. Arnold et al. do question whether unmet needs might drive the request for hastened death, and the authors encourage more research to develop interventions for the variety of challenges that emerge at end of life.

Several studies have been conducted to advance understanding of the ethical struggles that social workers face when dealing with a client's consideration to hasten death. In Oregon specifically, Harvath et al. (2006) conducted qualitative interviews with hospice social workers about hastened death and voluntary refusal of food and fluids. Many value conflicts were identified when patients decided to consider or actively pursue using ODDA. These conflicts revolved around issues such as patient autonomy, self-determination, quality of life, spiritual conflicts, and advocacy. The authors summarize the "opportunities and dilemmas" that the choice for assisted death has provided such as increased attention to concerns and fears about dying and attention to symptom management as well as the challenges to patient autonomy, professional standards of care, and quality of life (p. 203). Another study by Miller, Mesler, and Eggman (2002), which was also qualitative, found similar themes from hospice social work interviews. These social workers shared their struggles with self-determination, patient autonomy, advocacy, and empowerment. They also addressed four practice implications: unfinished business; religion/spirituality; fear; and how the legality of the option changed discussions with patients, families, and team members. In that regard, Miller, Hedlund, and Soule (2006) discussed four themes that had emerged from conversations with patients, families, team members, and health systems in hospice and oncology settings in Oregon. These themes were mental health, education, and choice; team concerns; family issues; and values, ethics, and restricted conversations. Social workers employed in religiously affiliated health systems were forbidden to discuss this option with patients and families in the early years of the law's implementation. This study's data was utilized to prepare for a mixed-methods survey of all hospice social workers in Oregon, which is discussed briefly later in this chapter.

Practical Guidelines

Yalom (1980) wrote many years ago that the exploration and consideration of ending one's life while dying "permits one to control that which controls one" (p. 122) and is part of how we, as humans, question our fate and our mortality. Although there are data and years of practice to guide hospice social workers in Oregon, the desire to discuss ending one's life while dying is not something that just happens in Oregon. There is the legal option to pursue this in Oregon (Miller & Hedlund, 2005) and, most recently, in the state of Washington

and the state of Montana. Most social workers practice in places where the choice to end life is not legal. Hudson et al. (2006) offer guidelines for desire-to-die statements based on a review of the literature and expert interprofessional consensus. Van Loon (1999) provides guidance specific to social workers about desire-to-die statements and requests and has created a flowchart that helps guide assessment and intervention within a mental health framework. These authors stress the importance of two major points in these two articles: (1) the professional must be aware of his or her

---

Box 71.2
Patient/Family Narrative: Dan

Dan is a 71-year-old Asian American man diagnosed with terminal cancer of the pancreas, who has been admitted to an Oregon hospice program. The patient is divorced and the only family member involved is one adult daughter. The policy of the hospice program is to have the patient bring up the topic of Death with Dignity, and this patient did so at the admission visit. The social worker was present at the admission visit and provided information to the patient and his daughter about Oregon's Death with Dignity Act (ODDA) and the steps that needed to occur in order to complete the process to obtain the prescription. The patient had already made both the oral and written requests as required by the law, and two physicians had certified their agreement on his diagnosis, prognosis, and capacity as required by the law. Dan was very strong in his Christian faith and so the chaplain of the agency was very involved and was present when the patient took the medication. (Agency policy allows this for team members, because some hospice programs in Oregon do not allow anyone from the hospice to be present.) The focus of the chaplain's work was on Dan's faith-based needs at end of life and this included having the chaplain and daughter present at the time of death. Dan was enrolled in hospice for 3 weeks during which the social worker made three home visits and numerous phone contacts with Dan and his daughter. The clinical work in these contacts was very similar to other hospice patients... active listening, tuning into concerns and feelings, assuring emotional and social support, checking resources that might be needed, ongoing mental health assessment, evaluation of cultural factors for the patient and family, and development of a care plan with the team. Dan's daughter believed that her father's decision was congruent with how he lived his life and how he would want to die. Although very sad about losing him, she supported his decision to use medication to end his life earlier than if he died from his disease and debilitation. The patient wanted a dignified death, which for him meant avoiding the suffering that would result from dependence, and losing the ability to enjoy life and take care of his own needs. He was firm, consistent, and unwavering in his decision. The social worker's role was to support the patient and family; educate about the Act; make a referral to a local agency with extensive knowledge about the law (this is common practice, although not mandated, when patients want to pursue use of the Act; see Compassion & Choices); keep the team informed of Dan's needs, desires, and care plan; and follow the tenets of client self-determination. The social worker did seek supervision for this case to assure best practices and to monitor self-awareness; the team process was essentially the same as with all other hospice patients.

own reactions to desire-to-die statements, because these will influence the conversations with the patient; and *(2)* it is imperative to find meaning in the patient's words and continue to assess concerns, mental health, and intent (see Box 71.2).

Conclusion

Social workers have never shied away from seeking the knowledge and skills to work with behaviors and actions that may be legal yet controversial, illegal, or difficult to manage, and assisted death is no exception (Miller, 2000). The evidence is clear that some dying patients will, no matter where they live, explore and possibly choose to end their lives before the natural course of events takes place. Social workers need to take the initiative to be prepared for the requests, both direct and indirect, and assist their team members and agencies with practices and policies to address these situations. This preparation means consideration of not only the content but also the process of how to handle desire-to-die statements. Social work is also the profession that would examine power, privilege, and vulnerable populations to insure that the agencies and institutions are using best practices to deliver quality palliative and end-of-life care to all patients and families who need them (Baines, 2007; Battin, van der Heide, Ganzinig, van der Wal, & Onwuteaka-Philipsen, 2007). This proactive stance provides protection and support to all involved in the dying experience.

LEARNING EXERCISES

- You are a hospice social worker in Florida and a patient asks you to "keep a secret:" he is considering a "way out of this," but he does not want anyone to know. How might you approach this? What kinds of questions come to mind? How could your agency and patient care team prepare for this kind of challenge? How does your team deal with patient "secrets"? What kind of practices and policies could be developed to deal with this situation?
- "Go Wish Values Sort Cards" (Coda Alliance, 2009) present few literacy barriers and offer an innovative way to examine personal values at end of life. Using the deck of 36 cards (including one wild card), each with a single value statement on it like "To be free from pain" or "To have my family prepared for my death," participants sort and prioritize, arriving at the 10 value statements most important to them. These statements can then be shared with a partner, discussed with one's doctor, or used to inform choices for an advance directive.

ADDITIONAL RESOURCES

Arnold, E. (2004). Factors that influence consideration of hastening death among people with life-threatening illnesses. *Health & Social Work, 29*(1), 17–26.

Breitbart, W., Rosenfeld, B., & Passik, S. (1996). Interest in physician-assisted suicide among ambulatory HIV-infected patients. *American Journal of Psychiatry, 153*(2), 238–242.

Callanan, M., & Kelley, P. (1992). *Final gifts: Understanding the special awareness, needs, and communications of the dying.* New York, NY: Simon & Schuster.

Chochinov, H., Wilson, K., Enns, M., Mowchun, N., Lander, S., Levitt, M. & Clinch, J. (1995). Desire for death in the terminally ill. *American Journal of Psychiatry, 152*(8), 1185–1191.

Emanuel, E., Fairclough, D., & Emanuel, L. (2000). Attitudes and desires related to euthanasia and physician-assisted suicide among terminally ill patients and their caregivers. *Journal of the American Medical Association, 284*(19), 2460–2468.

Foley, K., & Hendin, H. (2002). *The case against assisted suicide: For the right to end-of-life care.* Baltimore, MD: Johns Hopkins University Press.

Hillyard, D., & Dombrink, J. (2001). *Dying right: The death with dignity movement.* New York, NY: Routledge.

Madrid, E. (2007, September 28). Lovelle Svart, 1945-2007. *OregonLive.com,* Retrieved from http://blog.oregonlive.com/multimedia/2007/09/lovelle_svart_1945_2007.html

Ogden, R. D., Young, M. G. (2003). Washington State social workers' attitudes toward voluntary euthanasia and assisted suicide. *Social Work in Health Care, 37,* 43–70.

Quill, T., & Battin, M. (Eds.). (2004). *Physician-assisted dying: The case for palliative care and patient choice.* Baltimore, MD: Johns Hopkins University Press.

Rosenfeld, B. (2004). *Assisted suicide and the right to die: The interface of social science, public policy and medical ethics.* Washington, DC: American Psychological Association.

Schroepfer, T. A. (2006). Mind frames towards dying and factors motivating their adoption by terminally ill elders. *Journals of Gerontology: Social Sciences, 61B*(3), S129–S139.

Schroepfer, T. (2007). Critical events in the dying process: The potential for physical and psychosocial suffering. *Journal of Palliative Medicine,10*(1), 136–147.

Shavelson, L. (1995). A chosen death: The dying confront assisted suicide. New York, NY: Simon & Schuster Inc.

Task Force to Improve Care to Terminally Ill Oregonians. (2010). *The Oregon Death with Dignity Act. A guidebook for health care providers.* Retrieved from http://www.deathwithdignity.org/resources/physiciansquestions.asp

Washington State Department of Health. (2009). *Washington State Department of Health 2009 Death with Dignity Act report.* Retrieved from http://www.doh.wa.gov/dwda

Zaritsky, J. (Producer). (2010). *The suicide tourist.* [Web]. Retrieved from http://www.pbs.org/wgbh/pages/frontline/suicidetourist/

REFERENCES

Arnold, E. M., Artin, K. A., Person, J. L., & Griffith, D. L. (2004). Consideration of hastening death among hospice patients and their families. *Journal of Pain and Symptom Management, 27*(6), 523–532.

Association of Oncology Social Workers (AOSW). (2008). *The Association of Oncology Social Work position paper on active euthanasia and assisted suicide.*

Back, A., Wallace, J., Starks, H., & Pearlman, R. (1996). Physician-assisted suicide and euthanasia in Washington state: Patient requests and physician responses. *Journal of the American Medical Association, 275*(12), 919–925.

Baines, D. B. (2007). *Doing anti-oppressive practice.* Halifax, Canada: Fernwood Publishing.

Battin, M. P., van der Heide, A., Ganzini, L., van der Wal, G., & Onwuteaka-Philipsen, B. D. (2007). Legal physician-assisted dying in Oregon and the Netherlands: Evidence concerning the impact on patients in "vulnerable" groups. *Journal of Medical Ethics, 33,* 591–597.

Breitbart, W., Rosenfeld, B., & Passik, S. (1996). Interest in physician-assisted suicide among ambulatory HIV-infected patients. *American Journal of Psychiatry, 153*(2), 238–242.

Carr, M. F., & Mohr, G. J. (2008). Palliative sedation as part of a continuum of palliative care. *Journal of Palliative Medicine, 11*(1), 76–81.

Chochinov, H., Wilson, K. G., Enns, M., Mowchun, N., Lander, S., Levitt, M., & Clinch, J. J. (1995). Desire for death in the terminally ill. *American Journal of Psychiatry, 152*(8), 1185–1191.

Clark, D. (1998). Originating a movement: Cicely Saunders and the development of St. Christopher's Hospice, 1957–1967. *Mortality, 3*(1), 43–63.

Coda Alliance. (2009). *The Go Wish Game: Values sort cards.* Retrieved from http://www.codaalliance.org/gowishfaq.html

Csikai, E. (1999). Euthanasia and assisted suicide: Issues for social work practice. *Journal of Gerontological Social Work, 31*(3/4), 49–63.

Csikai, E. (2004). Advanced directives and assisted suicide: Policy implications for social work practice. In J. Berzoff & P. Silverman (Eds.), *Living with dying: A handbook for end-of-life health practitioners* (pp. 761–777). New York, NY: Columbia University Press.

Emanuel, E., Fairclough, D., Daniels, E., & Clarridge, B. (1996). Euthanasia and physician-assisted suicide: Attitudes and experiences of oncology patients, oncologists, and the public. *The Lancet, 347,* 1805–1810.

Emanuel, E., Fairclough, D., & Emanuel, L. (2000). Attitudes and desires related to euthanasia and physician-assisted suicide among terminally ill patients and their caregivers. *Journal of the American Medical Association, 284*(19), 2460–2468.

Ganzini, L., Goy, E. R., Dobscha, S. K., & Prigerson, H. (2009). Mental health outcomes of family members of Oregonians who request physician aid in dying. *Journal of Pain and Symptom Management, 28*(4), 306–315.

Ganzini, L., Harvath, T., Jackson, A., Goy, E., Miller, L., & Delorit, M. (2002). Experiences of Oregon nurses and social workers with hospice patients who requested assistance with suicide. *New England Journal of Medicine, 347*(8), 582–588.

Harvath, T. A., Miller, L. L., Smith, K. A., Clark, L. D., Jackson, A., & Ganzini, L. (2006). Dilemmas encountered by hospice workers when patients wish to hasten death. *Journal of Hospice and Palliative Nursing, 8*(4), 200–209.

Hudson, P. L., Scholfield, P., Kelly, B., Hudson, R., Street, A., O'Connor, M., & Aranda, S. (2006). Responding to desire to die statements from patients with advanced disease: recommendations for health professionals. *Palliative Medicine, 20,* 703–710.

Jacobson, J., Kasworm, E., Battin, M., Botkin, J., Francis, L., & Green, D. (1995). Decedents' reported preferences for physician-assisted death: A survey of informants listed on death certificates in Utah. *The Journal of Clinical Ethics, 6*(2), 149–157.

Lavery, J., Boyle, J., Dickens, B., Maclean, H., & Singer, P. (2001). Origins of the desire for euthanasia and assisted suicide in people with HIV-1 or AIDS: A qualitative study. *The Lancet, 358*(9279), 362–367.

Linder, J., & Meyers, F. J. (2009). End-of-life care in correctional settings. *Journal of Social Work in End-of-Life and Palliative Care, 5*(1–2), 27.

Mackelprang, R. W., & Mackelprang, R. D. (2005). Historical and contemporary issues in end-of-life decisions: Implications for social work. *Social Work, 50*(4), 315–324.

Manetta, A. A., & Wells, J. G. (2001). *Ethical issues in the social worker's role in physician-assisted suicide. Health and Social Work, 26*(3), 160.

Meier, E., Emmons, C., Wallenstein, S., Quill, T., Morrison, R., & Cassel, C. (1998). A national survey of physician-assisted suicide and euthanasia in the United States. *The New England Journal of Medicine, 338*(17), 1193–1201.

Miller, P. J. (2000). Life after death with dignity: The Oregon experience. *Social Work, 45*(3), 263–271.

Miller, P. J., & Hedlund, S. C. (2005). "We just happen to live here": Two social workers share their stories about Oregon's Death with Dignity law. *Journal of Social Work in End-of-Life and Palliative Care, 1*(1), 71–86.

Miller, P. J., Hedlund, S. C., & Soule, A. B. (2006). Conversations at the end of life: The challenge to support patients who consider Death with Dignity in Oregon. *Journal of Social Work in End-of-Life and Palliative Care, 2*(2), 25–43.

Miller, P. J., Mesler, M. A., & Eggman, S. T. (2002). Take some time to look inside their hearts: Hospice social workers contemplate physician-assisted suicide. *Social Work in Health Care, 35*(3), 53–64.

National Association of Social Workers (NASW). (2004). *NASW standards for palliative and end of life care.* Washington, DC: Author.

National Association of Social Workers (NASW). (2006). *End-of-life care.* Retrieved from http://www.socialworkers.org/practice/children/statements/129-135%20End-of-Life%20Care.pdf

National Hospice and Palliative Care Organization (NHPCO). (2000). *Standards of practice for hospice programs.* National Hospice and Palliative Care Organization. Retrieved from http://nhpco.org/i4a/pages/index.cfm?pageid=5308

Ogden, R. D., & Young, M. G. (2003). Washington state social workers' attitudes toward voluntary euthanasia and assisted suicide. *Social Work in Health Care, 37*(2), 43–70.

O'Mahony, S., Goulet, J., Kornblith, A., Abbatiello, G., Clarke, B., Kless-Siegel, S., …Payne, R. (2005). Desire for hastened death, cancer pain, and depression: Report of a longitudinal observational study. *Journal of Pain and Symptom Management, 29*(5), 446–457.

Oregon Department of Human Services. (2000). *Oregon's Death with Dignity Act The second year's experience.* Portland, OR: Oregon Health Division.

Oregon Department of Human Services. (2008). *Oregon's Death with Dignity Act: Three years of legalized physician-assisted suicide*. Portland, OR: Oregon Health Division.

Oregon Department of Human Services. (2010). *Twelfth annual report on Oregon's Death with Dignity Act*. Portland, OR: Oregon Health Division.

O'Reilly, K. B. (2010). Physician-assisted suicide legal in Montana, court rules. *American Medical News*. Retrieved from http://www.ama-assn.org/amednews/2010/01/18/prsb0118.htm

Quill, T. E., Lee, B., & Nunn, S. (2000). Palliative treatments of last resort: Choosing the least harmful alternative. *Annals of Internal Medicine, 132*, 488–493.

Schroepfer, T. (2006). Mind frames towards dying and factors motivating their adoption by terminally ill elders. *Journals of Gerontology: Social Sciences, 61B*(3), S129–S139.

Schroepfer, T. (2007). Critical events in the dying process: The potential for physical and psychosocial suffering. *Journal of Palliative Medicine, 10*(1), 136–147.

Schroepfer, T. (2008). Social relationships and their role in the consideration to hasten death. *The Gerontologist, 48*(5), 612–621.

Volker, D. (2001). Oncology nurses' experiences with requests for assisted dying from terminally ill patients with cancer. *Oncology Nursing Forum, 28*(1), 39–49.

Van Loon, R. A. (1999). Desire to die in terminally ill people: A framework for assessment and intervention. *Health and Social Work, 24*(4), 260–268.

Yalom, I. D. (1980). *Existential psychotherapy*. New York, NY: Basic Books.

72 *Terry Altilio*

Palliative Sedation: A View through the Kaleidoscope

For words, like Nature, half reveal and half conceal the Soul within.
—Alfred Lord Tennyson (In Memoriam, 1850)

Key Concepts

* *The decision to sedate an imminently dying patient requires a determination that consciousness must be sacrificed to achieve relief of intractable suffering.*
* *Palliative sedation is not euthanasia nor is it physician-assisted death.*
* *The intent in sedating a patient is to treat intractable symptoms, understanding that this medical intervention will influence the quality of interaction and communication at a time when each moment of life may be treasured by patients and their families.*
* *The process related to decision making requires weighing of medical information; psychosocial, spiritual, and cultural factors; and ethical principles in a clear and transparent process.*

Introduction

In 2007, palliative sedation moved front and center consequent to an invitation to write an article about the topic with Phil Higgins for the *Journal of Social Work in End-of-Life and Palliative Care* (Higgins & Altilio, 2007). In the course of reading the wealth of articles written on palliative sedation, we discovered that the notion of inducing sedation to treat an intractable symptom is laden with nuance, infused with ethical, moral, legal, psychosocial, and spiritual perspectives that inform the discussion and invite critical thinking, expertise, and personal reflection both as individuals and as a palliative care team committed to excellence in the care of patients and families. This chapter will focus on the questions and controversies and provide a lens into the thinking and discernment essential to a decision that involves the intentional loss of consciousness when days of life are limited.

Many essential elements of palliative care and social work practice are woven into this topic. They include an understanding of the unique values, beliefs, and goals of the patient and family; excellence in the assessment of symptoms and suffering; and careful consideration of the ethical and legal precepts and psychological, social, and spiritual factors that influence patients, families, and professional caregivers. Beyond the lived experience of the patient, a decision to sedate influences the bereavement process and the legacy of the death as it is woven into the fabric of a family history. Was a person helped to avoid a death with uncontrolled pain? Will a bereaved family feel robbed of the remaining time with their loved one because sedation changed the quality of their time together? These are some of the complex and rich aspects of palliative care that are reflected in the debate that surrounds palliative sedation. It is a decision that is made in the present, but it also has an impact for the future of the families as well as the clinicians who collaborated in decision making and provided care for the patient (Higgins & Altilio, 2007, p. 7).

As you read this chapter, imagine a kaleidoscope with loosely colored beads, pebbles, or other small colored objects. Look in one end and you will see that light enters and reflects off the mirrors contained within. Rotate the tube and the colored objects will tumble presenting you with changing and symmetrical patterns and colors reflected in the mirrors. The intent of this chapter is to shed light on the ideas and concepts, the beads and pebbles, which infuse this topic. In the actual practice of palliative care, each situation becomes a nexus of unique medical variables; the tube of the kaleidoscope rotates and the pattern changes. Yet there is expertise that needs to be acquired and principles that need to be explored to add some coherence to these ever-changing patterns.

Definitions That Inform the Discussion

While there is controversy and debate related to many aspects of this topic, there is some consensus about definitions. This discussion will use the term *palliative sedation*, but it is important to note that this description, for some, is controversial and viewed as a euphemism designed to avoid what some argue is an action that causes the death of "sentient life and the possibility for social interaction" and perhaps the death of biological life if artificial hydration and nutrition is withdrawn (Battin, 2008, pp. 27–28). Others suggest that the phrase "terminal sedation" adds further confusion because it may be interpreted as sedating a terminally ill patient or inferred that the purpose is to terminate a life (Chater, Viola, Paterson, & Jardis, 1998), which would be the act of euthanizing with the direct intention of causing death rather than sedating where the purpose and intent is to manage intractable symptoms.

Some of the words and phrases that pepper the literature include the following: continuous deep sedation (Seale, 2010); controlled sedation (Taylor & McCann, 2005); palliative sedation (Cherny & Portenoy, 1994; Cherny & Radbruch, 2009); respite sedation (Rousseau, 2005); sedation in the imminently dying (Carver & Foley, 2000); terminal sedation (Chater, Viola, Paterson, & Jardis, 1998; Simon, Kar, Hinz, & Beck, 2007; VanDelden, 2007); and lastly, total sedation (Rich, 2006).

The range of terminology reflects the complexity and controversy surrounding the sedation of imminently dying patients. Another tribute to the complexity and perhaps the incongruity of definition is the wide range of estimates as to how many patients are sedated at the end of life. Rousseau (2005) posits a range from 2% to 52%, whereas Cowan and Walsh (2001) estimate between 15% and 30%. Engstrom, Bruno, Holm, and Hellzen conducted a systematic review of the literature to describe the phenomena of palliative sedation from a nursing perspective (2007). They reviewed 15 studies from seven countries, nine from Japan, and one each from Israel, Norway, South Africa, Canada, Taiwan, and Germany. They found that the three most common symptoms leading to palliative sedation were delirium, agitation (13.8%–68%), dyspnea (10%–50%), and pain (2.5%–25%). In this review, the incidence of palliative sedation in palliative and hospice care ranged from 14.6% to 51% during the last 4 days of life. While there are limitations to any review

process, it is interesting to note that existential distress does not appear as a common precipitant for palliative sedation; this may be a reflection of the cultural influences or the ongoing dialogue about the appropriateness of this intervention to treat existential or psychological distress.

While none of these studies are based in the United States, it is important to the context of this discussion to realize that federal and state courts have had input into the understanding and parameters of palliative sedation to unconsciousness, differentiating the practice from physician-assisted suicide and removing criminal liability for physicians who *appropriately* provide this treatment to terminally ill patients. In 1997 the Supreme Court in *Washington v Glucksberg* and *Vacco v Quill* unanimously ruled that there is no constitutional right to physician-assisted suicide while unanimously affirming that "a patient who is suffering from a terminal illness and who is experiencing great pain has no legal barriers to obtaining medication, from qualified physicians, to alleviate that suffering, even to the point of causing unconsciousness and hastening death" (*Vacco v. Quill*, 117 S. Ct. 2293 U.S. 1997). The court was also unanimous in affirming that state laws are constitutionally valid in recognizing the distinction between prohibiting physician conduct that intentionally hastens death and that which may hasten death but is intended for other purposes such as relief of pain (Burt, 1997). For many, the ruling signaled a constitutional right to palliative care, but for others, the Court's endorsement of sedation, with the potential risk of hastening death, was akin to an endorsement of euthanasia. These differences of opinion reflect the richness and complexity of the subject. It is the intent of this chapter that readers not necessarily leave with answers but rather a deeper understanding of the questions.

The following are terms and ethical principles, pebbles and beads, frequently used in the discussion of palliative sedation. The definitions will be woven into a commentary that reflects the complexity of this aspect of care and invites social workers to enrich the dialogue and contribute skills and thoughtfulness to the decision-making process for each patient and family and to the evolving literature and research about this topic.

- *Palliative sedation* involves the administration of *nonopioid drugs* to sedate a terminally ill patient to unconsciousness as an intervention of last resort to treat *severe, refractory pain or other clinical symptoms* that have not been relieved by aggressive, symptom-specific palliation (National Ethics Committee, Veterans Health Administration, 2006). This *medical intervention* involves a decision, in consultation with an *informed patient, family, or agent* to provide sufficient doses of medications to reduce consciousness *in imminently dying* patients with *the goal of relieving physical symptoms, existential or psychological suffering,* deemed intractable after expert intervention. The intent is to relieve symptoms and suffering, not to hasten death (Cherny & Portenoy, 1994; Rousseau, 2005).

Commentary: You see in this definition that the term "nonopioid drug" is used. The purpose of sedation is not the treatment of pain; it is to induce sedation. This differentiation is important because it distinguishes this process from the management of symptoms at end of life, in which case one may achieve satisfactory symptom management and note sedation as either a side effect or an expected sign of an evolving dying process. The decision to consider sedation is a consequence of the inability to achieve symptom management, whether physical, existential, or psychological. While there is general consensus about the use of palliative sedation in the setting of intractable physical symptoms, there is much debate about its appropriateness in the setting of existential and psychological suffering. Some argue that treating existential suffering with a medical intervention is medicalization of the spiritual and psychosocial struggles that may arise at end of life (Davis & Ford, 2005); that this kind of distress may be dynamic, not necessarily indicative of imminent death; and that refractoriness is more difficult to establish (Cherny & Radbruch,2009). Others wonder whether this separation of physical symptoms from spiritual and psychological distress is a return to mind–body dualism that palliative care is intended to overcome and once again limits the focus of care to the body rather than the whole person. Is extinguishing consciousness to manage existential distress comparable to extinguishing the body to manage physical symptoms as one might do in euthanasia (Davis & Ford, 2005), where a practitioner is the agent who acts with the intent to cause the death of a patient to relieve the patient's suffering? This discussion naturally leads to the definitions of suffering and intractable symptoms.

- *Suffering* is a unique and personal experience of severe distress emanating from a threat to the integrity and intactness of the whole person (Cassell, 1991). To suffer, one must be conscious. Suffering can be consequent to a physical symptom or illness and be totally independent of a physical component. For example, the etiology may be based in the anticipation of death or the absence of meaning in life (Peppin, 2003). Suffering, like burden, is determined by the patient and in some situations, by proxy judgment of the family or the staff (van Bogaert & Ogunbanio, 2005).

Commentary: Proxy judgments of symptoms and suffering are complex because it is often difficult to differentiate distress of the patient, the family, caregivers, and staff. This assessment is essential to creating a care plan that includes interventions focused on the appropriate symptom and the appropriate person. Sedation of the patient is not the treatment for the suffering of family. How does one ensure that fatigue or impatience of the clinicians or suffering of the family does not dominate or determine the designation of intractable? All suffering, whether physical or existential, invites palliative

social work assessment, intervention, and collaboration, and the engagement of a palliative care team buffers against clinician and family factors driving the clinical judgment.

- *Intractable symptom* is one where aggressive and skilled efforts short of sedation have not provided relief. With physical symptoms the clinicians believe that additional invasive/noninvasive treatments are incapable of providing relief or they are associated with *unacceptable morbidity* and/or unlikely to provide relief within a *reasonable time frame.* (Salacz & Weissman, 2005). Determining "intractability" is in part dependent on the skill set of the practitioner. The lower the skill set, the more a clinician will encounter symptoms that he or she is unable to manage. In 2009, the European Association for Palliative Care (EAPC) published the Recommended Framework for the Use of Palliative Sedation within which authors Cherny and Radbruch write: "Extreme distress is a medical emergency and patient evaluation must be performed with due urgency. The patient must be evaluated by a clinician with sufficient experience and expertise in palliative care.... wherever possible the evaluation should be interdisciplinary" (p. 584). How does one ensure that the offer to sedate is not a reflection of inadequate training rather than a decision based in a thorough medical, psychosocial, spiritual, and ethical analysis? Does the perception of palliation as "comfort care," the antithesis of "aggressive" intervention, invite a less rigorous assessment and evaluation, which if done scrupulously might reduce the need for palliative sedation (Fainsinger, 1998; Peppin, 2003)?

Commentary: Within the concept of intractable or refractory symptom, there are implicit issues such as the mandate to develop expertise so that consciousness does not need to be sacrificed at a time when life is short and perhaps, for some, more precious. Consider the question of whose values might determine what is unacceptable morbidity and a reasonable time frame; how does one weigh the decision to preserve or sacrifice consciousness, and how much and how long does one suffer before "intractable" applies? The decision to diminish consciousness influences the end-of-life experience for both patient and family. When days of life are limited, the quality of time and the value of each exchange can be profoundly meaningful. The care team's role in facilitating the "loss of social selfhood" through diminished consciousness (Davis & Ford, 2005) is essentially different than this same loss occurring as a consequence of natural disease progression; this outcome also warrants ethical and professional justification. In weighing the risk and benefit, the losses to relationship and self-actualization are direct outcomes of sedation and require explicit consideration in clinical evaluation and discussions of informed consent (Lynch, 2003).

- *Imminently dying* is a determination that implies an ability to prognosticate and a responsibility to seek well-considered, informed professional judgment from practitioners with expertise in prognostication and in decision making about palliative sedation... The Veterans Administration report of 2006, concludes that palliative sedation is appropriate for patients who are "imminently dying" (p. 5); have "entered the final stage of the dying process" (p .8). Their discussion explores many considerations, including the sedation of those who are suffering but not imminently dying, the complexity and uncertainty of prognostication, and the concern that the trajectory of "terminal illness" in different diagnoses can make it difficult to distinguish when palliative sedation is or is not ethically permissible. The EAPC framework states, "Continuous deed sedation should only be considered if the patient is in the very terminal stages of their illness with an expected prognosis of hours or days at most" (Cherny & Radbruch, p. 584).

Commentary: Prognostication is essential to the decision making about palliative sedation. It informs the discussions with patients and families and creates the context in which a treatment is offered and in which consent is sought. Acknowledging that patients who are terminally ill but not imminently dying may experience refractory physical symptoms and the lack of consensus about the appropriateness of sedation for existential and psychological suffering begs a response from palliative care clinicians regardless of whether sedation is considered. The American Medical Association report Sedation to Unconsciousness in End-of-Life Care states: "… . the Council concurs with those who argue that existential suffering, distinct from previously listed clinical symptoms, is not an appropriate indication for treatment with palliative sedation to unconsciousness, because the causes of this type of suffering are better addressed by other interventions (Taylor & McCann, 2005). For example, palliative sedation to unconsciousness is not the way to address suffering created by social isolation and loneliness; rather such suffering should be addressed by providing the patient with needed social support" (p. 3).

The EAPC framework describes special considerations for the use of sedation in refractory existential or psychological distress, creating focused guidelines such as repeated, expert assessment and intervention by clinicians who have established relationships with the patient and family, and an interdisciplinary case conference including those providing care at the bedside. In many situations social workers have long-standing relationships with patients and families and need to represent that history and knowledge in these complex decision-making processes (p. 588). In situations where sedation may be seen as appropriate and proportionate, respite sedation might be initiated with a plan for lifting the sedation after an agreed-upon period of time. This leads to additional and essential concepts and principles; they are respite sedation, beneficence, and nonmaleficence.

- *Respite or intermittent sedation involves sedating for an agreed-upon, time-limited period to provide respite*

from suffering. Medication levels are gradually reduced to allow a return to consciousness. This option may be helpful for clinicians who struggle to assist patients who are not imminently dying or in settings where palliative sedation for existential and psychological suffering is not an option (Rousseau, 2005).
- *Beneficence* refers to actions that promote good and contribute to the well-being of patients. It is important to consider that interventions that are intended to be beneficent can become harmful over time as the patients and family contexts change.
- *Nonmaleficence* is interpreted as *first* do no harm, which mandates that clinicians weigh the potential risks and suffering that treatments or interventions may cause (Beauchamp & Childress, 2001).

Commentary: Ethical principles provide a framework within which to consider and weigh options. For example, a patient may ask to be sedated to create distance from his or her suffering and the suffering of his or her family. However, sedation in this person who is able to communicate and continues oral intake carries greater risk and ethical discernment because sedation will not only create a loss of consciousness, which impacts the quality of the remaining time with family, but will also interfere with oral intake, which may in fact hasten death. These deliberations require expert consultation; the weighing of the medical, legal, and ethical aspects; a comprehensive assessment of patient and family distress; and a plan of care that will include intensive palliative care and perhaps a short period of respite sedation. Alternately, considering sedation in a delirious person who has been unable to communicate and ceased eating and drinking does not have the same consequence but still requires purposeful deliberation. The medical condition may warrant expert assessment to determine whether this is an end-of- life delirium or caused by such things as changes in medications or metabolic disturbance. The treatment plan will depend on the goals of care, family input, and whatever is know about the wishes, values, and beliefs of the patient. Sedation may not be the treatment of choice after an expert clinical assessment that discovers that restoring the ability to interact is an important value for this patient and family. Other families will welcome the relief of a sedated imminently dying patient. Acts that are beneficent in one setting may cause harm in another. The option of respite sedation allows clinicians to respond to intractable suffering in a manner that does not result in permanent lack of consciousness but rather a respite from suffering. As with much decision making in life-threatening illness, this process involves converging ethical principles, such as autonomy, informed consent, double effect, and proportionality, all in the setting of an emerging understanding of the best medical information and the patient and family in their psychosocial-spiritual context.

- *Autonomy* recognizes an individual's right to self-determination. From this principle flow informed consent, confidentiality, privacy, and truth telling. It is important to note that individual autonomy in many families and cultures is not primary; rather, family decision making and process is valued (Blackhall, Murphy, Frank, Michel, & Azen, 2003). The cultural contexts that infuse a choice to delegate decision making to others and to waive informed consent are not stable or always harmonious; therefore, intracultural variability requires that we look beyond cultural norms to understand that dynamics of the individual family and the circumstances in which a patient defers these rights (Hyun, 2002).

- *Informed consent* recognizes the right of a patient and/or family to have sufficient information about palliative sedation provided in a manner that allows them to understand and appreciate the treatment or procedure being offered, including the nature and purpose, risks and benefits, and future consequences of both accepting or refusing the intervention.

- *Double effect:* this ethical principle makes the distinction between a direct and intended benefit and an unintended, indirect but possible and foreseeable negative outcome. An action may have two possible effects, one positive and one negative. The negative effect is not the means to the good effect. The positive effect is direct (relief of intractable pain and/or suffering) and is what is intended and sought, while the negative effect (possible hastened death) is indirect, foreseen but not intended. The good effect must outweigh the untoward outcome, and seeking this balance involves the concept of proportionality (Rousseau, 2005).

- *Proportionality:* this principle asserts that the correct test of an ethical obligation to recommend or provide an intervention is an estimate of benefit, the value attributed to the intervention, and the outcome for the patient. This principle, while not discussed often, informs decisions as to whether a treatment is appropriate to be offered and in what context. Patients and surrogates determine what they will accept as benefits and burdens, placing the duty on the physician to formulate this ratio for discussion with patients and families (Rousseau, 2005; Shannon & Walter, 1990; van Bogaert & Ogunbanio, 2005).

Commentary: These last principles and definitions bring us to a place of decision making and continued thoughtfulness about both the experience of the health care team and the patient and family when considering palliative sedation. The decision to offer sedation and the consent requires full discussion of the process, the risk and benefits, and especially the clinical intent of the intervention because it is in the neighborhood of intention where palliative care clinicians often struggle. Some of the questions that evolve when considering intention focus on whether sedation does in fact hasten death or whether the death is an expected outcome to the disease which is causing the symptoms. The few studies that provide some information

seem to indicate overall that sedation in the imminently dying was not associated with shortened life (Cherny & Radbruch, 2009; Claessens, Menten, Schotsmans, & Broeckaert, 2008; Maltoni et al., 2009; Sykes & Thorns, 2003). For this reason, some assert that the ethical principle of double effect does not apply because there is no unintended negative effect. They add that invoking of the principle in fact perpetuates a misconception that symptom control is associated with hastening death and thereby fosters a hesitation to provide relief to a very vulnerable group of patients. That said, when "intent" is the basis for the justification of an action, everyone's private thoughts, wishes, and words are considered. Patients may have the private goal of expediting their death; families may be fatigued, suffering, and overwhelmed by the demands of caring for a dying person, and they too may privately want the suffering to end. At the same time that physicians and other participating professionals are expected to have expert knowledge, there needs also to be a system in place which works to insure that the motives and needs of those other than the patients do not unduly impact recommendations and decisions or lead them to abandon patients through the act of sedation rather than confronting the implicit messages expressed. Just as patients and families can become exhausted and overwhelmed, professional caregivers experience complex responses and feelings in caring for patients at the end of life (Quill, 1993; Wein, 2000). These can have an unconscious influence on decisions. Creating transparent processes and the involvement of team members can enhance the shared nature of assessment, encourage introspection, and perhaps minimize the impact of unconscious feelings. Patients may be without physical symptoms, alert, and describing intractable psychological or existential suffering. They may or may not express a covert desire to hasten their death. The response would include an ethical and clinical assessment to determine whether the nature of the patient's circumstance meets the standard of proportionality (Jansen & Sulmasy, 2002). This process includes communication with patient, family, intimate network, and colleagues who have cared for the patient in the past and the present to assist as decisions are made, and an intensive treatment plan created to insure that patients are not abandoned to their suffering (Quill & Cassel, 1995; Rich, 2002).

Box 72.1.
Patient Family Narrative: Mr. Vann and His Family

The consent to sedation, under the best of circumstances, is a complex and profound discussion. Consider Mr. Vann, a 72-year-old, Episcopalian, married Englishman, father of three, grandfather of six, ages 7–16 years. He has stage 4 lung cancer and is extremely short of breath. In addition to pharmacologic management with opioids, steroids, and anxiolytics, he has been receiving nebulizer treatments and has been able to use focused breathing exercises and prayer to create a sense of calm in the setting of progressing illness and symptoms. His family has been helped to adapt their

Box 72.1 *(Contd.)*

conversation to seek yes or no answers expressed either verbally or by the nodding of his head. There is a fan in his room and most have learned that he is more comfortable with the curtains open and when they do not hover. They too have been taught to calm themselves by a simple focused breathing exercise and by monitoring their internal voices, which have the potential to either increase anxiety or to calm. (For more information on this subject, see Chapter 25.)

His physician anticipated respiratory symptoms at the end of life might be difficult to manage and had hoped to initiate a discussion about options for treatment during his next office visit. While he recognized that this discussion might be challenging, he knew also that it would be incongruous to believe that one could have an informed consent discussion if Mr. Vann were gasping for breath and in respiratory crises. In fact, some would assert that being highly symptomatic or having recently had an emergent medical event may compromise a patient's ability to truly give informed consent (Battin, 2007). Mr. Vann became highly symptomatic and was admitted to hospital, where he received morphine for symptomatic treatment of dyspnea, an anxiolytic for related anxiety, and a therapeutic thoracentesis to remove fluid from the pleural space; these provided temporary relief. Mr. Vann is receiving artificial nutrition and has consistently chosen to be resuscitated if he has a cardiac arrest. He has adapted over time to dyspnea and to his limited functional abilities. While others wonder about his quality of life, Mr. Vann continues to spend valued time with his grandchildren, enriching his and their lives with activities that do not burden him yet create shared and meaningful time and create memories. These activities include drawing, writing on a communication board to converse, and collaborating on an emerging family history. The grandchildren read to Mr. Vann. As his symptoms improve, his physician wishes to take this window of opportunity to help Mr. Vann and his family anticipate future symptom management needs and to create a care plan. In addition to the oncology clinicians, a palliative consultation is arranged to assist the team and family with options for symptom management and goals of care. Given the stage of disease, it is assumed that the fluid will reaccumulate in his lungs and that his death may involve intractable shortness of breath and may require sedation. The clinical teams work quickly to outline the options and information that will be helpful in the discussions with the patient, family, and staff.

- Consider the patient narrative in Box 72.1. Will sedation be necessary; if so, will it be continued until death, or is respite sedation more appropriate?

  - How will each of these options impact Mr. Vann and his family?
  - What are the patient's and family's beliefs and values about consciousness? What are their spiritual and philosophical influences?
  - How will sedation impact the family's process as they integrate Mr. Vann's death?
  - Will they feel robbed of precious time or at peace that his comfort was assured at the end of his life?

  - How can the clinicians involved in Mr. Vann's oncology care contribute to these deliberations?
  - How will the palliative care team collaborate to avoid duplication and confusion for the patient, staff, and family?

- Informed consent discussions need to consider the following:

  - Resuscitation status
  - A review of the continued benefit of artificial hydration and nutrition. A decision to sedate for intractable symptoms is not a decision to withdraw other modalities of treatment. These choices need to be assessed separately, with clearly articulated benefits, burdens, and values attributed to each.
  - What interests of the patient can be achieved? Will there be conflict between serving the interests and values of the patient and that of his family?
  - Clear discussion of the goals of care and the intent of sedation both to assist the patient and family decision making and to assist the clinical staff to develop a clear sense of the intent of the interventions being considered
  - Review of advance directives so this decision can be explored in the context of present realities and past directives
  - Which clinicians are most appropriate to lead discussions with the patient and family to insure that they receive the best information and do not feel abandoned during this difficult time?
  - How can staff create an environment to maximize Mr. Vann's ability to make a treatment choice based upon an honest and clear presentation of information that provides options and instills confidence in staff's ability to respond to his needs?

After a deliberate and expedient process of preparation, and with Mr. Vann's consent, a family meeting is organized including his wife and three adult children, the oncologist and palliative physician, a nurse practitioner, and social workers from the oncology and palliative care team. Mr. Vann chooses not to have his pastor or the palliative care chaplain in the meeting because he believes he is on "good terms with his God." While Mr. Vann is very aware that his disease is progressing, he appreciates the oncologist's offer to review the history and treatments provided since diagnosis 15 months ago. The process of prior decision making is also reviewed, and it is clear that the intent and goal of the artificial hydration and nutrition was to support Mr. Vann through chemotherapy; for Mr. Vann, if there is no chemotherapy that offers benefit, then hydration and nutrition are no longer necessary. There is also concern that the fluids are in fact contributing to shortness of breath and to swelling in Mr. Vann's legs and feet. This visible representation allows his family to actually "see" that an intervention which has been previously beneficial (beneficence) was now doing harm (nonmaleficence). This consensus informs the decision to discontinue this intervention. As the physicians presented medical information, it became clear to each family member that Mr. Vann was coming to the end of his life. The oncology social worker was able to enrich the review of medical history with prior psychosocial history and conversations that served to create a "life review" of the illness experience of this patient and family. The palliative social worker focused on the family process, observing nonverbal behaviors and working to respond to their individual and family reactions.

While Mr. Vann had previously requested resuscitation, in the setting of the current progression of his disease, this option was rediscussed. While considered medically inappropriate by the physicians, Mr. Vann's consent to a do not resuscitate (DNR) order emanated not from the physician's judgment, but from his knowledge that if he needed to be ventilator dependent, he would not be able to negotiate his own decisions or live with meaning and purpose. Decisions to sedate presume patients will choose to forego resuscitation because there is a seeming incongruity in choosing resuscitation to continue a life of intractable suffering. The inability of clinicians, patients, and families to agree on this topic is an invitation to begin anew the discussion of suffering, values, and options for treatment.

The principle of proportionality weighed heavily as Mr. Vann struggled to consider at what point he might relinquish consciousness and cognitive connection in exchange for relief of breathlessness. Respite sedation was discussed in an effort to provide an option other than complete and final loss of consciousness, what some have called the "loss of social selfhood" (Davis & Ford, 2005). Understanding that he was imminently dying it seemed torturous to allow sedation only to possibly come back to consciousness to see the suffering of family and to go through the same process again. Alternatives to sedation were discussed that included titrating medications with uncertain outcome and possible side effects, such as sedation or myoclonus. Immediate use of sedating medications might minimize the potential for crises and failed attempts at management and assure a semblance of comfort. Mr. Vann, having recently gone through a crisis of breathlessness, believed that he did not have to remain conscious to ensure that his wishes would be respected until his death and agreed that sedation would be most appropriate for him and his family. The palliative care team engaged family members to express their thoughts and feelings, suggesting that family members consider how to engage the grandchildren in visits, ritual, and legacy building as all considered the possibility of reduced consciousness. Mr. Vann and his family were assured that the clinical team would observe symptoms and physical findings that were predictive of increasing respiratory distress and proceed to sedate until his death. The palliative social worker encouraged family members to raise questions, repeating in clear and basic language the intent of the medical intervention, acknowledging that at any time breathlessness could develop and the patient and family might lose their ability to communicate. Validating the individual nature of each

relationship, the clinical team suggested that they each consider how they wished to share time with Mr. Vann. The palliative care team met with unit staff to provide information to help them to integrate the medical data and ethical and legal principles that informed each decision. The process and outcomes were documented and responsibility for follow-up determined. The palliative social worker was the clinician responsible to reach out to each family member to listen carefully and respond to any thoughts or worries that the intent of sedation was to shorten Mr. Vann's life and to reinforce the medical, ethical, and spiritual parameters that guided each of these decisions. The oncology social worker who represented a valued historical relationship visited patient and family to minimize any potential feelings of abandonment by the primary team. Both listened and responded to the complex feelings that often accompany end-of-life decisions such as regret, anger, guilt, or relief.

This same vigilance is often necessary for staff when decisions about discontinuing treatments and managing pain and symptoms at the end of life create complex feelings and perhaps cause moral distress. While there is some evidence that palliative sedation does not shorten survival, it continues to be important to express the intended purpose of sedating for refractory symptoms and suffering. Additionally, the palliative care physician and nurses continue to reach out to the staff to guide symptom assessment, level of sedation, and to listen for and respond to staff distress. Documentation reflects the critical thinking that informs each unique decision.

Conclusion: Where the Rubber Hits the Road

Clinicians who embrace the conversation about palliative sedation pose many questions: some seem certain; others challenge the basic premises and presumptions; and others build policy and guidelines seeking to guide clinicians who are compelled to act to manage symptoms in patients who are imminently dying and suffering. There are many aspects of discussion that shine light, as in the kaleidoscope, on some of the more philosophical and often unspoken conundrums implicit in palliative care. Conversations around this topic are profound and complex and demand a seriousness of thought, unbridled questioning, and openness in communication both to temper the rather ambiguous notion of intent and to foster decision making that is reflective of the myriad of issues that converge here.

As we turn the kaleidoscope again, consider the following:

- In a model of patient-centered care, how does one assess and balance the subjective nature of suffering with the objective process that seems essential to any decision to sedate to unconsciousness?
- Is it so that existential suffering and psychological distress are not the focus of medicine and therefore

a medical intervention is inappropriate and perhaps interferes in a person's ability to end his or her life grappling in an authentic, albeit less than peaceful manner?

- Is the decision to sedate just that of the physician who writes the "order"? How does one weigh a patient's willingness to give up consciousness against the physician's struggle to do what is right?
- How do social workers respond to their own conflicts and distress and ensure that they do not become moral accomplices to a team plan of care that they find ethically and morally unacceptable?
- What are the unique variables that need to be considered when considering palliative sedation in the home setting?
- How does one ensure that family is not sedating their own distress and suffering?
- How does the decision to sedate influence the bereavement process for family members?

At the risk of challenging a core belief of palliative clinicians, all members of the team do not carry the same responsibility. All need to grasp the complexity of analysis and decision making that this intervention demands. The social work contribution is essential because it is only with understanding the biopsychosocial-spiritual context that one can build understanding and consensus. While at our best we engage in the shared care of patients and families, understanding and respecting our common skill set as well as our unique expertise, in this aspect of practice our essential responsibilities differ. It is not the intent of social workers that is at the core of a decision to sedate a patient; it is not the action of a social worker that gives the medication to cease consciousness. These are the responsibilities of physicians and nurses. In the setting of palliative sedation at home, the participation of physicians and nurses is essentially different that that of social work clinicians. This is not to imply that we do not have responsibility; by our silence or participation we are moral accomplices, (Pellegrino, 1982) whether in hospital or at home, where actions may be left in the hands and hearts of family members. Social workers are essential participants as we assess; listen for exhaustion in our patients, families, and colleagues; explore the meaning of the decision for patients and families; and monitor the outcome, not only for the death experience itself but for the future integration of that experience in the legacy of the family, the team, and the professionals who participate. This responsibility requires expertise, thoughtfulness, and courage to question, raise doubt, and join the moral, medical, and ethical struggle that ought to accompany a decision to provide a medical treatment that intentionally takes consciousness. That said, the ultimate decision is not ours; the order comes from the physician, and the act of giving the sedating mediation in most instance rests with the nurse. This is a profound difference. It demands our respect and the best clinical wisdom and guidance that we can provide to ensure decisions that honor not only the needs of patient and families but that also value the struggles and needs of our colleagues.

ADDITIONAL RESOURCES

BioEthics.net: http://www.bioethics.net
Founded in 1993 as the first bioethics Web site, bioethics.net and *The American Journal of Bioethics* (AJOB) have grown to become the most read source of information about bioethics. AJOB is published in print and online by Taylor & Francis Group and housed at bioethics.net.

Center for Practical Bioethics offers Caring Conversations: http://www.practicalbioethics.org
A free publication and consumer education initiative that helps individuals and their families share meaningful conversations while making practical preparations for end-of-life decisions. Workbooks are available in English and Spanish, for young adults, and for veterans.

The Hastings Center: http://www.thehastingscenter.org
An independent, nonpartisan, and nonprofit bioethics research institute founded in 1969. The Center's mission is to address fundamental ethical issues in the areas of health, medicine, and the environment as they affect individuals, communities, and societies.

National Center for Ethics in Health Care: http://www.ethics.va.gov
Founded in 1991, it utilizes a multidisciplinary staff representing various fields, including medicine, nursing, philosophy, law, policy making, education, theology, social work, and health care administration. Center activities and initiatives support clinical ethics, organizational ethics, and research ethics throughout VHA. Under the Center's auspices, VHA's National Ethics Committee provides analysis and guidance on controversial ethics issues affecting patients, providers, health care managers, and health policy makers in concise, practical reports.

The President's Commission for the Study of Bioethical Issues: http://www.bioethics.gov
Advises the president on bioethical issues that may emerge from advances in biomedicine and related areas of science and technology. The Commission works with the goal of identifying and promoting policies and practices that ensure scientific research, health care delivery, and technological innovation are conducted in an ethically responsible manner.

The Stanford Encyclopedia of Philosophy (SEP): http://www.plato.stanford.edu
Designed so that each entry is maintained and kept up to date by an expert or group of experts in the field. All entries and substantive updates are refereed by the members of a distinguished Editorial Board before they are made public. The Table of Contents lists entries that are published or assigned.

REFERENCES

Battin, M. (2008). Terminal sedation: Pulling the sheet over our eyes. *Hastings Center Report, 38*(5), 27–30.

Beauchamp, T. L., & Childress, J. F. (2001). *Principles of biomedical ethics* (5th ed.). New York, NY: Oxford University Press.

Blackhall, L. J., Murphy, S. T., Frank, G., Michel, V., & Azen, S. P. (1995). Ethnicity and attitude toward patient autonomy. *Journal of the American Medical Association, 274*(3), 820-825.

Burt, R. A. (1997). The Supreme Court speaks–not assisted suicide but a constitutional right to palliative care. *New England Journal of Medicine, 337,* 1234-1236.

Carver, A.C., & Foley, K. (2000). The Wein article reviewed. *Oncology,* 598 & 601.

Cassell, E. (1991). *The nature of suffering.* New York,NY: Oxford University Press.

Chater, S., Viola, R., Paterson, J., Jardis, V. (1998) Sedation for intractable distress in thedying. *Palliative Medicine, 12,* 255-269.

Cherny, N. I., & Portenoy, R. K. (1994). Sedation in the management of refractory symptoms. *Journal of Palliative Care, 10,* 31-39.

Cherny, N.I. & Radbruch, L. (2009) European Association for Palliative Care (EAPC) recommended framework for the use of sedation in palliative care. *Palliative Medicine, 23*(7), 581-593.

Claessens, P., Menten, J., Schotsmans, P., & Broechaert, B. (2008). Palliative sedation: A review of the research literature. *Journal of Pain and Symptom Management, 36,* 310-333.

Cowan, J.D., & Walsh, D.(2001). Terminal sedation in palliative medicine – Definition and review of the literature. *Supportive Care in Cancer, 9,* 403-407.

Davis, M. P., & Ford, P. A. (2005). Palliative sedation definition, practice, outcomes and ethics. *Journal of Palliative Medicine, 8,* 699-701.

Engsrom, J., Bruno, E., Holm, B. & Hellzen, O. (2006). Palliative sedation at end of life – A systematic review. *European Journal of Oncology Nursing, 11*(1), 26-35.

Fainsinger, R. I. (1998). Use of sedation by a hospital palliative care support team. *Journal of Palliative Care, 14,* 51-54.

Higgins, P., & Altilio, T. (2007). Palliative sedation: An essential place for clinical excellence. *Journal of Social Work in End-of-Life & Palliative Care 2007, 3*(4), 3-30.

Hyun, I. (2003). Waiver of informed consent, cultural sensitivity and the problem of unjust families and traditions. *Hastings Center Report, 32*(5), 14-22.

Jansen, L. A. & Sulmasy, D. P. (2002). Sedation, alimentation, hydration and equivocation: Careful conversation about care at the end of life. *Annals of Internal Medicine, 136,* 845-849.

Maltoni, M., Pittureri, C., Scarpi, E., Piccinini, L., Martini, F., Turci, P.,… Amadori, D. (2009). Palliative sedation therapy does not hasten death: Results from a prospective multicenter study. *Annals of Oncology, 20*(7), 1163-1168.

National Association of Social Workers (NASW). (2003). *NASW standards for social work practice in palliative and end of life care.* Retrieved from http://www.socialworkers.org/practice/bereavement/standards/default.asp

National Ethics Committee, Veterans Health Administration. (2006). The ethics of palliative sedation as a therapy of last resort. *American Journal of Hospice and Palliative Care, 23,* 483-491. Retrieved from the Department of Veteran's Affairs Web site: http://www.ethics.va.gov/docs/necrpts/NEC_Report_20060301_The_Ethics_of_Palliative_Sedation.pdf

Pellegrino, E. D. (1982). The ethics of collective judgment in medicine and healthcare. *Journal of Medicine and Philosophy, 7*(1), 3-10.

Peppin, J. (2003). Intractable symptoms and palliative sedation at end of life. *Christian Bioethics, 9,* 343-355.

Quill, T. E. (1993). The ambiguity of clinical intentions. *Journal of the American Medical Association, 329,* 1039-1040.

Quill, T. E., & Cassel, C. (1995). Non-abandonment: A central obligation for physicians. *Annals of Internal Medicine, 122,* 368-374.

Rich, B. A. (2006). The ethical dimensions of pain and suffering. In K. Doka (Ed), *Pain management at the end of life* (pp. xx-xx). Washington, DC: Hospice Foundation of America.

Rousseau, P. (2001). Existential suffering and palliative sedation: A brief commentary with a proposal for clinical guidelines. *American Journal of Hospice and Palliative Care, 18,* 226-228.

Rousseau, P. (2005). Palliative sedation in the control of refractory symptoms. *Journal of Palliative Medicine, 8,* 8-12.

Salacz, M. E., & Weissman, D. E. (2005). Controlled sedation for refractory suffering: Part 1. *Journal of Palliative Medicine, 8*(1), 136-137.

Shannon, J. J., & Walter, T. A. (1990). Quality of life. In J. J. Shannon & T. A. Walter (Eds), *Quality of life: The new medical dilemma* (pp. 203-223). Mahwah, NJ: Paulist Press.

Simon, A., Kar, M., Hinz, J., & Beck, D. (2007). Attitude toward terminal sedation: An empirical survey among experts in the field of medical ethics. *Palliative Care, 6,* 4. doi:10.1186/1472-684X-6-4. Retrieved from http://www.biomedcentral.com/1472-684X/6/4

Sykes, N., & Thorns, A. (2003). The use of opioids and sedatives at the end of life. *The Lancet Oncology, 4,* 312-318.

Taylor, B. R., & McCann, R. M. (2005). Controlled sedation for physical and existential suffering? *Journal of Palliative Medicine, 8*(1), 144-147.

VanDelden, J. M. (2007). Terminal sedation: Source of a restless ethical debate. *Journal of Medical Ethics, 33,* 87-188. doi:10.1136/jme.2007.020446.

van Bogaert, G. A., & Ogunbanio, G. A. (2005). The principle of proportionality: Foregoing / withdrawing life support. *South African Family Practice, 47*(8), 66-67.

Wein, S. (2000). Sedation in the imminently dying. *Oncology, 14,* 585-592.

VIII
Professional Issues

"So the question remains–why do it? As much as anything, it's for the beauty. These vulnerable people are just beautiful … and there are those times when you see things that defy description because they're so beautiful. If you can avoid obsession with the dangers and the risks, the beauty comes through. Not everyone can see what you are privileged to see. Not everyone can see the illness and the injuries and still see the whole person. Not everyone can appreciate the beauty. But if you're still here, and if you're going back in again, then you can. The beauty draws you and you go in despite the risks. And the vulnerable people–living, dying, and dead–are glad you are there."

Greg Adams LCSW, ACSW, FT
Palliative Care and Center for Good Mourning
Arkansas Children's Hospital

Live your life with courage and serenity

Live your life with courage and serenity, trusting the universe to share its luminous gifts in unexpected moments.
Let curiosity and questions lead you through the mystery to wonder, awe, and greater love.
Be the instrument that shifts discord into harmony.
Let life teach you what you need to know.
Why despair? Be that light that you are.

Holly Nelson-Becker PhD., LCSW, ACSW
Loyola University of Chicago, IL

73

David M. Browning and Susan Gerbino

Navigating in Swampy Lowlands: A Relational Approach to Practice-Based Learning in Palliative Care

In the varied topography of professional practice, there is a high, hard ground where practitioners can make effective use of research-based theory and technique, and there is a swampy lowland where situations are confusing "messes" incapable of technical solution. The difficulty is that the problems of the high ground, however great their technical interest, are often relatively unimportant to clients or to the larger society, while in the swamp are the problems of greatest human concern.

—Donald Schön (1983, p. 42)

We need to move beyond the acquisition of formal logic to reasoning and sense-making that is concurrent with ongoing practice. In this way the conventional task of teaching as that of imparting knowledge can make room for the more dynamic process of facilitating learning. Imbued with learning, practitioners need not rely on old formulas as much as invent new tools with the help of their peers and teachers to find and work with current problems.

—Joseph Raelin (2007, p. 513)

Ring the bells that still can ring
Forget your perfect offering
There is a crack in everything
That's how the light gets in...

— "Anthem," Leonard Cohen (1992)

Key Concepts

- *Learning and teaching about palliative care should be tied to the challenges of everyday clinical practice.*
- *Learning and teaching about palliative care should be collaborative and relational.*
- *Learning and teaching about palliative care should be grounded in humility.*

Introduction

The passages that open this chapter convey three key concepts that frame the organization of this chapter, in which we explore the question of how postgraduate social workers best learn, and how social work educators best teach, palliative care practice: *(1)* learning and teaching about palliative care should be tied to the challenges of everyday clinical practice; *(2)* learning and teaching about palliative care should be user friendly and collaborative; and *(3)* learning and teaching about palliative care should be grounded in *humility.*

Learning and teaching about palliative care should be tied to the challenges of everyday clinical practice. Social work practice in palliative care takes place in swampy lowlands, areas of great human concern in which there is often suffering, in which technical solutions are of little help, and in which certainty about how to intervene is hard to come by. While theoretical approaches and evidence-based interventions can certainly be helpful, they do not "work" unless they "fit" with the uniquely messy lives of individual patients and families

673

who are negotiating their way through exceptionally challenging times. Formal logic and objective reasoning will not always suffice; the approach and set of responses that seemed to work so perfectly with the last patient or family may be entirely ineffective with the next. Optimal practice requires a practical kind of reasoning and flexible human engagement in the terrain of swampy lowlands that are themselves unique and constantly evolving for each patient and family.

Learning and teaching about palliative care should be user friendly and collaborative. Since the realities of practicing social work in the palliative care context involve practical reasoning and flexible human engagement, learning and teaching with social work practitioners needs to be user friendly. Since the core of palliative care practice is in relationships with patients and families, the learning process needs to be similarly collaborative and relational. Teaching aimed at helping practitioners navigate in swampy lowlands must involve helping them develop the tools, insights, and ways of thinking that will best help them with their navigation.

Learning and teaching about palliative care should be grounded in humility. Once we become clear about what it means to practice as social workers in palliative care, and once we define how to approach learning and teaching for and with these clinicians, there is a fundamental principle—a principle equally inherent in the practice, the learning, and the teaching—that must be honored. It is a core component of effective practice that may, at first glance, seem unrelated to concepts of expertise and competence. Navigating well in the swampy lowlands of palliative care means being comfortable with uncertainty and with not having answers while, simultaneously, being able to be present, compassionate, and responsive in the *midst* of that uncertainty. It is surely the case that having answers, being certain, and fixing problems are important components of professional competence. Nonetheless, palliative social workers who survive and prosper over time have internalized the humility that comes from realizing how imperfect their offerings are while appreciating, at the same time, how these less-than-perfect gifts can really matter in the lives of patients and families coping with life-threatening illness or the process of dying. With humility, we may allow ourselves as practitioners to make mistakes, to acknowledge them, and to keep trying. In situations where we are not at all sure what to do, we can do what we can. At the times when we are less than perfect, we can do our less-than-perfect best. We can ring the bells that still can ring, and in so doing, bear witness to the precious cracks in life—those places where the light gets in.

In this chapter, we will describe how these three key concepts inform our approach to teaching and learning with practicing social workers. Our observations are based on our experience teaching in the core clinical practice seminars of two postgraduate palliative care training programs: Smith College School for Social Work, in which the authors co-teach; and New York University Silver School of Social Work, in which one of the authors (SG) teaches solo. In both programs, the clinical practice seminar is part of a comprehensive curriculum that includes bereavement and palliative care theory, ethics, pain and symptom management, and leadership development (Berzoff, Dane, & Cait, 2006). We will outline the elements of relational learning and teaching we have found to be most salient and relevant from our work with these practitioners, and we will provide examples of how these elements are manifested in clinical practice seminars.

Ingredients of Relational Learning and Teaching

A collaborative and relational approach to practice-based learning shifts the idea of teaching as the imparting of knowledge or expertise, from one person who knows more to another who knows less, to a perspective in which the teacher's job is to structure and facilitate creative and meaningful ways for practitioners—including the teacher-practitioner—to learn from each other. The relational approach outlined in this chapter has been described in detail elsewhere as it applies to pediatric palliative care education (Browning & Solomon, 2006) and to interdisciplinary learning about difficult conversations in health care (Browning, Meyer, Troug, & Solomon, 2007). It builds upon relational approaches within social work education such as that of Rasmussen and Mishna (2003), who suggest that context is crucial to understanding learners, that the classroom should be understood as an intersubjective and relational field, that the teacher's experience of reality is only one of many, and that "disjunctions" in the learning process are both inevitable and potentially valuable. Similarly, Berry and Richards (2002) describe a relational approach to teaching as a growth-promoting process that fosters mutual engagement, mutual empathy, and mutual empowerment.

It is helpful to keep in mind the parallel process between the relational dynamics we hope to promote in learners as it applies to working with patients and families and the relational dynamics that need to be present in a learning environment to facilitate meaningful learning (Berzoff et al., 2006). In addition, we have found it important not to separate out learning about clinical work from learning about being a change agent in one's organization. Powerful clinical learning impacts one's sense of agency and responsibility, and inevitably has a felicitous impact on one's commitment to addressing the institutional constraints and possibilities that shape one's work life and the quality of care available to patients and families.

In our effort to carry out teaching and learning about palliative care that is tied to everyday practice, that is user-friendly and collaborative, and that is grounded in humility, we have found three categories of ingredients to be particularly salient and relevant: creating a safe and hospitable space for learning; validating experiential knowledge and already-existing competence; and inviting multiple perspectives while challenging fixed assumptions. As teachers, our job becomes how best to ensure that these ingredients will be "in the mix" throughout the learning process. In this section, we will describe each of these categories separately, then reflect on what happens in a learning setting when all of the ingredients are mixing well together.

Creating a Safe and Hospitable Space for Learning

A learning space needs to be hospitable not to make learning painless but to make the painful things possible, things without which no learning can occur—things like exposing ignorance, testing tentative hypotheses, challenging false or partial information, and mutual criticism of thought.

—*Parker Palmer (1993, p. 74)*

Working with patients and families confronting life-threatening illness or end-of-life challenges is an enormously demanding and complex practice that demands a lot from practitioners on cognitive, emotional, and spiritual levels. To create spaces for learning where practitioners can explore what it means to "show up" with patients and families, teachers need to commit themselves first and foremost to creating an atmosphere of psychological safety, respect, and mutual trust. The foundation for safety in learning is laid at the start by explicitly discussing the kind of learning environment that is necessary for the seminar to be successful, and by making it clear that the learners themselves are as responsible as the teacher(s) for establishing that environment. We normally begin our first contact with learners with a discussion of ground rules that we have found important for this kind of learning.

First, we review the importance of starting and ending on time, with beepers and cell phones turned off, and of letting the teacher(s) and the group know if there is a need to come to the session late or to leave early. We discuss the importance of treating each other—and each others' views—with respect. We describe our perspective on whole-person learning, in which learners will gravitate from cognitive, to emotional, to spiritual levels as necessary, and discuss how important it is to be open to learning on all of those levels. Very often, learners assume that professional educational activities will be conducted entirely in the cognitive realm; we find they are normally surprised and pleased to discover that "the rest of themselves" is invited into the learning. In this context, we remind learners of the importance of maintaining confidentiality with regard to the sharing of personal information.

Because our seminars normally enroll 18–24 participants, and we are invested in the learning occurring in a conversational and collaborative way, it is important to prepare learners for how we hope to accomplish this together. We discuss the normal tendency in any learning activity of this kind for there to be "loud voices," people who tend in group learning situations to talk a lot, and "soft voices," people who tend to

talk little or not at all. We suggest to the learners who talk a lot that they experiment with talking less, with the prediction that by so doing (and spending more time listening) they will have the opportunity to learn in new ways. Conversely, with learners who tend to be quiet, we propose that they try talking more, predicting that they may learn something new about themselves in the process. This initial conversation about loud and soft voices allows us as teachers to intervene throughout the seminars by respectfully curbing too much talk from some learners and inviting more verbal participation by others.

Creating an atmosphere of psychological safety and trust is important for its own sake, in terms of enabling learners to feel secure, but it also serves the larger educational goal, described by Palmer above, of "making the painful things possible." This is an especially apt phrase for practitioners who come together to learn about palliative care, in that the heart of learning about palliative care practice may be our collective capacity to talk about pain—physical, emotional, or spiritual—whether that pain is experienced by the patient, family members, or by us as practitioners. Making painful things possible can also mean examining cherished assumptions about oneself and one's practice that may need to be set aside or abandoned in order to become a more effective and engaged practitioner.

Validating Experiential Knowledge and Already-Existing Competence

When a person enters the culture of the professional disciplines they are confronted with a shift in what counts as knowledge ... In this culture, those ways of knowing the world that relate to the more popular and more local discourses of "lay" communities are marginalized—often categorized as quaint, folk and naïve—and frequently disqualified. These other ways of knowing, those that have been generated in the immediate contexts and intimate communities of a person's daily life, mostly don't count in terms of what might be taken for legitimate knowledge in the culture of the professional disciplines.

—*Michael White (1997, p. 11)*

Although a strong case can be made for the importance of appreciating experiential knowledge as part of professional practice in general, in the context of palliative care, the case is especially compelling. As has been true of many other spheres of social life, the practice of palliative care developed historically as a professional appropriation of what in the past was the domain of cultures, communities, and families. As White describes, professional training characteristically redefines what counts as knowledge, shifting from the community-based world of experience-based knowledge to the academic world of "abstract" or conceptual knowledge. In the process, professionals generally learn to distrust and/or invalidate experiential knowledge, whether that knowledge comes from the patients and families with whom they work or from their own personal experience.

As teachers, we have found that the majority of practitioners who enter our programs have little awareness or appreciation of the rich and deep storehouse of knowledge they already carry with them. They have generally been taught to see knowledge as the province of experts who have more power and are higher in the professional or academic pecking order than they are themselves. In addition, they have often practiced for years in contexts in which their accumulating practice knowledge has not been well validated, leading to a state of affairs in which, as practicing professionals, they literally *do not know what they know.*

Given these realities, we have found it important as teachers to take an explicit position that the knowledge that matters most in our time together is, first and foremost, that which comes from practitioners' own experience, both that which they have learned from the patients and families they serve, and that which they have learned from their personal lives. Through the course of the seminar, we encourage learners to "narrate" their emerging and developing "competence stories," to unearth all that they have come to know about palliative care practice from all the sources that have generated that knowledge. Academic sources of learning are often a part of that story, but the larger part of the narrative is generally tied to experiential learning that has heretofore been ignored or explicitly invalidated. Our learners generally find the unveiling of this larger story to be quite empowering, both in terms of their capacity to appreciate their own knowledge and expertise as they go forward professionally, but also because the larger story tends to remind them in an ongoing way of why working in palliative care *matters* to them.

Our emphasis on validating already-existing competence is tempered by a simultaneous appreciation that, when practitioners enroll in a program for social workers in palliative care, they expect to learn from the knowledge and expertise of the faculty. We have found it important to strike a balance between, on the one hand, cultivating respect and appreciation for the knowledge of the assembled group of practitioners, and on the other, knowing when and how to contribute to the conversation with our own knowledge and expertise. By keeping the focus on practice and by ensuring that the lion's share of air time in classes is devoted to learners connecting their own practice to the topic at hand, participants internalize a strong validation of their own knowledge and expertise.

There is another important dimension to the exploration of experiential knowledge. While we feel strongly that a full appreciation of one's practice knowledge is at the core of effective practice, we are not suggesting that this knowledge is inherently "right." Indeed, by creating an atmosphere of openness and respect, we make possible a learning climate in which assumptions or beliefs that may be narrow, faulty, or

limited by the extent or nature of one's experience, can come into the light of day and be critically reflected upon with colleagues.

Inviting Multiple Perspectives While Challenging Fixed Assumptions

If people don't engage across the divide of their differences, there is no learning.

—Ronald Heifetz, quoted in Flower (1995)

The creation of a safe and hospitable learning space makes possible certain kinds of learning that otherwise cannot occur. When a range of personal and professional perspectives are brought into a learning conversation, clinicians begin to learn across the boundaries of difference (Solomon, Browning, Dokken, Merriman, & Rushton, 2010). This is especially important in new and emerging fields like palliative care, in which there can develop a kind of "political correctness" regarding what devotees of the new paradigm assume they should think, feel and believe. We often make explicit the idea that we will know that we are learning well together when practitioners take the risk of sharing contrasting perspectives or opposing viewpoints with each other.

One way to cultivate an atmosphere in which clinicians are willing to take more risks in regard to learning is to play the role, as a teacher, of challenging or redirecting ideas presented that represent monolithic or unquestioned assumptions about what constitutes good palliative care practice. There are a myriad of such ideas that tend to emerge in conversations among palliative care practitioners. A few examples follow:

- It is best when people address unfinished business and say good-bye to loved ones before they die.
- Nearly all patients and families will choose hospice when they understand what it has to offer.
- It is better for people to be peaceful than to be angry when they die.
- Clinicians should never show strong feelings in the presence of patients and families because they will feel they have to take care of you.
- It is important for family secrets to be revealed before a loved one dies.

We have found it helpful, when these kinds of ideas are articulated, to present counter-examples of situations in which the assumption was not applicable. This has the effect of challenging myths and prescriptive models and cultivating more flexible and critical thinking. It also enhances the capacity of clinicians to make more accurate assessments and interventions that are appropriately linked to *this* particular patient and *this* particular family at *this* particular moment in time.

In addition to the multiple perspectives of learners in the room, teachers must give thought to the ways in which the perspectives of patients and families are represented in the learning process. It is important to include patient and family voices on their own terms, so that learners will be encouraged not only to think *about* patients and families, but to learn about what it means to learn *with* them. This can be accomplished by encouraging clinicians to contribute, when appropriate, their own experience as patients and family members vis-à-vis palliative and end-of-life care, as well as by the using film clips, patient and family narratives, and, when feasible, live presentations. Ann Hartman (1990), a leading social work educator, reminds us of our responsibilities in this regard:

> We must listen to our clients and bring forth their wisdom, their lived experience, their visions of the world. Because many of our clients are powerless and oppressed, their knowledge has been subjugated, and their insights have been excluded from the discourse by those who are empowered to define the "truth"— experts, professionals, and editorial boards. (1990, pp. 3–4).

It is very important, in the palliative care context especially, to remind each other as social workers about our professional obligation—one that is more clearly delineated for social workers than for other health care professionals—to present and represent the experience of the patients and families in ways that are faithful and empowering to them.

In addition to inviting philosophical and intellectual differences into learning conversations, it is also important to be alert to the wide range of differences—such as gender, ethnicity, race, class, sexual preference, personal experience, professional training, educational background—that shape how individual practitioners see the world.

> Just as we can be blind to the buildings and landmarks we pass daily on our way to the office—when our frame of mind is of getting to work rather than sightseeing—so too in professional practice our ways of looking, disciplined by personal and professional interests, bounded by institutionalized roles and routines, and rehearsed until they are second nature to us, determine what we can and cannot see. (McKee, 2003, p. 402)

When learners begin to assume a critical perspective on the ways in which their personal and professional positions have shaped how they see the world of palliative care, they are more likely, when they return to their workplaces, of "learning to what we do not see" (McKee, 2003, p. 402). One aspect of a critical perspective involves "problematizing" the very notion of expertise as it applies to helping others in the context of palliative care. In this regard, we like to share the advice of the Zen master Shunryu Suzuki, who told his students, "In the beginner's mind there are many possibilities, but in the expert's there are few."

Mixing the Ingredients Together

None of us is as smart as all of us.

—*Japanese proverb*

The most important parts of any conversation are those that neither party could have imagined before starting.

—*William Isaacs (1999)*

What happens when the core ingredients—creating a safe and hospitable space for learning, validating experiential knowledge and already-existing competence, and inviting multiple perspectives while challenging fixed assumptions— are all mixing well together in a seminar in which social workers come together to explore the swampy lowlands of palliative care practice? First, learners often tell us that they have never experienced this kind of learning before, either in their graduate training or in any professional work environment. They frequently describe an experience of trusting the learning process itself and of experiencing the learning as larger than the sum of the individuals in the room. They comment on the holistic nature of the learning—the fact that in a 30-minute period the conversation can travel, for example, through a sophisticated reflection on bereavement theory, to an emotional sharing of the pain of sitting with patients' suffering, to an exploration of the existential and spiritual insights that the work affords us. They describe "light bulb moments" in which they experienced insight into a long-held assumption that they have now rethought or revisioned. They express appreciation for having their accumulated grief—grief tied to doing this difficult work over many years—validated, and for the range of ways in which emotion—at times extremely powerful—was invited into the learning. They describe a different appreciation for the ethics of everyday practice—for the ways they talk about their patients and families, for how they and their colleagues treat each other, and for the importance of bringing their "whole persons" to their work with patients and families facing life-threatening illness or death.

Importantly, learners also comment on the joy of discovery in the way we have gone about learning together and reflect upon what they themselves—along with their fellow learners and the instructors—have contributed to making that learning happen. They recount new understandings of the many differences that are present in all professional settings that shape and sometimes limit the thinking and actions of professional caregivers. They describe a feeling of empowerment, of not having previously appreciated all that they know, and, concurrently, a sense of responsibility for carrying their learning forward in the form of new actions and endeavors in the hospitals, hospices, and other organizational settings in which they work. Finally, they reflect on aspects of the learning that are more difficult to pin down, perhaps because they are tied to mystery, an experience of interdependency, and even, at times, a sense of the sacred.

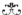

Illustrations of Relational Learning and Teaching

If we want a community of truth ... we must put a third thing, a great thing, at the center of the pedagogical circle ... Here, teacher and students have a power beyond themselves to contend with—the power of a subject that transcends our self-absorption and refuses to be reduced to our claims about it.

—*Parker Palmer (2007, pp. 119–120)*

The amazing and wonderful thing about bringing a group of clinicians together who have been practicing for some time in hospice or palliative care settings is that the subject we are learning about together—how human beings face, make sense of, and at times find meaning in the context of illness, death, and dying—is so innately *compelling*, pedagogically speaking. If there were ever a subject that, using Palmer's words, could transcend our self-absorption and refuse to be reduced to our intellectual claims about it, this surely must be it! As educators, one of our responsibilities in this regard is "keeping it real"—ensuring that the learning stays organized around the large and salient issues with which practitioners who do this work contend on a daily basis. In this section, we will offer three vignettes (see Boxes 73.1–73.3) that constitute composites of themes and practice challenges that we have found to be among the most common for practicing clinicians in hospice and palliative care.

Diana's dilemma (see Box 73.1) is one version of a common experience for clinicians working in hospice or palliative care. Because the work can be so challenging, and because it involves supporting patients and families at times in their lives when answers are hard to come by, we have found that clinicians often experience one version or another of

"not-enoughness." Diana feels less than sufficient because of the academic priorities that she feels shape practitioners' values and behavior in her work setting. Another learner might assume that if he just learns the proper theory and the proper technique, he will have the right words to say when a patient or family is facing a complex end-of-life decision. Still another might wonder why the work seems not to get any easier over the years, imagining this must represent some kind of deficit within her.

Not-enoughness takes a variety of forms—not smart enough, not strong enough, not compassionate enough, not resilient enough, not emotional enough, not spiritual enough, not courageous enough. Often paired with this self-disparaging notion is the belief that others *are* enough, that respected colleagues must *indeed* have what it takes, that they must somehow enjoy those special qualities that are lacking within oneself. Not-enoughness is a common belief structure for clinicians who do this very difficult work of sitting with patients and families who are suffering. It is an occupational hazard of sorts, and it is a no-win proposition unless the definition of enoughness incorporates the vulnerability and uncertainty that underlie this work and appreciates the central role of personhood—how practitioners bring their own unique humanness to the challenges at hand. We often try to bring home this truth in a humorous way, by sharing the words of Oscar Wilde, who is reputed to have said that you should be yourself, because everyone else is already taken.

While we believe it can be immensely helpful to learn relevant palliative care and bereavement theories and to develop new skills and techniques to improve one's practice, we have found those learning pursuits to be less than helpful if they are not built upon the more fundamental task of enabling practicing clinicians to identify, understand, articulate, and examine their already-existing competence, which is shaped by their unique personhood and embedded in their personal and professional experience. Many of our learners tell us at the end of our seminars that they came to realize, in retrospect, how little they heretofore have valued their own wisdom, especially when that wisdom is part of practice and rarely if ever articulated, honored, or celebrated. By taking seriously their own knowledge, and by integrating that knowledge into their own distinctive humanness, they begin to envision a different kind of professional identity as they prepare to return to their home institutions.

We have found the issues contained in Mark's dilemma (see Box 73.2) to be nearly universal among social workers who work in hospice and palliative care settings. Because of the intensity and intimacy of the work, there is often quite a bit of uncertainty about what it means to care and what happens to clinicians when they continue to care for patients and families over long periods of time. Not infrequently, as in Mark's example, social workers have learned to equate having feelings in the presence of patients and families with countertransference. In this light, we have found it important to help our learners distinguish between unconscious feelings and un-worked-through issues, on the one hand, and the depth

---

Box 73.1
Not-Enoughness

Diana shares her experience working for the past 7 years as a master-s-levelsocial worker on a palliative care team in a prominent teaching hospital. She has had a rich variety of professional experiences, but she lacks confidence and often feels that her personal anxiety about her level of competence translates into missed opportunities and prevents her from reaching out and being as effective as she is capable of being with patients and families. She is in an academic environment in which having a PhD or MD, conducting research, and publishing papers—while also doing clinical work—seem to be what really matters. Since she does not have these things, she assumes she must not be as bright or as competent as most of her colleagues. She often surmises that they have the right answers, and that she does not.

Box 73.2
Too Close or Too Distant?

Mark describes his work over the past 9 months with a middle-aged patient who has been battling an unusual type of breast cancer for 4 years. The patient is the single mother of three children, ages 5, 9, and 13 years; Mark's children are in the same age range. Mark feels very close to the patient and her children, and he has found his work with them to be particularly intense and meaningful. The patient is now facing the end of her life, and Mark fears he will be unable to conceal his feelings. He has worked in hospice for 5 years and, until now, has "always been able to care without getting too emotional."

Mark learned in his professional training that the display of feelings is inappropriate because it shifts attention from the patient's needs to your own. Also, he has a nursing colleague who recently discussed a case in team meeting in which she described feeling very sad and crying with a family at the bedside of a patient she had known a long time. Although the team seemed supportive at the time, Mark learned later that the nurse's supervisor (who is also Mark's supervisor) advised the nurse that her emotions were excessive, and that she should talk to a therapist "so she can get on top of her counter-transference."

---

of emotion clinicians often experience when working with very sick and dying patients and their families, on the other. The former we define as counter-transference, and the latter is perhaps best understood as the human experience of compassion. While it is undoubtedly the case that counter-transference can and does influence the clinical relationship in these contexts, we have found the wider challenge to be how to cultivate thoughtful conversations about the very strong and powerful feelings clinicians often experience in doing this work, feelings that much of the time have less to do with counter-transference and more to do with the human experience of being moved emotionally, on a regular basis, in one's day-to-day work.

Making a distinction between counter-transference and compassion lays the foundation for a deeper level of learning about how effective, caring clinicians sort out for themselves what it means to be too distant and what it means to be too close. When a safe and trusting environment is established, learners are willing to take the risk of describing scenarios that fall on various points along the closeness–distance spectrum. The dilemma posed by Mark above might fall somewhere in the middle of the spectrum. Another learner might pose a scenario describing a relationship with a patient and family that involves extra home visits, brooding about the patient all the time, and feeling closer to the patient's family than one's own. Still another might describe a rather bureaucratic, detached style with patients and families that she finds necessary in order to deal with so much suffering.

Conversations such as these about caring, compassion, and counter-transference lead naturally into a discussion of "professional boundaries." Similar to the way the term

counter-transference was used by Mark's supervisor in a way that may well have curtailed important learning for his nursing colleague and the interdisciplinary team, the concept and language of professional boundaries is often internalized by social workers in their training and work environments in a judgmental way that prevents them from talking openly with colleagues about strong feelings and experiences of intimacy. We emphasize two general rules as we explore these scenarios: first, whether the clinician's actions can be linked to the patient and family's best interest in a therapeutic sense; and second, whether the needs of the patient and family, as opposed to the needs of the clinician, remain paramount. We stress how important it is to describe and reflect upon these dilemmas of closeness and distance contextually as opposed to uncritically applying black-and white, rule-based thinking. We have found that only through a safe and thoughtful exploration of the actual situation faced by the clinician can the salient and relevant moral and ethical questions be brought to the surface and a therapeutic course of action identified.

It is common for professional caregivers to talk, as Regina does (see box 73.3), about the privilege of working with patients and families coping with serious illness and the end of life Indeed, sharing the particular positive meanings that clinicians encounter in this work is valuable and important to learning. However, it is equally important for clinicians to talk, as Sally does (see also box 73.3), about the times when theyexperience their work less in positive terms and more in terms of the emotional overload and exhaustion that it can bring. It is at times more socially acceptable and politically correct, in the cultures of hospice and palliative care, to talk about the work in terms of its blessings than to be able to talk frankly about its burdens. Moreover, it is possible, in some conversations, for the recounting of blessings to silence those

---

Box 73.3
Burdens and Blessings

Sally describes her concern about being able to maintain empathy with the patients and families with whom she works. She finds this to be particularly hard after a patient dies and she is expected to move right on to the next case. She was just assigned a new patient who is hopeful about her diagnosis, but Sally knows that the medical prognosis is poor and says, "I don't know if I can go there again." She has always loved her work with sick and dying patients, but she is beginning to dread going to work and fears that she is burning out.

Regina expresses surprise in response to Sally's account. She describes having worked in palliative care for many years, with what she believes is an optimal balance between being available to the patients and families with whom she works, but "never taking their problems home with me." She says it has always been an amazing privilege for her to be able to work with others at such difficult times in their lives, and she cannot understand how anyone could experience it as a burden.

who, for example, are not sure they can continue to sit with other people's suffering day after day, year after year.

When a group of learners feels permission to explore the entire range of experience and meanings attached to doing this work, there is the opportunity to move more deeply into the complex intersection of issues of meaning, purpose, spirituality, workload, the balancing of personal and professional demands, and efforts at self-care—all of which are directly relevant to working as a clinician in hospice and palliative care over a period of time. This conversation is often experienced by learners as invaluable, because it allows them to begin to identify the components of their particular personal and professional lives that require attention, nurturance, and revision.

Conclusion

Any genuine teaching will result, if successful, in someone's knowing how to bring about a better condition of things than existed earlier.
—*John Dewey (1916)*

In this chapter, we have proposed that palliative care practice for social workers takes place in swampy lowlands, a life terrain that is of utmost concern and significance to patients, families, and clinicians—a place where things *matter*. We have suggested that it is not easy, navigating in swampy lowlands, and that clinicians who practice in this landscape need and deserve opportunities for ongoing education that are tied to everyday practice, that are collaborative and user friendly, and that are grounded in humility. As teachers, we can do our best to thoughtfully craft this kind of learning; in return, we are given the special privilege of exploring, alongside our clinician-learner-colleagues, this messy, wondrous, challenging terrain. When the learning goes well, we are able to locate and reclaim our individual and collective bearings—as social workers and as human beings—and to go forward to make our worlds just a little bit better.

ADDITIONAL RESOURCES

WEB SITES

The American Academy of Hospice and Palliative Medicine: http://www.aahpm.org
Dedicated to expanding access of patients and families to high-quality palliative care and advancing the discipline of hospice and palliative medicine.
The Center to Advance Palliative Care: http://www.capc.org
Provides health care professionals with the tools, training, and technical assistance necessary to start and sustain successful palliative care programs in hospitals and other health care settings.

The Center for Courage & Renewal: http://www.couragerenewal.org
To nurture personal and professional integrity and the courage to act on it through supporting retreats that offer the time and space to slow down and reflect on life and work.
The Institute for Professionalism and Ethical Practice: http://www.ipepweb.org
An interdisciplinary educational initiative dedicated to cultivating relational competence in health care. The Institute specializes in developing and conducting innovative educational programs and interventions focused on difficult conversations in different settings.
The Initiative for Pediatric Palliative Care: http://www.ippcweb.org
Seeks to enhance the capacity of children's hospitals and related institutions.
The Social Work Hospice and Palliative Care Network: http://www.swhpn.org
An emerging network of social work organizations and leaders who seek to further the field of end-of-life and hospice/palliative care.

SUGGESTED READINGS

Csikai, E. L., & Jones, B. (2007). *Teaching resources for end-of-life and palliative care courses.* Chicago, IL: Lyceum Books.

Foyle, L., & Hostad, J.(Eds.). (2007). *Innovations in cancer and palliative care education.* Oxford, England: Radcliffe Publishing

Otis-Green, S., Ferrell, B., Spolum, M., Uman, G., Mullan, P., Baird, P., & Grant, M. (2009). An overview of the ACE project—Advocating for Clinical Excellence: Transdisciplinary palliative care education. *Journal of Cancer Education, 24*(2), 120–126.

Wee, B., & Hughes, N. (2007). *Education in palliative care–Building a culture of learning.* Oxford, England: Oxford University Press.

REFERENCES

Berry, J., & Richards, A. (2002). Relational teaching: A view of relational teaching in social work education. *Journal of Teaching in Social Work Education, 2*(1/2), 33–48.

Berzoff, J., Dane, B., & Cait, C. (2006). Innovative models for developing post-masters curriculum in end-of-life care. *Journal of Teaching in Social Work, 25*(3/4), 63–88.

Berzoff, J., Lucas, G., DeLuca, D., Gerbino, S., Browning, D., Foster, Z., & Chachkes, E. (2006). Clinical social work education in palliative and end of life care: Relational approaches for advanced practitioners. *Journal of Social Work in End-of-Life and Palliative Care, 2*(2), 45–63.

Browning, D., Meyer, E., Truoug, R., & Solomon, M. (2007). Difficult conversations in health care: Cultivating relational learning to address the hidden curriculum. *Academic Medicine, 82*(9), 905–913.

Browning, D., & Solomon, M. (2006). Relational learning in pediatric palliative care: Transformative education and the culture of medicine. *Child and Adolescent Psychiatric Clinics of North America, 15*(3), 795–813.

Cohen, L. (1992). Anthem. *The Future*, Track 5, Sony Records.

Dewey, J. (1916/1926). *Democracy and education.* New York, NY: Macmillan.

Flower, J. (1995). Ronald Heifetz: Leadership without easy answers. *The Healthcare Forum Journal, 38*(4), 30–34, 36.

Hartman, A. (1990). Many ways of knowing. Social Work, 35(1), 3–4.

Isaacs, W. (1999). *Dialogues and the art of thinking together.* New York, NY: Currency.

McKee, M. (2003). Excavating our frames of mind: The key to dialogue and collaboration. *Social Work, 48*(3), 401–408.

Palmer, P. J. (1993). *To know as we are known: A spirituality of education.* San Francisco, CA: Harper and Row.

Palmer, P. J. (2007). *The courage to teach: Exploring the inner landscape of a teacher's life. Tenth Anniversary Edition.* San Francisco, CA: John Wiley and Sons.

Raelin, J. A. (2007). Toward an epistemology of practice. *Academy of Management Learning and Education, 6*(4), 495–519.

Rasmussen, B., & Mishna, F. (2003). The relevance of contemporary psychoanalytic theories to teaching social work. *Smith College Studies in Social Work, 74*(1), 31–47.

Schon, D. (1983). *The reflective practitioner: How professionals think in action.* New York, NY: Basic Books.

Solomon, M., Browning, D., Dokken, D., Merriman, M., & Rushton, C. (2010). Learning that leads to action: Impact and characteristics of a professional education approach to improve the care of critically ill children and their families. *Archives in Pediatrics and Adolescent Medicine, 164*(4), 315–322.

White, M. (1997). *Narratives of therapists' lives.* Adelaide, South Africa: Dulwich Centre Publications.

74 *Mary Raymer and Gary Gardia*

Enhancing Professionalism, Leadership, and Advocacy: A Call to Arms

I really didn't want to see the palliative social worker. I didn't have a clue what he could do for me. Well, let me tell you, that social worker helped me negotiate a very large health care system where I often had felt lost during the weeks of tests and procedures to determine my diagnosis. He helped me practice what I wanted to say to the different physicians, located resources that I didn't know were available, and helped me identify my priorities and figure out where my energy was best spent.

—57-year-old palliative care client with pancreatic cancer

Key Concepts

◆ *Advocacy is not optional; it is one of our profession's ethical obligations and a cornerstone of social work practice.*

◆ *All social workers have the responsibility to cultivate and role-model leadership skills whatever their job title may be.*

◆ *Social workers at all levels of practice need to seek leadership opportunities in order to ensure that we are part of the decision-making process shaping palliative care.*

◆ *Elevating the professionalism of social work requires individual self-awareness and ongoing professional development and integrity.*

The Case for Renewing a Broader View of Advocacy

Clinical advocacy is a routine part of social work in palliative care. Social workers at the bedside advocate for the rights, needs, and decisions of clients on a daily basis. It is a key responsibility for the social work profession. Increasingly, however, there is concern in the field that while social workers embrace clinical advocacy they do not always view macro advocacy as their responsibility. In one study social work students substantially disagreed with the statement that "advocacy is the main thrust of social work" (Csikai & Rozensky, 1997). At a presentation by Edith Abbott at the Proceedings of the National Conference of Social Work, Abbott quotes Mary Richmond, "The good social worker, says Miss Richmond, doesn't go on mechanically helping people out of a ditch. Pretty soon she begins to find out what out to be done to get rid of the ditch." Social work has a responsibility and obligation to practice advocacy on a broader basis. The profession's person-in-environment approach requires that social workers intervene beyond the one-on-one level. Whether in our communities, institutions, or society at large, we cannot remain neutral when clients who need services are denied access to quality palliative care. We are charged with addressing organizational and public policy with special attention to disparities in care. Rejecting this obligation jeopardizes the psychosocial care of the people we serve.

The profession of social work grew out of a commitment to the pursuit of social justice and the development of the full potential of individuals, groups, communities, and the broader society. In the late 1800s the main focus of social work centered on fighting for basic human rights for some of the most vulnerable populations such as immigrants, minorities, women, children, the sick, and the poor. Palliative care patients and their families are a vulnerable population, and they are often unable to advocate for themselves.

One of the most concise definitions of advocacy is, "… the exclusive and mutual representation of a client(s) or a cause in a forum, attempting to systematically influence decision-making in an unjust or unresponsive system(s)" (Schneider & Lester, 2001, p. 65). This definition is inclusive of both clinical and macro advocacy. There are numerous reasons social workers may not view macro advocacy as their duty. They may see clinical practice as more gratifying or may feel overwhelmed with the demands placed on them by their job and direct practice. It may be that they have not received sufficient training for macro advocacy or they view it as too time consuming.

Social workers can practice macro advocacy in numerous everyday ways. Writing an e-mail or letter to politicians, joining national organizations, or participating in research are all forms of practicing macro advocacy that do not necessarily require significant amounts of additional time. Advocating for the greater good is a critical obligation inherent in social work practice. It sets us apart from many other professions. We are mandated by our code of ethics to "promote the general welfare of society, from local to global levels, and the development of people, their communities, and their environments. Social workers should advocate for living conditions conducive to the fulfillment of basic human needs and should promote social, economic, political and cultural values and institutions that are compatible with the realization of social justice" (National Association of Social Workers [NASW], pp. 26–27, 1996). The code goes on to address our professional obligation to social and political action. Additionally, the NASW Code under the Ethical Principles section states that "social workers pursue social change, particularly with and on behalf of vulnerable and oppressed individuals and groups of people" (p. 5). Our responsibility to participate in macro advocacy is highlighted in other places in our Code of Ethics, but clearly it is an ethical obligation, not a choice. Abdicating this responsibility minimizes our efficacy as a profession when it comes to shaping effective palliative care and ensuring access for all people.

An often neglected arena of advocacy is advocating for the profession itself and its role in palliative care. Many of our colleagues in other disciplines are confused about the role of social workers and all too often are unaware of what we are capable of contributing. We have a responsibility to educate our colleagues, the clients we serve, and the public at large. The ability to clearly articulate the difference between emotional support and psychosocial intervention is essential if we are to represent social work effectively. We need to document specific interventions and their outcomes, speak up in team meetings, and share our expertise. Many palliative care teams do not have full-time social work involvement. The assumption is often made that other disciplines can supply whatever a social worker would provide. By advocating for the profession of social work we are also advocating for the clients we serve. Psychosocial care is a stated priority in palliative care as evidence by the National Consensus Project Clinical Practice Guidelines for Quality

Palliative Care, and social workers need to provide a powerful clinical and leadership presence. To do this, it is critical that we visibly represent the profession's efficacy in our own daily work as well as teaching, writing, and participating in research. One of the first national studies of social work efficacy and palliative care was focused on hospice and the relationship between social work and hospice outcomes. That cross-sectional survey of 66 hospices found that increased social work involvement was significantly associated with lower hospice costs, better team functioning, reduced medical services, fewer visits by other disciplines, and increased client satisfaction (Reese & Raymer, 2004). This is the type of data that is needed if we are to effectively advocate for the profession. Just like other professions we have the responsibility to make sure that we are proving our effectiveness as well as choosing the optimal interventions for the people we serve.

What Social Work Brings to the Table

Palliative social workers are well suited to practicing macro advocacy for numerous reasons. Our professional values mesh well with the values espoused by palliative care. Keeping the stated values and ethics clear in our minds helps us problem-solve more effectively. Articulating and representing them well can influence decision makers as well as colleagues to strive for the best standards and policies. The training we receive in group process and systems helps us strategize more effective plans of action whether we are trying to facilitate collaborative work or we are negotiating or coalition building.

Problem-solving and communication skills are important parts of our education and make us more effective in many areas of macro advocacy, including research, public speaking, writing, testifying, or building alliances to improve services and benefits. Social workers in the trenches provide a direct link between policy, practice, and the life experience of patients, families, and clinicians. We bring a rich understanding of how society at large impacts everyday life for people in our palliative care programs. By collecting data and telling our stories we make an authentic and lasting impression on the people who have the power to improve policies and services.

Professionalism and Leadership

The two palliative social workers in Box 74.1 have very different approaches to dealing with change. Sarah was being a leader as she advocated for a positive way to integrate the change. Karen took a passive-aggressive approach, demonstrating unprofessional social work behavior. Professionalism is about character, the choices we make, how we intervene,

Box 74.1
Karen and Sarah: Laptops in the Home Electronic Documentation

Karen, a hospice social worker practicing in home care, could understand the importance of electronic documentation for nurses, but she believed that it could never be considered "good care" in social work practice. Although she had never used a laptop in her work, she imagined a computer would be too impersonal and create barriers to providing emotional support. When her supervisor said, "I see your point but electronic documentation is now the policy of the agency," Karen decided to organize the rest of the social workers. At this point, Karen was so committed to her belief that laptops would never work that she was unwilling to hear from her coworkers about the benefits of electronic documentation. She insisted that they all stick together and refuse to comply so that management would have to acquiesce to their demands.

Sarah worked for another agency that was converting to electronic documentation. She had heard the complaints about using laptops in patients' homes and quickly realized that with the right skills, they could be useful and effective. She approached her manager and said, "I realize that some of the people in our department are struggling with the concept of electronic documentation. How about if a couple of my social work colleagues and I put together a presentation on how to use this new format? We can demonstrate how to capture important information in a manner that does not interfere with providing effective and compassionate care."

and how we are perceived by others. Social workers display character by staying focused on the values that guide the profession, such as integrity and competence. Sarah demonstrated character when she sought the skills necessary to utilize electronic documentation in a way that would not interfere with quality care. As a result, it is likely that she will be perceived by others as effective in her role as a social worker.

In palliative care, the opportunities to link advocacy, professionalism, and leadership are numerous. It is not unusual for team members to become frustrated when one member of the family behaves in a way that disrupts care and draws attention away from the needs of the person who is ill. Team conversations may include judgmental and uninformed language such as "the crazy daughter" or "the controlling husband." The palliative social worker demonstrates leadership by redirecting these conversations. Educating team members about the features of specific types of personalities and how to intervene in an effective and respectful manner restores dignity to the family system and replaces clinician helplessness and judgment with clinical understanding and skills.

On the macro level, our ability to model and articulate the full scope of social work practice assists others to better understand our value. Offering to explore mechanisms to reach underserved populations or developing partnerships with disease-specific organizations falls under our area of expertise. These activities contribute to the goal of expanding

access to services while at the same time supporting the mission of the agency.

In the everyday world of practice, understanding the relationship between pain and suffering is another aspect of care that demands strong advocacy, expertise, and leadership from social workers. The inclination of many is to assess pain and treat only from a medical perspective. A critical role of palliative social work is to continually reinforce the nature of suffering as it relates to the biological, psychological, emotional, social, and spiritual dynamics that arise from serious illness. Educating people within our communities about the right to expert pain management and the nature of psychosocial suffering helps them to understand the comprehensive focus of palliative care. Calling attention to the difference between grief and depression and encouraging the critical thinking needed to understand the etiology and meaning of complex symptoms such as agitation demonstrates leadership and advocacy in the clinical realm. Without leadership and the confidence to speak up, there can be no advocacy.

In addition to the requisite need to "speak up," advocacy and leadership in palliative care also means that we continually seek the skills necessary to fulfill our role and enhance our effectiveness. Our actions are then professional and focused on providing excellent service to patients and families while supporting the mission and vision of the organizations for which we work. We are then solution focused and effective at maximizing the strengths of coworkers, patients, and families. Most important, we do not wait for others to define social work practice but rather we are shaping the unique and effective focus of social work in palliative care.

Getting to the Decision-Making Tables

Palliative social workers need to be at the decision-making tables. Instead of just responding to changes as they occur, social work involvement in designing change brings the values and expertise of the profession to the shaping of policy and the future of palliative care. It is during the decision-making process that advocating for the psychosocial needs of people who are ill and their loved ones is articulated and integrated into the organization's commitment to interdisciplinary practice. Decision making comes in various shapes, sizes, colors, and tones. Participating on committees, working on quality improvement initiatives, and program planning are examples of opportunities to actively contribute to enhanced care.

Each time a social worker contributes positively to meet challenges as they occur, he or she demonstrates to others that social workers are solution focused. When potential problems are avoided following a social worker's identification of areas that are out of compliance with regulations, they will be seen as proactive. Furthermore, by understanding the importance of balancing the needs of the organization with the needs of patients and families, social work input will be objective and focused on finding resolutions that build consensus and result in the best possible outcomes for all.

Getting to the decision-making tables is most likely to occur when it is clear the social worker possesses the knowledge and skills necessary to contribute at that level. A working knowledge of standards of care, regulations, and organizational policies that guide decision-making processes is one example of this critical knowledge base. At times, colleagues are unaware of the knowledge and training of social workers, and it is essential that we assert our willingness to contribute rather than passively waiting to be invited.

While palliative care clearly needs social workers involved in decision-making processes, more social workers are also needed in key management positions. Additionally, expanding the pool of mentors and identifying social work leaders as role models and teachers are positive steps and the mutual responsibility of practitioners, teachers, and students.

Looking to the Future

Professionalism, leadership, and advocacy are essential for social workers at both the micro and macro levels of palliative care. Social work has an opportunity and an obligation to advocate for the broader issues that impact the people we serve. We need to be at the decision-making tables to help design and shape the future. To ensure that we influence important decisions we need to consistently evaluate the quality of our professionalism, leadership, and advocacy skills. There is no paucity of issues to be addressed at the macro level. Culturally sensitive care, caregiver concerns, preserving interdisciplinary care, access to care, pain and symptom management, and keeping our values intact all need attention. To be good leaders we must be willing to engage in an ongoing process of self-awareness. We also need to continually seek education and training to enhance our levels of competence. It is crucial to the integrity of our profession that we lead in our everyday practice by role-modeling and inspiring others to carry out the important goals and objectives of palliative care. If we cannot concisely articulate a vision and mobilize others, we cannot exert positive influence. Effective social workers are assertive. They ask the necessary questions. They seek as individuals and as members of a team to explore answers. They challenge themselves and others to think critically. They do not complain but work toward finding solutions. They promote collaborative action to enhance care.

There are challenging times ahead for palliative care. Social workers need to participate at every level, both micro and macro. The challenge will be to look at palliative care as it exists today, assess its strengths and limitations, and deliver the best possible social work practice within those parameters. Then we are morally obligated to take it to the next step. We need to address those limitations and seek to enhance and preserve the existing strengths. Social workers need to be proactive not passive. We need to live our core values and use our skills to help shape the future of quality palliative care that lives up to its promise.

This is the true joy of life, the being used up for a purpose recognized by yourself as a mighty one; being a force of nature instead of a feverish, selfish little clod of ailments and grievances, complaining that the world will not devote itself to making you happy. I am of the opinion that my life belongs to the community, and as long as I live, it is my privilege to do whatever I can... Life is no "brief candle" to me. It is a sort of splendid torch which I have got to hold for a moment and I want to make it burn as brightly as possible before handing it on to future generations. (Shaw, 1903, p. xxxi).

LEARNING EXERCISES

I ADVOCACY/CORE VALUES

Consider the following values:

- Service
- Social justice
- Dignity and worth of the person
- Importance of human relationships
- Integrity
- Competence

1. Identify three specific actions you can take or have already taken that would fall in the realm of macro advocacy.
2. Which of our professional core values listed above are you putting into play with your advocacy efforts?

II LEADERSHIP EXERCISE

Identify one aspect of palliative care that you feel could use improvement. Now consider the following:

1. Which standards, regulations, and/or policies are related to this problem?
2. Who are the key players?
3. Is there something you could do to influence change, even minimally?
4. Develop a plan for action.

III PROFESSIONAL COLLABORATION

1) Think about a coworker you find difficult to work with. What is it about this person that is troubling for you? Make a list of those qualities and/or personality traits.
2) Now think about your own qualities and/or personality traits that have contributed to this dynamic. Make a list of those as well.

3) Now look at how you have responded to this struggle. Would you say your behavior has been professional or less than professional? What would other observers say?

4) Now determine whether this relationship interferes with the mission of your organization. If yes, is that acceptable to you? If it is not acceptable, what might you do about that? How can you assure that your behavior is professional at all times with this person?

5) Keep in mind that this is about you: your character, your integrity, and how others see you. This person may choose not to engage on a professional level with you. The point is that you behave professionally at all times, regardless of how others respond or interact.

ADDITIONAL RESOURCES

SUGGESTED READINGS

Agnew, E. N. (2004). *From charity to social work: Mary E. Richmond and the creation of an American profession.* Urbana, IL: University of Illinois Press.

Austin, D. M. (2002). *Human services management: Organizational leadership in social work practice.* Irvington, NY: Columbia University Press.

Chachkes, E., & Foster, Z. (2005). Taking charge: Social work leadership in end-of-life care. In J. Berzoff & P. R. Silverman (Eds.), *Living with dying: A handbook for end-of-life healthcare practitioners* (pp. 825–837). New York, NY: Columbia University Press.

Clark, E. (2005). The future of social work in end-of-life care: A call to action. In J. Berzoff & P. R. Silverman (Eds.), *Living with dying: A handbook for end-of-life healthcare practitioners* (pp. 838–847). New York, NY: Columbia University Press.

Goleman, D., Boyatzis, R. E., & McKee, A. (2004). *Primal leadership: Learning to lead with emotional intelligence.* Boston, MA: Harvard Business Press.

Haslam, S. A., Reicher, S. D., & Platow, M. J. (in press). *The new psychology of leadership: Identity, influence and power.* London, UK: Psychology Press.

Lawler, J. (2005). Leadership in social work: A case of caveat emptor? *British Journal of Social Work, 37*(1), 123–141.

Raymer, M. (1996). Revisiting the core values of hospice. *Caring, 15*(11), 52–55.

Raymer, M., & Reese, D. (2005). The history of social work in hospice. In J. Berzoff & P. R. Silverman. (Eds.), *Living with dying: A handbook for end-of-life healthcare practitioners* (pp. 150–160). New York, NY: Columbia University Press.

Roff, S. (2001). Analyzing end-of-life care legislation: A social work perspective. *Social Work in Health Care, 33*(1), 51–68.

Rosenberg, G., & Weissman, A. (1995). *Social work leadership in healthcare: Directors' perspectives.* New York, NY: Routledge.

Van Knippenberg, D., & Hogg, M. A. (2004). *Leadership and power.* Thousand Oaks, CA: Sage.

WEB RESOURCES

National Association of Social Workers. (2009). *NASW advocacy.* Retrieved from http://www.socialworkers.org/advocacy/Default.asp

National Association of Social Workers. (2009). *NASW blog.* Retrieved from http://www.socialworkblog.org/advocacy

National Consensus Project for Quality Palliative Care. (2009). *Clinical practice guidelines for quality palliative care.* Retrieved from http://www.nationalconsensusproject.org

Social Work Leadership Institute. (2009). Retrieved from http://www.socialworkleadership.org

Social Work for Social Work Leadership in Health Care. (2009). Retrieved from http://www.sswlhc.org

Social Work Today. (2009). *10 leadership strategies for women in social services management.* Retrieved from http://www.socialworktoday.com/archive/marapr2008p38.shtml

MEDIA

Borden, B., Eisner, E., Burg, M., & Baker, T. R., (Producers). (1995). *The cure.* [Motion Picture]. Hollywood, CA: Universal Studios.

Capra, F. (Producer). (1947). *It's a wonderful life.* [Motion Picture]. Hollywood, CA: Liberty Films.

Lustig, B., Molen, G. R., Glovin, I., Kennedy, K., & Rywin, L., (Producers). (1993). *Schindler's list.* [Motion Picture]. Hollywood, CA: Universal Studios.

Nichols, M., Hirsch, B., Tuber, J., Cano, L., & Hausman, M., (Producers). (1983) *Silkwood.* [Motion Picture]. Burbank, CA: ABC Motion Pictures.

REFERENCES

Csikai, C., & Rozensky, C. (1997). Social work idealism and students' perceived reasons for entering social work. *Journal of Social Work Education, 33*(3), 529–538.

National Association of Social Workers (NASW). (1996). *Code of ethics.* Washington, DC: Author.

National Conference on Social Welfare. (2005). Official proceedings of the annual meeting: 1918 [online]. Ann Arbor: University of Michigan Library. p 313. Available online at: http://good.lib.umich.edu/cgi/t/text/text-1dx?c=ncosw;iel=l;view=toc;idno=ACH8650.1918.001

Reese, D., & Raymer, M. (2004). Relationships between social work involvement and hospice outcomes: Results of the National Hospice Social Work Survey. *Social Work: A Journal of the National Association of Social Workers, 49*(3), 415–422.

Schneider, R. L., & Lester, L. (2001). *Social work advocacy: A new framework for action.* Belmont, CA: Wadsworth/Thompson Learning.

Shaw, G. B. (1903). *Man and superman: A comedy and a philosophy.* New York, NY: Brentano's.

75 *Terry Altilio*

The Power and Potential of Language

Words not only convey something, but are something; that words have color, depth, texture of their own, and the power to evoke vastly more than they mean; that words can be used not merely to make things clear, make things vivid, make things interesting ... but to make things happen inside the one ... who hears them.

—*Frederick Buechner, 1992, p. 15*

Key Concepts

- *Although intended to clarify, the words we choose in our verbal and written communication also have the potential to confuse and complicate matters for colleagues, patients, and families.*
- *Social workers are trained to listen for and raise consciousness of the implicit and explicit messages in palliative care communication.*
- *Palliative and end-of-life communication has integrated words and unique phrases that require clinical attention to insure that their meaning and intention are clear to patients and families.*
- *Illness and specific diseases such as cancer are replete with metaphors that may or may not be therapeutic and congruent with the values and personhood of patients and families.*
- *Metaphors may provide insight into the cognitive and emotional aspects of the illness experience and can help make sense of behaviors, emotional responses, and decisions.*
- *Vigilance to the language and metaphors used by patients, families, and professionals creates opportunities for a range of clinical interventions.*

Introduction

Social work as a discipline begins and ends in communication; listening to words, behaviors, and silence; choosing if, when, and how to respond; what words to use, to sit or stand, to touch or not. Often we focus on communication because similar to our colleagues in chaplaincy, psychology, and psychiatry, this is one of the core skills that allow us to serve patients, families, and our colleagues. Communication stretches far beyond "giving bad news"; it is central to all of our work. In many instances, our work is about words, even the ones we choose not to say.

This chapter is about language, the words that we hear in everyday communication, the phrases that have slipped into everyday palliative and end-of-life parlance. It is an invitation to listen as we are trained to do and to find ways in each unique encounter, whether as we speak or write, to become conscious of the implicit and explicit message and to become clearer about what we intend to communicate. While language can include gestures and actions, the focus of this discussion will be "the words, their pronunciation, and the methods of combining them used and understood by a community" (Language, n.d.), including both the health care community and those we are committed to serve.

A conversation about language cannot proceed without establishing the essential place of metaphor in the world of illness communication. Metaphor became a public focus of interest in 1978 when Susan Sontag (after being diagnosed with breast cancer) published *Illness as a Metaphor*. By discussing two diseases, tuberculosis and cancer, Sontag demonstrates how the public perception and the language chosen to describe disease and patients reflects an implicit message and attributed meaning that, in this conceptualization, included blaming the victim and associating disease to psychological traits. According to Sontag, the dynamics of this process serve to isolate and estrange patients and to create a false sense that those without illness can protect themselves from becoming an unfortunate victim of these diseases. Sontag pleads for discussion of disease free of metaphor. By 1989 when she published *AIDS and Its*

Metaphors (Sontag, 1989), cancer was being discussed more openly within clinical relationships and families and in the media but not necessarily without metaphor.

Metaphor is a figure of speech in which a word or phrase literally denoting one kind of object or idea is used in place of another to suggest a likeness or analogy between them (Metaphor, n.d.). Metaphors abound in clinical communication. Some are selected by patients and families and may be infused with expectations that are influenced by such variables as gender, culture, and role. Some are imposed, consciously or unconsciously, by the treatment team, advocacy groups, and the media. Generally they are not the focus of clinical inquiry, are not elicited or explored, nor tailored to the unique personal and illness-related circumstances of the patient. They often provide insight into the cognitive and emotional aspects of the illness experience and can help make sense of behaviors, emotional responses, and decisions. For example, a person who sees herself as a "fighter" engaged in a win-or-lose battle with a disease may be very reluctant to forego a resuscitation attempt because she equates such a decision with "giving up." Metaphors can be helpful if congruent with the values and personal characteristics of the patient; they can be isolating and dehumanizing when they are not responsive to the situation and the person on whom they are imposed (Reisfield & Wilson, 2004).

The fact that metaphors are contextual presents a curious dilemma. As patients and families move through transitions, they may discover that the metaphors that were useful and enabling at diagnosis become burdensome and diminishing as disease progresses. So, for example, the military and sports metaphors that infuse oncology create a win-or-lose construct and perhaps an experience of defeat and failure as disease progresses and end of life is anticipated. The metaphor of cancer as a journey, for some, is gentler and allows for twists and turns in the road, detours, hills, smooth or rocky roads, and many other variations along the way, including a period of feeling or being lost and changes in directions as the journey develops (Reisfield & Wilson, 2004). There may be a planned destination (such as cure of a disease), or the journey itself may be the source of meaning. Each variation implies an individualized approach to the illness experience.

While metaphors need to be respected, they can also be explored, reframed, or expanded when they do not allow for unintended consequences or the uncertainty that is implicit in living with life-threatening illness. Social workers who listen for metaphoric communication may intervene by joining the metaphor as in cultures where death and dying is approached through metaphor (for further discussion regarding this topic, see Chapter 63) or by gently exploring the meaning of metaphors that one anticipates will become less helpful as the illness experience evolves. Palliative care clinicians often work with patients through transitions, creating an opportunity to identify and adapt metaphor as a focus of intervention.

In addition to metaphor, this chapter will focus on words and phrases that pepper the care that palliative care clinicians provide to patients and families; what is said and what is heard. Some are setting specific and some are disease specific. To that end, this chapter will be divided into five sections: cancer, intensive care, palliative care, patients and families, and end of life. Of interest is that many patients and families within our fractured health care system move within and between these constructs very quickly. A patient in the intensive care unit (ICU) may go from being flooded with the language and technology of the ICU to the language and calm of a palliative care unit or transition from intense efforts to contain cancer to a suggestion that it is now time to focus on comfort, as though all efforts that came before did not have "comfort" as a concurrent goal. Patients may move from the "fight" mentality of oncology to a team of end-of-life clinicians who are focused on acceptance and do not perceive death to be a defeat. These transitions are often abrupt and incongruous and offer an opportunity for social work to identify and articulate this cacophonous experience and the confusion it sometimes engenders.

Words and Their Power

As well as consciousness about what words and phrases convey, Frederich Buechner's quote implies that words have power to make things happen, both inside the person who hears and the person who speaks. This speaks to the leadership potential that emanates from our communications whether they are spoken or written. "Care imitates language" (Sasser, 1999, p. 25). Consider that our relationships with people are influenced by the manner in which we write and speak of them. (Monroe, Holleman, & Holleman, 1992). Whether we depersonalize by identifying patients with their illnesses ("addict" or "sickler") or their emotional state ("overwhelmed," "in denial"), their behaviors ("noncompliant" or "nonadherent"), or their place in society (junkie), we risk losing their personhood and often cease our efforts to understand what informs their behaviors or emotional responses. In some instances the label of "addict" or "noncompliant" has grave impact on the willingness of medical staff to offer treatments. For example, chemotherapy may not be offered to someone who is labeled noncompliant for fear that he or she will be unable to follow up with the demands of treatment.

The words we select impact others physically, emotionally, cognitively, and behaviorally and may take the form of a cognitive-behavioral intervention. Just as we listen to the words and ideas expressed by patients and families to help us understand how we can best serve them, the words we use are suggestive; they can reframe, set expectation, bring forth memory, invite thoughts, and express a range of feelings (see Box 75.1).

Oncology and intensive care clinicians often say that patients have "failed" treatment or "failed" extubation to communicate with each other and with patients and families the

---

Box 75.1
Patient/Family Narrative: Jeanette

Jeanette is a 45-year-old single mother of two children, Jamal, age 6, and Tiffany, age 8. She is diagnosed with multiple myeloma and is referred to the palliative care consultation team for pain management and planning for the future care of Jamal and Tiffany. After a series of trials of pain medications, Jeanette is engaged in a discussion about a trial of methadone. She immediately refuses and breaks out in a sweat. Her anxiety is palpable. She asks the team to leave, refusing to try methadone. In an individual meeting with the palliative social worker, she shares that her mother struggled with addiction her entire life and attended a methadone maintenance clinic. Jeanette often came home from school and was greeted by her mother on the porch steps, nodding out. Her immediate visceral, cognitive and emotional response to the suggestion of methadone was infused with those memories, the identification and the associated painful emotions. Interventions included education about addiction and pain and assisting Jeanette to explore these early experiences in the safe setting of differentiating her life from that of her mother.

---

status of disease. While not intended to be judgmental, it implies that the patient has been unsuccessful or not made the grade, rather than making an objective statement about the outcome of treatments or simply stating that the person, due to his or her illness, is unable to breathe without assistance. In reading the rest of this chapter, consider cognitive-behavioral concepts such as overgeneralization, which are statements that are so general that they oversimplify reality (http://ksuweb.kennesaw.edu/~shagin/logfal-analysis-overgen.htm), and the all-or-nothing thinking that involves automatic thoughts which describe events in black-and-white categories, with no shades of gray (http://daphne.palomar.edu/di/allor.htm). It is useful to apply these concepts to phrases that have infused communication with patients, families, and each other, phrases that have the potential to cause inadvertent distress rather than affirming and suggesting possibility, no matter what the course of the illness.

Cancer

The language of oncology is replete with war and sports imagery. The National Cancer Act signed by Richard M. Nixon on December 23, 1971 (National Cancer Act of *1971*) launched what came to be called the war on cancer, a descriptive phrase which intended to bring "… . the same kind of concentrated effort that split the atom and took man to the moon … toward conquering this dread disease." (National Cancer Institute, n.d.) This public affirmation in the media of war imagery to describe cancer continues and was most vibrantly expressed on August 26, 2009, when much media coverage described Senator Edward Kennedy's death as a "lost battle with brain cancer." While many patients may

chose other metaphors to describe their cancer experience, it is difficult to protect oneself from the public discussion, which often uses imagery that projects a message of winning and losing, bravery and heroes. In addition to "body as battlefield," these metaphors do not represent a collaborative effort on behalf of the oncology clinicians and patient and family, but rather a hierarchal and authoritative relationship. The emphasis on the outcome, winning or losing, may deter patients and families from focusing on the process of living and valuing each day.

As one listens to the language that often surrounds cancer patients and their families, there is a delicate balance between a message of empowerment and a message of blame. "We will not be able to treat you unless your performance status improves; you need to eat and get out of bed." This statement can be the beginning of a dialogue designed to explore how the clinical team might assist the patient to meet these goals or the end of a conversation, leaving the patient demoralized, worried that he or she has disappointed the doctor, and the family wondering how to encourage the fighting spirit that might improve performance status and extend life. An unintended consequence of "battling cancer" is the related concepts of fighting to win and not giving up. It is as though a successful outcome is a matter of will obviating the uncertainty that is implicit when living with life-threatening illness. We will come back to this idea of how patients, families, and clinicians defend against uncertainty, magic, and mystery by presuming an ability to orchestrate the preferred outcome. Suffice to say that if cure or remission is a matter of will, then the responsibility for an unsuccessful outcome rests on the shoulders of the patient. In this context, family may struggle about their ability to motivate the patient or wonder whether their love and attachment lacked the power to fuel their fight for survival. In addition to the implication of failure, if there are no disease-modifying therapies that would be beneficial, there may also be an implied threat of abandonment exemplified by the infamous statement, "There is nothing more I can do for you." The utterance of this statement invites a clarification that the absence of additional disease-modifying therapies does not equate with the absence of ongoing care and intensive palliative interventions in collaboration with the oncology team. Patients may work with oncology clinicians for extended periods of time, and it is essential that these complex bonds be understood and respected to diminish a sense of abandonment and to create care plans that integrate the medical, psychosocial-spiritual history that is embedded within these relationships.

Palliative Care

Palliative care has its own complexity and challenges of language. We speak of life-threatening, life-limiting, or terminal illness; comfort or supportive care; withholding or withdrawing; futile or inappropriate; burden and barriers;

and do not resuscitate orders. It is often infused with what we "do not consider appropriate" rather than reinforcing what will be provided. Depending on the trajectory of illness, patients and families may engage with palliative clinicians as they are transitioning from the language of "aggressive care" to "comfort care" with neither phrase providing substantive information about the specific interventions that are no longer beneficial and the ones that they are to receive. Often families are asked, "Do you want everything done?" as though the choice is "everything" or "nothing." In the course of establishing goals of care and creating treatment plans, patients and families bring phrases that represent their worries and fears; "no hope," "starving the patient," "pulling the plug," and "giving up" are but a sample. There is conversation about withdrawing "care" when what we intend is to consider withdrawing "treatments" that are no longer helpful or have begun to cause harm. Often a patient and/or the patient's "body" will speak; the body's response to interventions will declare whether there is a positive effect and thereby inform those decisions.

Withholding care is a powerful phrase implying that clinicians are denying access as opposed to foregoing an intervention that is expected to be nonbeneficial. The language used in discussions about nutritional support provides opportunity for clarification. While infused with cultural and emotional significance, clinicians often complicate discussions by using the terms feeding and food. For many, feeding implies a shared social experience that is chosen and not forced. It involves taste and flavor. Artificial hydration and nutrition is a medical treatment void of the social attributes and pleasure that accompanies feeding and food (Shannon & Walter, 1990).

Patients and Families

Whether at home or in an institutional setting, social workers and palliative clinicians who work with family as the "unit of care" need to consider the clarity with which they communicate essential medical information. In the setting of technology, engaging distant and working family members becomes much more possible and allows medical staff to deliver medical information directly rather than through family members, who integrate and share through their own emotions and lay understandings.

The language used to describe patients and families, whether between clinicians, at team meetings, or in medical records is often as important as the language we listen for and use in our direct communications. Descriptors such as "dysfunctional," "noncompliant," "nonadherent," "in denial," "entitled," "unrealistic," and "overwhelmed" invite social work assessment and intervention; they often follow patients and family members through transitions and along the continuum of illness and elicit responses and biases from new staff based on the judgments, valid or not, of previous clinicians.

End of Life

Attending to the words and phrases that are often heard in end-of-life care requires a thoughtful vigilance. These include such concepts as "unfinished business," "giving permission to die," "letting go," and "hang a morphine drip" among others. Considering the implications of words and phrases that have been integrated into practice over the years raises consciousness, teaches, and encourages reflection and growth. For example, the infusion of cultural sensitivity and respect has challenged the idea that discussion of "death" must be free of euphemism. We have learned that the directness that some may value can be assaultive to others of another culture who speak of "passing," "crossing over," or "aged away." (For additional information, see Chapter 63.) The thought that an imminently dying person "holds on" or "lets go" with intention is not necessarily a cause-and-effect phenomenon and in some ironic way validates the idea that "will" may determine whether someone lives or dies. When we choose to engage and encourage patients and families in these concepts, it is important at the same time to affirm and recognize the uncertainty, magic, and mystery of life and death rather than projecting a "certainty" where there can be none. The idea that one might "give permission to die" is a complex emotional dynamic that in some spiritual systems may be viewed as presumptuous, and in some family systems may be incongruous with authentic feelings.

The Intensive Care Unit

Patients in the intensive care unit and their families are asked to learn a new language in the setting of an unfamiliar environment of sights, sounds, and machines that for many create an emotional and cognitive response that impacts integration of information. Essential decision making takes place in this setting as the staff cares emergently for patients at the same time they are engaging their families to guide the course of that care. In addition to a unique environment, there are often multiple consultants such as nephrologists or neurologists who are interested in one organ system or one set of lab values which may be improving. These consultants might observe a positive change and inform the family of "progress" at the same time the family receives information that the patient is getting sicker and might not survive.

Oftentimes consultants speak of one body part while intensivists give information about overall condition, a peculiar and confusing experience based not in language but more in the context from which clinicians speak. Of additional interest are discussions about "terminal extubation," which in some settings means that the ventilator will be removed and not replaced should the patient be unable to sustain himself or herself and perhaps more aptly described as final extubation; at other times this phrase means that the patient is expected to die soon after extubation. Equipment in the intensive care unit poses another challenge to clear and precise communication. Often referred to as "life support," there are times when families are asked to integrate brain death status at the same time that they are advised that "life support" equipment will be removed.

Conclusion

Vigilance about language is only a beginning. Many clinicians are completely unaware about the effect of the words they choose and would never intend to confuse, blame, or harm patients. Many patients and families integrate descriptors such as "terminally ill" and are never asked to consider what that descriptor means to them or to the person who first described their illness in those words. Perhaps it is in the land of extremes that we need to develop a caution. Breaking "all-or-nothing" communication into discrete parts is a beginning of dispelling the power of certain phrases and moving from a flurry of words to a conversation of meaning. "He would want everything done" moves from an exchange about "everything" to an understanding of what "everything" means in the setting of a unique person and a unique constellation of medical factors. "Everything" may mean any intervention that will return me to my former level of function, but not interventions that serve to extend life on a ventilator. Conversations that involve "black-and-white descriptors," "everything or nothing," or "hope or no hope" invite social work clinicians to explore meaning and intent; the world of palliative care is often gray and requires clinicians to join with patients and families in this land of uncertainty.

As palliative care continues to infuse medical culture and institutions, it behooves those of us who are able to follow patients and families through transitions over time to become aware of the fact that clinicians understand palliative care in different ways, some viewing the work as focused on end of life rather than care along the continuum of illness often in consultation with primary teams. Describing palliative care as providing support or comfort care may leave many patients and families confused and uncertain. This language does not equate with the expert and vigilant medical care they might expect as their family members lives with life-threatening illness. Clarity about the specialty of palliative care and the social work skill set that enriches the specialty will contribute to less ambiguous communication.

At times the task of vigilance in language requires that we listen for innuendo and move conversations from implicit to an explicit exchange. For example, in many settings the phrase "hang a morphine drip" has ominous meaning and equates with end of life and perhaps even hastened death. Palliative and hospice social workers who engage this conversation and begin a discussion of symptom management at end of life can assist practitioners to make decisions about a morphine infusion as a medical treatment for the management of symptoms, rather than as an intervention that is begun with no clinical assessment and critical thinking.

Listening for and eliciting metaphors invites clinical work that explores their coherence not only with the patients and their illness experience but also the implications for clinicians. Working in a world of "win/lose" metaphoric communication potentially leaves all participants in the war demoralized; patients, families, and clinicians who join together to "fight the good fight." It is interesting to consider how social workers might intervene to change language that is less than helpful. Sometimes the intervention involves partializing "all-or-nothing" communication; sometimes it is simply repeating the same information but in a manner that corrects or expands the focus from "nothing or all" to specifics that can be explored and considered in decision making and care planning.

Beyond the conversation with patients and families is the exchange during team meetings and the written record that often follows patients from team to team. Raising consciousness through shared learning has the potential to move the responsibility for vigilance in language and communication from social work to the entire team. This can only benefit patients and families and the systems in which we practice.

LEARNING EXERCISES

- In the safety of your interdisciplinary team or your class group, role play exchanges between medical practitioners, patients, and families that use some of the words and phrases in this chapter. Create a scenario in which you are working with a patient in the intensive care unit to determine goals of care and appropriate treatments that will provide benefit. As you have this exchange, make efforts to use language that has the following characteristics:

  - It is specific and clear.
  - It presents options that balance what will be provided as well as interventions that might have no benefit or do harm.

- Consider the most and least intimidating colleague in your practice setting. Imagine that they both continue to use the statement, "There is nothing more I can do for you" when speaking with patients whose illnesses are progressing. Work with a trusted colleague to create possibilities for leadership and intervention to mitigate the emotional impact on patients and their families. Project the risks and benefits of calling attention to the problematic statement in both the most and least intimidating of your colleagues. What direct and indirect approaches may be helpful? Consider practicing the intervention within a safe relationship while evaluating outcome and adapting approach.

ADDITIONAL SUGGESTED READINGS

Abratt, R. P. (2003). When the tumor is not the target: A title whose time is up? *Journal of Clinical Oncology, 21,* 4463–4468.

Casarett, D., Pickard, A., Fishman, J. M., Alexander, S. C., Arnold, R. M., Pollak, K. I., & Tulsky, J. A. (2010). Can metaphors and analogies improve communication with seriously ill patients. *Journal of Palliative Medicine, 13*(3), 255–260.

Gibbs, R. W., & Franks, H. (2002). Embodied metaphor in women's narratives about their experiences with cancer. *Health Communications, 14,* 139–165.

Lakoff, G., & Johnson, M. (1980). *Metaphors we live by.* Chicago, IL: University of Chicago Press.

Mabeck, C. E., & Olesen, F. (1997). Metaphorically transmitted diseases: How do patients embody medical explanations? *Family Practice, 14,* 271–278.

Sims, P. A. (2003). Working with metaphor. *American Journal of Psychotherapy, 57,* 528–536.

Skott, C. (2002). Expressive metaphors in cancer narratives. *Cancer Nursing, 25,* 230–235.

REFERENCES

Buechner, F. (1992). *Listening to your life: Daily meditations with Frederick Buechner.* New York, NY: Harper Collins Publishers.

Language. (n.d.). In *Merriam-Webster's online dictionary.* Retrieved from http://www.merriam-webster.com/dictionary/language

Metaphor. (n.d.). In *Merriam-Webster's online dictionary.* Retrieved from http://www.merriam-webster.com/dictionary/metaphor

Monroe, W., Holleman, W.L. & Holleman, M.C. (1992) "Is There a Person in This Case?", *Literature and Medicine, 11* (1), 45–63.

National Cancer Act of 1971, Pub. L. No. 92–218. Retrieved from http://dtp.nci.nih.gov/timeline/noflash/milestones/M4_Nixon.htm

National Cancer Institute. (n.d.). *Milestone (1971) National Cancer Act of 1971.* Retrieved from http://dtp.nci.nih.gov/timeline/noflash/milestones/M4_Nixon.htm

Reisfield, G. M., & Wilson, G. R. (2004) Use of metaphor in the discourse on cancer. *Journal of Clinical Oncology, 22*(19), 4024–4027.

Sasser, C. G. (1999). The interdisciplinary team. In S. K. Joishy (Ed.), *Palliative medicine secrets* (pp. 21–27). Philadelphia, PA: Hanley & Belfus Ins.

Shannon, J. J., & Walter, T. A. (1990). Quality of life. In J. J. Shannon & T. A. Walter (Eds.), *Quality of life: The new medical dilemma* (pp. 203–223). Mahwah, NJ: Paulist Press.

Sontag, S. (1978). *Illness as metaphor.* New York, NY: Farrar, Straus & Giroux.

Sontag, S (1989). *AIDS and its metaphors.* New York, NY: Farrar, Straus & Giroux.

76 *Ellen L. Csikai and Barbara L. Jones*

Professional Development: Educational Opportunities and Resources

A social worker builds your confidence and self-esteem.

—*11-year-old boy with cancer*

Key Concepts
- ◆ *A wide range of formal and informal educational resources is available for social work learners.*
- ◆ *Palliative social workers have many professional conferences and continuing education options available.*
- ◆ *Many social networking opportunities exist for palliative social workers.*

Introduction

A wide variety of opportunities exist that provide training for social workers interested in or already working in the field of palliative and end-of-life care. From social work students to practitioners with years of experience, such resources help to enhance the competence of social workers at all levels of practice. The resources discussed in this chapter include undergraduate- and graduate-level courses, certificate programs, fellowships, continuing education courses, and Webinars and seminars offered through professional organizations.

Schools of Social Work

Social work educational programs, at bachelor's, master's, and doctoral levels, may offer specific courses in end-of-life and palliative care or related courses in grief, loss, and bereavement. Social work students may also find some of this material covered in social work courses in health care. Many of these courses provide a beginning overview of the field for students who, as practitioners, will come into contact with people receiving end-of-life and palliative care or those who are grieving or in the bereavement process in any practice setting in which they will be employed. Courses at the bachelor's level tend to be more general in nature and provide an overview of death, dying, and bereavement issues. Those at the master's level range from general to specialty courses, such as end-of-life decision making, chronic illness, and pediatric palliative and end-of-life care. A few courses are also available through social work programs that are designed to involve students of other disciplines, including pastoral care, nursing, or medical students. One School of Social Work (University of Iowa) offers a Field of Practice specialization in the master's program. Another school (University of Texas at Austin) offers an Interdisciplinary Seminar in Psychosocial Oncology. Specialized courses may also be offered on the doctoral level depending on the expertise of faculty members in a particular school (Csikai & Jones, 2007)

Certificate Programs

Zelda Foster Studies in Palliative and End-of-Life Care

Zelda Foster was a pioneer in the development of the hospice movement in the United States. She was a true leader in the field of palliative and end-of-life care throughout her career. This program was named in her honor; its mission was modeled after her commitment to the field and to recognize her tremendous contributions to this social work specialty. The program currently has three initiatives: The Post-Master's Certificate Program, the Zelda Foster Fellowship, and in 2011, a Post-Master's Leadership Program, funded by a grant from the Fan Fox and Leslie R. Samuels Foundation, Inc. All of these programs are offered at the Silver School of Social Work at New York University.

The Post-Master's Certificate Program in Palliative and End of Life Care is offered annually and consists of four classes that integrate theory and practice. Classes meet every other week for 2 hours for 10 weeks and participants are eligible for 80 continuing education credits (CEUs). The program is open to social workers with at least 2 years of post-master's degree experience in palliative and end-of-life care. The program to date has had over 150 graduates, many of whom have gone on to assume leadership positions in palliative and end-of-life care. For more information, see: http://www.nyu.edu/socialwork/pdf/1241189616.pdf.

The Zelda Foster Fellowship Program enrolls current master's-level students. The selected student fellows participate in a 4-year program that begins in the final year of the master's in social work program and also includes 2 years of one-on-one mentoring after graduation. The fellows have a focused field placement in palliative and end-of-life care, attend monthly seminars, and receive financial support for conferences and advanced training.

The third initiative is the Post-Master's Leadership Certificate. It is a new program for social workers currently practicing in the field of palliative and end-of-life care who have leadership potential and at least 5 years post-master's degree experience in palliative and end-of-life care. It is a 3-year grant project that begins in 2010 with training for the first group of leaders in 2011. For more information on any of these initiatives, contact Dr. Susan Gerbino at susan. gerbino@nyu.edu.

Smith College/Bay State Medical Center End-of-Life Certificate Program

Another end-of-life certificate program is offered by Smith College and is sponsored by Bay State Medical Center in Northampton, MA. It is comprehensive and clinically focused and includes 14 courses and a 6-month clinically supervised internship. Participants are eligible for 63 CEUs. The program consists of two weekends of intensive coursework at the Smith College School for Social Work. Students must participate in a clinical internship in which they have an opportunity to work with at least three patients and families and lead one clinical group. Students participate in a monthly interdisciplinary peer supervision team so that they may incorporate what they learn in the coursework into their practices. Students also receive 2 hours of telephone clinical supervision each month and six sessions of telephonic group supervision. At the end of the internship, students write a final paper related to clinical theory, practice, and/or leadership. The program, now in its 10th year, has over 175 graduates. According to program leaders, graduates of the program have gone on to assume leadership positions in the field of palliative and end-of-life care, write successful grant proposals, develop needed community programs, teach, write, and conduct research. For more information, see: http://www.smith.edu/ssw/geaa/academics_cecertificate.php

Social Work Palliative Care Fellowships

Department of Veterans Affairs

A national interprofessional palliative care fellowship program was funded in 2002 by the Department of Veterans Affairs with the aim of providing the best possible care for the nation's veterans by transforming care of the seriously ill within their network. A total of six fellowships across the country are currently funded. Those eligible for this 1-year fellowship include physicians, nurses, psychologists, social workers, and pharmacists. Applicants must demonstrate motivation and the ability to assume leadership roles to promote palliative and end-of-life care, a commitment to interdisciplinary practice, and expressed interest in employment in the Veterans Health Administration system. One primary goal is to develop experts who demonstrate the clinical knowledge, skills, and attitudes to establish palliative care as the standard of care for veterans suffering from chronic, progressive, life-threatening illness. Teaching methods include classroom activities, clinical training, and interactive/participatory educational activities, including mentorship. Examples are programs at the Bronx Veterans Medical Center in New York (http://www.nynj.va.gov/grecc.asp) and the Veterans Administration Palo Alto Health Care System in California. For information about these fellowships, contact Sheila Kennedy at: sheila.kennedy@va.gov.

Beth Israel Medical Center

The Department of Pain Medicine and Palliative Care at Beth Israel Medical Center offers a postgraduate social work fellowship in palliative and end-of-life care. The social work fellowship was established in 2000, with a grant from the Open Society Institute Project on Death in America (PDIA) through their Social Work Leadership Award and receives ongoing support through the Barbara Zirinsky Fund. The fellowship program provides a supervised experience in the multidimensional assessment and care of patients. Fellows are involved in multiple practice sites (an inpatient pain, palliative care, and hospice unit; inpatient consultation service; and an ambulatory practice) and work with patients and families along the continuum of life-threatening illness. Fellows participate in various learning experiences, including interdisciplinary rounds, case discussions, didactic conferences, and departmental meetings. The primary focus is on multidimensional assessment and interventions in the management of symptoms and in the care of patients and families. The program is designed to develop role models, leaders, and mentors in social work practice in palliative care. The fellowship is 1 year in length and includes a stipend and benefits. For more information, see: http://www.stoppain.org.

University of Minnesota Medical Center, Fairview

A postgraduate Clinical Social Work Fellowship in Palliative Care is offered through the Transitions and Life Choices program of the University of Minnesota Medical Center, Fairview. Supervised clinical social work experience is provided on an inpatient interdisciplinary consultation service and in an outpatient palliative care clinic. Fellows participate in training experiences that include palliative care team rounds and case discussions, teaching rounds, journal club, palliative care training, and department planning meetings. Fellows are also expected to participate in clinical research. A goal of the program is to train leaders in palliative care clinical social work with a particular emphasis on advocacy. The fellowship is 9 months in length. For more information, see: http://www.fairview.org/tlc/social-workfellowship/index.asp.

Pediatric Palliative Care Fellowship

The Pediatric Advanced Care Team (PACT), the pediatric palliative care service at Children's Hospital Boston and the Dana Farber Cancer Institute, offer a full-time, academic year social work fellowship. PACT is an interdisciplinary team dedicated to improving symptoms and quality of life of children with advanced illness. The team includes physicians, nurses, chaplains, communication specialists, psychologists, child life specialists, social workers, and so forth. The fellowship provides the opportunity to offer clinical services to patients and families as well as work with related community services. PACT provides inpatient and outpatient services and care in the community. The fellow

functions as part of a multidisciplinary team and is responsible for consultation with other medical providers. This fellowship provides opportunities to attend PACT educational rounds featuring multidisciplinary experts in the field of pediatric palliative care, as well as other seminars offered at both the Children's Hospital and the Dana Farber Cancer Institute. For more information, see: http://www.children-shospital.org/clinicalservices/Site2266/mainpageS2266P8-sublevel9.html

The PACT fellowship is the only pediatric social work, end-of-life, and palliative care fellowship in the United States.

Conferences Sponsored by National Organizations

The National Hospice and Palliative Care Organization (NHPCO) sponsors several national conferences. For many years two annual conferences have been held: the Clinical Team and the Management and Leadership Conferences. Recently, more specialized or targeted conferences have been organized to focus on various topics such as diversity in palliative and end-of-life care and pediatrics. For more information, see: http://www.nhpco.org/templates/1/homepage.cfm

The American Academy of Hospice and Palliative Medicine (AAHPM) sponsors an Annual Assembly in conjunction with the Hospice and Palliative Nurses Association (HPNA). Social work presence in this organization is growing as is attendance at these conferences. A preconference session exclusively for social workers was held for the first time in 2008 and is ongoing. The pre-conference session is coordinated by the leaders of the Social Work Hospice and Palliative Care Network (SWHPN). For more information, see: http://www.swhpn.org or http://www.aahpm.org

Other professional membership organizations provide workshops and seminars at national meetings on topics related to palliative and end-of-life care. Organizations such as the Association of Pediatric Oncology Social Work (APOSW), the Association of Oncology Social Work (AOSW), the National Association of Perinatal Social Workers (NAPSW), and the National Organization for Hospice and Palliative Care (NHPCO) all offer national trainings for social workers. APOSW (http://www.aposw.org) and AOSW (http://www.aosw.org), specifically, have special interest groups for social workers interested in pediatric or adult palliative and end-of-life care. Each conference annually offers workshops and keynote and preconference sessions that focus on the needs of children, adults, and families receiving palliative and end-of-life care. Additionally, the Association of Death Education and Counseling (http://www.adec.org) and American Psychosocial Oncology Society (http://www.apos.org) offer annual conferences that are multidisciplinary and touch on a range of issues, including palliative, end-of-life care and grief and bereavement. ADEC is a professional membership organization that promotes excellence and diversity in death education, including a wide range of topics in thanatology, such as care for the dying, bereavement and grief issues, and cutting-edge research in the field. And APOS is a multidisciplinary membership organization dedicated to the psychosocial care of oncology patients, survivors, and families.

Continuing Professional Education Curricula

The Social Work End-of-Life Education Project

The Social Work End-of-Life Education Project began in 2001. The curriculum was based on the results of a national survey of social work clinicians working in palliative and end-of-life care in various practice settings (conducted by Ellen L. Csikai, MSW, MPH, PhD, and Mary Raymer, LMSW, ACSW, DPNAP). Data were collected regarding many aspects of professional practice, including previous education and perceptions of the educational content and skills needed to practice in this specialty area. The project, including the survey and educational curriculum development, was funded with a 2-year Social Work Leadership Development Award from the Soros Foundation, Open Society Institute's Project on Death in America. The project has become a full, 2-day curriculum presented by two experienced social work clinicians who practice in the field of palliative and end-of-life care. The curriculum has typically been offered as a preconference at the National Hospice and Palliative Care Organization's Clinical Team Conference and has been sponsored by social work groups around the country and in Singapore. Participants are eligible for 15 hours of CEUs. For more information, e-mail Mary Raymer: raymermsw@aol.com.

Promoting Excellence in Pain Management and Palliative Care for Social Workers

The Promoting Excellence course developed as a sister program to the National Cancer Institute–funded ACE Project: Advocating for Clinical Excellence—Transdisciplinary Palliative Care Education study (Otis-Green et al., 2009) as a social work–specific program to highlight the achievements of social work leaders in pain management and palliative care (Otis-Green, Lucas, Spolum, Ferrell, & Grant, 2008). This annual foundation-funded training was developed through the Southern California Cancer Pain Initiative (SCCPI) at the City of Hope to offer evidence-informed, clinically relevant continuing education using an interactive skills-building format. A two-track format allow learners an opportunity to customize their educational experience by selecting workshops that focus upon either advanced content or on the development of core competencies in pain

management and palliative care. The American Society on Aging recognized this course with the 2008 Healthcare and Aging Network Award for "innovation and quality." To learn more, see: http://sccpi.coh.org/.

Cancer Care for the Whole Patient: An Oncology Social Work Response

ExCEL in Social Work is a National Cancer Institute–funded leadership-training program that addresses the six critical aspects of psychosocial support necessary for oncology social workers to meet the standard of care recommended by the Institute of Medicine (IOM) 2008 Report. This is accomplished through a collaborative partnership between the City of Hope and the Association of Oncology Social Work (AOSW) and the Association of Pediatric Oncology Social Work (APOSW). A variety of evidence-based educational strategies were incorporated into this comprehensive educational effort to maximize impact and measure effectiveness, including intensive preconference trainings held in conjunction with the AOSW and APOSW annual organizational meetings. Shirley Otis-Green is the principal investigator for this national training program: sotis-green@coh.org. http://www.cityofhope.org/education/health-professional-education/nursing-education/excel/Pages/default.aspx

The Initiative for Pediatric Palliative Care

The Initiative for Pediatric Palliative Care (IPPC) is an evidence-based educational initiative that offers 2–3-day workshops for interdisciplinary teams and bereaved parents to learn together how to best provide pediatric palliative care. IPPC was started in 1998 as a "research, quality improvement, and education effort aimed at enhancing family-centered care for children living with life-threatening conditions" (http://www.ippcweb.org). This training has been offered to over 2000 participants in the United States to date and provides knowledge and skills to health care professionals in a collaborative learning environment. The IPPC sells its award-winning DVDs and training curriculum. For more information, see: http://www.ippcweb.org.

International Research Summer School

The International Research Summer School at Lancaster University's International Observatory on End-of-Life Care is an introduction (advanced) to social research methods used in end-of-life care research. The course is offered for those in any discipline involved in palliative and end-of-life care and is primarily geared toward those at an early stage in developing their own research. The course is taught by expert researchers in palliative and end-of-life care. The Summer

School takes place over a period of 2 weeks and participants may choose to attend one or both weeks. The first week consists of classroom-based learning using diverse teaching methods. In the second week, there is an opportunity for group discussion and individual sessions to help in the development of individual research ideas and projects. For further information, see: http://www.eolc-observatory. net/education/school.htm or contact Iris Cohen Fineberg, PhD, MSW, at: i.fineberg@lancaster.ac.uk.

Doctoral Training

School of Health and Medicine, Lancaster University, United Kingdom

The first doctorate in palliative care program began in June 2010 in the School of Health and Medicine at Lancaster University. It is an international part-time program designed for people working in palliative, hospice, and end-of-life care. The program's objectives are to create leaders in palliative care; to promote the development of advanced knowledge and practice; to foster critical approaches to evidence review; to enhance scholarship and research skills and to develop a critical unde rstanding of policy and practice. Teaching is primarily delivered through distance e-learning along with intensive sessions in Lancaster, United Kingdom. Research elements can be undertaken in the students' home environments and supervised by faculty from Lancaster. For more information, see: http://www.eolc-observatory.net/education/doctorate.htm.

Internet/Online Educational Resources

The National Association of Social Workers

Continuing education courses, developed by the National Association of Social Workers (NASW) national office, are offered by their WebEd program (online). Social workers who take courses and pass the exams will receive CEUs. Most courses are eligible for two CEUs. In the area of palliative and end-of-life care, two courses are offered: End-of-Life Care: The Social Worker's Role, and Achieving Cultural Competence to Reduce Health Disparities in End-of-Life Care. Both members and nonmembers of NASW may enroll in these courses. For more information, see: http://www.naswwebed.org.

Webinars

The National Hospice and Palliative Care Organization sponsors a host of Web-based continuing education courses.

NHPCO EDGE Webinars are offered twice a month on interdisciplinary and leadership topics. Individual or organizational members may participate. For more information, see: http://www.nhpco.org/i4a/pages/index.cfm?pageid=3268

The Center for the Advancement of Palliative Care (CAPC) is an excellent resource for all professionals working in end-of-life and palliative care. It is a clearinghouse of educational tools and also offers its own Webinars, online courses, audio conferences, and in-person seminars geared to an interdisciplinary audience. For more information, see: http://www.capc.org.

The Social Work Hospice and Palliative Care Network has worked with the Center to Advance Palliative Care (further description later) to sponsor Webinars and has also begun to offer its own Webinars to members. For more information, see: http://www.swhpn.org

The Association for Death Education and Counseling hosts a number of Webinars on topics such as Cultural Perspectives on Dying, Death and Grief, Complicated Grief, and Ethical Practice in Grief Counseling. For more information, see: http://www.adec.org/distance/webinars.cfm

Electronic Discussion Forums

The Social Work Network in Palliative and End-of-Life Care. The Social Work Network in Palliative and End-of-Life Care is an electronic (e-mail) discussion forum that began in 1999 to provide an opportunity for social workers interested in palliative and end-of-life care to communicate around issues that are important to patients, families, and professionals. The network links over 530 social workers around the world.

The listserv was initially supported by a Social Work Leadership Award from the Project on Death in America and the Department of Pain Medicine and Palliative Care, Beth Israel Medical Center, New York. It is currently supported by the Department and the Barbara Zirinsky Fund. The intention is to connect social workers with similar interests who work in a variety of practice settings, including geriatrics, hospice, oncology, nephrology, and pediatrics. The primary goal is to enhance communication, networking, and collaboration regarding clinical, education, research, policy, and professional issues. Over the years, the list has served to identify areas of commonality and unmet needs of social workers practicing in all aspects of palliative and end-of-life care. All messages are archived, which allows members to retrieve previous information. Those interested in joining this e-mail discussion group may send an e-mail request to Terry Altilio, LCSW, at: taltilio@chpnet.org.

My NHPCO. The National Hospice and Palliative Care Organization now has a social networking site: My.NHPCO. This online networking community is able to connect hospice and palliative care professionals and volunteers (members) from across the country. Through the site, members can share their experiences and knowledge with their peers. Features include the ability to use a blog that allows participants to engage in end-of-life care discussions, share documents, rank resources, and be involved in eGroups, e-mail discussion groups. There are eGroups that are already set up for discussion and others that are established based on suggested topics of interest to members. Members can search previous discussions and share documents through the eGroups. It is believed that this will allow for greater professional discussion that can enhance practice across the country (Radulovic, 2009).

*Social Work in Hospice and Palliative Care Network (SWHPN).*The Social Work in Hospice and Palliative Care Network is a network of social workers who seek to further the field of end-of-life and hospice/palliative care. The goal of the organization is to advance the role of the social worker in caring for the seriously ill, providing relief from pain, improving quality of life, supporting family and friends, assisting with difficult decision making, and coping with trauma, grief, and loss. This network grew out of the Social Work Leadership Development Awards Program, sponsored by the Open Society Institute's Project on Death in America, a project of the Soros Foundation. The organization offers members professional conferences, discussion forums, the Social Work Leadership Award, and opportunities for networking. The discussion forum offers information about issues relevant to social work in palliative and end-of-life care and sponsors a monthly "meet the expert" forum. SWHPN also hosts Webinars on topics relevant to the field of social work in end-of-life and palliative care. For additional information, see: http://www.swhpn.org/

Other Online Professional Educational Resources

Center to Advance Palliative Care

The Center to Advance Palliative Care (CAPC) is a national organization with a mission to increase the availability of quality palliative care services to people facing serious illness and their families and caregivers. To this end, health care professionals are provided with the tools, training, and technical assistance necessary to start and sustain successful palliative care programs in hospitals and other health care settings through its publications and Web-based resources, training seminars, and audio conferences. While it is a membership organization, membership is not required to access its resources. The official journal of the organization is the *Journal of Palliative Medicine.* Funding for the organization comes from several private foundations, and technical support is provided by the Mount Sinai School of Medicine in New York (CAPC, 2010). To access the organization's resources, go to: http://www.capc.org.

End-of-Life/Palliative Education Resource Center

The End-of-Life/Palliative Education Resource Center (EPERC) began in 2003, supported by a grant from the Robert Wood Johnson Foundation. The Center continues to have support from the Medical College of Wisconsin. The purpose of EPERC is to share educational resource materials among professional educators involved in palliative care education. It is an online resource where visitors to the site can search for and download educational materials. Users can find materials related to such content areas as pain, nonpain symptoms, communications skills, ethics, terminal care, and clinical interventions used near the end of life (EPERC, 2010). There are also suggested articles of interest and links to clinical and educational Web resource centers. Also offered is a monthly e-newsletter. Although the site was developed to assist those teaching in medical schools, it is a useful resource for all professionals and those not only involved in teaching, but in practice as well. For more information, see: http://www.eperc.mcw.edu

Conclusion

The educational resources and opportunities mentioned in this chapter are not meant to constitute an exhaustive list. As the field grows, so will the resources available to support and educate social work clinicians. Those discussed here are a sampling of some of the current educational, professional, and networking opportunities for social workers in palliative and end-of-life care. Together, these organizations, schools of social work, and various other programs and forums are creating an infrastructure that can provide needed education and training to enhance practice and to advance the specialty of palliative social work.

ADDITIONAL SUGGESTED READINGS

Csikai, E. L., & Chaitin, E. (2005). *Ethics and end-of-life decisions in social work practice.* Chicago, IL: Lyceum Books, Inc.

REFERENCES

Csikai, E. L., & Jones, B. (2007). *Teaching resources for end-of-life and palliative care.* Chicago, IL: Lyceum Books, Inc.
Center to Advance Palliative Care (CAPC). (2009). *Frequently asked questions.* Retrieved from http://www.capc.org/about-capc/faqs
End-of-Life/Palliative Education Resource Center (EPERC). (n.d.). *About EPERC.* Retrieved from http://www.eperc.mcw.edu/ EPERC
Otis-Green, S., Ferrell, B., Spolum, M., Uman, G., Mullan, P., Baird, P., & Grant, M. (2009). An overview of the ACE

project—Advocating for Clinical Excellence: Transdisciplinary palliative care education. *Journal of Cancer Education, 24*(2), 120–126.

Otis-Green, S., Lucas, S., Spolum, M., Ferrell, B., & Grant, M. (2008). Promoting excellence in pain management and palliative care for social workers. *Journal of Social Work in End-of-Life and Palliative Care, 4*(2), 120–134.

Radulovic, J. (2009). NHPCO steps boldly into the realm of social networking with MyNHPCO. *Newsline: Quarterly Insights Edition, September,* 39–42.

77 *Ellen L. Csikai*

Professional Connections for Palliative Social Workers

It was so helpful to meet with other like-minded peers. As the only palliative social worker in my institution, I often feel like a "lone ranger." Joining with other palliative social workers has been so energizing.

—Anonymous

Key Concepts

♦ *Opportunities are increasing for social workers to be engaged in palliative care education.*

♦ *a growing synergy of professional organizations exists from around the world that are interested in advancing the field of palliative social work.*

♦ *Social workers are welcome members in multidisciplinary palliative care organizations.*

Introduction

As palliative social workers, staying connected to the field, including keeping abreast of new knowledge, is part of our professional responsibility. One way to do so is through membership in professional organizations, several of which are available as a support for social workers in the field of palliative and end-of-life care. Membership organizations typically charge a fee in exchange for offering "member benefits" that may include opportunities for networking with fellow palliative care professionals, continuing education, and access to professional journals. As expected due to the interdisciplinary nature of palliative care practice, social work–specific membership organizations are joined by others which are interdisciplinary and some which are also international. This chapter focuses first on the various organizations and their specific links to palliative care practice and secondly on certification, another aspect of maintaining professional connection and credibility in the field. A certification, developed through a collaborative effort between the National Association of Social Workers (NASW) and the National Hospice and Palliative Care Organization (NHPCO), is now available for social workers practicing in hospice and palliative care environments.

Social Work–Specific Organizations

National Association of Social Workers

The largest membership organization of social workers in the United States is the National Association of Social Workers (NASW). All social workers, at all levels of social work education, in any field of practice, are encouraged to join and there are over 150,000 members. While the organization's membership is diverse, NASW develops practice resources and policy statements to meet the needs of this diverse membership. NASW members are also able to join a "specialty" practice section (SPS). Social workers working in palliative care may choose to join the Health Specialty Section, which is targeted toward social workers serving in both direct and indirect practice in health settings such as acute care, case management, pediatrics, chronic care, advocacy, administration, rehabilitation, and public health. Members of the specialty sections have an opportunity for practice-related chats, teleconferences (free continuing educational units), and they receive newsletters containing articles that may be of general interest to the members.

With respect to palliative and end-of-life care specifically, in 2004, NASW published "Standards for Social Work Practice in Palliative and End-of-Life Care." These standards were "designed to enhance social workers' awareness of the skills, knowledge, values, methods, and sensitivities needed to work effectively with clients, families, health care providers, and the community when working in end of life situations" (NASW, 2009a). There are 11 standards that cover the following areas: ethics and values; knowledge; assessment; intervention/treatment planning; attitude/self-awareness; empowerment and advocacy; documentation; interdisciplinary teamwork; cultural competence; continuing education; and leadership, supervision, and training. These practice standards are available through the NASW Web site. NASW policy statements on "End-of-Life Care" and "Hospice Care" can be found in the NASW Press publication, *Social Work Speaks, 8th edition, NASW Policy Statements 2009-2012*. In addition, NASW developed and currently offers (free of charge to members and nonmembers) two separate Web-ed courses to further social workers' continuing education needs in end-of-life and palliative care: Understanding End-of-Life Care: The Social Worker's Role and Achieving Cultural Competence in Reducing Health Disparities in End-of-Life Care. For more information, see: http://www.naswdc.org.

The Social Work Hospice and Palliative Care Network

The Social Work Hospice and Palliative Care Network (SWHPN) is a recently formed (2007) and emerging network of social work practitioners/leaders who seek to further the field of end-of-life and hospice/palliative care. The organization aims to advance the role of the social worker in caring for the seriously ill. The network is supported by funds from the Open Society Institute and membership fees and contributions. The network originally grew out of the Social Work Leadership Development Award Program (SWLDA), which was sponsored by the Open Society Institute's Project on Death in America (PDIA), a project of the Soros Foundation. The PDIA program helped coordinate the 1st Social Work Summit on End-of-Life and Palliative Care in 2002. At this meeting, a consensus process created a priority map for furthering the field. The 2nd Social Work Summit, held in June 2005, created a steering committee to coordinate next steps in the development of this field of practice for social workers. Goals of the network are to build consensus within

the profession; create intraprofessional and interprofessional partnerships; develop a social work specific knowledge base in palliative and end-of-life care; disseminate information to the social work community (national and international) and across professions; collaborate on program initiatives and resource sharing; and further development of capacity and advancement in the field (SWHPN, 2009a).

Currently this growing network has over 200 members. An annual meeting is held in conjunction with the American Academy of Hospice & Palliative Medicine Hospice & Hospice Palliative Nurses Association Conference. One member benefit is online access to the *Journal of Social Work in End-of-Life and Palliative Care*. The inaugural issue of this quarterly social work journal was published in 2004. It was developed in response to the priorities identified at the first Summit that articulated the need for increased professional development in palliative and end-of-life social work. The journal's primary goal is to be a premiere professional resource for both social work practitioners and academics, providing an opportunity to stay connected with the latest evidence-informed practice, clinical wisdom, and policy issues. In addition to access to the journal, other member benefits include online professional networking through LinkHealthPro, an interactive online community, that provides access to other health care professionals in hospitals and universities; newsletters and e-blasts on current developments in palliative and end-of-life care; information on professional conferences; access to data collected on professional interests in the field; and opportunities for collaborations with physicians, nurses, and multidisciplinary professional organizations (SWHPN, 2009b). For more information, see: http://www.swhpn.org and Chapter 76).

Oncology Social Work Organizations

Association of Oncology Social Work

Social workers who specialize in or have an interest in oncology may choose to join the Association of Oncology Social Work (AOSW). The AOSW, founded in 1984, has about 1000 members and provides a network for exchange of information, resources, and peer support. Some of the member benefits include a subscription to AOSW's official journal, the *Journal of Psychosocial Oncology*, and quarterly newsletters (AOSW, 2009a). Members can attend the annual conference at a reduced rate. A number of special interest groups (SIGs) are organized within AOSW and hold meetings at the annual conference in addition to communicating through listservs and newsletter features. There are three SIGs that pertain, directly or indirectly, to palliative social workers: End-of-Life Care, Pain and Palliative Care, and Ethics. The End-of-Life SIG is for members who are interested in end-of-life issues, including but not exclusive to, hospice care. The purpose is to keep members updated on current trends in end of life, to provide peer support, and to provide ongoing resources. There is a commitment to providing end-of-life educational opportunities at the annual conference and submitting regular features on current issues to the newsletter. The Pain and Palliative Care SIG encourages membership of social workers who are interested in learning and expanding the role of social work in the multidimensional aspects of cancer pain management and palliative care. It focuses on activities that will enhance and promote this role within social work and with interdisciplinary colleagues. The Ethics SIG addresses issues such as advance directives, treatment decisions, choices about end-of-life care, and communication with health care professionals (AOSW, 2009b). For more information, see: http://aosw.org.

Association of Pediatric Oncology Social Workers

The Association of Pediatric Oncology Social Workers (APOSW) has as its mission the advancement of pediatric psychosocial oncology care through clinical social work practice, research, advocacy, education, and program development (APOSW, 2009a). APOSW is a diverse organization with more than 380 members from nine countries. Membership includes social workers and allied health professionals working in hospitals, clinics, educational institutions, and organizations that provide support and treatment to children with cancer and their families. Among the member benefits is access to the APOSW listserv and to a "members only" Web site that contains information about special interest groups, advocacy and research information and other resources; and reduced registration fees at the annual APOSW conference (APOSW, 2009b). As with AOSW, APOSW has special interest groups pertaining to both end-of-life care and palliative care. For more information, see: http://aposw.org.

Multidisciplinary Organizations

National Hospice and Palliative Care Organization

The mission of the National Hospice and Palliative Care Organization (NHPCO) is "to lead and mobilize social change for improved care at the end of life." It was founded in 1978 as a charitable organization to advocate for the needs of people facing life-limiting illness. NHPCO is the largest membership organization specifically devoted to promoting access to hospice and palliative care and to maintaining quality care for persons facing the end of life and their families. Several types of memberships are available: Hospice Providers (programs that provide direct care to individuals with terminal illness and their families), Associate Providers (organizations that supply goods or services to hospice programs and professionals), State Hospice Organizations (state-based trade/advocacy organizations), International eAffiliate members (overseas programs, organizations, or individuals supportive of hospice and/or palliative care), and Individuals (professionals and volunteers) (NHPCO, 2009).

Individual members will be affiliated with NHPCO's professional organization: the National Council of Hospice and Palliative Professionals (NCHPP). This arm of NHPCO is for professionals working, studying, or volunteering in hospice or palliative care. NCHPP membership is complimentary for employees and volunteers of provider members. Benefits of membership include access to the NHPCO Web site, Newsbriefs, eNCHPP, monthly Newsline, quarterly Insights magazine, discounted subscription rate for the NHPCO's official journal, *Journal of Pain and Symptom Management*, and discounts for NHPCO-sponsored conferences and educational seminars. NHPCO sponsors two annual conferences: one focused on management and the other on direct practice. Within NCHPP, each professional discipline has a "section" and members choose affiliation (NHPCO, 2010). There are approximately 1700 members in the social work section. A section steering committee is appointed who will work together to set priorities for the section's work. A social work section leader is elected by the steering committee. The Social Work Section contributes to projects spearheaded by the steering committee and has worked on projects such as the hospice social work practice guidelines and the development of the Social Work Assessment Tool (SWAT).

In 2009, NHPCO launched a social networking community online called "MY NHPCO." This is accessible to all individual members as a professional communication tool. Through My NHPCO, members can create a personal profile, participate in preestablished eGroups and eGroups based on an area of interest, search the NHPCO directory for colleagues across the country, create a blog or follow other blogs, share documents, and view documents posted by others in an online library. For more information, see: http://www.nhpco.org/templates/1/homepage.cfm.

Academy of Hospice and Palliative Medicine

The Academy of Hospice and Palliative Medicine (AAHPM) is a professional organization for physicians and others who specialize in hospice and palliative medicine. Membership is also open to nurses and other health care providers, including social workers, who are committed to improving the quality of life of patients and families facing life-threatening or serious conditions. In 2010, there were over 50 active social work members. The AAHPM is "dedicated to expanding access of patients and families to high quality palliative care, and advancing the discipline of Hospice and Palliative Medicine, through professional education and training, development of a specialist workforce, support for clinical practice standards, research and public policy"

(AAHPM, 2009a). Among the membership benefits are subscription to the monthly *Journal of Pain and Symptom Management*, quarterly newsletters, and PC-FACS (Fast Article Critical Reviews for Clinicians in Palliative Care) distributed online. There is an annual conference held in conjunction with the Hospice and Palliative Nurses Association (HPNA). Within AAHPM, the College of Palliative Care (CPC) was formed to develop and support leaders in interdisciplinary palliative care research and education. The leadership of the CPC is interdisciplinary and includes representatives of the various disciplines that hold memberships in AAHPM, including social workers. The CPC's primary goal is to provide support for the development of leadership skills of junior, mid-level, and senior interdisciplinary practitioners who will advance palliative care as an academic and clinical discipline through educational and research endeavors. For example, to this end, the CPC hosts annual interdisciplinary retreats focused on education and research and offers opportunities for mentoring (AAHPM, 2009b). For more information, see: http://www.aahpm.org.

International Organizations

European Association for Palliative Care

The European Association for Palliative Care (EAPC) was established in 1988 to meet the needs of palliative care providers and professionals in Europe. Its mission is to "bring together many voices to forge a vision of excellence in palliative care that meets the needs of patients and their families." Its focus is to develop and promote palliative care in Europe through information, education, and research using multi-professional collaboration. The primary aim of the EAPC is to promote palliative care in Europe and to act as a centralizing organization for all of those who work, or have an interest, in the field of palliative care at the scientific, clinical, and social levels. Foci include training, networking, and promotion of information for practice (EAPC, 2009). Congress meetings and research forums are organized biannually along with other programs aimed at enhancing research capacity and education. Individual and provider organization memberships are encouraged. As of 2008 individual members represented 40 countries. *The European Journal of Palliative Care* is the official journal of the EAPC. Members received a discounted rate for subscription. For more information, see: http://www.eapcnet.org.

International Association for Hospice and Palliative Care

The International Association for Hospice and Palliative Care (IAHPC) focuses its work on program development, education, information dissemination, and policy change.

The expressed vision is to increase and optimize the availability of and access to hospice and palliative care for patients and their families throughout the world. The organization facilitates and provides palliative care education and training opportunities for care providers; acts as an information resource for professionals, health care providers, and policy makers; and develops collaborative strategies for hospice and palliative care providers, organizations, institutions, and individuals (IAHPC, 2009). IAHPC has both individual and provider organization memberships available. Programs offered for members include faculty development, recognition awards, traveling fellowships, and traveling scholarships. Reduced subscription rates are offered to members for selected journals. The Web site serves as a clearinghouse for information on publications and education/training seminars and conferences. Recently launched was a specialized online dictionary, Pallipedia, which will serve as a global educational resource. In addition, nonmembers may sign up to receive a free online monthly newsletter. For more information, see: http://www.hospicecare.com/ and http://pallipedia.org.

Social Work Credential in Hospice and Palliative Care

In 2008, the NASW and NHPCO collaborated to develop a social work credential in hospice and palliative care. It was designed by social work leaders in hospice and palliative care for social workers who meet the outlined national standards of excellence. The credential is administered by the NASW, and all materials needed for the application process are available at the NASW Web site. The credential is available for both the bachelor's degree in social work (BSW), certified hospice and palliative social worker (CHP-SW) and master's degree in social work (MSW), advanced certified hospice and palliative social worker (ACHP-SW) practitioners in the field. The basic requirements to qualify for the credential include the following:

- A degree in social work from an accredited university
- At least 2 years (3000 hours) of supervised social work experience in hospice and palliative care; for the ACHP-SW, qualifying supervision must be post-MSW
- A license to practice as a professional social worker (Note: BSWs who practice in states that do not license social workers at that level have additional experience [4 years] and CEU [40 contact hours] requirements [NASW, 2009b].)
- Twenty or more CEUs related specifically to the specialty practice
- A commitment to compliance with the *NASW Code of Ethics* and *NASW Standards for End of Life Care*
- Professional affiliations with both the NASW and the National Council of Hospice and Palliative

Professionals, a division of the National Hospice and Palliative Care Organization

The credential provides validation of professional competency because a national standard of social work practice has been verified and assured. The NASW credentials also provide confirmation of a renewable commitment to excellence and expertise in a specialized field of practice. The NASW credential demonstrates to the public that a practitioner has advanced knowledge in the specific field, and it also may offer leadership opportunities and recognition by peers and other health professionals in the field (NASW, 2009b). The NASW professional credentials must be renewed biannually, and this requires payment of a renewal fee and verification of at least 20 hours (from the initial date of credential) of continuing education or training specifically related to social work practice in hospice and palliative care. For more information, see: http://www.naswdc.org/

Conclusion

Opportunities for maintaining a professional connection in palliative care are available through a variety of professional organizations. The choice of organization(s) may depend on the particular setting or interests of the individual and the benefits that will be gained from the membership(s). Social workers may find that membership in more than one professional organization, social work specific and multidisciplinary, is necessary to meet professional goals and to stay current in all aspects of palliative care. In addition, certification of social work expertise in palliative care is becoming increasingly important for recognition by interdisciplinary colleagues and the public of social workers' capacity for specialized practice.

REFERENCES

American Academy of Hospice and Palliative Medicine (AAHPM). (2009a). *About AAHPM*. Retrieved from http://www.aahpm.org/about/index.html

American Academy of Hospice and Palliative Medicine (AAHPM). (2009b). *College of palliative care*. Retrieved from http://www.aahpm.org/about/college.html

Association of Oncology Social Workers (AOSW). (2009a). *Membership*. Retrieved from http://www.aosw.org/html/membership.php

Association of Oncology Social Workers (AOSW). (2009b). *AOSW special interest groups*. Retrieved from http://www.aosw.org/html/sigs.php

Association of Pediatric Oncology Social Workers (APOSW). (2009a). *About us*. Retrieved from http://www.aposw.org/index.php?option=com_content&task=view&id=33&Itemid=155

Association of Pediatric Oncology Social Workers (APOSW). (2009b). *Membership in APOSW*. Retrieved from http://www.aposw.org/index.php?option=com_content&task=view&id=35&Itemid=65

European Association for Palliative Care (EAPC). (2009). *About the EAPC*. Retrieved from http://www.eapcnet.org/about/about.html

International Association for Hospice and Palliative Care (IAHPC). (2009). *IAHPC: Who we are*. Retrieved from http://www.hospicecare.com/give

National Association of Social Workers (NASW). (2009a). *NASW standards for practice in palliative and end-of-life care*. Retrieved from http://www.naswdc.org/practice/bereavement/standards/default.asp

National Association of Social Workers (NASW). (2009b). *Certified Hospice and Palliative Social Worker (CHP-SW) and Advanced Certified Hospice and Palliative Social Worker (ACHP-SW)*. Retrieved from http://www.naswdc.org/credentials/credentials/chpsw.asp

National Hospice and Palliative Care Organization (NHPCO). (2009). *Join NHPCO*. Retrieved from http://www.nhpco.org/i4a/pages/index.cfm?pageid=3307

National Hospice and Palliative Care Organization (NHPCO). (2010). *National Council of Hospice and Palliative Professionals*. Retrieved from http://www.nhpco.org/i4a/pages/index.cfm?pageid=3628&openpage=3628

Social Work in Hospice and Palliative Care Network (SWHPN). (2009a). *Our story*. Retrieved from http://www.swhpn.org/our-story

Social Work in Hospice and Palliative Care Network (SWHPN). (2009b). *Welcome to SWHPN*. Retrieved from http://members.swhpn.org

78 *Jaime Goldberg and Michal Scharlin*

Financial Considerations for the Palliative Social Worker

Hospital-based palliative care services are typically justified to their parent institutions on the basis of quality issues and are supported through analyses of cost avoidance, improved hospital bed capacity, and other indirect benefits that accrue to the system. Maximizing billing opportunities for palliative care can tip the scale of the business plan in favor of the program's value and the system's willingness to allocate scarce resources to palliative care.

—Meier & Beresford, 2006, p. 250

Key Concepts

- ◆ *Social work opportunities to bill for services may affect palliative care team outcomes.*
- ◆ *Social work roots shape orientation toward current professionalization standards and compensation.*
- ◆ *Further research is required to better assess current financial practices and inform future advocacy efforts.*

Introduction

Skyrocketing and untenable health care costs in the United States require hospital administrators and clinicians alike to focus on quality care, fiscal responsibility, and institutional survival. Administrators are pressured to control spending by shrinking overhead, reducing the workforce, and streamlining hospital systems. Providers, in turn, are being scrutinized to control costs; palliative care providers in the hospital setting are particularly challenged to demonstrate their fiscal integrity while providing care that is informed by the National Consensus Project Guidelines for Quality Palliative Care (Meier & Beresford, 2006; von Gunten, Ferris, D'Antuono, & Emanuel, 2002).

Despite the fact that most people in the United States continue to die in hospitals (Field & Cassel, 1997; Tolle, Rosenfeld, Tilden, & Park, 1999; von Gunten et al., 2002; Weitzen, Teno, Fennell, & Mor, 2003), current regulatory and financial structures do not encourage comprehensive palliative care service delivery in the inpatient setting, because the acute care hospital system was not designed to provide comfort-oriented end-of-life care (von Gunten et al., 2002). With one-third of all health care dollars in the United States spent on care in the last 2 years of life, research has shown that palliative care teams are instrumental in lowering these costs by discouraging use of inappropriate end-of-life medical interventions, reducing intensive care unit admissions, and shortening hospital stays (Fromme et al., 2006; Hearn & Higginson, 1998; Payne, Coyne, & Smith, 2002; Smith et al., 2003; White, Stover, Cassel, & Smith, 2006). It is crucial for teams to provide evidence of this ability to improve patient care and cut unnecessary costs. The value of a palliative social worker, as with all professions, is measured by the ability to contribute to the patients, families, team, and setting in which he or she practices, whether that be a hospital, hospice, or extended care facility. Although data may be difficult to generate, further research is necessary to capture the palliative social worker's vital role in enhancing the financial well-being of interdisciplinary teams and institutions across practice settings.

In most palliative care teams, differential payment systems are employed, whereby physicians and nurse practitioners have provider status, meaning they are reimbursed for each service they provide, while social workers and chaplains are salaried. How is everyone impacted, positively and negatively, by this system? Does this reimbursement process affect the social worker's professional status and self-esteem? Research is necessary to examine how differential payment mechanisms mediate team dynamics, functioning, and effectiveness, as well as patient outcomes and overall costs.

While there are a host of issues surrounding the financing of palliative care, this chapter focuses more narrowly on these differential provider payment systems in acute care palliative teams. At the time of this writing, the U.S. health care system is in a state of flux, with some potential for major reforms. We are unable to predict how upcoming reforms will change the structural underpinnings of palliative care financing. We also do not discuss the relative strengths and weaknesses of general payment and billing systems for entire palliative care teams. Rather, we consider historical factors within and beyond the social work profession that inform current practices, whereby some palliative care specialists bill for their services, while others generally do not. This chapter is intended to explore various aspects of this phenomenon, including the implications for both palliative care as a specialty and for social work in particular. We consider the nuts and bolts of billing, the risks and benefits of change, and suggest directions for research and advocacy. We intend to stimulate thoughtful discussion within the palliative care and greater social work communities, promoting structural evaluation and self-assessment.

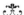

Historical Perspectives on Social Work Compensation

Much of the uniqueness of social work has stemmed from its singular commitment to advocacy and social action on behalf of its traditionally disempowered clients (Specht & Courtney, 1994). Social work's effort to convert its raison d'être into a concrete knowledge and practice base created tensions as it worked to professionalize. From its inception, social workers debated whether their commitment should be reflected in large-scale social reforms or in casework and community projects. These strains within the ranks of social workers can, to a great extent, be attributed to the pressure to establish occupational control over a particular sphere of helping activities and distinguish social work from charity and volunteerism (Haynes, 1998; Wenocur & Reisch, 2001).

While the profession of social work has grown and reinvented itself in response to rapid economic and social change, the historical tensions just described have become more entrenched as the profession has moved further toward a casework model, with psychotherapy for a primarily middle-class clientele as a hallmark of this shift (Haynes, 1998). Desire for professional recognition and autonomy, low salaries in nonprofit agencies, and poor working conditions in large public bureaucracies have also influenced this change (Wenocur & Reisch, 2001). Some argue that this shift to a more psychotherapeutic model of social work is an abandonment of the profession's original mission and core ethical principles (Specht & Courtney, 1994). In fact, the National Association of Social Workers (NASW) Code of Ethics states as its first Ethical Principle that, "Social workers' primary goal is to help people in need and to address social problems ... Social workers elevate service to others above self interest" (NASW, 2008, Ethical Principles). This debate pits the psychotherapeutic model and desire for professionalization as divergent from the profession's social justice roots (Reamer, 2006). The social work profession's complex relationship to finances and business is also reflected in this tension. Social workers are left both desiring compensation for hard work and skill, and perhaps wondering whether a desire for equitable remuneration is a compromise of the profession's commitment to marginalized populations.

Palliative social work has an ambiguous and evolving presence in this discussion. The specialty is in its infancy, yet its expansive scope of practice brings it squarely into the nexus of this debate, as palliative social workers participate in both macro social reform and individual counseling. Palliative social work extends from advocating for widespread changes in end-of-life service delivery, to ensuring access to medical care and medications, to working with patients and families struggling with mood disorders and adjustment to illness. Given the breadth of these activities, palliative social workers and similar specialists do not have a clear compensation model within the social work profession.

Palliative social workers have further challenges with regard to compensation because most fall under the umbrella of their respective social work departments, though they work most closely with non–social work palliative team members. Additionally, palliative social workers may be unclear where to identify within the social work field; while they are paid more than nonprofit employees, they are not compensated as much as private practitioners (NASW Center for Workforce Studies, 2006). Should palliative social workers look to their palliative care colleagues, social work colleagues, or both for compensation models? Perhaps we need to keep both fields in mind as we consider new models of palliative social work financing.

Social Work in Health Care

There are a number of challenges to creating an alternative framework for compensating palliative social workers that are related to their presence in the medical system. Examining intraprofessional issues, palliative social workers are often not involved in the core activities which define the jobs of most medical social workers. Medical social workers are financially supported by their institutions because of their role via "indirects," nonbillable, cost-saving measures, such as planning timely patient discharges and assisting patients and families with enrollment in state and federal entitlements (Auerbach, Mason, & LaPorte, 2007; Kadushin & Kulys, 1993). This role is an important clinical activity because transitions in health status and residence are symbolic of major life changes. They require careful social work interventions, often revolving around clinical issues such as grief and loss, as illness forces adaptation and change in the lives of patients and their families (T. Altilio, personal communication, March 9, 2010). Palliative social workers focus on a range of activities that differ from those of medical social workers. Complementing the medical social worker's role, the primary responsibilities of a palliative social worker lie in the areas of communication, psychosocial interventions, decision making, and evolving goals of care. While interventions such as family meetings, often run by palliative social workers, lead to decision-making that may impact disposition, palliative social workers generally rely on their medical social work colleagues to oversee the details of discharges. In considering payment models, research is needed to further articulate the distinction between medical and palliative social work roles and activities and investigate how palliative social workers contribute to both quality care and cost-saving measures.

More broadly, all social workers in the hospital setting are challenged by their adjunctive role as allied health professionals. Health care systems historically provided care within a hierarchical, paternalistic, medical model in which social workers were invited to contribute as "guests in host settings," working in institutions where the professional mission and decision making were defined and dominated by medical disciplines (Dane & Simon, 1991). This issue is still relevant for interdisciplinary team dynamics in the medical setting. Given that positive team dynamics are correlated with productivity and quality of performance (Gully, Incalcaterra, Joshi, & Beaubien, 2002), persistent differences in professional status between physicians and social workers can result in challenges to team functioning (Abramson & Mizrahi, 1996; Reese & Sontag, 2001). Even on hospice teams, where social workers are considered a necessary component to providing comprehensive care, equality, autonomy, and authority may be lacking for social

workers (Reese & Sontag, 2001). These differentials in status are reproduced by and mirrored in differentials in the existing payment systems. One focus of research might be to investigate status differentials within the interdisciplinary team and the resulting effects on performance and compensation.

Differential Payment within Palliative Care Teams

The complex issues of identity and history described earlier are both causes and reflections of payment structures within interdisciplinary teams. Differential payment systems among professionals within a single palliative care team are the norm in acute care settings with third-party billing. Health care professionals and agencies with third-party payers utilize three basic types of payment methods: salary, fee for service, and capitation. Briefly, employees who work on salary are paid a fixed daily, weekly, monthly, or annual amount—regardless of the number of patients they see or what services they provide. In a fee-for-service model, providers or institutions bill the client or insurance company for each service rendered, including tests and medication. In a capitation system, providers or institutions are paid a fixed amount per patient or per diagnosis, which is not dependent on service provision (Gosden et al., 2006).

A differential in payment systems occurs in palliative care teams when physicians and nurse practitioners have provider status, meaning that they can be reimbursed on a fee-for-service basis, while social workers and chaplains are considered part of the bundle of services (Coleman, 2010). The "bundle" is a per diem inpatient bed fee, which takes into account hospital overhead, as well as nursing, administrative, and janitorial staff. While differential payment systems do not exist in government-run facilities such as the Veterans Administration, where all professionals on the palliative care team are salaried, differentials do exist in many teams located in fee-for-service acute care settings (Meier & Beresford, 2006).

In the context of fiscally responsible institutions and a political and economic climate where palliative care teams are asked to prove their worth by their cost-saving capacity, clinicians who work on a fee-for-service basis are able to market themselves as visibly generating additional revenue to the hospital system on behalf of the palliative care team. This revenue-generating ability may be viewed by some providers as a demand that restricts the content and duration of patient interactions. However, when serving on an interdisciplinary team, the ability to bill fee for service may also be viewed as a relative advantage, as hospitals look to providers' financial solvency when allocating resources to various specialties (Meier & Beresford, 2006).

There is a dearth of information about how or whether the differential in payment structures influences the direct care of patients and families, as well as the functioning and long-term survival of teams. It is a shared responsibility to ensure that fiscal stability and patient-family care are equally considered in treatment planning. In settings where a palliative care team does not have financial support to hire a social worker, or the social worker is required to cross-cover other hospital departments, psychosocial work best done by a mental health clinician may be done by a physician or nurse because of availability and ability to bill. In environments where money equates with value, social workers may need to be very articulate about the nature of their psychosocial, ethical, and decision-making contributions, as well as the effect of these contributions on the fiscal well-being of the institution. This is necessary to ensure that the inability to bill is not equated with lack of skill or clinical involvement in outcomes. Research is necessary to explore how asymmetries in payment systems may influence whether finances, rather than best practices, drive team structure, decision making, and patient-family care.

Given these considerations, what are possibilities for reform? It is important to note that this discussion of modifying social work compensation is directed at the palliative social worker, but it has implications for social workers in various practice settings. Many in the health care industry are in favor of radical change that would alter the entire domestic health care system (Blendon & Benson, 2009; Larson et al., 2004). However, given the unlikelihood of a complete overhaul of the fee-for-service model, what are the pros and cons of the current system for social work compensation? Despite the challenges described earlier, the current system gives the palliative social worker the flexibility to engage in a wide variety of tasks, ranging from concrete resource referral to team management, administration, and psychotherapy. Palliative social workers are also able to truly embrace the patient and family as a unit of care, often working with family members longitudinally in multiple areas, including adaptation, treatment options, caregiver concerns, finances, psychological distress, goals of care, anticipatory grief, and bereavement. As part of the "bundle" of services, palliative social workers may not be as driven by volume of patient visits as are other providers, thereby allowing the time to provide quality and comprehensive services while being protected from the financial pressures of billing.

In weighing the status quo, it is worthwhile to imagine what alternatives within the fee-for-service model might look like. Examining advocacy efforts that led to restructuring and provider status in another discipline may assist social workers in discerning the risks and benefits of engaging in such a process and potentially serve as a model for change. Before any broad-based campaign is undertaken, it is important to build a body of research documenting current palliative social work practices and promote demonstration projects to investigate alternative models. Without the availability of this evidence, we turn to our nurse practitioner colleagues for guidance in the process of advocating for professional standardization and provider status, which led to their ability to bill for services.

Provider Status

The Nurse Practitioner Model

The nurse practitioner (NP) or advance practice nurse (APN) has come to serve an important role on inpatient palliative care consultation teams, combining nursing's focus on treating the whole patient and the medical provider's expertise in diagnosing and prescribing—all while recouping salary costs through billing for consultations (Meier & Beresford, 2006).

It was only through advocacy work during the 1980s and 1990s that nurse practitioners gained provider status and thus the ability to bill for their services (Buppert, 1999). Prior to this change in reimbursement structure, NPs, who were salaried under hospital nursing departments or billed under physicians in the outpatient setting, had an ill-defined role in patient care. In the mid-1980s, organizations such as the American Academy of Nurses and the National Organization of Nurse Practitioners began lobbying the Center for Medicare & Medicaid Services (CMS, at that time the Health Care Financing Agency [HCFA]) around the issue of reimbursement. There was widespread disagreement within the NP community about these proposed changes. Many NPs, much like social workers, held the philosophy that they earned a salary for "taking care of people" and thus could not be concerned with money. There was also resistance from physicians who asserted that NPs were practicing medicine without a license (M. McHugh, personal communication, December 22, 2009).

HCFA proposed that in order to receive reimbursement, the NP's education and credentials must be better defined and standardized. As a result, there was a national shift to create uniformity in the education and credentialing of nurse practitioners. The Balanced Budget Act of 1997 significantly changed the reimbursement structure for Medicare Part B by redefining physicians' services. This redefinition also allowed for direct reimbursement to NPs regardless of geography, as opposed to earlier legislation which allowed for NP reimbursement only in rural and underserved areas (M. McHugh, personal communication, December 22, 2009).

Nurse practitioners can currently only bill for palliative care services delivered in the hospital if they are not paid from the hospital's nursing department (Buppert, 1999). If NPs are salaried from that source, their services, like hospital social workers, are considered part of the bundle and not reimbursed on a fee-for-service basis. Billing for the services of NPs who fall under the nursing department would be seen as double dipping and therefore insurance fraud. If, however, the NP is salaried from a non-hospital budget source, such as a faculty practice or education line, then the clinician may bill Medicare Part B or other insurers in exactly the same way as a physician (M. McHugh, personal communication, December 22, 2009). Currently, Medicare reimburses NPs at a rate of 85% of what a physician would receive for the same visit (Buppert, 1999). Medicare billing numbers are available for NPs who meet CMS requirements, which include being certified by an approved certification agency. As the palliative care specialty is not yet recognized as a stand-alone certification, NPs must receive certification in one of several approved fields (such as family medicine) in order to be able to bill (M. McHugh, personal communication, December 22, 2009). Of note, NPs employed under hospice are not eligible for direct reimbursement as a result of Medicare Part A billing, except when the NP serves as the patient's hospice attending of record (Buppert, 1999).

The recognition of NPs as primary health care providers is a principal example of a field's efforts to professionalize, legitimize, and command recognition for itself. Several key strategies were influential in attaining this success, which may be useful for the social work profession:

1. Embracing the idea that the nursing profession had the potential to expand its role
2. Conducting evidence-informed research validating the worth of the nurse practitioner
3. Establishing national professional standards for education and credentialing
4. Uniting and empowering individual practitioners through professional organizations
5. Championing incremental steps to achieve the goal of provider status recognition (Buppert, 1999).

Palliative Social Work Professionalization and Standardization

The structure of advocacy employed by nurse practitioners can serve as a potential model for specialist social workers who may consider pursuing provider status. To achieve this goal, there is increasing support in palliative social work for determining standards of practice that would inform billing and better define the specialty (Loscalzo, 2007). Here we discuss changes to forward the attainment of provider status through professionalization and specialization and also describe some concerns regarding pursing these goals.

Social work currently has systems for licensure and certification, which may provide a structure upon which to build a similar process to that of our nurse practitioner colleagues. Social work licensure is regulated by individual state-licensing bodies, which in most states are overseen by the Association of Social Work Boards (ASWB). In general, licensure for post-master's advanced general and advanced clinical practice social work can be obtained after 2 years of supervised practice and successful completion of an examination.

The National Association of Social Workers (NASW) has not established specializations beyond clinical licensure. However, NASW does have several certifications, including the Advance Certified Hospice and Palliative Social Worker certification, which is a joint venture with the National Hospice and Palliative Care Organization (NHPCO) (NASW, n.d.; NHPCO, 2008). This certification calls for one to have worked in the field a certain number of hours, but it does not require a standardized educational curriculum, testing mechanism, nor advanced practice clinical social work licensure. The creation of national standards would need to accompany the creation of a more robust credentialing process, if the social work profession follows the model and evolution of our nurse practitioner colleagues.

To establish national standards, an evidence-informed consensus would need to be reached about the nature of services provided by palliative social workers. These may include individual or family psychotherapy or counseling, family meetings, initial assessments, patient advocacy, communication and problem-solving related to treatment options or placement decisions, resources and referral, bereavement, and assistance making final arrangements. To establish provider status, the next step in this process would be to determine which of these services would be considered billable, create a value hierarchy, and assign a monetary value to each (i.e., how much each service might be billed for). Further research, collaboration, and advocacy among social workers and palliative care professionals are necessary to establish broad-based support for this type of change.

It is important to consider that palliative social work specialization has financial and status-related implications for social work colleagues. Of particular concern is how the partnership between palliative and other social workers would be affected. While collaboration in a setting of mutual professional respect can serve to enhance quality of care and the self-worth of each professional, in a setting of competition and worry about professional survival, it can create conflict and diminished self-esteem. Where broad cultural values equate money with worth, would colleagues who do not bill be marginalized? We must attend to whether advocating for specialization and reimbursement for one segment of the social work profession enhances or disenfranchise other social workers.

Current Fee-for-Service Practices

Despite these challenges, social workers are already billing for outpatient psychotherapy, and it is becoming increasingly common for palliative social workers to consider billing Medicare and private insurance companies for their services in hospital outpatient clinics (Landis, 2008). Of note, social workers billing for psychotherapy in the outpatient setting must hold a clinical license, bill under Medicare Part B, obtain a National Provider Identifier Number, acquire malpractice insurance, and follow the Center for Medicare & Medicaid Services (CMS) application guidelines (Coleman, 2010). In addition, outpatient clinicians can also apply for inclusion on other managed care provider panels, which allow them to bill non-Medicare third-party payers (Coleman, 2005). Currently, clinical social workers are unable to bill for inpatient services, although the National Association of Social Workers (NASW) is advocating for change on this front in skilled nursing facilities (Coleman, 2010). One explanation for this difference in billing is that interactions with patients and families in the outpatient setting are more discrete and circumscribed, making it easier to account for amount of time spent and services provided. This is much more difficult on an inpatient palliative care service where social workers' tasks on the team are more varied and fluid. However, having addressed similar concerns, systems have been developed that allow for physician and nurse practitioner billing, even where education and counseling are their primary activities (von Gunten, Ferris, Kirschner, & Emanuel, 2000).

To set standards for billing in palliative outpatient clinics, as well as consider expanding billing to the inpatient setting, it is helpful to become familiar with the system of terminologies currently employed by medical providers to describe and bill for services. Medicare guidelines detailed in the next section set the standards for billing practices, though Medicare carriers and other insurance companies vary widely in their interpretation of CMS regulations, sometimes causing confusion among providers and payers (Mezzocco, 2001).

HCPCS and CPT Codes

Level I Healthcare Common Procedure Coding System (HCPCS) or Current Procedural Terminology (CPT) codes assign a five-digit number to all diagnostic and medical services performed by health care providers. CPT codes, created by the American Medical Association (AMA), are used to determine the amount of reimbursement that a practitioner or institution will receive from an insurer. They are also used by hospitals/clinics to code the kind of intervention that occurs between provider and patient, even when third-party billing is not employed. Hospitals and clinics in the United States almost all use a combination of International Classification of Diseases (ICD) and HCPCS/CPT codes, facilitating the ease with which population-based morbidity and mortality can be tracked and the provision of services reimbursed and monitored (Hammond & Cimino, 2006; Mezzocco, 2001).

Many social workers in inpatient and outpatient settings are more familiar with the ICD or Diagnostic and Statistical Manual (DSM) codes used for diagnosis and billing purposes. The current version of the ICD in use is the ICD-9-CM. Unlike the HCPCS and CPT codes, ICD and DSM are diagnostic, not procedural terminologies (Hammond & Cimino, 2006). If clinical social workers are to consider

expanding their billing practices, understanding how to use the procedural codes is essential. There are three types of CPT procedural codes: Evaluation and Management (E&M) codes (99201–99499), Health and Behavior Assessment/Intervention (HBAI) codes (96150–96155), and Psychiatric codes (90801–90899). Currently, clinical social workers in outpatient clinics may only bill CPT Psychiatric codes and in some instances use HBAI codes reimbursed by select carriers and private insurance companies (Gordon, 2009; Substance Abuse and Mental Health Services Administration [SAMHSA], 2009).

CPT Evaluation and Management (E&M) Codes
Physicians bill using CPT E&M codes when the patient's primary diagnosis is a physical or mental disorder. Medicare will also reimburse for E&M services provided by nurse practitioners, clinical nurse specialists, certified nurse midwives, and physician assistants (SAMHSA, 2009). E&M codes are typically determined by the amount of time a provider spends with a patient, where the provider saw the patient, the type of visit (e.g., initial vs. follow-up), and level of visit complexity . E&M codes are used to report services including, but not limited to, patient history, focused exam, and decision making (Meier & Beresford, 2006; von Gunten et al., 2000). Until 2010, Medicare reimbursed a primary diagnosis of mental illness at a rate of about 50%, while primary physical illnesses were reimbursed at 80% of the negotiated visit cost (Mauch, Kautz & Smith, 2008). However, as delineated by the Medicare Improvements for Patients and Providers Act of 2008 (MIPPA), the differential between mental health and physical health copayments will be phased out beginning in 2010, until complete mental health parity is achieved in 2014 (Coleman, 2008). Neither clinical social workers nor psychologists may bill using these codes (SAMHSA, 2009).

CPT Health and Behavior Assessment/Intervention (HBAI) and Psychiatric Codes

CPT HBAI codes do not require an ICD-9 code for a psychiatric disorder; they only require a physical disorder that has psychosocial consequences. HBAI codes identify interventions that improve patient adherence with regimens for physical health problems. While considered within their scope of practice, clinical social workers cannot bill Medicare using HBAI codes because of restricted reimbursement guidelines for clinical social work practice (Center for Medicare & Medicaid Services, 1998; M. Coleman, personal communication, May 6, 2010). However, some third-party payers do allow clinical social workers to bill using HBAI codes.

CPT Psychiatric codes are combined with ICD-9-CM codes 290–319 for the diagnosis and treatment of patients with primary mental, psychoneurotic, and personality disorders (Mauch, Kautz & Smith, 2008). Mental health specialists, including physicians, clinical psychologists, clinical social workers, nurse practitioners, clinical nurse specialists, and physician assistants may bill using these codes. These are the only codes that clinical social workers can bill under with all third-party payers, including Medicare. In order to use these codes, social workers must diagnose the patient with a mental disorder, hold a clinical license, and perform clinical duties in an outpatient setting.

Alternative Billing Models

Health and Behavior Assessment/Intervention (HBAI) Code Billing Model

One of the simplest and most immediate ways to create a billing terminology for palliative social workers is to consider revising current Medicare standards to match many other third-party payers and allow clinical social workers to bill using HBAI codes. Clinical social workers are only authorized under Medicare guidelines to bill services for the diagnosis and treatment of mental illnesses and they therefore are not eligible to bill using CPT E&M or HBAI codes (Center for Medicare & Medicaid Services, 1998),; however, psychologists, even those without board certification in the health psychology subspecialty, are allowed to bill with HBAI codes (SAMHSA, 2009).

While HBAI codes seem to best reflect the whole-person focus of palliative social work, there are pros and cons in considering the potential use of these codes for social work billing. On the one hand, the codes describe an encounter between social worker and patient-family that is centered around a health event, rather than a psychopathology, as would be indicated by using a DSM code. There are no DSM codes that can be used for life review, suffering that is not considered pathological, and uncomplicated grief and bereavement. Moreover, the HBAI codes might allow palliative social workers to capture some of the case management and other services they provide that do not qualify as psychotherapy. On the other hand, HBAI codes primarily value psychosocial interventions only in their power to increase treatment adherence and improve medical outcomes. This perspective might encourage a view of psychosocial-spiritual care as a handmaiden to bio-physical interventions, instead of honoring them in their own right.

A practical challenge in using HBAI codes is that behavioral health providers largely cannot bill Psychiatric codes (CPT 90801–90899) and Health and Behavior Assessment/Intervention (HBAI) codes (96150–96155) for the same patient on the same day (Mauch, Kautz & Smith, 2008). For services rendered to patients who require both psychiatric and HBAI services, only one provider may report the principal service given, even if services are provided by two distinct practitioners. In a palliative care setting where clinical social workers might use HBAI codes, this might become problematic if any combination of psychiatrists, psychologists, and social workers see a patient in the same day. Further, Medicare only reimburses for one service per day, regardless of the codes presented (M. Coleman, personal communication, May 6, 2010). This would limit Medicare reimbursement of clinical social workers on interdisciplinary teams; a social worker using an HBAI code and a physician using an E&M code could not bill for a patient on the same day.

Incident-to Billing Model

Under many health plans, physicians and nurse practitioners can currently bill at a higher rate if they see a patient with a social worker, billing for a "dyad" or "triad" visit (M. Coleman, personal communication, May 6, 2010). In this practice, the primary provider makes the diagnosis and bills for interventions, with the social worker's services incidental to the primary practitioner. This type of billing is currently only possible through Medicare in outpatient settings where the social worker is employed directly by a physician(Mauch, Kautz & Smith, 2008, von Gunten et al., 2000). However, other third-party payers may have differing guidelines for applying the "incident-to" practice (Mazzocco, 2001). Incident-to billing might be adapted for palliative care inpatient and outpatient settings where social workers are employed directly by a large institution, rather than an individual physician. This model might also be altered to allow for some flexibility regarding who is the primary provider, and perhaps be adapted to consider billing for patient services as an interdisciplinary team. In this last scenario, when two or more providers see a patient, perhaps none of them would need to be identified as the "primary" provider, instead using an augmented team billing code.

Hospice Capitation Billing Model

Home hospice agencies are reimbursed by Medicare Part A through capitation, whereby the agency receives a daily flat fee per patient to cover salaries (direct service and administration), medication, tests, and overhead. In this model, all health care providers are salaried and the hospice is paid as a team, avoiding the payment differential described earlier in acute care settings with third-party billing. The hospice billing model may be considered by policy makers as a template for use by inpatient and/or outpatient palliative care teams. Of note, Medicare hospice regulations require the inclusion of a social worker on all hospice teams. Policy makers might look to this requirement as a gold standard for interdisciplinary care and as a goal for inpatient palliative care teams, as well. One complication in the use of this model is that even under hospice capitation where physicians are salaried, physicians are additionally reimbursed for in-home visits. Hospice has traditionally been a nurse-driven team and physicians have only recently increased their involvement in home visits (S. Etzioni, personal communication, February 4, 2010). It is unclear whether the enhanced role of hospice physicians in direct patient care will create similar tensions within hospice teams as we have hypothesized exist in acute care settings.

Conclusion

Social work and palliative care have a natural synergy because they both favour whole-person and person-in-environment approaches, embracing the patient and family as the unit of care. With the emergence of social workers as core members of palliative care teams, concerns related to team dynamics and viability set the stage for all team members to consider financial concerns. For many, the value of their work is measured in financial compensation and the degree to which they contribute to the solvency of their organization. The time has come to consider the benefits and risks implicit in the traditional view of social workers, who largely have not concerned themselves with remuneration and expect to be supported for the intrinsic value of their work. As with other helping professions, changes in social work financing must be supported by research focused on establishing evidence for the quality and effectiveness of our work and our role in overall hospital cost-savings.

As clinical social workers have already achieved provider status in the outpatient setting for psychotherapy, future research and advocacy efforts must focus on the influence of expanded specialization, standardization, and provider status on patients, families, and fellow palliative care and social work practitioners. NASW has already begun advocacy efforts aimed at altering the Medicare reimbursement regulations to allow clinical social workers to bill under Medicare Part A in nursing home settings (Coleman, 2010). To move forward, palliative social workers must join with other specialized social workers and leadership organizations to consider these issues, refining the current system with new and valid evidence to create lasting change. Finally, with this discussion of finances and billing, we must underscore that in palliative social work encounters, the patient and family must remain the focus; ultimately, the contribution of the palliative social worker must be measured by the quality of his or her contribution to care.

LEARNING EXERCISES

- Locate U.S. Senators and Congresspeople with a social work background. Contact them via phone, letter, or e-mail to begin advocacy efforts aimed at examining options for changes in Medicare and other third-party payment systems for social workers.
- This chapter focuses on billing practices in the United States. What are the implications of this discussion for countries where there is socialized medicine? What about resource-challenged countries?
- In this chapter, we discuss implications for changing the compensation structure established by Medicare and other third-party payers. How would these changes affect treating those without any insurance? What about those enrolled in Medicaid?

ADDITIONAL RESOURCES

SUGGESTED READINGS

Cassel, E. J. (2001). Forces affecting caring by physicians. In L. E. Cluff & R. H. Binstock (Eds.), *The lost art of caring: A challenge to health professionals, families, communities, and society*. Baltimore, MD: The Johns Hopkins University Press.

Specht, H., & Courtney, M. E. (1994). *Unfaithful angels: How social work has abandoned its mission*. New York, NY: The Free Press.

Wenocur, S., & Reisch, M. (2001). *From charity to enterprise: The development of American social work in a market economy*. Urbana, IL: University of Illinois Press.

WEB SITES

The Association of Social Work Boards (ASWB): http://www.aswb.org

The association of boards that regulate social work. ASWB develops and maintains the social work licensing examinations used across most of the United States and in several Canadian provinces.

Center to Advance Palliative Care (CAPC): http://www.capc.org

Provides health care professionals with the tools, training, and technical assistance necessary to start and sustain successful palliative care programs in hospitals and other health care settings.

Center for Medicare and Medicaid Services (CMS): http://www.cms.hhs.gov

Ensures effective, up-to-date health care coverage and promotes quality care for beneficiaries. Policy related to financial concerns for social workers is available on the website, including The Mental Health Parity and Addiction Equity Act of 2008 (MHPAEA), which expanded the Mental Health Parity Act (MHPA) of 1996. In addition, for details on the website regarding Medicare reimbursement regulations for specific professions, see Chapter 12 (Sections 210, 150 and 160) and Chapter 15 (Sections 160 and 170) of the Medicare Claims Processing Manual.

National Association of Social Workers (NASW): http://www.socialworkers.org

The largest membership organization of professional social workers in the world, with 150,000 members. It works to enhance members' professional growth and development, create and maintain professional standards, and advance social policies.

Social Work Network in Palliative and End-of-Life Care Listserv: http://www.stoppain.org/for_professionals/content/information/listserv.asp

Provides a forum for social workers in various fields to network and discuss multidimensional aspects and issues related to palliative and end-of-life care.

REFERENCES

Abramson, J. S., & Mizrahi, T. (1996). When social workers and physicians collaborate: Positive and negative interdisciplinary experiences. *Social Work, 41*(3), 270–281.

Auerbach, C., Mason, S. E., & LaPorte, H. H. (2007). Evidence that supports the value of social work in hospitals. *Social Work in Health Care, 44*(4), 17–32.

Blendon, R. J., & Benson, J. M. (2009). Understanding how Americans view healthcare reform. *NEJM Health Care Reform Center*, doi:10.1056/NEJMp0906392.

Buppert, C. (1999). *Nurse practitioner's business practice and legal guide.* Gaithersburg, MD: Aspen Publishers.

Center for Medicare & Medicaid Services (1998). *Clinical social worker services.* (Code of Federal Regulations No. 63 FR 20128). Retrieved from The United States Printing Office Web Site: http://ecfr.gpoaccess.gov/cgi/t/text/text-idx?c=ecfr&sid=d3e203191cc28c1830403d31c6176326&rgn=div8&view=text&node=42:2.0.1.2.10.2.35.53&idno=42

Coleman, M. (2005). *Managed care companies with provider panels for clinical social workers.* Retrieved from the National Association of Social Workers Web site: http://www.socialworkers.org/practice/clinical/csw0405.pdf

Coleman, M. (2008). *Revised 2008 Medicare fee schedule for clinical social workers.* Retrieved from the National Association of Social Workers Web site: http://www.socialworkers.org/practice/clinical/2008/csw091708.asp

Coleman, M. (2010). *Enrolling in Medicare as a clinical social work provider.* Retrieved from the National Association of Social Workers Web site: http://www.socialworkers.org/assets/secured/documents/practice/clinical/WKF-MISC-38710.ClinicalSW.pdf

Dane, B. O., & Simon, B. L. (1991). Resident guests: Social workers in host settings. *Social Work, 36*(3), 208–213.

Field, M. J., & Cassel, C. K. (Eds.). (1997). *Approaching death: Improving care at the end of life.* Washington, DC: National Academy Press.

Fromme, E. K., Bascom, P. B., Smith, M. D., Tolle, S. W., Hanson, L., Hickam, D. H., & Osborne, M. L. (2006). Survival, mortality, and location of death for patients seen by a hospital-based palliative care team. *Journal of Palliative Medicine, 9*(4), 903–911.

Gordon, C. (2009, July 23). Billing codes for Medicare and other insurance companies. [Online forum comment]. Retrieved from

Gosden, T., Forland, F., Kristiansen,I. S., Sutton, M., Leese B., Giuffrida, A.,... Pedersen, L. (2006). Capitation, salary, fee-for-service and mixed systems of payment: Effects on the behaviour of primary care physicians. *Cochrane Database of Systematic Reviews, 3*, doi:10.1002/14651858.CD002215.

Gully, S. M., Incalcaterra, K. A., Joshi, A., & Beaubien, J. M. (2002). A meta-analysis of team-efficacy, potency, and performance: Interdependence and level of analysis as moderators of observed relationships. *Journal of Applied Psychology, 87*(5), 819–832.

Hammond, W. E., & Cimino, J. J. (2006). Standards in medical informatics. In E. H. Shortliffe, L. E. Perreault, G. Wiederhold, & L. M. Fagan (Eds.), *Medical informatics: Computer applications in health care and biomedicine* (3rd ed., pp. 278–285). New York, NY: Springer.

Haynes, K. S. (1998). The one hundred-year debate: Social reform versus individual treatment. *Social Work, 43*(6), 501–509.

Hearn, J., & Higginson, I. J. (1998). Do specialist palliative care teams improve outcomes for cancer patients? A systematic literature review. *Palliative Medicine, 12*, 317–332.

Kadushin, G., & Kulys, R. (1993). Discharge planning revisited: What do social workers actually do in discharge planning? *Social Work, 38*(6), 713–726.

Landis, D. (2008, May 7). Outpatient palliative care questions [Electronic mailing list message]. http://peach.ease.lsoft.com/archives/sw-pall-eol.html

Larson, E. B., Fihn, S. D., Kirk, L. M., Levinson, W. Loge, R. V., Reynolds, E., ...Williams, M. (2004). The future of general internal medicine. *Journal of General Internal Medicine, 19*, 69–77.

Loscalzo, M. J. (2007). Social workers: The connective tissue of the health care system. In L. Emanuel & S. L. Librach (Eds.), *Palliative care: Core skills and clinical competencies.* Philadelphia, PA: Saunders.

Mauch, D., Kautz, C., & Smith, S. A. (2008). *Reimbursement of mental health services in primary care settings* [Electronic version]. (HHS Pub. No. SMA-08-4324). Rockville, MD: Center for Mental Health Services, Substance Abuse and Mental Health Services Administration.

Mazzocco, W. (2001). Key elements of reimbursement coding: A guide for nurse practitioners. *Advance for Nurse Practitioners, 9*(9). Retrieved from Advance for NPs and Pas Web site: http://nurse-practitioners.advanceweb.com/Article/Key-Elements-of-Reimbursement-Coding.aspx

Meier, D. E., & Beresford, L. (2006). Billing for palliative care: An essential cost of doing business. *Journal of Palliative Medicine, 9*(2), 250–257.

National Association of Social Workers (NASW). (n.d.). *Certified Hospice and Palliative Social Worker (CHP-SW) and Advanced Certified Hospice and Palliative Social Worker (ACHP-SW).* Retrieved from http://www.socialworkers.org/credentials/credentials/chpsw.asp

National Association of Social Workers Center for Workforce Studies (2006). *Assuring the sufficiency of a frontline workforce: A national study of licensed social workers. Executive Summary.* Retrieved from National Association of Social Workers Web Site: http://workforce.socialworkers.org/studies/nasw_06_execsummary.pdf

National Association of Social Workers. (2008). *Code of Ethics.* Retrieved from National Association of Social Workers. Retrived from: http://www.socialworkers.org/pubs/Code/code.asp

National Hospice and Palliative Care Organization (NHPCO). (2008). *NHPCO and NASW announce the first Advanced Certified Hospice and Palliative Care Social Worker credential.* Retrieved from National Hospice and Palliative Care Organization Web site: http://www.nhpco.org/i4a/pages/index.cfm?pageid=5765

Payne, S. K., Coyne, P., & Smith, T. J. (2002). The health economics of palliative care. *Oncology, 16*(6), 801–808.

Reamer, F. G. (2006). *Social work values and ethics.* New York, NY: Columbia University Press.

Reese, D. J., & Sontag, M. (2001). Successful interprofessional collaboration on the hospice team. *Health and Social Work, 26*(3), 167–175.

Shortliffe, J., & Cimino, J. (2006). Biomedical informatics: Computer applications in health care and biomedicine. New York, NY: Springer Science and Business Media.

Smith, T. J., Coyne, P., Cassel, B., Penberthy, L., Hopson, A., & Hager, M. A. (2003). A high-volume specialist palliative care unit and team may reduce in-hospital end-of-life care costs. *Journal of Palliative Medicine*, 6(5), 699–705.

Specht, H. & Courtney, M. E. (1994). *Unfaithful angels: How social work has abandoned its mission*. New York, NY: The Free Press.

Substance Abuse and Mental Health Services Administration (SAMHSA). (2009). *Mental health codes and payers*. Retrieved from SAMHSA Web site: http://www.hipaa.samhsa.gov/pdf/Table_MH_Codes_Payers.pdf

Tolle, S. W., Rosenfeld, A. G., Tilden, V. P., & Park, Y. (1999). Oregon's low in-hospital death rates: What determines where people die and satisfaction with decisions on place of death? *American College of Physicians*, 30(8), 681–685.

von Gunten, C. F., Ferris, F. D., Kirschner, C., & Emanuel, L. L. (2000). Coding and reimbursement mechanisms for physician services in hospice and palliative care. *Journal of Palliative Medicine*, 3(2), 157–164.

von Gunten, C. F., Ferris, F. D., D'Antuono, R., & Emanuel, L. (2002). Recommendations to improve end-of-life care through regulatory change in U.S. health care financing. *Journal of Palliative Medicine*, 5(1), 35–41.

Weitzen, S., Teno, J. M., Fennell, M., & Mor, V. (2003). Factors associated with site of death: A national study of where people die. *Medical Care*, 41(2), 323–335.

Wenocur, S., & Reisch, M. (2001). *From charity to enterprise: The development of American social work in a market economy*. Urbana, IL: University of Illinois Press.

White, K. R., Stover, K. C., Cassel, B., & Smith, T. J. (2006). Nonclinical outcomes of hospital-based palliative care. *Journal of Healthcare Management*, 51(4), 260–273.

79 Social Work Research Agenda in Palliative and End-of-Life Care

Guadalupe R. Palos

You know, uh, because medicine says, there's really no hope and because you guys know what you're doing and, from a science standpoint, this is how it's gonna end. You know, there's still— God Almighty, who could step in and intervene at any time and I stand on that hope, you know, but I don't know that she has the same relationship. So that's difficult for me to see her there and not have the same tools that I have [pause] from God, and so it's difficult besides the stress that it puts on a family.

—37-year-old, married, Caucasian woman caring for her dying 64-year-old mother

Key Concepts

- *Palliative and end-of-life care is an emerging specialty area with an evolving science providing multiple opportunities to design studies that link social work practice and research questions.*
- *Social workers practitioners across all settings must integrate critical thinking in the selection and evaluation of interventions that will meet the needs and values of patients and families requiring palliative and end-of-life care.*
- *Social workers across all settings can build partnerships with community stakeholders, palliative care specialists, and skilled research teams to plan research studies that will promote the growth of palliative and end-of-life social work.*

Introduction

Research in palliative social work has a promising yet challenging future. In the past decade, the demand for professional social workers with specific knowledge, skills, and expertise in palliative and end-of-life care has dramatically increased. Professional organizations such as the Project on Death in America, National Association for Social Workers, the Social Work in Hospice and Palliative Care Network, and others have responded to this demand by *(a)* conducting national summits to develop action plans and networks to continue the growth in palliative and end-of-life care (Altilio, Gardia, & Otis-Green, 2007; Blacker, Christ, & Lynch, 2005; Christ & Blacker, 2002); *(b)* developing professional standards for social work practice (Gingerich, 2007; Gwyther et al., 2005; National Association of Social Workers [NASW], 2009; Payne, 2009; Walsh, Corbett, & Whitaker, 2005); and *(c)* creating a national agenda for coordinating social work research (Bern-Klug, Kramer, & Linder, 2005; Christ & Blacker, 2006; Kramer, Christ, Bern-Klug, & Francoeur, 2005). The strong combined efforts, collaboration, and dedication of these professionals and organizations led to the development of a proactive research agenda specific to palliative and end-of-life care. This social work research agenda is a comprehensive approach that *(a)* prioritizes key areas to develop and support social work research; *(b)* outlines specific steps to build a strong research infrastructure; *(c)* presents strategies for educating the next generation of social work researchers; and *(d)* promotes the dissemination of evidence-based research to enhance education, practice, policies, and program development in palliative and end-of-life care.

The primary goal of this chapter is to increase the social work professional's knowledge about social work research. A secondary goal is to raise the social worker's awareness on how to link their practice with research methodology to develop evidence-informed (i.e., evidence-based) social work interventions and treatment models. To achieve these goals, the chapter begins with a review of the federal and Congressional mandates implemented to advance the science of social work research in palliative and end-of-life care and follows with a discussion of the vision and commitment social work leaders and experts demonstrated in creating a national agenda for social work research. Next, the chapter will discuss methodological challenges in designing palliative and end-of-life clinical trials for patients and families. The chapter will close by presenting strategies for linking practice and scientific evidence and to continue building a solid foundation for social work research.

Highlights of Social Work Research Initiatives

Significant progress has been made to address the national research priorities outlined in *The National Agenda for Social Work Research in Palliative and End-of-Life Care* (Kramer et al., 2005), yet the efforts must continue. The timing of the proposed research agenda complemented several initiatives from Congress and the National Institutes of Health (NIH) such as the mandate from the Congressional Appropriations Committee to "develop a social work research plan that outlined research priorities, as well as a research agenda across NIH Institutes and Centers" (NASW, 2010, p. 1) and the Social Work Reinvestment Initiative that "is a collaborative effort comprised of leading social work organizations and other stakeholders committed to securing federal and state investments related to the recruitment, training, retention and research that strengthens the profession and communities it serves" (Senate Report 107-216, 2002, p. 155). These initiatives were strongly supported by the *NIH Social Work Plan for Social Work Research* (National Institutes of Health, 2003). The NIH Plan included various activities such as *(a)* providing NIH funding calling for investigator-initiated research grant applications specifically from social work researchers; *(b)* building the research infrastructure with centers across the nation to train and educate social workers in research; and *(c)* obtaining input from the social work community on the needs of social worker researchers.

Evidence of the support and momentum created by the social work research initiatives was demonstrated with the development of the Dorothy I. Height and Whitney M. Young, Jr. Social Work Reinvestment Act. The 111th Congress mandated the establishment of the National Center for Social Work Research (Inouye, 2009). The creation of the center was based on three significant Congressional findings:

(1) Social workers focus on the improvement of individual and family functioning and the creation of effective health and mental health prevention and treatment interventions in order for individuals to become more productive members of society.

(2) Social workers provide front-line prevention and treatment services in the areas of school violence, aging, teen pregnancy, child abuse, domestic violence, juvenile crime, and substance abuse, particularly in rural and underserved communities.

(3) Social workers are in a unique position to provide valuable research information on these complex social concerns, taking into account a wide range of social, medical, economic, and community influences from an interdisciplinary, family-centered, and community-based approach.

In 2009, the National Association of Social Workers (NASW) proactively established a think tank or institute entitled the Social Work Policy Institute (SWPI) to increase the visibility and strength of social workers in forming public policy, monitoring social work effectiveness, and creating a forum for examining issues in social service and health care delivery. Since its inception, the SWPI has hosted symposiums on comparative effectiveness research (CER) and on hospice social work (http://www.socialworkpolicy.org/press-releases/social-work-policy-institute-holds-think-tank-symposium-on-hospice-social-work.html. The SWPI think tanks are essential to identify current issues, identify gaps in practice and research, and create action plans for future policy and research. The institute is also a key stakeholder in strengthening the linkages between research and practice as evidenced by its role in supporting a change in philosophy from evidence-based practice to evidence-informed social work interventions and treatment models.

One critical area absent, yet applicable to each of the three significant findings, evolves from palliative and end-of-life care. Illness and death is an outcome regardless of the social problem identified, the geographic area, or other demographics. This omission indicates that work in this area, however, is far from complete. Potential challenges to implementing the social work research agenda in palliative and end-of-life care need to be identified and examined.

Creating a National Social Work Research Agenda in Palliative and End-of-Life Care

In 2002, the First Summit on End-of-Life and Palliative Care was held in Durham, North Carolina, to unite social work leaders and experts in developing a proactive initiative for social work in palliative and end-of-life care. This landmark summit culminated in the creation of a *Priority Map of the Social Work Agenda for Palliative, End-of-Life Care, and Grief Work* (Blacker et al., 2005; Christ & Blacker, 2002; Kramer et al., 2005). (For additional information, see Chapter 3.) In this priority map, two of the ten priority items for advancing social work focused on building funding and training for research on palliative and end-of-life care and developing a national research agenda. In the Second Summit held in 2005, research was once again identified as a priority action item (Blacker et al., 2005). During this summit, the deep commitment to advancing the science of social work in this specialty was represented in the national research agenda for social work (Bern-Klug et al., 2005; Kramer et al., 2005). Table 79.1 summarizes the priority research items outlined at the 2005 Summit.

Social Work Practice with Scientific Evidence

Since its inception the profession of social work and its practice has been guided by the use of various social science theories and models of practice. The purpose of social work

Table 79.1. Social Work Research Priority Action Items for Examining Palliative and End-of-Life Care	
Priority 1	Increasing the quality and quantity of social work research by building research capacity, training, mentoring, and leadership
Priority 2	Developing standard outcomes to measure the effectiveness of social work interventions in palliative and end-of-life care
Priority 3	Conducting research on the cost-effectiveness and efficacy of social work practice models that address palliative and end-of-life care
Priority 4	Promoting the social work research agenda through inter- and intradisciplinary practice-oriented collaborations and representation on national research advisory councils, organizations, and federal agencies
Priority 5	Establishing a strong research infrastructure for palliative and end-of-life social work research
Priority 6	Building commitment to funding social work research initiatives in palliative and end-of-life care
Priority 7	Advancing the science of social work research in palliative and end-of-life care through systematic, well-planned dissemination of research findings

Source: Adapted from Blacker, Christ, & Lynch, 2005.

practice models is to assist social workers in synthesizing the existing theories, assessing their models of practice, and determining how theories may be used to implement the most effective intervention needed for a particular situation. Examples of social work practice models include the cognitive-behavioral model, the biopsychosocial-spiritual model, the family-centered care model, and others. Several of these models were more often based on practice or theory rather than scientific research evidence.

In the early 1990s, a new philosophy for teaching and practice of medicine began to appear in medical journals and was termed *evidence-based medicine* (EBM). This new approach emphasized new knowledge and skills such as developing questions based on practice, searching and retrieving the best available evidence, and conducting a critique of the research methods presented in the evidence to determine the reliability and validity of the findings. Over time, EBM has proven to be a valuable approach in basing clinical decisions on scientific evidence. The EBM approach has evolved in other ways such as developing better access and retrieval of evidence-based data and increasing the integration of patient's preferences and values into clinical and practice decision making (Gambrill, 1999; Gambrill, 2007; Gibbs & Gambrill, 2002; Jenson, 2007; NASW, 2009). In fact, it has been integrated into other professions such as mental health, nursing, and health policy to guide clinical practice and decision making (Gambrill, 1999; Sackett, Straus, Richardson, Rosenburg, & Haynes, 2002).

Despite the adoption of EBM by many professions, the EBM model often does not readily fit the ethics and values embedded in the social work profession. For example, randomized clinical trials and meta-analyses may not be available, ethical, or practical in certain areas of social work practice. Our society recognizes that the social work profession is based "on ethical standards, clinical judgments, and practice wisdom" (Barker, 2003, p. 149). Although other professional disciplines may consider these factors in designing research studies, the core values of the social work profession—service, social justice, dignity and worth of the person, importance of human relationships, integrity, and competence—reflect the uniqueness of the social work profession (NASW, 1996). Thus, the core values and their principles unique to social work may not always be balanced within the complexity of an evidence-based medicine approach.

In response to this dilemma, this approach has been adapted to a model called evidence-based practice (EBP). The Institute for the Advancement of Social Work Research defines evidence-based practice "as a process that combines well-researched interventions with clinical experience, ethics, and client practices, and cultures to guide and inform the delivery of treatments and services" (Social Work Policy Institute, 2010, p. 10). This approach seems to fit the values, ethics, and practice of social work practice, education, and research. Much of the literature in EBP social work indicates that the overall goal of the EBP model is to guide social work practice and interventions based on scientific evidence from social work research (Howard, McMillen, & Pollio, 2003; Jenson, 2007; NASW, 2009). The benefit in using this approach is recognized by social workers in all types of settings and practice. The National Association of Social Work (NASW) believes that EBP will help practitioners meet their ethical responsibilities to "fully utilize evaluation and research evidence in their profession" (NASW, 1996).

A major initiative was launched under the American Recovery and Reinvestment Act of 2009, which provided generous funding for the National Institutes of Health, the Department of Health and Human Services, and the Agency for Healthcare Research and Quality to develop an agenda for comparative effectiveness research (CER). One major goal of CER is to assess the effectiveness of health care treatments and strategies of health care delivery. Because of the critical role the social work profession has in working with people who are vulnerable, oppressed, and living in poverty, the leadership of the CER initiative partnered with the Social Work Policy Institute (SWPI) of the NASW to host a research symposium with the goals of strengthening collaborations between the social work profession and federal agencies; to use CER methodology to build the research base of effective social work interventions and treatment; and most important, to strengthen linkages between research and practice that would lead to standards of practice (Social Work Policy Institute, 2010).

A major transformation, which occurred during the summit, was a change in philosophy regarding the evidence-based practice model previously used in social work. Participants at the summit concluded that a more appropriate term for social work would be *evidence-informed practice* (EIP). The adaptation of the model was based on the observations that the social work practice has not always integrated the results from research into practice and planning. The NASW report, *Comparing Effectiveness Research (CER) and Social Work*, lists three major outcomes of the EIP approach: *(1)* ability to locate the best practice and evidence-informed treatments by reviewing and synthesizing the most current research findings; *(2)* base practice and planning on established guidelines and standards; and *(3)* use outcomes research to guide one' own practice (2010). Hence, a major goal of our social work profession is to use evidence-informed practice (clinical research) to guide future social work practice, interventions, and treatment models.

Two of the most valuable tools used to determine the effectiveness of interventions are *(1)* the rating system for the hierarchy of the different levels of evidence and *(2)* the systematic approach used to identify the best available evidence (Gibbs, 2003; Reitsma et al., 2009; Sackett et al., 2002). These tools provide a necessary foundation for comparative effectiveness research (CER), which seeks to guide practitioners in selecting the most appropriate intervention for a specific patient or client situation.

For example, the EBM levels of evidence range from Level 1 to Level 9 (University of Washington Health Sciences Libraries, n.d.). In this framework, meta-analyses and systematic reviews, such as those provided in the Cochrane Collaboration Web site, are grouped into Level 1. These are considered the best evidence. Randomized clinical trials such as those published in scientific journal and listed on databases such as Pub MED fall into Level 4. Clinical guidelines and standards of practice such as those used by the National Quality Forum or the Agency for Healthcare Research and Quality are considered Level 3. The system assigns each type of evidence a numerical value to rank their usefulness as evidence.

The Cochrane Collaboration and Review, however, warns that this approach has several limitations. For example, each level uses different items to rate the quality, which makes it hard to determine which individual item has been met in a specific study (Reitsma et al., 2009). However, the model provides a summary of the types of evidence used in determining evidence-based practice. In social work, the sources of "evidence" may include the social worker's experience, the client/family values and preferences, the mission and values of an agency or organization, and the research available in social work.

According to the SWPI CER report (2010), multiple sources of information or evidence are available in the scientific world. However, each method has certain challenges when used in comparative effectiveness research. For example, the best evidence valued by scientific world values is systematic reviews or meta-analyses, or evidence-based clinical guidelines. Then there are research studies such as randomized clinical trials (RCTs), case control studies, or cohort studies. The CER initiative identified priority populations, conditions, and environments to test the effectiveness of the interventions. In hope of developing individually personalized interventions, the priority research populations were expanded to include ethnically and racially diverse populations, those with comorbid conditions, or those that differed by linguistic, cultural, or other demographic characteristics. While inclusion of these heterogeneous groups will make important advances in social work and CER research, this is a complex and challenging task. As a result, researchers who choose this area of research will need to be creative in the use of research designs and methods. For example, randomized clinical trials may need to focus on the group or community level rather than the individual level. Community-based participatory research models may be more appropriate to determine the effectiveness of service delivery and program planning. The effectiveness of service delivery and programs can also be evaluated using economic research methods, such as cost-effectiveness, cost-utility, or cost–benefit analysis. One of the most unique methods will be the use of qualitative and quantitative methods research to better understand the perspective of the client/patient/family in his or her own words. There is no question that the next generation of social work researchers will have multiple unique and challenging methods to determine future practice standards and guidelines.

Gibbs (2006) points out that the EBP approach can be adapted for social work research. He developed the Clinical Oriented Practical Evidence (COPES), which combines pieces of the EBM model such as the rating system and the process for identifying the best available scientific evidence. The COPES model adapts the EBM tools to reflect the reality of social work practice. The tools of the model are the Clinical Oriented Practical Evidence Search (COPES) and the Methodology Oriented Locaters for Evidence Search (MOLES). Table 79.2 provides examples of how the COPES

approach may be used in developing social work research in palliative and end-of-life care. The COPES approach is similar to the P process in that it may be grouped into different steps. The steps are based on a similar problem-solving process used in social work practice. Although the steps appear to be simple, the process is systematic, methodological, and comprehensive. If a step is omitted or taken out of sequence, it will increase the risk of limitations and erroneous conclusions when linking practice with research.

The examples provided in the COPES worksheet focus on areas that a social worker would encounter in his or her daily practice. The worksheet begins by providing three types of potential research areas: assessment, evaluation, and risk.

Table 79.2.
Evidence-Based Practice for Social Work Research Palliative and End-of-Life Care

Four Elements in a Well-Formulated Question

Question Types	Client Type and Problem	What You Might Do	Alternative Course of Action	What You Want to Accomplish
	How would I describe a group of clients of a similar type? Be specific.	Apply a treatment; act to prevent a problem; measure to assess a problem; survey clients; screen clients to assess risk.	What is the main alternative other than in the box to the left?	Outcome of treatment or prevention? Valid measure? Accurate risk estimation, prevented behavior, accurate estimation of need?
Example: Assessment	If family caregivers of patients who are receiving end-of-life care report feeling tired, sleepy, and sad	Are given three different assessment tools to evaluate them for fatigue, sleep disturbances, and distress	OR Are given one tool that assesses for multiple symptoms, including fatigue, sleep disturbances, and distress	Which method would provide a better assessment of the caregiver's emotional and physical status?
Evaluation	If seriously ill or dying patients are referred to an inpatient palliative care unit (hospital)	Are given an opportunity to participate in a family conference, which includes the entire team	OR Are given an opportunity to have a conference with only the social worker of the unit	Which approach would result in better outcomes for the patient and his or her family? Which method would lead to better client satisfaction?
Risk	If patients are receiving palliative care at home	Are monitored for their risk to increased distress and sadness using a telephone call by a social work once a week	OR Are monitored by a telephone voice system twice a week	Will the telephone call or the voice system provide better monitoring of the patient's increased risk for distress and sadness?

Source: Adapted with permission from Gibbs, L. (2003). *Evidence-based practice for the helping professions: A practical guide with integrated multimedia.* Pacific Grove, CA: Brooks/Cole—Thomson Learning.

Gibbs' (2003) approach uses four pieces to develop an appropriate research question. These areas include *(1)* describing the type of client and the client's problem; *(2)* identifying the standard strategies used in social work practice, *(3)* identifying an alternative approach, and *(4)* stating the desired outcomes for the client.

The COPES model integrates the MOLES process to further develop the research question. As shown in the example on Table 79.3, the process guides the researcher (novice or expert) through the research process. First, the researcher uses the data from the COPES planning form; next, the instructions on the MOLES planning sheet ask the person to identify terms that will help when a search for the scientific evidence is conducted. The MOLES process even provides examples of the types of evidence that may be used to support the research questions. For further discussion on this model, the reader is referred to the Web site resource list at the end of this chapter.

Table 79.3.
MOLES Search Planning Sheet: Social Work Research in Palliative and End-of-Life Care

	Column 1: Client Type and Problem	Column 2: What You Might Do	Column 3: Alternate Course of Action	Column 4: Intended Result	Column: MOLES Appropriate to Question Type (Effectiveness, Prevention, Risk, Assessment, Description)
Row 2: Determine Your Question Type, Then Insert Elements of Your Question in Spaces on Right	If seriously ill or dying patients are referred to an inpatient palliative care unit (hospital)	Are given an opportunity to participate in a family conference, which includes the entire team	OR Are given an opportunity to have a conference with only the social worker of the unit	Which approach would result in better outcomes for the patient and their family? And which method would lead to better patient/client satisfaction?	Leave blank
Row 3: Insert Key Terms from above, Synonyms, or Terms from Thesaurus or Controlled Language Vertically Connecting Terms by OR	Palliative care AND social work OR end-of-life care	AND family conferences	OR social work in inpatient unit or hospice AND end-of-life care	Qualitative research OR client satisfaction research AND family conferences AND palliative care AND social work	**In this box insert appropriate MOLES for your question type.** Client or patient satisfaction survey OR in-depth interview OR participant observation

MOLES, Methodology Oriented Locaters for Evidence Search.
Source: This table follows Sackett, D. L., Richardson, W. S., Rosenberg, W., & Haynes, R. B. (1997). *Evidence-based medicine: How to practice and teach EBM.* New York, NY: Churchill Livingstone.
Adapted with permission from Gibbs, L. (2003). *Evidence-based practice for the helping professions: A practical guide with integrated multimedia.* Pacific Grove, CA: Brooks/Cole—Thomson Learning.

By developing and implementing each step in the model, the social worker will be able to answer the question about a social work intervention using best available scientific evidence. When social work practice is linked with empirical research, the science of palliative social work will contribute to building evidence-based practice. The desired outcome is advance evidence-informed social work practice and research in palliative and end-of-life care.

Palliative and end-of-life care is a fairly new specialization and evolving science for social workers practitioners, educators, and researchers. As a result, there are multiple opportunities to link social work practice and research areas in the design of studies that will contribute to evidence-informed practice social work models for palliative and end-of-life care. The guidelines of the National Quality Forum (NQF) Preferred Practice for Palliative and Hospice Care were developed to promote quality palliative and end-of-life care. Clinicians, researchers, and policy makers support the NQF's efforts to promote excellence in this emerging specialty (Ferrell et al., 2007; Lynch & Dahlin, 2007; National Quality Forum, 2006). The NQF framework consists of eight broad domains and 38 practices that may be used to guide clinicians in their daily practice. The eight domains are as follows:

- Structure and processes of care
- Physical aspects of care
- Psychological and psychiatric aspects of care
- Social aspects of care
- Spiritual, religious, and existential aspects of care
- Cultural aspects of care
- Care of the imminently dying patient
- Ethical and legal aspects of care.

Further information on the domains and preferred practices may be obtained from the National Consensus Project for Quality Palliative Care Web site (http://www.nationalconsensusproject.org) and the NQF Web site: http://www.qualityforum.org

A well-documented example of linking the NFQ practice guidelines with the social work agenda is presented in an article by Altilio and colleagues (Altilio, Otis-Green, & Dahlin, 2008). The authors explain how Domain 4 of the *Guidelines, Social Aspects of Care* can be linked to several areas of practice and research related to care planning and communication. They center much of their discussion on the NQF Preferred Practice 18 (Conduct regular patient and family care conferences with the team) and Preferred Practice 19 (Develop and implement a comprehensive social plan). As one compares the NFQ domains and preferred practices, it is evident that social workers' standards, ethics, and practice complement the NFQ framework. Combining the NFQ standards with social work standards will provide a strong foundation for social research and practice in palliative and end-of-life care.

The purpose, process, and outcomes of each area of family conferences and social plans is thoroughly discussed, and case studies provide excellent examples of how social workers actualize their unique and essential roles and functions in palliative and end-of-life care. The value of family conferences in palliative and end-of-life care has been well documented (Fineberg, 2005; Heyman & Gutheil, 2006; Jones, 2005; Owen, Goode, & Haley, 2001; Teno & Claridge, 2004). (For additional information, see Chapter 22.) There are several unanswered research questions surrounding the family conference and social work practice. For example, certain research questions may emerge from the practice of a social work practitioner in an adult palliative care unit. Examples of appropriate questions that would examine areas not well studied may include research questions such as the following:

- When is the family conference the most effective in the trajectory of the palliative care experience?
- Do the needs of the patient, caregiver, and family differ; if so, how, and what interventions would be most effective?
- How do cultural background, values, and expectations of the patient and family affect decision making and delivery of social work intervention?
- What type of skill set is required of a palliative social worker to facilitate a family conference?
- What types of ethical conflicts do social work researchers encounter when their studies are conducted with patients who are dying and their families, whose values, attitudes, and practices may differ or conflict with those of the Western biomedical health care system?

Advancing Social Work Research in Palliative and End-of-Life Care

The long-term goals of the national research agenda for palliative and end-of-life social work is to advance the field and provide a scientific foundation for improving practice and outcomes for patients, families, and providers. Changes in social problems, health care settings, patient and family populations, combined with the growing attention to having a "good death," whatever that may mean in different cultures, are opening up opportunities for new research questions and studies. Table 79.4 provides a brief summary of research domains and objectives outlined in the *National Agenda for Research in Social Work in Palliative and End-of-Life Care* (Kramer et al., 2005). Potential areas of research, which may advance evidence-informed practice for social workers, are also listed and linked to each domain and objectives. Most researchers, regardless of background, agree that evidence-informed practice is essential for a profession to survive and that applies to social work in palliative and end-of-life care. Eduardo Bruera, M.D., a world-renowned palliative care physician noted that "research is not just useful but it is essential for the survival of social work in palliative and end-of-life care" (Interview with Eduardo Bruera, M.D.).

Table 79.4.
Domains and Objectives of Social Work Research Agenda for Palliative and End-of-Life Care

Research Domain	Selected Objective(s)	Potential Area of Research
Domain 1: Fragmentation, gaps, transition, and continuity of care	Develop and test innovations and interventions that *(a)* identify and prevent unnecessary transitions and *(b)* facilitate smooth necessary transitions	In collaboration with other team members, design a pilot study to identify the areas with the most severe fragmentation and gaps occurring along the trajectory of palliative and end-of-life care
Domain 2: Health care disparities and care	Investigate variations in the illness and death trajectory among diverse populations with attention to comorbidities	Develop descriptive studies with multiethnic, underserved patients who have more than one chronic diseases to better understand the impact on patients and family systems when dealing with symptoms of more than one disease
Domain 3: Financing and policy	Conduct descriptive research on financing practices across states to identify Medicaid and other coverage/reimbursement policies for palliative and end-of-life care for diverse populations	Design feasibility studies to determine the effectiveness of social work interventions that identify clients who may face financial barriers to care before they encounter the difficulties
Domain 4: Mental health services and issues	Develop reliable, valid, and practical rapid symptom assessment instruments and measures to examine the prevalence and severity of psychological symptoms among diverse care recipients with advanced disease	Develop clinical trial interventions that assess the prevalence of depression, distress, and other psychological symptoms in both patients and their caregivers and provide unique interventions (access to licensed social work counselors in the clinic) and test the effectiveness of that intervention
Domain 5: Individual and family needs, experiences, and care	Assess spiritual growth and other valued/positive experiences/conditions that contribute to resiliency, meaning making, and stress-related growth among diverse care recipients and family members	Conduct descriptive studies to examine the effects of positive coping skills of racially and cultural diverse patients, their caregivers, and families during the trajectory of illness and at end of life
Domain 6: Communication across the trajectory of palliative and end-of-life care	Identify and evaluate the social worker's contributions to the interdisciplinary team and the efficacy of team processes in influencing care outcomes	Design randomized clinical trials that compare the outcomes of patients and families who receive a systematic social work assessment and intervention and those who do not receive the social worker's intervention
Domain 7: Quality of care and services	Develop valid and reliable measures to assess social work processes and outcomes important to palliative and end-of-life care	Design and evaluate a social work–based intake form that assesses preferences for advance care planning, family presence during resuscitation, withdrawing nonbeneficial treatments, and other similar sensitive topics
Domain 8: Individual, caregiver, and family decision making, support, and care	Develop and test family conferencing models appropriate to different settings and diverse populations; consider cost as well as outcomes	Identify the unique contributions and evaluate the effectiveness of the social worker's role and practice in interdisciplinary palliative care family conference
Domain 9: Grief and bereavement	Develop age-specific and culturally sensitive measures of grief and bereavement outcomes	Conduct qualitative interviews to understand the experience of diverse groups towards grief and bereavement and use the data to develop user-friendly questionnaires that meet health-literacy criteria and universally understood concepts of grief and bereavement

Table 79.4. *(Contd.)*

Domain 10: Pain and symptom management	Develop and test social work interventions and practice guidelines to address pain and other symptoms	Identify innovative approaches (e.g., use trained community lay volunteers as educators) to educate patients and families about the barriers associated with using opioids for pain management
Domain 11: Curriculum development, education, and training	Develop and evaluate training initiatives to assist in the cultural transformation of death in America (e.g., community workshops on grief, advance directives, family caregiving, and navigating health care systems)	Use participatory research methods to gain trust and input from community-based organizations to develop culturally and linguistically appropriate strategies that will address specific values, attitudes, and practices about illness, dying, death, and issues related to this area

EoL, end of life.

Source: Domains and objectives adapted from Blacker, Christ, and Lynch (2005) and Kramer, Christ, Bern-Klug, *and* Francoeur (2005).

Challenges in End-of-Life Research Designs and Methods

Research involving palliative or end-of-life care continues to challenge patients, their families, researchers, and other health care providers. Complex challenges include *(a)* determining eligibility criteria for patient populations appropriate for the study sample; *(b)* identifying simple and user-friendly data collection tools and methods; *(c)* defining constructs such as a grief, bereavement, "good or bad death"; and *(d)* integrating values, decision making, and ethics into the research design and methods. The standards used to measure meaningful clinical research in the biomedical world include *(a)* using randomized clinical trial design; *(b)* establishing sufficient power; *(c)* having minimal attrition and missing data; and *(d)* relying on objective, measurable outcomes to measure success or effectiveness of a particular intervention or treatment (Cohen, 1988; Friedman, Furberg, & DeMets, 1998; Harman, 1967; Lynn, 1986). Unfortunately, when people require palliative or end-of-life care, theories or gold standards are not always ethical, feasible, or practical. For instance, randomized clinical trials are considered the "gold standard" in clinical research; however, certain groups such as the disabled, the incarcerated, the homeless, or ethnic and racial minorities have been excluded from participating in these trials. Yet these populations are often the most vulnerable and require interventions from experienced social work practitioners, particularly when they face a chronic, debilitating disease or pending death.

In fact, the social worker will often uncover the existence of social problems the family experienced before their need for palliative and end-of-life care. Bruera, a palliative care physician notes that "social workers in palliative specialization have not studied (in great depth) the impact of these social morbidities on the dying and the way the palliative care team

manages that entire experience" (Interview with Eduardo Bruera, M.D.). Social workers recognize that when a family has a serious history of social problems such as criminal behavior, substance abuse problems, and other similar social problems, these issues must also be addressed in the assessment, planning, and delivery of comprehensive, social work interventions. Unfortunately, there are no studies that have identified the best strategies for assisting those patients and families as they live with life-threatening illness and when they are dying. And more important, there is a lack of evidence to prove which strategies are the most effective for social workers to use in these sensitive circumstances. To close these gaps, social workers in palliative care must create a demand for evidence-informed research that will empower the practice. The narrative discussed in this chapter (see Box 79.1) is an excellent example of the types of social problems seriously ill patients and their families face during the illness experience.

Barriers that influence the linking of research to social work practice have been well documented and include factors such as lack of training or education in research methodology, lack of mentors, lack of administrative support, or lack of research infrastructure. A National Cancer Institute (NCI)-funded NASW study examined how social workers incorporate new research findings into their daily practice. Their results indicated that the two major barriers were lack of time and a lack of easy access to research findings (NASW, 2003). Fortunately, the study also identified strategies for improving the linkage between practice and research. Table 79.5 lists a few simple strategies that would help improve practice and research collaborations. Diane Benefiel, an expert social work practitioner in palliative and end-of-life care states, "to advance palliative care social work, we must educate ourselves about research and collaborate with our team members to design research studies so we can provide solid evidence to support our social work models" (Palos, 2009). (Interview with Diane Benefiel, 2009).

Table 79.5.
Strategies to Improve Practice and Research Collaboration in Palliative and End-of-Life Social Work

Involve community-based social work practitioners in the design and implementation of a new research study

Increase the knowledge and use of Web-based research resources by social workers in all settings (practitioners, educators, administrators, and researchers) by increasing access to Web-based databases, PDF publications, and other electronic resources

Develop methods to coordinate, consolidate, and disseminate resources, information, and education via the Web, social work journals, or newsletters from professional association or organizations

Continue collaborations with other professional organizations such as the National Quality Forum, the National Association for Social Workers, the Council on Social Work Education, Society for Social Work and Research, the National Hospice and Palliative Care Organization, the American Academy of Hospice and Palliative Medicine, and other key groups

Partner with community-based social work practitioners to brainstorm about potential areas of research with vulnerable populations often forgotten but who also need palliative and end-of-life care (e.g., social workers who deliver services to the disabled, homeless, the incarcerated, military families, and children)

Conducting research with patients and families who are living with life-threatening illness or dying requires innovative approaches that meet unique parameters yet maintain strong scientific rigor. George (2002) identified four major issues related to the research design. First, the researcher must determine whether the study will be cross-sectional or longitudinal; second, the investigator must decide whether surrogates may be used when the patient is too ill or unable to participate in the research; third, the research must choose appropriate data collection methods; and last, the researcher must make a decision whether to collect retrospective data in the study. George (2002) noted that gaps in palliative and end-of-life research include the following:

- Insufficient attention to psychological and spiritual issues
- The prevalence of psychiatric disorders and the effectiveness of the treatment of such disorders among dying persons
- Providers and health system variables
- Social and cultural diversity
- The effects of comorbidity on trajectories of dying (p. 86).

Table 79.6 illustrates the methodological challenges that social work researchers need to consider when designing and conducting palliative and end-of-life research trials (Engelberg, 2006; Field & Cassel, 1997; George, 2002; Lorenz et al., 2008; Pritchard et al., 1998; Sage, 2006; Steinhauser et al., 2006; Straus & Sackett, 1999). Despite these challenges, there is a vast supply of research tools and new opportunities emerging to assist social workers interested in conducting their own research studies. Table 79.7 illustrates how a mixed-methods approach was used in a study funded by the National Cancer Institute (NCI). In this study, a social work investigator chose to combine qualitative (semi-structured interviews) with quantitative (surveys) methods to ask specific research questions that evolved from her practice in working with highly symptomatic patients, their caregivers, and families. As illustrated in this example, a mixed-methods

Table 79.6.
Methodological Challenges in Conducting Palliative and End-of-Life Research

Challenge	Rationale
Inadequate sample size	Sampling techniques are not representative or adequate contributing to a small pool of eligible patients
Inadequate power	Incomplete data or decrease in study participants as the trial progresses
Respondent burden	Patients or study participants are too ill or debilitated to complete self-report assessment or study forms
Missing data	High withdrawal or dropout due to personal preferences, complicated or lengthy trials, progression of disease, or death
Tailored palliative and end-of-life interventions	Clinical trials rely on standard interventions and procedures while palliative and end-of-life interventions meet the individual's needs and use an interdisciplinary approach
Cultural, spiritual, or personal values	Clash of worldviews between biomedical researchers and patient/family Family members may wish to protect dying patient and attempt to convince a loved one not to participate in research

Table 79.7.
Illustration of a Mixed-Methods Research Study: Effects of Cancer Symptoms on Minority Caregivers

The general aim of this descriptive, longitudinal research study is to determine the effects of cancer patients' symptoms on the physical and mental health of poor, minority caregivers.

Domain	Problem	Research Question	Method
(1) Disparities and multicultural (2) Physical and psychological health status	Little understanding of the experience of being a caregiver to a patient who has limited resources and advanced cancer	What is the experience of being a minority or nonminority person caring for an underserved patient with advanced cancer over the patient's treatment?	Qualitative method: use a standardized script to ask caregivers specific questions about their experience
(3) Family and caregiver's physical and emotional health	Little evidence of the types of poor physical and mental health outcomes caregivers of underserved patients experience	What is the prevalence and severity of symptoms experienced by the patient's caregiver?	Quantitative methods: use valid and reliable tools to measure symptoms (fatigue, distress, depression, stress, sleep disturbances, and others)

Note: Funded by the National Cancer Institute, K07 CA102482—Effects of Cancer Symptoms on Minority Caregivers, Principal Investigator: Guadalupe R. Palos, RN, LMSW, DrPH.

approach provides an innovative way to examine a sensitive area with groups who may not be familiar or comfortable with the usual questionnaire studies (Creswell, Plano, & Vicki, 2007; Ell, Nishimoto, Mantell, & Hamovitch, 1988; Field & Cassel, 1997; Gibbs, 2007; Green et al., 2007; Lobchuk & Degner, 2002; Owen et al., 2001; Pierson, Curtis, & Patrick, 2002; Thornton, Pham, Engelberg, Jackson, & Curtis, 2009; Vincent, 2001).

The social work practitioner in palliative and end-of-life care frequently uses a "mixed-methods approach" in his or her daily practice. Practitioners use qualitative methods to understand or describe the meaning of key events or crisis in a client's life. To collect data (so to speak), the practitioner listens, observes, and responds to the client's verbal and nonverbal behavior. Once the interaction is terminated, the social worker begins his or her documentation or field notes of the meeting. Practitioners also use quantitative methods to assess a client's behavior, attitudes, or affect using more objective methods. The quantitative methods may include assessing the client for certain psychological concerns by using standardized scales or tools to measure depression, anxiety, and other similar mental health conditions. Social workers in palliative and end-of life care settings have recognized the benefits in using both methods in their practice with clients and their families. For example, the narrative in Box 79.1 provides an example of how the research process may be integrated into a social worker's daily practice in a palliative care setting.

There are many clinical issues as well as social service needs that are evident in this narrative. In this chapter, we will focus on the research aspects of the situation. Based on the need for a referral to another hospital for palliative

care, there are gaps and fragmentation in Clara's care and the potential for Clara to feel abandoned by her primary oncology team. Emily's history illustrates the critical need to schedule a team family conference as soon as possible and to include the caregiver in family assessments. Another area of concern is the anticipation of escalating pain and further physical decline as Clara's disease progresses.

This is an excellent opportunity for the social worker to integrate practice with research. For example, the social worker's is aware of a study that is tracking changes in the effects the patient's cancer symptoms has on the caregiver's physical and mental health over a 20-week period. The social worker may determine that participation of the patient/caregiver in this particular study may provide the family

---

Box 79.1
Patient/Family Narrative: Clara

Clara, age 58, is an African American matriarch of her nuclear and extended family who is diagnosed with incurable metastatic breast cancer. Her oncology team has referred Clara to another hospital to receive outpatient palliative care, anticipating that she will need active palliative intervention as she comes to the end of her life. There are three major concerns related to Clara's needs: (1) declining functional status; (2) developing a plan to address transportation to and from her appointments to the clinic; and (3) determining whether Clara's primary caregiver and daughter, Emily, has the physical and emotional strength to be the primary caregiver. Emily was diagnosed with schizophrenia years ago. Currently, she is not taking her medications because she believes the medicine will impair her ability to function as a caregiver.

additional support. The outcome, in this example, led to an integration of social work practice (assessment and observations) and research methods to evaluate the emotional and physical health of the caregiver and patient.

The combination of a family conference (qualitative methods) with more formal assessment through validated questionnaires will provide a comprehensive database of information that can be used to triage interventions and assess outcomes for any family in crisis.

Social workers who believe they may not have the skills or knowledge needed to conduct research in their settings must be reminded that their profession has prepared them with basic skills in gathering data. As noted in the narrative, the social worker integrated the same knowledge and problem-solving skills used in daily practice with the research process. Social workers must recognize the critical need to integrate practice and research into their daily routine, despite the competing demands. In choosing to become a researcher (novice or expert), social workers will formalize their knowledge and expertise in research methodology to link research with their practice.

Changing the Future

At this time, research in social work palliative care is a frontier that will provide new opportunities for research collaboration with other disciplines on the palliative care and end-of-life team. The unique body of skills, knowledge, and experience that a social worker brings to the team are highly valued by other members of the team. Social workers who step forward to conduct research in this subspecialty area will be the future leaders in palliative and end-of-life research, practice, education, and policy initiatives. Fortunately, the profession had the vision to develop a strong palliative social work research agenda, the voice to disseminate the goals and objectives of the plan to key partners in palliative and end-of-life care, and the commitment to provide the best evidence-informed model for changing the future of social work practice and research in palliative and end-of-life care.

Summary

The specialization of social work research in palliative and end-of-life care is rapidly evolving. The response to the development of a research agenda from the social work profession and leadership continues to contribute to the growing interest in palliative and end-of-life care. Dr. Bruera believes, "the future of palliative social work is very bright … because it impacts the field in a way no other profession impacts palliative care" (Interview with Eduardo Bruera, M.D.).

Despite the growth, the field is primed for continuing pioneer work that will link practice, education, and research to address the gaps in palliative care and end-of-life care. Social workers willing to be the pioneers of research will find there are many rewards, advantages, and disadvantages to conducting this type of research.

For example, education and training in conducting rigorous empirical research is limited in schools of social work, funding to support future research in palliative care is severely restricted, and to date, social work research lacks the foundation of scientific evidence needed to support the models of practice and interventions currently employed. Despite these challenges, there are innovative ways to move palliative social work to the next level. The timing is perfect to reach out to social work colleagues working in diverse community settings—those working in settings such as hospitals, agencies, nursing homes, and hospices. Establishing partnerships with community-based social workers will provide an avenue to reach groups who reflect our most vulnerable and diverse populations. By reaching out and becoming visible, trust and cooperation between researchers and social workers may be built, and that will have a positive effect on future research efforts. Ultimately, the goal is to build an evidence-informed social work practice model that will advance the science of palliative and end-of-life care for the next generation of patients and their families.

LEARNING EXERCISES

- To become familiar with the databases available to search for relevant research:
  a. Go to your library or library's Web site and locate the menu of databases.
  b. Enter a search term for a topic or intervention related to social work palliative and end-of-life care.
  c. Once the search results are available, review the various citations. Examine their date, journal, and authors. Then determine whether the citation is a review paper or original research. Rate each piece of information using the seven levels of evidence.
  d. Summarize the evidence provided in each source and describe how the citations would influence your social work practice or intervention.
  e. Provide a brief rationale for your outcomes.
- To raise awareness of the lived experiences of researchers who currently conduct studies with patients who require palliative and end-of-life care:
  a. Develop a list of 3–4 questions that you can use to interview a researcher in palliative or end-of-life care.
  b. Ask the researcher whether you may interview him or her and tape his or her views toward designing and conducting research in palliative care settings.

The researcher may be a social worker, nurse, physician, or other allied health provider.

c. Take field notes during the interview (who was present, the setting, time started).

d. Listen to your taped interview and identify research topics that are applicable to palliative care and end-of-life care research, social work practice, or key topics identified in the national agenda for social work research in palliative and end-of-life care.

- To become familiar with Internet Resources that will link you to social work list-serv sites that provide "latest news," data, or lists of researchers that may be interested in collaborating on research studies.

a. Go to the Web site resource list provided in this chapter and select a Web site under Professional Organizations to visit.

b. For example, go to the Social Work Research Network SWRnet Web site: http://www.bu.edu/swrnet/

c. Review the different resources available to the user such as subscribing to the SWRnet newsletter, signing up on the listserv, or checking the funding site for potential sources to fund your research.

d. Another excellent resource is the Social Work Hospice and Palliative Care Network (SWHPN) Web site. This Web site is designed specifically for social workers interested in end-of-life and palliative care. Visit the Web site and view the benefits available to members: http://www.swhpn.org/.

ADDITIONAL RESOURCES

SUGGESTED READINGS

Aday, L. A. (2001). *At risk in America: The health and health care needs of vulnerable populations in the United States.* San Francisco, CA: Jossey-Bass.

Ferrell, B. R., & Coyle, N. (Eds.). (2010). *Textbook of palliative nursing* (3rd ed.). New York, NY: Oxford University Press.

Field, A. (2009). *Discovering statistics using SPSS* (3rd ed.). Thousand Oaks, CA: Sage Publications.

Gibbs, L. (2003). *Evidence-based practice for the helping professions: A practical guide with integrated multimedia.* Pacific Grove, CA: Brooks/ Cole an Imprint of Wadsworth Publishers.

Glanza, K., Rimer, B. K., & Viswanath, K. (Eds.). (2008). *Health behavior and health education: Theory, research, and practice.* (4th ed.). San Francisco, CA: John Wiley & Sons.

Hair, J. F., Black, W. C., Babin, B. J., & Anderson, R. E. (2010). *Multivariate data analysis* (7th ed.). Upper Saddle River, NJ: Prentice-Hall.

Hales, S., Zimmermann, C., & Rodin, G. (2008). The quality of dying and death. *Archives of Internal Medicine, 168*(9), 912–918.

Jones, J. H. (1981). *Bad blood: The Tuskegee syphilis experiment.* New York, NY: The Free Press.

Jordan, C., & Franklin, C. (2003). *Clinical assessment for social workers: Quantitative and qualitative methods.* Chicago, IL: Lyceum Books, Inc.

Lewins, A., & Silver, C. (2007). *Using software in qualitative research: A step-by step guide.* Thousand Oaks, CA: Sage Publications.

Miller, W. R., & Rollnick, S., (2002). *Motivational interviewing: Preparing people for change.* New York, NY: The Guilford Press.

Rubin, A., & Babbie, E. R. (2008). *Research methods for social work.* Belmont, CA: Brooks/Cole, Cengage Learning.

RESOURCES AND WEB SITES

FEDERAL AGENCIES

Government Web sites that provide clinical information, funding opportunities, research findings, current funded studies, instructions for completing grant applications, training and research programs, and other pertinent resources related to research.

Agency for Healthcare Research and Quality: http://www.ahrq.gov/

National Institutes of Health: http://www.nih.gov/

National Institutes of Health Research Portfolio Reporting Tool (RePORT): http://www.ahrq.gov/

National Quality Forum (NQF): http://qualityforum.org/

PROFESSIONAL ORGANIZATIONS

National Association of Social Workers: Promoting Excellence in Pain Management and Palliative Care for Social Workers: National Association of Social Workers Research Web site: http://www.socialworkers.org/research/researchMore.asp

Social Work Hospice & Palliative Care Network: http://www.swhpn.org/

Social Work Research Network (SWRnet): http://www.bu.edu/swrnet/

Society for Social Work and Research (SSWR): http://www.sswr.org/

EVIDENCE-BASED PRACTICE RESOURCES

Clinical Oriented Practical Evidence Search—COPE Planning Sheet: http://www.evidence.brookscole.com/copse.html

Evidence-Based Practice for the Helping Professions: http://www.evidence.brookscole.com/index.html

Evidence Based Clinical Practice Tutorial—University of Rochester: http://www.urmc.rochester.edu/hslt/miner/resources/evidence_based/index.cfm

Evidence Based Practice & Policy Online Resource Training Center, William & Albert Musher Program at Colombia University School of Social Work: http://www.columbia.edu/cu/musher/Website/Website/EBP_Resources_WebEBPP.htm

Institute for the Advancement of Social Work Research (2007)– Partnerships to Integrate Evidence-Based Mental Health Practices into Social Work Education and Research:

http://login.npwebsiteservices.com/iaswr/ EvidenceBasedPracticeFinal.pdf

Introduction to Evidence-Based Medicine—Duke and University of North Carolina Chapel Hill: http://www.hsl.unc.edu/ services/tutorials/ebm/index.htm

Journal of Evidence-Based Social Work—The Haworth Press: http://www.informaworld.com/smpp/ title~content=t792303996 ~db=all

Methodology Oriented Locaters for Evidence Searching—MOLES Planning Sheet: http://www.evidence.brookscole.com/search. html

CLINICAL TRIALS WEB SITE

Education Network to Advance Cancer Clinical Trials (ENACCT): http://www.enacct.org/yourrole

INTERNET PROFESSIONAL DATABASES FOR SEARCHES

Campbell Collaboration: http://www.campbellcollaboration.org/ CINAHL

Cochrane Collaboration: http://www.cochrane.org/docs/ campbell.htm

Cochrane Library: http://mrw.interscience.wiley.com/cochrane/ cochrane_search_fs.html

Expert Consensus Guidelines: http://www.psychguides.com/

Google Scholar: http://scholar.google.com/

ISI Web of Science: http://apps.isiknowledge.com/WOS_ GeneralSearch_input.do?product=WOS&search_mode=Gener alSearch&SID=1E6ABOoCbiIeGoHE6@L&preferencesSaved

Note: You may need a subscription from your library to access the database.

MEDLINE—PubMed: http://www.ncbi.nlm.nih.gov/sites/entrez? myncbishare=mdacclib&holding=mdacclib_fft&dr=abstract

Plus with Full Text (Cumulative Index to Nursing and Allied Health Literature)—EBSCO: http://web.ebscohost.com/ehost/ search?vid=1&hid=11&sid=0a20298e-8d9b-40a0-b3a7-e81748d4e2ab%40sessionmgr14

Psychology and Behavioral Sciences Collection—EBSCO: http:// web.ebscohost.com/ehost/ search?vid=1&hid=11&sid=03fcc287-5d2f-48e7-80db-546ad21501e9%40sessionmgr13

Scopus: http://www.scopus.com/home.url

Note: You may need a subscription from your library to access the database.

REFERENCES

Altilio, T., Gardia, G., & Otis-Green, S. (2007). Social work practice in palliative and end-of-life care: A report from the summit. *Journal of Social Work in End-of-Life and Palliative Care, 3*, 68–86.

Altilio, T., Otis-Green, S., & Dahlin, C. M. (2008). Applying the National Quality Forum preferred practices for palliative and hospice care: A social work perspective. *Journal of Social Work in End-of-Life and Palliative Care, 4*, 3–16.

Barker, R., (Ed.). (2003). *The social work dictionary* (5th ed.). Washington, DC: NASW Press.

Bern-Klug, M., Kramer, B. J., & Linder, J. F. (2005). All aboard: Advancing the social work research agenda in end-of-life and palliative care. *Journal of Social Work in End-of-Life and Palliative Care, 1*, 71–86.

Blacker, S. & Christ, G. (March 20-22, 2002). *Designing an agenda for social work in end-of-life and palliative care. Unpublished Executive summary of Interactive workshop report from Social Work Summit on End-of-Life and Palliative Care, Duke University.* Durham, NC.

Blacker, S., Christ, G., & Lynch, S. (2005). *Charting the course for the future of social work in end-of-life and palliative care: A report of the 2nd social work summit on end-of-life and palliative care.* The Social Work in Hospice and Palliative Care Network. Retrieved from :http://www.swhpn.org/monograph.pdf.

Christ, G., & Blacker, S. (2006). Shaping the future of social work in end-of-life and palliative care. *Journal of Social Work in End-of-Life and Palliative Care, 2*, 5–12.

Cohen, J. (1988). *Statistical power analysis for the behavioral sciences* (2nd ed.). Hillsdale, NJ: Lawrence Erlbaum Associates.

Creswell, J. W., Plano, C., & Vicki, L. (2007). *Designing and conducting mixed methods research.* Thousand Oaks, CA: SAGE Publications.

Ell, K., Nishimoto, R., Mantell, J., & Hamovitch, M. (1988). Longitudinal analysis of psychological adaptation among family members of patients with cancer. *Journal of Psychosomatic Research, 32*, 429–438.

Engelberg, R. A. (2006). Measuring the quality of dying and death: methodological considerations and recent findings. *Current Opinion in Critical Care, 12*, 381–387.

Ferrell, B., Connor, S. R., Cordes, A., Dahlin, C. M., Fine, P. G., Hutton, N., …Zuroski, K. (2007). The national agenda for quality palliative care: The National Consensus Project and the National Quality Forum. *Journal of Pain and Symptom Management, 33*, 737–744.

Field, M. J., & Cassel, C. K. (1997). *Approaching death: Improving care at the end of life [Report of the Institute of Medicine].* Washington, DC: National Academy Press.

Fineberg, I. C. (2005). Preparing professionals for family conferences in palliative care: Evaluation results of an interdisciplinary approach. *Journal of Palliative Medicine, 8*, 857–866.

Friedman, L. M., Furberg, C., & DeMets, D. L. (1998). *Fundamentals of clinical trials.* (3rd ed.) New York, NY: Springer.

Gambrill, E. (1999). Evidence-based clinical practice, evidence-based medicine and the Cochrane collaboration. *Journal of Behavioral Therapeutic Experimental Psychiatry, 30*, 1–14.

Gambrill, E. (2007). Views of evidence-based practice: Social workers' code of ethics and accreditation standards as guides for choice. *Journal of Social Work Education, 43*, 447–462.

George, L. K. (2002). Research design in end-of-life research: State of science. *Gerontologist, 42*, 86–98.

Gibbs, L. (2003). *Evidence-based practice for the helping professions: A practical guide with integrated multimedia.* Pacific Grove, CA: Brooks/ Cole, an imprint of Wadsworth Publishers.

Gibbs, L. (2007). Applying research to making life-affecting judgments and decisions. *Research on Social Work Practice, 17*, 143–150.

Gibbs, L., & Gambrill, E. (2002). Evidence-based practice: Counterarguments to objections. *Research on Social Work Practice, 12*, 452–476.

Gingerich, B. S. (2007). Quality and competence in end of life/ palliative care. *Home Health Care Management and Practice, 19*, 402–403.

Green, J., Willis, K., Hughes, E., Small, R., Welch, N., Gibbs, L., & Daly, J. (2007). Generating best evidence from qualitative research: the role of data analysis. *Australian and New Zealand Journal of Public Health, 31*, 545–550.

Gwyther, L. P., Altilio, T., Blacker, S., Christ, G., Csikai, E. L., & Hooyman, N. (2005). Social work competencies in palliative and end-of-life Care. *Journal of Social Work in End of Life and Palliative Care, 1*, 87–120.

Harman, H. H. (1967). *Modern factor analysis*. (2nd ed., text rev.) Chicago, IL: University of Chicago Press.

Heyman, J. C., & Gutheil, I. A. (2006). Social work involvement in end of life planning. *Journal of Gerontological Social Work, 47*, 47–61.

Howard, M. O., McMillen, C. J., & Pollio, D. E. (2003). Teaching evidence-based practice: Toward a new paradigm for social work education. *Research on Social Work Practice, 13*, 234–259.

Jenson, J. M. (2007). Evidence-based practice and the reform of social work education: A response to Gambrill and Howard and Allen-Meares. *Research on Social Work Practice, 17*, 569–573.

Jones, B. L. (2005). Pediatric palliative and end-of-life care: The role of social work in pediatric oncology. *Journal of Social Work in End-of-Life and Palliative Care, 1*, 35–62.

Kramer, B. J., Christ, G. H., Bern-Klug, M., & Francoeur, R. B. (2005). A national agenda for social work research in palliative and end-of-life care. *Journal of Palliative Medicine, 8*, 418–431.

Lobchuk, M. M., & Degner, L. (2002). Symptom experience: Perceptual accuracy between advanced stage cancer patients and family caregivers in the home care setting. *Journal of Clinical Oncology, 20*, 3495–3507.

Lorenz, K. A., Lynn, J., Dy, S. M., Shugarman, L. R., Wilkinson, A., Mularski, R. A., … Shekelle, P. G. (2008). Evidence for improving palliative care at the end of life: A systematic review. *Annals of Internal Medicine, 148*, 147–159.

Lynch, M., & Dahlin, C. M. (2007). The National Consensus Project and National Quality Forum preferred practices in care of the imminently dying. *Journal of Hospice and Palliative Nursing, 9*, 316–322.

Lynn, M. R. (1986). Determination and quantification of content validity. *Nursing Research, 35*, 382–385.

National Association of Social Workers (NASW). (1996). *NASW code of ethics*. Washington, DC: Author.

National Association of Social Workers (NASW). (2003). *Barriers of translating oncology research to social work practice*. Retrieved from http://www.naswdc.org/research/NCI-Report.pdf

National Association of Social Workers (NASW). (2009). *Evidence-based practice*. Retrieved from http://www.socialworkers.org/ research/researchMore.asp

National Association of Social Workers (NASW). (2010). *Social work reinvestment fact sheet: A mandate for action*: Retrieved from http://socialworkreinvestment.org/Content/overview.pdf

National Institutes of Health (NIH). (2003). *NIH plan for social work research*. Retrieved from http://obssr.od.nih.gov/pdf/ SWR_Report.pdf

National Quality Forum. (2006). *A national framework and preferred practices for palliative and hospice care quality: A consensus report*. Washington, DC: Author.

Owen, J. E., Goode, K. T., & Haley, W. E. (2001). End-of-life care and reactions to death in African American and white family caregivers of relatives with Alzheimer's disease. *Omega, 43*, 349–361.

Payne, M. (2009). Developments in end-of-life and palliative care social work: International issues. *International Social Work, 52*, 513–524.

Pierson, C. M., Curtis, J. R., & Patrick, D. L. (2002). A good death: A qualitative study of patients with advanced AIDS. *AIDS Care, 14*, 587–598.

Pritchard, R. S., Fisher, E. S., Teno, J. M., Sharp, S. M., Reding, D. J., & Knaus, W. A. (1998). Influence of patient preferences and local health system characteristics on the place of death. *Journal of the American Geriatrics Society, 46*, 1242–1250.

Reitsma, J. B., Rutjes, A. W. S., Whiting, P. V. V., Leeflang, M. M. G., & Deeks, J. J. (2009). Assessing methodological quality. In J. J. Deeks, P. M. Bossuyt, & C. Gatsonis (Eds.), *Cochrane handbook for systematic reviews of diagnostic test accuracy version 1.0.0.*(pp. xx–xx). The Cochrane Collection.

Sackett, D. L., Straus, S. E., Richardson, W. S., Rosenburg, W., & Haynes, R. B. (2002). *Evidence-based medicine: How to practice and teach EBP* (2nd ed.). New York, NY: Churchill Livingstone.

Sage, M. R. (2006). Linguistic competence/language access services (LAS) in end-of-life and palliative care: a social work leadership imperative. *Journal of Social Work in End-of-Life and Palliative Care, 2*, 3–31.

Senate Report. (2002) Department of labor, health, and human services, and education, and related agencies appropriation bill, 2003. Report 107-216 (page 155). Retrieved from

Social Work Policy Institute. (2010). *Comparative effectiveness research and social work: Strengthening the connection*. Washington, DC: National Association of Social Workers.

Steinhauser, K. E., Clipp, E. C., Hays, J. C., Olsen, M., Arnold, R., Christakis, N. A., …Tulsky, J. A. (2006). Identifying, recruiting, and retaining seriously-ill patients and their caregivers in longitudinal research. *Palliative Medicine, 20*, 745–754.

Straus, S. E., & Sackett, D. L. (1999). Applying evidence to the individual patient. *Annals of Oncology, 10*, 29–32.

Teno, J. M., & Claridge, B. R. (2004). Family perspectives on end-of-life care at the last place of care. *Journal of the American Medical Association, 291*, 88–93.

Thornton, J. D., Pham, K., Engelberg, R. A., Jackson, J. C., & Curtis, J. R. (2009). Families with limited English proficiency receive less information and support in interpreted intensive care unit family conferences. *Critical Care Medicine, 37*, 89–95.

University of Washington Health Sciences Libraries. (n.d.). *Evidence-based practice tools summary*. Retrieved from http:// healthlinks.washington.edu/ebp/ebptools.html

Vincent, J. L. (2001). Cultural differences in end-of-life care. *Critical Care Medicine, 29*, N52–N55.

Walsh, K., Corbett, B., & Whitaker, T. (2005). Developing practice tools for social workers in end-of-life care. *Journal of Social Work in End-of-Life and Palliative Care, 1*, 3–9.

80

Debra Parker Oliver and Karla T. Washington

Merging Research and Clinical Practice

A lot of [the] time the social workers will come out and ... say, "What can I do for you?" [The caregiver is] in this position, "Well, I don't know what you can do for me. I don't know what you have to offer. I don't know what your agency encompasses. I need you to tell me what you can do for me." There are so many decisions. You are so overwhelmed that all of a sudden somebody asks you a question like that, and it's like, "I don't know. I don't even know my own name half the time. What do you want?" But [this intervention] had a structured way. It had steps to follow and think about, and think back, and move forward.
—Response from Sara Smith, a hospice caregiver participating in a problem-solving intervention study (Demiris et al., in review)

Key Concepts

There are three key concepts that are important to highlight when reviewing this chapter. These three concepts are defined as follows:

◆ *Practice evaluation refers to a systematic assessment of the effectiveness of interventions to bring about positive outcomes for patients and families to ensure that they receive the most appropriate services available. The assessment of interventions and their outcomes is a key component of evidence-based practice.*

◆ *Evidence-based practice refers to the integration of the best available research and clinical expertise with client values to direct care. In addition to improving outcomes for patients and families, an advantage of using evidence-based interventions in palliative social work is that those findings can be used to demonstrate the value of social work on interdisciplinary palliative care teams.*

Evidence-informed practice is a term used to describe a way of merging research and practice that is different from more rigid conceptualizations of evidence-based practice. Evidence-informed practice honors multiple ways of knowing and stresses the important roles of judgment and critical thought in determining the appropriate use of research in decision making.

Introduction

The purpose of this chapter is to educate palliative social workers about the importance of research and its relationship to practice. Palliative social workers participate in research to improve care for patients and families and advocate for patient and family participation in research of new interventions. Equally important is the reading and evaluation of research studies highlighting interventions and the integration of evidence from that research into clinical practice. After reading this chapter, social workers will be able to describe strategies to evaluate social work practice in palliative care and, in turn, practice palliative social work that is informed by a solid evidence base.

Merging Research and Clinical Practice

Social Work and Research

How many social work students appreciate the connection between research and effective practice? How many practitioners do? How might research help answer the question asked by the medical director? The consensus among many social work students appears to be that research skills are something learned in order to be successful in research class, nothing

735

As a hospice social worker, you provided services to Mrs. Jones and her husband for 6 months prior to her death. Today you are attending an interdisciplinary team meeting during which Mrs. Jones' death is being discussed. The discussion is focused primarily on pain and symptom management and the events surrounding the death. The following conversation occurs:

The registered nurse who was on call the night of the death reports, "Mrs. Jones died Sunday morning at 3:00 a.m. Mr. Jones phoned me at 1:30 a.m. and told me his wife had changed and asked me to come and check on her. Upon arriving at the home, Mr. Jones greeted me and we went to the living room to see his wife. Her respirations were very shallow, and he could not awaken her. I noticed the Signs and Symptoms of Impending Death handout at the bedside, and I asked Mr. Jones if he had discussed the information in the handout with his wife's nurse case manager. He reported that they had reviewed the information earlier in the week, which was why he had called. I assured him that he had done the right thing and told him I felt her passing was nearing. Mrs. Jones was peaceful, and Mr. Jones was accepting of the events. I encouraged him to say his final words and give his wife reassurance, which he did beautifully. She passed peacefully and he seemed to be handling things quite well, expressing tremendous appreciation. I feel we did an outstanding job considering where they were when we started."

The medical director then asks the nurse case manager, "So all pain and symptoms were under control and the goals of care were met?" The nurse case manager responds, "Yes. When she came to us, her pain was out of control. At that time, she rated her pain as a 7 on a scale from 1 to 10. Mr. Jones was very nervous when we started the morphine and getting him to understand the importance of giving it regularly, especially for breakthrough pain, was very challenging." The medical director turns to you and asks, "So, how did your work with the patient and family go? Do you feel the goals of care were achieved?"

How Do We Know?

The discussion in Box 80.1 presents an interesting question. How do we know what we know? Richard Grinnell and Yvonne Unrau (2008) describe five ways we acquire knowledge: authority, tradition, experience, intuition, and research. The first way we might answer the question presented by the medical director in Box 80.1A is based on what someone in authority tells us. Perhaps you know you did a good job and the family was satisfied because the family told you so or perhaps the doctor or nurse told you so. This can be quite gratifying but then, of course, you must decide how they know. A second way you might know you were successful is based on tradition. Tradition is a very common approach to the dissemination of knowledge, especially early in the life of a new and emerging knowledge base. When hospice emerged in the United States, the primary way American providers learned about hospice was through the traditions in the United Kingdom. A third way to acquire knowledge is through experience. Perhaps you are a very experienced social worker and have worked with hundreds of families and think you know when you are being effective and when you are not. Similarly, social workers tend to "know" they did a good job by intuition. We may use "practice judgment" or "practice wisdom" to define a problem or implement and evaluate an intervention.

A fifth way social workers acquire knowledge is by implementing research methods and using data. A systematic and ongoing process of psychosocial assessment would

When I started working with the patient's husband, he was terrified that he would kill his wife if he gave her the pain medication as ordered. After I helped him sort through those fears and used facts to challenge some common myths about pain medications, he grew to understand why his wife's pain medication was ordered and how to assess her pain. He eventually felt comfortable administering the medicine in accordance with the guidelines the nurses provided. When we began working together, Mr. Jones expressed strong agreement with many inaccurate statements about pain medication on the Caregiver Pain Medicine Questionnaire (CPMQ) (Letizia, Creech, Norton, Shanahan, & Hedges, 2004). His level of agreement with inaccurate beliefs gradually decreased. On his most recent CPMQ, he indicated strong disagreement with such potentially harmful statements as, "It's better for hospice patients to wait to take pain medication until it is really needed or else it will not work later." As Mr. Jones grew more comfortable responding to his wife's pain, her pain ratings decreased from a 7 out of 10 to 2 out of 10. At the same time, Mr. Jones' caregiver quality of life scores increased dramatically. The goals of improved adherence with pain medication administration, increased quality of life, and lowered pain for the patient all seem to have been achieved.

more. Research's applicability beyond the educational arena goes largely unexplored. Most students develop a professional identity as a practitioner, not a researcher and while the need for evidence-based practice is increasingly emphasized in social work education, too few students recognize their professional responsibility to contribute to the evidence base from which they supposedly structure their practice. The same can be said of many social work practitioners who decline to participate in research or who become informed of emerging evidence only when time permits or when professional or administrative bodies require continuing education.

The social work profession is composed largely of individuals with a strong and sincere commitment to helping others, yet, as social workers, we often devote little time to determining whether our efforts have been effective. We dedicate even less time to systematically evaluating innovative social work strategies in order to expand our existing professional knowledge base. Our goal is helping others, but do we? How do we know?

allow you to answer the medical director's question by providing data that support your efforts as a social worker. Familiarity with research about the ways social workers can impact pain management, using tested instruments to assess how to intervene, measuring the results of the intervention, and reporting the outcome data allows you to arrive at conclusions based on evidence. For example, a social worker employed by an agency that uses an ongoing interdisciplinary assessment of caregivers and of pain might respond to the medical director as exemplified in Box 80.1B.

This answer to the medical director's question is what this chapter is all about. It is about using data to show what we know, measure what we need to do, assess how well we did it, and find a way to communicate with other members of the interdisciplinary team in a way that highlights the social work role and the potential outcomes of social work practice. Using data to support palliative social work at all stages of the process from assessment to termination and follow-up begins with understanding and using evidence. The question then shifts from whether palliative social workers should participate in research to a discussion of how participation in research can best be supported.

Research Participation

Research impacts social work practice in many significant ways, especially in palliative care. There are a number of ways social workers can use the interconnectedness of research and clinical practice to their advantage. Minimally, palliative social workers must be good consumers of research, reading the published literature on a regular basis, keeping abreast of what is happening in the field, and learning new skills and information. We can also implement strategies to evaluate our own effectiveness either as individual workers (using a single subject design, for example) or as part of a larger agency-based evaluation effort. In addition, social workers in the field can directly support the efforts of researchers by volunteering to participate in studies or by helping researchers connect with other potential study participants. Finally, we can conduct research either independently or as part of a research team. While undertaking research endeavors may be daunting to novice social workers, mentorship is made readily available through local universities or organizations such as the Social Work Hospice and Palliative Care Network (http://www.swhpn.org), National Hospice and Palliative Care Organization (http://www.nhpco.org), and the American Academy of Hospice and Palliative Medicine (http://www.aahpm.org).

Gate Keeping

Any discussion of social work's involvement in research is incomplete without a discussion of gate keeping. The term gatekeeper is used in a variety of contexts to refer to an individual who accepts responsibility for granting or denying access to someone or something (Holloway & Wheeler, 2002). Researchers commonly use the term gatekeeper to describe someone who controls access to potential research participants. Many gate-keeping decisions are based on ethical considerations and rightfully so. Palliative care research can be an ethical landmine; however, there are a number of guidelines available to assist social workers in conducting or supporting ethical research.

Recruitment into palliative care research has historically been very challenging. Reasons for poor recruitment have been linked to gate keeping by health care providers who believe that patients and family members ought not be burdened with making decisions about participation in research (Hudson, Aranda, Kristjanson, & Quinn, 2005; McMillan & Weitzner, 2003; Ross & Cornbleet, 2003; Sherman et al., 2005). Despite the hesitation expressed by many palliative care providers, findings show that when given the opportunity to be involved in research, palliative care patients and their family members are often interested. A recent study by David Casarett and colleagues (2004) found that when a standard screen was used to determine research interest, 54% of patients of two community-based hospices were willing to participate in survey-based research, 40% were willing to enroll in clinical trials, and 65% said they would enroll in family-focused research.

Ethical social work practice requires a commitment to clients. We are obligated to place the interests of our clients above our own interests and above the interests of other professionals, including researchers (National Association of Social Workers [NASW], 1999). Some social workers erroneously interpret this ethical directive and conclude that it is our role to "protect" patients and families from research activities. That conclusion is flawed. First, our professional commitment is to promote our clients' interests, not to define our clients' interests. To deny patients and families the opportunity to decide for themselves if they want to participate in research is in direct opposition to our ethical obligation to promote clients' self-determination (NASW, 1999). Certainly informed consent and full disclosure of any associated risks and benefits must be discussed prior to initiating any study (Institutional Review Boards and most agency policies prohibit research if these conditions are not met), but clients are entitled to weigh the pros and cons for themselves. If the social work evidence base in palliative care is to be strengthened, we must remain aware of the fact that gatekeepers can facilitate access as readily as they can impede it.

Evidence-Based Practice

In many ways, the current emphasis on evidence-based social work is influenced by similar movements in other disciplines, particularly medicine. David Sackett is considered by many to be the father of evidence-based medicine in England. He and his colleagues (Sackett, Rosenberg, Gray, Haynes, & Richardson, 1996) define evidence-based practice as "the conscientious, explicit and judicious use of current best evidence in making decisions about the care of individual patients. [It] means integrating individual clinical expertise with the best available external clinical evidence from systematic research" (p. 71). Similarly, the Institute of Medicine (2001) defines evidence-based medicine as "the integration of best research evidence and clinical expertise with patient values" (p. 147). The consistent theme in these definitions is the application of evidence and clinical expertise to patient care. Joan Zlotnik and Colleen Galambos (2004) have challenged social workers to be active in organizing social work evidence through systematic reviews and meta-analyses in order to help social workers determine which evidence is most appropriate to consult in a given client situation.

In exploring the use of evidence-based practice (EBP) in social work, Angela Murphy and John McDonald (2004) examined how EBP changed the professional status of social workers in multidisciplinary teams in Australia. Unfortunately, they found that social workers had the least knowledge and experience in applying EBP. Participants in their study reported that social work was not as influential in multidisciplinary teams, often having less power and influence than nurses or physicians. Murphy and McDonald suggest that the lack of scientific evidence used by social workers may facilitate the marginalization of the profession.

Social workers in palliative care settings have been found to suffer from the marginalization to which Murphy and McDonald refer in their study. MacDonald's (1991) research revealed that hospice social workers often feel disempowered because end-of-life care can be dominated by professional nurses. Furthermore, the research found that social workers' roles on the hospice team are frequently blurred with those of nurses and chaplains. More recent research suggests social workers' roles continue to be unclear to other members of the palliative care team, as evidenced by the following comments provided by a hospice medical director: "I didn't even know what a clinical social worker did. We talked about a young, gay man dying with AIDS … I was practically in tears. I didn't realize all that the social worker offered the patient" (Parker Oliver, Tatum, & Kapp, in review). While the reasons for these perceptions and experiences may vary, it is clear that using language that articulates our skill set and evidence is important in demonstrating the value of social work on the palliative care team.

Approaches to Assessing Evidence in Palliative Care

H. Stephen Leff and Jeremy Conley (2006) outline three approaches to assessing evidence in mental health: narrative reviews, systematic reviews (including meta-analyses),

and registries. These strategies are also quite useful when assessing evidence in palliative care. Narrative reviews summarize multiple studies about a focused topic or group of interventions. The focus of narrative reviews is broad, making them useful when building conceptual or theoretical models. Narrative reviews are typically considered to be more subjective and susceptible to bias than systematic reviews in which a focused clinical research question is answered by collecting and synthesizing all relevant evidence generated by an explicit search strategy. Researchers conducting systematic reviews typically establish firm criteria used to determine whether a study is included in the review. Every study generated by the review's search strategy is included in the review, providing a more comprehensive and arguably less biased overview of the existing evidence about a specific topic or the effectiveness of a particular type of intervention. This makes them extremely useful to practitioners committed to EBP. A systematic review in which the studies' quantitative results are statistically synthesized is called a meta-analysis. Research registries are established systems used to collect and maintain information on studies of specific research topics. Registries typically store information in a structured fashion, often in an online database.

Systematic Reviews and Meta-Analyses

Systematic reviews are seen as an objective way to consider all established evidence and answer a specific clinical question. The process involves the retrospective synthesis of studies in a systematic way to answer a predetermined, focused research question. Systematic reviews apply predefined strategies to identify, analyze, and synthesize research findings from primary studies in an effort to answer specified clinical questions. Meta-analyses are systematic reviews in which statistical procedures are used to essentially combine the quantitative results of different studies to determine which interventions were most effective as well as which factors contributed to the interventions' success. To be included in a meta-analysis, the combined studies must all address the same hypothesis using similar methodology (Greenhalgh, 1997). Majolein Gysels and Irene Higginson (2007) explain that systematic reviews and meta-analyses are particularly important in research areas that are relatively new, young, or underdeveloped because they are often able to overcome problematic issues associated with studies that are underpowered due to low sample sizes. As a result, they may be more relevant in palliative care than in many other areas of health care.

Systematic reviews and meta-analyses are excellent additions to any palliative social worker's toolkit. They provide a comprehensive review of all the available evidence about a given topic while controlling for much of the bias that can be present in a less rigorously developed literature review. However, like all research, they have limitations and some are of a better quality than others. The methodology and findings of any systematic review need to be critically evaluated before using the results to support or reject practice interventions.

Social workers must evaluate the validity of a systematic review in much the same way they evaluate the validity of a single research study. The review must begin by stating the clear and focused question that initiated the study. It must explicitly identify the criteria used to decide which studies would be included, and it should provide a detailed description of the search strategy and databases used to identify studies. The quality will only be as good as the studies it includes; therefore, it is necessary to consider characteristics of the individual studies included in the review (often summarized in a table).

While systematic reviews provide an excellent resource for practice, they are made up of individual studies and pieces of evidence. It is important to note that not all evidence is equal. There are many different ways research is "graded" or evaluated. Each study within a systematic review is evaluated in some manner. The evaluation method used should be outlined and documented clearly. Generally evidence is graded based on the type of study (randomized controlled trials are often considered strongest; expert opinion is typically considered weakest), the length of the study, the size of the study, and whether the study has a qualitative or statistical analysis. Many scoring strategies have been developed, but what is most important is ensuring that a clearly explicated evaluation system was used when conducting the review.

Other quality issues related to systematic reviews include bias, timeliness, and applicability. Although systematic reviews are far less subjective than narrative reviews, they are not completely without bias. Two of the most common biases are journal and author bias. Reviews that contain a significant number of studies from the same author or same journal are prone to bias; their results must be carefully examined. Assuring that the research is current is also an important consideration when assessing the quality of reviews. Interventions are developed and tested regularly, especially in a new and emerging field like palliative care. Ideally, a review will contain the most recent evidence available; however, the time lag between the review preparation and publication, which is often considerable in social work, must be taken into account as a potential threat to the review's quality. It is possible, if not probable, that new studies will have appeared in the professional literature since a published review was originally conducted. Finally, the applicability of any systematic review must be determined based on each social worker's individual practice. Each social worker must decide whether the results are applicable to his or her specific client group and address all clinically relevant information. A recent article by Anderson, McNamara, and Arnold (2009) outlines the use of systematic reviews and meta-analyses in palliative care and provides a useful list of examples of each.

Important Concepts for Evidenced-Based Practice: Intervention, Effectiveness, and Evidence

The EBP movement in social work is based upon the belief that we must commit to determine which interventions are most effective for given populations facing various situations. According to Debbie Plath (2006), fundamental to understanding EBP is the clear understanding of three key terms: intervention, effectiveness, and evidence. Despite the fundamental nature of these concepts, their application in practice is not always straightforward.

Interventions are core to social work practice, yet identifying and defining them is often a great challenge. For members of the palliative care team from non–social work disciplines, it may be fairly easy to define what is meant by an "intervention." For example, in medicine, an intervention may be the writing of a prescription. In social work, determining what constitutes an intervention is more arduous. Furthermore, it may be difficult to clearly articulate the goals of an intervention. In introductory social work coursework, we are taught that intervention is the stage in the generalist practice model in which social workers behave in a way designed to help clients reach their goals (Zastrow & Kirst-Ashman, 2010). Plath (2006) notes that social work interventions are rarely discretely defined or labeled. This can present a significant challenge to studying and conducting EBP.

The second concept related to EBP is effectiveness. Plath (2006) explains that effectiveness is measured by answering one basic question: "Does it work?" (p. 61). If there is a clearly defined intervention outcome being measured, then effectiveness is more easily assessed. If, however, our goals are broader as is often the case in palliative care (e.g., establishing "improved quality of life" as a positive outcome of social work intervention), measuring effectiveness can be quite challenging. Plath also notes that psychosocial client goals, even within the practice setting, may be in conflict with the goals of other disciplines represented on the palliative care team. For example, the social worker may be intervening as an advocate for the patient or caregiver in a team discussion related to their overall care. Using our opening scenario, it is not uncommon for nurses or physicians to become quite frustrated with caregivers who do not give pain medication "as ordered," resulting in ineffective pain control for the patient. In this case, the social worker may need to advocate for the caregiver by explaining to the nurses and physicians that the caregiver is not trying to be difficult, but rather is afraid; thus, the medical intervention (the medication) will not be successful until the social worker can work with the caregiver to understand the bases of their fears about administering pain medications. The effectiveness of social work intervention then may be measured not only with decreased caregiver fear of administering pain medications, but it is also seen in increased adherence with the pain management protocol and, subsequently, better pain management.

The third concept critical to EBP is evidence. Plath (2006) states that evidence is most often thought of as a legal term used to suggest authority or legitimacy. The agreed-upon sources of evidence in social work are often broader and less tangible than in other disciplines represented on the palliative care team. Plath notes that contributors to the social work literature appear to agree that the selection of evidence-generating research methods should be based on what is most likely to adequately answer the research question being explored; both qualitative and quantitative research methods can contribute to the advancement of social work knowledge. Support for the use of mixed-methods approaches in social work research is growing, as many argue that such a design provides for the strongest evidence, allowing researchers to take advantage of the strengths of both qualitative and quantitative approaches. This is in contrast to more traditional understandings of research (such as in medicine) in which randomized clinical trials using strictly quantitative measures area often regarded as the gold standard for generating evidence.

Evidence is generated to establish an intervention's effectiveness. Social work researchers determine which outcomes an intervention is designed to address and then decide how to best verify to what degree that outcome has been achieved. Evidence provides that answer.

Social work researchers and the consumers of social work research (i.e., social work practitioners) can benefit from assessing the evidence (commonly referred to as data) collected in any study used to inform or shape practice. Specifically, social workers can determine which individuals or groups are represented by the data. Members of racial and ethnic minority groups tend to be underrepresented in palliative care (Crawley et al., 2000; Krakauer, Crenner, & Fox, 2002). It is not surprising, then, that they are also underrepresented in palliative care research. It is erroneous to assume that the results of studies conducted with minimal minority participation can effectively inform practice with minorities. Similarly, it is erroneous to assume that patients and family members share the same perspectives or that male caregivers face the same issues identified in research conducted with female-only samples. Social work's commitment to social justice is equally applicable in practice and research. We must continually work to promote greater diversity in both palliative care practice and research.

Evidence-Informed Practice

This chapter's endorsement of EBP is not intended to minimize the very complex discussion occurring among social workers with regard to the integration of research and practice. Some practitioners view EBP as incompatible with the way social workers have traditionally approached practice. Critics of EBP stress that it has the potential to ignore the important interactional and interpretive elements of practice

and overemphasize the standardization of interventions. They further contend that grading systems and so-called hierarchies of evidence often employed by those supporting EBP do little to highlight the significant value of qualitative research and practice wisdom (Haynes, Devereaux, & Guyatt, 2002; Webb, 2001). Others adopt a more inclusive definition of EBP, such as the one provided in this chapter, which stresses the importance of coupling research with clinical expertise to provide services in accordance with the values of individual patients and families. A similarly broad definition of EBP is offered by Leonard Gibbs and Eileen Gambrill (2002). Furthermore, as previously discussed, support for EBP does not necessarily translate into a disparaging view of qualitative research or expertise gained from practice.

However, given the contentious nature of the discourse concerning the merging of research and social work practice, some advocate for the promotion of evidence-informed models that are more explicitly inclusive (Epstein, 2009). Evidence-informed practice (EIP) emphasizes that research be used in a manner that strengthens but does not limit practice. It honors multiple ways of knowing and acknowledges the unique strengths and limitations of both practice wisdom and research-based knowledge. Irwin Epstein (2009) provides a useful discussion of EIP and its potential for moving the social work profession beyond a "dualistic" (p. 216) understanding of research and practice toward a more "synergistic" (p. 217) integration of these two complementary aspects of our work.

An additional argument for adoption of EIP in palliative social work is that the research base for practice in this area is currently quite limited relative to other disciplines and to social work in other settings. Furthermore, research in palliative care is plagued with significant barriers to generating widely generalizable results (Cook, Finlay, & Butler-Keating, 2002; Jordhoy et al., 1999; O'Mara, St. Germain, Ferrell, & Bornemann, 2009). As a result, palliative social workers may struggle to find empirically supported guidance for certain practice decisions. Adherence to EIP principles allows practitioners to draw from many different bodies of knowledge to inform their work, thereby addressing current limitations in the evidence base.

Additional Ways to Utilize Research in Social Work Practice

Conducting Your Own Review of the Evidence

Being an informed critical consumer of existing research is not the only way to infuse current evidence into your palliative social work knowledge base. In a field as young as palliative social work, it may be necessary for individual practitioners to conduct their own systematic reviews and build the necessary evidence to answer research questions relevant to their area of practice. While the focus of this chapter is not on how to conduct an evidence-based systematic review, being an excellent critical consumer of research is an appropriate start. Several resources provided at the conclusion of this chapter have been developed to help guide those interested in performing a systematic review.

Using Peer-Reviewed Journals in Practice

The importance of keeping abreast of current research is critical to delivering quality palliative social work services. While finding relevant research in one comprehensive source is not always feasible, we are fortunate to have numerous journals related to our practice, many sponsored by our professional organizations and specific to social work in palliative care. A list of journals known to publish research that is often applicable to social work practice is provided at the end of this chapter. This is not by any means an exhaustive list, but rather an example of the broad range of professional literature that is available to social workers in palliative care settings.

Social workers in many settings face limited access to professional journals after they complete their formal education and no longer enjoy the benefits of university libraries. Access to professional journals can be promoted in a number of ways. Membership to professional organizations is often accompanied by a complimentary subscription to one or more journals. Social work colleagues can join together and commit to reading a select number of articles each week or month during meetings or in agency-supported journal clubs. It is likely that studies published in journals directed at other disciplines represented on the palliative care team are of interest to social workers as well. Learning about current research alongside other members of the care team is an excellent way to grow professionally. While shrinking budgets and other financial constraints may limit an agency's ability to subscribe to several journals, proposals for agency subscriptions to one or two key journals may be successful, especially if employees provide a description of how the information will be used to improve patient care. Online resources are also valuable sources of information. One example is PubMed Central, a free archive of medically oriented journal literature managed by the National Center for Biotechnology Information in the National Library of Medicine (http://www.ncbi.nlm.nih.gov/pmc/). Finally, members of palliative care teams associated with major hospitals (especially university-affiliated hospitals) may be surprised to learn the extent of their ability to utilize the institution's health sciences libraries.

Participating in Research

As mentioned earlier, social workers are often able to take advantage of opportunities to work with researchers to help build our evidence base. Research in palliative care is very challenging, and the support and participation of social workers in palliative care settings is critical to the success of any research study in this environment. The Population Based Palliative Care Research Network (PoPCRN) (http://www.uchsc.edu/popcrn/) is a network of palliative care providers who understand the value of research and volunteer to help researchers obtain the sample sizes necessary to advance the science of palliative care. Contacting authors of journal articles, sharing your opinions, or offering to assist in future research is yet another way to be involved in building the evidence base for social work practice in palliative care. Author contact information is made available in nearly all journal articles. Practitioners should never hesitate to contact an author. Most would be excited to hear your comments and consider your help in their future work.

Conducting Research

Another less popular and more involved way to participate in research as a practitioner is to conduct your own research. Given all the discussion regarding the assessment of evidence, it is clear that knowledge of research methodology is critical if you desire to do primary research of your own. Having access to knowledgeable methodologists as well as analysts and Institutional Review Boards to assess ethical concerns are critical supports that practitioners might engage for mentorship and assistance. Collaborating with local university-based or established palliative care researchers is a helpful way to get specific answers to your practice questions and share the excitement that can occur in assessing interventions. Collaboration between social work practitioners and researchers is often mutually beneficial. It allows researchers to remain grounded in the real-world issues facing palliative social workers and allows practitioners to incorporate cutting edge, evidence-based strategies into their daily practice. In addition, strong partnerships ensure that palliative social workers and researchers alike are equipped with up-to-date evidence that can be used to inform policies that influence social work in palliative care settings. Recognition of the interconnectedness of practice, policy, and research is vital to the social work profession and is widely regarded as one of its key strengths. The references at the end of this chapter can be helpful in conducting research in palliative care settings.

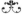

Conclusion

Although some social workers almost seem to view practice and research as incompatible, many others successfully merge the two, often in a way that strengthens both. The palliative social work research base is limited but is growing every day as a result of the efforts of practitioners and researchers partnering to generate and disseminate knowledge that nourishes professional growth. By using data to improve care delivered to patients and families, palliative social workers deliver on their commitment to the ethical imperatives of competence and service and increase the likelihood that future generations of social workers will be equipped to serve patients and families in the most effective manner possible.

LEARNING EXERCISES

- *Critique a study in palliative care.* Locate an original article on a study in palliative care. Read the article and respond to the following questions:

  a. Has the researcher defined the problem? Is there at least one research question guiding the study?

  b. Are there any obvious sampling problems? Explain.

  c. Are there any obvious methodological problems?

  d. Using the grading criteria outlined in the additional suggested reading by Anderson and colleagues (2009), how would you grade this research?

  e. Overall, do you think the research makes an important contribution to the advancement of social work practice? Explain.

- *Review a systematic literature review.* Using the Social Work Abstracts database, identify a systematic review that is of interest to palliative social workers. Answer the following questions:

  a. Does the review clearly identify the research question? Have the authors specified the search criteria, the criteria for including studies in the sample, and the data extracted from each study?

  b. Have the reviewers interpreted and critiqued the literature or merely summarized it?

  c. Is the study a meta-analysis? How do you know?

  d. Overall, do you think the review makes an important contribution to the palliative social work knowledge base? Why or why not?

- *Conduct a systematic review.* Using the additional suggested readings provided at the end of this chapter, develop a focused research question, outline a specific search strategy, define your specific study inclusion criteria, and develop a data extraction tool for a systematic review of the literature to answer your research question.

ADDITIONAL RESOURCES

SUGGESTED READINGS

Addington-Hall, J., Bruera, E., Higginson, I. J., & Payne, S. (Eds.). (2007). *Research methods in palliative care*. Oxford, England: Oxford University Press.

Anderson, W., McNamara, M. C., & Arnold, R. (2009). Systematic reviews and meta-analyses. *Journal of Palliative Medicine, 12*(10), 937–946.

Counsell, C. (1997). Academia and clinic: Formulating questions and locating primary studies for inclusion in systematic reviews. *Annals of Internal Medicine, 127*(5), 380–387.

Galvan, J. (2006). *Writing literature reviews: A guide for students of the social and behaviorial sciences* (3rd ed.). Glendale, CA: Pyrczak Publishing.

Jadad, A. R., Moher, D., & Klassen, T. P. (1998). Guides for reading and interpreting systematic reviews: II. How did the authors find the studies and assess their quality? *Archives of Pediatrics and Adolescent Medicine, 152*(8), 812–817.

Klassen, T. P., Jadad, A. R., & Moher, D. (1998). Guides for reading and interpreting systematic reviews: I. Getting started. *Archives of Pediatrics and Adolescent Medicine, 152*(7), 700–704.

Ling Pan, M. (2008). *Preparing literature reviews: Qualitative and quantitative approaches* (3rd ed.). Glendale, CA: Pyrczak Publishing.

Moher, D., Jadad, A. R., & Klassen, T. P. (1998). Guides for reading and interpreting systematic reviews: III. How did the authors synthesize the data and make their conclusions? *Archives of Pediatrics and Adolescent Medicine, 152*(9), 915–920.

Mullen, E. J. (2006). Choosing outcome measures in systematic reviews: Critical challenges. *Research on Social Work Practice, 16*(1), 84–90.

MODEL SYSTEMATIC REVIEWS APPLICABLE TO SOCIAL WORK PRACTICE IN PALLIATIVE CARE

Grady, P. (2005). Introduction: Papers from the National Institutes of Health State of the Science Conference on Improving End-of-Life Care. *Journal of Palliative Medicine, 8*(Suppl. 1), S1–S3.

Harding, R., & Higginson, I. J. (2003). What is the best way to help caregivers in cancer and palliative care? A systematic literature review of interventions and their effectiveness. *Palliative Medicine, 17*(1), 63–74.

Stolz, P., Uden, G., & Willman, A. (2004). Support for family carers who care for an elderly person at home—a systematic literature review. *Scandinavian Journal of Caring Sciences, 18*(2), 111–119.

PEER-REVIEWED JOURNALS IN PALLIATIVE CARE

Journal of Social Work in End-of-Life and Palliative Care
American Journal of Hospice and Palliative Medicine
Journal of Pain and Symptom Management
Journal of Palliative Care
Journal of Palliative Medicine
Palliative Medicine

REFERENCES

Anderson, W., McNamara, M. C., & Arnold, R. M. (2009). Systematic reviews and meta-analyses. *Journal of Palliative Medicine, 12*(10), 937–946.

Casarett, D., Kassner, C. T., & Kutner, J. S. (2004). Recruiting for research in hospice: Feasibility of a research screening protocol. *Journal of Palliative Medicine, 7*(6), 854–860.

Cook, A., Finlay, I., & Butler-Keating, R. (2002). Recruiting into palliative care trials: Lessons learnt from a feasibility study. *Palliative Medicine, 16*(2), 163–165.

Crawley, L., Payne, R., Bolden, J., Payne, T., Washington, P., & Williams, S. (2000). Palliative and end-of-life care in the African American community. *Journal of the American Medical Association, 284*(19), 2518–2521.

Demiris, G., Parker Oliver, D., Washington, K., Doorenbos, A., Wechkin, H., & Berry, D. (2010). Problem solving therapy for hospice caregivers: A pilot study. *Journal of Palliative Medicine. 13*(8), 1005–1011. doi: 10.11089/jpm.2010.0022

Epstein, I. (2009). Promoting harmony where there is commonly conflict: Evidence-informed practice as an integrative strategy. *Social Work in Health Care, 48*(3), 216–231.

Gibbs, L., & Gambrill, E. (2002). Evidence-based practice: Counterarguments to objections. *Research on Social Work Practice, 12*(3), 452–476.

Greenhalgh, T. (1997). Papers that summarise other papers (systematic reviews and meta-analyses). [Review]. *BMJ, 315*(7109), 672–675.

Grinnell, R. M., & Unrau, Y. A. (2008). *Social work research and evaluation: Foundations of evidence-based practice.* New York, NY: Oxford University Press.

Gysels, M., & Higginson, I. J. (2007). Systematic reviews. In J. M. Addington-Hall, E. Bruera, I. J. Higginson, & S. Payne (Eds.), *Research methods in palliative care* (pp. 115–136). Oxford, England: Oxford University Press.

Haynes, R. B., Devereaux, P. J., & Guyatt, G. H. (2002). Clinical expertise in the era of evidence-based medicine and patient choice. *Evidence-based Medicine for Primary Care and Internal Medicine, 7*(2), 36–38.

Holloway, I., & Wheeler, S. (2002). *Qualitative research in nursing* (2nd ed.). Oxford, England: Blackwell Publishing.

Hudson, P., Aranda, S., Kristjanson, L., & Quinn, K. (2005). Minimising gate-keeping in palliative care research. *European Journal of Palliative Care, 12*(4), 165–169.

Institute of Medicine. (2001). *Crossing the quality chasm: A new health system for the 21st century.* Retrieved 25 August, 2010 from http://iom.edu/Reports/2001/Crossing-the-Quality-Chasm-A-New-Health-System-for-the-21st-Century.aspx .

Jordhoy, M. S., Kaasa, S., Fayers, P., Overness, T., Underland, G., & Ahlner-Elmqvist, M. (1999). Challenges in palliative care research; Recruitment, attrition and compliance: Experience from a randomized controlled trial. *Palliative Medicine, 13*(4), 299–310.

Krakauer, E. L., Crenner, C., & Fox, K. (2002). Barriers to optimum end-of-life care for minority patients. *Journal of the American Geriatrics Society, 50*(1), 182–190.

Leff, H. S., & Conley, J. A. (2006). Desired attributes of evidence assessments for evidence-based practices. *Administration Policy in Mental Health, 33*(6), 648–658.

Letizia, M., Creech, S., Norton, E., Shanahan, M., & Hedges, L. (2004). Barriers to caregiver administration of pain medication in hospice care. *Journal of Pain and Symptom Management, 27*(2), 114–124.

MacDonald, D. (1991). Hospice social work: A search for identity. *Health and Social Work, 16*(4), 274–280.

McMillan, S. C., & Weitzner, M. A. (2003). Methodologic issues in collecting data from debilitated patients with cancer near the end of life. *Oncology Nursing Forum, 30*(1), 123–129.

Murphy, A., & McDonald, J. (2004). Power, status and marginalization: Rural social workers and evidence-based practice in multidisciplinary teams. *Australian Social Work, 57*(2), 127–136.

National Association of Social Workers (NASW). (1999). *Code of ethics.* Retrieved from http://www.naswdc.org/pubs/code/code.asp

O'Mara, A. M., St. Germain, D., Ferrell, B., & Bornemann, T. (2009). Challenges to and lessons learned from conducting palliative care research. *Journal of Pain and Symptom Management, 37*(3), 387–394.

Parker Oliver, D., Tatum, P., & Kapp, J. (2010). The narrative experiences of hospice medical directors. *American Journal of Hospice and Palliative Medicine.* doi: 10.1177/1049909110366852

Plath, D. (2006). Evidence-based practice: Current issues and future directions. *Australian Social Work, 59*(1), 56–72.

Ross, C., & Cornbleet, M. (2003). Attitudes of patients and staff to research in a specialist palliative care unit. *Palliative Medicine, 17*(6), 491–497.

Sackett, D. L., Rosenberg, W. M., Gray, J. A., Haynes, R. B., & Richardson, W. S. (1996). Evidence based medicine: What it is and what it isn't. *BMJ, 312*, 71–72.

Sherman, D. W., McSherry, C. B., Parkas, V., Ye, X. Y., Calabrese, M., & Gatto, M. (2005). Clinical methods. Recruitment and retention in a longitudinal palliative care study. *Applied Nursing Research, 18*(3), 167–177.

Webb, S. A. (2001). Some considerations on the validity of evidence-based practice in social work. *British Journal of Social Work, 31*(1), 57–79.

Zastrow, C. H., & Kirst-Ashman, K. K. (2010). *Understanding human behavior and the social environment.* Belmont, CA: Brooks/Cole.

Zlotnik, J. L., & Galambos, C. (2004). Evidence-based practices in health care: Social work possibilities. *Health and Social Work, 29*(4), 259–261.

81 *Barbara Ivanko*

Quality Improvement and Organizational Change

We always thought we were doing such a great job; we knew we had to be, because "the patients and families loved us!" Imagine how surprised we were when we started collecting real data about outcomes and found that we could do so much better.
—*Regina Di Pietro, hospice social worker (personal communication, May 15, 2009)*

Key Concepts

- *Despite a national agenda for outcome measurement, benchmarking, and quality improvement in health care, relatively little is known empirically about the quality of social work in palliative care.*
- *Numerous validated tools that can be useful in measuring outcomes in social work at the patient level are now available. The data collected can be aggregated and used as part of larger process-improvement initiatives.*
- *Organizational change is a more global approach to process change and quality improvement. Strategic change is necessary for organizations to remain viable and relevant and must be executed in a systematic manner to be successful.*

Introduction

Social workers are familiar with the concept of change. Our training is largely geared toward helping individuals, organizations, and communities evaluate their current status, assess the need for change, learn new skills, and sometimes shed maladaptive or archaic thoughts and behaviors and replace them with newer, more productive tactics. Typically, this involves an approach that recognizes and mobilizes the strengths that exist within the individuals and/or system and honors their right to self-determination as they decide what and how to change. However, comparatively little attention has been paid to the analysis of data to evaluate what to change, and then, whether the new way of doing things is better—or simply different. This chapter provides an overview of the use of data to evaluate clinical outcomes in both individual and systemic social work practice in palliative care, with the goal of improving the quality of care. We will also examine the necessity and process of change at the organizational level, a key component in the sustainability and effectiveness of palliative care agencies and other health care providers.

Quality Improvement and Social Work

Palliative care and hospice care typically include social workers as part of an interdisciplinary team. When the goal of care is improved quality of life, social workers are uniquely suited to assess psychological and social factors that impact well-being, and they can intervene with the ineffective coping and emotional stress that can further impair physical function. They also provide important education and linkage with community resources. Social workers are trained in the ecological perspective, which views individuals as functioning within a larger system of family, community, and service providers. This allows social workers to assess and intervene with palliative care goals from a personal and environmental view and to evaluate treatment interventions in terms of quality of life.

Randolph Markey (2001) eloquently captured the powerful effect of his social worker's intervention of empathic, nonjudgmental listening while he was undergoing treatment for a congenital brain condition:

> The doctors write in my chart. They don't write that my brother is dead, or that I love Rachmaninoff. They don't write that my son doesn't walk yet, or that I am missing Hanukkah, his first Hanukkah. They don't write that my parents won't visit me in the hospital because they are terrified that I will die. The doctors know the inside of my brain, but they don't know my middle name ... I have no words here for the late nights, the darkness, the begging for a hand to hold, the terror, the resignation, the relationship to the pain, the calling for someone to blame ... At the hospital, a major American teaching hospital, no comfort was offered. I had to ask for a social worker to come to my room and talk with me. And when the social worker came, do you know what she did? She listened. She witnessed. In the meetings I spent with her, just a handful, she mostly just sat there and listened. For reasons I don't completely understand, it was the only time I was able to just let go and cry. I wept all the fear and pain and regret and frustration and she witnessed and had the wisdom not to interfere ... I went back to see her maybe a year after the surgeries, and again I wept in her office. The empathy that is inherent in respectful witnessing was the most powerful emotional experience of my illness to date. Aside from the birth of my child, it was the most powerful emotional experience of my life. (p. HE01)

Historically, social workers have used a professional model of self-monitoring to ensure high-quality service provision; relying on self-awareness, clinical supervision, continuing education, ethics, and general licensing requirements (Morris, 2000). The social services literature has lacked a framework for assessing quality in specific practice settings (Megivern et al., 2007). Social workers have not quantified their contributions in health care within a medical model, despite the fact that social workers frequently function as part of an interdisciplinary medical team. Social worker Douglas MacDonald (2001), in his last "Hospice vignette" in the *American Journal of Hospice and Palliative Care*, writes of how he misses the early days of hospice:

> When there was more time and fewer rules, when there was less concern with documentation and regulatory oversight, the staff was smaller and close knit, and it was easier to make meaningful contributions by just being yourself and being guided by your intuition. (p. 419)

An outcome-driven model of social work would ask how "meaningful contributions" are defined and measured from the patient's point of view, what evidence there is that those contributions add to the patient's overall well-being, and

what systems can be developed to ensure favorable quality outcomes across palliative care teams and organizations. Indeed, the days of intuitive practice and fewer rules are over, and social workers must begin in earnest to identify and measure the high-quality care they provide. Furthermore, such evidence must demonstrate that the favorable patient outcomes are produced by interventions that only a professional social worker can provide. Making a contribution to a health care team by "just being yourself" begs the question of whether a volunteer or nonprofessional team member could produce the same outcome.

Quality improvement through outcome evaluation and evidence-based practice is now a significant focus of most health care providers. One example of this can be found in the home health industry. For years, the Centers for Medicare and Medicaid Services (CMS) has required certified home health agencies to collect outcome data using a standardized tool. Since 2003, CMS has posted this performance and outcome data on the "Home Health Compare" (Medicare, 2008) Web site so that consumers and other stakeholders can review their quality record. Among the outcomes reported are the percentage of patients who get better at walking or moving around, the percentage of patients who get better at getting in and out of bed, and the percentage of patients who have less pain when moving around. Higher percentages signify better performance by the agency. Home health agencies also use this data to evaluate their results against other agencies and to market themselves if their results are better than their competitors. In late 2009, CMS announced a pilot project called Hospice Assessment, Intervention, and Measurement (AIM), intended to similarly promote the effective collection of outcome data from hospice agencies, using a uniform collection tool. The measures selected by the project include palliative social work issues such as anxiety, family education, cultural sensitivity, and advance directives (National Hospice and Palliative Care Organization [NHPCO], 2009). In addition to a trend toward mandatory, standard outcome measures, there has been discussion for years about linking payment to home health and other agencies based on the quality of their outcomes. The better the care, the more the agency will earn. CMS has already had success with a pilot "pay-for-performance" program in which physician groups received reimbursement based on outcome measures. The goal of this and other value-based purchasing initiatives is to tie performance to costs—part of CMS's "drive to transform Medicare from a passive payer to an active purchaser of higher quality, more efficient health care" (Centers for Medicare and Medicaid Services [CMS], 2007). Eventually, a pay-for-performance system will link most provider compensation with the quality of their outcomes (CMS, 2009).

Despite this national agenda for quality improvement and national benchmarking, and the value social workers can add to patient outcomes in palliative care, research evidence about the quality of social services in the United States is sparse (McMillen et al., 2005).

Social workers, like all clinicians, have a responsibility to continuously renew and improve themselves, to ensure their ability to provide excellent clinical services, and to maintain regulatory compliance. The old adage "What got you here won't keep you here" is true for individuals as they evolve personally and professionally, as well as social workers. The environmental and internal systems that frame social workers and their workplace are continuously changing; thus, individuals and organizations must detect and respond to those changes strategically to remain relevant. The last point becomes vitally important for social workers' employment prospects and pay scale in an era when health care reimbursement is being tied to quality.

Models of Quality Improvement

Total quality management (TQM) is a management philosophy created by W. Edwards Deming. It gained momentum beginning in 1962 with Japanese "quality circles" (QCs). Quality circles brought workers together weekly to discuss improvements to the workplace and the quality of their work. Its focus is on the internal and external customer, and it is aimed at continuous improvement through the use of data collection and statistical analysis. After success in Japan, QCs moved to the United States in the 1970s and became so popular in American industry in the 1980s that *Business Week* described them as a fad (Byrne, 1986). The migration of quality management into health care has followed.

The Plan-Do-Check-Act (PDCA) cycle was adapted by Deming from the work of statistician Walter Shewhart. The PDCA cycle, comprised of the following steps, remains a common model for process and performance improvement in health care and industry:

- *Plan* to improve your quality first by identifying what things are going wrong and come up with ideas for solving these problems.
- *Do* changes designed to solve the problems on a small scale first. This minimizes disruption to routine activity while testing whether the changes will work.
- *Check* whether the changes are resulting in the desired outcome.
- *Act* to implement changes on a larger scale if the experiment is successful. This usually requires the involvement of other departments affected by the changes and whose cooperation will be needed to implement them on a larger scale. Of course, if the changes do not result in improved outcomes, the cycle must begin again at the "Do" stage, as another hypothesis for what might create improvement is considered and tested.

Both TQM and PDCA are described in various levels of detail by numerous authors including Deming himself (1989) and Mary Walton (Walton, 1986). One criticism of TQM is

that it does not offer guidance on isolating the root cause of quality deficiencies, nor does it offer recommendations for which specific steps to take to improve quality.

Another improvement methodology that is increasingly used in health care organizations is Lean Six Sigma. The foundation of Lean Six Sigma is the use of data, facts, and teamwork to delight customers with quality and speed, and to improve processes by improving flow and eliminating variation and defects (George, Rowlands, & Kastle, 2004). Samuels and Adomitis (2003) recommend the following Six Sigma process:

1. Define the purpose and scope
2. Create a performance baseline to compare data
3. Analyze root causes quantified by actual data
4. Implement procedures to eliminate root causes of errors to improve performance
5. Evaluate the performance of the process (pp. 70–75)

Quality assessment performance improvement (QAPI) has become an integral part of hospice and palliative care since the Centers for Medicare and Medicaid Services (CMS) incorporated QAPI as a Condition of Participation for Hospices in 2008 (Department of Health and Human Services, 2008). Condition 418.58 requires that hospices show measurable improvement in indicators that will improve palliative outcomes and end-of-life services. While CMS does not specify which indicators should be evaluated or which measurement tools and methodology are used, it does require that data are used so that problem identification and outcome evaluation are evidence based. QAPI further requires that the performance improvement projects focus on areas that are high risk, high volume, and problem prone. Possible sources of data collection would include assessments performed by clinicians, and patient and family satisfaction surveys. Data collection at the patient level should be done in a systematic way, using validated tools by trained evaluators to ensure interrater reliability. The absence of a standardized tool for hospice quality measurement makes interagency and national benchmarking of outcomes challenging. The hospice AIM pilot mentioned earlier seeks to address this deficit.

Outcome Measurement

Important metrics in the evaluation of palliative social work outcomes focus on the perceptions and satisfaction of the patient, and often, the patient's family. Ideally, the metrics used can be compared with previous points in time within the social worker's own organization and/or with national data on best practice and outcomes.

Wensing and Elwyn (2002) outline four components for using the patient's perspective on their care in the performance improvement process:

1. *Provide information about their outcomes to stakeholders.* People seeking health care can then

decide based on the outcomes whether to pursue care with any given provider. This makes quality care a competitive advantage. The "Home Health Compare" Web site is a perfect example of this use of data.

2. *Provide the data to patients and allow them to evaluate options and outcomes in their care.* A social worker could share data with a patient or family member about the outcome of a medical intervention to open a discussion about whether to continue a particular treatment. Outcome data on psychosocial interventions might be shared to motivate and reinforce progress.

3. *Improve upon organizational weaknesses.* Later in this chapter organizational change and social workers' potential value in that process are discussed.

4. Engage patients and families in improving health care systems.

Clinical outcomes for social work in palliative care would focus on such issues and symptoms as pain, fear, anxiety, well-being, mental status, powerlessness, anger, exhaustion, caregiver fatigue, suicide risk, understanding of advance directives, understanding of educational material, hopelessness, body image, quality of life, interpersonal support, isolation, sadness, depression, grief, and suffering.

One of the barriers to measuring outcomes in palliative social work has been the lack of reliable, validated measurement tools. Without these, identification of opportunities for improvement and the evaluation of interventions and quality of care are impossible. Social work education has typically focused on the process and relationship between social worker and client, rather than the quantitative value of the discipline. Despite the inclusion of research and statistics in the social work course work, the practice has remained more of an art than a science. In recent years, a number of patient-focused, family-centered survey instruments that address the needs and concerns of patients and their families have allowed social workers to "cross this measurement barrier" (Teno, 2004). The importance of validated measurement cannot be overstated. Measurement enables social workers to evaluate the effectiveness of their interventions with each patient and family, in areas identified by the patient and family, affording them the opportunity to improve outcomes on a case-by-case basis. Focusing and adjusting interventions to maximize optimal outcomes is good clinical care and responsibly patient centered. Measurement also compels palliative care organizations to evaluate the effectiveness of their common practices, processes, and systems in the aggregate. This holds providers accountable for their quality of care and allows providers to maintain their positions relative to competitors. These tools also hold the potential to identify cultural differences in patients' and families' response to social work interventions and to develop culturally appropriate clinical practices. Notably, outcome measures also allow social workers to validate their effectiveness in the palliation of the multidimensional

aspects of suffering along the continuum of illness and at end of life.

There are now dozens of instruments available, with a focus on issues that are relevant to social work practice, such as The Missoula-VITAS Quality of Life Index (MVQOLI) (Byock, 1998), The Edmonton Symptom Assessment Scale (ESAS), (Chang, Hwang, & Feuerman, 2000; Kaasa, Loomis, Gillis, Bruera, & Hanson, 1997), The Caregiver Strain Index (Robinson, 1983), and The Meaning of Life Scale (Warner & Williams, 1987). The Social Work Outcomes Task Force of the Social Work Section of the NHPCO developed the Social Work Assessment Tool (SWAT) specifically to document social work effectiveness in hospice and palliative care programs (Reese et al., 2006).

The NHPCO Family Evaluation of Hospice Care (FEHC) provides national benchmarks on families' retrospective ratings of hospice care with questions about "Help with the patient's feelings of anxiety/sadness," "Hospice emotional support to family after patient's death," and "Hospice emotional support to family prior to patient's death" (2009). There are similar questions on NHPCO's Family Evaluation of Palliative Care (2008). However, when an interdisciplinary team is caring for a patient and family, these surveys do not isolate the interventions of the social worker as correlated with the support to the family; the nurse, chaplain, or volunteer may have been the source of the support. Since surveys are administered after the patient dies, the evaluation of help with the patient's anxiety or sadness is assessed by someone other than the patient and does not allow modification of ineffective interventions with an individual patient or family in real time.

Suncoast Hospice in Florida is one of the nation's largest hospices, serving more than 2500 patients a day. This hospice is meeting the need for social work outcome data by incorporating the ESAS into their Suncoast Solutions documentation software. The ESAS identifies and measures the severity of common symptoms in patients receiving palliative care. The tool asks the patient to rate symptoms such as pain, depression, anxiety, and well-being on a 0 to 10 scale. Capturing consistent data about psychosocial issues like anxiety and well-being establishes a baseline assessment that will prompt individualized interventions by the team social worker. The efficacy of the interventions can be evaluated on a patient-by-patient case by readministering the ESAS, and they can be adjusted if the outcomes are not consistent with the patient's goals. At the aggregate level, success in alleviating suffering linked to depression, anxiety, and well-being can be used by Suncoast Hospice to evaluate the quality performance of specific clinicians and teams. The data can also identify which interventions work best in various settings, with different ethnic and demographic groups, and at different levels of care. Suncoast Solutions software is used by hundreds of hospices nationwide, which will ultimately allow for national benchmarking of outcomes for social work (H. Stellrect, personal communication, November 11, 2009).

Organizational Change

As we have discussed, health care providers are compelled to evaluate information about their clinical outcomes in order to make the changes necessary to meet the needs of their patients, families, and community with appropriate, quality services. Since providers also have an interest in maintaining market share and in meeting revenue and expense goals, they must also analyze external influences on health care. These influences include reimbursement and regulatory changes, as well as the larger economic and social environment. In "How the Mighty Fall," Jim Collins (2009) outlines the stages of organizational decline and complacency that result from inattention to internal and external variables. Collins builds a dramatic case for staving off complacency and cultivating an organization that recognizes the need for and is capable of change. Collins has identified five avoidable stages of decline:

1. *Hubris born of success.* In this early stage, people become arrogant and begin to view their success as a product solely of their own merit and as an entitlement. They begin to forget the context, processes, and factors that supported that early success. Palliative care providers receive deep appreciation from those they serve, and many clinicians regard their work as a calling. The often sacred nature of palliative care must not lull those involved into thinking this renders them impervious to universal business principles.
2. *Undisciplined pursuit of more.* Success—however it is defined by the organization or the clinician—acclaim, growth, and recognition are pursued greedily in this stage. This results in overextension without the discipline and preparation that went into building the foundation for the initial success.
3. *Denial of risk and peril.* Despite evidence that suggests that improvement is required, people in this stage continue to behave in the same ways, resisting change. Outcomes suffer, but the poor results are excused away or minimized.
4. *Grasping for salvation.* The momentum of decline thrusts people into quick-fix moves that may produce short-term improvement, but do not result in the foundational change that will result in sustained excellence.
5. *Capitulation into irrelevance or death.* The organization remains in a downward spiral and ultimately fails.

Building and sustaining a successful palliative care program and keeping the program off the path to irrelevance requires the ability to recognize the need for change and avoid the slope of decline before it is too late. Then, the ability to successfully manage and execute positive change is essential.

Despite the requisite need for change, more than 70% of organizational change efforts fail (Judge & Douglas, 2009). Retired Harvard Business School professor John P. Kotter (2007) developed an effective eight-step model for change management. Kotter asserts that the reason most change initiatives fail is that organizations do not adhere to the eight steps, or they do them in the wrong order. At each step in Kotter's model, the skills and abilities of social workers can be mobilized to achieve the desired change:

Step One: Establish a Sense of Urgency
People within the palliative care organization must look hard at the organization's competitive position, trends in funding, regulatory scrutiny, and ability to attract skilled clinicians. This information must be communicated broadly in order to mobilize and motivate the organization to change. This stage shakes individuals out of their comfort zones. An important component of social work education and training is the ability to motivate and facilitate change, either through empathy, reward, or confrontation. This skill, along with the ability to assess systems on multiple levels, makes social workers potentially powerful allies and leaders in the change process.

Step Two: Form a Powerful Guiding Coalition
Creating a shared commitment to renewal involves a small group, usually outside the traditional chain of command. This group grows over time, and the involvement of constituents at a grassroots level builds the trust and vision required to produce change. Social workers' training in communication and group formation lends itself to this coalition building.

Step Three: Creating a Vision
The vision clarifies the direction in which an organization needs to move. It inspires the coalition to make the change. Kotter's rule of thumb is that if you cannot communicate the vision to someone in 5 minutes or less and get a response that indicates understanding and interest, then this step in the process needs more work.

Step Four: Communicating the Vision
Communicating the vision by every vehicle possible and the teaching of new behaviors by coalition members are the keys to this phase. Here again in steps three and four, social workers' skills in effective communication and removing barriers to communication can be a critical asset in change management.

Step Five: Empowering Others to Act on the Vision
This involves eliminating barriers, creating new systems and structures that support change, and encouraging risk and new ideas. A fundamental concept in social work education is the empowerment of individuals and groups to gain the capacity to interact in a new way, in the direction of new goals. It is a core social work belief that a sense of power is linked with self-esteem, and that individuals alone or acting in collaboration with others can make significant changes.

Step Six: Planning for and Creating Short-Term Wins
Early success and the recognition of that success reinforce the change and provide motivation for further change and inspire others to join the change agents. Social workers can support their organization through this phase of the change process by using their ability to provide positive feedback and increasing the group's focus on the future.

Step Seven: Consolidating Improvements and Producing Still More Change
The enhanced credibility from the early successes energizes the process and allows for new projects and continuing change.

Step Eight: Institutionalizing New Approaches
In this phase, the connection between the organization's success and the new way of doing things is communicated, and the development of new leaders and succession planning ensures sustained success. The change becomes anchored in the organization. Social workers can be an asset in steps seven and eight as they leverage their ability to model new behaviors and continually assess the effectiveness of the various systems within the organization and how they work together in service of the vision. The account in Box 81.1 of one hospice's change initiative demonstrates a refusal to be complacent, adherence to Kotter's steps, and the integration of outcome measures to ensure that the changes being made are the right changes, and that they are done well.

Box 81.1
Organizational Narrative: Hospice of Palm Beach County

Hospice of Palm Beach County followed this process during a time of intentional cultural and operational change. This hospice had consistently earned high scores on the FEHC surveys returned to them by grateful families, and it was the provider of choice in its service area. The hospice enjoyed strong employee retention and an excellent compliance history. In 2009, after years of steady growth to a census of more than 1200 patients per day, the hospice was beginning its final step in the transition to an electronic medical record. Along with other hospices nationwide, Hospice of Palm Beach County was also facing decreased Medicare reimbursement, increased scrutiny, and the looming nursing shortage. The chief operating officer (COO) and the vice-president of patient services (VP) knew that the same way of delivering care that had served them so well for decades would need to evolve in order to adapt to the changing health care environment. They interviewed and visited other large hospices and began to see an emerging pattern of a "new" model of care, driven by the intertwined concepts of truly interdisciplinary teams (not merely multidisciplinary) and patient/family-driven care. The new models were less dependent on nurses, using the strength of the team's collaboration and the increased involvement and higher expectations of social workers and chaplains to facilitate a more seamless, service-oriented hospice experience. Among the key

variables to the success of the new model of care were as follows: lower social worker-to-patient ratios (hence increased participation in care by social workers); delegation of nonnursing tasks to non–nursing team members (to unburden nurses from needless overfunctioning); the use of technology (point of care, computerized documentation, text messaging, voicemail, and e-mail); evidence-based care planning; and training in communication, teamwork, and problem solving for the teams.

After engaging the support of the chief executive officer and the executive leadership team, the COO and VP began to share some of the new ideas with direct patient care clinicians, their supervisors and managers, and various other stakeholders within the organization, including physicians and finance personnel. Over a period of several months, a coalition of 12 employees was formed. They were chosen for their enthusiasm, receptivity to change, and inherent leadership ability, though not all were formal leaders. Four members of that coalition, including the COO, were social workers.

The group of 12 went on a retreat, where they worked on the vision for the new evolution in care delivery and technology. On this retreat, additional training about outcome measures, visit design, and enhancing the hospice experience for patients and families was provided. The group also worked on a script for communicating the vision to all 16 hospice teams and all other departments at the hospice, including the two teams that would pilot the new model of care. A formal communication structure devoted to sharing information about the change process over time was also created, to be branded throughout the hospice so that all employees would know that information was available and where to look for updates. They gave the communication a "Heard It through the Grapevine" theme to allow for some fun with graphics and music. The receptivity and openness of the group to new ideas, and the energy and fun of this retreat, was a short-term win, propelling the change forward and eliciting the interest of others.

Members of the coalition recruited additional members of the hospice's leadership team and clinical staff to become experts in various areas related to the transitions, so that they could train others. Another early success was the long-awaited introduction of laptop computers and the availability of text-messaging to one of the pilot teams. This prompted the following e-mail from the team supervisor:

Everyone loves the computers. Only one concern so far: air card being replaced on Kim's computer today. Susan was able to do her Plan of Care updates while driving as a passenger in her car on visits! There were multiple laptops up and running on the table at IDG! People are looking at their e-mail! The chaplain is writing on the computer notepad and feels it will be a great help with the hearing impaired families. He has been able to pull up some scripture verses for patients to read! It is a great thing! People are beginning to text. We have not had any group texts but everyone is encouraged to try a text if they have a message to get to their coworker. I think everyone will become more confident with computers and texting. It is nice to have time to get used to the computers and text messages. Again, it is a great thing! Thank you to everyone who is involved in this endeavor! (C. McCormack, personal communication, November 4, 2009)

> **Box 81.1** *(Contd.)*
>
> *This e-mail, and others like it, was posted on the hospice's intranet home page, and it was widely forwarded to share the excitement of change with the other teams. This created an atmosphere of anticipation and motivation to move forward.*
>
> *As the evolution in this hospice's care model continues, new employees are being oriented only to the changed way of doing things in order to institutionalize the change. The success with the two pilot teams with the changes in technology and the numerous new expectations of the team members is being measured across numerous planes and compared with teams still operating under the old model. These measures include the following: financial performance (the expectation is that the changes will be budget neutral); employee satisfaction as measured by the NHPCO Survey of Team Attitudes and Relationships (STAR); patient outcomes as measured by the Functional Assessment of Chronic Illness Therapy - Palliative Care (FACIT-pal); and family satisfaction as measured by the NHPCO FEHC survey. The number of after-hours calls will also be tracked, under the assumption that tighter team collaboration will result in a drop in avoidable evening and weekend calls. If these outcome measures demonstrate that the changes in care delivery and technology result in improved outcomes, more teams will be converted. This is the "Check" step in the PDCA process discussed earlier in the chapter. Of course, if any outcomes suffer, the root cause will be analyzed and adjustments made until the desired outcomes are attained. (J. Lopez-Devine, personal communication, November 27, 2009)*

Conclusion

The transition to a focus on outcome measures and a more evidence-informed style, at both the clinical and system levels, is for many social workers a step into a foreign land. It does not mean that social workers must abandon the values of genuineness, caring presence, and positive regard. Nor does it signal the end of intuition, "being yourself," or social work as a calling. These are fundamental to social work and rather than abandoned, must be infused with evidence. This will enrich the critical thinking that informs how we maximize the benefits to those we seek to serve. Fortifying these fundamentals with empirical evidence and the flexibility and accountability required to continually improve is best for patients and families, and it is essential to the future of the discipline of social work.

LEARNING EXERCISES

- Consider your own practice setting and work with clients. Write down five specific social work interventions that you routinely use with patients and families. Describe how you would specifically and measurably evaluate whether the social work interventions are resulting in the desired outcome. Which measurement tools would you use? What would

you do if the interventions did work? What would you do if they did not?
- Using the same interventions from Exercise 1, identify the reasons that an individual trained in social work must perform those interventions, as opposed to another discipline or a well-trained nonclinician. Differentiate between which tasks require a bachelor's-level education and which require master's-level education.
- Think of a process at your school or workplace that is not resulting in favorable outcomes. Design a performance improvement process using the Plan-Do-Check-Act model. Consider carefully which variables in the process to change in order to achieve improvement, and how you would evaluate whether those changes are working well. Assuming you have success and decide to implement the change on a larger scale, what other systems and people would have to be involved? How would you engage them in the coalition for change?
- Assume that you are providing social work services as part of an interdisciplinary team to a cancer patient with the goal of alleviating his or her anxiety. After 3 weeks of weekly meetings with the patient, facilitating and teaching relaxation through guided imagery, there is no improvement in the patient's level of anxiety, as measured by the Beck Anxiety Inventory. What are some of the best ways to proceed to help the patient achieve the desired outcome of less anxiety? How will you know whether the changes you make are helping the patient?
- Think of a change initiative in your school or workplace that was not successful. Which, if any, of Kotter's steps was missed? What could the organization have done better to achieve success?
- Are you, or have you ever been, part of an organization that became complacent and slid into irrelevance? Describe the process using Collin's model of decline.

ADDITIONAL RESOURCES

Collins, J. (2001). *Good to great.* New York, NY: Harper Collins.

Hepworth, D., Rooney, R., & Larsem, J. (2001). *Direct social work practice: Theory and skills* (6th ed.). Pacific Grove, CA: Brooks/Cole.

Lynn, J., Chaudhry, E., Simon, L. N., Wilkinson, A. M., & Schuster, J. L. (2007). *The Common Sense Guide to Improving Palliative Care.* New York, NY: Oxford University Press.

Reed, A. (2009). *The MVI clinical leader program.* Multi-View Incorporated Systems. Hendersonville, NC

Studer, Q. (2003). *Hardwiring excellence: Purpose, worthwhile work, making a difference.* Gulf Breeze, FL: Fire Starter Publishing.

Williams, R. L. (1994). *Essentials of Total Quality Management.* New York, NY: American Management Association.

HELPFUL WEB SITES

Brown University Center for Gerontology and Healthcare Research: http://www.chcr.brown.edu

"Improving quality of life for chronically ill persons through basic and applied research."

Multi-View International: http://www.multiviewinc.com
Provides resources for benchmarking and measurement for hospices.

National Palliative Care Research Center: http://www.npcrc.org
"Committed to stimulating, developing, and funding research directed at improving care for seriously ill patients and their families."

REFERENCES

Byock, I. M. (1998). Measuring quality of life for patients with terminal illness: The Missoula-VITAS quality of life index. *Journal of Palliative Medicine, 12*, 231–244.

Byrne, J. (1986). Business fads: What's in-and out. *Business Week, 60*, 40–47.

Centers for Medicare and Medicaid Services (CMS). (2007). *Media release database*. Retrieved from http://www.cms.hhs.gov/apps/media/press/release.asp

Centers for Medicare and Medicaid Services (CMS). (2009). *Home health quality initiatives*. Retrieved from http://www.cms.hhs.gov/homehealthqualityInits/

Chang, V.T., Hwang, S. S., & Feuerman, M. (2000). Validation of the Edmonton Symptom Assessment Scale. *Cancer, 88*(9), 2164–2171.

Collins, J. (2009). *How the mighty fall: And why some companies never give in*. New York, NY: HarperColllins.

Deming, W. E. (1989). *Out of crisis*. Cambridge, MA: MIT Press.

Department of Health and Human Services (DHHS). (2008). Hospice conditions of participation: Final rule. Retrieved from http://edocket.access.gpo.gov/2008/pdf/08-1305.pdf

George, M., Rowlands, D., & Kastle, B. (2004). Foundations of Lean Six Sigma. In M. George, D. Rowlands, & B. Kastle, *What is Lean Six Sigma?* (pp. 8–10). New York, NY: McGraw-Hill.

Judge, W., & Douglas, T. (2009). Organizational change capacity: The systematic development of a scale. *Journal of Organizational Change Management, 22*(6), 635.

Kaasa, T., Loomis, J., Gillis, K., Bruera, E., & Hanson, J. (1997). The Edmonton Functional Assessment Tool: Preliminary development and evaluation for use in palliative care. *Journal of Pain and Symptom Management, 13*, 9–10.

Kotter, J. P. (2007). Leading change: Why transformation efforts fail. *Harvard Business Review, 85*, 96–103.

MacDonald, M. (2001). Thank you, I'm sorry, and goodbye. *American Journal of Hospice and Palliative Care, 18*(6), 417–419.

Markey, R. (2001, October 23). A piece of my mind. *The Washington Post*, HE01.

McMillen, C. J., Proctor, E. K., Megivern, D., Striley, C. W., Cabassa, L. J., Munson, M., & Dickey, B. (2005). Quality of care in the social services: Research agenda and methods. *Social Work Research, 29*(3), 181–191.

Medicare. (2008). *Home health compare*. Retrieved from http://www.medicare.gov/HHCompare/Home.asp?version=default&browser

Megivern, D. M., McMillan, J. C., Proctor, E. K., Striley, C. L. W., Cabassa, L. J., & Munson, M. R. (2007). Quality of care: Expanding the social work dialogue. *Social Work, 52*(2), 115–124.

Morris, R. (2000). Social work's century of evolution as a profession: Choices made, opportunities lost. In R. Morris & J. G. Hopps (Eds.), *Social work at the millenium: Critical reflections on the future of the profession* (pp. 42–70). New York, NY: Free Press.

National Hospice and Palliative Care Organization (NHPCO). (2008). *FEPC survey materials*. Retrieved from http://www.nhpco.org/i4a/pages/Index.cfm?pageID=4936

National Hospice and Palliative Care Organization (NHPCO). (2009). *Family evaluation of hospice care*. Retrieved from http://www.nhpco.org/files/public/Statistics_Research/NHPCO_FEHC_Template.pdf

Reese, D., Raymer, M., Orloff, S., Gerbino, S., Valade, R., Dawson, S.,… Huber, R. (2006). The Social Work Assessment Tool (SWAT). *Journal of Social Work in End-of-Life and Palliative Care, 2*(2), 65–95.

Robinson, B. C. (1983). Validation of a caregiver strain index. *Journal of Gerontology, 38*(3), 344–348.

Samuels, D. I. & Adomitis, F. L. (2003). Six Sigma can meet your revenue cycle needs: Six Sigma is far from being the latest quality improvement fad; It is a proven technique grounded in principles that will endure as long as there are processes that require improvement. *Health-Care Financial Management, 57*(11), 70–75.

Teno, J. (2004). *TIME: Toolkit Instruments to Measure End-of-life care*. Retrieved from the Brown University Center for Gerontology and Health Care Research Web site: http://www.chcr.brown.edu/pcoc/toolkit.htm

Walton, M. (1986). *The Deming management method*. New York, NY: Putman Publishing Group.

Warner, S. C., & Williams, J. I. (1987). The meaning of life scale: Determining the reliability and validity of a measure. *Journal of Chronic Disease, 40*(6), 503–512.

Wensing, M. A. & Elwyn, G. (2002). Research on patient's views in the evaluation and improvement of quality of care. *Quality and Safety in Health Care, 11*(2), 153–157.

82 *Judith R. Peres*

Public Policy in Palliative and End-of-Life Care

Laws, like sausages, cease to inspire respect in proportion as we know how they are made.
—*John Godfrey Saxe, 1869*

Key Concepts

- *Advance health care directive or advance directive (AD): A written health care directive and/or appointment of an agent, or a written refusal to appoint an agent or execute a directive.*
- *Life-sustaining treatment: Medical procedures that replace or support an essential bodily function. Life-sustaining treatments include cardiopulmonary resuscitation, mechanical ventilation, artificial nutrition and hydration, dialysis, and certain other treatments.*
- *Medicare: The federal program that provides health care to persons 65 years of age and older and to others entitled to Social Security benefits. Medicare is administered at the federal level, as contrasted with Medicaid, which is administered by the states. Medicare was established in 1965 by amendment to the Social Security Act (Public Law 89-97), the pertinent section of the amendment being "Title XVIII–Health Insurance for the Aged."*
- *Original Medicare Plan: The term used by the Center for Medicare and Medicaid Services (CMS) (formerly HCFA) to describe the basic "fee-for-service" Medicare plan, offered by the federal government, and available nationwide. Unless the beneficiary chooses an alternate plan such as Medicare managed care plan or a private fee-for-service plan, the original plan will be the one in effect.*
- *Medicaid: The federal program that provides health care to indigent and medically indigent persons. While partially federally funded and managed by CMS, the Medicaid program is administered by the states, in accordance with an approved plan for that state, and each state has considerable flexibility in designing requirements. This is in contrast with Medicare, which is federally funded and administered at the federal level by CMS. The Medicaid program was established in 1965 by amendment to the Social Security Act, under a provision entitled "Title XIX–Medical Assistance."*
- *MedPAC: The Medicare Payment Advisory Commission (MedPAC) is an independent Congressional agency established by the Balanced Budget Act of 1997 (P.L. 105-33) to advise the U.S. Congress on issues affecting the Medicare program. The Commission's statutory mandate is quite broad: In addition to advising the Congress on payments to private health plans participating in Medicare and providers in Medicare's traditional fee-for-service program, MedPAC is also tasked with analyzing access to care, quality of care, and other issues affecting Medicare.*

- *Patient Self-Determination Act (PSDA): An amendment to the Omnibus Budget Reconciliation Act of 1990, the law became effective December 1991 and requires most U.S. hospitals, nursing homes, hospice programs, home health agencies, and health maintenance organizations to give adult individuals, at the time of inpatient admission or enrollment, information about their rights under state laws governing advance directives. These include the following: (1) the right to participate in and direct their own health care decisions; (2) the right to accept or refuse medical or surgical treatment; (3) the right to prepare an advance directive; and (4) information on the provider's policies governing use of these rights. The act prohibits institutions from discriminating against a patient who does not have an advance directive. The PSDA further requires institutions to document patient information and provide ongoing community education on advance medical care.*
- *Public policy: The body of principles that underpin the operation of legal systems. This addresses the social, moral, and economic values that tie a society together: values that vary in different cultures and change over time. Law regulates behavior either to reinforce existing social expectations or to encourage constructive change, and laws are most likely to be effective when they are consistent with the most generally accepted societal norms and reflect the collective morality of the society.*

Introduction

Note: Policies are fluid and evolve. With that in mind, new legislation has been or will be enacted that may potentially impact the programs throughout this chapter.

Social workers, trained to be client advocates and change agents, can assist in mediating the prevailing challenges and barriers that individuals and their families face in understanding, seeking, and obtaining palliative and end-of-life care. All too often, U.S. public policies concerning palliative and end-of-life care fail to reflect the diversity of values and preferences that frame individual and family concerns (Field & Cassel, 1997; Lynn & Adamson, 2003; National Institutes of Health, 2004; Shugarman, Lorenz, & Lynn, 2005; SUPPORT Principal Investigators, 1995). As advocates, social workers seek to understand the strengths and needs of the individual while identifying the assets and overcoming the barriers present in the physical, social, and political environment that affect individual well-being (Bern-Klug et al., 2009; Roff, 2001).

In 2009, the public policy debate on palliative and end-of-life care was fraught with highly charged rhetoric, fears, mistrust, and suspect motives. In a society that is capable of misunderstanding the need for frank and open communication about values, goals, and preferences for care near the end of life, by labeling those efforts as "death panels," the social work perspective becomes not just important but critical in promoting a thoughtful and measured dialogue about the importance of respecting a person's values and goals for care (Clark, 2009).

Many people fear living with advanced illness and dying, in part because of the inadequacies of the current system of financing and organizing palliative and end-of-life care. When asked, most people state a preference to die at home surrounded by their friends and family at all stages along the illness trajectory (Dinger, 2005; Last Acts Coalition, 2002; Pritchard et al., 1998); instead they too often die without loved ones in hospitals and nursing homes (SUPPORT Principal Investigators, 1995; Teno, Kabumoto, & Wetle, 2004). Many frail individuals need additional social supports, such as personal care, at home, but these services are often not available or affordable, especially to persons not eligible for Medicaid (Tilly & Wiener, 2001; Wiener & Tilly, 2003).

Pain near the end of life is widespread, despite the availability of effective pain management techniques (Morrison & Meier, 2004; Teno, Kabumoto, & Wetle, 2004). Life-prolonging treatments and diagnostic studies continue for many patients, even when physicians know that there is little chance of prolonging quality life, often resulting in additional discomfort, suffering, and pain. Many observers question whether these illness-specific treatments near the end of life are what patients want (Curtis, 2005; Hawkins, Ditto, Dinks, & Smucker, 2005; Shah et al., 2008) or whether offering them are cultural, automatic responses to physicians' training in saving and extending lives and perceiving death both as avoidable and as a failure. Physicians, nurses, and social workers receive little training in palliative and end-of-life care, and many are ill at ease in discussing these issues (Cherlin et al., 2007; Csikai & Raymer, 2003).

In addition to the lack of training, misunderstandings and lack of information about Medicare and Medicaid program rules concerning coverage, quality of care, and reimbursement policies (Gage et al., 2000), as well as federal and state laws regarding controlled substances (Joranson, Gilson, Dahl, & Haddox, 2002; Jost, 2000), all play into the policy debate about palliative and end-of-life care.

Into this mix steps the social worker, who is grappling with palliative and end-of-life care at the individual, family, and societal levels. Despite emerging competencies and standards of practice, social work responsibilities in palliative and end-of-life care vary widely, depending upon the setting and their role(s) in that setting. Regardless of setting, social

workers can advocate for financing policies that can improve timely access to supportive palliative care services and represent the concerns and needs of their clients and families living with advanced illness.

This chapter reviews the role of U.S. public policy on palliative and end-of-life care as governed by federal programs and policies (e.g., Medicare, Medicaid, Veterans Administration), and state laws (e.g., prescription drugs) and the Patient Self-Determination Act (PSDA). Supplementary resources and key terms are found at the end of this chapter.

Public Policy

Palliative care is one of the many neglected public policy issues of our time. Being aware of the influences public policy plays in the delivery of palliative care allows the practicing social worker to be an effective advocate for the client and family living with advanced illness. In fact, in developing the National Association of Social Worker's (NASW) standards for social work practice in palliative and end-of-life care, empowerment and advocacy are included as important components for successful practice:

Standard 6: Empowerment and Advocacy

The social worker shall advocate for the needs, decisions, and rights of clients in palliative and end-of-life care. The social worker shall engage in social and political action that seeks to ensure that people have equal access to resources to meet their biopsychosocial needs in palliative and end-of-life care. (NASW, 2003)

Public policy in palliative care provides the social worker the perfect opportunity to advocate at both the micro and macro level. Policy issues have long been the focus of intense societal debate, as providers, medical ethicists, policy makers, legislators, and the public have considered essential questions concerning patient autonomy, quality of life, and withdrawal of life-sustaining treatments (Rao et al., 2005). Policies in general emanate from two sources: the private sector or the public sector. Private policies such as in a hospital or nursing home can support a service by increasing or redirecting monetary and human resources to palliative care programs. Public policy refers to the government or a political party decision, actions, and other matters that will prove advantageous to society in general (Oliver, 2006). Both types of policy strive to develop a plan or course of action designed to define issues, select goals and a means for reaching them, and allocate resources to address identified needs.

The development of policy depends on partnerships between many stakeholders, including governmental and private agencies, public health agencies, employers, health care providers and community-based organizations, providers, and citizens. As we saw in the heath insurance reform efforts of 2009–2010, however, policy making is not always a rational and orderly process; instead, it is a political process, which is propelled by dynamic negotiations between groups with competing societal priorities and conflicting social ideologies.

Public policies are enacted through many government venues as state and federal laws, regulations, and manuals. Statutes are formal, written laws enacted by a legislature. Federal and state laws specific to social work practice in palliative care can be found in Medicare; Medicaid; state pain, insurance, and licensure statutes; and the PSDA. An excellent resource for understanding statutes and the policy process can be accessed through the Library of Congress "Thomas" Site: http://thomas.loc.gov/home/abt_thom.html.

Regulations fill in the details of the laws. For instance, federal law requires psychosocial services be covered for nursing home residents, and regulations define who is qualified to deliver the services (Bern-Klug et al., 2009). When a notice of proposed rule making is issued, the public is given an opportunity to comment on the issues. Electronic comments on rules governing Medicare and Medicaid can be submitted and searched at: http://www.cms.hhs.gov/eRulemaking/01_Overview.asp

Both state and federal policies have helped to lay the foundation for current approaches to palliative and end-of-life care.

From a public policy perspective, health care providers are subject to an overwhelming amount of regulation and oversight by a plethora of federal and state agencies. Consequently, a tangle of coverage, financing, regulation, and oversight rules influences and interferes with the palliative and end-of-life services that people and their families with advanced illness ought to receive. To be effective advocates on behalf of persons with advanced illness, social workers need a clear understanding of the policies impacting palliative and end-of-life care. This is especially true in understanding both the influences that regulations have in access to palliative care through hospice as well as the lack of coverage and regulation allowing people to access palliative care in nursing facilities, hospitals, and the community.

Palliative Care and Public Policy

Over the past 20 years, a series of research, reports, and discussions helped define current palliative care issues in public policy. In the 1990s, the Supreme Court ruling on the Cruzan case affirmed the constitutional right to refuse life-sustaining medical treatment (Sabatino, 2007). The court's decision was quickly followed by the passage of the federal Patient Self-Determination Act and durable power of attorney for health care statutes in many states (*Patient Self-Determination Act of 1990*). In 1995, the groundbreaking Study to Understand Prognoses and Preferences for Outcomes and Risks of Treatments (SUPPORT) documented serious deficiencies in care

for dying patients (SUPPORT Principal Investigators, 1995). SUPPORT was quickly followed by a number of reports undertaken by the Institute of Medicine (IOM), including *Approaching Death: Improving Care at the End of Life* and various National Institute of Health (NIH) and private foundation initiatives, including the Robert Wood Johnson Foundation, supporting research programs and public engagement activities associated with end-of-life care (Field & Cassel, 1997; Lorenz et al., 2004). In addition, the Soros Foundation Open Society Institute's (OSI) Project on Death in America (PDIA) supported many social workers who generated and translated research and created programs to enhance the skills of social work in the emerging specialty of palliative care (Open Society Institute, n.d.). (For more information see Chapter 3)

During this same time period, standards of practice for palliative and hospice care have developed through professional medical, nursing, social work, hospice organizations, and regulatory bodies. In April 2009, the National Consensus Project (NCP) issued the second edition of the *Clinical Practice Guidelines* (NCP, 2009), which encompass the core essential elements of quality palliative care delineated within eight specific domains. The Social Aspects of Care are included as Domain 4 in the NCP Clinical Practice Guidelines for Quality Palliative Care. While social workers are essential participants in all domains, social workers have a unique perspective and ability to enhance the social and community aspects of a care plan (Altilio, Otis-Green, & Dahlin, 2008).

Of particular interest to social workers are the NASW Standards for Social Work Practice in Palliative and End of Life Care, outlining 11 key guiding principles for social workers practicing in this arena with the following specific acknowledgment:

Social workers also have expertise in analyzing, influencing, and implementing policy change and development at local, state and federal levels that can be used to make important improvements in the care of patients living with life-limiting illness and the dying. (NASW, 2003)

Table 82.1.
Domains of High-Quality Palliative Care

1. Structure and processes of care
2. Physical aspects of care
3. Psychosocial and psychiatric aspects of care
4. Social aspects of care
5. Spiritual, religious, and existential aspects of care
6. Cultural aspects of care
7. Care of the imminently dying patient
8. Ethical and legal aspects of care

Source: National Consensus Project, 2009, Second Edition.

The creation of national standards, the development of a specialty in palliative medicine, and the growing unmet needs of patients with serious illness and their families are fueling growth in palliative care despite the lack of official status of public policy.

Increases in Palliative Care Services

Palliative care programs serve Medicare beneficiaries and others who are ineligible for hospice, have difficulty accessing the Medicare hospice benefit, or Medicare beneficiaries who do not want to forgo life-prolonging treatments related to their terminal illness. Palliative care serves persons along the continuum of illness and may be provided concurrently with active curative directed toward the disease but is not considered a covered Medicare benefit outside of hospice. However, availability of these services varies widely across geographic regions, and fee-for-service Medicare reimbursement for physicians, nurse practitioners, and social workers does not cover the interdisciplinary team (Wennberg, Fisher, Goodman, & Skinner, 2008). The prevalence of hospital palliative care programs in the United States has steadily increased since 2000, with 53% of hospitals reporting a palliative care program in 2006 compared to 25% in 2003 (Goldsmith, Deitrich, Du, & Morrison, 2008). Yet it is not clear that all these programs have congruity of staffing or mission.

It is becoming clear that there is not a boundary between when life-prolonging therapy ends and palliative care begins and that both can be provided concurrently. One response to this growing need for concurrent palliative care has been the growth of palliative care hospital units. Financial support for inpatient palliative care units appears to be growing with evidence that these units may both improve the quality of care and reduce the cost of care for seriously ill patients by critical decision making and by controlling the costs of drugs and nonbeneficial services provided to dying patients while improving quality (Norton et al., 2007). One recent study demonstrated that patients receiving palliative care consultation had significantly lower costs than usual care patients (Morrison, Maroney-Galin, Kralovec, & Meier, 2005).

However, since palliative care outside of hospice is not a formally recognized public policy, in-hospital palliative care programs need to be subsidized by their institutions to survive (Shugarman et al., 2005). In profiling the most innovative and successful hospital-based palliative programs, one study identified a series of challenges that were identified by program staff. These challenges include cumbersome billing for palliative care services, receipt of payment from multiple sources, denial of claims, and the need to patch together resources from multiple funding streams.

Even though the number of hospital-based palliative care programs is increasing, a major barrier to their expansion is that they do not easily fit into the coverage and payment policies of Medicare and other insurers. Resources, such as Center to Advance Palliative Care (CAPC), National Hospice and Palliative Care Organization (NHPCO), National Association of Social Workers (NASW), and the Social Work Hospice and Palliative Care Network (SWHPN) exist to assist social workers in understanding how to advocate for these palliative care services (see Resource section for Web links).

Lack of Public Palliative Care Policy. The lack of a clear public policy for palliative and end-of-life care complicates the delivery of seamless palliative and end-of-life care because there are conflicting goals among the health and long-term care systems (e.g., hospitals, nursing facilities, and hospice and community services). The health care venue is primarily curative; long-term care is primarily convalescent, rehabilitative, or restorative; hospice is palliative; and community services can provide a bridge or support for maintaining function but not necessarily for dying at home. Care providers in each of these settings are often influenced by specialized training that emphasizes certain skill sets, institutional protocols and culture, regulatory issues, and funding streams. As a result, the goals of treatment for persons with similar conditions may vary widely depending upon the setting they are in. This inconsistency and lack of continuity is well documented in having a negative impact on care planning and communication, for the general population and especially so for the seriously ill and those coming to the end of their lives.

Social workers have the comprehensive knowledge needed to lead the necessary systemic reforms to identify and overcome these incongruities so that palliative and end-of-life care is accessible to persons and their families living with advanced illness.

Medicare

Although a great deal of attention has focused on care for persons with advanced illness near the end of life (Lorenz et al., 2004; NIH State-of-the-Science Conference Statement on Improving End-of-Life Care, 2004), the role of Medicare's reimbursement and coverage rules in shaping care for persons with advanced illness has received much less attention (Buntin & Huskamp, 2002). This is surprising because 83% of all people who die in a year are covered by Medicare (Hogan, Lunney, Gabel, & Lynn, 2001), and spending in the last year of life consistently accounts for about 27% of total Medicare expenditures (Hogan et al., 2001; Lubitz & Riley, 1993). Medicare is the dominant payer and what it covers and how it reimburses providers has a profound effect on what and how care is provided for persons with advanced illness.

Coverage and Payment

Medicare covers a broad array of services needed by beneficiaries with advanced illness, including hospital care, physician services, home health care, skilled nursing facility care, durable medical equipment (including air fluidized beds, canes, commode chairs, crutches, hospital beds, etc.), prescription drugs, rehabilitation services, outpatient mental health services, nonphysician health services, and hospice (Gottlich, 2003; Morrison & Meier, 2004). Custodial care is not covered, except within the hospice benefit and Program for All-Inclusive Care of the Elderly (PACE; Eng, 2002). PACE admits beneficiaries to receive end-of-life services based on their functional status and acuity level so they enter a coordinated care program (with many palliative services available) earlier than beneficiaries enrolling in Medicare hospice. Such a program may better serve people with advanced illness because they are more likely to receive coordinated services to prevent avoidable and/or unnecessary hospitalizations. Medicare provides some help with activities of daily living through the skilled nursing facility and home health benefits, but only for persons who need skilled care. Medicare requires its providers to query patients about advance directives and to implement them when necessary; it recently added an advance care planning discussion to the "Welcome to Medicare" visit (*Medicare Improvements for Patients and Providers Act of 2008*). Medicare however does not reimburse for the time that quality advance directive conversations require.

In most cases, Medicare coverage is dependent on whether care meets "medical necessity" criteria, which usually allow payment for services only for as long as the person is improving (Centers for Medicare & Medicaid Services [CMMS], 2005). As a result, coverage for services such as physical therapy ends once the person ceases to improve. For persons receiving palliative care, however, functional improvement may or may not be the goal. Although physical therapy may be important for quality of life and to maintain function and to prevent deconditoning, if there is no improvement, chances are that it will not be reimbursed. One challenge of our current "system" is that the same patient with the same physical condition and same response or lack of response to physical therapy will qualify or not qualify for coverage depending upon the venue he or she is in—the community, hospice, nursing facility, or hospital. Because of the acute care focus, the following components of quality palliative and end-of-life care are not covered: interdisciplinary care, on-call services, home health aides for personal care, patient/family education regarding advance directives or self-care, support and training of family caregivers, bereavement counseling, and continuity of care across time, place, and providers.

Medicare *payment policies* are also focused on medically necessary acute care treatment in hospitals and skilled nursing services, which are not always aligned with the goals of advanced illness management (Gottlich, 2003). With the exception of the Medicare Hospice Benefit and PACE program, original Medicare's financial incentives promote hospitalization and the use of skilled nursing facilities (Schamp & Tenkku, 2006).

The 2009 MedPAC Report to Congress documents that over the last two decades, the 5% of beneficiaries who die in a given year account for roughly one-quarter of Medicare spending in that year, which amounts to roughly $40,000 or more in spending in their last year of life (MedPAC, 2009). Yet much of this spending is not ultimately of benefit to the patient. According to the Dartmouth Atlas Project, which studied data on 4.7 million Medicare beneficiaries, a fundamental problem is that most acute care hospitals have become the first-line providers of services to chronically ill elders, whose care would be better managed, safer, and less expensive outside the hospital setting. The study demonstrated that Medicare could have realized substantial savings—$40 billion or nearly one-third of what it spent for enrollees' care over the 4 years—if all U.S. hospitals practiced high-quality/low-cost standards of care at the end of beneficiaries' lives (Wennberg, Fisher, Goodman, & Skinner, 2008).

The Medicare Hospice Benefit statute and the regulations developed by CMS represented the best available model when hospices were introduced in this country almost 30 years ago. They serve well those patients who have conditions for which disease-modifying therapy can be sharply distinguished from therapies with palliative intent. For others, however, the approach to palliative care has been altered by the fact that medical advances have blurred the line between treatment directed at the underlying disease and treatment directed at the relief of suffering. For many cancer patients, treatments including radiation therapy, chemotherapy, blood transfusions, and surgery are not just curative but can now be used to prolong the symptom-free period and enhance the quality of remaining life.

Over a decade of research on palliative care for Medicare beneficiaries indicates the following:

- Few physicians are trained in geriatrics as a specialty or even as a topic of medical education. The current Medicare fee-for-service program lacks incentives for case management, a critical part of end-of-life care, paying instead for episodic interventions, such as surgery and diagnostic tests, while providing inadequate coverage for supportive services (Fins, Peres, & Schumacher, 2003).
- Many patients die in hospitals, despite their desire to die at home. The number of palliative care units has grown, but they face financial difficulties (Shugarman et al., 2005).
- Medicare covers home health services for dying patients through hospice, but it does not provide services to people without a skilled care need. The use of Medicare home health care has risen and fallen in response to Medicare payment incentives. Little is known about the provision of end-of-life care by home

health agencies (McCall, Korb, Petersons, & Moore, 2002).

- Medicare's skilled nursing facility benefit is geared toward short-term, post-acute care, but substantial proportions of Medicare beneficiaries die in nursing homes. Substantial numbers of nursing home beneficiaries are in pain and have had feeding tubes inserted, raising questions of quality of care. Interaction between the Medicare hospice care and the Medicare skilled nursing facility benefit is complex and does not always work well (Gage et al., 2000; Miller, Gozalo, & Mor, 2001; Teno, 2004).
- Hospice is the principal Medicare benefit geared to addressing the needs of people who are dying, but despite the growth in recent years, the limitation of coverage to people with only 6 months to live and the requirement that beneficiaries receive all acute care treatment directed toward their life-threatening illness before enrolling creates an access barrier for many.
- Although managed care organizations potentially have the flexibility to provide the broad range of services needed by Medicare beneficiaries with advanced illness and emphasize care management, few health plans have focused on palliative and end-of-life care. Hospice services remain a "carve-out" in Medicare Advantage plans (Emanuel et al., 2002). Under the Medicare carve-out mechanism for hospice utilization, when the Medicare Advantage patient elects to enroll in hospice care with a Medicare certified hospice, the plan's monthly payment from Medicare is reduced. The elected hospice assumes responsibility for all of the patient's care related to the terminal condition and receives Medicare reimbursement through its usual channels, just as it would for a Medicare beneficiary not enrolled in a Medicare Advantage plan.
- While the Patient Self-Determination Act of 1990 requires Medicare providers to inform beneficiaries about advance directives, a large research literature finds that advance directives, as currently constituted, are not effective. As a result, there has been a movement toward advance care planning, which embodies a broader approach for beneficiaries to control their care.

Medicare Part B Services

Medicare provides for outpatient physicians and other practitioners such as social workers through Part B payments. As the gateway to almost all other services, physicians are some of the most important players in palliative and end-of-life care. There are a growing number of community palliative care programs, and Medicare Part B billing can contribute to some of the funding (Meier & Beresford, 2006). Medicare covers 80% of the cost of unlimited physician services after payment of the Part B deductible ($155 in 2010). Critics argue that physicians provide care that is overly specialized,

continue aggressive curative treatments beyond the point when they are likely to be effective, fail to adequately address pain, and fail to have caring interactions with patients and their families (Lynn, 2004). However, as in other disciplines, the growing specialty of palliative medicine may produce specialist physicians who will influence the quality and focus of care working in consultation with the referring team and interdisciplinary palliative clinicians who together can meet the holistic needs of palliative care patients and their families.

For social workers and other health care providers, the clinical payment rate is set at the beginning of each year. Clinical social workers may receive reimbursement for outpatient psychotherapy, individual and group to individuals with mental illness ICD-9-CM diagnosis, but these codes often have no applicability to patients and families who are struggling to manage life- threatening illness over time. Medicare pays on a Resource-Based Relative Value Scale (RBRVS). Social workers are paid 75% of the physician rate. Only services rendered face to face may be billed (42 CFR §410.73); hence, the telephone work done by clinicians in follow-up and to support continuity of care is not reimbursed.

It is useful to be aware of the billing code for physicians providing palliative care. Code V66.7 is approved for diagnosis of palliative care (ICD-9, 1996). This code was designed to help legitimize and encourage the use of palliative care. This code also provided the opportunity to create a new diagnosis-related group to allow payment for care of patients who die in hospitals or otherwise require hospitalizations for hospital-based palliative care. Unfortunately, lack of consistency in using this code may lead to either underestimation or overestimation of the number of patients receiving hospice and palliative care (Wolfsfeld, Zhu, & Hendricks, 2004).

In its 2008 report, *Retooling for an Aging America: Building the Health Care Workforce*, the Institute of Medicine (IOM) concluded that the nation's elder health care workforce is too small and too unprepared to meet the health care needs of the rapidly growing number of older Americans. By 2030, there will be just 8000 geriatricians, despite the fact that the United States will need about 36,000 to cover the workload as the number of Americans 65 years and older mushrooms. The report also found that social workers have essential skills needed to help an aging population but these skills go unrecognized by older adults and their families and that the cost effectiveness of social work services needs to be made explicit to public payers, such as Medicaid and Medicare (IOM, 2008).

Hospital Services

Medicare pays the full amount of hospital care for 60 days after payment of the Part A deductible ($1100 in 2010). For days 61–90, there is a daily coinsurance that amounts to one-quarter of the Part A deductible ($275 in 2010) and from days 91–150, that co-insurance rises to one-half of the Part A deductible ($550 in 2010). Medicare pays for hospital care prospectively, using the diagnosis-related group (DRG) system, which does not specifically provide for palliative care. This system is developed on a weighted mean, ignoring actual length of stay as well as the actual cost of providing care, and it pays a fixed amount based on diagnosis. Consequently, hospitals make more money when stays are short, break even when the length of stay equates with payment, and lose money when lengths of stay exceed the reimbursement.

When in the hospital, dying patients receive services that are often inconsistent with their desires and those of their families (SUPPORT Principal Investigators, 1995). Death in the inpatient care setting often means acute care and expensive diagnostic procedures (Barnato, McClellan, Kagay, & Garber, 2004; Gillick & Mitchell, 2004; Rady & Johnson, 2004). About 10% of Medicare beneficiaries spend 7 or more days in an intensive care unit (ICU) in the last 6 months of their lives (Last Acts Coalition, 2002), and patients with poor prognoses who die in an ICU often do not have prior discussions of alternative treatment options or palliative care approaches (Rady & Johnson, 2004). Acute inpatient care is associated with inadequate pain control and lack of supportive services (Bryce et al., 2004; Clarke et al., 2003).

Even though the number of hospital-based palliative care programs is increasing, a major barrier to their expansion is that they do not easily fit into the coverage and payment policies of Medicare and other insurers. While hospital-based palliative care programs seek to provide comprehensive end-of-life care, they often cannot deliver the complete package of services available through many hospice programs due to the lack of reimbursement and coverage for family support and bereavement services, caregiver training, care coordination, and family counseling. Outpatient patient counseling is covered under the Medicare fee-for-service plan, but this service is not commonly billed and does not recognize a social worker's role in an interdisciplinary team. The Medicare Improvements for Patients and Providers Act of 2008 provides Medicare coinsurance parity for mental health services, reducing beneficiaries' copayments by 5% per year, and finally reaching 20% in 2014—achieving full parity with Medicare outpatient benefits. However, for Medicare coverage, the focus of family therapy must be the treatment of the patient's condition. Family therapy is generally not covered if directed to the effects of the patient's condition on the family.

Home Health Care

Medicare home health services include skilled nursing, physical, speech, and occupational therapy, social work services, and aide services for assistance with functional needs. These services could enable the provision of good end-of-life care at home, but Medicare limits coverage to beneficiaries who meet the definition of "homebound" and who have a part-time (fewer than 8 hours per day) or intermittent skilled need (MedPAC, 2006). No deductible or coinsurance is required.

In response to extremely rapid increases in Medicare home health use and expenditures during the early 1990s, the Balanced Budget Act of 1997 (BBA) mandated the implementation of a prospective payment system for home health

that was designed to return the benefit to a more skilled care focus. The initial impact of the BBA was to substantially reduce spending for the Medicare home health benefit (Komisar, 2002). Several studies examined the effects of the changes in the home health payment system and did not find any substantial increases in the rates of potentially adverse outcomes such as hospitalizations, skilled nursing facility admissions, emergency room visits, and death (McCall, Petersons, Moore, & Korb, 2003). On the other hand, MedPAC (2006) documented a dramatic drop in the number of visits provided during a 60-day episode of care, which may have a negative impact on Medicare beneficiaries with multiple chronic disabilities and those needing palliative and end-of-life care. There are a growing number of agencies providing home-based palliative care programs, which are discussed in Chapter10.

Nursing Facilities

Nursing facilities are the final residence for many frail dying Medicare beneficiaries, precisely those individuals who might not want acute medical interventions and who are at risk of suffering iatrogenic complications from such interventions. Currently in the United States, one in four persons dies in a nursing home, and in six states the rate is more than one in three; projections show that by 2020 the proportion of elderly Americans who will die in nursing facilities will reach 40% (Brown University Center for Gerontology and Health Care Research, n.d.c). There is increasing documentation that the experience of dying in nursing facilities is problematic (Miller & Mor, 2006). Despite the frequency of death in nursing facilities, the end-of-life experience has been studied less there than in other sites of death (Thompson & Chochinov, 2006), and much existing research has focused on deficits in care, such as inadequate pain management, the absence of emotional and spiritual support (Kayser-Jones, 2002), lack of advance directives (Teno & Gruneir, 2007), and the need for improvement in palliative end-of-life care treatment strategies (Huskamp, Stevenson, Chernew, & Newhouse, 2010; Miller, Mor, & Teno, 2003; Teno, Weitzen, & Wetle, 2001).

Although Medicare pays for some skilled nursing facility care, Medicaid is the dominant payer. Medicare's skilled nursing facility benefit is limited to 100 days of care for beneficiaries who have a 3-day prior hospitalization and need skilled care. While there is no cost sharing for the first 20 days of care, beneficiary coinsurance is one-eighth of the hospital deductible per day ($137.50 in 2010) for days 21 to 100. Nursing facility residents who receive care through Medicare's Part A skilled nursing facility (SNF) benefit cannot simultaneously receive hospice care reimbursed by Medicare. Once they are no longer on a skilled Part A Medicare stay in the nursing facility, they can choose to elect their Part A hospice benefit and still reside in the nursing facility.

Dying SNF residents often need complex medical management, which is more available in a SNF bed than non-skilled custodial care, but they also require the symptom management expertise and psychosocial and spiritual support available through specialized palliative care/hospice. However, the decision to enroll in hospice often comes down to a financial choice because there are financial disincentives associated with hospice choice for both residents/families and nursing facilities (Miller et al., 2003). Medicare does not cover the cost of room and board services associated with a nursing facility stay once the beneficiary is no longer eligible for skilled nursing facility care. Often times, families do not have the funds to cover the room and board costs.

Potential Barriers to Good Palliative Care in Nursing Facilities
Some researchers have found that good palliative care in skilled nursing facilities may not be available for several reasons. First, attending physicians and staff lack specific education and training in the provision of palliative care (Fins et al., 2003). Second, curative, restorative, maintenance, or preventive care goals in skilled nursing facilities may conflict with palliative care goals (Fins et al., 2003; Jennings, Ryndes, & D'Onofrio, 2003; Johnson, 2005). Travis et al. (2001) examined patterns of care during the last year of life using retrospective chart review of 41 nursing home residents and found that while most residents died receiving palliative care, their progression toward a palliative care plan was often slowed by indecision or inaction on the part of key decision makers and sometimes interrupted by acute care until the last few days of life.

Unnecessary transfers from skilled nursing facilities to hospitals greatly disrupt the continuity of care. Huskamp, Buntin, Wang, and Newhouse (2001) reported that they were told of instances in which skilled nursing facilities transferred dying Medicare patients to hospitals in part to avoid the additional staffing and other costs associated with their care. Quality of care is also affected by inadequate communication between hospitals and skilled nursing facilities, lack of time for teams to discuss and refine goals upon transfers, structural disincentive to refer to hospice until Medicare Part A coverage and reimbursement days are exhausted, and bed-hold regulations (Miller & Mor, 2006).

Some analysts have suggested that a stronger palliative physician presence and oversight of physicians knowledgeable in palliative care are needed to improve the quality of end-of-life care in these facilities (Miller et al., 2004). In addition, training of staff, including nurses, social workers, and home health aides and attendants might create environments in which residents and their families can be cared for in a familiar and consistent setting as they come to the end of life.

Intersection of Medicare Hospice and Nursing Facility Care
While most hospice patients are in the community, a substantial portion of beneficiaries receive their care in nursing facility. A recent Office of Inspector General (OIG) report found that 31% of Medicare hospice beneficiaries resided in nursing facilities in 2006. Nursing facilities mostly contract with community-based hospices, and almost half of nursing home residents choosing hospice were dually eligible for Medicare and Medicaid. A decade of research has demon-strated that hospice can have a positive effect on the process of dying for nursing facility residents because it is associated with better pain management, less use of feeding tubes, fewer physical restraints, and lower hospitalization rates (Miller et al., 2001; Miller et al., 2003; Mitchell, Teno, Roy, & Lapane, 2003). Notably, there is evidence of a "diffusion effect" for non–hospice enrollees in nursing facilities where there is hospice presence (Miller et al., 2001). A better collaborative relationship between hospice and nursing facility staff has the potential to improve end-of-life care for frail elders.

Unfortunately, the potential for fraud and abuse in arrangements between nursing facilities and hospices has been an area of increasing concern since the mid-1990s. According to two recent OIG reports, a growing number of Medicare beneficiaries are receiving hospice care in nursing facilities, but most of these services do not meet Medicare requirements. The first report, *Medicare Hospice Care: Services Provided to Beneficiaries Residing in Nursing Facilities*, found that the number of beneficiaries receiving hospice care in nursing facilities has risen dramatically over the last few years, expanding from 580,000 in 2001 to 939,000 in 2006, an increase of 62%. The 31% of Medicare hospice beneficiaries who lived in a nursing facility during 2006 cost the government approximately $2.59 billion. The most commonly provided hospice services included nursing services, home health aide services, and medical social services (U.S. Department of Health and Human Services [DHHS] OIG, 2009a). An accompanying report, *Medicare Hospice Care for Beneficiaries in Nursing Facilities: Compliance with Medicare Coverage Requirements*, shows that 82% of the services provided in nursing facilities do not meet Medicare coverage requirements (DHHS OIG, 2009b). The Centers for Medicare and Medicaid Services ([CMS], 2008) responded to the reports and stated that the new conditions of participation issued on June 5, 2008 addresses the interaction and care of beneficiaries choosing hospice in nursing facilities.

Hospice
The existing Medicare Hospice Benefit provides one opportunity to help shape a better care system for beneficiaries near the end of their lives. Currently, the only Medicare program tailored to the end of life, in general, hospice programs do not provide costly disease-modifying treatments; thus, most beneficiaries consider hospice only when these have been exhausted or patients choose to forgo access to other acute care services. Pioneered in England, hospice took root in the United States during the 1970s and was added as a benefit to the Medicare program in 1982 (*Tax Equity and Fiscal Responsibility Act of 1982*).

Currently, for Medicare beneficiaries electing the hospice benefit, palliative care services related to the terminal illness are covered. A primary care physician and the hospice medical director must certify that the patient has an expected prognosis of 6 months or less if the patient's disease trajectory follows its normal course. This prognosis rule was designed to restrict access to the hospice benefit to control overall costs and to target beneficiaries in the terminal stages of cancer, and it does not fit the end-of-life trajectories of most other diseases (Gage et al., 2000; Jennings et al., 2003). Attempts to comply with this rule delay enrollment, preventing beneficiaries from receiving the full scope of benefits (Foley, 2005).

The Medicare Hospice Benefit is one of the only Medicare benefits with mandated interdisciplinary team-based care. Under the Medicare Hospice Benefit, hospices provide a package of services that include the following: physician, nursing, social work, home health aide, volunteer, physical therapy, occupational therapy, speech therapy, counseling, dietary, and spiritual professionals; medications related to the terminal illness; medical supplies and equipment; short general inpatient and respite care; 13 months of bereavement follow-up; and any other services reasonable and necessary for palliation of the terminal illness (CMS, 2008). The hospice benefit does not cover curative treatment related to the terminal illness nor room and board payment for staying in a facility. Medicare pays hospice agencies on a per-diem basis, paying fixed inpatient and outpatient reimbursements regardless of services provided. Payments are made according to four different categories of care: routine home care (RHC), continuous home care (CHC), inpatient respite care (IRC), and general inpatient care (GIC).

Despite adjustments for inflation, the fees have not kept up with the cost of cutting-edge palliative treatments. The basic routine home care payment was $142.91 per day in fiscal year 2010. Many patients who meet the criterion for hospice care—having less than 6 months to live—are offered and choose treatments that palliate symptoms and prevent disease progression such as oral chemotherapies, radiation, or blood transfusions. These treatments vary greatly in cost, some costing more than $10,000 per month—too much for most hospice programs, despite the statute allowing for such coverage if it is considered "palliation."

Medicare hospice spending has more than tripled between 2000 and 2008, when it reached $11.2 billion. Over this time, the number of Medicare-participating hospices increased by more than 1000 providers, nearly all of which were for-profit entities (MedPAC, 2009). Recent MedPAC reports found several distinct patterns underlying broader spending and utilization trends in hospice. These patterns include a pronounced shift in patients' terminal diagnoses, the profitability of longer stays, and gaps in accountability for appropriate benefit use. Hospice now provides care to beneficiaries with a wide range of terminal conditions, in contrast to the earlier years of the benefit. Consequently, in 2009, MedPAC recommended changes to the Medicare Hospice Benefit in reimbursement, increasing hospice organizations' accountability, and ensuring greater involvement by physicians in recertifying the need for end-of-life care. The recommended reimbursement rates would decrease over the length of a patient's stay but would include a payment for higher costs of care near time of death. Developing a payment system that closely matches the actual costs of the first and last periods of care

was designed to align payment incentives with the needs of beneficiaries.

In 2007 hospice use was found to significantly reduce Medicare costs during the last year of life by an average of $2309 per hospice user (Taylor et al., 2007). In addition, Medicare costs were reduced further the longer an individual was enrolled in hospice. Cost savings were more pronounced for patients with cancer than for patients with other diagnoses, especially for longer stays. Despite the benefits in terms of both quality of life and cost effectiveness, hospice referrals have historically been made too late. The barriers to timely referral have been researched and well documented and are related to physician and patient attitudes as well as the reimbursement structure itself. Among the most commonly cited patient-related barriers are denial of health status, desire to exhaust all treatment options, a negative perception of hospice, and patient demographics (McCarthy, Burns, Davis, & Phillips, 2003).

Managed Care and Medicare Advantage. Over the last two decades, Medicare has provided options for beneficiaries to enroll in managed care organizations. Potential advantages of managed care systems for end-of-life care include coordinated care across delivery sites, the use of interdisciplinary teams and integrated services, and the opportunities to develop innovative programs, service arrays, utilization controls, and quality assurance systems (Lynn, Wilkinson, Cohn, & Jones, 1998). Nonetheless, managed care plans generally have not taken advantage of the flexibility of capitation to develop high-quality end-of-life care, although there are exceptions (Fox, 1999; National Task Force on End-of-Life Care in Managed Care, 1999). In its June 2004 report to Congress, MedPAC observed that the current funding mechanism for hospice care under Medicare managed care "works against the goal of fully integrated healthcare delivery... (and) discourages plans from continuing efforts to coordinate their care" (MedPAC, 2004, pp. 149–150).

Managed care enrollment is associated with higher hospice utilization among seriously ill Medicare beneficiaries than in the fee-for-service system (Emanuel et al., 2002; McCarthy, Burns, Davis & Phillips, 2003; MedPAC, 2004; Riley & Herboldsheimer, 2001; Virnig, Fisher, McBean, & Kind, 2001). Analysts have suggested several reasons for this difference: (1) people who join managed care organizations may be more inclined to use hospice care; (2) there is some evidence that managed care organizations have a higher percentage of cancer deaths, diagnoses that account for a high proportion of hospice users; and (3) managed care organizations may be better able to identify Medicare beneficiaries with terminal illness who may benefit from a palliative approach to care (Riley & Herboldsheimer, 2001).

Private insurers such as Aetna, Kaiser Permanente, United Healthcare, and others, have developed and implemented new palliative care models. They use an interdisciplinary team of providers to manage symptoms and pain, provide emotional and spiritual support, and educate patients and family members on an ongoing basis about changes in the patient's condition. New benefit options being tested by these payers include a palliative care benefit that is separate from hospice and does not involve sacrificing ongoing disease treatment, an extended eligibility period for hospice benefits to encourage patients to enter hospice earlier, and a concurrent care model that allows patients who are continuing to pursue curative care to access hospice benefits at the same time. The results of a Kaiser Permanente study showed that the program increased patient satisfaction and the proportion of patients dying at home rather than in the hospital, and it reduced emergency department visits, inpatient admissions, and costs (Spettell, Rawlins, Krakauer et al., 2009). For a complete discussion of these emerging programs, see Chapter 8

Medicaid

Medicaid is available only to certain low-income individuals and families who fit into an eligibility group that is recognized by federal and state law. Hospice is an optional benefit for state Medicaid programs. Individuals who live in states that choose to provide a Medicaid Hospice Benefit may be able to obtain payment for hospice services even if coverage is not available under Medicare. (For example, if the individual does not have Medicare Part A.) Limitations on copayments and deductibles would be reflected in the state's Medicaid plan in accordance with Medicaid law.

Services for hospice care under Medicaid must be provided by a public agency or private organization that is primarily engaged in providing care to terminally ill individuals, that meets the Medicare conditions of participation for hospices, and that has a valid provider agreement. The Centers for Medicare and Medicaid Services (CMS) has taken the position that states may provide a more limited benefit under Medicaid than is available under Medicare. At a minimum, however, Medicaid hospice coverage must be available for at least 210 days. The services to be covered under Medicaid are essentially those described earlier for Medicare-covered hospice.

Hospice care is available for individuals who live in Medicaid-reimbursed nursing facilities. Under these circumstances, Medicare Part A will pay the hospice program to provide palliative care. The state Medicaid agency will pay the hospice program a daily rate for the hospice patient's room and board, which is then reimbursed to the nursing facility. Room and board services include the performance of personal care services, assistance in the activities of daily living, socializing activities, administration of medications, maintaining the cleanliness of the resident's room, and supervising and assisting in the use of durable medical equipment and prescribed therapies.

State Medicaid nursing facility reimbursement policies have varying effects on hospice use, which can greatly influence access to care. According to regulations, when dual-eligible nursing facility residents elect their Medicare Hospice Benefit, 95% of the Medicaid nursing facility per diem is paid to the hospice which, in turn, pays the nursing home. This "pass-through" payment process in some cases is considered a barrier (Gage et al., 2000, Miller & Mor, 2006). This complexity of bureaucratic arrangements required social workers to have clear understanding to ensure that people with advanced illness can access the care and benefits they need.

For Medicare beneficiaries who are eligible for both Medicare and Medicaid, Medicare-covered hospice beneficiaries can simultaneously receive Medicaid-covered personal care attendant services. In this case, Medicaid coverage of personal care services is the equivalent of a non-dual-eligible Medicare beneficiary paying out of pocket for custodial care. The hospice must coordinate its hospice aide and homemaker services with the Medicaid personal care benefit to ensure that the patient receives all the hospice aide and homemaker services he or she needs while avoiding duplication of services. The Medicare acute care statute and policy limitations prohibit coverage of personal care attendant services.

Home health services—both skilled and unskilled—are also covered through other funding sources such as Medicaid, Older Americans Act, and locally funded programs, but availability varies greatly by state, reinforcing the challenges in creating policy that provides for equal access of care for all who need it (Wiener & Tilly, 2003).

Public Policy and Pain Management

Social workers need to learn about government drug control policy and engage in advocacy to facilitate patient access to pain management (Joranson et al., 2002). There are many effective treatments for pain, but opioid analgesics are often essential for the relief of pain in the 50 million Americans who suffer from chronic pain associated with cancer and other serious diseases. Unrelieved pain is oftentimes crippling; it triggers a range of problems that include depression, social isolation, disturbed sleep, decreased mobility, falls, difficulty in thinking clearly, and loss of appetite (Joranson et al., 2002; Portenoy, 1996).

The high level of pain among dying persons is one of the major problems in end-of-life care (Miller et al., 2003; Teno et al., 2004). Historically, the primary Medicare barrier to pain control for people near the end of life involved lack of coverage for prescription drugs (Wiener & Tilly, 2003). In 2003, Congress created a new broad, outpatient prescription drug benefit under Part D of Medicare, through the enactment of the Medicare Prescription Drug, Improvement, and Modernization Act (P.L. 108–173). Coverage of prescription drugs began on January 1, 2006.

Medicare Part D provides coverage that many beneficiaries did not previously have, but drug plans have great latitude in establishing formularies. While plans are required to cover at least two drugs in each therapeutic class, some analgesic medications may be excluded. In addition, certain medications, including opioid analgesics and high-cost drugs, may require prior authorization, creating a barrier to using certain medications and leading to delays and increasing physicians' administrative burden.

Other barriers to adequate pain control—unrelated specifically to Medicare—arise because the drugs commonly used are narcotics, such as morphine, which are controlled substances. Some patients, family members, and providers fear addiction, misunderstand the effect of opioids on normal functioning, and believe their use hastens death (Dahl, 2003; Dinger, 2005; NCP, 2009). Physicians may also be reluctant to prescribe opioids because of complicated state and federal rules and law enforcement oversight (Quill & Meier, 2006). The primary focus of these regulations and statutes is to reduce the abuse of drugs rather than to discourage appropriate medical use of opioids (Wilson, 1999).

All states have statutes or regulations that address pain management. About half the states have some form of law that tries to ensure adequate efforts, including the use of controlled substances to manage pain if done in accordance with accepted medical standards. These laws are sometimes criticized as reinforcing the misperception that treating persons with pain with opioids is outside the normal professional practice of medicine. Some of these laws also exclude chemically dependent people from access to treatment rather than reinforcing the need to develop the skill set necessary to treat pain in patients with complex problems and medical needs. Other state laws and regulations provide that a charge of unprofessional conduct can be based simply on the number of doses or the duration of an opioid prescription. Existing clinical standards for pain management, however, recognize that the number of doses or duration cannot be used as litmus tests for appropriate care (Fins et al., 2003; Last Acts Coalition, 2002). While some state policies are useful and effective at decreasing the chance that these drugs will be misused or diverted, some create formidable barriers to good pain management (Joranson et al., 2002).

Reasons for ineffective pain management include lack of knowledge of patients and health care professionals, negative attitudes toward the use of medication, fear of drug addiction, drug regulations, concerns about cost, and reimbursement barriers. Additionally, cultural, ethnic, and religious factors inform the experience of pain and are a focus of assessment and intervention by palliative care clinicians. In the United States, certain groups face higher risks of unrelieved pain. Minorities, females, children, elders, those who speak a language other than English, and the traditionally underserved face a significant risk for undertreatment of pain. Factors that may be responsible for this disparity include lack of access to pain specialists, lower rates of insurance coverage, limited access to prescribed pain medications, cultural differences between patients and professionals, language barriers, and the short amount of time spent with professionals (Payne, 2001).

Medical experts agree that at least 90%–95% of all serious pain can be safely and effectively treated, yet at least half of dying patients report being in pain. Unrelieved pain is costly to society in both direct and indirect ways, and it can ruin the quality of life of patients and their families (American Pain Society, 2009). Social workers who understand the relationship between policy, regulation, and care at the bedside as related to the undermanagement of pain can become expert advocates, both at the micro and macro level, because it is a shared responsibility to intervene in aspects of care that create unnecessary suffering.

The Patient Self-Determination Act

The Patient Self-Determination Act (PSDA) was an amendment to the Omnibus Budget Reconciliation Act of 1990 (P.L. 101–508). The law became effective December 1991 requiring most U.S. hospitals, nursing homes, hospice programs, home health agencies, and health maintenance organizations to provide to adult individuals, at the time of inpatient admission or enrollment, information about their rights under state laws governing advance directives, including the following: (1) the right to participate in and direct their own health care decisions; (2) the right to accept or refuse medical or surgical treatment; (3) the right to prepare an advance directive; and (4) information on the provider's policies that govern the utilization of these rights. The Act prohibits institutions from discriminating against a patient who does not have an advance directive. The PSDA further requires institutions to document patient information and provide ongoing community education on advance directives.

Patient autonomy and individual choice are core values in Western bioethics and important components of end-of-life decision making. They are not always the values that our patients and families ascribe to, however, because culture and spiritual values and beliefs are just two of the variables that influence how one approaches this aspect of life. Ensuring the centrality of the patient's and the family's voice in medical decision making and honoring patient preferences for end-of-life care are at the heart of social work and often requires that we advocate for a culturally sensitive approach in the setting of a system that is essentially based on Western values.

More than a decade after the Patient Self-Determination Act was enacted, only about 20%–30% of Americans have an advance directive (Hickman, Hammes, Moss, & Tolle, 2005). However, there is a clear age difference in the proportion of people who have advance directives. A study of nursing home residents found that approximately 60% had some type of advance directive (McAuley & Travis, 2003); a recent study by the Pew Research Center found that 54% of individuals age 65 or older said they had a living will (Pew Research Center for the People and the Press, 2006); and an AARP (formerly the American Association of Retired Persons) survey of its members (55 and older) found that 60% had named a health care proxy or durable power of attorney (Dinger, 2005).

Recently, a Department of Health and Human Services (DHHS) Report to Congress (responding to PL 109-103, 2006 Appropriations), *Advance Directives and Advance Care Planning*, summarizes findings from a multidimensional effort; the report reflects the perspectives of experts in palliative end-of-life care and advance care planning, individuals with disabilities, and other nationwide stakeholders. Three key findings of the study are as follows:

- Effective advance care planning and discernment of end-of-life care preferences is an ongoing process best accomplished through continuing communication among individuals, clinicians, and family members.
- Interventions that involve a range of professionals and other stakeholders in advance care planning have been successful in increasing the number of advance directives and concordance with patients' wishes. Health information technology holds promise for replication of these efforts.
- The focus of advance care planning must shift from a focus on formal written advance directive forms to a developmental discussion process. Specific attention could be given to models that translate into immediate medical orders to guide specific treatment decisions such as the POLST (Physician Orders for Life-Sustaining Treatment) program paradigm (Shugarman & Wenger et al, 2008).

For further discussion of these issues, see Chapter 69.

Veterans Administration and Palliative Care

Many Americans are unaware that more than 50,000 veterans die each month, roughly 28% of all deaths in the United States. The Department of Veterans Affairs provides hospice and palliative care to a growing number of veterans at each of its medical centers and inpatient hospice care in many of its nursing homes throughout the country. Nearly 9000 veterans were treated in designated hospice beds at Veterans Administration (VA) facilities in 2007, and thousands of other veterans were referred to community hospices to receive care in their homes. VA partners with community hospice programs in 35 states to promote hospice services that are not provided directly by VA staff.

Hospice care is part of the basic eligibility package for veterans enrolled in the Veterans Health Administration (VHA). In 2002, the VA embarked on a major initiative to improve veterans' care at the end of life through a coordinated plan to increase access to hospice and palliative care services. Within 3 years, the number of veterans receiving VA-paid home hospice tripled, all VA hospitals have a palliative care team, and a nationwide network of VA

partnerships with community hospice agencies was established (Edes, Shreve, & Casarett, 2007).

Most recently a new effort between the National Hospice and Palliative Care Organization (NHPCO) and the Department of Veterans Affairs Hospice and Palliative Care Program has been launched to reach the nearly 40% of enrolled veterans who live in areas that are considered rural, where community hospices and VA palliative care programs are often not readily available. On any given night, more than 200,000 veterans are without shelter and lack basic health care. These policy initiatives may be a beginning effort to reach those veterans who are disenfranchised and suffering with life-threatening illness.

Recently, grants have been awarded to 18 providers that represent a range of community-based organizations. These providers are working collaboratively with their own community partnerships on innovative programs that aim to provide care and services to veterans at the end of life. The grants will contribute funding to each grantee provider for 9 months to not only support the success of individual programs but to ultimately assist the VA in discovering new ways to reach homeless veterans and veterans living in rural areas (NHPCO, 2009). (See Chapter 12 for additional discussion of palliative care for veterans.)

Conclusion

As the baby boom generation ages and struggles to address the needs of persons living with life-threatening illness and coming to the end of life, attention will continue to focus on care options, costs, and the personal and policy decisions that will drive access to care and the quality of the services that are provided. The principles of palliative care—such as the alleviation of pain and other physical symptoms and respect for the patient and family, their values and preferences—are appropriate for all patients, not only those with chronic or fatal illnesses, and are at the core of social work values. However, people who are either actively dying or living with an advanced illness are in particular need of improvements in their treatment both on a daily basis and individual level over the long term. This vulnerable population is most in need of the care coordination and interdisciplinary focus that is the essence of palliative care. Palliative and end-of-life care policy issues are and will continue to be a public-interest focal point, and it is critical that social workers keep the needs of seriously ill people on the policy forefront.

LEARNING EXERCISES

- Reflect upon a recent patient experience with a colleague and discuss the impact of various public policies upon this patient's care.
- Identify an advocacy opportunity in your local area of influence and take steps to improve the issue.

ADDITIONAL RESOURCES

Center to Advance Palliative Care: http://www.capc.org/
about-capc

The Center to Advance Palliative Care (CAPC) provides health
care professionals with the tools, training, and technical
assistance necessary to start and sustain successful palliative
care programs in hospitals and other health care settings.
CAPC is a national organization dedicated to increasing the
availability of quality palliative care services for people facing
serious illness.

Center for Medicare and Medicaid Resources (CMS):
http://www.cms.hhs.gov/
http://www.cms.hhs.gov/center/snf.asp
http://www.cms.hhs.gov/center/hospice.asp

Compilation of Social Security Laws: http://www.ssa.gov/OP_
Home/ssact/title18/1862.htm

Growth House: http://www.growthhouse.org/

Growth House, Inc., provides resources for life-threatening illness
and end-of-life care. The primary mission is to improve the
quality of compassionate care for people who are dying through
public education and global professional collaboration.
Provides free access to over 4000 pages of reviewed educational
materials from over 40 major health care organizations.

The Library of Congress: THOMAS: http://www.thomas.gov/

THOMAS was launched in January of 1995, at the inception of the
104th Congress. The leadership of the 104th Congress directed
the Library of Congress to make federal legislative information
freely available to the public. Since that time THOMAS has
expanded the scope of its offerings to include bills, resolutions,
activities in Congress, Congressional Record, Schedules,
Committee Information, Government Resources, and learning
sections for teachers.

Medicare Learning Network: http://www.cms.hhs.gov/
MLNGenInfo/

The Medicare Learning Network (MLN) Web site was established
by CMS in response to the increased usage of the Internet as a
learning resource by Medicare health care professionals. This
Web site is designed to provide you with the appropriate
information and tools to aid health care professionals in
learning about Medicare. For courses and information, visit the
Web site. For a list of the training programs, Medicare Learning
Network Matters articles, and other education tools available,
visit the Web site.

Pain and Policy Studies Group: http://www.painpolicy.wisc.edu/

The Pain and Policy Studies Group provides technical assistance
and monitors progress to improve the availability of opioid
analgesics for pain management and palliative care. This group
coordinates programs of national and international policy
studies to identify and address barriers to opioid availability in
national policy and national health care systems.

Physician Orders for Life-Sustaining Treatment Paradigm
(POLST): http://www.ohsu.edu/ethics/polst/

POLST paradigm forms are available in many states. The form is
designed to help health care professionals honor the end-of-life
treatment desires of their patients. The form has physician
orders that follow patient wishes and treatment intentions, and
it enhances the appropriateness and quality of patient care.

Social Work Hospice and Palliative Care Network: http://www.
swhpn.org/

SWHPN was created to bridge the gaps in social work's access to
information, knowledge, education, training, and research in
hospice and palliative care.

REFERENCES

American Pain Society. (2009). *Treatment of pain at the end of life.*
Retrieved from http://www.ampainsoc.org/advocacy/
treatment.htm

Altilio, T., Otis-Green, S., & Dahlin, C. M. (2008). Applying the
National Quality Forum Preferred Practices for Palliative and
Hospice Care: A social work perspective. *Journal of Social Work
in end-of-life and Palliative Care, 4*(1), 3–16.

Barnato, A. E., McClellan, M. B., Kagay, C. R., & Garber, A. M.
(2004). Trends in inpatient treatment intensity among
Medicare beneficiaries at the end-of-life. *Health Services
Research, 39*(2), 363–375.

Bern-Klug, M., Kramer, K., Chan, G., Kane, R., Dorfman, L., &
Saunders, J. B. (2009). Characteristics of nursing home social
services directors: How common is a degree in social work?
Journal of American Medical Directors Association, 10, 36–44.

Brown University Center for Gerontology and Health Care
Research. (n.d.c). *Facts on dying.* Retrieved from http://www.
chcr.brown.edu/dying/2001DATA.HTM

Bryce, C. L., Loewenstein, G., Arnold, R. M., Schooler, J., Wax, R.
S., & Angus, D. C. (2004). Quality of death: Assessing the
importance placed on end-of-life treatment in the intensive-
care unit. *Medical Care, 42*(5), 423–431.

Buntin, M., & Huskamp, H. (2002). What is known about the
economics of end-of-life care for Medicare beneficiaries?
Gerontologist, 42(Special Issue III), 40–48.

Centers for Medicare & Medicaid Services. (2005). *Hospice
Medicaid manual: Publication 21.* Retrieved from http://www.
cms.hhs.gov/Manuals/PBM/itemdetail.asp?filterType=dual,%2
0keyword&filterValue=Hospice&filterByDID=0&sortByDID=1
&sortOrder=ascending&itemID=CMS021923&intNumPerPag
e=10

Centers for Medicare and Medicaid Services. (2008). Medicare and
Medicaid programs: Hospice conditions of participation.
Federal Register, 73(109), 32089–32220. Retrieved from http://
edocket.access.gpo.gov/2008/pdf/08-1305.pdf

Centers for Medicare and Medicaid Services. (2009). *Update to the
hospice payment rates, hospice cap, hospice wage index and the
hospice price for FY 2010.* CMS Manual System, Pub 100-004,
Medicare Claims Processing, Transmittal 1796. Baltimore, MD:
Centers for Medicare and Medicaid Services.

Cherlin, E., Morris, V., Morris, J., Johnson-Hurzeler, R., Sullivan,
G. M., & Bradley, E. H. (2007). Common myths about caring
for patients with terminal illness: Opportunities to improve
care in the hospital setting. *Journal of Hospital Medicine, 2*(6),
357–365.

Clark, E. (2009, October). "Death panel" rhetoric sets us back.
NASW News, 54(9). Retrieved from http://www.socialworkers.
org/pubs/news/2009/10/clark.asp

Clarke, E. B., Curtis, J. R., Luce, J. M., Levy, M., Dans, M., Nelson,
J., & Soloman, M. Z. (2003). Quality indicators for end-of-life
care in the intensive care unit. For The Robert Wood Johnson
Foundation Critical Care End-of-Life Peer Workgroup
Members. *Critical Care Medicine, 31*(9), 2399–2340.

Connor, S., & Adams, J. (2003). Caregiving at the end-of-life. *Hastings Center Report, 33*(2 Suppl.), S8–S9.

Csikai, G., & Raymer, M. (2003). The social work end of life care education project: An assessment of educational needs. (NASW EOL-p.12).

Curtis, J. R. (2005). Interventions to improve care during withdrawal of life-sustaining treatments. *Journal of Palliative Medicine, 8*(1), S116–131.

Dahl, J. L. (2003). The myths and realities of pain control with opioids. *Wisconsin Medical Journal, 102*(5), 19–20.

Dinger, E. (2005). *AARP Massachusetts end-of-life survey.* Washington, DC: AARP.

Edes, T., Shreve, S., & Casarett, D. (2007). Increasing access and quality in department of veterans affairs care at the end of life: A lesson in change. *Journal of American Geriatric Society, 55*(1), 1645–1649.

Education in Palliative and End-of-Life Care (EPEC) Project (2006). Home page. Retrieved from http://www.epec.net/EPEC/Webpages/index.cfm

Emanuel, E. J., Ash, A., Yu, W., Gazella, G., Levinsky, N. G., Sayina, O., McClennan, M., & Moskowitz, M. (2002). Managed care, hospice use, site of death, and medical expenditures in the last year of life. *Archives of Internal Medicine, 162*, 1722–1728.

Eng, C. (2002). Future considerations for improving end-of-life care for older persons: Program of All-inclusive Care for the Elderly (PACE). *Journal of Palliative Medicine, 5*(2), 305–309.

Field, M. J., & Cassel, C. K. (Eds.). (1997). *Approaching death: Improving care at the end of life.* Washington, DC: National Academy Press.

Fins, J. J., Peres, J. R., & Schumacher, J. D. (2003). *On the road from theory to practice: A resource guide to promising practices in palliative care near the end-of-life.* Washington, DC: Last Acts National Program.

Foley, K. (2005). Improving end-of-life care: Why has it been so difficult? *Hastings Center Report Special Report, 35*(6), S42–S46.

Fox, P. (1999). *End-of-life care in managed care organizations.* Washington, DC: AARP.

Gage, B. J., Bartosch, W. J., & Osber, D. S. (2005). *Medicare post-acute care: Evaluations of BBA payment policies and related changes. Report* prepared for Centers for Medicare & Medicaid Services). Waltham, MA: RTI International.

Gage, B., & Dao, T. (2000). *Medicare's hospice benefit: Use and expenditure.* Report to the Office of the Assistant Secretary for Planning and Evaluation, U.S. Department of Health and Human Services. Washington, DC: U.S. Department of Health and Human Services.

Gage, B., Miller, S. C., Coppola, K., Harvell, J., Laliberte, L., Mor, V., & Teno, J. (2000). *Important questions for hospice in the next century.* Report to the Office of the Assistant Secretary for Planning and Evaluation, U.S. Department of Health and Human Services. Washington, DC: U.S. Department of Health and Human Services.

Gillick, M., & Mitchell, S. (2004). A framework for meaningful Medicare reform. *Journal of Aging Social Policy, 16*(3), 1–12.

Goldsmith, B., Deitrich, J., Du, Q., & Morrison, R. S. (2008). Variability in access to hospital palliative care in the United States. *Journal of Palliative Medicine, 11*(8), 1094–1103.

Gottlich, V. (2003). Medical necessity determinations in the Medicare program: Are the interests of beneficiaries with chronic conditions being met? Washington, DC: Center for Medicare Advocacy Inc.

Hawkins, N. A., Ditto, P. H., Danks, J. H., & Smucker W. D. (2005). Micromanaging death: Process preferences, values, and goals in end-of-life medical decision making. *Gerontologist, 45*(1), 107–117.

Hickman, S. E., Hammes, B. J., Moss, A. H., & Tolle, S. W. (2005). Hope for the future: Achieving the original intent of advance directives. Improving end-of-life care: Why has it been so difficult? *Hastings Center Special Report, 35*(6), S26–S30.

Hogan, C., Lunney, J., Gabel, J., & Lynn, J. (2001). Medicare beneficiaries' costs of care in the last year of life. *Health Affairs, 20*(4), 188–195.

Huskamp, H. A., Buntin, M. B., Wang, V., & Newhouse, J. P. (2001). Providing care at the end of life. Do Medicare rules impede good care? *Health Affairs, 20*(3), 204–211.

Huskamp, H. A., Stevenson, D. G., Chernew, M. E., & Newhouse, J. P. (2010). A new Medicare end-of-life benefit for nursing home residents. *Health Affairs, 29*(1), 130–135.

Institute of Medicine. (2008). *Retooling for an aging America: Building the health care workforce.* Washington, DC: Academic Press.

Jennings, B., Ryndes, T., & D'Onofrio, C. (2003). Access to hospice care: Expanding boundaries: Overcoming barriers. *Special Supplement to the Hastings Center Report, 35*(6), S3–S7, S9–S13, S15–S21.

Johnson, S. H. (2005). Making room for dying: End-of-life care in nursing homes. Improving end-of-life care: Why has it been so difficult? *Hastings Center Report Special Report, 35*(6), S37–S41.

Joranson, D. E., & Ryan, K. M. (2007). Ensuring opioid availability: Methods and resources. *Journal of Pain and Symptom Management, 33*(5), 527–532.

Joranson, D. E., Gilson, A. M., Dahl, J. L., & Haddox, J. D. (2002). Pain management controlled substances, and state medical board policy: A decade of change. *Journal of Pain and Symptom Management, 23*(2), 138–147.

Jost, T. (2000). Medicare and Medicaid financing of pain management. *The Journal of Pain, 1*(3), 183–194.

Kayser-Jones, J., (2002). The experience of dying: An ethnographic nursing home study [Special issue]. *The Gerontologist, 42,* 11–19.

Komisar, H. L. (2002). Rolling back Medicare home health. *Health Care Financing Review, 24*(2), 33–55.

Last Acts Coalition. (2002). *Means to a better end: A report on dying in America today.* Washington, DC: Partnership for Caring.

Lorenz, K., Lynn, J., Morton, S. C., Morton, S. C., Maglione, M., Dy, S.,…Rolon, C. (2004). *End-of-life care and outcomes. Summary, evidence report/technology assessment: Number 110* (AHRQ Pub. No. 05-E004-1). Rockville, MD: Agency for Healthcare Research and Quality.

Lubitz, J. D., & Riley, G. F. (1993). Trends in Medicare payments in the last year of life. *New England Journal of Medicine, 328*(15), 1092–1096.

Lynn, J. (2004). *Sick to death and not going to take it anymore! Reforming health care for the last years of life.* Berkeley, CA: University of California Press; and New York, NY: Milbank Memorial Fund.

Lynn, J., & Adamson, D. M. (2003). *Living well at the end-of-life: Adapting health care to serious, chronic illness in old age. Rand health white paper WP-137.* Washington, DC: The Washington Home Center for Palliative Care Studies.

Lynn, J., Wilkinson, A., Cohn, F., & Jones, S. B. (1998). Capitated risk-bearing managed care systems could improve end-of-life care. *Journal of the American Geriatrics Society, 46*(3), 322–330.

McAuley, W. J., & Travis, S. S. (2003). Advance care planning among residents in long-term care. *American Journal of Hospice and Palliative Care, 20*(5), 353–359.

McCall, N., Korb, J., Petersons, A., & Moore, S. (2002). Constraining Medicare home health reimbursement: What are the outcomes? *Health Care Financing Review, 24*(2), 57–76.

McCall, N., Petersons, A., Moore, S., & Korb, J. (2003). Utilization of home health services before and after the balanced budget act of 1997: What were the initial effects? *Health Services Research, 38*(1), 85–106.

McCarthy, E. P., Burns, R. B., Davis, R. B., & Phillips, R. S. (2003). Barriers to hospice care among older patients dying with lung and colorectal cancer. *Journal of Clinical Oncology, 21*, 728–735.

McCarthy, E. P., Burns, R. B., Ngo-Metzger, Q., Davis, R. B., & Phillips, R. S. (2003). Hospice use among Medicare managed care and fee-for-service patients dying with cancer. *Journal of the American Medical Association, 289*(17), 2238–2245.

Medicare regulations found at 42 CFR §410.73 and the Medicare Carriers Manual Part 3, Chapter II, §2152 for the covered services of a clinical social worker.

Medicare Exclusions from Coverage. See "for items and services… not reasonable and necessary for the diagnosis or treatment of illness or injury or to improve the functioning of a malformed body member." S.S.A. 1862(a)(1)(A), 42 U.S.C. 1395y(a)(1)(A). http://www.ssa.gov/OP_Home/ssact/title18/1862.htm

Medicare Improvements for Patients and Providers Act (MIPPA) of 2008, Pub. L. No. 110-275 (2008). Retrieved from http://www.cms.hhs.gov/WelcometoMedicareExam/

MedPAC. (2003, November). *Report to the Congress: Impact of the resident caps on the supply of geriatricians.* Washington, DC.

MedPAC. (2004, June). *Report to Congress: New approaches in Medicare.* Washington, DC.

MedPAC (2006, March). *Report to Congress: Medicare Payment Policy.* Washington, DC.

MedPAC (2009, March). *Report to Congress: Reforming Medicare's hospice benefit.* Washington, DC.

Meier, D., & Beresford D.L. (2006). Billing for palliative care: An essential cost of doing business. *Journal of Palliative Medicine, 9*(2), 250–257.

Miller, E., & Mor, V. (2006). *Out of the shadows: Envisioning a brighter future of long-term care in America.* Brown University Center for Gerontology and Health Care Research.

Miller, S., Gozalo, P., & Mor, V. (2000). *Use of Medicare's hospice benefit by nursing facility residents.* Washington, DC: U.S. Department of Health and Human Services.

Miller, S., Gozalo, P., & Mor, V. (2001). Hospice enrollment and hospitalization of dying nursing home patients. *The American Journal of Medicine, 111*, 38–44.

Miller, S., Intrator, O., Gozalo, P., Ray, J., Barber, J., & Mor, V. (2004). Government expenditures at the end-of-life for short- and long-stay nursing home residents: Differences by hospice enrollment status. *Journal of the American Geriatrics Society, 52*, 1284–1292.

Miller, S., Mor, V., & Teno, J. (2003). Hospice enrollment and pain assessment and management in nursing homes. *Journal of Pain and Symptom Management, 26*(3), 791–799.

Miller, S., Mor., V., Wu, N., Gozalo, P., & Lapane, K. (2002). Does receipt of hospice care in nursing homes improve the management of pain at the end of life? *Journal of the American Geriatrics Society, 50*, 507–515.

Mitchell, S., Teno, J., Roy, J., & Lapane, K. (2003). Clinical and organizational factors associated with feeding tube use among nursing home residents with advanced cognitive impairment. *Journal of the American Medical Association, 290*, 73–80.

Morrison, R. S., Maroney-Galin, C., Kralovec, P. D., & Meier, D. E. (2005). The growth of palliative care programs in United States hospitals. *Journal of Palliative Care, 8*(6), 1127–1134.

Morrison, R. S., & Meier, D. E. (2004). Clinical practice-palliative care. *New England Journal of Medicine, 350*, 2582–2590.

National Association of Social Workers (NASW). (2003). *Standards for social work practice in palliative and end of life care.* Retrieved from http://www.socialworkers.org/practice/bereavement/standards/default.asp

National Association of Social Workers (NASW). (2009). *End-of-life care.* Retrieved from https://www.socialworkers.org/research/naswResearch/EndofLifeCare/default.asp

National Consensus Project for Quality Palliative Care (NCP). (2009). *Clinical practice guidelines for quality palliative care, second edition.* Retrieved from http://www.nationalconsensusproject.org

National Hospice and Palliative Care Organization (NHPCO). (2009). *Reaching out: Quality hospice and palliative care for rural and homeless veterans.* Grants to Increase Access to Hospice and Palliative Care for Rural and Homeless Veterans Awarded by National Hospice and Palliative Care Organization, February 25, 2009.

National Institutes of Health. (2004). *State of the science conference statement: Improving end-of-life care.* Bethesda, MD: Author.

National Task Force on End-of-Life Care in Managed Care. (1999). *Meeting the challenge: Twelve recommendations for improving end-of-life care in managed care.* Newton, MA: Center for Applied Ethics and Professional Practice, Education Development Center.

Norton, S. A., Hogan, L. A., Holloway, R. G., Temkin-Greener, H., Buckley, M. J., & Quill, T. E. (2007). Proactive palliative care in the medical intensive care unit: Effects on length of stay for selected high-risk patients. *Critical Care Medicine, 35*(6), 1530–1535.

Oliver, T. R. (2006). The politics of public health policy. *Annual Review of Public Health, 27*, 195–233.

Open Society Institute. (n.d.). *Project on Death in America: January 2001–December 2003 report of activities.* Retrieved from http://www.soros.org/resources/articles_publications/publications/report_20041122

Payne, R. (2001). Palliative care for African Americans and other vulnerable populations: Access and quality issues. In K. M. Foley & H. Gelband (Eds.), *Improving palliative care for cancer* (pp. 153–160). Washington, DC: National Academy Press.

Patient Self-Determination Act of 1990, 42 U.S.C. §1395 cc (a) (1990).

Pritchard, R. S., Fisher, E. S., Teno, J. M., Sharp, S. M., Reding, D. J., Knaus, W. A., Wennberg, J. E., & Lynn, J. (1998). Influence of patient preferences and local health system characteristics on the place of death. SUPPORT Investigators. Study to Understand Prognoses and Preferences for Risks and Outcomes of Treatment. *Journal of American Geriatric Society, 46*(10), 1242–1250.

Portenoy, R. K., (1996). Opioid therapy for chronic nonmalignant pain: A review of critical issues. *Journal of Pain and Symptom Management, 11*(4), 203–217.

Pew Research Center for the People and the Press. (2006). *Strong public support for right to die: More Americans discussing–and planning–end-of-life treatment.* Washington, DC: Author. Retrieved from http://people-press.org/reports/display.php3?ReportID=266

Quill, T., & Meier, D. (2006). The big chill—Inserting the DEA into end-of-life care. *New England Journal of Medicine, 354*(1), 1–3.

Rady, M., & Johnson, D. (2004). Admission to intensive care unit at the end-of-life: Is it an informed decision? *Journal of Palliative Medicine, 18*(8), 705–711.

Rao, J. K., Alongi, J., Anderson, L. A., Jenkins, L., Stokes, G. A., & Kane, M. (2005). Development of public helath priorities for end-of-life initiatives. *American Journal of Preventative Medicine, 29*(5), 453–460.

Riley, G., & Herboldsheimer, C. (2001). Including hospice in Medicare capitation payments: Would it save money. *Health Care Financing Review, 23*(1), 137–147.

Roff, S. (2001). Analyzing end-of-life care legislations: A social work perspective. *Social Work in Healthcare, 33*, 51–68.

Sabatino, C. (2007). *Advance directives and advance care planning: Legal and policy issues.* Washington, DC: ABA Commissioin on Law and Aging.

Schamp, R., & Tenkku, L. (2006). Managed death in a PACE: Pathways in present and advance directives. *Journal of the American Medical Directors Association, 7*(6), 339–344.

Shah M., Quill T., Norton S., Sada Y., Buckley M., & Fridd C. (2008). "What bothers you the most?" Initial responses from patients receiving palliative care consultation. *American Journal of Hospice and Palliative Care, 25*(2), 88–92.

Shugarman, L., Campbell, D., Bird, C., & Lynn, J. (2004). Differences in Medicare expenditures during the last three years of life. *Journal of General Internal Medicine, 19*, 127–135.

Shugarman, L. R., Lorenz, K., & Lynn, J. (2005). End-of-life care: An agenda for policy improvement. *Clinics in Geriatric Medicine, 21*(1), 255–272.

Shugarman, L., Wenger, N., Wilkinson, A., & Peres, J. R. (2008). *Report to Congress on advance directives and advance care planning.* Office of the Assistant Secretary for Planning and Evaluation, U.S. Department of Health and Human Services. Washington, DC: U.S. Department of Health and Human Services.

Spettell, C. M., Rawlins, W. S., Krakauer, R., Fernandes, J., Breton, M. E., Gowdy, W., Brodeur, S., MacCoy, M., & Brennan, T. A. (2009). A comprehensive case management program to improve palliative care. *Journal of Palliative Medicine, 12*(9), 827–832.

SUPPORT Principal Investigators. (1995). A controlled trial to improve care for seriously ill hospitalized patients: The Study to Understand Prognoses and Preferences for Outcomes and Risks of Treatment (SUPPORT). *The Journal of the American Medical Association, 274*, 1591–1598.

Taylor, D. H., Jr, Ostermann, J., Van Houtven, C. H., Tulsky, J. A., & Steinhauser, K. (2007). What length of hospice use maximizes reduction in medical expenditures near death in the US Medicare program? *Social Science & Medicine, 65*, 1466–1478.

Tax Equity and Fiscal Responsibility Act of 1982, Pub. L. No. 97-248 (1982).

Teno, J., Clarridge, B., Casey, V., Welch, LC., Wetle, T., Shield, R., & Mor, V. (2004). Family perspectives on end-of-life care at the last place of care. *Journal of the American Medical Association, 291*, 88–93.

Teno, J. M., Gruneir, A., Schwartz, Z., Nanda, A., & Wetle, T. (2007). Association between advance directives and quality of end-of-life care: A national study. *Journal of the American Geriatrics Society, 55*, 189–194.

Teno, J., Kabumoto, K., & Wetle, T. (2004). Daily pain that was excruciating at some time in the previous week: Prevalence, characteristics, and outcomes in nursing home residents. *Journal of the American Geriatrics Society, 52*, 762–768.

Teno, J., Lynn, J., Wenger, N., Phillips, R. S., Murphy, D. P., Connors, A. F., Jr.,...Knaus, W. A. (1997). Advance directives for seriously-ill hospitalized patients: Effectiveness with the Patient Self-Determination Act and the SUPPORT intervention. *Journal of the American Geriatric Society, 45*, 500–507.

Teno, J. M., Weitzen, S., & Wetle, T. (2001). If you build more nursing home beds, more persons will die in them. *Journal of the American Geriatrics Society, 49*, S11.

Thompson, G. N., & Chochinov, H. M., (2006). Methodological challenges in measuring quality care in the long-term care environment. *Journal of Pain and Symptom Management, 32*, 378–391.

Tilly, J., &Wiener, J. (2001). *Medicaid and end-of-life care.* Washington, DC: Last Acts Financing Committee.

Travis, S. S., Loving, G., McClanahan, L., & Bernard, M. (2001). Hospitalization patterns and palliation in the last year of life among residents in long-term care. *Gerontologist, 41*(2), 153–160.

U.S. Department of Health and Human Services. Office of the Inspector General. (1997). *Hospice patients in nursing homes.* DHHS Publication No. OEI-05-95-00250. Washington, DC: U.S. Department of Health and Human Services.

U.S. Department of Health and Human Services, Office of the Inspector General. (2006). *Effect of the home health prospective payment system on the quality of home health care.* OEI-01-04-00160. Washington, DC: U.S. Department of Health and Human Services.

U.S. Department of Health and Human Services, Office of the Inspector General. (2009a). *Memorandum report: Medicare hospice care: Services provided to beneficiaries residing in nursing facilities.* OEI-02-06-00223. Washington, DC: U.S. Department of Health and Human Services.

U.S. Department of Health and Human Services, Office of the Inspector General. (2009b). *OIG report: Medicare hospice care for beneficiaries in nursing facilities: Compliance with Medicare coverage requirements.* OEI-02-06-00221. Washington, DC: U.S. Department of Health and Human Services.

U.S. Department of Veterans Affairs. (2008). *VA offers hospice care.* Retrieved from http://www.military.com/veterans-report/va-offers-hospice-care

U.S. National Center for Health Statistics. (2009). *Deaths: Final data for 2006.* Retrieved from http://www.cdc.gov/nchs/data/nvsr/nvsr57/nvsr57_14.pdf

Virnig, B. A., Fisher, E. S., McBean, A. M., & Kind, S. (2001). Hospice use in Medicare managed care and fee-for-service systems. *American Journal of Managed Care, 7*(8), 777–786.

Wennberg, E., Fisher, F., Baker, L., Sharp, S. M., & Bronner, K. K. (2005). Evaluating the efficiency of California providers in caring for patients with chronic illnesses. *Heath Affairs 543.* Retrieved from http://content.healthaffairs.org/cgi/content/abstract/hlthaff.w5.526

Wennberg, J. E., Fisher, E. S., Goodman, D. C., & Skinner, J. S. (2008). Tracking the care of patients with severe chronic illness: The Dartmouth Atlas of Health Care 2008, executive summary, April 2008. Lebanon, NH: The Dartmouth Institute for Health Policy and Clinical Practice.

Wennberg, J., Fisher, E. S., & Skinner, J. S. (2002). Geography and the debate over Medicare reform. *Health Affairs.* Retrieved from http://www.chelationtherapyonline.com/articles/p119.htm

Wennberg, J., Fisher, E., Stukel, T., Skinner, J. S., Sharp, S. M., & Bronner, K. K. (2004). Use of hospitals, physician visits, and hospice care during last six months of life among cohorts loyal to highly respected hospitals in the United States. *British Medical Journal, 328,* 607.

Wiener, J. M., & Tilly, J. (2003). Long-term care and American federalism: Can states be the engine of reform? In J. Holahan, A. Weil, & J. M. Wiener (Eds.), *Federalism and health policy* (pp. 249–292). Washington, DC: The Urban Institute Press.

Wilson, C. H. (1999). Establishing the right of the terminally ill to adequate palliative care: The litigation alternative. *Journal of Palliative Medicine, 2*(1), 15–22.

Wolfsfeld, L., Zhu, A., & Hendricks, A. (2004). *Hospice and palliative care for VA Patients.* Health Care Financing and Economics Data Brief No. 2004-06.

83 *Elizabeth J. Clark*

Self-Care as Best Practice in Palliative Care

I had been looking forward to seeing Mary at her appointment this afternoon. She was to finish her chemotherapy last week, and I was sure she would be upbeat. I was shocked when she walked into my office and immediately started crying. It appears her chemo wasn't successful and her cancer has spread. She was devastated. So was I. It is getting harder and harder for me to witness such suffering. Maybe it's time I thought about closing my private practice and doing something that doesn't hurt as much.

—Palliative social worker

Key Concepts:

◆ *For all palliative care professionals, self-care is critical to professional quality of life.*

◆ *Those working in palliative care are at high risk for compassion fatigue and professional grief.*

◆ *Witnessing suffering can lead to vicarious trauma.*

◆ *Losing hope as a professional caregiver is a symptom of burnout.*

◆ *Professional self-care requires a variety of positive self-care strategies at both the personal and organizational levels.*

Introduction

Palliative and end-of-life care is a rapidly expanding and changing field (Mackelprang & Mackelprang, 2005), and social work has an important role in its delivery (Blacker, 2004). Social workers focusing on palliative care services are usually employed in settings such as a hospital, hospice, or nursing home. Since one of the hallmarks of palliative care is an interdisciplinary team approach, a private clinical practice for palliative care might be difficult to maintain. There are, however, some exceptions that should be taken into account. Social workers who do contract services for nursing homes or hospices might find that they are providing palliative care outside the usual framework. They also may lack the support of a palliative care team but integrate the clinicians and staff in these settings into an informal team that works together to care for patients. Likewise, social workers who specialize in bereavement counseling in their solo clinical practice might lack an adequate peer support network. Social workers in human service agencies and settings may also witness loss, suffering, and trauma. Those working in child welfare, school social work, mental health centers, homeless shelters, or prisons may recognize the need for palliative care across the continuum of illness but may be unable to provide the care or find the needed resources.

Regardless of work setting, professionals who have a palliative care function and work in high-loss situations are at greater risk for professional grief, burnout, and/or difficulty maintaining hope. For all palliative care professionals, self-care is critical.

In 2008, the Delegate Assembly of the National Association of Social Workers (NASW), the policy-setting body for the Association, passed a new policy statement titled "Professional Self-Care and Social Work." In the introduction, the policy states that professional self-care is an essential underpinning to best practice in social work and that it has relevance in every setting (NASW, 2009). We give credence to many of the difficulties faced by social workers: a lack of resources, long hours, high caseloads, inadequate staffing and supervision, and safety concerns. Yet we rarely talk about the stress implicit as we witness suffering or repeatedly hear themes of helplessness and hopelessness from those we serve (Cunningham, 2003). Some researchers refer to this as vicarious traumatization or as secondary traumatic stress (See Box 83.1.) (Adams, Boscarino, & Figley, 2006; Stamm, 2009). Figley coined the term "compassion fatigue," and defined it "as the natural, predictable, treatable, and preventable unwanted consequence of working with suffering people" (Figley, 2002, p.124).

Witness to Suffering

Although the world is full of suffering, it is full also of the overcoming of it.

—Helen Keller

Palliative care seeks to prevent or relieve suffering for any serious illness. Palliative care is not only the assessment and treatment of pain and other symptoms (Kramer, 2008), but a broad concept that spans the continuum of care and the holistic experience of the patient and family. The World Health Organization (WHO) defines palliative care as "an approach that improves the quality of life of patients and their families facing the problems associated with life-threatening illness" (WHO, 2009). When we think of suffering, we often think in terms of physical factors such as pain and shortness of breath and the failure to relieve such symptoms. What may not be as obvious is psychological or emotional pain or suffering related to spiritual and existential issues. There are many contributing factors to suffering, and

---

Box 83.1
Patient and Family Narrative: Mrs. Simon

Mrs. Simon was admitted to the hospital in excruciating pain. Her diagnosis was late-stage mycosis fungoides, and her body was covered with deep open sores. Every small movement was painful. Due to her condition, Mrs. Simon was assigned a private room. Her husband of 40 years was with her constantly. The medical team was not having great success in controlling Mrs. Simon's pain. Her suffering was visible and almost palpable to those who went into her room. In a short time, no one wanted to be assigned to care for Mrs. Simon. This staffing issue was addressed at a team meeting. Mrs. Simon's distress was so great that they all felt helpless and overwhelmed so they were unable to stay in Mrs. Simon's room for very long. To respond to this reaction, her physical care was divided among various staff during each shift and her pain management care plan was readdressed. What most amazed the staff was that Mr. Simon rarely left his wife's room. No one could understand how he could withstand such suffering.

---

the interplay between the causes may not be clear. For example, patients experiencing significant physical pain may also be suffering emotionally, not only from their pain but also from watching their family's sense of helplessness (See Box 83.2). Spiritual suffering may be related to unsolved life dilemmas, the search for meaning, or the fear that one has been abandoned by his or her God.

Witnessing suffering leaves an emotional legacy, and watching others suffer changes us in subtle ways (Cunningham, 2003). Arbore, Katz, and Johnson (2006, pp. 24–25) state that "being present to suffering on a daily basis places huge demands on our psyches, our souls, and our very being."

Professional Grief

By the very nature of their work, palliative care teams usually practice in high-loss environments such as hospitals, medical centers, nursing homes, and hospices. Similar to learning to deal with suffering, palliative care clinicians must learn to deal with multiple losses and the eventual deaths of many of their patients.

Box 83.2
Patient and Family Narrative: Ellen

Ellen was a 54-year-old single woman who had been diagnosed with a life-threatening cancer at age 41. Since her diagnosis, she had had numerous surgeries, had been on many chemotherapy protocols, and had undergone several rounds of radiation therapy. She had survived a second, unrelated cancer. Ellen had been treated in her small local community, and she and her family knew many of her health care team well. She was an easy patient, uncomplaining, agreeable, strong—a fighter—a model patient who had "beaten the odds." Her family also had come to believe that Ellen could get through anything. After a long remission for her original cancer, Ellen presented with a third cancer, acute leukemia that was caused by her previous treatments. She was admitted to the hospital in September for therapy. No matter what her doctors tried, a complete remission eluded Ellen. She went home with a partial remission in December, to be readmitted within a week. Day after day, Ellen lay in her hospital bed with a 10-pound sand bag on her left shoulder because the area around her port bled without the weight. After being hospitalized for almost 5 months, Ellen announced to her family, and then to her health care team, that what she was doing "was no longer living—that it was really just prolonging dying." She wanted all transfusions and treatments stopped. Her wishes were reluctantly honored. Some staff seemed angry that Ellen was "giving up," and her family wanted her to keep fighting. Ellen did not change her mind, and she died a short time later. The health care team was saddened by the death of a patient they had cared about for 13 years, and at the same time they acknowledged that they were also somewhat relieved. Watching Ellen and her family suffer for 5 months had been extremely difficult for everyone.

Almost half a century ago, Aries noted that "some form of mourning, whether spontaneous or obligatory, has always been mandatory in human society." He further noted that "it is no longer fitting to manifest one's sorrow or even give evidence of experiencing any" (1967, p. 16). This is particularly true in high-loss work environments where professional grief is often hidden and its expression unsanctioned. It generally is internalized and unexpressed; it has no natural outlet; and work demands may quickly overshadow the loss. There are few organizational or societal norms for dealing with professional grief.

Doka has used the phrase "disenfranchised grief" to describe grief that is not recognized (2002). Much earlier, Fulton and Fulton (1980) discussed nursing home staff who hid their grief because they were not "legitimately bereaved." In a study of gravediggers, Petrillo (1990) referred to "distant mourners," gravediggers who witness the suffering of the bereaved at the cemetery but have no claim to share in the bereavement. These concepts of "disenfranchised grief" and "distant mourning" appear applicable to professional practice in palliative care. We are not supposed to become "attached" to our patients and their families. We are warned against countertransference issues. We are told we should keep "an emotional distance" and an emotional balance. Yet Egnew (2004, p. xxv) claims that "palliative care social work cannot be done at arm's length, behind the protection of a professional role. Rather, it must be done through a personal connection." He further notes that palliative care social work is personal in nature, and that we are all vulnerable to the helplessness that accompanies death.

Burnout

Have courage for the great sorrows of life and patience for the small ones. And when you have finished your daily tasks, go to sleep in peace.

—*Victor Hugo*

The concept of "burnout" was coined in 1973 by psychologist Herbert Freudenberger. He defined "burnout" as "a depletion of energy experienced by professionals when they felt overwhelmed by others' problems" (Freudenberger, 1980, p. 90). Freudenberger's concepts evolved from his work in the free clinic movement of the 1960s, which was developed as an alternative model of general health care to serve people—hippies—who had rejected the "establishment" (Freudenberger, 1974). Interestingly, the term was used to refer to the professionals who worked with the young people, not the hippies themselves who often had chronic drug use problems. One researcher wrote that the professionals quickly lost much of their idealism and became less trusting and sympathetic toward their clients (Cherniss, 1980).

Another well-known pioneer in the study of the burnout syndrome was Christina Maslach who developed the Maslach Burnout Inventory (Maslach & Jackson, 1986), which allowed us to begin to quantify and measure variables. The assumption was that burnout is a type of job stress that arises from interaction between helper and recipient. The most widely used definition of burnout comes from Maslach and Jackson (1986, p. 1): "Burnout is a syndrome of emotional exhaustion, depersonalization and reduced personal accomplishment that can occur among individuals who do 'people work' of some kind." In the time since its earliest definition, burnout has been used as a generic concept. Other researchers use different terminology, but the underlying idea is the same. It has been attributed to the individual, to the workplace, and to their interaction. It can be considered as prolonged job stress—demands at the workplace that tax or exceed the individual's resources.

Additionally, the work setting and institutional practices can be a source of ethical stress and job dissatisfaction (O'Donnell et al., 2008). Ethics stress, defined by Raines (2000) as "the stress associated with ethical issues and/or dilemmas," can lead to job dissatisfaction and burnout (Mackelprang & Mackelprang, 2005; Ulrich et al., 2007). Social workers confront major ethical issues in end-of-life and palliative care. Among others, these may include life and death decisions, quality of care and quality of life issues, health disparities, and lack of resources.

Stamm (2009) has developed a Professional Quality-of-Life Scale that uses three concepts of compassion satisfaction, compassion fatigue, and secondary traumatic stress. In this model, burnout is one element of the negative effect of compassion fatigue. It is associated with hopelessness and difficulties in doing a job effectively, which results in the sense that one is not making a difference.

Burnout is usually a gradual process with clusters of symptoms. Cox, Kuk, and Leiter (1999, p. 179) identified three clusters of symptoms that are usually present:

- Exhaustion (intellectual, emotional, or physical) and lack of enthusiasm
- Desperation or emotional detachment
- Reduced personal accomplishment, helplessness, and low self-esteem

Other symptoms may include physical symptoms such as fatigue or sleeplessness, psychological symptoms such as depression, anger, or guilt; and behavioral symptoms such as working longer hours and feeling indispensible. An additional effect of burnout is difficulty in maintaining hope.

Maintaining Hope

Weeping may endure for a night, but joy cometh in the morning.

—*Psalms 30:5*

Most health care professionals have never given much thought to the concept of hope. In fact, most of us assume that other people hope like we do. Social workers are seldom taught about hope as a clinical concept. Instead, hope is based on the medical model, or what maybe called therapeutic hope—hope that is based on the outcome of the treatment(s) or the amelioration of the disease or physical problem (Nuland, 1995). We also fail to recognize that hope is a universal concept and that people hope differently. Some use religion or spirituality as the basis for their hope. Others might use science and look for research data to underpin their outlook. Still others use a combination of cultural and personal values and individual experiences. We do know that each person's hope is unique, and that as health care professionals, we have an obligation to support individual hopes and to build a community of hope for our patients and their families.

We sometimes worry that we will "give patients false hope." There is the danger of giving patients and families false reassurances, but, by definition, hope can never be false (Clark, 2008). Hope changes as an individual's situation changes, and hope often transcends reality. We may at times need to help patients and their loved ones reformulate broken hopes. Social workers are expert at reframing and helping patients set realistic goals. What is most important to remember is that no matter how dire the situation, hope can always be found. At the end of life, hope may center around living to participate in a special event, having the opportunity to say "good-bye," or having a peaceful, pain-free death. Twaddle, a palliative care physician, contends that many patients in hospice programs define hope as "trust and reliance in the people and process of support" rather than any expectation of cure. She notes that individuals and families in hospice are "hopeful in living well despite advanced disease" (Twaddle, 2007, p. 503).

Losing hope as a professional caregiver is a symptom of burnout and results from suffering and loss. It undermines feelings of effectiveness and even the capacity to care. Walsh-Burke (2006) notes that at times social workers can abuse themselves or others with manipulative strategies, or avoidance tactics, such as overworking, shutting in emotions, or using substances such as alcohol or drugs. Another major clue to burnout is feeling indispensible, a belief that no one else can, or will, do your job or do it as well as you can. These are warning signs that are important to address. Meisinger, in her book *Stories of Pain, Trauma, and Survival* describes the importance of being constantly self-aware: "The black hole becomes deep and overwhelming and the way out can be painful for the social worker who doesn't have the ability to critically self-assess and ask for help" (Meisinger, 2009, p. 75). While there is an essential resiliency and hopefulness about social workers, these traits can be diminished when work stress and emotional demands become overwhelming (Cunningham, 2003).

The concept of resiliency continues to evolve (Greene & Conrad, 2002). For the purpose of this chapter, resiliency is defined as a balance between stress and one's ability to cope with repeated stress. Certain psychological traits are associated with resilience and are thought to be protective factors. These include a sense of self-esteem and self-efficacy, hope, personal control, and self-understanding (Greene & Conrad, 2002).

The first step toward managing feelings of hopelessness, helplessness, and professional grief is to acknowledge that they exist. Not only do they exist, but they are common and normal in high-loss settings.

Another way to combat burnout in palliative and end-of-life care is to move beyond "therapeutic hope" and to focus instead on extending hope beyond the medical aspects of disease to the successes you have had in the other domains of your caregiving, what might be identified as psychosocial successes. Psychosocial successes are identifiable and significant things you do that contribute to the emotional and physical well-being of the patient and family regardless of the ultimate outcome of the illness. These things can be as simple as purchasing a card for a bed-ridden patient who wants to send a loved one a birthday wish, or as complex as spending hours assisting a patient in completing a life review process. Sometimes these activities may not become part of the patient's medical record, but they contribute to his or her quality of life and well-being. Take note of the things you do that make a positive difference.

Bernice Harper, one of the foremost experts on hospice social work, believes that experience helps to mitigate burnout. As early as 1977, she developed "A Schematic Comfort–Ability Growth and Development Scale in Coping with Professional Anxieties in Death and Dying," which delineates the development sequence of the health professional as one learns to work in the area of death and dying. Based on stage theory, it operates on a continuum of growth and development as health care workers develop coping mechanisms for their feelings. Harper begins with the premise that working in the areas of death and dying necessitates both psychological and emotional skill. Her guiding framework is (1) working with dying patients and their families is a traumatic experience; (2) excessive anxieties are a deterrent to healthy adaptation; and (3) anxiety is inherent in working with the dying (1977, pp. 18–19).

The Comfort–Ability Scale represents a normative sequence of emotional and psychological progress. It covers a 24-month period and has five stages that advance along a line of comfortability that forms the backdrop for the growth process. The stages are intellectualization, emotional survival, depression, emotional arrival, and deep compassion (p. 28). In Harper's first printing (1977), Stage 5, with component parts of self-realization, self-awareness, and self-actualization, is the culminating point. In her later edition (Harper, 1994) she adds a Stage 6 to represent the mature, seasoned professional who possesses inner knowledge, wisdom, power, and strength.

Harper contends that "The Burned-Out Syndrome" is not an issue when a social worker reaches Stage 6 because his or her professional growth and development has reached a point of self-awareness, self-empowerment, and comfort in working with the dying patient and family. This maturity and "line of comfort-ability" forms the essential coping mechanism and serves as an antidote to burnout.

Another antidote to burnout is good self-care. Renzenbrink (2004, p. 848) urges social workers to practice relentless self-care and notes that "dealing daily with intense emotion can be extremely challenging and may even be dangerous to health and well-being." Bailey, Koney, McNish, Powers, and Uhly (2008) use the concept of radical self-care to describe activities such as yoga, meditation, or other hobbies that center a person and bring balance to life. Radical self-care leads to personal resilience and to regaining a sense of purpose.

Self-care has both personal and professional components. Professional self-care is an essential component of social work practice that reflects a choice and a commitment to be actively involved in maintaining one's effectiveness as a social worker (NASW, 2009). In fact, social workers have an ethical obligation for self-care. The profession's Code of Ethics (NASW, 2008) has a section dedicated specifically to this issue:

> *Social workers should not allow their own personal problems, psychosocial distress, legal problems, substance abuse, or mental health difficulties to interfere with their professional judgment and performance or to jeopardize the best interests of people for whom they have a professional responsibility. (4.05)*

Professional self-care requires the development of a variety of positive self-care strategies for prevention of burnout, compassion fatigue, and loss of hope. It might be helpful to develop your own written self-care plan and find ways to maintain it. The following strategies are only a starting point. To be successful, they must be tailored to both the individual and the work setting.

Strategies for Self-Care at the Personal Level

- Know your own strengths and weaknesses.
- Be aware of your own beliefs, values, and feelings and how they may influence your social work practice.
- Understand the relationship between self-care and excellent social work practice.
- Keep a balance between the personal, professional, and spiritual areas of your life.
- Build a personal support system both inside and outside your work setting.
- Allow time to deal with your emotions.
- Participate in a peer support network.
- Keep a journal of psychosocial successes.
- Attend a retreat or conference on self-care.
- Seek counseling if needed.

Strategies for Self-Care at the Professional Level

- Recognize that palliative and end-of-life care will encompass ethical dilemmas and value conflicts.
- Ensure effective interdisciplinary teamwork that values the contributions of each discipline.
- Encourage requirements for basic and continuing professional education about palliative and end-of-life care.
- Increase your skill level through advanced training and supervision.
- Identify barriers to offering effective palliative and end-of-life care at the macro level such as access to and inequities of care.
- Join others in your organization or community who are trying to bring about positive change regarding palliative and end-of-life care practice and education.
- Lobby for needed workplace supports such as extra leave time and split shifts.
- Establish rituals and grieving practices for professional staff and the workplace.
- Maintain a community of hope that fosters trust and compassion, and that respects individual differences, including different visions of hope.
- Advocate for sound institutional ethics practice and adequate ethics resources.

Social work practice and involvement are crucial to the provision of quality palliative and end-of-life care for patients with serious or life-limiting illness. Professional self-care is equally crucial to assure that the practitioner can function effectively in palliative and end-of-life care settings as well as in personal and family life.

C. Murray Parkes, one of the world's foremost experts in loss and bereavement has stated:

> *With proper training and support, we shall find that repeated griefs, far from undermining our humanity and our care, enable us to cope more confidently and more sensitively with each succeeding loss. (1986, p. 7)*

LEARNING EXERCISES

- Most health care professionals do not enter their fields prepared to deal with suffering and loss. Many spend years trying to develop the right balance of compassion and involvement, of engagement and detachment, and the need to protect oneself from personal hurt and burnout while supporting and counseling clients. This balance requires an ongoing self-monitoring. Your personal history—especially your personal loss history—plays a major role in keeping a healthy balance in your professional practice. If a similar loss in your own life has not been adequately resolved, you may have greater difficulty managing your response to your client's situation. If a situation reminds you of one of your own fears, you may become overly involved, and your clinical effectiveness may be diminished.

Take a few moments to think about clients whose suffering or death has affected you in a significant way. Two or three may immediately come to mind. Write a paragraph about each person. Then look for similarities. Why did these particular clients have such an impact? Did they remind you of someone you love or of a personal fear? How do you assess your interaction with each of them? Was it appropriate? Guarded? Overinvolved? How can you be more effective when you are working with future clients with similar characteristics or histories?

- Most people never think about how they hope or how they learned to hope. Yet families and professionals usually have well established hoping patterns. Some families use a religious hope constellation: "It's out of my hands; only God knows what will happen and I just have to trust in Him; there is no use in planning or completing advance care documents because some greater force will decide; or my fate is already determined." Other families rely on science or medical facts in determining how and for what to hope. They may get numerous opinions, search the Internet, analyze statistics, and rely on the testimony of others in similar situations.

  Health care professionals usually think in terms of therapeutic hope—hope for a cure or the efficacy of a treatment or procedure. Sometimes they have difficulty in relating to the broader hopes of their clients. These different hoping patterns can be the cause of conflict among the various professionals on a palliative care team, or between the professionals and the patient or the patient's family. Identify a situation where there was a difference of opinion about hope. Did your own hoping style play a role in the conflict? Who taught you how to hope? Can you accept all forms of hope?

- At the time Mrs. Simon, in the first patient and family narrative (see Box 83.1), was admitted, there were questions that should have been asked and discussed. For example, did the team think that Mrs. Simon was unaffected by their reluctance to be in her room? Was she really in too much pain to notice that the same staff person rarely came in twice in one day? Did the team use her husband's presence to excuse their own? Most important, what could the team have learned from Mr. and Mrs. Simon about their worldview and how Mr. Simon could be a steadfast companion while witnessing such terrible agony? What could the team have learned about themselves and their own humanity? Were there other interventions that might have been responsive to Mrs. Simon's physical and emotional suffering? Consider your answers to these questions. Can you think of other questions that might have been relevant?

ADDITIONAL RESOURCES

American Academy of Bereavement (AAB): http://www.bereavementacademy.com
A nonprofit organization founded in 1993, AAB is a national association devoted to the education, preparation, and advancement of bereavement specialists.
American Trauma Society (ATS): http://www.amtrauma.org
A leading spokes-organization for trauma care and trauma prevention in the United States. ATS has been the foremost advocate for trauma victims and their families for the past 30 years and continues to seek optimal care for all trauma victims.
Association for Death Education and Counseling (ADEC): http://www.adec.org
An interdisciplinary organization in the field of dying, death, and bereavement. ADEC offers numerous educational opportunities through its annual conference, courses and workshops, its certification program, and its newsletter, *The Forum*.
Compassion Fatigue Awareness Project (CFAP): http://www.compassionfatigue.org
A project with the mission of promoting an awareness and understanding of compassion fatigue and its effect on caregivers.
Hospice Foundation of America (HFA): http://www.hospicefoundation.org
Assists those who cope either personally or professionally with terminal illness, death, and the process of grief.
National Hospice and Palliative Care Organization (NHPCO): http://www.nhpco.org
The largest nonprofit membership organization representing hospice and palliative care programs and professionals in the United States.
Professional Quality of Life (PQL): http://www.proqol.org
A scale that uses three concepts of compassion satisfaction, compassion fatigue, and secondary traumatic stress.

REFERENCES

Adams, R. E., Boscarino, J. A., & Figley, C. R. (2006). Compassion fatigue and psychological distress among social workers: A validation study. *American Journal of Orthopsychiatry, 76*(1), 103–108.
Arbore, P., Katz, R. S., & Johnson, T. A. (Eds.). (2006). *When professionals weep: Emotional and countertransference responses in end-of-life care*. New York, NY: Routledge.
Aries, P. (1967). *The hour of our death*. London, England: Vintage Books.
Bailey, D., Koney, K. M., McNish, M. E., Powers, R., & Uhly, K. (2008). *Sustaining our spirits: Women leaders thriving for today and tomorrow*. Washington, DC: National Association of Social Workers.
Blacker, S. (2004). Palliative care and social work. In J. Berzoff & P. R. Silverman (Eds.), *Living with dying: A handbook for end-of-life healthcare practitioners* (p. 419). New York, NY: Columbia University Press.
Cherniss, C. (1980). *Professional burnout in human service organizations*. New York, NY: Praeger Publishers.

Clark, E. J. (2008). *You have the right to be hopeful* (4th ed.). Silver Spring, MD: National Coalition for Cancer Survivorship.

Cox, T., Kuk, G., & Leiter, M.P. (1993). *Burnout health, work stress and organizational healthiness*. In W. B. Schaufeli, C. Maslach, & T. Marek (Eds.), *Professional burnout: Recent developments in theory and research* (pp. 177–193). Washington, DC: Taylor & Francis.

Cunningham, M. (2003). Impact of trauma work on social work clinicians: Empirical findings. *Social Work, 48*(4), 451–459.

Doka, K.J. (2002). *Disenfranchised grief: New directions, challenges and strategies for practice*. Champaign, IL: Research Press.

Doka, K. J. (2007). Section IV: The importance of self-care. In K. J. Doka (Ed.), *Living with grief: Before and after the death* (pp. 299–300). Washington, DC: Hospice Foundation of America.

Egnew, T. R. (2004). Foreword. In J. Berzoff & P. R. Silverman (Eds.), *Living with dying: A handbook for end-of-life healthcare practitioners* (p. xxv). New York, NY: Columbia University Press.

Figley, C. R. (Ed.). (2002). *Treating compassion fatigue*. New York, NY: Brunner-Routledge.

Fink-Samnick, E. (2007). Fostering a sense of professional resilience. *The New Social Worker, 14*(3), 24–27.

Freudenberger, H. J. (1974). Staff burnout. *Journal of Social Issues, 30*, 159–165.

Freudenberger, H. J. (1980). *Burn-out: The high cost of high achievement*. New York, NY: Anchor Press.

Fulton, R., & Fulton, J. (1980). *Caring relationships: The dying and the bereaved*. Amityville, NY: Baywood Publishing.

Greene, R., & Conrad, A. (2002). Basic assumptions and terms. In R. R. Greene (Ed.), *Resiliency: An integrated approach to practice, policy, and research*. Washington, DC: NASW Press.

Harper, B. (1977). *Death: The coping mechanism of the health professional*. Greenville, SC: Southeastern University Press.

Harper, B. (1994). *Death: The coping mechanism of the health professional*. (2nd ed.). Greenville, SC: Southeastern University Press.

Kramer, B. J. (2008). Palliative care. In T. Mizrahi & L. E. Davis (Eds.). *Encyclopedia of social work* (20th ed., pp. 337–340). Washington, DC: National Association of Social Workers.

Mackelprang, R. W., & Mackelprang, R. D. (2005). Historical and contemporary issues in end-of-life decisions: Implications for social work. *Social Work, 50*(4), 315–324.

Maslach, C., & Jackson, S. E. (1986). *Burnout inventory*. Palo Alto, CA: Consulting Psychologists Press.

Meisinger, S. E. (2009). *Stories of pain, trauma and survival*. Washington, DC: National Association of Social Workers.

National Association of Social Workers (NASW). (2004). *Standards for palliative and end-of-life care*. Washington, DC: Author.

National Association of Social Workers (NASW). (2008). *Code of ethics*. Washington, DC: Author.

National Association of Social Workers (NASW). (2009). *Family policy. Social work speaks, National Association of Social Workers policy statements, 2009-2012* (8th ed., pp. 134–139). Washington, DC: NASW Press.

Nuland, S. B. (1995). *How we die. Reflections on life's final chapter*. New York, NY: Random House.

O'Donnell, P., Farrar, A., BrintzenhofeSzoc, K., Conrad, A. P., Danis, M., Grady, C.,… Ulrich, C. M. (2008). Predictors of ethical stress, moral action and job satisfaction in health care social workers. *Social Work in Health Care, 46*(3), 29–51.

Parkes, C. M. (1986). Orienting the caregiver's grief. *Journal of Palliative Care, 1*: 5–7.

Petrillo, G. (1989-90). The distant mourner: An examination of the American gravedigger. *Journal-of-Death-and-Dying, 20*(2), 139–148.

Raines, M. L. (2000). Ethical decision making in nursing: Relationships among moral reasoning, coping style, and ethics stress. *Journal of Nursing Administrative Law, Ethics and Regulation, 2*(1), 29–41.

Renzenbrink, I. (2004). In Relentless Self Care. J. Berzoff & P. R. Silverman, *Living with dying: A handbook for end-of-life healthcare practitioners* (p. 848). New York, NY: Columbia University Press.

Stamm, B. H. (2009). *Professional quality of life scale (ProQOL) [PQL Scale]*. Retrieved from http://proqol.org/ProQol_Test.html

Twaddle, M. L. (2007). Hospice. In A. M. Berger, J. L. Shuster Jr., & J. H. Von Roenn, *Palliative care and supportive oncology* (3rd ed., p. 503). Philadelpha, PA: Lippincott Williams & Wilkins.

Ulrich, C., O'Donnell, C., Taylor, C., Farrar, A., Danis, M., & Grady, C. (2007). Ethical climate, ethics stress, and the job satisfaction of nurses and social workers in the United States. *Social Science and Medicine, 65*, 1708–1719.

Walsh-Burke, K. (2006). *Grief and loss: Theories and skills for helping professionals*. Boston:, MA Pearson Education.

World Health Organization (WHO). (2009). *WHO definition of palliative care*. Retrieved from http://www.who.int/cancer/palliative/definition/en/

84 *Shirley Otis-Green*

Legacy Building: Implications for Reflective Practice

Working with those facing end of life has taught me much about how I want to live my life and how I want to leave this world.

—Retiring palliative social worker

Key Concepts

- ◆ *Reflective palliative social work practice offers rich opportunities for vicarious learning.*
- ◆ *Intentional legacy building implies conscious awareness of our transient nature.*
- ◆ *Reflective palliative social work shows us how lessons learned have application in our personal life and leads to increased authenticity in practice.*
- ◆ *A commitment to "professionalism" asks that palliative social workers have the courage to seek excellence in their delivery of care, which is enhanced when we regularly and intentfully reflect upon the impact that we are having and the legacy that we are creating.*

Introduction

Palliative social workers work with individuals and families facing serious and often life-threatening illness or injury. The impact of this is often life altering for all involved. Patients frequently report that from the time of diagnosis they begin to consider the possibility of their own mortality and that this visceral awareness that they may die has lasting implications on the way that they live the rest of their lives. A reflective practitioner has opportunities to vicariously learn from the experiences of others and can apply these lessons both personally and professionally (Otis-Green, in press).

Every major faith tradition offers guidance regarding proper preparations for one's death (Corr, Nabe, & Corr, 2003; Puchalski, 2006; Walsh, 1999) and despite sometimes radical differences between these traditions, the concept of legacy work is often explicitly addressed. A common theme throughout is the intentional use of the time prior to dying as an opportunity to minimize regrets. Another commonality is the suggestion that we benefit from not waiting until we are on our death-bed to begin these preparations. It is from this perspective that this chapter is written. I belief that there is wisdom in contemplating the legacy that we are building within our homes, institutions, and communities while we are well enough to influence it.

Working with oncology patients at a Southern California comprehensive cancer center, I have been privileged to witness both dying done well and to sit at the bedside of those whose deaths still haunt me. It was from these experiences that we developed the Transitions Program to offer comprehensive psychoeducational support services to our advanced cancer patients, their families, and to the professionals who cared for them (Otis-Green, 2006). Through this work we found that a menu approach to services offered individualized and more culturally nuanced care. We learned that we benefit from examples of how others have managed under similar circumstances. It was through developing programs to support those facing end of life that I learned the importance of conscious legacy building (see Box 84.1).

Box 84.1
Patient/Family Narrative: Maria

Maria was a 42-year-old second-generation Mexican American woman who came to our medical center immediately after being diagnosed with widely metastatic breast cancer. Because of the aggressive nature of her disease and her young age, she was tested to determine whether there was a genetic predisposition to her illness. As a mother of two young daughters, she was overwhelmed with concern regarding the impact her illness would have on her family. She wept upon learning that she was positive for a BRCA1 (breast cancer susceptibility gene-1) genetic mutation. Her genetic counselor helped her to understand that historically, a number of Jewish people of Ashkenazy heritage carried this genetic mutation, and that many of the Jewish population in Spain during the Middle Ages faced expulsion or forced conversions to Catholicism (Weitzel, et al, 2005). Many of these converts subsequently migrated to South and Central America. Maria was amazed to learn that her inherited genetic susceptibility to this illness was possibly linked to these events from so long ago. It was her concern about the impact of her illness and the genetic implications of her disease upon her children that led her to see a social worker and regularly attend a Transitions Program support group.

In the group, Maria shared her story and reflected upon the lasting legacy of these events and how they have influenced her current situation. She voiced fear that she would die and explored with others ideas about how to prepare her family for her eventual passing. She was encouraged to consider how she could intentionally build a positive legacy for her children. Her social worker recommended several books that offered suggestions regarding preparations for end of life and she found insights from Living with the End in Mind (Kramp & Kramp, 1998) particularly meaningful due to its immediate applicability to her situation.

In the support group, she shared the steps she had taken to create a series of scrapbooks for each of her daughters. She also got ideas from the group about creating a video life review to allow her to share more about her childhood history and to offer an opportunity to pass on her values and dreams for her children (Elgin & Ledrew, 2001). Reluctantly, Maria voiced concern that she may have passed on her "defective genes" to her daughters. The group encouraged her to consider the many positive attributes that she had also likely passed on to them, such as her strength of character, her courage, and her sense of humor. A group member reminded her that by being tested, she was also passing on information helpful to her children's future medical care, because they would benefit from a heightened awareness of what to look for in health screenings. Another member reminded her that no parent's genes are "perfect" and that she had given her children the gift of life, and that they, like all of humanity, would need to someday face illness and death, but that she now had an opportunity to model strategies for them to better face these challenges when the time came.

At her next visit with her social worker, they talked in depth about a parent's desire to protect children from harm whenever possible as well as a parent's obligation to prepare children when they cannot be fully protected. Maria had come to realize that although she would not be able to protect her children from suffering following her death, there were many things that she could do to better prepare them for this eventuality.

Professionalism in Clinical Practice

Because "we don't know what we don't know," it can be especially beneficial for patients to hear how others have faced these types of situations. By sharing how others have left lasting legacies, we can generate ideas that may be adapted to the specific needs of the patient and family in front of us (Otis-Green, 2003; Spence, 1997). Palliative social workers are well positioned to pass on strategies that have been useful to others.

A thoughtful practitioner soon realizes the importance of anticipatory guidance as a core palliative social work intervention. Our patients will be facing their medical situation for the first time, whereas we have the benefit of past experiences that can greatly assist our patients and families as they navigate this uniquely personal journey. Examples of how others have faced difficult circumstances can be immensely inspiring, for example, Randy Pausch's account of his legacy-building strategies has become meaningful for many (Pausch, 2008). Facilitating bereavement support groups reminds us that the work that we do is long lasting. The bereaved are able to recount vividly the details of losses that occurred decades ago with breathtaking detail. The time surrounding a meaningful loss will be remembered by the survivors for the rest of their lives, and memories made during this period are deeply treasured (Chochinov, 2002). It is humbling to reflect upon the significance of this work. Being with those who are at their most vulnerable emphasizes the urgency of delivering compassionate, competent care (Puchalski & Ferrell, 2010; Rumbold, 2002). It is this responsibility that underscores the need for palliative social workers to hold themselves accountable to the highest standards of professionalism and leadership.

Professionalism requires that we have the courage to commit to seeking excellence in our delivery of care that can only be achieved when we regularly pause to reflect upon the impact that we are having and, thus, the legacy that we are leaving. Professionalism of this caliber has both personal and professional ramifications. In this integrated model of professionalism, palliative social workers would be expert clinicians, skillful educators, proficient in basic research concepts and tireless patient advocates. The assimilation of these core skills requires a commitment to lifelong learning. Clearly, the balance of these abilities would be unique to each individual and would evolve over time within each practitioner's career. Unfortunately, social workers (like other health care professionals) may see one or more of these key competencies as "optional" to their career.

Although it can be initially overwhelming to imagine developing basic proficiency in each of these areas, it is my belief that it is not only possible, but necessary if we are to be the voice of the patients and families that we serve. In the same way that palliative social workers recognize the value of transdisciplinary education (Otis-Green et al, 2009) to meet the biopsychosocial-spiritual needs of those within our care, professionalism from this perspective demands a basic proficiency within each of these core elements (practice, research, education, and advocacy). Moreover, as with other areas of practice, we need acute awareness of our limitations and knowledge of where we can turn for expert assistance when we find ourselves outside of our skill set.

Transdisciplinary education identifies the core competencies that all members of the health care team need to address the multidimensional concerns of those we serve. From this view, all team members would be required to be at least minimally able to identify psychosocial distress, to complete a spiritual screening, to assess for pain and symptom management needs, and to have culturally sensitive interpersonal communication skills. Each member would also be well versed in the skill set of his or her colleagues and able to refer to the appropriate discipline for further assistance when indicated. Team members would not work beyond their identified scope of practice, but they would be expected to develop the necessary skills to allow them to competently identify the patient and family's basic physical, social, psychological, and spiritual needs. Because we cannot be "all things to all people," individual practitioners need an accurate assessment of the limits of our generalist skills and a clear awareness of when and where to refer when more specialized skills are called for.

If we are to strive for excellence in care, we need to continually develop and refine our skill set. Patients who are facing the end of life do not have the luxury to wait until we hone our skills. There is an urgency to this work that calls for a willingness to "roll up our sleeves and do what needs to be done." There may not be a second chance to address a particular patient issue or fill a particular family need.

Skillful clinical care demands critical thinking to determine what intervention is most appropriate for this particular situation at this particular time. Ideally, such decisions would be made following a careful review of the existing evidence base. A commitment to evidence-informed practice holds practitioners accountable to contribute to building a strong evidence base for future generations to more effectively and efficiently deliver expert care.

If we are to be effective members of a well-functioning team, we need to be able to educate our colleagues about what services palliative social workers provide and our patients and families about their plan of care. If we are to be congruent with our core social work values, we need to engage policy makers and administrators about what is needed to deliver quality whole-person care. Palliative social workers are called to be change agents, pursuing equal access and representing the voices of the traditionally underserved and most vulnerable members of our society. Advocacy is needed at all levels of care from the individual/family level, to the institutional, regional, state, national, and global spheres. We, like other health professionals, have an obligation to be activists representing the conscience of our communities regarding social justice in health care.

Developing these vital skills allows us to feel better at the end of the day, knowing that we did the best we could for those we serve (Palmer, 2000). Professionalism of this magnitude becomes a way of being within the world and offers an internal consistency that builds a lasting legacy of change. Palliative social workers are needed who are committed to doing what matters and doing it well.

Personal Implications

If we are to avoid hypocrisy in our practice, we are invited to see that what is "good" for our patients is often "good" for us as well. If we are to be credible when we talk with our patients about making advance directives, we would do well to have had these discussions with our own families and complete the forms ourselves. Working with those who are dying reminds us that we too will someday die. Talking with families about a loss reminds us of our past losses. The separations that we often make between "us" and "them" have no meaning in palliative social work practice (Berzoff, et al, 2006). We are all in this together. It is from the recognition of our shared humanity that our greatest contributions are made—contributions that create a lasting legacy of effective social work practice.

Summary

Intentional legacy building implies conscious awareness of our transient nature and offers frequent reminders that we need to "practice what we preach." I am mindful of a patient who said that following her diagnosis she had redoubled her efforts to "make her mark" on the world. That language conjured up an image for me of how bears reach high upon a targeted tree to scratch their "mark" indelibly on the bark for other animals to note their passing. Perhaps this urgency to leave our "mark" speaks to this nearly universal desire to leave a legacy of our having been. This textbook is an example of an intentional act of legacy building by the editors as we seek together with our contributors to "make our mark" in the field of palliative social work.

LEARNING EXERCISES

- Reflect upon the last two patient deaths that you experienced.

  a. How were the ways that these two individuals approached their deaths similar? How were they different?

  b. How did their deaths impact their loved ones? What steps had they taken to prepare others for their dying? Were there missed opportunities? What lessons do these deaths offer you? There are opportunities to learn from all death experiences. Notice your responses to those who appear to have accepted their dying and to those who have wished and worked to extend every last breath. What judgments do we make about how "well" or "not well" others have died, and how might these judgments influence our practice?

c. Were there things that you witnessed that you would want to emulate in your own life and in your own dying? Were there things that you identified that you might wish to do differently?

d. How might you apply these observations with future patients and families?

e. What steps can you take to apply these lessons in your personal life?

- This exercise can be done either individually or in small groups. Think about a colleague who has recently left your organization. What was the institutional impact from that person's departure? Were people relieved that he or she was no longer there? Has that person's professional legacy been positive or negative? Now, imagine that you will be leaving your current place of employment. Reflect upon the legacy that you have built with the following questions:

a. How is your institution different for you having been there?

b. Do you have any regrets?

c. How lasting is your influence likely to be?

d. How would you like to be remembered by your peers?

e. What opportunities exist for you to build a stronger legacy?

ADDITIONAL RESOURCES

Borneman, T., & Brown-Saltzman, K. (2010). Meaning in illness. In B. R. Ferrell & N. Coyle (Eds.), *Textbook of palliative nursing* (3rd ed., pp. 673–683). New York, NY: Oxford University Press.

Byock, I., (1997). *Dying well: Peace and possibilities at the end of life.* New York, NY: Riverhead Books.

Byock, I. (2004). *The four things that matter most.* New York, NY: Free Press.

Calhoun, L. G., & Tedeschi, R. G. (Eds.). *Handbook of posttraumatic growth: Research and practice.* Mahwah, NJ: Lawrence Erlbaum Associates.

Davey, J. (2007). *Writing for wellness: A prescription for healing.* Enumclaw, WA: Idyll Arbor, Inc.

Dolan, S. R., & Vizzard, A. R. (2007). *From the start consider the finish: A guide to excellent end-of-life care.* Denver, CO: Outskirts Press Inc.

Ersek, M.& Cotter, V. (2010). The meaning of hope in the dying. In B. R. Ferrell & N. Coyle (Eds.), *Textbook of palliative nursing* (3rd ed., pp. 579–595). New York, NY: Oxford University Press.

Faas, A. I. (2004). A personal reflection: The intimacy of dying an act of presence. *Dimensions in Critical Care Nursing, 23*(4), 176–178.

Ferrell, B. R., & Coyle, N. (2008). *The nature of suffering and the goals of nursing.* New York, NY: Oxford University Press.

Ferrell, B.R. (1996). Humanizing the experience of pain and illness. In B. R. Ferrell (Ed.), *Suffering* (pp. 3–27). Sudbury, MA: Jones and Bartlett Publishers.

Frankl, V. E. (1984). *Man's search for meaning.* New York, NY: Washington Square Press.

Halifax, J. (2008). *Being with dying: Cultivating compassion and fearlessness in the presence of death.* Boston, MA: Shambhala Publications, Inc.

Hansen, M. J. (2009). A palliative care intervention in forgiveness therapy for elderly terminally ill cancer patients. *Journal of Palliative Care, 25*(1), 51–60.

Hedlund, S. (2007). Hope and communication in cancer care: What patients tell us. In P. Angelos (Ed.), *Ethical issues in cancer patient care* (2nd ed., pp. 67–77) New York, NY: Springer.

Kearney, M. (2000). *A place of healing: Working with suffering in living and dying.* New York, NY: Oxford University Press.

Baird, P. (2010). Spiritual care interventions. In B. R. Ferrell & N. Coyle (Eds.), *Textbook of palliative nursing* (3rd ed., pp. 663–671). New York, NY: Oxford University Press.

Keyes, C. L. M., & Haidt, J. (2003). *Flourishing: Positive psychology and the life well-lived.* Washington, DC: American Psychological Association.

Kleinman, A. (2006). *What really matters: Living a moral life amidst uncertainty and danger.* New York, NY: Oxford University Press.

Knight, S. J., & Emanuel, L. (2007). Process of adjustment to end-of-life losses: A reintegration model. *Journal of Palliative Medicine, 10*(5), 1190–1198.

Lee, V. (2008). The existential plight of cancer: Meaning making as a concrete approach to the intangible search for meaning. *Supportive Care in Cancer, 16*(7), 779–785.

Levey, J., & Levey, M. (1998). *Living in balance.* Berkeley, CA: Conari Press.

Levine, S. (1997). *A year to live: How to live this year as if it were you last.* New York, NY: Random House, Inc.

Levoy, G. (1997). *Callings: Finding and following an authentic life.* New York, NY: Three Rivers Press.

Lynn, J., Schuster, J. L., & Kabcenell, A. (2000). *Improving care for the end of life: A sourcebook for health care managers and clinicians.* New York, NY: Oxford University Press.

Merrill, A. R., & Merrill, R. R. (2003). *Life matters: Creating a dynamic balance of work, family, time and money.* New York, NY: McGraw-Hill.

Palmer, P. J. (2004). *A hidden wholeness: The journey toward an undivided life.* San Francisco, CA: Jossey-Bass.

Perry, B. (2008). Why exemplary oncology nurses seem to avoid compassion fatigue. *Canadian Oncology Nursing Journal, 18*(2), 87–99.

Remen, R. N. (1996). *Kitchen table wisdom.* New York, NY: Riverhead.

Riemer, J., & Stampfer, N. (1994). *So that your values live on.* Woodstock, VT: Jewish Lights Publishing.

Schacter-Shalomi, Z., & Miller, R. (1995). *From age-ing to sage-ing.* New York, NY: Warner Books, Inc.

Seligman, M. E. P. (2002). *Authentic happiness: Using the new positive psychology to realize your potential for lasting fulfillment.* New York, NY: Free Press.

Stanley, K. J. (2002). The healing power of presence. *Oncology Nursing Forum, 29*(6), 935–940.

Taylor, E. J. (2007). *What do I say? Talking with patients about spirituality*. Philadelphia, PA: Templeton Foundation Press.

Tolstoy, L. (2004). *The death of Ivan Ilych and other stories*. New York, NY: Barnes & Noble Books.

INTERNET RESOURCES

Following are several Web sites to help with legacy-building exercises and resources:

A Legacy to Remember: http://alegacytoremember.com

All about Aging: http://allaboutaging.com

Association of Personal Historians: http://www.personalhistorians.org

The Legacy Center: http://thelegacycenter.net

Chapters of Life: http://chaptersoflife.com

REFERENCES

Berzoff, J., Lucas, G., Deluca, D., Gerbino, S., Browning, D., Foster, Z. & Chatchkes, E. (2006). Clinical Social Work Education in Palliative and End-Of-Life Care, Journal of Social Work in End-Of-Life & Palliative Care, 2(2), 45–63.

Chochinov, H. M. (2002). Dignity-conserving care: A new model for palliative care. *Journal of the American Medical Association*, 287(17), 2253–2260.

Corr, C. A., Nabe, C. M., & Corr, D. M. (2003). *Death and dying, life and living* (4th ed.). Belmont, GA: Wadsworth/Thomson Learning.

Elgin, D., & Ledrew, C. (2001). *Living legacies: How to write, illustrate and share your life stories*. Berkeley, CA: Conari Press.

Kramp, E. T., & Kramp, D. H. (1998). *Living with the end in mind: A practical checklist for living life to the fullest by embracing your mortality*. New York, NY: Three Rivers Press.

Otis-Green, S. (2003). Legacy building. *Smith College Studies in Social Work, Special Issue: End-of-Life Care*, 73(3), 395–404.

Otis-Green, S. (2006). The transitions program: Existential care in action. *Journal of Cancer Education*, 21(1), 23–25.

Otis-Green, S., Ferrell, B., Spolum, M., Uman, G., Mullan, P., Baird, P., & Grant, M. (2009). An overview of the ACE Project-Advocating for Clinical Excellence: Transdisciplinary palliative care education. *Journal of Cancer Education*, 12(10), 885–905.

Otis-Green, S. (in press). Embracing the existential invitation to examine care at the end of life. In Quall & Kasl-Godley (Eds.), *Gero-psychology series: End-of-life and bereavement care*. Hoboken, NJ: John Wiley and Sons, Inc.

Palmer, P. J. (2000). *Let your life speak: Listening for the voice of vocation*. San Francisco, CA: Jossey-Bass.

Pausch, R. (2008). *The last lecture*. New York, NY: Hyperion.

Puchalski, C. (2006). *Time for listening and caring: Spirituality and the care of the chronically ill and dying*. New York, NY: Oxford University Press.

Puchalski, C., & Ferrell, B. (2010). Making Health Care Whole: Integrating spirituality into patient care. West Conshohocken, PA: Templeton Press.

Rumbold, B. (2002). Spirituality and Palliative Care: Social and Pastoral Perspectives. South Melbourne, Australia: Oxford University Press.

Spence, L. (1997). *Legacy: A step by step guide to writing personal history*. Athens, OH: Swallow Press/Ohio University Press.

Walsh, R. (1999). *Essential spirituality*. New York, NY: Wiley & Sons.

Weitzel, J., Lagos, V., Blazer, K., Nelson, R., Richer, C., Herzog, J., McGuire, C., & Neuhausen, S. (2005). Prevalence of *BRCA* mutations and founder effect in high-risk Hispanic families. *Cancer Epidemiology, Biomarkers and Prevention*, 14, 1666. doi:10.1158/1055-9965.

Epilogue: Lessons Learned Along the Yellow Brick Road

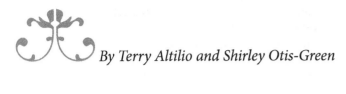

By Terry Altilio and Shirley Otis-Green

Lessons Learned Along the Yellow Brick Road

We invited our social work colleagues who are members of a variety of professional listservs™ to contribute unique motivational words, wisdom and anecdotes. The following were selected from over 200 submissions by practicing social workers who on a daily basis move this specialty forward. This collection reflects the attributes of *Wisdom, Heart, and Courage* as sought by the Scarecrow, the Tinman and the Lion on their adventures along the yellow brick road (Baum, 1900). We offer these thoughts to inform and inspire your journey.

Wisdom

"Palliative care education does not have to teach clinicians to have all the answers but rather provides knowledge and inspires courage to know when there is a question to be raised and to raise it. Discovering answers is often shared work."
Terry Altilio, LCSW, ACSW
Social Work Coordinator
Department of Pain Medicine & Palliative Care
Beth Israel Medical Center, NY

Reflect
Enjoy
Laugh
Educate
Allow…
Spiritual growth
Encourage
Christine A. Betros, MSW, LSW
Palliative Care Social Worker
Lyons, NJ

"Not everything is black and white. Social Work lives within the gray."
Leora Botnick, LCSW
Social Work Supervisor
Oncology & Palliative Care
Lincoln Medical & Mental Health Center

"It's their journey, not ours;" after all our guidance, education and support, people have to navigate their journey in their own way."

"Keep showing up" that is, don't make assumptions too quickly about the uncommunicative, guarded, reserved patient or family member in favor of those instantly engageable and articulate people. I have found that by continuously "showing up" relationships can be developed that pave the way for the most important and profound work."
Susan Conceicao, LCSW-R
Metropolitan Jewish Hospice
Brooklyn, NY

"Let everyone know, she said,
This tall, dignified, black woman in her sixties.
I resisted hospice for so long,
But, now I have my freedom.
They take care of my pain,
While I tend to my garden.
Let everyone know."

An experience with one of my favorite lung cancer patients. I will always remember her.
Annemarie Conlon, MBA, LCSW
Doctoral Student, American Cancer Society
Doctoral Grantee
University of Texas at Austin

"There is nothing more important than being fully present; the easiest and hardest place to be. It is the foundation of all the work that follows."
Richard Dickens, LCSW-R
Blood Cancers Program Coordinator &
Mind/Body/Spirit Project Coordinator
CancerCare

"Expect change, embrace uncertainty, and ensure self care."
Lori Eckel, LCSW
Portland, OR

"Just because we can, doesn't mean we should."
Fran Heller, LMSW
Senior Social Worker, Palliative Care Consult Service
NY Presbyterian, CUMC

"Whose agenda is it?"
Odette M. Joseph, LCSW
Sentara Virginia Beach General Hospital Palliative Care

"Never forget the bigger picture."
Andrea Karoff LCSW, OSW-C
Coordinator, Psychosocial Oncology
Creticos Cancer Center
Advocate Illinois Masonic Medical Center

"I often feel like I live with a cast of characters in my head (both dead and alive) that supply me with wisdom about how to prioritize my life on a daily basis."
Amanda Moment, LICSW
Palliative Care Social Worker
Dana Farber/Brigham and Women's Cancer Center
Boston, MA

"Assess deeply, intervene discretely, refer widely."
Christopher Onderdonk, MSW, LCSW
Access Center Social Worker
San Diego Hospice and the Institute for Palliative Medicine

"Increase your tolerance of ambiguity."
Shirley Otis-Green, MSW, LCSW, ACSW, OSW-C
Senior Research Specialist
City of Hope National Medical Center
Duarte, CA

"When I reflect upon what has been most significant in my work the word LISTEN is the first and most important skill that I have relied upon consistently. If you master the skill of listening you will learn what you need to be effective in most situations. Listening will usually allow you to develop a healthy working relationship. I know this works by the many years of experience in the hospital/acute care setting and from being exposed to patients of all ages and backgrounds. Listening usually allows you as the practitioner to abstract that piece of information that may make the difference. LISTEN TO LEARN."
Debbie Rex, MSW
St. Luke's Hospital Bethlehem Campus

"Meaning and purpose are the sworn enemies of stress and distress."
Brahms E. Silver, MA, MSW, PSW, OSW-C
Oncology Social Worker
Jewish General Hospital
Segal Cancer Centre, Montreal, Quebec, Canada

"Believe in the innate wisdom of children:. Recently, I was working with a woman whose father was dying in the palliative care unit. She was struggling with how to tell her nine year-old son that his grandfather was dying, and requested my assistance in doing so. As the child snuggled on her lap, his mom started to try to tell him but was overwhelmed by tears. The child climbed off her lap, got a cup of water, crawled back into his mom's lap, saying, "Mom, what I need from you is to take a deep breath and a small sip." Ah, believe in the children, they know best how to comfort us."
Wendy Walters, LCSW, OSW-C
Family Support Coordinator
UAB Health System
Birmingham, AL

Heart

"What does it mean to be loving, faithful and merciful in this situation?"
Greg Adams, LCSW, ACSW, FT
Palliative Care and Center for Good Mourning
Arkansas Children's Hospital

"We all love, we all grieve - and soothing that grief and sadness takes the same things: care, understanding, respect for what matters to the patient and loved ones, and time."
Joanne B. Glusman, MSW, LSW

"I find hearts with hope amidst the hopelessness."
Judith Lacy Hewes, MSW, RCSWI
Florida Hospital Cancer Institute

"I consider my job to be a high privilege. I enter into patients' and families' lives when they are at their most vulnerable."
Kelly C. Markham, LCSW
Palliative Care Coordinator
Baptist Hospital
Pensacola, FL

"Learning to maintain professional boundaries with patients and families is a process. It doesn't mean we don't cry with them, because we sometimes may."
Cindy Miller, LMSW
Social Worker, Pediatric Oncology
Monroe Carell Jr. Children's Hospital at Vanderbilt

"I keep reminding myself that while I have chosen this path, the people that I love have not. This helps me to keep from bringing my work home to them."
Amanda Moment, LICSW
Palliative Care Social Worker
Dana Farber/Brigham and Women's Cancer Center
Boston, MA

"Take time to Play. Sit with toddlers when they are thrilled to play and want everyone to join them or when they laugh and it's a whole body laugh. Watch, listen, be where they are, let yourself laugh with them, and keep the image. On the really bad days at work, take time to resurrect that image of joy and use it as a tool for hope."
Sue Stephens, LCSW, ACSW
Social Worker, Pediatric Hematology/Oncology
Cancer Institute of New Jersey

"Sometimes in all the good work we do, we become forgetful....we forget that not everyone is as used to the dying process as we are. Sometimes, unless there are loud emotive outbursts, we deem families as 'doing ok'....Yet, isn't this the first time their mom, or dad, or spouse is dying? Do we forget the emotional impact that signing on to hospice services might mean for someone? We may become so comfortable with not forcing food and fluids that we forget that in extended care facilities the young caregivers feel lost; as if they've abandoned their resident when we tell them it's "ok" for someone not to eat and do not give them some other manner of caring for their charge. We forget that using morphine every hour is not the 'norm' in someone's home. These are the thoughts that have been parts of recent conversations. We need to remind ourselves that this is the first time this patient and family have had this experience of dying for a particular family member. It matters that they know about hospice and yet it doesn't matter, as each situation is as unique as the individuals we serve. It is the social worker's job, charge, role, call if you will, to bring these reminders to the team when others forget."
Kris Vanags Rilling, LCSW
Social Work Discipline Leader
HospiceCare Inc. NY

"If I'm 100% emotionally present and listen carefully to the client, the rest will unfold exactly as it should."
Ashley Varner, MSW, MBA, LCSW-C
Senior Director, Caregiving Programs
Cancer Support Community
Uniting The Wellness Community & Gilda's Club Worldwide

"The relationship with the families, our words and our feeling about what they are experiencing, are our tools. Let families know: "I am with you.""
Lynda Walker, LCSW

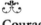

Courage

"The history and tradition of social work rests in the embracing and overcoming of obstacles. Labels such as noncompliance and nonadherence invite social work assessment; it is where we begin while for others it is where the conversation ends.

Terry Altilio, LCSW, ACSW
Department of Pain Medicine & Palliative Care
Beth Israel Medical Center, NY

"Hope is too often underestimated—it is resilient and diverse. We can hope for many different and sometimes mutually exclusive things at the same time."

"The human spirit is boundless; use your humanity to fearlessly unearth this"
Erin Columbus, LMSW
Program Director of Online Services
CancerCare of NY

"To work in end-of-life care one must be willing to dance with mystery."
Richard Dickens, LCSW-R
Blood Cancers Program Coordinator &
Mind/Body/Spirit Project Coordinator
CancerCare

"Don't be afraid of silence... words aren't always necessary. Families may or may not remember what you said, but most often remember your presence."
Carolyn McCarley, LCSW
HemOnc Social Worker
Arkansas Children's Hospital

"Think of a metaphor for your work and remind yourself of it when you're feeling depleted. For example, I visualize palliative care as a team expedition...with preparation, divisions of labor, obstacles, opportunity for replenishment and abundant rewards."
Elizabeth A. Rohan, PhD, MSW
Health Scientist
Centers for Disease Control and Prevention
Division of Cancer Prevention and Control, Atlanta, GA

"Get in there and do what needs to be done. They don't call it social **work** for nothing!"
Lynda Walker, LCSW

REFERENCES

Baum, L. F. (1900). *The wonderful wizard of Oz* . Chicago, IL: George M. Hill Company.

Appendix: Patient Narratives

Section II Social Work Practice: Setting Specific

Chapter 5: Palliative Care Consultation
Goals of Care Narratives: Vignettes illustrate the range of goals of care possible within complex medical illness. Clinical focus: Decision making which supports patient values and preferences, p. 45.

Female, age 60. Clinical focus: Supporting family system through a transition from critical care to a palliative care unit, trust-mistrust with health care system in the face of a missed diagnosis, p. 48.

Chapter 6: Palliative Social Work in the Intensive Care Unit
Mrs. Amalu, age 73 and family. Clinical focus: Unresponsive woman being cared for in the intensive care unit, family decision-making in the setting of perceived suffering and cultural variables, p. 56.

Mr. Taylor, age 87 and daughters. Clinical focus: brain injured man with an advance directive, supporting family in advocating for their father and educating them to the emotional and medical process of withdrawing life-sustaining treatment, p. 59.

Chapter 7: Palliative Social Work in the Emergency Department
Anne, age 52, an actively dying, unresponsive daughter of Rosemary, age 80. Clinical focus: Discovering Anne's beliefs and values related to end of life and assisting her mother's process for honoring her wishes through targeted clinical assessment, selective interventions and liaison activity between the Emergency Department staff, family and palliative care team, p. 65.

Chapter 8: Social Work and Palliative Care in Hospice
Dean, age 75, Lydia and family. Clinical focus: Assessment in a home hospice setting, blended family, varied emotional and cognitive responses to illness, financial distress and physical symptoms present upon admission, p. 74.

Chapter 9: Pediatric Hospice and Palliative Care: The Invaluable Role of Social Work
Maria, age 12, two siblings and her mother. Clinical focus: Core concepts of pediatric hospice and palliative care, including care coordination between the hospital and home based hospice provider, p. 80.

Chapter 10: Home Based Palliative Care
Mrs. Carson, age 52, with heart failure. Clinical focus: Patient confined to home, receiving team home visits. Mrs. Carson gradually improves and as the social worker begins to develop a plan of care in response to this improvement, Mrs Carson dies suddenly, p. 90.

Edward, age 68, visits the hospital emergency room on multiple occasions to request care. Clinical focus: Primary issues of anxiety and depression are identified as contributing factors, social work interventions include improving Edward's support system and coping skills in order to diminish ineffective use of the emergency room, p. 93.

Native American Tribal Partnerships. Clinical focus: A home palliative care program in the mid-west uses a start-up grant to form partnerships with two area Native American tribes. Over time, as the social worker continued to reach out to families and various tribal subgroups, trust in the partnership increased and led to culturally congruent access to palliative care, p. 97.

Mr. Harrison. Clinical focus: A home based palliative social worker developed an initiative to provide care to persons experiencing homelessness in the midst of advancing illness. Clinical intervention, advocacy and perseverance result in Mr. Harrison's becoming able to accept care which met his needs for safety, nutrition and comfort at end of life, p. 97.

Sara, age 64 married, male-to-female transgender client with heart failure. Clinical focus: Advocacy and education about transgender aspects of care assists the team to address verbal abuse by Sarah's partner of 20 years and clinical interventions help Sarah to increase her sense of inner peace as her health deteriorates, p. 98.

Mr. Carlos Santiago and family, age 55 with end stage renal disease (ESRD). Clinical focus: Cultural and spiritual aspects of care and family conference intervention, p. 244.

Chapter 23: The Doctor Within: Integrative Medicine, Social Work and Palliative Care
Ms R. age 62. Clinical focus: Use of breathing exercises, guided imagery and meditation, gentle stretches and aromatherapy to work with chronic pain and despair, p. 253.

Ms. S, age 102. Clinical focus: Hand massage: finding a way to connect, p. 255.

Cathy age 40. Clinical focus: Biofield energy work in conjunction with radiation for cancer, p. 255.

Drum circle. Clinical focus: Intervention for elders in a nursing home providing connection, creative expression and emotional release, physical activity and joy, p. 256.

Chapter 24: Sexuality, Sensuality and Intimacy in Palliative Care
Couple, Rita age 54 and Carmen, age 52. Clinical focus: Rita who was paralyzed from the waist down due to her spinal cord injuries and Carmen demonstrated the use of bathing in physical intimacy, p. 262.

Lilly, age 46, married to Herman age 55. Clinical focus: Lilly with congestive heart failure (CHF) and Herman learn erotic massage, p. 265.

James, age 32 and his partner of 5 years, Gary age 29. Clinical focus: James is diagnosed with cancer of the tongue and Gary learns strategies to enhance intimacy and their relationship, p. 266.

Jerry age 71 and his wife of 50 years, Rita, age 68. Clinical focus: Jerry diagnosed with chronic obstructive pulmonary disease (COPD) learns the use of the C.A.R.E.S.S. evaluation model, p. 266.

Esther, age 46 married to Kelvin, age 47. Clinical focus: Esther diagnosed with recurrent ovarian cancer and Kelvin learn the use of non-verbal communication of sexual interest, sensual bathing techniques, and written erotica, p. 267.

Henry, age 26 married to Sharda. Clinical focus: Henry diagnosed with end-stage hepatitis integrates the use of enhanced appearance to address low self-esteem Additionally, addresses the importance of learning to time the release of medical information to manage negative self observation (spectatoring), p. 268.

Chapter 25: The Social Work Role in Pain and Symptom Management
Mitchell, age 57, diagnosed with melanoma. Clinical focus: Assessment in a palliative pain clinic, interventions for pain, coping with pain, social engagement and anxiety, p. 277.

Chapter 26: The Whys and Wherefores of Support Groups: Helping People Cope
Lisa, age 43 widowed mother of 5 children. Clinical focus: Bereavement counseling and support for young widow and children, value and meaning of support groups in filling this need, p. 288.

Mary, age 45, bereaved woman who is deaf. Clinical focus: Cultural aspects of appropriate and respectful program planning, recognizing need to be flexible and creative in serving varying populations, p. 291.

Advisory Committees. Clinical focus: Cultural aspects of providing appropriate care, creative opportunities to incorporate and utilize community members to develop credibility, provide and access resources, p. 295.

Chapter 27: Social Work and Technology: The Software and Hard Drive of Patient and Family Care
Junior social worker Martin and Mrs. Mosely. Clinical focus: Internet information related to management of pain, patient's desire for control, use of alternative medicine, evaluation of information obtained, opportunity for enhanced teamwork, p. 301.

Palliative social worker Mike counsels patient Mr. Jaminson. Clinical focus: On-line anonymity concerns.

Social worker Amy and use of Facebook within her professional role. Clinical focus: Communication with patients and their families, appropriate boundaries, confidentiality, p. 302.

Chapter 28: Bereavement in the Beginning Phase of Life: Grief in Children and their Families
Series of narratives. Clinical focus: Assessment and intervention with grief and loss in children and adolescents who are seriously ill, dying and/or bereaved, their families, parents and siblings.

Chapter 29: Holding On and Letting Go: The Red Thread of Adult Bereavement
Hannah, bereaved partner. Clinical focus: Continuing bonds theory, p. 321.

Laura, bereaved mother, son died on 9/11. Clinical focus: Complicated and traumatic mourning, prolonged grief disorder, stage theory and construction of meaning, p. 321.

Sarah, bereaved spouse. Clinical focus: Avoidant grief, p. 321.

Jerry and Joan, bereaved parents. Clinical focus: Dual process model of bereavement, p. 321.

Miss Havisham, bereaved fiancé. Clinical focus: Prolonged grief reaction, p. 323.

Section IV Population-Specific Practice

Chapter 30: Palliative Social Work and Oncology Care
Doug age 69, a single old sailor with atypical caregivers. Clinical focus: Utilizing knowledge of the person in the social environment to develop a discharge plan for Doug who is diagnosed with advanced prostate cancer, p. 333.

Shu. Clinical focus: Calligraphy aids family communication, integrating an art activity using a young mother's knowledge of Japanese calligraphy opens communication with her children at the end-of-life, p. 334.

Children's group narrative. Clinical focus: What's hardest when a parent has cancer, young children in a support group share their losses when a parent has cancer, p. 335.

Mr. Jones, age 26. Clinical focus: Social worker provides education and assistance to the patient related to advance care planning and collaborates with interdisciplinary team to plan for a Do Not Resuscitate (DNR) order in the dialysis unit, p. 344.

Chapter 31: Palliative Care in Chronic Kidney Disease
Mrs. Blake, a widow age 74 & family. Clinical focus: Family conflict and decision-making process related to discontinuing hemodialysis treatment. Social worker, in collaboration with the dialysis and hospice teams, helps the patient and family with supportive counseling, education, empathetic listening, referral and collaboration with hospice, p. 346.

Chapter 32: Emerging Opportunities for Palliative Social Workers: Organ Failure and Neurological Disease
Mr. Payton, age 68 and Mrs. P, married for 41 years. Clinical focus: Clinical picture of congestive heart failure patients, symptom management of dyspnea and anxiety and caregiver distress, p. 353.

Mr. Nesbit, age 70 and Mrs. Nesbit. Clinical focus: Communication issues regarding information on prognosis, advance care planning for acute stroke patient, cognitive behavioral therapy, p. 355.

Chapter 33: Social Work, HIV Disease and Palliative Care
Miss J, age 34. Clinical focus: Poor adherence, mental health issues, fragile sobriety and declining health in the setting of complex family dynamics, p. 363.

Louis, age 25. Clinical focus: End-of- life issues complicated by complete dependence on family because of paralysis, p. 363.

Nancy, age 59. Clinical focus: End-of-life issues, failure of HAART, complicated grief, limited support system and impaired trust of medical system – reason unknown, p. 364.

Chapter 34: Palliative Care with Vulnerable Populations
James, age 35. Clinical focus: Patient with bipolar I disorder, liver failure and homelessness; social work in a homeless shelter, p. 370.

Olivia, age 22. Clinical focus: Patient with stage IV-B cervical cancer who is uninsured and living in a rural area, p. 375.

Chapter 35: Palliative Care with Lesbian, Gay, Bi-Sexual and Transgender Persons
Lucy is being treated for cancer, her life partner is Jennifer. Clinical focus: Jennifer is invalidated when staff ask if she is a family member. A social worker acknowledges and validates Jennifer as the same-sex partner with the goal of diminishing the impact of disenfranchised grief and with Lucy's consent, clinical Interventions are tailored to include Jennifer in treatment discussions, p. 380.

Chapter 36: Social Work in Pediatric Palliative Care
Alex, age 9 months, and her young family. Clinical focus: Coping with Alex's complex cardiac condition, adjustment to diagnosis, anticipatory guidance for long term coping, family advocacy, complex decision making, ethics, uncertainty and challenges of coordinating care across settings and over time, p. 392.

Chapter 37: Palliative Social Work with Older Adults and their Families
Sylvia, age 84. Clinical focus: An older adult living in an urban setting, recently discharged to home following hospitalization related to multiple leg fractures, illustrates how development of multiple co-morbid chronic conditions can threaten autonomy and lead to increased isolation and dependency, p. 398.

Walter, age 71 and Olivia, age 68, a married couple living in the community with three adult children who live nearby. Clinical focus: Family caregiving with chronically ill older parents, including one parent with early-stage dementia, family decision making about day-to-day care and long-term care alternatives, p. 401.

Section V Collaborations in Palliative Care

Chapter 38: Teamwork in Palliative Care: An Integrative Approach
Mrs. Green, age 42 and family. Clinical focus: Husband and teenage children's adjustment to patient's advanced illness, interventions targeted at reducing anxiety, claustrophobia and fears, p. 419.

Mrs. Xiong, age 54. Clinical focus: Facilitation of cultural awareness and treatment decision making, p. 420.

Mr. Jones, age 78. Clinical focus: African-American worldview regarding advance directives and end-of-life decision making, p. 420.

Mr. Smith, age 43. Clinical focus: Cultural factors, primary team and family ethical dilemma concerning decision making in the intensive care unit related to withdrawal of non-beneficial treatments decision making in the intensive care unit, p. 421.

decision making capacity; family is comforted as patient dies in a manner coherent with her values, p. 485.

Chapter 49: Social Work and Genetics
Ms. B., age 35, and her teenage daughter, homeless and undocumented. Clinical focus: Basic survival issues in context of highly penetrant autosomal dominant condition in which surgery may prevent cancer, p. 490.

Julia, a newborn and her family. Clinical focus: Lethal chromosome condition with familial inheritance, cultural elements of family communication and decision making, perinatal hospice, p. 492.

Mrs. Hughes middle-aged women with mother with dementia. Clinical focus: Family communication about genetic susceptibility; clinical and ethical challenges for social worker, p. 493.

Chapter 50: Social Work and Spiritual Care Professionals
Eric, age 44, HIV-positive, gay male living in rural state. Clinical focus: Grief and loss, bereavement, social isolation and loneliness, substance abuse, suicidal ideation, financial and spiritual issues, p. 499.

Chapter 51: Social Work and Bioethics: Enhanced Resolution of Ethical Dilemmas and the Challenges along the Way
Mr. Smith age 72, clarifying a living will. Clinical focus: Conflict resolution among family members related to clarification of a patient's written wishes for end-of-life care, p. 505.

Mr. G. and his eldest son. Clinical focus: Understanding cultural and family dynamics and how they impact end-of-life decision making for patients, p. 505.

Section VI Palliative Social Work: Regional Voices from a Global Perspective

Chapter 53: The Need for Global Capacity Building for Palliative Social Work
South Africa: St. Luke's Hospice, Cape Town: Differences in palliative care within a small geographic region, p. 519.

Hungary: Rebuilding social work education and providing a specialty in health social work, p. 521.

Foundation for Hospices in Sub-Saharan Africa (FHSSA): An international model for matching resources between organizations in the United States and Sub-Saharan Africa, p. 521.

Cambodia: Providing palliative care with limited resources and continuing to build capacity, p. 521.

Chapter 54: Palliative Care, Culture and the Pacific Basin
Mrs. I, age 65 and family from American Samoa, visiting family in Hawaii. Clinical focus: Cultural differences creating family conflict related to decision making and causing conflict between heath care workers and family over family's desire to have 24 hour support for the patient, p. 529.

Chapter 57: Palliative Social Work in Buenos Aires, Argentina
Yolanda, age 53. Clinical focus: Woman with advanced breast cancer who benefits from attending the day treatment center, p. 546.

German, age 70. Clinical focus: Man with pancreatic cancer coping with existential suffering and life regrets who benefits from music workshops at the day treatment center, p. 547.

Juan, age 43. Clinical focus: Man with metastatic colon cancer who struggles with how to express the emotional impact of his illness, p. 547.

Chapter 58: Australian Palliative Social Work
Ivan, age 76. Clinical focus: Disconnection and reconnecting; the importance of unfinished business, p. 551.

Mrs. K, age 66. Clinical focus: Cultural issues and long term care; social work interventions through the transition from palliative care to residential aged care for a patient and family, p. 552.

Chapter 59: Palliative Social Work: An African Perspective
Palliative Care in Africa: The Reality. Clinical focus: Mrs. D and her three children living with multiple AIDS related deaths, poverty, lack of access to medication and a decimated extended family unable to provide financial and emotional support, p. 558.

Zimbabwean rural family. Clinical focus: Balancing practical and emotional needs that arise from multiple deaths and illness, p. 558.

Chapter 61: Palliative Social Work in Japan
Shinobu, age 50, youngest daughter of K family. Clinical focus: anticipatory grief of a family member and the notion of "dignity conserving care", p. 568.

Tazuko, age 58, cancer patient with severe pain. Clinical focus: difficulty accessing the palliative care team in a timely manner, p. 571.

Chapter 62: Palliative Social Work in a Chinese Context: An Integrated Framework for Culturally Respectful Practice
Mr. Ma aged 59, with terminal lung cancer. Clinical focus: Living life to the fullest, participation in self-help group, maintenance of high level of social and physical activities until the end of life, p. 576.

Thomas, age 70 and his father with terminal lung cancer. Clinical focus: Life review, extreme filial devotion, father's desire to protect his son from awareness of his impending death, importance of creating a video of patient's life which serves as a legacy and opportunity for father and son to talk openly about dying, p. 576.

Mr. Shek, age 64 with metastatic lung cancer. Clinical focus: Seeking pardon and relationship closure, use of guided imagery, establishing contact with estranged wife, a plea for posthumous forgiveness, p. 577.

goals; Exploring meaning, purpose, spirituality, balancing work and professional life and self care, p. 679.

Chapter 74: Advocacy and Leadership in Palliative Social Work: A Call to Arms

Karen, social work advocacy and leadership. Clinical focus: Professionalism as a pathway to resolve challenges and obstacles; principles: professionalism, leadership, advocacy interventions: critical thinking, assertive/positive approach to addressing challenges, role modeling social work values, peer support and mentoring, interdisciplinary team coordination and education, p. 685.

Chapter 75: The Power and Potential of Language

Jeanette, age 45, single mother of Jamal age six and Tiffany, age eight. Clinical focus: Diagnosed with multiple myeloma, Jeanette is referred to the palliative care consultation team for pain management and planning for the future care of Jamal and Tiffany, p. 691.

Chapter 80: Merging Research and Clinical Practice

Sara Smith, a hospice family caregiver participating in a pilot intervention study, describes her frustration when social workers make vague offers of help. Clinical focus: The importance of skilled, focused interventions and the impact research can have on social work practice, p. 735.

Mrs. Jones' death is reviewed by the hospice interdisciplinary team. Clinical focus: The narrative is designed to help social workers to provide specific responses based upon empirical outcomes showing the benefits of interventions and their knowledge of evidence-based practice, p. 736.

Chapter 81: Continuous Quality Improvement and Organizational Change

Institutional Narratives - Suncoast Hospice: Incorporating outcome measures in the electronic medical record to facilitate outcome evaluations at the patient, organization and national levels, p. 748.

Hospice of Palm Beach County: Systematic organizational change and the use of outcome evaluation to assess the outcomes of the change initiatives, p. 750.

Chapter 83: Self-Care as Best Practice in Palliative Care

Mr. and Mrs. Simon. Clinical focus: Impact on staff of witnessing great physical suffering, p. 772.

Ellen, age 54. Clinical focus: Challenges in deciding when disease modifying treatments are no longer effective, p. 772.

Chapter 84: Legacy Building: Implications for Reflective Practice

Maria, age 42, with metastatic breast cancer, mother of two daughters. Clinical focus: Genetic testing and participation in support services as Maria confronts the impact of her illness upon her family, p. 780.

INDEX

Ethical issues/dilemmas (*continued*)
confidentiality and privacy, 608–9
conflict of interest, 609–10
cultural conflict, 620–21
decision making, 622–23
in dialysis decision making, 341
faced by volunteers, 510–11
genetics and genetic counseling, 490–92
hastened death and, 654–55
interdisciplicary collaboration, 406
online healthcare services, 301–2
pain management, 66–67, 272–73
palliative care and, 89, 94, 98–99, 116, 162,
334, 421–22, 605–6
in palliative care consultation team (PCCT),
421–22
in palliative sedation, 664–67
pediatric palliative care and, 388–90, 637–47
professional level, 131, 150, 418–22, 479–80,
674, 677, 679, 684, 700, 704–5, 710, 712,
721–22, 725, 727, 737, 773, 775
recommendations for, 610–11
stress, 773
team work, 497
truth telling, 607–8
use of advanced medical technologies,
616–19
Ethical practice, 737
for elderly, 406
Europe, palliative care development in, 538
European Association for Palliative Care
(EAPC), 538, 706
European Journal of Palliative Care, 706
Evidence-based medicine (EBM), 721
Evidence-based practice, 371, 721–22
definition, 738
important concepts for, 739–40
in social work, 737–38
Evidence-informed practice (EIP), 722, 740
Evidence-informed psychosocial strategies, 271
Exosystem-level dynamics, of social workers, 35
Experiment Perilus, 7
Expression of emotions, among patients in
Singapore, 581–82
Expressive arts activities, 292
Extended care facilities, 241, 403–4, 416, 709

Facebook, 301
FACES. *See* Family Adaptability Cohesion
Evaluation Scale (FACES)
Facilitator-led discussions, 292
FACIT-F. *See* Functional Assessment of Chronic
Illness Therapy-Fatigue Scale (FACIT-F)
Fairbairn, W. R. D., 261
Faith and trust in nursing care, 82
Families. *See also* Family communication
assessment of, 236–37
bereavement care, 242
biopsychosocial-spiritual assessment, 236–37
caregiving, 241
conferences, 242–43
culture, language, and the health care system,
240, 544, 563, 574, 580, 600, 619–20,
628–30
definition, 236
developmental and life course issues, 237–38
discord, 239

effective family responses and adaptive
relationships, 237
facilitating care for, 241–44
family systems theory to clinical practice, 236
financial issues, 240–41
geographic distribution, determination of, 237
and geriatric palliative care, 401–3
immigration, acculturation, and
assimilation, 240
importance of, 235
narratives, 238–39
in palliative care, 236, 402
patients' views of, 236
resilience of, 237
social environment outside of family,
240–41
social work skills for working with, 241–42
and substance abuse, 239–40
Western and non-Western cultures, 240
Family Adaptability Cohesion Evaluation Scale
(FACES), 175
Family caregivers, 128, 130, 171, 175, 177, 223,
224–26, 280, 402
Family-centered care, 48–49, 387, 398, 420, 453,
465–66, 495, 557, 720
for cancer patients, 334–36, 570
for elderly, 405
Family communication, 692
confidentiality issues, 422
genetics and, 492–93
in geriatric palliative care, 402–3
palliative social work in United Kingdom
and, 589
with SLP, 483–84
Family conference concepts, 730
Family Conference Toolkit, 419
Family decision-making process, 419
for cancer patients, 175–76
for dialysis patients, 342–43
for ED patients, 64–65
geriatric population, 402–3
hastening death, 652
for ICU patients, 56–60
intervention approaches, 282
pediatric palliative care, 640–43
Family factors, and Indian patients, 563
Family-focused care, 48–49
Family genogram, 580–81, 584
Family Medical Leave Act (FMLA), 383Family
memory, 313–14
Family-oriented society, in Singapore, 580
Family therapy, to Indian patients, 563
Family Therapy Clinic, 462
Fatigue, 271, 281–82
assessment, 282
Fatigue Symptom Inventory (FSI), 282
Federated States of Micronesia (FSM), 527
Feifel, H., 7
Feldman, D., 121
Field, L., 343
Field, S., 64
Financial support, for capacity building, 520–21
Five Remembrances, 256
FMLA. *See* Family Medical Leave Act (FMLA)
Foley, K., 300, 303
Food and palliative social work in Singapore, 583
Foster, Z., 8

Four-box method, pediatric palliative care and,
643–45
Fox, R., 7
Frailty, in elderly, 398
Francoeur, R. B., 27, 133
Freud, S., 261
Freudenberger, H. J., 773
Friending, 302
FSI. *See* Fatigue Symptom Inventory (FSI)
Fulton, J., 773
Fulton, R., 773
Functional Assessment of Chronic Illness
Therapy-Fatigue Scale (FACIT-F), 282
Functional impairments, 354
cognitive impairment, 356–57
Rogers and Addington-Hall's work, 356
Fund-raising, 433–36
benchmarking of organizations, 435
guiding principles for, 433–35
lessons learned in, 435
making personal connection and, 434
overview, 433
potential donors, 434
tax status and, 434–35

Galambos, C., 738
Gambrill, E., 740
Ganzini, L., 653
Gardia, Gary, 27
Garland, E. L., 252
Gate keeping, 737
General Social Care Council, 444
GeneReviews Web site, 492
Genetic Information Nondiscrimination
Act, 490
Genetic practice, social work and, 490–91
Genetics
DNA banking, 492
and family communication, 492–93
genetic practice across life span, 489–90
historical perspective, 490
and perinatal death, 492
social work, palliative care and, 491–92
Genograms, 238, 632
George, L. K., 728
Gerbino, S., Dr., 696
Geriatric depression, in older cancer
patients, 461
Geriatric health care workforce, lack of
skilled, 404
Geriatric palliative care, 398
ageism and marginalization, 401
chronic illnesses and conditions, 398
clinical case management and care transitions
in, 405
comprehensive geriatric assessment, 404–5
cultural diversity and promoting social
justice, 405–6
family caregiving and, 402
family-centered practice for, 405
family communication and decision-making,
402–3
family roles and dynamics in, 401–3
health care disparities and, 403
health care financing and delivery, 403
implications for, 404–6
interdisciplinary and ethical practice, 406